Saunders
Review of Dental Hygiene

Saunders

Review
of
Dental
Hygiene

Debralee McKelvey Nelson, R.D.H. M.A.

Associate Professor
Department of Dental Hygiene
University of South Dakota
Vermillion, South Dakota

W.B. SAUNDERS COMPANY

A Division of Harcourt Brace & Company
Philadelphia London Toronto Montreal Sydney Tokyo

W.B. SAUNDERS COMPANY
A Division of Harcourt Brace & Company

The Curtis Center
Independence Square West
Philadelphia, Pennsylvania 19106

Library of Congress Cataloging-in-Publication Data

Nelson, Debralee McKelvey.
    Saunders review of dental hygiene/Debralee McKelvey Nelson. —
1st ed.

        p.   cm.

    Includes bibliographical references.

    ISBN 0–7216–7576–X

    1. Dental hygiene. 2. Dental hygiene—Case studies. 3. Dental
hygiene—Examinations, questions, etc. I. Title. II. Title:
Review of dental hygiene.
    [DNLM: 1. Dental Prophylaxis Case Report. 2. Dental Prophylaxis
Examination Questions.   WU 18.2 N425s 2000]

    RK60.7.N44 2000   617.6′01′076—dc21

    DNLM/DLC   99-27192

SAUNDERS REVIEW OF DENTAL HYGIENE   ISBN 0–7216–7576–X

Printed in the United States of America

Last digit is the print number: 9   8   7   6   5   4   3   2   1

Contributors

EDITH J. APPLEGATE, M.S.
Professor of Biology
Kettering College of Medical Arts
Kettering, Ohio
Chapter 2: Anatomy, Biochemistry, and Physiology

GERRY BARKER, R.D.H. M.A.
Associate Professor
Department of Dental Public Health & Behavioral Science
Coordinator of Oncology Education
University of Missouri—Kansas City
School of Dentistry
Kansas City, Missouri
Chapter 15: Special Needs Patient Care

ROBIN APPLEBEE BEILBY, R.D.H., M.A.
Private Practice in Colorado;
Assistant Professor
Department of Dental Hygiene
School of Dentistry
University of Colorado
Denver, Colorado
Chapter 11: Clinical Treatment

KIMBERLY KRUST BRAY, R.D.H., M.S.
Associate Professor
Division of Dental Hygiene
School of Dentistry
University of Missouri—Kansas City
Kansas City, Missouri
Chapter 15: Special Needs Patient Care

JACQUELINE N. BRIAN, R.D.H., M.S.Ed.
Professor
Department of Dental Hygiene
Indiana University-Purdue University Fort Wayne
Fort Wayne, Indiana
Chapter 7: Radiology

WILLIAM CAFRUNY, PH.D.
Professor
Molecular Microbiology and Immunology Group
Department of Basic Biomedical Sciences
School of Medicine
University of South Dakota
Vermillion, South Dakota
Chapter 4: Microbiology and Immunology

MARY DANUSIS COOPER, R.D.H., M.S.Ed.
Professor
Department of Dental Hygiene
Indiana University-Purdue University Fort Wayne
Fort Wayne, Indiana
Chapter 6: Nutrition
Chapter 17: Ethics and Jurisprudence

MARGARET J. FEHRENBACH, R.D.H., M.S.
Educational Consultant
DH Forum, Online Continuing Education Program
Dental Hygiene Program
Marquette University
Milwaukee, Wisconsin
Chapter 3: Head, Neck, and Dental Anatomy

ALISA D. FEUGATE, R.D.H., M.A.
Associate Professor of Dental Hygiene
Department of Dental Hygiene
College of Health Professions
Northern Arizona University
Flagstaff, Arizona
Chapter 13: Pain Management

CINDY C. GADBURY-AMYOT, R.D.H., M.S.
Associate Professor
Division of Dental Hygiene
School of Dentistry;
Director, Graduate and Degree
Completion Studies
University of Missouri—Kansas City
Kansas City, Missouri
Chapter 10: Dental Biomaterials

KEVIN GYOLAI, M.S.
Assistant Professor
Department of Mathematics and Science
North Dakota State College of Science
Wahpeton, North Dakota
Chapter 5: General and Oral Pathology

CARRIE CARTER-HANSON, R.D.H., M.A.
Private Practice in Missouri;
Formerly Assistant Professor
Division of Dental Hygiene
School of Dentistry
University of Missouri—Kansas City
Kansas City, Missouri
Chapter 16: Community Oral Health

KAM M. HOFFMANN, B.S.
PhD Candidate, Biochemistry
Department of Molecular Biosciences
University of Kansas
Lawrence, Kansas
Chapter 2: Anatomy, Biochemistry, and Physiology

JANIS KEATING, R.D.H., M.A.
Independent Educational Consultant and Professional Lecturer;
Clinical Associate Professor
Department of Dental Hygiene
School of Dentistry
University of Colorado Health Sciences Center
Denver, Colorado
Chapter 11: Clinical Treatment

BEVERLY J. KENNEDY, R.D.H., M.A.
Assistant Professor
Department of Dental Hygiene
University of South Dakota
Vermillion, South Dakota
Chapter 14: Medical and Dental Emergencies

THOMAS A. LANGWORTHY, Ph.D.
Professor
Molecular Microbiology and Immunology Group
Department of Basic Biomedical Sciences
School of Medicine
University of South Dakota
Vermillion, South Dakota
Chapter 4: Microbiology and Immunology

SALME E. LAVIGNE, R.D.H., M.S.
Associate Professor and Director
School of Dental Hygiene
Faculty of Dentistry
University of Manitoba
Winnipeg, Manitoba
Canada
Chapter 12: Periodontology

DEBRALEE MCKELVEY NELSON, R.D.H., M.A.
Associate Professor
Department of Dental Hygiene
University of South Dakota
Vermillion, South Dakota
Chapter 15: Special Needs Patient Care

DONAL SCHEIDEL, D.D.S.
Assistant Professor
Department of Dental Hygiene
University of South Dakota
Vermillion, South Dakota
Chapter 8: Infection Control

EVELYN H. SCHLENKER, Ph.D.
Professor
Department of Physiology & Pharmacology
School of Medicine
University of South Dakota
Vermillion, South Dakota
Chapter 2: Anatomy, Biochemistry, and Physiology

KIMBERLY A. STABBE, R.D.H., M.S.
Professor
Dental Hygiene Program
Johnson County Community College
Overland Park, Kansas
Chapter 9: Pharmacology

DONNA STACH, R.D.H., M.Ed.
Associate Professor
School of Dentistry
University of Colorado Health Sciences Center
Denver, Colorado
Chapter 11: Clinical Treatment

SUSAN SWANSON, D.D.S.
Associate Professor
Allied Dental Education Department
North Dakota State College of Science
Wahpeton, South Dakota
Chapter 1: Histology and Embryology
Chapter 5: General and Oral Pathology

I dedicate this book to my parents,
Jim and Maxcine McKelvey, who devoted a lifetime
to teaching us respect, honesty, and diligence.

To my husband, Mark, who never complained about
countless evenings and weekends spent interacting
with my computer rather than him.

To my children, Kam and Mike, who remained
forever loving, forgiving, and helpful
during the development of this text.

Acknowledgments

A heartfelt thank you goes to all of the contributors to this new review text. Without your enthusiasm, diligence, and attention to detail, none of this would be possible. A special thanks goes to Robert F. Nelson and all of the contributing authors who provided questions and cases for the simulated board examination and the clinical case studies.

Thanks, also, to my students who willingly reviewed parts of this book and offered their suggestions.

Preface

This review textbook is intended to guide the dental hygiene student or graduate through the process of preparing for professional licensure examinations. It was developed by educators with experience teaching dental hygiene students. While particularly helpful in preparing readers for the National Board Dental Hygiene Examination (NBDHE), this review text will also prove useful when preparing for many regional and state dental hygiene board examinations, as well as for clinical practice. Dental hygiene faculty will find this text particularly useful for course development. The numerous clinical case scenarios found in each chapter and in the simulated national board examination provide valuable examples of "real-life" situations that students and practitioners may expect to experience. These cases can be used by faculty to illustrate course content and to test for learning.

Saunders Review of Dental Hygiene is composed of 17 content-review chapters followed by a full-length simulated national board examination. Topics covered in the content-review chapters include histology, embryology, general and head anatomy, biochemistry, physiology, microbiology, immunology, general and oral pathology, nutrition, radiology, infection control, pharmacology, dental biomaterials, clinical treatment, periodontology, pain management, medical and dental emergencies, special needs patient care, community oral health, and ethics and jurisprudence. The introductory section contains information on preparing for the National Board Dental Hygiene Examination (NBDHE) and other licensure examinations. It includes study strategies and advice on taking multiple-choice, stand-alone, and case-based questions.

Each chapter begins with a clinical case study and continues with numerous clinical case studies scattered throughout the content review. The case studies are related to the chapter content and are included to encourage the reader to test and apply their knowledge of the chapter topics. The content review is in outline format and contains a basic review of current dental hygiene knowledge. Following the case studies and content review for each chapter are a series of review questions and an answer key with rationale. The rationale for each question includes the reason why each answer choice is either correct or incorrect so that the reviewer is able to clarify knowledge and improve reasoning ability. Additional reading and reference material lists are provided in each chapter.

The final section of *Saunders Review of Dental Hygiene* is a simulated national board examination that resembles the NBDHE in content, format, and length. Whether taken before or after studying the review material in each chapter, the simulated examination will help the reader identify subject weaknesses. An answer key with rationale for each answer choice follows the simulated examination.

Debralee M. Nelson

Preparing For Dental Hygiene Licensure Examinations

In the United States and other countries, jurisdictions governing the licensure of dental hygienists require at least three measures of competency before granting professional licensure. The three measures are successful completion of (1) an educational program, (2) a written examination, and (3) a practical examination. The written and practical (clinical) examinations were developed to test basic professional and clinical knowledge and are thus used to determine examiners' competency to practice the profession. This review book was developed to help students and graduates prepare for written professional examinations required by national, regional, and local licensing jurisdictions. The book will also prove valuable for review of topics covered on clinical examinations.

TYPES OF DENTAL HYGIENE BOARD EXAMINATIONS

The three types of board examinations taken by those seeking licensure in dental hygiene are (1) the national written examination (National Board of Dental Hygiene Examination [NBDHE]); (2) the regional clinical examinations (given by the Central Regional Dental Testing Service, Inc [CRDTS], the Northeast Regional Board of Dental Examiners, Inc [NERB], the Southern Regional Testing Agency, Inc [SRTA], and the Western Regional Examining Board [WREB]); and (3) the state jurisprudence examinations (given by State Boards of Dentistry or Dental Examiners).

National Board Dental Hygiene Examination (NBDHE)

The NBDHE is developed and administered by The Joint Commission on National Dental Examinations of the American Dental Association. This examination fulfills or partially fulfills the written examination requirement in all 50 states of the United States and the District of Columbia, Puerto Rico, and the Virgin Islands. Individual states determine acceptance of the examination as a requirement, the time period before expiration of results, and the percentage score accepted as passing.

The purpose of the NBDHE is to determine the professional competency of applicants for licensure. The candidate's ability to recall, analyze, and apply basic information and concepts typically taught in the dental hygiene curriculum is assessed.

The NBDHE is written in the English language and is comprised of 350 multiple-choice questions. Of the total, approximately 200 questions are traditional (stand-alone) multiple-choice questions and the remaining 150 questions are based on approximately 12 to 15 dental hygiene cases. The examination is comprehensive in that it covers topics taught to enable competency to perform dental hygiene care as determined by delegated functions of dental hygienists in the majority of states. More specifically, Component A of the examination, the stand-alone multiple-choice section, is composed of the following:

  Scientific Basis for Dental Hygiene Practice (approximately 30%)
  Provision of Clinical Dental Hygiene Services (approximately 60%)
  Community Health Activities (approximately 10%)

Multiple-choice questions contain a question stem and 4 to 5 answer choices. There is only one correct answer per question. Component B of the examination contains case-based problems with comprehensive scenarios that describe a specific situation and require the examinee to demonstrate skill in the following areas:

Assessment and interpretation of patient characteristics

Radiographic techniques, procedures, and interpretation

Planning and management of dental hygiene treatment

Selection and proper use of preventive agents

Determination of suitable supportive services

The case-based scenario may include written descriptions, photographs, illustrations, radiographs, dental and periodontal data, or other information necessary to present the case. Each case is followed by 10 to 12 multiple-choice test items related to the scenario.

Scoring is based on the number of correct answers given and a conversion scale for the examination. Because the examination is given to numerous dental hygiene students at one time, the first-time test-takers become the reference group. Their performance is equated to those of previous reference groups. Using a conversion scoring system such as this regulates the pass rate for the NBDHE to approximately 90% or greater. Passage of the NBDHE requires a score of 75 or greater. Although only one score is given for the entire examination, examinees receive printed reports on their results for subsections of the examination. Examination scores are released to the candidates approximately 6 to 8 weeks after the test date. If candidate permission is given, score reports can also be mailed to dental hygiene program directors and to licensing boards at no additional cost. To request the Candidate Guide for the National Board Dental Hygiene Examination, please contact The Joint Commission on National Dental Examinations of the American Dental Association at 312-440-2678.

Regional Clinical Examinations

Regional Clinical (Practical) Examinations are typically administered by corporate testing agencies. The four agencies that develop and administer regional clinical examinations are the CRDTS, NERB, SRTA, and WREB. The agencies are not licensing services; however, state licensing agencies (State Boards of Dentistry or Dental Examiners) often use the results of these examinations as qualifiers for state licensure. Since most state licensing agencies subscribe to a particular regional testing service, the scores of that particular regional test are often required of those seeking licensure in the state.

The major purpose of regional testing is to asses clinical competency of dental hygiene graduates for licensure purposes. Clinical procedures tested are those generally taught in the region. Regional clinical examinations typically require the examinee to perform clinical procedures (data collection, debridement procedures, radiographs, and so on) that are then evaluated by calibrated examiners. A written component may be included in some regional examinations. Clinical examiners are generally practicing dental hygienists and dental clinicians and educators.

Scoring of regional clinical examinations is determined by each individual testing agency. In most instances, clinical procedures are categorized and given point values. The examinee must successfully pass most, if not all, of the categories to pass the examination. Each agency determines which individual competencies examinees must have in order to be considered clinically competent. For more information on a specific regional testing agency, contact the state board of dentistry or dental examiners for the state in which licensure is sought. They can provide contact and other information regarding the particular regional examination required by the agency.

State or Local Dental Hygiene Licensure Examinations

In most states and locales, a board of dentistry or dental examiners is responsible for determining competency for dental hygiene licensure in that practice area. The dental boards often use results of national, regional, and state examinations as criteria for granting licensure. For each type of examination, the state licensing agencies must determine what score(s) meets their individual state requirements for acceptable competency. These competency scores are usually equivalent to, but may differ from, the national or regional testing agency's minimum passing score.

The usual purpose of state or local licensure examinations is to assess the candidate's knowledge of state law relating to the practice of dentistry and/or dental hygiene. A few states may also administer their own clinical examination. Most local licensure examinations are short, written tests. Some are taken at specific test sites, while others are mailed to the applicant for completion at home. To obtain information regarding state licensure examinations, contact the state board of dentistry or dental examiners for the state where licensure is desired. Scoring of local licensure examinations is determined by individual state testing agencies.

PREPARING FOR PROFESSIONAL EXAMINATIONS

Standardized testing attempts to assess knowledge and comprehension of specific subject matter along with the ability to analyze information and apply the knowledge in practical ways. Examination questions therefore tend to run the gamut of easy (rote memory or recall) to difficult (analysis or case study). While memorization is adequate to answer simple questions, the student must have a deeper understanding of concepts and theory to answer questions that assess higher level learning.

The best preparation for professional board examinations is thorough study throughout the course of the professional program. Review for the NBDHE and other professional examinations can refresh the memory and help clarify materials not understood well previously.

1. Proper preparation is essential for successful test-taking. The more time the student initially spends learning the material, the less time is needed when reviewing material for competency testing. Conversely, those who have not mastered a subject will need to spend more time reviewing for a competency examination, since they must "relearn" much material.

2. Becoming familiar with the examination is vitally important in test-taking. Examine the testing materials and sample booklets. Have a general knowledge of which topics are covered and in what depth, the type or style of questions on the examination and their depth and number, the sections or parts of the examination, the amount of time allowed to answer each question or section on the test, common directions or instructions used, materials that can be used during the examination, and how the examination is scored.

3. Schedule study time. Begin studying for national board examinations approximately 3 to 6 months in advance. Schedule study time into the weekly calendar, preferably setting aside the same time period each week (for example, set aside Thursday mornings from 8:00 AM to 10:00 AM for review). In this way, the review is organized, manageable, and unforgettable. Set up a schedule of study topics (use the REVIEW SCHEDULE at the end of this section). If inadequate time remains for a thorough review of all subject matter, select a few (3–5) of the weakest subjects or those subjects that appear in greatest concentration on the examination and learn them well. Trying to review the entire curriculum in too short of time period will only serve to frustrate and seldom leads to much learning.

   a. Plan study time in 2 to 5 hour segments. Be sure to take planned, frequent breaks. The breaks should occur every 30 to 60 minutes and last less than 10 minutes. Set a timer to ring whenever a break is due. This technique is helpful for training to concentrate on the task rather than on the clock. When a break arrives, use the time to visit the restroom, refill beverages, or take a brisk walk or exercise before sitting down to study again. Do not turn on the television, pick up a novel, or do anything that may interfere with the resolve to study.

   b. Make it a rule to always study the most difficult subject first, saving easier subjects for later in the study period. This avoids procrastination and provides an immense sense of accomplishment.

    c. Studying in groups or individually is a personal preference. For those persons who find it difficult to set a study schedule and follow through, group study may be the answer. While group study is more difficult to organize and somewhat more time consuming, it is particularly beneficial in that it allows members to learn from each other, leads to less boredom, and allows for discussion of topics. A study group should be limited to 6 or fewer members, have a set time and place for meeting, and should require members to prepare for the meetings. Keeping members on the task of reviewing is the most difficult part of the group study. All members should be informed before the study period of what the topic of review is and how they should prepare for it. This can help bring members to a similar level of knowledge and will lead to more meaningful discussion. Studying individually has its benefits and detriments, also. Individual study sessions are easier to organize, less time consuming, and allow one the ability to review at his/her own pace. This type of studying is best for the self-directed learner who is able to set a study schedule and follow through. Like the study group, study sessions should be held at specific times in specific locations.

    d. Set a specific start and end time for each review session. This helps motivate participants to stay on task. Planning the study period to end when a favorite television program or other event begins can be a good incentive and reward.

    e. After every review sessions, check off the subject matter studied on the REVIEW SCHEDULE and plan the next review topic. Charting of progress on a form such as the REVIEW SCHEDULE provides a sense of accomplishment and further incentive to continue reviewing.

4. Getting enough rest is essential before a big examination. This is much easier to accomplish when one feels comfortably prepared for the examination. Not surprisingly, the ability to sleep well before a stressful event is made much easier when one feels up to the task that awaits him/her. It is extremely important that the reviewer not study the evening before a big examination. Instead, do something relaxing to relieve anxiety—take a long walk, watch a favorite movie, prepare a nice meal—and go to bed at the usual time.

5. Proper nutrition is also essential while reviewing for the examination and before taking the test. The diet should be well balanced and provide enough calories for sustenance. Eating a good breakfast before the examination is vitally important, since brain cells need nutrition to function effectively.

6. Attitude is probably the single most important factor in successful test-taking, besides thorough studying. Taking the test with the attitude that one is prepared and capable of success is extremely important. Many people can attest to the fact that the pressure they put on themselves before an examination can adversely affect their performance. Think positively. Having a clear and relaxed mind is very important. A little anxiety is normal and can be beneficial during an examination.

USING SAUNDERS REVIEW OF DENTAL HYGIENE

The material contained in the NBDHE is primarily applicable to dental hygiene practice. Success on the national board examination (NBDHE) means you have an adequate understanding of the concepts and applications of the dental hygiene knowledge base. *Saunders Review of Dental Hygiene* consists of 17 chapters and a simulated NBDHE. The chapters provide a comprehensive review of the basic knowledge of dental hygiene scientific subjects that are likely to appear on the NBDHE.

Each chapter in *Saunders Review of Dental Hygiene* begins with a clinical case study. As many as six clinical case studies are interspersed within each review chapter. They are used to illustrate important applications of content in the chapter and contain a problem situation followed by a series of questions with answers and rationale. Case studies are helpful in improving analytical and application skills. A careful study of these cases will help prepare the graduate for the types of cases that appear on the NBDHE and for situations that arise in clinical practice.

After each clinical case study is a comprehensive review of the subject of the chapter. It is recommended that each clinical case study be read both before and after reviewing the chapter content that follows. After the entire chapter content review and clinical cases have been studied, the review questions should be answered and the answers compared with those in the rationale section that follows. Questions included in *Saunders Review of Dental Hygiene* were specifically developed to be similar in format, content, and depth to those that appear on the NBDHE. The rationale with answer key is particularly useful because it contains discussion of why certain answers are correct or incorrect and can help the reader better understand why one answer choice is better than another.

The final section of this book, the Simulated National Board Dental Hygiene Examination, is comparable in length, format, and difficulty to the NBDHE. Part A contains 200 randomly ordered, multiple-choice questions over basic dental hygiene science, provision of clinical dental hygiene services, and community health activities. Part B consists of 15 case-based studies developed to help the student assess, plan, integrate, evaluate, and analyze clinical information. The case studies were selected to imitate "real" situations the dental hygienist may encounter in practice and requires the reader to carefully assess given medical and dental information, photographs, and radiographs to answer case-specific questions. A careful study of this section of the simulated examination will help the graduate develop the knowledge and skills necessary to successfully manage cases presented on the NBDHE and in clinical practice.

Types of Questions on the NBDHE

There are seven basic question formats on the NBDHE. These include the paired true-false, cause-and-effect, question, completion, negative, testlet, and case study question formats. Each question stem is followed by four to five answer choices. Following is a brief description and example of each.

Paired True-False questions contain two statements about a related topic. The reader will be asked to determine if either one or both of the statements is true. Like multiple-choice questions with four answer choices, the reader has a 25% chance of selecting the correct answer by guessing. Following is an example:

Gingival inflammation always precedes periodontal disease. Periodontal disease always follows gingival inflammation.
A. both statements are true.
B. both statements are false.
C. the first statement is true, the second is false.
D. the first statement is false, the second is true.

Cause-and-Effect questions are similar in format to paired true-false questions. They consist of a single statement that is divided into cause-and-effect portions. The two portions are separated by the word "BECAUSE." The reader will be asked to determine if the statement and reason are correct and related. Like multiple-choice questions with four to five answer choices, the reader has a 20% to 25% chance of selecting the correct answer by guessing. Following is an example:

Obesity is often associated with Type I Diabetes Mellitus because obesity affects insulin resistance.
A. both the statement and reason are correct and related.
B. both the statement and reason are correct but not related.
C. the statement is correct, but the reason is not.
D. the statement is not correct, but the reason is correct.
E. neither the statement nor the reason is correct.

Question-Type questions are the simplest to read and understand. They ask a specific question for which there is one BEST answer. An example is:

Which one of the following collimator types can most effectively reduce scatter radiation to the patient?

A. long round
B. pointed plastic
C. rectangular
D. short round

Completion-Type questions are also simple and easy to read and understand. The question stem consists of a partial statement that the BEST answer completes. An example is:

Opsonins are
A. cytokines produced by B cells
B. antigens that directly neutralize viruses
C. antibodies deficient in the Fc region
D. molecules that stimulate phagocytosis

Negative-Type questions ask the reader to determine which answer does NOT pertain to information in the question stem. It usually includes the words "NOT," "LEAST LIKELY," or "EXCEPT."

Candida albicans is known or suspected to cause all of the following denture-related problems, EXCEPT one. Which one is the exception?
A. denture stomatitis
B. epulis fissuratum
C. papillary hyperplasia
D. angular cheilitis

Testlet-Type questions include a brief description of a situation or case study (usually one to two paragraphs in length) and a series of five or more situation-related questions. This type of question is commonly used on the NBDHE to test Community Health Activity items. Refer to the Community Health Testlet on the simulated NBDHE in the final section of *Saunders Review of Dental Hygiene*.

Case-Based-Type questions contain patient information (health and dental history, significant oral findings, radiographs, periodontal probe readings, photographs, and so on) followed by a series of 10 to 12 case-based questions. This type of question requires that the case information be carefully studied, paying particular attention to its focus. Information useful for answering the case questions must be identified and analyzed. Refer to the final section of this book for examples of case-based questions.

Test-Taking Strategies for Multiple-Choice Style Tests

Multiple-choice style questions tend to be more time consuming than other questions. They require careful reading and analysis of the question stem for content and meaning. Following are some standard guides for taking multiple-choice style tests.

1. Read each question carefully for meaning.
   a. The words "never," "always," and "all" are so restrictive that they seldom appear in the correct answer.
   b. When the words "except," "not," or "but" appear in the question stem, the focus of the question stem changes.
2. At the examination site, quickly preview the questions in the examination before beginning to answer them. Try to answer each question before looking at the possible answer choices. Find an answer choice that parallels yours. If the correct answer can't be determined easily, begin eliminating answer choices, with the most obviously wrong answer first. Once choices are limited to two or three, attempt to clarify the question by redefining or restating it or drawing on other knowledge. When unsure, choose the answer that was instinctively the first choice.
3. Answer all questions while going through the examination and record the answers on the answer form. Rather than waste time on a difficult question, select what was instinctively the first choice and mark it on the answer form. Also mark the question (circle the question number in the test booklet, not on the answer form) so that more time can be spent on the question once easier questions are

answered. Many times, difficult questions will seem easier once other questions have jogged the memory.

Text Anxiety

Test anxiety has affected nearly everyone at some time in his or her life. It is often described as an extreme anxiety that causes shaky legs, sick stomach, jittery hands, chaotic thinking, and outright panic. If unmanaged, it can result in wasted time and ineffective test taking. Being prepared for an examination, plus having a positive attitude (confidence in oneself) and a strategy to deal with the jitters allows the examinee to take control of the anxiety and makes test taking a success. Mild anxiety is normal and is actually helpful because it increases alertness. When faced with the panicky feeling of high anxiety, however, the ability to concentrate is poor. Following are several effective ways to prevent and control test anxiety.

1. Careful preparation for an examination is essential in preventing test anxiety. Knowing the material over which one is being tested provides one with confidence to pass the test. Procrastination and poor time management are usually the culprits in poor test preparation. Use the REVIEW SCHEDULE in this section to plan study times and stick with them.

2. Confidence in oneself is vital to success. A positive attitude, along with careful test preparation, is essential to success. The type of careful test preparation that increases self-confidence includes a thorough review of test subjects, adequate study time, familiarization with the test format and instructions, and an understanding of test scoring (whether wrong answers are penalized or not). Plan to arrive at the test site early, with appropriate materials (pens, pencils, identification, wristwatch, and so on) so that there is time to relax.

3. Take the night off. Be confident in your preparation. Studying the evening prior to a big examination serves only to focus attention on what hasn't been learned rather than what has and increases anxiety.

4. Relaxation techniques can help relieve anxiety. Practice deep breathing (breathe in deeply, hold breath a few seconds, then release) whenever muscle tension is felt—when studying or during the examination. Visualization is another relaxation technique that can relax tenseness. To visualize, close one's eyes and sit comfortably. Use as many senses (hearing, vision, smell, taste, feel) as possible to relive a pleasant experience. Imagine floating on water in warm sunlight or the sounds of nature on a hike in the woods.

5. Once the test begins, answer the easier questions first. Read each question carefully and formulate an answer before looking at the answer choices given. Select the correct answer from the choices given. If unsure, mark the question so it can be returned to at a later time. (If unanswered questions are penalized, select an answer, mark the question, and return to it later, as time allows.) Often, answering easier questions first helps jog the memory and can provide clues to answering the more difficult questions. When unsure of an answer, select the one intuitively felt to be accurate. Never change an answer unless sure the change is the correct choice.

Review Schedule

Chapter	Content Review	Clinical Cases	Questions	Rationale
1 Histology and Embryology				
2 Anatomy, Biochemistry, and Physiology				
3 Head, Neck, and Dental Anatomy				
4 Microbiology and Immunology				
5 General and Oral Pathology				
6 Nutrition				
7 Radiology				
8 Infection Control				
9 Pharmacology				
10 Dental Biomaterials				
11 Clinical Treatment				
12 Periodontology				
13 Pain Management				
14 Medical and Dental Emergencies				
15 Special Needs Patient Care				
16 Community Oral Health				
17 Ethics and Jurisprudence				
Simulated NBDHE				

Contents

Chapter ONE

Histology and Embryology

Susan Swanson, D.D.S.

Clinical Case STUDY

A 60-year-old patient reports to the office for a new patient exam. The radiographs reveal endodontic treatment of tooth #30. The clinical exam reveals that the distal-buccal cusp of tooth #30 has fractured off. The patient indicates that he has no pain associated with any of his teeth.

Clinical Case QUESTIONS

1. Why is tooth #30 not painful?
2. Which cells are no longer active in tooth #30?
3. Discuss possible causes of the distal–buccal cusp fracture.

Clinical Case RATIONALE

1. Although the tooth exhibits a fractured cusp, the patient feels no pain because its nerve tissues were removed during endodontic therapy.
2. The cells associated with pulp tissue (odontoblasts, fibroblasts, histiocytes, and undifferentiated mesenchymal cells) are no longer present after endodontic therapy.
3. The endodontic treatment of tooth #30 increased the likelihood of the tooth fracturing. Posterior teeth often are crowned to reduce the chance of a tooth fracturing. Age-related changes also may cause a tooth to become more brittle.

Content Review

General Terminology

Embryo refers to the stage of human development that occurs between the second and eighth weeks of gestation.

Fetus refers to the stage of human development that occurs after 8 weeks' gestation.

Growth is the increase in weight and/or spatial dimension caused by an increase in the cell size, cell number, and/or cell products.

Development refers to aging and maturation.

Histodifferentiation is the process by which a primitive cell develops into a more specialized cell (e.g., the cells of the inner enamel epithelium of the enamel organ become the ameloblast cells that form enamel).

Histology is the science and study of tissues.

Morphodifferentiation is the stage of development in which cells align and a structure takes form (e.g., after the four layers of the enamel organ are defined, the basement membrane becomes fixed and becomes a template for the dentinoenamel junction).

General Histology

Histology is the study of the structure, composition, and function of tissues. Tissues consist of a group of similar cells that combine in a characteristic pattern and perform a specific function. In addition to cells, tissues also comprise intercellular substance and tissue fluid.

Tissue Components

Tissue components include cells, cell products (known as intercellular substance), and fluids derived from blood plasma (known as tissue fluid).

I. Tissue cells vary considerably in size, shape, structure, and function.

II. Intercellular substance consists of fibrous elements, such as collagen, and ground substance, known as mucopolysaccharides.

III. Tissue fluid is a component of blood plasma that serves to carry nutrients to the cells of the tissue.

Tissue Types

Tissues may be grouped into four main types: epithelial, connective, nerve, and muscle. All four tissues are found in the oral cavity.

I. Epithelial Tissues
  A. May be tissues that act as a surface covering (e.g., skin) or as a lining tissue (e.g., mucous membrane tissue that lines the oral cavity).
  B. May be very specialized tissues, such as salivary glands and tooth enamel.
  C. May be further classified according to the type and arrangement of epithelial cells (see Table 1–1).
  D. Are vascular and rely on neighboring connective tissue for nutrients and the removal of cell waste.
II. Connective Tissues
  A. May be classified as loose, dense, cartilage, bone, or fluid (bone and lymph).
  B. Contain a variety of cells, such as fibroblasts, macrophages, and mast cells.
  C. Provide a variety of functions, such as transporting material (vascular tissue), providing structural support (cartilage and bone), forming ligaments, and supporting and surrounding other tissues (tissues located below the basement membrane of the skin and mucous membrane).
III. Muscle Tissues
  A. Consist of specialized fibers that allow contraction.
  B. May be further divided into three tissue types: skeletal, smooth, and cardiac.
  C. Are considered involuntary (such as heart muscle, which contracts in response to body controls) or voluntary (such as muscles of the arms, legs, and trunk).
IV. Nerve Tissue
  A. Is part of the central (brain and spinal cord) and peripheral (associated with other body organs) nervous systems.
  B. Of the central nervous system is soft and fragile; nerve tissue of the peripheral nervous system is tough.

Embryonic Development

Embryology is the study of gestational development and begins the moment the sperm and ovum unite. This development often is divided into three stages: the zygote stage (week 1), the embryonic stage (weeks 2 through 8), and the fetal stage (weeks 9 through birth).

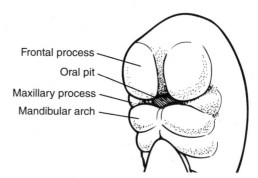

Figure 1.1 Embryonic development of the midface.

General Embryonic Layers

The general embryonic layers are the ectoderm, the mesoderm, and the endoderm. These layers are important because they are all precursors to the structures of the face and oral cavity.
  I. The ectoderm forms the enamel and the lining of the nasal and oral cavities.
  II. The mesoderm forms the skeletal system, muscles, vascular and lymphatic systems, and some internal organs.
  III. The endoderm forms the lining of the GI system, lungs, and genitourinary system.

Embryonic Development and Histology of the Oral Cavity

The face and structures of the oral cavity begin development early in the embryonic period. It is important to understand not only the development of these structures but also their minute structure, composition, and function. The following information provides a review of the embryonic development and histology of the midface, palate, oral mucous membrane, salivary glands, and the dentition and its associated structures.
I. The Midface
  A. Develops from the first brachial arch and the frontal process.
    1. The frontal process develops the forehead.
    2. The brachial arch forms the maxillary processes, which form the cheeks, and the mandibular arch, which forms the mandible (Fig. 1–1).

TABLE 1.1	Types of Epithelium		
Cell Type	**Cell Shape**	**Cell Arrangement**	**Location**
Simple squamous	Flat	Single layer	Vascular system, heart, pleura, mucous membrane
Simple cuboidal	Square	Single layer	Kidney, glands, respiratory tissue
Simple columnar	Rectangular	Single layer	Most glands, small intestines
Simple pseudostratified	Triangular	Single layer	Respiratory passages
Stratified squamous	Polyhedral	Several layers	Skin, lining of mouth, pharynx
Stratified columnar	Columnar over other cells	Several layers	Oropharynx, larynx
Stratified transitional	Square- to pear-shaped	Several layers	Urinary passages, bladder

B. Centers around development of the primitive mouth or stomodeum and occurs by the end of the third week.

C. Development takes place above the stomodeum, where the frontal process forms the median and lateral nasal processes.

   1. The median nasal process forms the center of the nose, the nasal septum, and the globular process.

   2. The lateral process forms the sides of the nose and the infraorbital areas.

D. Structures such as the philtrum are derived from an extension of the median nasal process called the globular process.

E. May exhibit abnormalities, such as a cleft lip, due to a failure of the median nasal process to merge with the globular process.

II. The Palate

A. Develops from the first brachial arch and the frontal process.

B. Is derived from the right and left palatine processes and the globular process.

C. Soft tissue fuses between 8 and 12 weeks' gestation.

D. May exhibit abnormalities, such as a cleft, due to an incomplete fusion of the palatine processes, either with each other or with the premaxillary area of the palate.

III. The Tongue

A. Is formed from brachial arches I to IV; the anterior part of the tongue is derived from the first brachial arch and the posterior part is derived from brachial arches II to IV.

B. Is formed by three anterior swellings: two lateral lingual swellings and the tuberculum impar; these three swellings form the anterior portion of the tongue.

C. A posterior swelling called the copula forms the posterior portion or root of the tongue.

D. Also plays a role in the development of the thyroid gland; the thyroid gland develops from epithelial tissue in the center of the tongue at a site termed the foramen caecum.

IV. The Dentition

A. Develops from the first brachial arch and the frontal process.

B. Formation is referred to as odontogenesis and begins at 6 weeks' gestation.

C. Formation begins at the anterior part of the mandible.

D. Does not begin calcification until approximately the fourth month.

E. Develops from a narrow strand of thickened epithelium called the primary lamina dura.

F. Develops from the tooth germ, which consists of three layers: the enamel organ, the dental papilla, and the dental sac.

G. Form is a reflection of the outer enamel epithelium, which determines the shape of the crown, and Hertwig's epithelial sheath, which determines the shape of the roots.

H. May exhibit abnormalities, such as taurodontism, which is caused by an incomplete invagination of Hertwig's root sheath. Taurodontism is best noted on a radiograph, where the bifurcation area is positioned more apically.

I. Consists of several tooth layers

   1. The enamel

      a. Formation is referred to as amelogenesis and begins at the cusp tips or incisal edge.

      b. Develops from the enamel organ.

      c. Is formed by specialized cells called ameloblasts, which begin forming enamel soon after the beginning of dentin formation.

      d. Is the hardest human tissue, is composed of 96% inorganic and 4% organic material, and is much more difficult to abrade with a toothbrush than cementum or dentin.

      e. Consists of a rod, a rod sheath, and an inter-rod substance.

      f. Cannot repair itself because ameloblasts are lost during tooth eruption.

      g. In cross-section may exhibit dark and light bands (Hunter-Schreger bands) that run perpendicular to the dentinoenamel junction (DEJ), which are caused by a change in the direction of enamel rods.

      h. In cross-section may exhibit fine lines called lines of Retzius from the DEJ to the cusp tips and are caused by the layering process of enamel formation.

      i. May exhibit fine horizontal lines called perikymata, which are a reflection of the lines of Retzius.

      j. May exhibit fine cracks extending into the enamel from the facial surface, which are termed enamel lamellae.

      k. Caries are a reflection of the orientation of the enamel rods and are influenced by hypomineralized areas of enamel, such as enamel lamellae and enamel tufts located at the DEJ.

      l. May form an enamel pearl when a group of cells from Hertwig's root sheath becomes displaced to dentin on the root surface, causing cells to differentiate into ameloblasts and form enamel. The enamel pearl is significant in that it extrudes from the root surface and may feel much like calculus.

   2. The dentin

      a. Formation is referred to as odontogenesis; dentin is the first tissue to be mineralized during tooth development.

      b. Develops from the dental papilla.

      c. Is formed by specialized cells called odontoblasts.

d. Forms first at the cusp tip or incisal edge and progresses toward the root.

e. Located closest to the pulp is the newest and is called predentin; this dentin is initially noncalcified but calcifies within 24 hours.

f. Is composed of 30% organic and 70% inorganic material and is easier to abrade than enamel.

g. Is weaker than enamel and harder than cementum and bone.

h. Consists of tubules that contain the odontoblastic process or Tomes fibers of the odontoblast.

i. Tubules are oriented perpendicular to the DEJ and the dentinocemental junction (DCJ).

j. Exhibits a less mineralized layer below the cementum, called Tomes granular layer, which can cause root sensitivity.

k. That forms secondary to attrition, caries, or trauma is termed reparative dentin.

l. Tubules that do not contain the odontoblastic process and are filled with mineral salts are referred to as sclerotic dentin. Sclerotic dentin is common in older teeth and may decrease the rate of caries spread.

3. The cementum
   a. Formation is referred to as cementogenesis.
   b. Develops from the dental sac.
   c. Is formed by cells of the periodontal ligament called cementoblasts.
   d. Consists of cellular cementum, which is located primarily in the apical and furcation areas, and acellular cementum, which is located in the more cervical portion of the root.
   e. Is composed of 50% organic and 50% inorganic material and has a hardness similar to bone; is easier to abrade than enamel or dentin.
   f. Is normally 0.05 mm wide, is widest at the root apex and furcation areas, and is thinnest at the cervical third of the tooth.
   g. Serves as an attachment site for Sharpey's fibers.
   h. Contains cementocytes housed in lacuna and connected by nutritional pathways called canaliculi.
   i. That forms excessively in localized areas is termed hypercementosis and may be an indicator of chronic inflammation or Paget's disease.
   j. Does not meet enamel approximately 10% of the time, just meets enamel 30% of the time, and overlaps enamel 60% of the time.

4. The pulp
   a. Is formed from the dental papilla of the tooth germ.
   b. Is the only nonmineralized tissue of the tooth.
   c. Consists of three histologic zones: the odontoblastic zone, the cell-free zone, and the cell-rich zone.
   d. Primary cell is the fibroblast.
   e. Contains the nuclei of the odontoblast, which is the cell responsible for dentin formation.
   f. Contains corkscrew-like fibers called Korff fibers, which lie between the odontoblasts.
   g. Contains cells associated with nerve tissue and the vascular system.
   h. May exhibit calcifications, which are referred to as pulp stones or denticles.
   i. May exhibit age-related changes, such as a decrease in pulp size, an increase in mineralization of the pulp, and a decrease in tooth sensitivity.

5. Periodontal ligament
   a. Is a thin layer of connective tissue that surrounds the root of the tooth.
   b. Principal fibers have a characteristic orientation reflective of their location (Fig. 1–2 and Table 1–2).
   c. Width decreases with a decrease in tooth function; for example, the periodontal ligament (PDL) width of tooth #30 would decrease with the loss of tooth #3. The PDL width may increase as a result of excessive tooth function. A tooth abutment for a large bridge may receive excessive forces and the PDL space may enlarge.
   d. Fibers are made up of collagen, a product of fibroblast cells.
   e. Also contains specialized cells such as cementoblasts, cementoclasts, osteoblasts, and osteoclasts.
   f. May contain epithelial rests (epithelial rests of Malassez), which are remnants of Hertwig's root sheath and may have later pathologic significance (tumor formation).

V. Bone and Alveolar Process
   A. Of the mandible and maxilla are derived from the frontal process and the first brachial arch.
   B. Consist of an outer dense layer of bone called compact bone and an inner spongelike bone called trabecular bone.
   C. Are composed of 50% mineralized tissue and 50% nonmineralized tissue.
   D. Of the mandible and maxilla form primarily without a cartilaginous template; this process is known as intramembranous bone formation. The bones of the mandible (excluding the cartilaginous mandibular condyle) and maxilla form directly from connective tissue, which initially exhibits tiny centers of ossification.
   E. Form when tension is placed on the periodontal

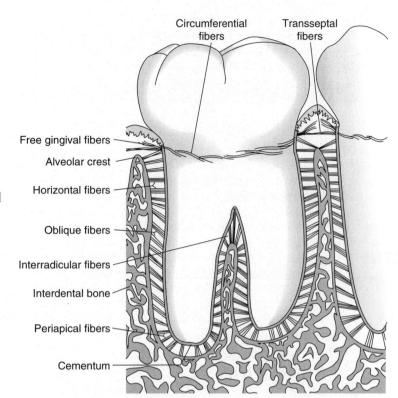

Figure 1.2   Principal fibers of the periodontal ligament.

ligament and resorb when pressure is placed on the periodontal ligament; bone formation and bone resorption are both necessary processes for tooth movement by orthodontics (e.g., a tooth that is moved mesially causes compression of the PDL fibers on the mesial side of the tooth, leading to bone resorption); the tension on the PDL fibers on the distal side of the tooth leads to bone formation.

F. Form as a result of osteoblastic activity and resorb as a result of osteoclastic activity.
G. Decrease in trabecular number and size if tooth function is decreased.
H. Contain internal vascular canals, which nourish the bone and surrounding tissues, such as the PDL.
I. Contain internal cellular channels and spaces called lacunae and canaliculi, respectively.

TABLE 1.2 Principal Fibers			
Principal Fiber Groups	**Location**	**Attachments**	**Function**
Free gingival fibers	Cervical	Cementum to gingiva	Hold gingival tissues tightly against tooth during occlusal pressures
Transseptal fibers	Apical to gingival fiber group; on mesial and distal surfaces	Cementum of one tooth to cementum of adjacent tooth	Maintain proper tooth relationships
Alveolar crest fibers	Alveolar crest	From cementum to alveolar crest in periodontal ligament	Resist horizontal movements of tooth
Horizontal fibers	Apical to alveolar crest	Cementum of tooth root to bone of tooth socket	Resist horizontal pressures to tooth
Oblique fibers	Apical to horizontal group	Cementum of tooth to bone of tooth socket in oblique direction	Resist vertical pressures to tooth
Apical fibers	Apex of tooth	Cementum to bone in bottom of tooth socket; radiate around apex	Resist lifting and tilting forces on tooth
Interradicular fibers	Root furcation	Crest of interradicular septum to cementum of the furcation	Stabilize tooth

VI. Oral Mucous Membrane
  A. Is the lining of the oral cavity that opens to the outside of the body and is derived from the germ layer referred to as the ectoderm.
  B. Consists of the outer epithelial tissue layer and the underlying layer of connective tissue or lamina propria.
  C. Contains an outer layer of stratified squamous epithelial cells.
  D. If located in areas of trauma, may exhibit an outer protective layer of epithelial cells without nuclei, called keratinized tissue.

 Clinical Case **STUDY**

A 49-year-old patient presents in the office with a complaint of tooth pain. The medical and dental history reveal the patient received radiation treatment for a tumor associated with the submandibular gland. The intraoral exam reveals a number of carious lesions, and the oral mucosa appears quite dry. The patient complains that her tissues are sore when she eats.

Clinical Case QUESTIONS

1. What is the cause of the patient's xerostomia?
2. What are the recommendations for treatment of xerostomia?
3. What types of secretory cells were most damaged during the radiation treatment provided for this patient?

Clinical Case RATIONALE

1. The primary cause of her xerostomia is the radiation treatment received for the tumor. Radiation treatment causes glandular tissue fibrosis or atrophy, resulting in partial or total loss of secretory function of the glands. Discomfort and difficulty speaking and swallowing are common complaints of those suffering from inadequate saliva production.
2. The patient may utilize a salivary substitute throughout the day to provide moisture for the mouth when speaking and swallowing. Drinking water frequently, sucking on sugar-free lozenges, and humidifying air in the home have also been found to be beneficial. Daily use of a prescription fluoride gel or rinse helps prevent the formation of caries.
3. The secretory cells that make up the submandibular glands are serous and mucous cells, and both types of cells are damaged by radiation treatment.

E. That covers the gingiva and hard palate is keratinized and is called masticatory mucosa.
F. That lines the nonmasticatory areas typically is nonkeratinized and is called lining mucosa.
G. Of the dorsum of the tongue is considered a specialized mucosa.
H. Of the majority of the tongue is referred to as filiform papillae and is highly keratinized.
I. Contains specialized epithelial cells called taste buds that are most often associated with the circumvallate papillae; however, taste buds also may be associated with the fungiform and filiform papillae.
J. Tissue referred to as gingival epithelium may vary histologically, depending on whether it is outer, sulcular, or junctional epithelium.
K. In the gingival sulcus, exhibits a histologic pocket depth that is determined by the distance from the gingival crest to the point of attachment of the junctional epithelium. The probing depth may be greater than the histologic pocket depth because the probe slightly penetrates tissues at the base of the gingival sulcus.

VII. Salivary Glands
  A. Tissues develop from the epithelium that lines the early oral cavity.
  B. Cells are duct or secretory cells.
    1. When containing serous cells, glands secrete amylase, which contributes to the breakdown of starches.
    2. When containing mucous cells, glands secrete mucin, which acts as a lubricant.
  C. Include the following major glands:
    1. The parotid gland is bilateral and located slightly inferior and anterior to the ear and is a serous gland commonly associated with the childhood infection known as mumps.
    2. The submandibular gland is bilateral and located on the medial posterior part of the mandible and is a serous and mucous gland.
    3. The sublingual gland is bilateral and located in the floor of the mouth and is a serous and mucous gland.
  D. Include minor salivary glands that are located on the lips, cheeks, palate, and tongue and contain serous cells, mucous cells, or a combination of both.

 CONTENT REVIEW QUESTIONS

1. The midface and all structures of the oral cavity except the posterior part of the tongue develop from the:
   A. frontal process and first brachial arch
   B. frontal process and second brachial arch
   C. stomodeum and buccopharyngeal membrane
   D. forebrain and tuberculum impar

2. The formation of an ameloblast from cells of the inner enamel epithelium is an example of:
   A. histodifferentiation
   B. morphodifferentiation
   C. odontogenesis
   D. dentinogenesis
3. Which structure becomes a template for the dentino-enamel junction of the fully formed tooth?
   A. outer enamel epithelium
   B. stellate reticulum
   C. basement membrane
   D. dental papilla
4. Tooth development begins when a localized growth of cells on the jaw ridge produces a strand of epithelium. What is this stand called?
   A. tooth germ
   B. tooth bud
   C. dental lamina
   D. enamel organ
5. The posterior third of the tongue develops from the:
   A. Meckel's cartilage
   B. copula
   C. tuberculum impar
   D. lingual swellings
6. Which of the following determines the shape of the tooth root?
   A. rests of Malassez
   B. stellate reticulum
   C. Hertwig's sheath
   D. dental lamina
7. Enamel contains which percentage of inorganic substance?
   A. 4%
   B. 38%
   C. 74%
   D. 96%
8. The changes in direction of enamel rods create:
   A. lines of Retzius
   B. Hunter-Schreger bands
   C. perikymata lines
   D. neonatal lines
9. Perikymata are external manifestations of:
   A. lines of Retzius
   B. Hunter-Schreger bands
   C. lines of Ebner and Owen
   D. enamel spindles
10. An enamel pearl is often:
    A. found on the occlusal surface, causing discomfort during chewing
    B. confused with calculus because of its location
    C. seen as an opacity ring on the facial surface of anterior teeth
    D. found within the pulp chamber, obliterating the blood supply
11. Odontoblast nuclei are located in the:
    A. predentin
    B. dentinal tubules
    C. pulp
    D. periodontal ligament
12. Cellular cementum is most likely found:
    A. at the apical portion of the tooth
    B. at the CEJ
    C. equally throughout the root surface
    D. closest to the dentin
13. A chronic inflammation of a tooth may cause a localized thickening of cementum referred to as:
    A. a cementicle
    B. hypercementosis
    C. cementogenesis
    D. a cementoid
14. What percentage of the time does cementum NOT meet enamel at the CEJ?
    A. 10
    B. 20
    C. 40
    D. 50
15. Rank the following tissues from most to least abrasion resistant:
    A. dentin, enamel, cementum
    B. enamel, cementum, dentin
    C. enamel, dentin, cementum
    D. cementum, enamel, dentin
16. Which of the following is NOT true as the pulp ages?
    A. vascularity decreases
    B. pulp chamber size decreases
    C. mineralization decreases
    D. sensitivity increases
17. At which location does cementum have the greatest thickness?
    A. at the apex or furcation areas
    B. closest to the CEJ
    C. at Sharpy's attachment sites
    D. at mesial root surfaces
18. Which cells are most active on the mesial side of a tooth being translated mesially during orthodotic treatment?
    A. fibroblasts
    B. osteoblasts
    C. cementoblasts
    D. osteoclasts
19. The most common type of epithelium found in the oral cavity is classified as:
    A. stratified squamous
    B. cuboidal
    C. transitional
    D. simple squamous
20. Which of the following is NOT considered a primary location for taste buds?
    A. circumvallate papillae
    B. fungiform papillae
    C. filiform papillae
    D. foliate papillae
21. Epithelial rests of Malessez are associated with which of the following?

A. the dental sac
B. the dental papilla
C. the enamel organ
D. the lamina dura

22. Which of the following tissues is MOST keratinized?
    A. circumvallate papillae
    B. filiform papillae
    C. foliate papillae
    D. fungiform papillae

23. Which of the following increase in response to an increase in occlusal activity?
    A. cortical bone
    B. trabecular bone
    C. circumferential bone
    D. lamellar bone

24. The histologic pocket depth is:
    A. less than the probing depth
    B. equal to the probing depth
    C. greater than the probing depth
    D. lessened as periodontal disease increases

25. Which of the following is NOT true of sclerotic dentin?
    A. caries will progress more rapidly than in normal dentin
    B. is found in most older teeth
    C. is where odontoblasts have degenerated
    D. is where calcium salts have filled dentinal tubules

26. Corkscrew-shaped structures that lie among dentin are called:
    A. Tomes fibers
    B. Korff's fibers
    C. enamel spindles
    D. dentinal tubules

REVIEW QUESTION RATIONALES

1. **A** The frontal process and first brachial arch are responsible for the formation of the face and oral cavity, not including the base of the tongue. Brachial arches II, III, and IV merge to form the base of the tongue. The stomodeum and buccopharyngeal membranes are important in the formation of the primitive mouth. The tuberculum impar is important in the formation of the anterior portion of the tongue.

2. **A** Histodifferentiation is the formation of a more specialized cell from a primitive cell. Primitive cells are the cells of the inner enamel epithelium and specialized cells are the ameloblasts. Morphodifferentiation is the development of a different form, such as occurs when cells of Hertwig's root sheath align themselves to dictate the shape of the root. Odontogenesis refers to the formation of teeth; dentinogenesis refers to the formation of dentin.

3. **C** The basement membrane marks the junction where the dentin and enamel will meet. The outer enamel epithelium and stellate reticulum are cell layers of the enamel organ. The dental papilla forms the pulpal tissue.

4. **C** The strand of epithelial cells that marks the beginning of tooth formation develops along the jaw ridge and is called the dental lamina. The primary dental lamina forms the primary teeth and the secondary dental lamina is responsible for the formation of permanent teeth. The tooth germ or bud refers to later stages of tooth development. The enamel organ and dental papilla refer to tissues associated with tooth development after the initial localized growth of cells.

5. **B** The copula is a posterior swelling that forms the base of the tongue. The lingual swellings and tuberculum impar form the anterior portion of the tongue. The first brachial arch is responsible for the formation of the maxilla, mandible, and midface. Meckel's cartilage is important in the formation of the alveolar bone.

6. **C** The shape of the developing root is determined by Hertwig's root sheath, which forms when the outer and inner epithelial tissues join. Rests of Malassez are epithelial remnants of Hertwig's sheath and are trapped in the tissues of the periodontal ligament. The dental lamina and stellate reticulum are structures associated with the developing tooth and are not responsible for the shape of the root.

7. **D** Enamel is the hardest tissue in the body and contains 96% inorganic material. Dentin contains 76% inorganic material and cementum contains 50% inorganic material.

8. **B** The light and dark bands of Hunter-Schreger are oriented perpendicular to the DEJ and are caused by curvature of the enamel rods. Neonatal lines, lines of Retzius, and perikymata also are lines found in the enamel.

9. **A** Perikymata are fine horizontal lines that may be visible on the enamel surface. The lines are a manifestation of the lines of Retzius, which are seen microscopically as narrow lines that extend from the DEJ to the cusp tips. Hunter-Schreger bands and enamel spindles are features of the enamel that would not be visible on the external enamel surface.

10. **B** Enamel pearl often is confused with calculus because of its location and shape. Enamel pearls often form near the CEJ and are rounded structures that protrude from the tooth surface. They are never found on the occlusal surface of teeth and are never seen as opacity rings on facial surfaces of anterior teeth. Denticles (pulp stones) commonly are found within the pulp chamber, unlike enamel pearls.

11. **C** The nuclei of the odontoblast cell, the cell responsible for dentin formation, is found in the pulp. The dentinal tubules may contain cytoplasmic extensions of the odontoblast. The newly formed dentin, referred to as predentin, would not contain odontoblast nuclei.

12. **A** The apical as well as the furcation areas are the sites associated with cellular cementum. Cemento-

cytes are not located equally throughout the root surface. The thin cervical cementum has few or no cementocytes. The region closest to dentin contains few cementocytes.

13. **B** A thickening of apical cementum is referred to as hypercementosis. This thickening may be a result of persistent inflammation. A cementicle is a calcification found in the PDL. Cementogenesis refers to the normal formation of cementum. Cementoid is the most recently formed cementum by cementoblasts.

14. **A** Cementum does not meet the enamel approximately 10% of the time at the CEJ. This situation may have clinical significance in terms of root sensitivity and the development of root caries.

15. **C** Enamel is the hardest and therefore the most abrasion resistant tissue, followed by dentin and cementum. The strength of enamel is important in the longevity of tooth structure.

16. **C** Mineralization of the pulp increases as the tooth ages, which has clinical significance when endodontic therapy is indicated. Vascularity decreases and the pulp chamber size decreases as a result of aging. Heavy occlusal function may cause the pulp to completely fill with reparative dentin. As the pulp shrinks, patients may also note a decrease in tooth sensitivity.

17. **A** The apex and the furcation areas are the sites where cementum is thickest (>0.05 mm), while the cervical third is thinnest (0.02 to 0.05 mm). Cementum is approximately 0.05 mm thick on the remaining portions of the root surface.

18. **D** The cells most active on the mesial side of a tooth being moved mesially would be the cells responsible for bone removal or the osteoclasts. The osteoblasts would become active on the distal side of a mesially moved tooth. Fibroblasts and cementoblasts would not experience a great change in activity.

19. **A** Stratified squamous epithelium is the most common type of soft tissue of the oral cavity. Cuboidal or simple squamous epithelial and transitional cells are not considered primary cell layers of the oral cavity.

20. **C** Taste buds are not associated with the filiform papillae. Taste buds are associated with the fungiform, foliate, and circumvallate papillae.

21. **C** Epithelial rests are trapped epithelial cells associated with the inner and outer enamel epithelium that is associated with the enamel organ. The dental sac and dental papilla are mesenchymal components of the tooth germ and would not be associated with trapped epithelial cells.

22. **B** Filiform papillae are more keratinized than fungiform, foliate, or circumvallate papillae.

23. **B** When tooth function increases, the amount of trabeculae also increases. Cortical, lamellar, and circumferential bone do not appear to show significant changes as a result of increased occlusal forces.

24. **A** The histologic depth is less than the probing depth. The probe will slightly penetrate the junctional epithelium leading to a greater probing depth. As tissue health decreases we would expect the probe to penetrate more easily.

25. **A** The presence of sclerotic dentin may decrease the rate at which caries spreads. The sclerotic dentin is a site where odontoblasts have degenerated and may be noted in older teeth. The dentin tubules associated with sclerotic dentin contain calcium salts.

26. **B** Korff's fibers are corkscrew-like collagen structures that lie among the cytoplastic extensions of the odontoblasts. Enamel spindles are extensions of the odontoblastic process into enamel. Dentinal tubules contain the odontoblastic process. Tomes layer is also associated with dentin and is a band of unmineralized spots that may be associated with root sensitivity.

Additional Readings

Bath-Balogh M, Fehrenbach M: Illustrated Dental Embryology, Histology and Anatomy, 1st ed. Philadelphia, WB Saunders Company, 1997.

Enlow DH, Hans MG: Essentials of Facial Growth, Philadelphia, WB Saunders Company, 1996.

Melfi RC: Permer's Oral Embryology and Histology, 9th ed. Philadelphia, Lea and Febiger, 1994.

Taber's Cyclopedic Medical Dictionary, 16th ed. Philadelphia, FA Davis, 1993.

Chapter TWO

Anatomy, Biochemistry, and Physiology

Evelyn H. Schlenker, Ph.D. • Edith J. Applegate, M.S. • Kam M. Hoffmann, B.S.

 ## Clinical Case STUDY

Twenty-three year old Alvin Zana is seated for his oral prophylaxis appointment. During oral inspection, a hard, fixed mass, approximately 6 mm wide by 36 mm long by 6 mm deep, is noted on the right side of his neck. The enlargement is visible. Mr. Zana mentions that the swelling has been there for at least 6 months and is getting larger, but that he has no discomfort. Further inspection of the mouth reveals poor oral hygiene, moderate gingivitis, and no evidence of caries. The patient states that he feels fine, although he tires easily.

Clinical Case QUESTIONS

1. What is the enlargement along the right side of the neck?
2. What would cause such a severe enlargement?
3. Identify treatment planning procedures for Mr. Zana.

Clinical Case RATIONALE

1. The enlargement along the right side of the neck is most likely a tumor or enlarged cervical lymph nodes along the sternocleidomastoid muscle. Other lymphadenopathy may be detected in the armpit and groin areas.
2. Such a severe enlargement is indicative of severe infection (local or systemic) or a malignancy.
3. Treatment planning procedures for Mr. Zana should include a thorough examination of the oral cavity for possible causes of the swelling (e.g., pulpal infection, periodontal infection) and a panoramic radiograph. If no evidence suggests dental causative factors, his dental prophylaxis should be rescheduled until he has seen his physician. It is imperative that the patient seek immediate medical consultation.

Content Review

Gross Anatomy

Gross anatomy is the study of the structure of the body from its simplest structure, the cell, to its most complex, the organ system.

Basic Concepts, Organization, and Definitions

I. Organization Summary
   A. Anatomy is the study of structure; physiology is the study of function.
   B. Structures and associated functions are organized in an interacting hierarchy from simple to complex (chemicals, cells, tissues, organs, body systems, total organism).
   C. Organ systems of the body include integumentary, skeletal, muscular, nervous (including sense organs), endocrine, cardiovascular, lymphatic, respiratory, digestive, urinary, and reproductive.

II. Anatomic Terms
   A. Directional terms describe the relative position of body parts in anatomical position.
      1. Superior is toward the head or upper part.
      2. Inferior is away from the head or toward the lower part.
      3. Anterior is nearer to the front of the body.
      4. Posterior is nearer to the back of the body.
      5. Medial is nearer to the midline of the body or structure.
      6. Lateral is away from the midline of the body or structure.
      7. Proximal is nearer to the point of origin or nearer to the attachment of an extremity.
      8. Distal is away from the point of origin or farther from the attachment of an extremity.
      9. Superficial is toward or on the surface.
      10. Deep is away from the surface.
   B. The body and its parts may be sectioned (cut) along imaginary planes (Fig. 2–1).

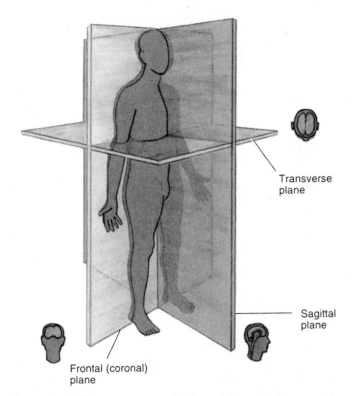

Figure 2.1 Transverse, sagittal, and frontal planes of the body.
(From Applegate EJ: The Anatomy and Physiology Learning System, Philadelphia, WB Saunders, 1995, p. 14.)

1. Sagittal planes divide into right and left parts.
2. Transverse (horizontal) planes divide into upper and lower regions.
3. Frontal (coronal) planes divide into front and back portions.
  C. The human body has two major cavities:
1. The dorsal cavity includes the cranial cavity and spinal cavity.
2. The ventral cavity is subdivided by the diaphragm into the thoracic cavity and the abdominopelvic cavity.
  D. Some terms that refer to specific body regions are: antebrachial, antecubital, axillary, brachial, buccal, carpal, cephalic, cervical, costal, cranial, ophthalmic, oral, otic, pectoral, plantar, and sternal (Fig. 2–2).
III. Homeostasis
  A. Refers to the relative constancy of the body's internal environment.
  B. Typically is maintained by negative feedback mechanisms under regulation from the nervous and endocrine systems.
  C. When lacking, is manifest in illness or disease.

Cell Structure

Cells differ in size, shape, and function, but all have a membrane, cytoplasm, nucleus, and various organelles (Fig. 2–3).

I. Cell (Plasma) Membrane
  A. Is a selectively permeable double layer of phospholipid molecules with scattered proteins and carbohydrates in a fluid mosaic.
  B. Proteins function as receptors, transport channels, carriers, enzymes, support, and immunological identifiers.
II. Cytoplasm
  A. Is a gel-like fluid (approximately 90% water) inside the cell.
  B. Has a variety of organelles suspended in it.
III. Nucleus
  A. Is the control center of the cell.
  B. Chromatin threads, consisting largely of DNA, condense into chromosomes just before cell division; DNA codes for the production of proteins in the cytoplasm through transcription and translation.
  C. Nucleolus is a dense region of RNA within the nucleus and is the site of ribosome formation.
IV. Organelles
  A. Are suspended in the cytoplasm.
  B. Membranous organelles are surrounded by a phospholipid membrane.
1. Endoplasmic reticulum (ER) with ribosomes is rough endoplasmic reticulum (RER) and is involved in protein synthesis; without ribosomes, it is smooth endoplasmic reticulum (SER) and is involved in lipid and carbohydrate synthesis.
2. Golgi apparatus packages secretory products for exocytosis.
3. Lysosomes contain enzymes to rid the cell of bacteria and debris.
4. Mitochondria produce ATP, which provides energy for cellular activities.
  C. Nonmembranous organelles.
1. Cytoskeleton provides strength and flexibility; consists of microfilaments and microtubules.
2. Centrioles are paired, near the nucleus, and direct movement of chromosomes during cell division.
3. Cilia are short, hair-like projections that move substances across the surface of the cell.
4. Flagella are long, thread-like projections that move the cell.
5. Ribosomes are granules of RNA involved in protein synthesis; may be attached to the endoplasmic reticulum or may be free in the cytoplasm.

Tissues

Tissues are groups of similar specialized cells that are connected by an intercellular matrix. There are four main tissue types in the body: epithelial, connective, muscle, and nerve.
I. Epithelial Tissues

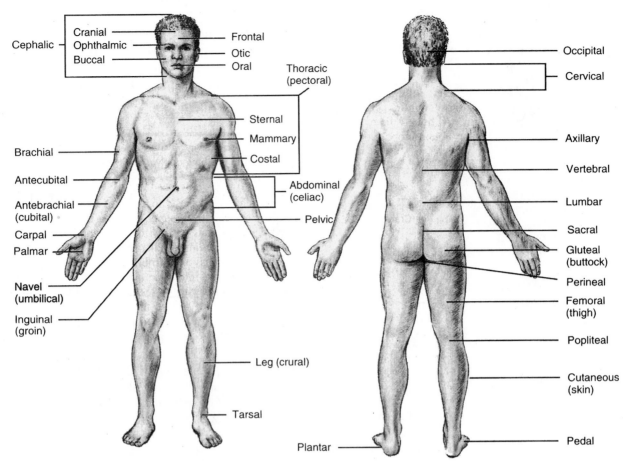

Figure 2.2   Terms for the regions of the body.
(From Applegate EJ: The Anatomy and Physiology Learning System, Philadelphia,
WB Saunders, 1995, p. 16.)

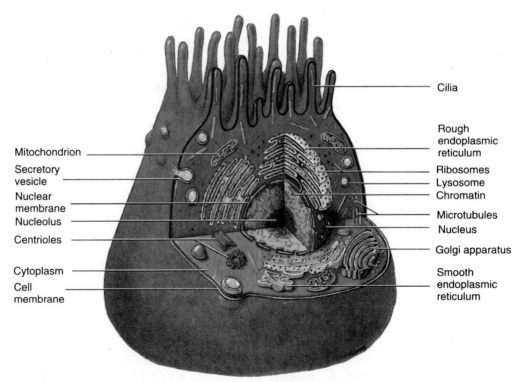

Figure 2.3   Generalized cell.
(From Applegate EJ: The Anatomy and Physiology Learning System, Philadelphia,
WB Saunders, 1995, p. 44.)

A. Consist of tightly packed cells with little intercellular matrix, are avascular, reproduce readily, cover the body, line body cavities, and cover organs within the body.

B. Cells may be squamous, cuboidal, or columnar in shape, may be arranged in single (simple) or multiple (stratified) layers, and may have cilia.

 1. Simple squamous epithelium, which is suited for diffusion and filtration because it is very thin, is found in lungs and capillaries.

 2. Simple cuboidal epithelium is found in kidney tubules (absorption) and glandular epithelium (secretion).

 3. Simple columnar epithelium lines most of the digestive tract for absorption and secretion; it may have cilia, goblet cells (secrete mucus), and/or microvilli.

 4. Pseudostratified columnar epithelium appears stratified but actually forms a single layer; it is found in the respiratory tract, where it has cilia and goblet cells.

 5. Stratified squamous epithelium has many layers of cells for protection; it covers the body (keratinized) and lines the mouth, anus, and vagina (nonkeratinized).

 6. Transitional epithelium has several layers but can be stretched in response to tension; it lines the urinary bladder.

II. Connective Tissues

A. Have an abundance of intercellular matrix, which contains fibers and relatively few cells.

B. Functions include structural framework, transporting materials, protecting internal organs, supporting and surrounding other tissues, storing energy reserves, and defending the body against microorganisms.

C. Connective tissue proper contains a variety of cells (including fibroblasts, macrophages, and mast cells) and fibers in the matrix. Fibers, produced by fibroblasts, are either collagenous, elastic, or reticular.

D. Connective tissue proper is classified as loose connective tissue, which includes areolar and adipose (fat) tissue, and dense connective tissue, which has an abundance of fibers in the matrix and is found in tendons and ligaments.

E. Fluid connective tissue includes blood and lymph. Specialized cells in the blood include red blood cells (erythrocytes), white blood cells (leukocytes), and platelets (thrombocytes).

F. Supporting connective tissue includes cartilage and bone.

G. Cartilage consists of chondrocytes in a firm matrix that contains fibers. A fibrous membrane, the perichondrium, surrounds cartilage. Cartilage is classified as hyaline, elastic, or fibrocartilage, depending on the type of fibers in the matrix.

H. Bone, or osseous tissue, consists of osteocytes in a matrix that contains collagen fibers and calcium salts to make it hard. Periosteum surrounds bone.

III. Muscle Tissue

A. Consists of muscle fibers and is specialized for contraction; the three types are skeletal, cardiac, and smooth muscle.

 1. Skeletal muscle fibers are cylindrical, multinucleated, striated, under voluntary control, and attached to the skeleton.

 2. Cardiac muscle has branching fibers, one nucleus per cell, striations, and intercalated disks; is involuntary; and is located in the wall of the heart.

 3. Smooth muscle cells are spindle-shaped, have a single, centrally located nucleus, lack striations, are involuntary, and are found in walls of internal organs and blood vessels.

IV. Nerve Tissue

A. Is specialized to conduct electrical impulses that transmit information from one body part to another.

B. Neurons are the conducting cells; each neuron consists of a cell body with one or more afferent processes called dendrites and a single efferent process called an axon.

C. Several types of neuroglial cells function in support and defense of the nervous system; these cells do not conduct impulses.

Membranes and Glands

Body membranes are sheets of epithelial tissue that cover body and organ surfaces, line body cavities, and separate and support visceral organs. Glands are specialized masses of epithelial tissue that have a secretory function.

I. Epithelial Membranes form a barrier or interface and typically have a connective tissue base with a covering of epithelium.

A. Mucous membranes line body cavities that open to the exterior, such as the mouth, stomach, intestines, urinary bladder, and respiratory tract; they secrete mucus for lubrication and protection.

B. Serous membranes line internal cavities and cover organs; they always consist of two layers: parietal and visceral; they are delicate and moist and secrete a serous fluid for lubrication.

C. Cutaneous membranes are epithelial membranes that cover the body surface, are relatively thick, waterproof, and typically dry; they also are called the integument or skin.

II. Glandular Epithelium

A. Consists of two types of glands: exocrine, which secrete their product onto a free surface through a duct, and endocrine, which secrete their product directly into the blood.

B. Glands are classified as merocrine (most common), apocrine, or holocrine, depending on the method of secretion.

1. Merocrine glands produce a thin, watery product that is secreted by exocytosis through the cell membrane.
2. Apocrine glands produce a product that accumulates at the surface of the cell; subsequently a portion of the cell membrane is pinched off and discharged with the product.
3. Holocrine glands produce a product that fills the cell; the entire cell is discharged with the enclosed product.

C. Exocrine secretions may be serous (watery, typically containing enzymes), mucous (thick and slippery), or mixed (containing mucus and enzymes).

Integumentary System

The integumentary system consists of the skin (cutaneous membrane), including its glands, hair, and nails. The skin has an outer epidermis and an inner dermis anchored to underlying tissues by the hypodermis or subcutaneous tissue (Fig. 2–4).

I. Epidermis
   A. Is stratified squamous epithelium that has five distinct layers in thick skin and four layers in thin skin.
      1. Stratum corneum is the outermost layer of dead cells, which are continually sloughed off and replaced by cells from deeper layers.
      2. Stratum lucidum, which is absent in thin skin, is a thin, clear layer just beneath the stratum corneum.
      3. Stratum granulosum appears granular because organelles are shrinking and keratin is being deposited in this layer.
      4. Stratum spinosum is located next to the stratum basale and undergoes limited mitosis.
      5. Stratum basale is innermost and closest to blood supply. It is an actively mitotic layer; it also contains pigment cells called melanocytes, which produce a dark pigment called melanin.
   B. Color of epidermis depends on the activity of melanocytes, amount of carotene (yellow pigment), and blood supply in the dermis.
II. Dermis (Stratum Corium)
   A. Upper papillary layer is fibrous connective tissue that contains vessels, nerves, and embedded accessory structures.
   B. Lower reticular layer is a meshwork of collagen and elastic fibers.
III. Hypodermis (Subcutaneous Tissue)
   A. Anchors the skin to underlying organs.
   B. Is composed of loose connective tissue and adipose tissue, which acts as a cushion and insulates the body from heat and cold.
IV. Accessory Structures (Glands, Hair, Nails)
   A. Are derived by cell division in the stratum basale of the epidermis.
   B. Include two types of sweat glands: merocrine glands (numerous and widely distributed) and apocrine glands (larger and less numerous).
   C. Sebaceous glands are oil glands associated with hair follicles.
   D. Hair is divided into a visible shaft and a root, which is embedded in the skin and surrounded by a follicle. The central core of hair is the medulla, which is surrounded by a cortex and cuticle. Arrector pili muscles associated with hair contract

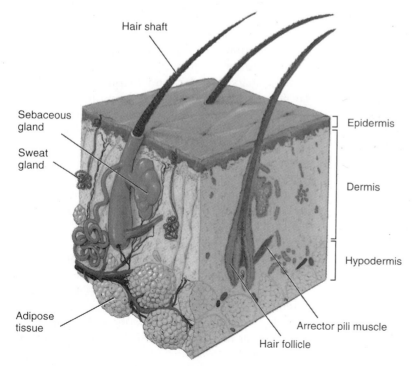

Figure 2.4 Structure of the skin.
(From Applegate EJ: The Anatomy and Physiology Learning System, Philadelphia, WB Saunders, 1995, p. 85.)

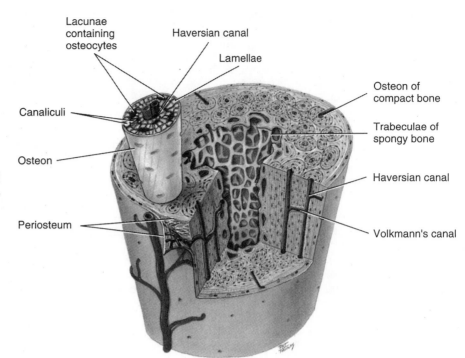

Figure 2.5 Structure of bone tissue. (From Applegate EJ: The Anatomy and Physiology Learning System, Philadelphia, WB Saunders, 1995, p. 97.)

in response to cold and fear to make the hair stand on end.

E. Nails are thin plates of hardened stratum corneum; each has a free edge, nail body, root, eponychium, nail bed, nail matrix, and lunula.

Skeletal System

The skeletal system is made up of the 206 bones in the body, including 80 in the axial skeleton, which forms the axis of the body, and 126 in the appendicular skeleton, which consists of the appendages and their attachments. This system functions to provide support, protect soft body parts, produce movement with muscles, store minerals (calcium), and form blood cells.

I. Osseous Tissue consists of osteons (haversian systems). In compact bone, the osteons are packed closely together. Spongy bone is less dense; it consists of bony plates called trabeculae around irregular spaces that contain red bone marrow (Fig. 2–5).

II. Long Bones, such as the femur, humerus, and phalanges, have a diaphysis around a medullary cavity, with an epiphysis at each end. The epiphysis is covered with articular cartilage; the remainder of the bone is covered with periosteum.

III. Surface Markings on bones include those for articulation, those for muscle attachment, and depressions and openings.

IV. Axial Skeleton consists of the skull, hyoid, vertebral column, and thoracic cage.

A. Skull comprises 28 bones: 8 bones in the cranium (frontal, occipital, 2 parietal, 2 temporal, ethmoid, and sphenoid); 14 bones in the face (2 maxillae, 2 zygomatic, 2 nasal, 2 inferior nasal conchae,

2 lacrimal, 2 palatine, 1 mandible, and 1 vomer); and 6 auditory ossicles (malleus, incus, and stapes in each ear).

B. Hyoid bone is a single U-shaped bone that supports the tongue.

C. Vertebral column consists of 26 bones separated by intervertebral disks (7 cervical, 12 thoracic, 5 lumbar, 1 sacrum, 1 coccyx). Four curvatures add strength and resiliency to the column. Thoracic and sacral curvatures are concave anteriorly; cervical and lumbar curvatures are convex anteriorly.

D. Thoracic cage comprises 25 bones: one sternum and 24 ribs (12 pairs).

V. Appendicular Skeleton consists of the upper and lower extremities and their pectoral and pelvic girdles, which attach the extremities to the axial skeleton (Figs. 2–6).

A. Upper extremities comprise a total of 60 bones; each extremity consists of 30 bones (1 humerus in the arm, 1 lateral radius and 1 medial ulna in the forearm, 8 carpals in the wrist, 5 metacarpals in the hand, and 14 phalanges in the fingers).

B. Pectoral girdle includes the clavicle (collar bone) and the scapula (shoulder blade) on each side, for a total of four bones.

C. Lower extremities comprise a total of 60 bones— 30 bones in each extremity (1 femur in the thigh, 1 medial tibia and 1 lateral fibula in the leg, 7 tarsals in the ankle and instep, 5 metatarsals in the foot, 14 phalanges in the toes, and 1 patella or kneecap).

D. Pelvic girdle includes two bones, the os coxae or innominate bones; each is formed from the ilium,

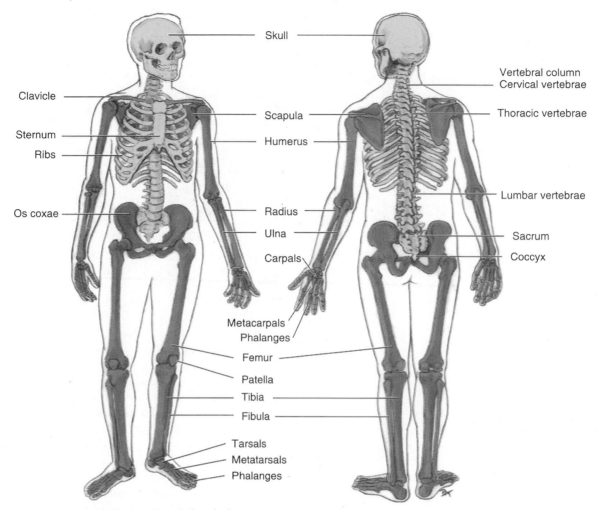

Figure 2.6 Bones of the skeleton.
(From Applegate EJ: The Anatomy and Physiology Learning System, Philadelphia, WB Saunders, 1995, p. 101.)

ischium, and pubis, which are fused together; a large depression, the acetabulum, provides the socket for the head of the femur.

VI. Articulations or Joints

A. Synarthrosis refers to an immovable fibrous joint; an example is a suture in the skull.

B. Amphiarthrosis refers to a slightly movable joint, in which bones are connected by hyaline cartilage or fibrocartilage; examples include the symphysis pubis and intervertebral discs.

C. Diarthrosis (synovial joint) refers to a freely movable joint with motion limited only by surrounding tendons, ligaments, and bones. Bones are held together by a fibrous joint capsule lined with synovial membrane that secretes synovial fluid for lubrication. Types include gliding, condyloid, hinge, saddle, pivot, and ball-and-socket; examples include the hip, knee, shoulder, elbow, and wrist.

Muscular System

The muscular system includes all skeletal muscle tissue that can be controlled voluntarily. The functions of these muscles are to produce skeletal movement, maintain posture, support soft tissues, and produce heat to maintain body temperature.

I. Structure of Skeletal Muscle (Fig. 2–7)

A. Muscles and muscle fibers are surrounded by connective tissue coverings, which extend beyond the muscle to form tendons; endomysium surrounds individual muscle fibers; perimysium surrounds each fasciculus; epimysium covers the entire muscle.

B. Each skeletal muscle fiber represents a single muscle cell, which has a sarcolemma, sarcoplasm, sarcoplasmic reticulum, mitochondria, and myofibrils composed of the myofilaments actin and myosin.

C. Actin and myosin are organized in repeating

sarcomeres and the arrangement is responsible for the striations that are evident in skeletal muscle fibers.

II. Attachments and Actions
   A. Muscles are attached to bones by tendons. The origin is the less movable attachment; the insertion is the more movable attachment.
   B. Primary muscle action is classified as agonist, which refers to the muscle that is the "prime mover"; synergist, which refers to muscles that assist the prime mover; or antagonist, which refers to muscles that move in opposition to the prime mover.
   C. Muscle contraction is either isometric or isotonic. During isometric contraction, the tension in the muscle increases, but the length does not change. Isotonic contraction results in movement because the muscle fibers shorten; however, the muscle tension remains unchanged.

III. Major Axial Muscle Groups (according to their site of action)
   A. Head and neck: muscles of facial expression (frontalis, orbicularis oris, orbicularis oculi, and buccinator); muscles of mastication (temporalis, masseter, and lateral and medial pterygoids); muscles in neck (sternocleidomastoid and trapezius).
   B. Spine: erector spinae, which form a mass on either side of the vertebral column.
   C. Trunk: thoracic wall (external and internal intercostals); abdominal wall (external and internal oblique, transversus abdominis, rectus abdominis); and diaphragm.
   D. Pelvic floor: superficial (bulbospongiosus, ischiocavernosus, and transversus perinea) and deep (levator ani and coccygeus).

IV. Major Appendicular Muscle Groups (according to their site of action; Fig. 2–8, *A* and *B*)
   A. Shoulder and arm: shoulder (trapezius and serratus anterior); arm (pectoralis major, latissimus dorsi, deltoid, and rotator cuff muscles).
   B. Forearm and hand: forearm (triceps brachii, biceps brachii, brachialis, and brachioradialis); hand (extensor muscles on posterior surface of forearm, flexor muscles on anterior surface, and pronator and supinator muscles).
   C. Thigh: muscles that abduct and rotate (gluteus maximus, gluteus medius, gluteus minimus, and tensor fasciae latae); muscles that adduct (adductor longus, adductor brevis, adductor magnus, gracilis); muscles that flex (iliopsoas).
   D. Leg: extensors are the quadriceps femoris in the anterior compartment (vastus lateralis, vastus medialis, vastus intermedius, and rectus femoris); flexors are the hamstrings in the posterior compartment (semimembranosus, semitendinosus, and biceps femoris).
   E. Ankle and foot: muscles for dorsiflexion (tibialis anterior in the anterior compartment); plantar flexion (gastrocnemius and soleus in the posterior compartment); and eversion (peroneus in lateral compartment).

Nervous System

The nervous system includes all neural tissue (neurons and neuroglia) in the body. The region of communication between neurons is the synapse, which occurs through the effects of neurotransmitters. The nervous system is divided into the central nervous system (brain and spinal cord) and the peripheral nervous system (cranial and spinal nerves), which function together to integrate and coordinate body activities and to assimilate experiences to assist memory and learning.

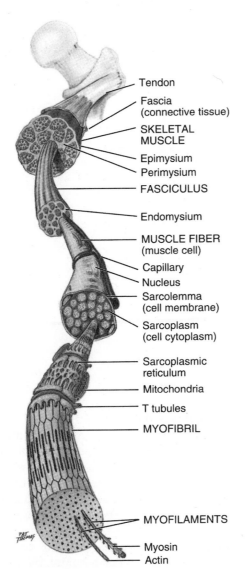

Tendon
Fascia (connective tissue)
SKELETAL MUSCLE
Epimysium
Perimysium
FASCICULUS
Endomysium
MUSCLE FIBER (muscle cell)
Capillary
Nucleus
Sarcolemma (cell membrane)
Sarcoplasm (cell cytoplasm)
Sarcoplasmic reticulum
Mitochondria
T tubules
MYOFIBRIL
MYOFILAMENTS
Myosin
Actin

Figure 2.7 Structure of muscles.
(From Applegate EJ: The Anatomy and Physiology Learning System, Philadelphia, WB Saunders, 1995, p. 127.)

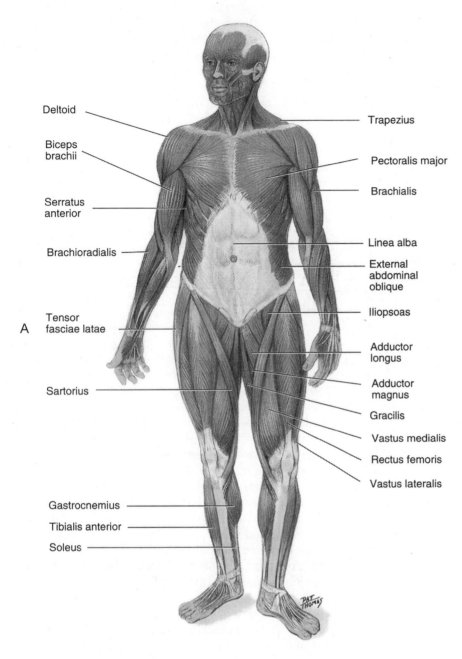

Deltoid

Biceps brachii

Serratus anterior

Brachioradialis

A Tensor fasciae latae

Sartorius

Gastrocnemius

Tibialis anterior

Soleus

Trapezius

Pectoralis major

Brachialis

Linea alba

External abdominal oblique

Iliopsoas

Adductor longus

Adductor magnus

Gracilis

Vastus medialis

Rectus femoris

Vastus lateralis

Figure 2.8 General view of body musculature. *A,* Anterior view.
(From Applegate EJ: The Anatomy and Physiology Learning System, Philadelphia, WB Saunders, 1995, p. 145, 146.)

I. Functions
A. Sensory functions transmit information to the brain and spinal cord.
B. Motor functions transmit information from the brain and spinal cord to effectors, such as muscles and glands.
C. Integrative functions interpret the sensory information and act by stimulating motor pathways.
II. Central Nervous System (CNS)
A. Is composed of the brain and spinal cord (Figs. 2–9 and 2–10).
B. Is covered by membranes called meninges, which comprise an outer layer (dura mater), middle layer (arachnoid), and innermost layer (pia mater); the subarachnoid space between the arachnoid and

pia mater contains blood vessels and cerebrospinal fluid.
C. Components of the brain
1. Cerebrum is the largest portion, is divided into two hemispheres by the longitudinal fissure, and is connected by a band of white fibers, called the corpus callosum. The outer surface is the cerebral cortex, which is composed of gray matter and is marked by gyri (raised folds or convolutions on the cerebrum surface) and sulci (grooves or furrows between convolutions). Each hemisphere has a frontal, parietal, occipital, and temporal lobe, and an insula. The primary somatosensory area is in the parietal lobe, the primary somatomotor area is in the

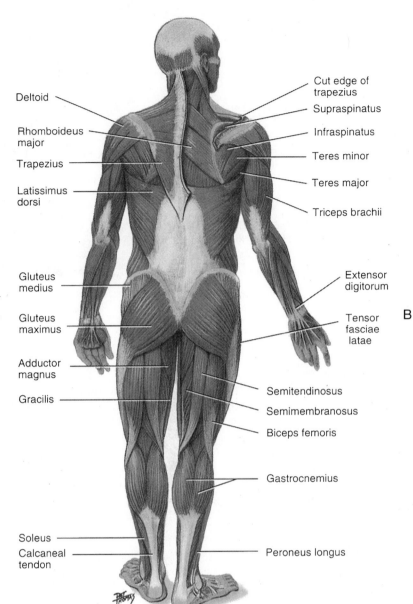

Deltoid

Rhomboideus major

Trapezius

Latissimus dorsi

Cut edge of trapezius

Supraspinatus

Infraspinatus

Teres minor

Teres major

Triceps brachii

Gluteus medius

Gluteus maximus

Adductor magnus

Gracilis

Extensor digitorum

Tensor fasciae latae

Semitendinosus

Semimembranosus

Biceps femoris

Gastrocnemius

Soleus

Calcaneal tendon

Peroneus longus

B

Figure 2.8 *Continued. B,* Posterior view. (From Applegate EJ: The Anatomy and Physiology Learning System, Philadelphia, WB Saunders, 1995, p. 145, 146.)

frontal lobe, the visual cortex is in the occipital lobe, the auditory and olfactory areas are in the temporal lobe, and taste is in the parietal lobe.

2. Diencephalon is surrounded by the cerebrum and includes the thalamus and hypothalamus. The thalamus serves as a relay station for sensory impulses that travel to the cerebral cortex; the hypothalamus plays a key role in maintaining homeostasis.

3. Brainstem is the region between the diencephalon and spinal cord. It consists of the midbrain, pons, and medulla oblongata. The midbrain contains voluntary motor tracts and visual and auditory reflex centers; the pons contains the pneumotaxic and apneustic areas that help regulate breathing movements; the medulla oblongata contains ascending and descending tracts and vital cardiac, vasomotor, and respiratory centers.

4. Cerebellum is the second largest portion of the brain; it is a motor area that coordinates skeletal muscle activity and is important in maintaining muscle tone, posture, and balance.

5. Spinal cord is a continuation of the medulla oblongata and extends from the foramen magnum to the first lumbar vertebrae. It acts as a conduction pathway and reflex center. Ascending tracts in the cord conduct sensory impulses to the brain; descending tracts carry motor impulses from the brain to effectors.

III. Peripheral Nervous System (PNS)

A. Includes all cranial and spinal nerves.

B. Consists of an afferent (sensory) division and an efferent (motor) division. The efferent division

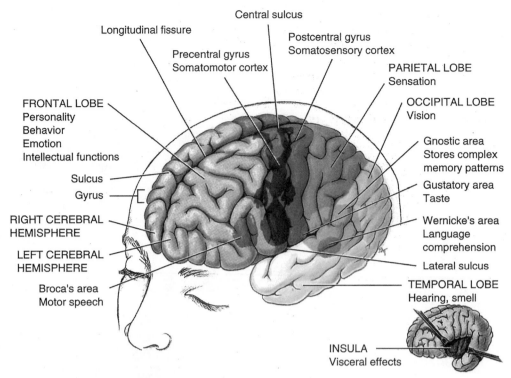

Figure 2.9 Lobes of the cerebrum.
(From Applegate EJ: The Anatomy and Physiology Learning System, Philadelphia, WB Saunders, 1995, p. 167.)

includes the somatic nervous system, which enables voluntary control over skeletal muscle contraction, and the autonomic nervous system, which regulates smooth and cardiac muscle contraction and glandular activity.

C. Components include:

1. Bundles of nerve fibers (axons and dendrites).
2. Twelve pairs of cranial nerves that emerge from the inferior surface of the brain; these are designated by Roman numeral and name.
   a. I—Olfactory
   b. II—Optic

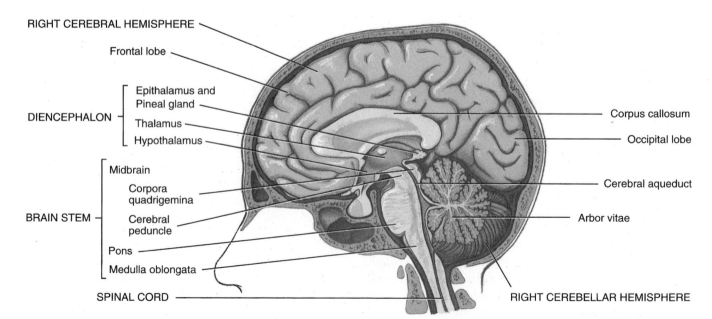

Figure 2.10 Midsagittal section of the brain.
(From Applegate EJ: The Anatomy and Physiology Learning System, Philadelphia, WB Saunders, 1995, p. 168.)

   c. III—Ophthalmic
   d. IV—Trochlear
   e. V—Trigeminal
   f. VI—Abducens
   g. VII—Facial
   h. VIII—Vestibulocochlear
   i. IX—Glossopharyngeal
   j. X—Vagus
   k. XI—Accessory
   l. XII—Hypoglossal

3. Spinal nerves contain both sensory and motor fibers; 31 pairs emerge from the spinal cord and are grouped according to origin. In all but the thoracic region, the main portions of the nerves form complex networks called plexuses (cervical, brachial, lumbar, sacral); nerves emerge from the plexuses to supply specific regions of the body.

IV. Autonomic Nervous System (ANS)
  A. Is a visceral efferent system that is part of the peripheral nervous system; it innervates smooth muscle, cardiac muscle, and glands.
  B. Has two divisions, the sympathetic and parasympathetic, with most organs being innervated by both to maintain homeostasis.
    1. Sympathetic division (thoracolumbar division) of the ANS is an energy expending system that prepares the body for emergencies or stressful conditions. Most of the postganglionic neurons in this division release norepinephrine.
    2. Parasympathetic division (craniosacral division) of the ANS is an energy conserving system that is most active when the body is in a normal relaxed condition. Most of the postganglionic neurons in this division release acetylcholine.

Sense Organs

Sense organs include the widely distributed general senses and the localized special senses of taste, smell, vision, hearing, and equilibrium.

I. General Senses are widely distributed in the body and include touch, pressure, proprioception, thermoreception, and pain.
  A. Touch and pressure—free nerve endings, Meissner corpuscles, Pacinian corpuscles.
  B. Proprioception (sense of position or orientation)—Golgi tendon organs and muscle spindles.
  C. Thermoreception (temperature changes)—thermoreceptors are free nerve endings, some of which are sensitive to heat, others to cold; extremes in temperature stimulate pain receptors.
  D. Pain (nociceptors)—free nerve endings that are stimulated by tissue damage.

II. Gustatory (taste) and Olfactory (smell) Senses are localized special senses, closely related, and complementary.
  A. Taste receptors are located on the papillae on the surface of the tongue. Salty, sweet, sour, and bitter are the four taste sensations. Cranial nerve VII (facial) transmits taste impulses from the anterior two thirds of the tongue and cranial nerve IX (glossopharyngeal) transmits impulses from the posterior one third of the tongue; impulses are interpreted in the parietal lobe.
  B. Receptors for smell are located in the olfactory epithelium of the nasal cavity. Cranial nerve I (olfactory) transmits impulses from the olfactory epithelium; impulses are perceived as odors in the temporal lobe.

III. Visual Sense is a localized special sense.
  A. Protective features of the eye: eyebrows, eyelids, and eyelashes protect the eye from foreign particles and irritants. Lacrimal glands produce tears that moisten and cleanse the eye and destroy bacteria.
  B. Structure of the eyeball: sclera (white) and cornea (clear) form the outermost fibrous layer; choroid (absorbs excess light), ciliary body (changes shape of lens), and iris (regulates size of pupil) form the middle vascular layer; retina is the innermost, or nervous, layer and contains the visual receptors; aqueous humor fills the anterior cavity and vitreous humor fills the posterior cavity of the eye (Fig. 2–11).
  C. Refraction (bending of light rays) is necessary to focus light rays on the retina. The four refractive media are the cornea, aqueous humor, lens, and vitreous humor. In the normal relaxed eye, refractive media are sufficient to focus light rays from 20 or more feet on the retina; closer objects require accommodation to focus. Accommodation involves change in the shape of the lens, convergence of the eyes, and constriction of pupil.
  D. Photoreceptors are rods for vision in dim light and cones for color and acuity in bright light; cones are concentrated in the fovea centralis and rods are located peripherally in the retina.
  E. Visual pathway begins with impulses that are triggered by chemical reactions in the rods and cones that are transmitted to the optic nerve.

IV. Auditory Sense is a localized special sense (Fig. 2–12).
  A. Regions of the ear include the outer ear (auricle and external auditory meatus), which ends at the tympanic membrane; the middle ear, which contains the auditory ossicles (malleus, incus, and stapes); and the inner ear, which contains the vestibule, semicircular canals, and cochlea.
  B. Receptors for hearing are located in the organ of Corti in the cochlea.
  C. Sound waves cause the tympanic membrane to vibrate; vibrations are transmitted to inner ear by the ossicles. As fluids in the inner ear vibrate, the organ of Corti moves and hairs on the receptor cells bend, triggering an impulse that is transmitted on the cochlear branch of cranial nerve VIII to

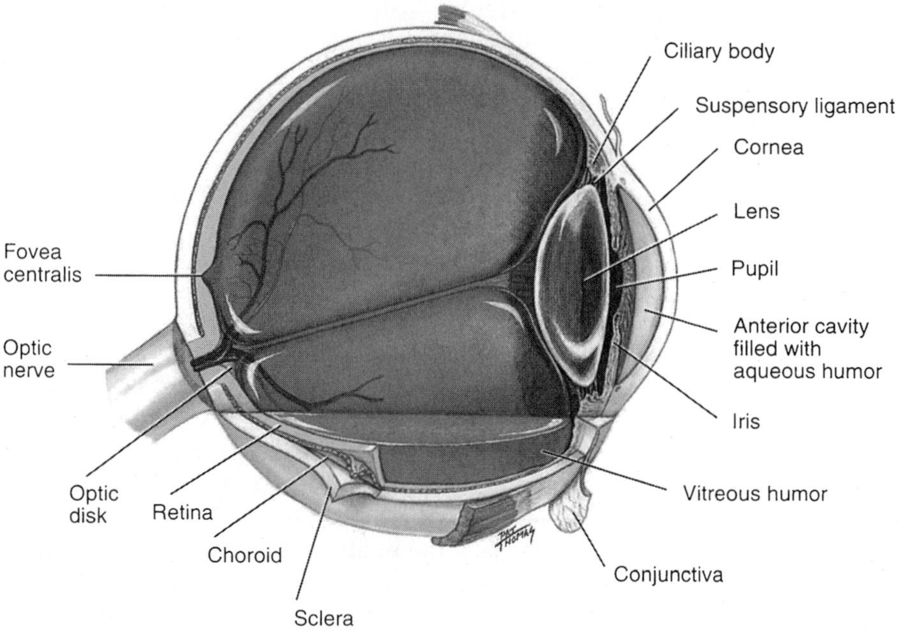

Figure 2.11   Anatomy of the eye. (From Applegate EJ: The Anatomy and Physiology Learning System, Philadelphia, WB Saunders, 1995, p. 191.)

the temporal lobe, where the impulses are interpreted as sound.

V. Sense of Equilibrium is a localized special sense.
1. Receptors are located in the vestibule and semicircular canals of the inner ear.
2. As fluids in the inner ear move relative to the force of gravity, hairs on the receptor cells bend, triggering an impulse that is transmitted

on the vestibular branch of cranial nerve VIII; the brain interprets the impulses in terms of acceleration and position.

Endocrine System

The endocrine system consists of endocrine glands and the hormones they produce. The endocrine system acts with the nervous system to regulate body activities to

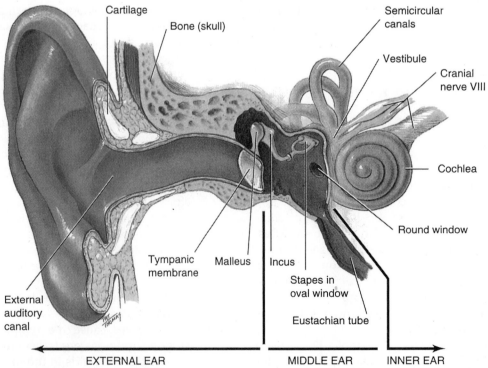

Figure 2.12   Anatomy of the ear. (From Applegate EJ: The Anatomy and Physiology Learning System, Philadelphia, WB Saunders, 1995, p. 196.)

maintain homeostasis. The nervous system acts through electrical impulses and neurotransmitters, and its effects are localized and of short duration; the endocrine system acts through chemicals called hormones and its effects are more generalized and of longer duration.

I. Chemical Classes of Hormones
   A. Proteins and polypeptides, which are long chains of amino acids; includes most of the hormones in the body.
   B. Amines, which are derivatives of amino acids; includes epinephrine, norepinephrine, and thyroxine.
   C. Steroids, which are derivatives of cholesterol, a lipid; includes sex hormones and hormones from the adrenal cortex.
II. Mechanisms of Hormone Action
   A. Hormones react with specific receptor sites on or in cells; cells with appropriate receptors make up the target tissues.
   B. Protein hormones react with receptors on the cell membrane; amines and steroids react with receptors in the cytoplasm or nucleus.
   C. Most hormone action is regulated by negative feedback; stimulus may be other hormones, substances in the blood, or direct neural stimulation.
III. Endocrine Glands and Their Hormones (Fig. 2–13)
   A. Anterior pituitary (adenohypophysis)—growth hormone (GH), adrenocorticotropic hormone (ACTH), thyroid stimulating hormone (TSH), follicle stimulating hormone (FSH), luteinizing hormone (LH), and prolactin.

   B. Posterior pituitary (neurohypophysis)—antidiuretic hormone (ADH) and oxytocin.
   C. Thyroid gland—thyroxine and calcitonin.
   D. Parathyroid gland—parathyroid hormone.
   E. Adrenal (suprarenal) cortex—mineralocorticoids (aldosterone), glucocorticoids (cortisol), and sex steroids.
   F. Adrenal (suprarenal) medulla—epinephrine and norepinephrine.
   G. Pancreas (islets of Langerhans)—insulin and glucagon.
   H. Testes—androgens (testosterone).
   I. Ovaries—estrogen and progesterone.

Cardiovascular System

The cardiovascular system includes the blood, heart, and blood vessels.

I. Blood (liquid connective tissue)
   A. Volume and characteristics: measures about 5 liters; 8% of body weight; pH = 7.35 to 7.45; four to five times heavier than water; is the transport medium in the body.
   B. Composition: plasma is approximately 55% of blood volume, formed elements compose approximately 45% of the volume.
      1. Plasma is primarily water; it also contains plasma proteins, nutrients, gases, electrolytes, and some nitrogenous waste compounds.
      2. Formed elements include:
         a. Erythrocytes (RBCs or red blood cells), which are anucleate, biconcave disks that contain hemoglobin and transport oxygen and some carbon dioxide. A normal erythrocyte count is 4.5 to 6 million/mm^3.
         b. Leukocytes (WBCs or white blood cells), which have a nucleus and do not have hemoglobin. The five types of leukocytes include neutrophils (most numerous), eosinophils, basophils, monocytes, and lymphocytes. Leukocytes provide defense against disease and mediate inflammatory reactions. A normal WBC count ranges between 5,000/mm^3 and 9,000/mm^3.
         c. Thrombocytes (platelets), which are small fragments of cells and aid in blood clotting. A normal count is between 250,000 and 500,000/mm^3 of blood.
   C. Blood types (ABO and Rh)
      1. ABO blood types are based on agglutinogens (antigens), which are present on the surface of RBCs. Type A has A agglutinogens and anti-B agglutinins (antibodies); type B has B agglutinogens and anti-A agglutinins; type AB has both agglutinogens and neither agglutinin; and type O has neither agglutinogen and both agglutinins.
      2. In transfusion reactions, the recipient's agglutinins react with the donor' agglutinogens; type

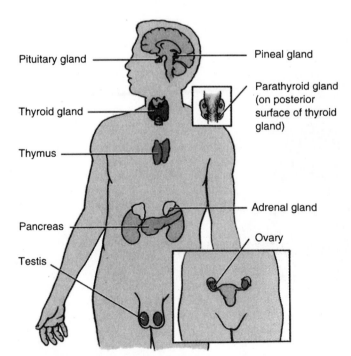

Figure 2.13 Endocrine glands.
(From Applegate EJ: The Anatomy and Physiology Learning System, Philadelphia, WB Saunders, 1995, p. 208.)

Labels for Figure 2.13:
Pituitary gland
Thyroid gland
Thymus
Pancreas
Testis
Pineal gland
Parathyroid gland (on posterior surface of thyroid gland)
Adrenal gland
Ovary

AB is called universal recipient and type O is called universal donor.

3. People with Rh+ blood have Rh agglutinogens; those with Rh– blood do not. Normally neither type has anti-Rh agglutinins. Exposure to Rh+ blood causes an Rh– individual to develop anti-Rh agglutinins and subsequent exposures may result in a transfusion reaction.

II. Heart (Fig. 2–14)

A. Is located in the middle mediastinum, between the second and sixth ribs. The apex points downward and to the left so that two thirds of the heart mass is on left. The heart is approximately the size of a closed fist; is enclosed in a fibrous pericardial sac that is lined with a serous membrane.

B. Heart wall: outer layer is the epicardium (serous membrane); middle layer is the myocardium, which is the thickest layer and is composed of cardiac muscle; innermost layer is the endocardium, which is composed of simple squamous epithelium.

C. Chambers: atria are thin-walled receiving chambers; ventricles are thick-walled pumping chambers.

1. Right atrium receives oxygen poor blood from the systemic circulation through the inferior and superior venae cavae; left atrium receives oxygen rich blood from the lungs through pulmonary veins.

2. Right ventricle pumps blood to the lungs through the pulmonary trunk; left ventricle pumps blood to the systemic circulation through the aorta; left ventricle has the thickest myocardium.

D. Valves

1. Atrioventricular valves are located between the atria and ventricles; the tricuspid valve is on the right and the bicuspid (mitral) valve is on the left.

2. Semilunar valves are located at the exits from the heart; the pulmonary semilunar valve regulates flow from the right ventricle into pulmonary trunk; the aortic semilunar valve is between the left ventricle and the ascending aorta.

III. Blood Vessels

A. Arteries carry blood away from the heart; arterial wall consists of tunica intima (simple squamous epithelium), tunica media (smooth muscle), and tunica externa (connective tissue).

B. Veins carry blood toward the heart; walls are composed of the same three layers as arterial walls, but they are thinner and have valves to prevent the backflow of blood.

C. Capillaries form the connection between arteries and veins. Capillary walls are simple squamous epithelium, which makes them an ideal site for the exchange of materials between blood and cells.

D. Circulatory pathways (Fig. 2–15)

1. Pulmonary circulation transports oxygen-poor

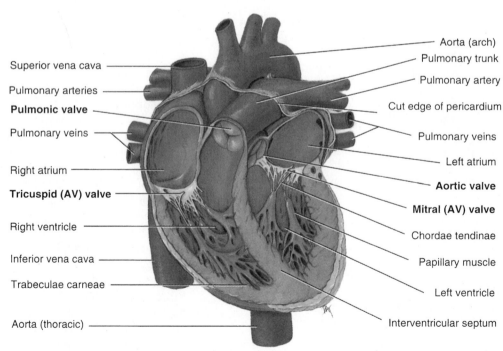

Figure 2.14 Internal view of the heart.
(From Applegate EJ: The Anatomy and Physiology Learning System, Philadelphia, WB Saunders, 1995, p. 248.)

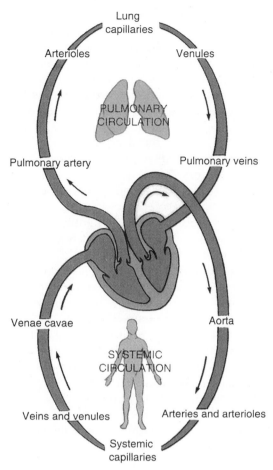

Figure 2.15 Circulatory pathways.
(From Applegate EJ: The Anatomy and Physiology Learning System, Philadelphia, WB Saunders, 1995, p. 262.)

blood from the right ventricle through the pulmonary arteries to the lungs, where the blood picks up a new oxygen supply; subsequently pulmonary veins return the oxygen rich blood to the left atrium.

2. Systemic circulation carries oxygen-rich blood from the left ventricle through the systemic arteries to the capillaries in the tissues of the body for oxygen and carbon dioxide exchange; systemic veins transport oxygen-poor blood containing carbon dioxide from the capillaries to the superior and inferior venae cavae, and subsequently into the right atrium.

3. Hepatic portal circulation carries venous blood from the digestive system to the liver, where it filters through sinusoids and subsequently enters the hepatic veins to the inferior vena cava (IVC).

Lymphatic System

The lymphatic system is composed of the lymph, lymphatic vessels, and lymphatic organs. It functions to return excess interstitial fluid to the blood, absorb fats

and fat soluble vitamins from the digestive system, and provide defense against invading microorganisms and disease.

I. Lymph is interstitial fluid that has entered lymph vessels.

II. Lymphatic Vessels carry fluid from interstitial spaces and return it to subclavian veins, where it becomes part of blood plasma. The vessels have thin walls and valves; small lymphatic vessels merge to form larger ones until there are two main ducts that empty into the subclavian veins. The right lymphatic duct drains the upper right quadrant of the body and the thoracic duct drains the remainder of the body.

III. Lymphatic Organs include the lymph nodes, tonsils, spleen, and thymus (Fig. 2–16).

   A. Lymph nodes consist of dense masses of lymphocytes separated by spaces called sinuses; they filter and cleanse the lymph before it enters the blood. Nodes tend to cluster in three areas: the inguinal nodes cluster in the groin, the axillary nodes in the armpit, and the cervical nodes in the neck. No lymph nodes exist in the CNS.

   B. Tonsils are aggregates of lymphatic tissue that provide protection against pathogens that may

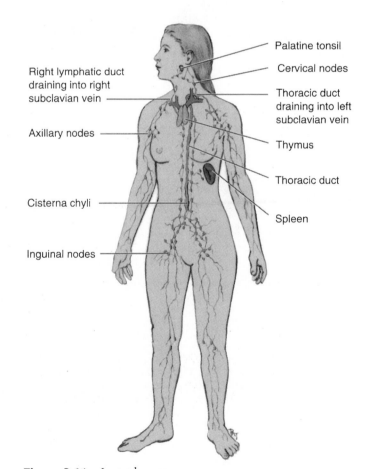

Figure 2.16 Lymph organs.
(From Applegate EJ: The Anatomy and Physiology Learning System, Philadelphia, WB Saunders, 1995, p. 290.)

enter through the nose, mouth, and throat. Pharyngeal tonsils (adenoids) are located in the nasopharynx; palatine tonsils are located in the oropharynx; and lingual tonsils are located at the posterior portion of the tongue.

C. The spleen is posterior to the stomach and consists of large masses of lymphocytes and macrophages supported by a reticular fibrous framework. It is similar to a lymph node but is larger and filters blood instead of lymph; also acts as a reservoir for blood.

D. Thymus is anterior to the ascending aorta and posterior to the sternum; its principal function is the processing and maturation of T-lymphocytes, which are involved in the body's defense against pathogens; also produces the hormone thymosin.

Respiratory System

The respiratory system (Fig. 2–17) includes the upper and lower respiratory tracts and the lungs. It functions to move gases to and from exchange surfaces, where diffusion can occur. It also defends body against pathogens, permits speech, and helps regulate the acid-base balance in the body.

I. Upper Respiratory Tract
   A. Nose (nasal cavity) warms, moistens, and filters air; opens to the outside through the external nares and into the pharynx through the internal nares; separated from the oral cavity by the palate.

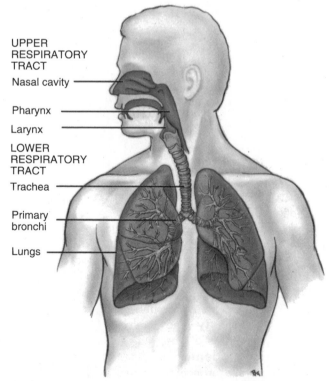

Figure 2.17   Respiratory tract.
(From Applegate EJ: The Anatomy and Physiology Learning System, Philadelphia, WB Saunders, 1995, p. 306.)

B. Pharynx (throat) is the passageway for air; is divided into the nasopharynx, oropharynx, and laryngopharynx (hypopharynx); opening from the oral cavity into the oropharynx is the fauces.

C. Larynx (voice box) is formed by nine cartilages that are connected by muscles and ligaments. The three largest cartilages are the thyroid, cricoid, and epiglottis. Vocal folds (cords) are present in the central region of larynx; air passing through the larynx vibrates vocal folds to produce sound.

II. Lower Respiratory Tract
   A. Trachea (windpipe) framework is supported by 15 to 20 c-shaped pieces of hyaline cartilage. The mucous membrane lining has goblet cells and cilia; goblet cells secrete mucus that traps inhaled particles; cilia provide cleansing action to remove mucus with trapped particles. Trachea divides into right and left primary bronchi at the carina.
   B. Bronchial tree
      1. Primary bronchi enter the lungs and subdivide into secondary (lobar) bronchi, which branch into tertiary (segmental) bronchi.
      2. Branching pattern continues into smaller and smaller passages until the branches terminate in tiny air sacs called alveoli.
      3. Alveoli are composed of simple squamous epithelium, which permits rapid diffusion of oxygen and carbon dioxide.
   C. Lungs
      1. Are formed by the bronchial tree and alveoli and are covered by pleura, a serous membrane.
      2. Right lung has three lobes; is shorter, broader, and has a greater volume than the left lung.
      3. Left lung has two lobes and an indentation—the cardiac notch—to accommodate the apex of the heart.
      4. Air flows into and out of the lungs through the conducting passages because of pressure differences between the atmosphere and the gases inside the alveoli.

Digestive System

The digestive system (Fig. 2–18) includes the digestive tract (oral cavity, pharynx, esophagus, stomach, small intestine, large intestine, rectum, and anus) and the accessory organs (liver, gallbladder, and pancreas). Its functions include ingestion, mechanical digestion, chemical digestion, secretion, mixing and propelling movements, absorption, and elimination of waste products.

I. Histology of the wall of the digestive tract features a mucosal lining (simple columnar epithelium and connective tissue), submucosa (connective tissue with blood vessels and nerves), muscularis externa (smooth muscle), and outermost serosa (serous membrane) (Fig. 2–19).

II. Oral (buccal) Cavity
   A. Hard and soft palates form the roof; tongue forms the floor.

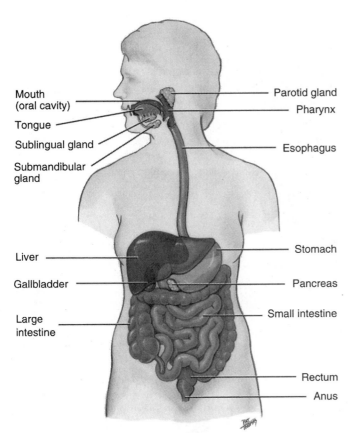

Figure 2.18 Organs of the digestive system.
(From Applegate EJ: The Anatomy and Physiology Learning System, Philadelphia, WB Saunders, 1995, p. 328.)

A. Located in upper left quadrant of the abdomen, anterior to the spleen.

B. Divided into a fundus, cardiac region, body, and pyloric region.

C. Mucosal lining has folds, called rugae, and glandular cells.

D. Parietal cells secrete hydrochloric acid and intrinsic factor; chief cells secrete pepsinogen, which is converted to pepsin by acids; and endocrine cells secrete the hormone gastrin.

E. Chyme is the semifluid mixture of ingested food, liquids, and gastric juice that passes through the pyloric sphincter into the small intestine.

F. The pH of the luminal contents may be as low as 2.

VI. Small Intestine extends from the pyloric sphincter to the ileocecal valve; materials require approximately 5 hours to pass through the small intestine and into the large intestine.

A. Is divided into a duodenum, jejunum, and ileum.

B. Absorptive surface area of the mucosa is increased by plicae circulares, villi, and microvilli; each villus contains a blood capillary network and a lymph capillary called a lacteal.

C. Glandular cells in the mucosa produce peptidase, which acts on proteins; maltase, sucrase, and lactase, which act on disaccharides; and lipase, which acts on neutral fats.

D. Hormones produced by the small intestine are

B. Parotid, submandibular, and sublingual salivary glands discharge secretions into the oral cavity; saliva from these glands lubricates the mouth, dissolves chemicals, moistens food, and helps control bacteria.

C. Mastication (chewing) is accomplished by the action of the teeth; 20 teeth in the deciduous dentition are replaced by 32 teeth in the permanent dentition.

III. Pharynx (throat) serves as a passageway for solid food, liquids, and air; muscles in the wall contract during deglutition (swallowing) to propel food along the passageway into the esophagus and subsequently into the stomach.

IV. Esophagus carries liquids and solids from the pharynx to the stomach; is located posterior to the trachea and anterior to the vertebral column; passes through the diaphragm at vertebral level T-10 through the esophageal hiatus; and enters the cardiac region of the stomach. Lower esophageal (cardiac) sphincter controls passage of food from esophagus into stomach.

V. Stomach functions include temporary storage of ingested food, maceration and mixing of ingested materials, secretion of enzymes that begin breaking chemical bonds (digestion), and production of intrinsic factor.

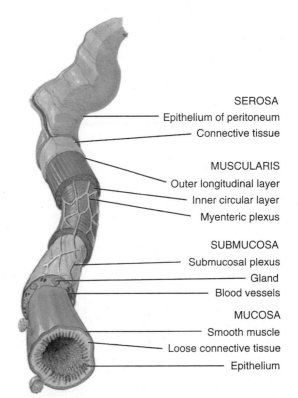

Figure 2.19 Basic histology of the digestive tract.
(From Applegate EJ: The Anatomy and Physiology Learning System, Philadelphia, WB Saunders, 1995, p. 329.)

secretin and cholecystokinin. Secretin stimulates the pancreas to produce a fluid rich in bicarbonates; cholecystokinin stimulates the gallbladder to secrete bile and stimulates the pancreas to secrete digestive enzymes.

VII. Large Intestine is divided into cecum, colon, rectum, and anal canal.
   A. Main functions are to absorb water, electrolytes, and vitamins; compact the feces; store fecal material prior to defecation.
   B. Cecum is the short region inferior to the ileocecal valve; vermiform appendix is attached to the cecum.
   C. Colon is divided into ascending (right), transverse, descending (left), and sigmoid regions; teniae coli, haustra, and epiploic appendages are characteristics of the colon.

VIII. Rectum and Anal Canal are terminal portions of the digestive system; distention of the rectal wall stimulates the defecation reflex.

IX. Accessory Organs
   A. Pancreas is retroperitoneal and extends from the duodenum to the spleen. Most of the pancreas is composed of exocrine cells, which produce the enzymes amylase, trypsin, peptidase, and lipase; pancreatic enzymes are carried to the duodenum by the pancreatic duct (of Wirsung). The endocrine cells (islets of Langerhans) produce insulin and glucagon.
   B. Liver is located in the upper right quadrant of the abdomen. The functional unit is the liver lobule, which consists of hepatocytes arranged like spokes of a wheel around a central vein and separated by sinusoids. Blood is brought to the liver by the portal vein and hepatic artery, where it flows through the sinusoids into the central vein and subsequently into the hepatic veins. Functions of the liver include the production of bile, production of plasma proteins, detoxification of harmful substances, filtering of blood, and nutrient metabolism.
   C. Gallbladder is attached to the visceral surface of the liver by the cystic duct, which joins the hepatic duct to form the common bile duct; common bile duct empties into the duodenum. Functions to store, concentrate, and secrete the bile produced by the liver.

Urinary System

The urinary system consists of the kidneys, ureters, urinary bladder, and urethra (Fig. 2–20). It functions to rid the body of wastes, regulate fluid volume, maintain electrolyte concentrations, control blood pH, and secrete renin and erythropoietin.

I. Kidneys are located behind the peritoneum between the twelfth thoracic and third lumbar vertebrae. They are enclosed by a capsule and surrounded by perirenal fat. Blood vessels enter and the ureter leaves

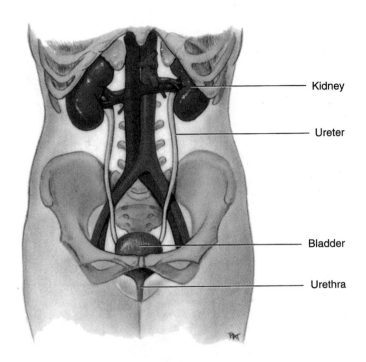

Figure 2.20 Components of the urinary system. (From Applegate EJ: The Anatomy and Physiology Learning System, Philadelphia, WB Saunders, 1995, p. 372.)

the kidney at an indentation called the hilum on the medial side. The peripheral region is granular in appearance and is called the cortex; the inner region is striated in appearance and is called the medulla. The left kidney generally is higher than the right one.
   A. Functional unit is the nephron, which consists of a renal corpuscle and a renal tubule. Renal corpuscle, located in the cortex, includes the glomerulus and renal capsule. Blood filtration occurs in the glomerulus and filtrate passes into the capsule (Fig. 2–21).
   B. Reabsorption of water and electrolytes to adjust volume and content of urine occurs in the renal tubule; the straight portions of the tubule are located in the medulla and the convoluted portions are in the cortex.
   C. Juxtaglomerular apparatus associated with the nephron secretes renin.

II. Ureters enter the urinary bladder on the posterior and inferior surface; urine is formed in the kidney and leaves the kidney through the ureters, which transport it to the urinary bladder.

III. Urinary Bladder is posterior to the symphysis pubis in the pelvic cavity and stores urine until micturition.
   A. Lining is mucous membrane (consisting of transitional epithelium) with folds, called rugae, that allow for expansion.
   B. Trigone, a triangular region in the floor of the bladder, is outlined by the two ureters and the urethra.
   C. Detrusor muscle (smooth muscle) in the wall

compresses the bladder to expel urine into the urethra for micturition.

IV. Urethra transports urine from the urinary bladder to the exterior; opens to the exterior through the external urethral orifice.

   A. Urine flow is controlled by an internal sphincter (smooth muscle), where the urethra leaves the bladder, and by an external sphincter (skeletal muscle), where the urethra penetrates the pelvic floor.

   B. Female urethra is short; male urethra is long and extends the entire length of the penis. Male urethra is divided into prostatic, membranous, and spongy (penile) portions.

   C. Urine is the fluid produced by the nephrons of the kidney; composition is approximately 95% water and 5% solutes from cellular metabolism; volume varies but typically is 1 to 2 liters per 24 hours; color is yellow or amber, but varies with concentration and diet; appears clear or transparent when freshly voided, but becomes cloudy upon standing; pH ranges between 4.6 and 8.0, with an average of approximately 6; specific gravity ranges between 1.001 to 1.035, thus urine is slightly heavier than water.

Reproductive System

The reproductive system consists of the gonads (testes), ducts, accessory glands, and penis in the male and the gonads (ovaries), uterine tubes, uterus, vagina, external genitalia, and mammary glands in the female.

I. Male (Fig. 2–22)

   A. Testes begin development in the abdominal cavity and subsequently descend into the scrotum shortly before birth.

      1. Dartos muscle (smooth) gives the scrotum a wrinkled appearance; cremaster muscle (skeletal) draws the scrotum closer to the body.

      2. Testes are composed of seminiferous tubules, which produce sperm, and interstitial cells, which produce testosterone.

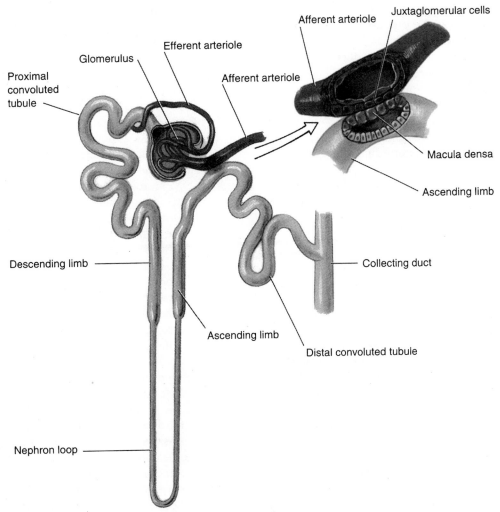

Figure 2.21 Structure of the nephron.
(From Applegate EJ: The Anatomy and Physiology Learning System, Philadelphia, WB Saunders, 1995, p. 375.)

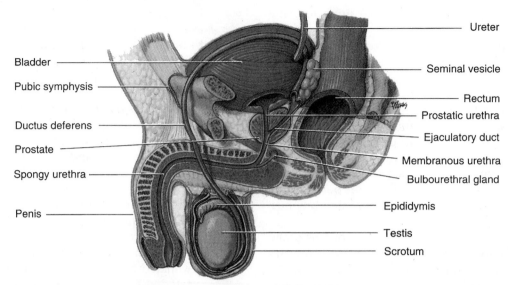

Figure 2.22 Structures of the male reproductive system.
(From Applegate EJ: The Anatomy and Physiology Learning System, Philadelphia, WB Saunders, 1995, p. 392.)

3. Spermatogenesis is the process by which spermatids are formed in the seminiferous tubules; spermiogenesis is the process by which spermatid becomes mature sperm.

B. Ducts include the epididymis, ductus deferens, ejaculatory duct, and urethra.
   1. Epididymis is a convoluted tube on the margin of the testes; sperm mature and become fertile in the epididymis.
   2. Ductus deferens begins at the epididymis and extends to the ejaculatory duct posterior to the urinary bladder.
   3. Ejaculatory duct is a short tube formed by the ductus deferens and the duct leading from the seminal vesicles; penetrates the prostate gland and empties into the urethra.
   4. Urethra is the passageway for both urine and seminal fluid (sperm plus glandular secretions); seminal fluid enters the prostatic section of the urethra.

C. Accessory glands include the seminal vesicles and the prostate and bulbourethral glands.
   1. Seminal vesicles are paired with saccular glands posterior to the urinary bladder; secretion contains fructose, prostaglandins, and coagulation proteins; secretion accounts for 60% of the volume of seminal fluid.
   2. Prostate gland is a dense gland, inferior to the urinary bladder, that encircles the proximal portion of the urethra; secretion empties into the prostatic urethra and accounts for 40% of seminal fluid.
   3. Bulbourethral glands (Cowper's glands) are located near base of penis and secrete a viscous fluid that cleanses the urethra and lubricates the penis; does not contribute to seminal fluid.

D. Penis
   1. Is three columns of erectile tissue bound together and encircled by skin; two dorsal columns are corpora cavernosa and the single ventral column is corpus spongiosum, which encircles the urethra; expanded distal portion of corpus spongiosum is the glans penis.
   2. Dilation of erectile spaces with blood causes an erection.

II. Female (Fig. 2–23)
A. Ovaries are located in the pelvic cavity on each side of the uterus.
   1. Numerous ovarian follicles make the ovaries appear granular.
   2. Oogenesis (ovum production) occurs monthly in the ovarian follicles as part of the ovarian cycle; follicle cells produce estrogen.
   3. At ovulation, an oocyte and surrounding cells (corona radiata) are released through the ruptured ovarian wall.
   4. After ovulation, the follicle cells are transformed into a corpus luteum that produces progesterone; later, corpus luteum degenerates into a corpus albicans.

B. Uterine tubes (fallopian tubes or oviducts)
   1. Extend laterally from the uterus.
   2. The portion near the ovary expands to form the infundibulum, with fimbriae around the periphery.
   3. Are the normal site for fertilization.

C. Uterus consists of a fundus, body, and cervix.
   1. Fundus and body normally anteflex over the superior surface of the urinary bladder.
   2. Cervix is the narrow end that projects into the vagina; opening from the body into the cervix is the internal os; opening from the cervix into the vagina is the external os.

3. Wall consists of an outer perimetrium, a middle myometrium (smooth muscle), and an inner endometrium (mucous membrane).
4. Endometrium is further divided into stratum basale (deep layer) and stratum functionale (superficial layer); stratum functionale is the portion that is sloughed off and shed during menstruation.

D. Vagina is a muscular tube that extends from the cervix to the exterior.

E. External genitalia are collectively referred to as the vulva or pudendum.
   1. Includes the labia majora, labia minora, clitoris, vestibule, and vestibular glands.
   2. Labia majora are lateral fat-filled folds that protect the other genitalia; labia minora are narrow folds that enclose the vestibule.
   3. Clitoris is erectile tissue at the anterior end of the vestibule; posterior to the clitoris, the urethra and the vagina open into the vestibule.
   4. Vestibular glands secrete fluids for lubrication.

F. Mammary glands
   1. Are located in the breast; consist of lobules of glandular units that produce milk. Lactiferous ducts transport milk to the nipple.
   2. Suspensory ligaments (cords of connective tissue) help support the breast.
   3. Estrogen and progesterone stimulate development of mammary glands and adipose deposition to form the breast; prolactin stimulates milk production; oxytocin causes the ejection of milk.

 ## Clinical Case STUDY

Emma Brown, a 78-year-old woman, is in the office to have tooth #31 extracted. The tooth crown is badly decayed. Root resection prior to removal is anticipated. Her dental history indicates an allergy to a local anesthetic. During a previous dental office visit, Mrs. Brown experienced swollen lips and oral mucous membranes and difficulty breathing after receiving an injection.

Clinical Case QUESTIONS

1. Did Mrs. Brown have an allergic reaction to a local anesthetic or was her reaction psychosomatic? Explain.
2. Identify the common types of local anesthetic agents used in dentistry. Which agent(s) are least likely to cause an allergic reaction? Which are most likely to cause an allergic reaction?
3. Before Mrs. Brown is given a local anesthetic, what precautions should be taken?
4. Discuss the type of injection(s) that are needed to adequately anesthetize tooth #31 for extraction. Identify the anatomical landmarks associated with the area.

Clinical Case RATIONALE

1. Mrs. Brown showed signs of a delayed allergic reaction to a local anesthetic—namely swelling of the oral tissues and respiratory difficulty.
2. Common local dental anesthetic agents include the amides, which are least likely to cause an allergic

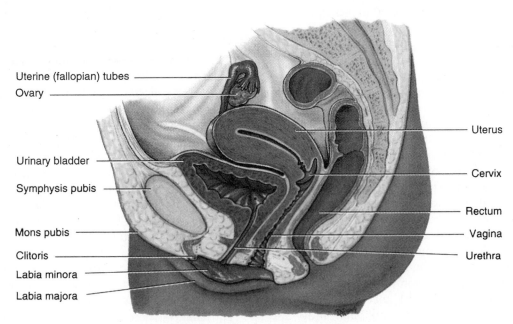

Figure 2.23   Organs of the female reproductive system.
(From Applegate EJ: The Anatomy and Physiology Learning System, Philadelphia, WB Saunders, 1995, p. 400.)

reaction, and the esters, which are most likely to cause an allergic reaction.

3. The following precautions should be taken: a) consult with her former dentist about the type of anesthetic that was given when she experienced the reaction or refer her for allergy testing, and b) avoid the use of topical or local agents that contain the offending agent (either ester or amides).

4. For the extraction of tooth #31, a 25-gauge long needle should be used. Injections should include an inferior alveolar nerve block, a lingual nerve block, and a buccal nerve block. Anatomical landmarks associated with the area include the retromolar pad, the pterygomandibular raphe, and the coronoid notch.

Biochemistry

Biochemistry is the study of living matter or organisms at a molecular level. It requires an understanding of how molecules are structured, how they bond and form more complex structures, and how they affect living matter.

Organic Chemistry

Hydrocarbons are carbon- and hydrogen-based molecules that exist in several different forms and have various properties. Hydrocarbons are found within several of the products we use daily and they also make up the major components of our bodies.

I. Parent Hydrocarbons
  A. Have chemical characteristics that can be greatly influenced by the replacement of hydrogen atoms with one or more functional groups.
  B. Functional groups include:
    1. Alcohols, which are components of several natural products, including menthol, which is used in throat lozenges.
    2. Ethers, which have a long history of use as anesthetics.
    3. Aldehydes, which have a variety of uses. Formaldehyde, which is used for the preservation of biological samples, is one type.
    4. Ketones, which include progesterone and testosterone, two important sex hormones.
    5. Carboxyl groups, which are found in salicylic acid, a constituent of aspirin.
    6. Organohalogens, which have several uses; are found in insecticides and are used in the treatment of brain cancer.
    7. Amines, which are used in the treatment of several ailments, including migraine headaches, hypertension, and inflammation.
    8. Esters, which are commonly used in the production of topical and local anesthetics such as those used in dentistry; although they are available, frequent allergies to ester agents have reduced their use.
    9. Amides, which are commonly used in the production of topical and local anesthetics used in dentistry; also are known for their polymerizing capabilities (are used to make nylon).

II. Saturated Hydrocarbons
  A. Are molecules that contain hydrogen atoms and carbon atoms, which are connected by single bonds.
  B. Structure can be straight chain, branched, or cyclic: Straight chain hydrocarbons have higher boiling points than branched hydrocarbons because more surface contact is allowed between straight chain hydrocarbons.

III. Unsaturated Hydrocarbons
  A. Are carbon- and hydrogen-based molecules that contain at least one double or triple bond between carbon atoms; Vitamin A is an example of an unsaturated hydrocarbon.

Cells

Cells are living units that can exist either independently or within a network of other cells.

I. Prokaryotic cells are simple cells that do not contain a true nucleus.

II. Eukaryotic cells are more complex cells that exist either as a single-celled organism or in a multicellular organism; these cells do contain a true nucleus.

III. Membranes
  A. Are bilayer structures that separate the environment within the cell or organelle from the outside environment.
  B. Consist of a variety of lipids and proteins whose nonpolar parts are protected within the lipid bilayer; the polar parts of these structures are exposed either to the inside of the cell or to the extracellular environment.

Biomolecules

Biomolecules are found in living organisms and are classified as belonging to one of four major groups: carbohydrates, lipids, proteins, or nucleic acids.

I. Carbohydrates are important for transport, energy, and the structure of the cell.
  A. Monosaccharides are the basic units of complex carbohydrates (e.g., glucose).
  B. Oligosaccharides consists of two to ten monosaccharides (e.g., sucrose).
  C. Polysaccharides consist of many monosaccharides (e.g., starch).

II. Lipids are important for energy and for the structure of the cell.
  A. Fatty acids are carboxylic acids with hydrocarbon side chains; they exist as a major component of other naturally existing lipids.
  B. Triacylglycerols consist of three fatty acids that are esterified to a glycerol molecule; they exist as a form of energy storage.

C. Saponifiable lipids are amphipathic molecules that consist of a polar head group and a nonpolar tail; they exist as structural lipids that are found in biological membranes and also play a role in the transport of other lipids in the circulatory system.

D. Nonsaponifiable lipids do not contain fatty acid molecules; the three major classes are steroids, prostaglandins, and leukotrienes. They are involved in the regulation of body functions.

III. Amino Acids, Peptides, and Proteins are important components in the development of molecules used by the body for forming cell structure, catalyzing reactions, and transmitting signals.

A. Amino acids
1. Are the building blocks of peptides and proteins.
2. Consist of an amino group, a carboxylic acid group, and an R group; the R group varies from one amino acid to another and is the component that determines the characteristics of each amino acid.

B. Peptides
1. Are molecules that consist of more than one amino acid linked by a peptide bond.
2. Bonds link amino groups of one amino acid to the carboxylic acid group of another amino acid (peptide bond); formation of a peptide bond results in the release of a water molecule.

C. Proteins
1. Are present in the cells of all living organisms.
2. Are functional molecules that consist of one or more peptide molecules.
3. Are important components in the chemical and physical functioning of the cell.

IV. Nucleic Acids
A. Encode genetic information; are the molecular basis of heredity.

B. Are made up of nucleotides, which consist of a nitrogenous base, a sugar, and a phosphate.
1. Adenosine monophosphate (AMP)
2. Guanosine monophosphate(GMP)
3. Cytosine monophosphate (CMP)
4. Thymidine monophosphate (TMP); found only in deoxyribonucleic acid (DNA)
5. Uridine monophosphate (UMP); found only in ribonucleic acid (RNA)

C. Include RNA and DNA; located in the nucleus (DNA and RNA) and in the cytoplasm (RNA).
1. Structure and replication of DNA
a. Basic structure of deoxyribonucleic acid (DNA) is a double helix with two strands of DNA that run antiparallel to one another.
1) The two strands are held together by formation of hydrogen bonds between a nucleotide on one strand of DNA and a nucleotide on the other strand of DNA.
2) Deoxy AMP forms a base pair by forming two hydrogen bonds with deoxy TMP.
3) Deoxy GMP forms a base pair by forming three hydrogen bonds with deoxy CMP.
b. Semiconservative replication
1) During replication, the two complementary strands of DNA are separated.
2) The separation allows the protein DNA polymerase to synthesize a new strand of DNA that is complementary to each of the original strands of DNA.
3) Replication of one double-stranded DNA molecule results in two double-stranded molecules of DNA, which are identical to the original molecule of DNA.
4) The process of DNA replication is necessary for cell division. When the cell divides into two, each of the daughter cells receives one of the DNA molecules.

2. Structure and function of RNA
a. RNA is similar to DNA in structure except that:
1) RNA contains a ribose sugar instead of a deoxyribose sugar.
2) RNA contains uridine monophosphate (UMP) instead of deoxythymidine monophosphate (TMP).
3) RNA is a single-stranded molecule rather than a double-stranded molecule.
b. The overall function of mRNA, tRNA, and rRNA is the synthesis of proteins.

3. Transcription is the process of transferring genetic information from DNA to a messenger RNA (mRNA) transcript; Genetic information from an mRNA transcript is used as a guide for protein synthesis.

4. Translation is the process of transferring genetic information from mRNA to the synthesis of proteins.

5. Mutagenesis is an alteration in the DNA that changes the encoded genetic information; chemicals, viruses, and radiation are three classes of agents that cause mutation.

6. Gene expression is regulated by a number of proteins called transcription factors, which are in turn regulated by other internal and external stimuli.

7. Genetic engineering is the process of using specific techniques for manipulating genetic information; for example, the gene for human insulin can be placed in bacteria, allowing expression of a large quantity of human insulin. This protein can then be purified from the bacteria and used for diabetic treatment.

8. Gene therapy is a type of genetic engineering; it involves compensating for a damaged gene that is responsible for causing an illness by expressing a foreign gene in the affected cells.

Metabolism

Metabolism is the process of producing and using energy. Catabolism and anabolism are important parts of the process.

I. Catabolism
   A. Is the process of breaking down large complex molecules into simpler molecules.
   B. Produces energy for physical activity; helps maintain body temperature and elimination of body waste.

II. Anabolism
   A. Is the process of building larger, more complex molecules from smaller, simpler units.
   B. Is important in new cell development and in older cell maintenance.

III. Enzymes (most) are functional proteins involved in catalyzing specific reactions.

IV. Adenosine Triphosphate (ATP) is the main form of energy storage.
   A. The energy released from exothermic reactions can be stored in the form of ATP by the addition of an inorganic phosphate (P_i) to a molecule of ADP ($ADP + P_i = ATP$).
   B. Energy stored in the form of ATP can be donated to an endothermic reaction by hydrolysis of the inorganic phosphate (P_i) from the ATP molecule, resulting in a molecule of ADP ($ATP = ADP + P_i$).
   C. The use of ATP can be compared to a farmer's buying and selling of food. When a farmer has more food (energy) than his family can eat, he can sell it to get money (ATP). When his family needs more food (energy), he can use his money (ATP) to buy more food (energy).
   D. Glycolysis is the pathway for catabolism (breakdown) of the simple sugar glucose.
      1. 1 glucose + 2ADP + $2P_i$ + 2NAD = 2 pyruvate + 2ATP + 2NADH; One NADH molecule can be used to make approximately 3 ATP molecules.
   E. Pyruvate dehydrogenase is an enzyme that catalyzes the conversion of a molecule of pyruvate into acetyl CoA, which can be used in the tricarboxylic acid cycle (TCA cycle) for further production of energy.
      1. Pyruvate + CoA + NAD = Acetyl CoA + CO_2 + NADH
   F. Tricarboxylic acid cycle (TCA) is the pathway for further breakdown of glucose to produce energy.
      1. Acetyl CoA + 1FAD + 1GDP + P_i + 3NAD = $2CO_2$ + $1FADH_2$ + 1GTP + 3NADH
   G. Electron transport and oxidative phosphorylation is the pathway by which electrons are donated from NADH and $FADH_2$ to a series of proteins found in the mitochondrial membrane. The elec-

trons proceed down the electron transport chain and result in the reduction of O_2 to H_2O and eventually the production of ATP.
   1. NADH ~ 3ATP
   2. FADH ~ 2ATP
   H. The overall goal of these metabolic pathways is to use the food we take into our bodies for the production of ATP, which enables our bodies to store energy for later use.

 Clinical Case **STUDY**

John Rivers is a 14-year-old who has Duchenne muscular dystrophy. He is wheelchair bound and recently developed an upper respiratory infection (URI) with symptoms of cough, sore throat, fever, and dyspnea. As a consequence of the URI, his end tidal Pco_2 increased from 45 to 55 mm Hg, his maximal inspiratory pressure (MIP) and maximal expiratory pressures (MEP) dropped from 30 cm H_2O to 10 cm H_2O, and his vital capacity dropped. As the URI improved, his symptoms gradually improved. His recovery took more than 2 weeks.

Clinical Case QUESTIONS

1. Why would the Pco_2 increase?
2. What could be the reason for the decreased respiratory muscle strength exemplified by the decrease in MIP, MEP, and vital capacity?
3. The decrements in lung function were reversible: what does this say about the effects of the URI on the patient?

Clinical Case RATIONALE

1. An increase in the Pco_2 indicates alveolar hypoventilation, which may be associated with the marked respiratory weakness (normal values of MIP and MEP would be more than double the pre-URI values in this case) and increased airway resistance (decreased airway diameter) caused by inflammation and edema. Increased Pco_2 also may occur because of increased metabolism (fever) and an inability of the weakened ventilatory muscles to compensate.
2. The marked decrease in respiratory muscle strength during the URI may be caused by the release of cytokines, muscle injury from free radical production, and/or anorexia, all of which affect respiratory muscle performance.
3. Resolution of the increased Pco_2 and decreased respiratory muscle strength occurs as the URO clears up and the factors mentioned in #2 disappear.

Physiology

Physiology is the study of the function of organ systems. It includes the structural-functional hierarchy of molecules → cells → tissues → organs → organ systems → individual → population.

Cell Physiology

Cell physiology is the study of the general and specific functions of cells and requires an understanding of the cell structure and its environment.

I. Cell Structure

   A. Structure (Fig. 2–24) includes cell components, such as organelles, plasma, and cytoskeletal elements, and their importance in cell function.

   B. Plasma membrane surrounds each cell, selectively allows movement of water and other substances into and out of cells, and is involved in cell-to-cell recognition.

      1. Components include:

         a. phospholipids, which are polar and have charged heads.

         b. lipids, which are hydrophobic.

         c. cholesterol, which affects membrane fluidity.

         d. proteins, such as channels, enzymes, receptors, and carbohydrates.

      2. Fluid mosaic model is the current working model of a membrane.

   C. Endoplasmic reticulum is a fluid-filled membrane organelle found within cells. It consists of two types:

      1. Rough endoplasmic reticulum

         a. Contains large amounts of ribosomes.

         b. Is involved in synthesis of proteins for cell structure and function.

         c. Is found in large amounts in growing cells and in cells that make digestive enzymes.

      2. Smooth endoplasmic reticulum

         a. Is involved in the production of steroid hormones.

         b. Detoxifies harmful substances.

         c. Produces lysosomes.

         d. Uses calcium in muscle cells for contraction and relaxation.

   D. Golgi apparatus or complex

      1. Consists of layers of membranes and enclosed sacs.

      2. Is involved in processing substances made in the endoplasmic reticulum.

      3. Directs finished products to intra- or extracellular locations.

   E. Vesicles

      1. Are membrane-surrounded buds.

      2. Are formed from the Golgi complex.

      3. Coated vesicles contain chemicals for intracellular use.

      4. Secretory vesicles are used for export (exocytosis).

      5. Also are involved in trafficking substances into the cell from the environment (endocytosis, pinocytosis, phagocytosis).

   F. Lysosomes

      1. Are membrane-enclosed organelles derived from the Golgi complex.

      2. Contain enzymes to digest unwanted debris or foreign matter.

      3. Are involved in apoptosis (tissue regression).

   G. Peroxisomes

      1. Are membrane-enclosed organelles that contain oxidative enzymes (such as catalase) for detoxifying chemicals.

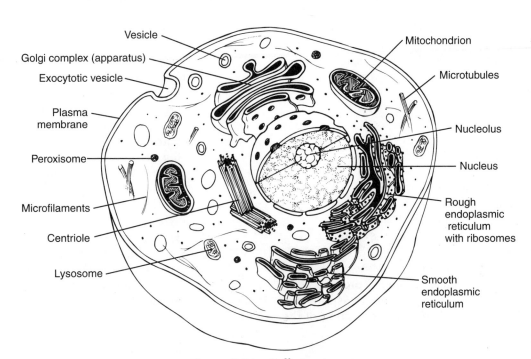

Figure 2.24 Cell structure.

H. Mitochondria
1. Are organelles with an inner membrane (containing cristae or respiratory enzymes) and an outer membrane.
2. Produce energy for the cell in the form of adenosine triphosphate or ATP.
3. Produce heat (especially mitochondria found in brown fat).
4. Are found in large numbers within metabolically active cells such as cardiac and skeletal muscles.

I. Ribosomes
1. Consist of granules of RNA and proteins that are found on the endoplasmic reticulum or are free in the cytoplasm.
2. Are involved in protein production.

J. Nucleus
1. Contains DNA molecules that act as the genetic "blueprint" for the cell's protein production.
2. Has inner and outer bilayers that make up the nuclear envelope, which contains pores for transporting substances across the membranes.
3. Contains a nucleolus that is involved in the assembly of ribosomes.

K. Cytoskeletal structures
1. Microtubules are long, slender, hollow tubes involved in cell movement, transport of vesicles within the cell, and the formation of mitotic spindles in cellular reproduction.
2. Microfilaments are composed of helically intertwined chains of actin and myosin found in muscles (contraction) and microvilli.
3. Intermediate filaments or rods are made of protein and form the scaffolding (skeleton) of the cell (cytoskeleton).

II. Environmental Milieu of Cells
A. The cell environment consists of intracellular and extracellular compartments separated by the plasma membrane. The kidneys regulate water and electrolyte content of the extracellular compartment.
1. Extracellular fluid
a. Is located outside of the cell and includes the interstitial fluid and plasma
b. Is high in Na^+, Cl^-, Ca^{+2}
c. Is low in K^+
d. Has a pH close to 7.4
2. Intracellular fluid
a. Is located within the cell
b. Is low in Na^+, Cl^-, Ca^{+2}
c. Is high in K^+
d. Has a pH close to 7.0.
B. The plasma membrane contains proteins that consist of channels, pumps, and transport systems, which help regulate the composition of the intracellular fluid.
C. Kidneys help regulate the composition and volume of the plasma and interstitial fluid (see section on functional anatomy of the urinary system).

III. Common Cell Functions
A. Five major physiologic functions of the cell.
1. Response to the environment, which includes:
a. Production of substances (e.g., mucus in response to tobacco smoke).
b. Movement (involving part of a cell, such as cilia, or entire cell, such as lymphocyte).
c. Ingestion of substances (e.g., nutrients or bacteria).
d. Generation of electrical impulses (e.g., action potential).
2. Synthesis of proteins for structural and functional requirements.
3. Use of membrane transport for:
a. Separation of internal and external cell environments.
b. Communication between cells.
c. Intracellular communication.
d. Fluid volume regulation.
4. Duplication for:
a. Growth (mitosis).
b. Reproduction (meiosis).
5. Differentiation and specialization as:
a. Muscle cells (skeletal, smooth, and cardiac).
b. Nervous cells (neurons).
c. Epithelial cells (lining of organs and tissues).
d. Connective tissue cells (fibroblasts, white blood cells).

IV. Specific Cell Functions
A. Transport of substances across the plasma membrane
1. Permeability or the ability of a substance to move across the membrane
a. Totally permeable—anything can cross.
b. Impermeable—nothing can cross.
c. Semipermeable—only some substances can cross.
2. Diffusion mechanism of transport
a. Random movement of molecules from a higher to a lower concentration gradient. Once concentrations differences are eliminated, no net movement occurs. The following factors affect the diffusion rate:
1) The higher the temperature, the greater the diffusion.
2) The smaller the molecule, the faster it diffuses.
3) The shorter the distance across the membrane, the faster the rate of diffusion.
4) The greater the available surface area for diffusion, the higher the rate of diffusion.
5) The more lipid soluble the substance, the more readily it moves across the membrane.
b. Movement of ions depends on their charge (different charges attract, similar

ones repeal) and their concentration gradients.

  c. Osmosis is the net movement of water down its concentration gradient.

    1) The amount of water that moves depends on the concentration of water relative to the solute and the relative permeability of the membrane to the solute.

    2) An isotonic solution has the same osmotic characteristics on both sides of the membrane. No net movement of water occurs.

    3) A hypotonic solution contains more water outside the cell than inside the cell. Water moves into the cell and exerts a pressure, increasing the volume of the cell, and may cause the cell to burst.

    4) A hypertonic solution contains less water outside than inside the cell. Movement of water out of the cell makes it shrink (crenation).

3. Carrier-mediated transport

  a. Uses a molecule to move substances across the plasma membrane.

  b. Exhibits selectivity for a substance, saturation, or a transport maximum (a limit to how much can be moved), and competition for transporting substances that are closely related chemically.

  c. Includes the following types:

    1) Facilitated diffusion for molecules like glucose

      a) Moves down a concentration gradient.

      b) Uses no energy.

    2) Primary active transport

      a) Moves substances against their concentration gradients.

      b) Uses energy in the form of ATP.

      c) An example is the Na^+-K^+ ATPase pump.

    3) Secondary active transport (more than one molecule is moved)

      a) Uses energy.

      b) Moves molecules against their concentration gradients.

      c) Creates a gradient to move a second substance with the energy used to move one ion.

      d) An example is the coupled transport of sodium with amino acids in the intestine.

B. Cell communication

  1. Communication between cells

    a. Hormones are made by one cell type, are transported in blood, and affect cells at a distant site.

    b. Neurotransmitters are chemicals, produced by one neuron, that affect neurons or muscle cells.

    c. Paracrine secretion involves one cell secreting a chemical (e.g., a neurotransmitter, cytokine, or gas such as NO) that affects a nearby cell.

    d. Tight junctions are specialized connections between cells that restrict the movement of substances between cells.

  2. Communication from the outside of a cell to its interior

    a. Channels allow fluxes of ions (e.g., Na^+, Cl^+, K^+) or water into or out of a cell.

    b. Receptors

      1) Bind chemicals from outside of the cell that couple to membrane-bound enzymes (e.g., adenosine cyclase), which affect intracellular second messenger systems (e.g., elevate calcium levels).

      2) A large intracellular response occurs (amplification) when only a small number of membrane receptors are activated.

C. Membrane potential

  1. Occurs when there is a difference in the numbers and charges of ions across the plasma membrane.

  2. Does not exist when the number and charge characteristics of ions are the same on either side of the membrane.

  3. Is greater as both the concentration gradient and difference in charge across the membrane increase.

  4. Is affected by the permeability of a membrane for an ion.

    a. Membranes are "leaky" for K^+ but "tight" for Na^+.

    b. Proteins have a negative charge and are trapped within the cell; the leakiness for K^+ that leaves the cell results in a relative negative charge inside the cell compared to outside of the cell.

Neurophysiology

Neurophysiology is the study of the nervous system, which comprises the central and peripheral nervous systems. These systems are responsible for sensing and responding to both external and internal stimuli.

I. Organization of the Nervous System

  A. Central nervous system (CNS) includes the brain and the spinal cord.

  B. Peripheral nervous system (PNS)

    1. Afferent fibers receive information obtained from sensory stimuli and direct information to the CNS.

    2. Efferent fibers direct commands from the CNS to target tissues, such as to muscles and glands.

a. Somatic nervous system consists of efferent fibers that innervate skeletal muscles and is voluntary. Primary neurotransmitter is acetylcholine (acting on nicotinic receptors).

b. Autonomic nervous system innervates glands, cardiac and smooth muscles, and is involuntary. Consists of two branches: the sympathetic nervous system (primary neurotransmitter is norepinephrine) and the parasympathetic nervous system (primary neurotransmitter is acetylcholine, which acts on muscarinic receptors).

c. Excitable tissues that transfer information by means of changes in membrane potential include neurons and cardiac, smooth, and skeletal muscles.

II. Structural and Functional Anatomy of the Neuron

A. Dendrites are branching structures that direct electrical information to the cell body.

B. Cell body or soma is the integrating center of the neuron; also is involved in protein synthesis.

C. Axon consists of a specialized region called the hillock and a tube-like structure that may or may not be myelinated.

D. Endplate is the last segment of the axon and has vesicles containing neurotransmitters for release into the synapse, a region between a dendrite or cell body of another (postsynaptic) neuron.

III. Information Transfer in the Nervous System

A. Graded potential

1. Is a form of information that is transferred in the nervous system by changes in membrane potential proportional to the strength of the stimulus.

2. Travels only small distances, in any direction, in decrements (dies out gradually).

3. May result from an outflow of positively charged ions (K^+) from the cell or an inflow of negatively charged ions (Cl^-) into the cell (hyperpolarization).

4. May result from an influx of positively charged ions (Na^+ or Ca^{+2}), which leads to depolarization.

5. Involves changes in membrane potential because of the rapid opening of specific channels and the increase in membrane permeability for an ion.

B. Action potential (Fig. 2–25)

1. Is created as a result of a rapid (1 msec), large change in membrane potential.

2. Includes the following associated events:

a. Sodium channels open and increase the influx of Na^+.

b. If enough Na^+ enters through channels ("flood gates"), the membrane reaches its threshold, the membrane potential becomes positive (inside vs. outside), and an action potential is initiated:

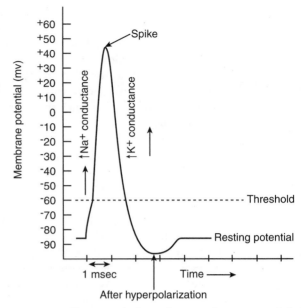

Figure 2.25 Characteristics of an action potential in a neuron. During the spike Na+ conductance decreases rapidly, thus making another action potential impossible to initiate (absolute refractory period). During the after hyperpolarization, another action potential can be initiated using a stronger stimulus (relative refractory period).

1) Na^+ channels become inactivated while K^+ channels are open, countering the influx of positive charges.

2) The outflow of K^+ leads to a subsequent hyperpolarization, decreasing membrane potential below the resting membrane potential.

3) The Na^+-K^+ ATPase pump helps return the membrane potential back to the resting potential.

3. Is not decrementally conducted and can travel over long distances on axons.

4. The strength of a stimulus is coded in the nervous system by the number of action potentials that occur (frequency).

5. Has refractory periods.

a. Absolute refractory period occurs when no additional action potential can be generated, regardless of the stimulus strength. This is caused by an inactivation of Na^+ channels.

b. Relative refractory period occurs when a stronger than normal stimulus can initiate an action potential. This may occur when the cell is hyperpolarized.

c. Refractory periods help ensure that the propagation of action potentials occurs in one direction; also help limit the frequency of action potentials.

6. The velocity of action potential conduction is affected by the:
   a. Amount of myelination. Myelinated fibers propagate action potentials faster.
   b. Diameter of the axon. Larger fiber diameter axons conduct faster.
   c. Presence of nodes of Ranvier; their presence results in saltatory (jumping) conduction from one node to the next.

C. Synapses
   1. Are areas between neurons and target cells (e.g., other neurons, muscle, glands).
   2. Are formed by the following components:
      a. Presynaptic neurons that contain vesicles loaded with a variety of neurotransmitters.
      b. Postsynaptic neurons or effector tissues that contain specific receptors for released neurotransmitters.
      c. Synaptic cleft, which is the area between two neurons or between a neuron and a target cell.
   3. Have excitatory postsynaptic potentials (EPSPs) that are the result of an influx of positive ions, through either ionic channels or receptor-activated channels in the postsynaptic cell. The EPSP results in a graded depolarization.
   4. Have inhibitory postsynaptic potentials (IPSPs) that are the result of either an efflux of K^+ or an influx of negatively charged ions. The IPSP results in a graded hyperpolarization.
   5. Each neuron has a number of other neurons and synapses impinging upon it. The net response of a neuron depends on the:
      a. Number and frequency of inputs (spatial and temporal summation).
      b. Chemical characteristics of the neurotransmitters released presynaptically and of the postsynaptic receptors.
         1) Some neurotransmitters cause an IPSP (glycine or GABA) or an EPSP (glutamate).
         2) Decreased numbers of acetylcholine receptors on muscle are found in myasthenia gravis.
      c. The rate and amount of neurotransmitters released.
         1) Too little dopamine is released in Parkinson's disease.
         2) Too little acetylcholine is released presynaptically in myasthenic syndrome.
         3) Decreased oxygen levels are a result of decreased neurotransmitter release caused by lowered ATP availability.
      d. The termination of the interaction between a neurotransmitter and its receptor.
         1) Availability of breakdown enzymes (such as acetylcholinesterase)
         2) Reuptake of neurotransmitters

         3) Ability of a chemical to dissociate from its receptor (some pesticides do not dissociate and cause persistent depolarization)

Skeletal Muscle Physiology

Skeletal muscles are relatively large cells and are involved in locomotion, work, and heat production.

I. Basic Structural Components of Skeletal Muscle (Fig. 2–26)
   A. Muscles are surrounded by connective tissue (epimysium).
   B. Each muscle consists of fascicles surrounded by a perimysium.
   C. Muscle fibers are surrounded by an endomysium.
   D. Individual muscle cells or fibers are surrounded by a sarcolemma, which invaginates into the cell, forming "T" tubules.
      1. Muscle cells are multinucleated.
      2. They can be large (as much as 2.5 feet in length).
      3. The endoplasmic reticulum is well-developed.
      4. Actin and myosin filaments make up the myofibrils.
   E. The contractile unit of the muscle is the sarcomere.
      1. "A" band consists of myosin (thick filaments composed of heads and tails) and actin (thin filaments). "M" line consists of only myosin.

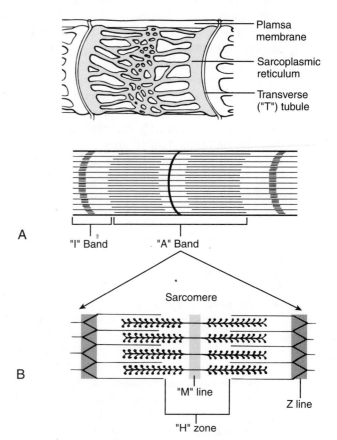

Figure 2.26 The muscle cell (A) and its components and the sarcomere (B), the contractile unit.

2. Actin filaments are surrounded by tropomyosin, to which troponins are attached. These molecules interact with calcium ions and allow actin to bind to myosin heads; also allow filaments to slide (causing contraction of the muscle).
3. "I" Band contains actin filaments and other proteins linked to "Z" Line.
4. "H" zone contains only myosin filaments.

II. Skeletal Muscle Function
A. Neuromuscular junction and excitation-contraction coupling.
   1. Motoneurons release acetylcholine, which binds to receptors on the muscle endplate.
   2. Receptors form channels that respond to the binding of acetylcholine by allowing an influx of cations into the muscle cell, resulting in an action potential that travels along and into the muscle fiber by means of the "T" tubules.
   3. Action potential causes the release of calcium from the sarcoplasmic reticulum.
   4. Calcium binds to troponin and results in a conformational change of tropomyosin, allowing actin to bind to myosin heads activated with ATP.
   5. Interaction of actin and myosin results in sarcomere shorting (contraction).
   6. Actin and myosin filaments require ATP to separate.
   7. If calcium levels continue to be high within the cell, contraction continues. If not, relaxation occurs because of calcium reuptake in the sarcoplasmic reticulum.
B. Factors involved in muscle contraction
   1. Active tension develops from the interaction of actin and myosin against connective tissue outside and proteins within the muscle fibers.
   2. Motor unit consists of a motoneuron and all of the muscle fibers it innervates.
      a. A small motor unit (one motoneuron for only a few fibers) is characteristic of muscles that perform fine motor tasks.
      b. A large motor unit (one motoneuron that innervates many fibers) is characteristic of larger fibers involved in throwing or locomotion.
   3. The smallest amount of tension that a muscle can generate is a twitch.
      a. The time needed to obtain the maximum twitch tension is the contraction time (may last 50 to 80 msec). This includes the time needed for excitation-contraction coupling and is influenced by the amount of connective tissue it has to contract against.
      b. The time needed for total relaxation of a contracted muscle is the relaxation time (approximately 80 msec). This involves the time needed for the dissociation of actin and myosin and the sequestration of calcium by the sarcoplasmic reticulum.
4. Summation of individual twitches occurs if the frequency of action potentials from the motoneuron to the muscle is high enough; may lead to tetanus, the maximum tension the muscle can obtain.
5. Types of muscle contractions
   a. Isometric contraction results in the generation of force by a muscle without a change in its length (e.g., trying unsuccessfully to lift a very heavy suitcase).
   b. Isotonic contraction results in muscle shorting in the process of moving a load. The lighter the load, the greater the rate of shortening.
   c. Some activities that a muscle performs consist of both types of contraction (e.g., lifting a weight that is not too heavy. Initially there is an isometric contraction, then an isotonic contraction when the weight actually moves).
   d. The work of a muscle is determined by the force moved per unit distance.
6. Types of fatigue
   a. Muscle fatigue
      1) The inability of a muscle to continue to work at a given level.
      2) May be caused by the following:
         a) Accumulation of waste products (lactic acid).
         b) Depletion of energy stores (phosphates).
         c) Muscle disease (muscular dystrophy).
   b. Neuromuscular junction fatigue
      1) The inability to manufacture enough acetylcholine presynaptically.
   c. Central fatigue
      1) The inability of the CNS to drive the muscles; may occur in response to muscle fatigue.
7. Muscle fiber types differ and are found in differing proportions in many muscles, such as those in the diaphragm and the gastrocnemius muscles.
   a. Slow oxidative fibers (e.g., in soleus muscle)
      1) Slow contracting.
      2) Fatigue resistant.
      3) Contain many mitochondria.
      4) Small in diameter.
      5) Develop a low level of tension.
   b. Fast glycolytic fibers (e.g., in extensor digitorium longus)
      1) Fast contracting.
      2) Fatigue sensitive.
      3) Have few mitochondria.
      4) Large in diameter.
      5) Develop a high level of tension.

c. Fast oxidative fibers (e.g., in arm muscles)
   1) Fast contracting.
   2) Have an intermediate level of fatigue resistance.
   3) Have many mitochondria.
   4) Intermediate in diameter.
   5) Develop an intermediate level of tension.

Endocrinology

Endocrinology is the study of endocrine glands, the hormones they secrete, and their effects on the body.

I. Endocrine System
  A. Consists of the pineal, hypothalamus, pituitary, thyroid, and adrenal glands; the pancreas, testes, and ovaries; and the hormones they secrete.
  B. Is generally a slower control system compared with the nervous system.
  C. Produces hormones with wide-reaching effects on many body processes (Fig. 2–27).
  D. Produces some hormones in the periphery and some in the central nervous system, but their functions differ in each location.
  E. Produces many hormones in a rhythmic manner (e.g., circadian, monthly).

II. Chemical Categories of Hormones
  A. Peptide and protein hormones
    1. Hydrophilic (water soluble).
    2. Transported as free hormones.
    3. Produced in the hypothalamus, pineal gland, pancreas, parathyroid gland, gastrointestinal tract, kidneys, liver, thyroid glands, and heart.
  B. Amines (tyrosine derivatives)

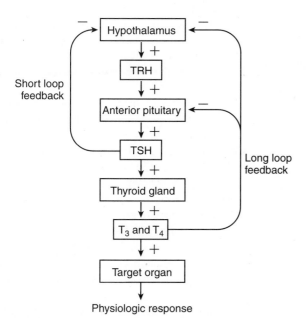

Figure 2.27 Negative feedback in the endocrine system. *TRH,* thyroid releasing hormone; *TSH,* thyroid stimulating hormone; T_3, triiodothyronine.

    1. Include catecholamines (hydrophilic), which are produced in the adrenal medulla.
    2. Include thyroid hormones (iodinated tyrosine derivatives), which are lipophilic (lipid soluble) and act at the genomic level to produce new proteins.
    3. Bind to plasma proteins.
  C. Steroid hormones (cholesterol derivatives)
    1. Are lipophilic and easily enter cells.
    2. Bind to both membrane and intracellular receptors.
    3. Can activate genes to initiate protein synthesis and may activate second messengers.
    4. Are produced in the adrenal cortex, the gonads (testes and ovaries), and the placenta.

III. Hormones Produced by the Central Nervous System
  A. Pineal gland hormone
    1. Melatonin
     a. Induces sleep.
     b. Affects reproduction (↑ high levels depress reproduction).
     c. Acts as an antioxidant.
     d. Enhances the immune system.
     e. Is involved in modulation of body rhythms.
  B. Hypothalamic hormones
    1. Thyrotropin-releasing hormone (TRH) stimulates the release of thyroid-stimulating hormone (TSH) from the anterior pituitary gland, which then regulates the production of thyroid hormones.
    2. Corticotropin-releasing hormone (CRH) stimulates the release of adrenocorticotropin hormone (ACTH), which acts on the adrenal cortex to produce cortisol in response to stress.
    3. Gonadotropin-releasing hormone (GnRH) stimulates the release of follicle-stimulating hormone (FSH) and luteinizing hormone (LH) from the anterior pituitary gland.
     a. FSH in females stimulates the growth of ovarian follicles and the production of estrogen.
     b. FSH in males is needed for sperm development in the testes.
     c. LH in females helps promote the formation of the corpus luteum and the production of estrogen and progesterone.
     d. LH in males stimulates the production of testosterone from Leydig cells in the testes.
  C. Pituitary hormones
    1. Growth hormone–releasing hormone (GH-RH)
     a. Stimulates the release of growth hormone (GH) by the anterior pituitary gland.
     b. GH acts directly or through the production of somatomedins to:
      1) Increase the influx of amino acids into cells.
      2) Increase protein synthesis.

3) Decrease cellular uptake of glucose and elevate blood glucose levels.
4) Stimulate insulin secretion.
5) Stimulate cartilage and bone growth.
2. Somatostatin inhibits the release of GH.
3. Prolactin-releasing factor (PRF) stimulates the anterior pituitary to release prolactin, which affects development of the breast and milk production.
4. Prolactin-inhibiting hormone inhibits the release of prolactin.
5. Vasopressin or antidiuretic hormone (ADH) and oxytocin are produced by the hypothalamus but are stored in and released from the posterior pituitary.
   a. ADH decreases water excretion from the kidney, is involved in stress responses, and contracts blood vessels (except in the lungs).
   b. Oxytocin increases uterine contractions and aids in milk ejection by the breast in response to suckling.

IV. Hormones Produced by the Peripheral Nervous System
   A. Thyroid hormones
      1. Are produced and stored in the thyroid gland.
      2. Include both thyroxine (T4) and triiodothyronine (T3).
         a. T4 also can be converted to T3 by diiodinases in the brain, kidneys, liver, and brown fat.
         b. The major systemic source of T3 is derived by conversion from T4 in liver and kidneys.
         c. Production is regulated in a feedback manner by TSH.
      3. Are transported in blood bound to plasma proteins.
      4. Major functions in the body include:
         a. Regulation of metabolic rate.
         b. Regulation of heat production and body temperature regulation.
         c. Intermediary metabolism of carbohydrates and fats.
         d. Increasing the number of catecholaminergic receptors on cells.
         e. Increasing heart rate and the force of heart muscle contraction.
         f. Stimulating growth, teeth eruption, and CNS development by its interaction with growth hormone.
      5. Thyroid hormone disorders
         a. Include hypothyroidism and hyperthyroidism.
         b. Consequences are dictated by the severity of the disorder, its duration, and the time of onset.
   B. Hormones that affect calcium metabolism

1. Calcium levels in plasma are tightly regulated. The active form is free (1.3 mmol/L), not bound to plasma proteins. The largest body store is in bone.
2. Deviations from a relatively normal range can affect:
   a. Neuromuscular excitability; low levels (hypocalcemia) result in contraction and twitching of skeletal muscles.
   b. Excitation-contraction coupling in cardiac and smooth muscles.
   c. CNS excitability.
   d. Stimulus-secretion coupling of hormones and neurotransmitters.
   e. Maintenance of tight junctions between epithelial cells.
   f. Clotting of blood.
3. Calcium is regulated by the parathyroid hormone, which is produced in the parathyroid glands, and vitamin D (cholecalciferol), which is produced by the skin.
   a. Decreased plasma calcium levels stimulate the release of parathyroid hormone.
   b. Parathyroid hormone stimulates the kidney to conserve calcium and phosphate.
   c. In conjunction with vitamin D, parathyroid hormone promotes intestinal reabsorption of calcium and phosphate.
   d. Parathyroid hormone promotes bone reabsorption.
   e. Low levels of parathyroid hormone can affect tooth development and may result in delayed tooth eruption and defects in the matrix, mineralization of enamel, and dentin production.
4. Calcitonin also affects calcium and phosphate handling. It is produced by thyroid C cells within the thyroid gland.
   a. Elevated levels of calcium promote the release of calcitonin.
   b. Calcitonin (short-term increase) decreases the movement of calcium from bone into plasma.
   c. Calcitonin (long-term increase) decreases bone reabsorption by inhibiting osteoclasts, thereby decreasing plasma calcium and phosphate levels.
   C. Hormones of the pancreas
      1. Pancreas is located in the left posterior abdominal wall and has many functions related to regulation of metabolism.
      2. Pancreas has both exocrine and endocrine functions.
         a. Exocrine glands (acini) secrete enzymes (proteases, amylase, and lipases) and an aqueous bicarbonate-rich fluid into the intestine.

b. Cells in the isles of Langerhans produce insulin, glucagon, somatostatin, and pancreas polypeptide.
   1) Insulin produced in β cells:
      a) Lowers blood glucose, fatty acid, and amino acid levels.
      b) Promotes the storage of these nutrients as glycogen, triglycerides, and protein.
      c) Promotes uptake of glucose.
      d) Release is primarily stimulated by elevations in blood glucose levels.
      e) Release also occurs with elevated blood amino acid levels and parasympathetic nervous system stimulation.
   2) Glucagon is produced in α cells and counteracts many of the effects of insulin.
      a) Increases the breakdown of glycogen to glucose.
      b) Produces ketone bodies from the breakdown of fatty acids.
      c) Inhibits liver protein synthesis and promotes protein degradation.
      d) Excess glucagon exacerbates the effect of insulin deficiencies (e.g., in diabetes mellitus).

D. Hormones of the adrenal glands
  1. The cortical and medullary regions of the adrenal glands have different endocrine functions.
    a. Cortex secretes various hormones.
      1) Mineralocorticoids (mainly aldosterone)
        a) Promote sodium retention and potassium elimination by the kidney.
        b) Are involved in long-term regulation of blood volume and pressure.
        c) Secretion is stimulated by the renin-angiotensin system, decreased plasma sodium levels, and increased potassium levels.
      2) Glucocorticoids, such as cortisol, are regulated by ACTH and:
        a) Promote gluconeogenesis.
        b) Stimulate protein degradation in muscle (wasting).
        c) Facilitate lipolysis.
        d) Have a permissive effect on the actions of catecholamines.
        e) Exert antiinflammatory and immunosuppressive effects.
      3) Sex steroid hormone production includes:
        a) Low levels of androgens.
        b) Low levels of estrogens.
        c) Dehydroepiandrosterone (DHEA), the most important form of androgen, whose production peaks at 25 to 30 years of age and then declines.

b. Medulla secretes mainly epinephrine and some norepinephrine. Control of medullary secretion is through the sympathetic nervous system.

E. Testicular hormones
  1. Testosterone
    a. Is produced by Leydig cells in the testes under the stimulation of LH.
    b. In conjunction with FSH, stimulates the production of sperm.
    c. Production is regulated by negative feedback of LH production.
    d. Promotes growth and maturation of male reproductive organs at puberty.
    e. Induces the development of secondary male sexual characteristics.
    f. Increases protein production in muscles.
    g. Promotes long bone growth.
    h. Promotes the production of red blood cells.
  2. Inhibin
    a. Is produced by Sertoli cells.
    b. Inhibits FSH production.

F. Ovarian hormones and the menstrual cycle
  1. Hormones
    a. Estrogens (estradiol [most important], estrone, estriol)
      1) Are essential for follicular (egg) maturation and release.
      2) Stimulate the development and maintenance of the female reproductive tract.
      3) Induce the production of progesterone and oxytocin receptors.
      4) During pregnancy estrogen inhibits the milk-secreting action of prolactin, but stimulates development of breast ducts.
      5) Promote fat deposition.
      6) Decrease blood cholesterol levels.
      7) Promote bone density and close epiphyseal plates.
      8) Act as an antioxidant.
      9) Promote vasodilation.
    b. Inhibin inhibits the production of FSH during the follicular phase of the menstrual cycle.
    c. Progesterone
      1) Prepares the uterus for the developing fetus and suppresses uterine contractions during pregnancy.
      2) Inhibits GnRH production.
      3) Stimulates alveolar development in breasts and inhibits the milk-secreting action of prolactin.
      4) Stimulates ventilation.
  2. Hormonal changes during the menstrual cycle
    a. Ovarian cycles begin at puberty (approximately 12 years of age) and typically

continue until menopause (approximately 50 years of age), with breaks during pregnancy and lactation.

   b. When the follicular phase begins and menstruation occurs:
1) Estradiol, progesterone, FSH, and LH levels are low.
2) The outer layer of the endometrium sheds.
3) Follicles begin to mature.

   c. When the follicular phase continues:
1) Estradiol levels increase and progesterone, LH, and FSH levels are low.
2) The follicle matures.
3) The endometrium develops.

   d. When ovulation occurs:
1) Estradiol levels fall and LH and FSH rise sharply.
2) The follicle is released.
3) Cervical mucus thins.

   e. During the luteal phase:
1) Both estradiol and progesterone levels increase but FSH and LH levels are low.
2) The corpus luteum develops.
3) The endometrium develops.

G. Hormones involved in fluid volume and blood pressure regulation
1. Renin is produced by the kidney and stimulated by:
   a. Low plasma sodium levels.
   b. A decreased extracellular fluid volume.
   c. A decrease in blood pressure.
   d. Sympathetic nervous system stimulation.
2. Angiotensin I and II
   a. Renin converts angiotensinogen (made in the liver and released into the plasma) into angiotensin I (AI).
   b. In the lungs, angiotensin-converting enzyme (ACE) coverts AI to angiotensin II (AII).
   c. Are potent vasoconstrictors and promote the production of aldosterone.
3. Antidiuretic hormone (ADH) or vasopressin is produced by the hypothalamus in the central nervous system, not peripherally).
   a. Stimuli for its release include AII, ↓ extracellular fluid volume, stress, and ↑ extracellular fluid osmolarity.
   b. ADH increases water retention by the kidney and is a potent vasoconstrictor.
4. Atrial natriuretic peptide is produced in the right heart and in the lungs.
   a. Its production is influenced by an increase in extracellular fluid volume.
   b. It increases water excretion (diuretic).
   c. It increases sodium excretion (natriuretic).
   d. Elevated plasma levels are found in patients with congestive heart failure.

H. Hormones that regulate satiety (food intake)
1. Leptin is produced peripherally by white adipose cells
   a. Is transported in the blood across the blood-brain barrer by selective carriers; in the brain it acts on receptors located in the hypothalamus and brainstem regions to effect a number of physiological functions.
   b. Also regulates reproductive behaviors and sleep.
2. Other neuromodulators and neurotransmitters associated with feeding include opioids, galanin, and neuropeptide 4.

Respiratory Physiology

Respiratory physiology is the study of the respiratory system, which controls gas exchange, acid-base balance, and vocalization and enhances venous return.

I. Respiratory Functional Anatomy
  A. Structures involved with gas exchange
1. Nose and mouth act as ports into the respiratory system.
2. Gases travel through the nasopharnyx into the glottis and larynx.
3. Gases enter the lungs by means of the trachea, a large-diameter tube that contains cartilaginous rings, connective tissue, smooth muscle, and mucous glands and is lined with epithelial cells and goblet cells.
4. Bronchi, the next branched structures that air passes through, subdivide into bronchioli, which resemble a tree. Bronchioli contain less cartilage and more smooth muscle than bronchi.
5. Respiratory bronchioli branch to form ducts that connect to alveolar sacs.
6. Alveolar sacs constitute the gas exchange portions of the lung and consist of:
   a. Type-I cells: flat, large, thin cells.
   b. Type-II cells, which produce surfactant (keeps lungs dry, decreases surface tension, decreases work of breathing) and can divide and differentiate to form Type-I cells.
   c. Pulmonary capillaries, which are metabolically active.
7. The entire gas exchange region of the lung is approximately the size of a tennis court!
  B. The thoracic cavity is the home of the lungs and heart.
1. The inner portion of the chest wall is covered by a lining (the visceral pleura).
2. The lungs consist of five lobes and are covered by the parietal pleura.
3. In between the linings is the "pleural space," which contains a small amount of fluid (approximately 2 mL).
   a. The fluid is constantly exchanged.

b. It helps lubricate the lungs as they move in the thoracic cavity.

c. The fluid helps "attach" (or couple) the lungs to the chest wall (like two microscope slides with a drop of fluid in between).

d. Pressures within the pleural space are below atmospheric level during normal breathing.

C. The chest wall consists of skeletal muscles and bony elements.

1. Helps to maintain normal posture; important in ventilation and in locomotion.

2. Chest wall muscles are the ventilatory pump.

3. Muscles forming the pump consist of the diaphragm, internal and external intercostals, abdominal muscles, and accessory muscles (sternocleidomastoids and scalenes).

D. Diseases of the chest wall skeleton (e.g., osteoporosis) and muscles (e.g., muscular dystrophy) decrease breathing capacity.

II. Functions of The Respiratory System

A. Respiratory system performs a number of vital functions to help maintain homeostasis.

B. Gas exchange: oxygen and carbon dioxide

1. Exchange with the environment in the lungs (ventilation).

2. Exchange between the lungs, circulatory system, and the cells (diffusion and transport).

3. Exchange in cells (respiration) involves the use of oxygen and the production of carbon dioxide.

C. Acid-base balance: the maintenance of a blood pH of approximately 7.4.

1. Respiratory system is a rapid response system that alters plasma levels of carbon dioxide.

2. It works in conjunction with other buffering systems including blood, kidneys, bones, and other cells.

D. Regulation of air flow involved in vocalization.

E. Metabolism and elimination of substances via the pulmonary circulation (e.g., conversion of AI to AII).

F. Defense against inhaled particles (airways and nose) and emboli (pulmonary circulation).

G. Means for drug delivery because of the lung's large surface area and ready access to the circulation.

H. Enhancement of venous return.

III. Specific Functions of the Respiratory System

A. Process of ventilation.

1. Tidal volume is the volume of a breath that depends on the force of respiratory muscle contractions and the elasticity of the lung.

a. Part of a breath goes to the alveolar sacs for gas exchange.

b. Part of a breath remains in the conducting branches of the lung, forming the "dead space" volume.

c. During inspiration, alveolar pressures are below atmospheric pressure and suck air into the lung. The lungs are stretched like a rubber band.

d. During expiration, alveolar pressures are above atmospheric pressures and push the air out of the lungs. The "stretched rubber band" is released.

e. The frequency of breathing in adults is approximately 15 breaths per minute.

f. Minute ventilation is the product of the tidal volume and the frequency of breaths per minute.

2. Multiple factors drive ventilation.

a. Elevated levels of carbon dioxide in plasma are sensed primarily by neurons within the ventral medulla.

b. Decreased levels of oxygen are sensed by the carotid bodies.

c. Increased levels of hydrogen ions are sensed by the carotid bodies.

d. Within the airways and lung, receptors are sensitive to stretch, congestion (e.g., pneumonia or pulmonary emboli), and irritation (e.g., smoke).

3. Ventilation increases with:

a. Increased metabolic demands, such as occur during exercise.

b. Use of stimulants such as caffeine and progesterone.

c. Decreased levels of oxygen found at high altitudes and in patients with cardiopulmonary disease.

d. Acidosis that occurs in patients with poorly controlled diabetes mellitus.

4. Ventilation decreases with:

a. Metabolic alkalosis.

b. Overdoses of some drugs (e.g., morphine, heroin).

c. Respiratory muscle failure.

d. Use of supplemental oxygen by patients with chronic obstructive lung disease (low levels of oxygen provide their only chemical drive to breathing; for healthy people, the major drive is elevations in carbon dioxide levels).

B. Lung mechanics and volumes.

1. Compliance is a measure of the distensiblity of the lung (Δvolume/Δpressure).

a. It increases in emphysema because of the destruction of connective tissue.

b. It decreases in pneumonia (increased lung water) and in diseases that decrease levels of lung surfactant (e.g., adult respiratory distress syndrome [ARDS]).

2. Resistance is a measure of the ease with which air moves in and out of the lung and is related to the radius of the airways (Resistance α 1/radius^4). Thus small decreases in radius have large effects on airways resistance.

a. Resistance is increased by agents that cause contraction of airway smooth muscles (e.g., acetylcholine, histamine, leukotrienes).

b. Resistance is increased by excess mucus (bronchitis), airway edema, and tumors within or around airways.

c. Changes in mechanics, such as decreasing compliance (lung fibrosis) or increasing resistance (asthma), increase the work of breathing and can induce breathlessness when a patient is performing a minor task such as brushing hair.

d. Lung volumes (Fig. 2–28) are influenced by lung and chest wall mechanics.

  1) Lungs volumes are smaller in patients with fibrosis.

  2) Lung volumes are larger in patients with hyperinflation caused by emphysema.

C. Oxygen and carbon dioxide handling by the body.

  1. Source of gases and transport processes.

    a. The major sources of oxygen are the lungs and the blood (approximately 8 L).

      1) Approximately 0.3 mL of oxygen per 100 mL of blood is transported as dissolved.

      2) 19.9 mL of oxygen per 100 mL of blood is transported bound to hemoglobin.

      3) A small amount of oxygen is in muscle, bound to myoglobin.

    b. Carbon dioxide is produced by aerobic metabolism and is transported in blood.

      1) Some is transported as dissolved carbon dioxide (2.9 mL CO_2 per 100 mL blood).

      2) Some is bound to proteins in blood (2.1 mL per 100 mL blood) as carbaminohemoglobin.

      3) The majority is transported as bicarbonate (42 mL per 100 mL blood): $CO_2 + H_2O \xrightarrow{CA} H_2CO_3 \rightarrow HCO_3^- + H^+$, where CA is the enzyme carbonic anhydrase. At the level of the lung, this reaction is reversed and CO_2 is released by the lungs.

      4) Total body stores of carbon dioxide are approximately 120 L.

D. Diffusion of gases across the lungs.

  1. Occurs in areas that are both ventilated and perfused with blood.

  2. Depends on the solubility of the gas in plasma membranes.

    a. CO_2 is 20 times more soluble than O_2.

    b. The partial pressure of arterial O_2 is 100 mm Hg and that of CO_2 in arterial blood is 40 mm Hg.

  3. Is affected by the thickness of the alveolar-capillary barrier.

    a. Normally about 0.5 μm

    b. Increases during lung edema.

E. Normal values for arterial and venous partial pressures of gases:

  1. Arterial P_{CO_2} is 40 mm Hg; P_{O_2} is 100 mm Hg.

  2. Mixed venous P_{CO_2} is 45 mm Hg; P_{O_2} is 40 mm Hg.

F. Regulation of acid-base balance by the lungs occurs by increasing or decreasing ventilation of CO_2: $CO_2 + H_2O \xleftarrow{CA} H_2CO_3 \leftarrow HCO_3^- + H^+$ (the acid).

  1. If the amount of CO_2 produced by the body is equal to the ventilation, the pH remains constant (7.4).

  2. If the amount of CO_2 produced by the body is greater than the ventilation, the pH decreases and an acidosis results (pH < 7.35).

  3. If ventilation is greater than the amount of CO_2 produced by the body, the pH increases and an alkalosis results (pH > 7.45).

  4. Hydrogen ions are produced by metabolism or during periods of low oxygen and are buffered by the bicarbonate ions (HCO_3^-) produced from the reaction of CO_2 and H_2O (see above).

  5. The resulting decrease in bicarbonate ions can be restored ONLY by the kidneys.

G. Decreased delivery to or use of oxygen occurs when:

  1. The alveolar P_{O_2} is decreased (hypoxic hypoxia).

    a. In high altitudes (decreased barometric pressure).

    b. During lung disease or respiratory failure.

  2. The amount of functional hemoglobin decreases (anemic hypoxia).

    a. In anemia caused by decreased red blood cell production, abnormal forms of hemoglobin (sickle cell anemia), or blood loss.

    b. In carbon monoxide poisoning, which prevents hemoglobin from binding to O_2 (CO

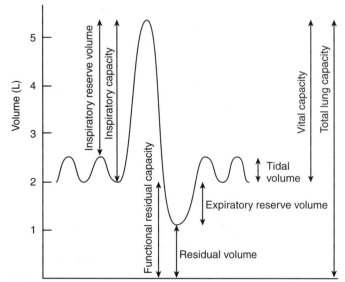

Figure 2.28 Lung volumes and capacities in a normal adult. Residual volume and any capacities containing residual volume cannot be determined using a spirometer.

binds to hemoglobin 150 times greater than does oxygen.)

3. Blood flow to the tissues decreases (ischemia or stagnant hypoxia) as a result of:
   a. Heart failure.
   b. The effect of diabetes mellitus on blood vessels.
   c. Stroke.
   d. Arteriosclerosis.
4. Poisoning of enzymes involved in using oxygen to form ATP (histotoxic hypoxia).
   a. Carbon monoxide.
   b. Cyanide.

Renal Physiology

Renal physiology is the study of the urinary system, which consists of the kidneys, ureter, bladder, and urethra. Kidneys selectively excrete substances, reabsorb nutrients and water, affect blood pressure, and influence acid-base balance.

I. Functional Anatomy of the Urinary System
   A. Kidneys
      1. Renal cortex contains the cortical nephrons.
      2. Renal medulla contains juxtamedullary nephrons that concentrate urine.
      3. Renal pelvis is the collecting region for urine produced by the nephrons.
      4. Renal artery is the major source of oxygen and nutrients for the kidney.
      5. Renal vein carries blood that has been "conditioned" by the kidneys.
      6. Ureter is the conduit for transporting urine from the kidney to the bladder.
      7. Bladder stores urine and empties it by the process of micturition, which involves autonomic nervous system reflexes.
      8. Urethra is a conduit for excreting urine from the body.
      9. Blockages along any of these structures result in increased pressure, which may damage the kidneys.
II. Major Functions of the Kidneys
   A. Conservation of water, electrolytes (especially sodium), and nutrients.
   B. Regulation of acid-base balance in conjunction with other systems (lungs, blood, bone).
   C. Secretion of erythropoietin (a hormone that stimulates the production of red blood cells).
   D. Elimination of waste and foreign products.
   E. Regulation of plasma volume, which affects blood pressure.
   F. Secretion of renin, an enzyme that produces angiotensin I from angiotensinogen.
   G. Production of the active form of vitamin D involved in calcium handling by the body.
   H. Function unit of the kidney is the:
      1. Nephron (Fig. 2–29)
         a. Short nephrons are called cortical nephrons;

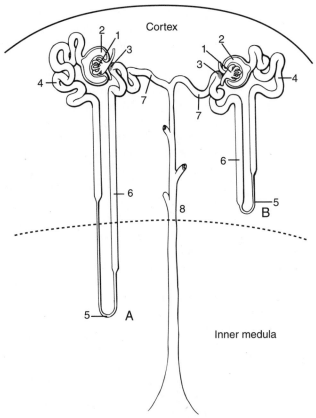

Figure 2.29 Nephrons in the kidney. *A* denotes a juxtamedullary nephron, and *B* denotes a cortical nephron. Parts of the nephron are: *1*, glomerulus; *2*, Bowman's capsule; *3*, macula densa; *4*, proximal tubule; *5*, tip of the loop of Henle; *6*, ascending portion of the loop of Henle; *7*, distal convoluted tubule; and *8*, collecting duct.

longer nephrons involved in concentrating urine are juxtamedullary nephrons.
         b. Basic components of nephrons include:
            1) Vascular components.
               a) The afferent arteriole delivers blood to the nephron.
               b) The glomerulus is a dense capillary bed formed from the arteriole that acts to filter the plasma, allowing all substances in the blood except proteins and cells to enter the nephron.
               c) The efferent arteriole carries blood from the glomerulus.
               d) All three structures listed are in series.
               e) The peritubular capillaries are formed from the efferent arteriole and supply blood to the rest of the nephron.
               f) The juxtamedullary apparatus (JMA) consists of the vascular and nephron tubular components, macula densa, and the juxtaglomerular cells of the afferent arteriole. The JMA produces chemicals that affect blood flow to the kidneys.

2) Tubular components.
   a) Bowman's capsule is the portion of the nephron into which filtered plasma enters.
   b) The proximal tubule is primarily involved in reabsorption of most filtered constituents. Secretion of H^+ and organic ions may occur.
   c) Loop of Henle is involved in concentration of urine in conjunction with the distal tubule and the collecting duct. The loops are especially long in medullary nephrons.
   d) Distal tubule and collecting duct have variable control (by means of hormones such as aldosterone, vasopressin, and atrial natriuretic peptide) of sodium, potassium, hydrogen ions, and water.

c. Processes performed by the nephron.
   1) Handling filtered plasma and urine production.
      a) Glomerular filtration and the glomerular filtration rate (GFR) involves indiscriminate filtration of plasma; depends on:
         (1) Blood pressure.
         (2) Leakiness of the glomerular capillaries and Bowman capsule.
         (3) Afferent versus efferent vasoconstriction.
            (a) Afferent constriction leads to ↓ GFR and decreased perfusion of the rest of the nephron.
            (b) Efferent constriction leads to ↑ GFR and decreased perfusion of the rest of the nephron.
         (4) Tubular reabsorption—selective, high-volume process dependent on:
            (a) Energy—Na^+ reabsorption (water and Cl^- follow passively; glucose, phosphate, and amino acids are transported secondarily).
            (b) Concentration—normally there is a higher concentration of substances in the proximal tubule than in the peritubular vessels.
            (c) Hormones—aldosterone (for sodium), vasopressin (for water), and atrial natriuretic peptide (for both sodium and water).
            (d) Tubular maximum for the substance—once this is reached, a substance is 'dumped' into the urine (e.g., high plasma glucose levels in diabetes mellitus result in glucose in the urine; typically all glucose in the nephron is reabsorbed back into the blood).
         (5) Tubular secretion results in the movement of substances from the peritubular capillaries into the nephron for excretion.
            (a) Secretion of hydrogen and bicarbonate ions depend on the acid-base status of the body.
            (b) Potassium secretion is dependent on the amount of aldosterone present.
            (c) Organic ions and cations (especially some drugs and endogenous substances such as histamine, epinephrine and creatinine) are secreted.
         (6) Plasma clearance and urinary excretion.
            (a) Clearance of a substance by the kidneys refers to the volume of plasma that is completely cleared of the substance per unit of time.
            (b) Inulin is filtered, not reabsorbed or secreted. It is completely cleared by the kidney and is used to measure GFR.
            (c) Glucose in a healthy person is filtered but completely reabsorbed. Therefore none is cleared by the kidney.
      b) Excretion is a measure of the amount of urine that leaves the body per unit of time.
         (1) It is the difference between what is filtered and what is reabsorbed plus what is secreted. Normal excretion rates are 1 mL/min.
         (2) Excretion rates depend on the concentration of the urine, which is modulated by the osmolarity of the plasma and the hormonal status of an individual.
         (3) Excretion rates fall during dehydration, decreased blood pressure, and renal disease.
         (4) Acid-base handling by the kidney involves reabsorption or secretion of H^+ and HCO_3^-. If the disturbance is caused by the kidney or a metabolic source, the respiratory system tries to compensate.

(5) Normal—metabolically produced acids are buffered by HCO_3^-, which is replaced by the kidneys.

(6) Metabolic acidosis—H^+ is secreted and HCO_3^- is reabsorbed; an increase in ventilation eliminates the CO_2 produced by combining the excess H^+ with HCO_3^-.

(7) Respiratory acidosis (hypoventilation)—HCO_3^- and H^+ are generated from CO_2 and H_2O. H^+ is secreted and HCO_3^- is reabsorbed.

(8) Respiratory alkalosis (hyperventilation)—the excess HCO_3^- is secreted by the kidneys and H^+ is retained. CO_2 levels in the blood are low.

(9) Metabolic alkalosis—handled by the kidney in a similar manner to respiratory alkalosis, but metabolic alkalosis depresses ventilation and CO_2 builds up in the plasma to compensate.

Blood Pressure

Blood pressure is the force that drives blood through vessels to carry nutrients and oxygen to tissues, and waste products and metabolized substances away from tissues. Mean blood pressure = cardiac output × total peripheral resistance.

I. Factors That Affect Mean Blood Pressure
   A. Cardiac output is the amount of blood pumped by the heart per minute.
      1. Heart rate (beats per minute) is:
         a. Increased by sympathetic nervous system (NS) stimulation and by the release of norepinephrine and epinephrine.
         b. Decreased by parasympathetic NS stimulation.
      2. Stroke volume (amount of blood ejected by the heart per beat) is influenced by:
         a. Amount of blood returning to the heart (venous return), which is increased by increases in blood volume, decreased right atrial pressure, skeletal muscle contractions, and increased venous tone.
         b. Contractility of heart muscle is increased by the same factors that increase heart rate.
         c. Condition of the heart; as the heart fails, cardiac output decreases.
   B. Total peripheral resistance of blood vessels is influenced by:
      1. Diameter of blood vessels, especially "resistance" vessels or arterioles that have a large amount of smooth muscles. Diameter is affected by:
         a. Sympathetic nervous system stimulation, which leads to constriction.

b. Local conditions (e.g., decreased O_2 and increased metabolites, cytokines, adenosine, and histamine) increase dilation.

c. Circulating hormones (vasopressin and angiotensin are constrictors and atrial natriuretic peptide is a dilator).

      2. Blood viscosity, which is affected by:
         a. Dehydration, which leads to increased viscosity and resistance.
         b. Number of red blood cells (RBC) (viscosity is increased in polycythemia [increased RBCs] and decreased in anemia).

II. Short-Term Regulation Of Blood Pressure
   A. The central nervous system (CNS) regulates blood pressure for the short term.
      1. Pressure and volume sensors are located in the:
         a. Carotid sinus and aortic arch (pressure).
         b. Right atrium and lungs (volume).
   B. Afferent pathways to the CNS include the medulla oblongata, hypothalamus, and cortex.
   C. CNS responses to decreased blood pressure include:
      1. Increased sympathetic nervous system outflow.
      2. Release of hormones such as vasopressin from the pituitary gland.
      3. Stimulation of renin release by the kidneys.
   D. Systemic consequences include:
      1. Increased cardiac output.
      2. Increased total peripheral resistance.
      3. Production of angiotensin II and aldosterone.

III. Long-Term Regulation of Blood Pressure
   A. Is influenced by the kidney, which either retains or excretes sodium and water.
   B. Involves measurement of arterial blood pressures (systolic, diastolic, and mean blood pressures) by means of:
      1. Direct use of an indwelling catheter.
      2. Indirect use of a pressure cuff, sphygmomanometer, and stethoscope as follows:
         a. Occlude the brachial artery with an inflated cuff to a pressure greater than systolic pressure.
         b. As pressure within the cuff is reduced, turbulent sounds are heard that indicate the SYSTOLIC PRESSURE (SP, which normally is approximately 120 mm Hg).
         c. When the sound disappears, the DIASTOLIC PRESSURE is reached (DP, which normally is approximately 80 mm Hg).
         d. MEAN ARTERIAL PRESSURE = DP + ⅓ (SP-DP).

IV. Blood Pressure Abnormalities
   A. Hypertension (systolic/diastolic 160/100 mm Hg; borderline is 140/90 mm Hg)
      1. May be caused or potentiated by:
         a. Excess fluid retention cause by hormonal abnormalities (e.g., increased levels of aldosterone).

b. Stress.

c. Renal disease.

d. Obesity.

e. Diabetes mellitus.

f. Aging (which also may result in hypotension).

2. Consequences of hypertension include:

a. Increased work by the heart, which may lead to failure.

b. Stresses on blood vessels, which may lead to atherosclerosis and stroke.

B. Hypotension (low blood pressure)

1. May be caused by:

a. Heart disease that leads to decreased cardiac output.

b. Decreased sympathetic nervous system function or β-adrenergic receptor blockade (use of drugs that cause this, such as propranolol).

c. Shock related to:

1) Blood loss.

2) Septic (bacterial) infections.

3) Neurogenic causes (fainting).

4) Anaphylactic reactions (e.g., bee stings in susceptible individuals cause release of mediators like histamine).

Gastrointestinal (GI) Physiology

Gastrointestinal physiology is the study of the GI tract, which consists of the mouth, esophagus, stomach, and small and large intestines, and is primarily responsible for the digestion of food into more usable forms of nutrients for cells of the body.

I. General Structure of Digestive Organs (from the lumen to the outside)

A. Mucosal membrane is composed of specialized cells, including:

1. Exocrine cells, which produce digestive juices and contain enzymes for intracellular digestion of foodstuffs.

2. Endocrine cells, which produce hormones.

3. Epithelial cells, which are involved in absorption of digested food stuffs and water.

B. Lamina propria is a thin layer of connective tissue on which the mucous membrane rests. It contains small blood vessels, lymph vessels, and nerves.

C. Muscularis mucosa is a smooth muscle layer that alters the surface area of the digestive organ.

D. Submucosa is a thick layer of connective tissue that gives the digestive organ distensiblity and elasticity. It contains:

1. Blood vessels.

2. Lymph vessels.

3. Submucous plexus (an intrinsic nervous system of the gut).

E. Muscularis externa consists of:

1. Longitudinally arranged smooth muscles.

2. The myenteric plexus (another intrinsic nervous system).

3. Circular smooth muscles.

F. Serosa is a thicker outer layer of connective tissue.

II. Functions of the GI Tract

A. Include the digestion of food stuffs to nutrients that can be absorbed and used by cells for energy, growth, repair, heat production, and differentiation.

1. Digestive processes

a. Motility—movement and mixing of food stuffs along the GI tract.

b. Secretion—production and release of enzymes, hormones, fluids, mucus, or electrolytes that aid in digestion.

c. Digestion—breakdown of injected food stuffs to nutrients that may be used by the body.

d. Absorption—uptake of digested materials across the GI tract into the blood or lymphatics for delivery to cells.

B. Include defense against ingested substances that may be harmful to the body.

III. Anatomic Structures and Functions of Digestion

A. The mouth ingests foods and contains the:

1. Tongue, which mixes food with saliva and contains taste buds. The fluid in saliva helps dissolve foods so that they may be 'tasted.'

2. Teeth, which chew food to decrease its size and to allow better mixing of food with saliva, which acts as a lubricant.

B. Salivary glands and accessory digestive glands produce secretions that contain:

1. Saliva (fluid, mucous, lysozyme, and bicarbonate).

a. Saliva production is tonically stimulated by the parasympathetic nervous system.

b. Production can be stimulated by the smell or sight of food or an anticipatory reflex.

c. The fluid and lysozyme have antibacterial actions that help prevent the formation of caries.

2. Salivary amylase, which begins to digest starches.

C. Pharynx allows movement of gases into the lungs and chewed foodstuffs into the esophagus. During swallowing the glottis closes to prevent foodstuffs from entering the lungs.

D. Esophagus is tubelike and consists of both smooth and skeletal muscles.

1. It moves chewed food from the mouth toward the stomach by peristaltic contractions.

2. Mucus produced by cells lining the lumen is protective and helps movement of food.

3. After the gastroesophageal sphincter relaxes, food enters the stomach.

E. Stomach consists of three regions: fundus (thin walled), body (thin walled), and antrum (thick muscular wall).

1. Functions of the stomach include:
   a. Storage of ingested food until it is emptied into the small intestine.
   b. Secretion of HCl and enzymes that initiate digestion.
   c. Pulverization and mixing of food to produce chyme (thick liquid mixture).

2. Major secretions of the stomach and their locations.
   a. Oxyntic mucosa (in fundus and body)
      1) Mucous neck cells produce a thin mucus.
      2) Chief cells produce pepsinogen, which is converted to the enzyme pepsin under the influence of HCl to initiate protein digestion.
      3) Parietal (oxyntic) cells produce HCl and intrinsic factor, which help absorb vitamin B_{12} in the ileum.
      4) Epithelial cells secrete a thick mucus to protect the stomach from autodigestion.
   b. Pyloric area contains G cells that secret gastrin, a hormone that stimulates parietal and chief cells.

3. Emptying of chyme from the stomach.
   a. Depends on the volume and fluidity of the chyme, which initiates gastrin production and reflexes (via the vagus nerve and the intrinsic nervous system) that stimulate antrum contraction → emptying.
   b. The presence of acid and/or fat in the duodenum initiates the enterogastric reflex and the release of secretin, cholecystokinin, and a gastric inhibitory peptide that prevent emptying.
   c. Vomiting is caused by active contraction of respiratory muscles that act on the stomach → emptying.

4. Gastric secretion is stimulated during various phases.
   a. Cephalic phase—smell or thought of food leads to secretion of HCl, gastrin, and pepsinogen.
   b. Gastric phase—large volume of food, caffeine, or alcohol leads to gastrin and HCl secretion.
   c. Intestinal phase—chyme enters into the duodenum, leading to decreased gastrin and HCl secretion.

F. Functions of the pancreas and liver (accessory organs)

1. The exocrine pancreas produces enzymes (e.g., trypsin [activated by enterokinase], chymotrypsin, amylase, lipase) and an alkaline watery solution, which are secreted into the small intestine.

2. The pancreas also is an endocrine organ that produces insulin, glucagon, and somatostatin (see section on endocrinology).

3. The liver produces bile, cholesterol, and lecithin; these aid in the formation of micelles, which facilitate absorption of fats.

4. Bile produced by the liver is stored in the gall bladder.

5. Additional functions of the liver not associated with digestion include:
   a. Storage of glycogen.
   b. Production of fibrinogen and prothrombin, which are involved in blood clotting.
   c. Detoxification of waste products and foreign substances.
   d. Synthesis of amino acids and proteins.
   e. Production of red blood cells in the fetus and destruction of RBCs in the adult.

6. All blood that leaves the gut passes through the liver via the portal vein, allowing additional processing of nutrients and blood detoxification.

G. The role of the small intestine (duodenum [8 inches], jejunum [8 feet], and ileum [20 feet]) in digestion and absorption.

1. Segmentation, which results in mixing and moving of chyme:
   a. Is initiated by pacemaker cells in the gut.
   b. Responds to the presence of chyme in the stomach and the production of gastrin by the duodenum.
   c. Is stimulated by the parasympathetic NS and inhibited by the sympathetic NS.

2. Digestion of chyme occurs by
   a. Pancreatic enzymes released into the small intestine.
   b. Intracellular enzymes.
   c. Crypts of Lieberkuhn secrete water and electrolytes and constantly replace epithelial cells that secrete mucus.

3. The small intestine has a large surface area for absorption because of the presence of villi and microvilli.

4. Absorption of most nutrients occurs in the duodenum and the jejunum.

5. Absorption of vitamin B12 and bile salts occurs in the terminal ileum.

6. Absorption of calcium and iron depends on the body's needs.

H. Processing of substances not absorbed in the small intestine by the large intestine (colon, cecum, appendix, and rectum).
   a. The primary substances absorbed in the large intestine are electrolytes and water.
   b. Matter in the colon consists of feces and an alkaline mucus for protection.
   c. Movements (haustrations) are slow contractions and mass movements.

d. The gastrocolic reflex: mass movements in response to food in the stomach lead to movement of feces into the rectum.

e. Elimination of feces occurs by means of the defecation reflex.

1) The internal anal sphincter (smooth muscle) under involuntary control relaxes and the rectum and sigmoid colon contract.

2) The external sphincter (skeletal muscle) is under voluntary control.

3) Relaxation of both sphincters leads to defecation.

4) Increased intraabdominal pressure leads to ejection of feces from the body.

5) Control of defecation develops with age.

CONTENT REVIEW QUESTIONS

1. Some cells that line the respiratory tract produce mucus, which traps inhaled particles and subsequently is propelled upward for expectoration. This upward movement is produced by the action of:
   A. ribosomes
   B. cilia
   C. flagella
   D. centrioles

2. The tissue that lines the oral cavity is:
   A. simple squamous epithelium for diffusion of fluids
   B. simple columnar epithelium for absorption
   C. pseudostratified columnar epithelium with goblet cells for production of mucus
   D. stratified squamous epithelium for protection from abrasion

3. Which of the following is NOT a type of connective tissue?
   A. blood
   B. bone
   C. cartilage
   D. muscle

4. The lining of the respiratory tract is described as:
   A. a mucous membrane
   B. a cutaneous membrane
   C. a serous membrane
   D. a parietal membrane

5. An abrasion on the surface of the skin heals when new cells form to replace the damaged cells. The layer of skin that produces the replacement cells is the:
   A. stratum lucidum
   B. stratum corneum
   C. stratum granulosum
   D. stratum basale

6. A fracture of the radius:
   A. is a fracture in the axial skeleton
   B. is a fracture on the medial side of the forearm
   C. is a fracture of the brachium or arm
   D. is a fracture on the lateral side of the forearm

7. Diarthrotic joints (diarthroses):
   A. have a fibrous joint capsule lined with a synovial membrane
   B. are immovable joints
   C. include the intervertebral discs
   D. are fibrous joints

8. Which of the following muscles is NOT associated with the lower extremity?
   A. adductor longus
   B. sternocleidomastoid
   C. biceps femoris
   D. gastrocnemius

9. Which of the following is NOT a part of the central nervous system?
   A. cranial nerves
   B. cerebrum
   C. cerebellum
   D. spinal cord

10. The cerebellum:
    A. contains centers that help regulate breathing movements
    B. regulates heart rate and blood pressure
    C. is important in maintaining posture and equilibrium
    D. contains centers for hearing and vision

11. The afferent division of the peripheral nervous system:
    A. consists entirely of cranial nerves
    B. consists entirely of spinal nerves
    C. carries sensory impulses to the central nervous system
    D. carries motor impulses from the central nervous system to the effectors

12. Which of the following is NOT true about the autonomic nervous system?
    A. it is a visceral efferent system
    B. it is divided into sympathetic and parasympathetic divisions
    C. its effectors are skeletal muscles
    D. it is part of the peripheral nervous system

13. Taste and smell:
    A. are general senses
    B. are localized and closely related
    C. are a type of proprioception
    D. are detected by Meissner's and Pacinian corpuscles

14. The rods and cones of the eye are located:
    A. in the innermost layer of the eye
    B. in the cornea
    C. in the ciliary body
    D. in the lens

15. The organ of Corti:
    A. is located in the middle ear
    B. contains the malleus, incus, and stapes
    C. functions to provide equilibrium
    D. contains the receptors for hearing

16. The hormone aldosterone:
    A. reacts with receptors on the surface of the cell membrane
    B. is one of the sex hormones
    C. is produced by the adenohypophysis
    D. is a derivative of cholesterol

17. The formed elements of the blood that contain hemoglobin and transport oxygen are the:
    A. thrombocytes
    B. leukocytes
    C. monocytes
    D. erythrocytes

18. A person with type A blood may be given a transfusion of:
    A. type A or type AB blood
    B. type A or type O blood
    C. type B or type AB blood
    D. type AB or type O blood

19. An Rh factor reaction called hemolytic disease of the newborn may occur when:
    A. anti-Rh agglutinins of the fetus come in contact with agglutinogens from an Rh– mother
    B. Rh+ agglutinogens of the fetus come into contact with anti-Rh agglutinins from an Rh– mother
    C. Rh+ agglutinogens of the fetus come into contact with Rh– agglutinogens from an Rh– mother
    D. anti-Rh agglutinins of the fetus come into contact with anti-Rh agglutinins from an Rh– mother

20. Blood in the hepatic portal vein:
    A. has a lower oxygen content than blood in the hepatic artery
    B. has a higher oxygen content than blood in the descending aorta
    C. has a higher oxygen content than blood in the left atrium
    D. has a lower glucose content than blood in the hepatic artery

21. Lymph from the right inguinal lymph nodes:
    A. flows into the thoracic duct, then into the right subclavian vein
    B. flows into the thoracic duct, then into the left subclavian vein
    C. flows into the right lymphatic duct, then into the right subclavian vein
    D. flows into the right lymphatic duct, then into the left subclavian vein

22. Most diffusion of oxygen and carbon dioxide occurs across the walls of the:
    A. trachea
    B. bronchi
    C. alveoli
    D. hypopharynx

23. One of the differences between the right lung and the left lung is that the:
    A. the left lung has a greater volume because it is longer than the right lung
    B. the right lung is covered by a serous membrane but the left lung is not

24. C. the right lung has an indentation for the base of the heart but the left lung does not
    D. the right lung has three lobes but the left lung has two

24. An incision into the stomach from the outside passes through the histologic layers of the wall in the following sequence:
    A. serous membrane, smooth muscle, connective tissue with blood vessels and nerves, simple columnar epithelium
    B. smooth muscle, simple columnar epithelium, serous membrane, connective tissue with blood vessels and nerves
    C. simple columnar epithelium, smooth muscle, connective tissue with blood vessels and nerves, serous membrane
    D. serous membrane, simple columnar epithelium, connective tissue with blood vessels and nerves, smooth muscle

25. Mucosal cells of the stomach secrete all of the following EXCEPT:
    A. hydrochloric acid
    B. gastrin
    C. pepsinogen
    D. amylase

26. The small intestine is divided into the following three regions:
    A. proximal jejunum next to the stomach, middle duodenum, and distal ileum
    B. proximal ileum next to the stomach, middle duodenum, and distal jejunum
    C. proximal duodenum next to the stomach, middle jejunum, and distal ileum
    D. proximal jejunum next to the stomach, middle ileum, and distal jejunum

27. Cells of the small intestine secrete both enzymes and hormones. Secretin is a hormone produced by the small intestine that:
    A. stimulates contraction of the gallbladder
    B. stimulates production of pancreatic enzymes
    C. stimulates secretion of an alkaline fluid from the pancreas
    D. stimulates secretion of hydrochloric acid from the stomach

28. Which of the following is NOT true about the liver?
    A. blood is drained from the liver by the hepatic portal vein
    B. liver produces bile
    C. liver is located in the upper right quadrant of the abdomen
    D. oxygenated blood is brought to the liver by the hepatic artery

29. Which of the following sequences BEST describes the flow of urine?
    A. urinary bladder, urethra, ureter, kidney
    B. kidney, urethra, urinary bladder, ureter
    C. kidney, ureter, urinary bladder, urethra
    D. urinary bladder, ureter, urethra, kidney

30. Which of the following describes the correct sequence for the passage of spermatozoa through the male reproductive tract?
    A. urethra, seminiferous tubules, epididymis, ejaculatory duct, ductus deferens
    B. seminiferous tubules, ejaculatory duct, epididymis, ductus deferens, urethra
    C. epididymis, seminiferous tubules, ejaculatory duct, ductus deferens, urethra
    D. seminiferous tubules, epididymis, ductus deferens, ejaculatory duct, urethra

31. Most of the volume of seminal fluid is composed of:
    A. sperm from the testes
    B. fluid from the seminal vesicles
    C. fluid from the prostate gland
    D. fluid from the penis

32. The portion of the uterine wall that is sloughed off during menstruation is the:
    A. perimetrium
    B. stratum basale of the endometrium
    C. stratum functionale of the endometrium
    D. myometrium

33. The basic structure of DNA is:
    A. a single helix
    B. a double helix
    C. a triple helix
    D. a quad helix

34. RNA is dissimilar to DNA in all of the following ways, EXCEPT one. Which of the following is the exception?
    A. is single-stranded
    B. contains uridine monophosphate
    C. assists in protein translation
    D. is involved in transcription

35. The process of breaking large, complex molecules into smaller, simpler units is called:
    A. anabolism
    B. catabolism
    C. electron transport
    D. oxidative phosphorylation

36. Products of aerobic metabolism include all of the following, EXCEPT:
    A. H_2O
    B. heat
    C. lactic acid
    D. ATP
    E. CO_2

37. According to Fick's law of diffusion, the greatest net movement of a substance across a membrane will occur if:
    A. the concentration gradient is small
    B. the thickness of the membrane is great
    C. the temperature is low
    D. the available surface area is large
    E. the membrane permeability for a substance is low

38. Osmosis:
    A. is associated with movement of H_2O across a membrane
    B. is unrelated to membrane permeability
    C. is associated primarily with movement of solutes across a membrane
    D. is unrelated to the concentration gradient

39. Carrier-mediated transport is characterized by all of the following, EXCEPT:
    A. movement of substances across a membrane
    B. specificity
    C. saturation or transport maximum
    D. competition
    E. requirement of energy (ATP)

40. In a neuron, an action potential:
    A. is a local event
    B. is small in amplitude
    C. travels down an axon toward the synapse
    D. is caused by an influx of negative ions

41. Which of the following four types of nerve fibers has the fastest conduction velocity?
    A. an unmyelinated small fiber
    B. an unmyelinated large fiber
    C. a myelinated small fiber
    D. a myelinated large fiber

42. During the absolute refractory period:
    A. additional stimulation produces a small action potential
    B. summation of inhibitory post-synaptic potentials will elicit another action potential
    C. no action potential can be produced, no matter how strong the stimulus
    D. the action potential that is produced moves toward the dendrites

43. The autonomic nervous system:
    A. is not part of the peripheral nervous system
    B. innervates only smooth and cardiac muscles
    C. comprises the sympathetic and parasympathetic nervous systems
    D. innervates skeletal muscles
    E. uses the neurotransmitter glutamate

44. All of the following are true of skeletal muscles, EXCEPT:
    A. they contain actin and myosin microfilaments
    B. they require external Ca^{+2} for contraction
    C. they use acetylcholine as the neurotransmitter
    D. they contain an extensive sarcoplasmic reticulum
    E. they need energy for both contraction and relaxation

45. Cardiac muscles:
    A. need no external Ca^{+2} for contraction
    B. have action potentials that last more than 200 msec
    C. contain few mitochondria
    D. contract in response to acetylcholine
    E. exhibit summation

46. Hormones can be divided into the following three classes of chemicals:
    A. amines, peptides, and steroids
    B. free fatty acids, peptides, and amines
    C. steroids, free fatty acids, and phospholipids
    D. amines, phospholipids, and steroids

47. Parathyroid hormone:
    A. decreases Ca^{+2} plasma levels in response to hypocalcemia
    B. acts on the kidney to conserve Ca^{+2}
    C. acts with Vitamin D to decrease intestinal absorption of Ca^{+2}
    D. affects only phosphate metabolism in muscle

48. The pancreas:
    A. is only an endocrine gland
    B. produces glucagon, which decreases glucose levels
    C. produces insulin, which promotes cellular uptake of plasma glucose
    D. secretes hormones that breakdown carbohydrates and proteins

49. Aldosterone:
    A. is produced in the adrenal medulla
    B. is stimulated by increased Na^+ plasma levels
    C. is involved in regulation of blood volume by means of its effects on the kidneys
    D. is stimulated by a rise in blood pressure or a fall in K^+ plasma levels
    E. is stimulated by high estrogen levels only

50. Glucocorticoids such as cortisol have all of the following characteristics, EXCEPT:
    A. promote muscle breakdown
    B. promote gluconeogenesis
    C. are involved in stress responses
    D. stimulate the immune system
    E. are regulated by ACTH

51. Testosterone:
    A. is produced by Leydig cells in testes through stimulation of follicle stimulating hormone (FSH)
    B. stimulates production of sperm in Sertoli cells
    C. decreases red blood cell production
    D. decreases protein production in muscles

52. Estrogen:
    A. induces production of testosterone receptors in the uterus
    B. is essential for follicular maturation
    C. promotes oxygen production
    D. decreases bone density

53. Hormones involved in fluid volume regulation include all the following, EXCEPT:
    A. angiotensin II
    B. aldosterone
    C. antidiuretic hormone
    D. inhibin
    E. atrial natriuretic peptide

54. Gas exchange across the lung:
    A. depends on alveoli that are ventilated and perfused by blood
    B. is similar for oxygen and carbon dioxide
    C. occurs in the bronchi
    D. depends on a large pressure gradient for CO_2
    E. occurs primarily in the pulmonary artery

55. The pleural "space":
    A. normally contains a large amount of fluid
    B. contains positive (above atmospheric) pressure
    C. helps "attach" the chest wall and lung for ventilation
    D. produces surfactant

56. Ventilation:
    A. is determined by the product of tidal volume and frequency of breathing
    B. is little influenced by the body's O_2 demands
    C. is stimulated by high levels of CO_2
    D. is stimulated by anoxia

57. Most CO_2 that is transported in blood is:
    A. in the form of bicarbonate ions
    B. dissolved
    C. bound to plasma proteins
    D. bound to hemoglobin
    E. in the form of H_2CO_3

58. Decreased access to O_2 by cells of the body can occur in all of the following conditions, EXCEPT:
    A. inhalation of carbon monoxide
    B. decreased hemoglobin levels
    C. high altitude
    D. increased blood flow to the cells
    E. cyanide poisoning

59. Alveolar hyperventilation:
    A. decreases O_2 levels in blood
    B. increases CO_2 levels in blood
    C. decreases the pH of blood
    D. decreases H^+ in blood

60. Substances produced by the stomach include all of the following, EXCEPT:
    A. mucus
    B. hydrochloric acid (HCl)
    C. intrinsic factor
    D. Vitamin B_{12}
    E. pepsinogen

61. Functions of the liver include:
    A. detoxification of wastes
    B. production of red blood cells in adults
    C. synthesis of steroid hormones
    D. production of vitamin A
    E. synthesis of fats

62. The layer of the intestine that contains both longitudinal and circular muscle layers is the:
    A. lamina propria
    B. muscularis mucosa
    C. serosa
    D. muscularis externa

63. Functions of the small intestine include all of the following, EXCEPT:
    A. absorption of digested food stuffs
    B. production of fluids and electrolytes
    C. production of enzymes that are released into the intestine
    D. movement of chyme through the intestine
    E. absorption of Vitamin B_{12} and bile salts

64. The large intestine:
    A. absorbs food
    B. produces water and electrolytes

C. produces mucus for protection and lubrication
D. absorbs hormones
E. produces intrinsic factor

65. Major functions of the kidneys include all of the following, EXCEPT:
   A. production of erythropoietin
   B. production of renin
   C. production of angiotensin II
   D. regulation of blood volume
   E. acid-base regulation

66. A blockage of the ureter may:
   A. increase pressure within the kidney
   B. increase urine excretion
   C. increase the size of nephrons
   D. cause prostatic hypertrophy

67. Components of a nephron include all of the following, EXCEPT:
   A. the glomerulus
   B. juxtaglomerular apparatus
   C. Bowman's capsule
   D. urethra
   E. Loop of Henle

68. The glomerular filtration rate (GFR):
   A. is increased by an increase of blood pressure
   B. is decreased by constriction of the efferent arteriole
   C. is decreased by increasing the leakiness of the Bowman's capsule
   D. is increased by constriction of the afferent arteriole

69. In respiratory acidosis:
   A. kidneys play no role
   B. kidneys compensate by producing chloride
   C. kidneys compensate by reabsorbing HCO_3^-
   D. kidneys compensate by reabsorbing H^+

70. Cardiac output is:
   A. increased by an increase in contractility of the heart
   B. increased when the heart rate decreases
   C. decreased by an increase in venous return
   D. decreased by an increase in stroke volume

71. Total peripheral resistance:
   A. increases as the diameter of blood vessels decrease
   B. is decreased by angiotensin II
   C. is independent of blood viscosity
   D. increases by increased production of metabolites
   E. decreases with dehydration

72. Blood pressure or volume is sensed by receptors in all of these locations, EXCEPT:
   A. the right atrium
   B. the carotid sinus
   C. the carotid body
   D. the aortic sinus

73. A decrease in blood pressure results in:
   A. the release of acetylcholine
   B. increased sympathetic nervous system discharge
   C. decreased heart rate
   D. decreased cardiac output

74. Hypertension:
   A. decreases the work of the heart
   B. contributes to the formation of atherosclerotic plaques
   C. affects only the pulmonary circulation
   D. is age independent
   E. is lower in obese people

75. Hypotension may occur in all the following situations, EXCEPT:
   A. when heart failure occurs
   B. when there is a rapid release of epinephrine
   C. when blood is lost
   D. when septic shock occurs
   E. when sympathetic nervous system-blocking drugs are taken

76. Functions of the plasma membrane include all of the following, EXCEPT:
   A. selectively allows movement of substances into the cell interior
   B. contains receptors that allow communication between cells
   C. synthesizes proteins
   D. is involved in cell division
   E. forms vesicles for endocytosis

77. Organelles that produce ATP are:
   A. mitochondria
   B. Golgi apparatus
   C. peroxisomes
   D. lysosomes
   E. vesicles

78. An influx of chloride ions (Cl^-) into a neuron results in:
   A. depolarization
   B. hyperpolarization
   C. an excitatory post synaptic potential
   D. repolarization

79. The effectiveness of synaptic transmission is decreased during all the following, EXCEPT:
   A. hypoxia
   B. administration of tetanus toxin
   C. blocking of a post-synaptic receptor
   D. decrease in neurotransmitter release during moderate exercise

---

REVIEW QUESTION RATIONALES

1. **B** Both cilia and flagella are involved in movement. Flagella move the cell and cilia move substances across the cell surface. Ciliary action moves the mucus with trapped particles upward for subsequent removal from the body. Ribosomes are involved in protein synthesis and centrioles function in cell division.

2. **D** Diffusion and absorption do not occur across the tissue that lines the oral cavity. Mucus in the oral

cavity is a component of the saliva produced by the salivary glands. The lining of the oral cavity is subject to abrasion by food during mastication, therefore the lining consists of many layers of cells—primarily stratified squamous epithelium—to provide protection from the abrasive action.

3. **D** The four main categories of tissue are epithelial, connective, muscle, and nervous. Blood, bone, and cartilage, along with areolar tissue, adipose, tendons, and ligaments, are examples of connective tissue.

4. **A** Serous membranes line body cavities that do not open to the outside and consist of parietal and visceral layers. The cutaneous membrane is the skin. Mucous membranes line body cavities that open to the exterior, such as the respiratory and digestive tracts.

5. **D** Stratum basale is the actively mitotic layer that produces new cells. The other layers consist of dead or dying cells and have no mitotic ability, with the exception of stratum spinosum, which has limited mitotic ability.

6. **D** The radius is a bone of the appendicular skeleton and is located on the lateral side of the forearm. The humerus is the bone in the brachium or arm.

7. **A** Diarthrotic joints are freely movable joints whose range of motion is limited by adjacent muscles, bones, and ligaments. They have a fibrous joint capsule lined with a synovial membrane that secretes synovial fluid into the joint cavity for lubrication. Immovable joints are synarthroses. Intervertebral disks are located between the vertebral bodies to form slightly movable joints, or amphiarthroses.

8. **B** The adductor longus, biceps femoris, and gastrocnemius are associated with the lower extremity. The adductor longus adducts the thigh at the hip joint; the biceps femoris is one of the hamstrings on the posterior side of the thigh and flexes the knee; the gastrocnemius is located on the posterior leg and plantar flexes the foot. The sternocleidomastoid is a neck muscle.

9. **A** The central nervous system includes the brain and spinal cord; the cerebrum and cerebellum are parts of the brain. The peripheral nervous system comprises 12 pairs of cranial nerves and 31 pairs of spinal nerves.

10. **C** The pons in the brainstem contains the apneustic and pneumotaxic centers, which regulate rate and depth of breathing. Heart rate and blood pressure are established by vital centers in the medulla oblongata. The auditory cortex is in the temporal lobe, and the visual cortex is in the occipital lobe; both are in the cerebrum. The cerebellum is a motor area that coordinates skeletal muscle activity and is important in maintaining muscle tone, posture, and equilibrium.

11. **C** The afferent division of the peripheral nervous system carries sensory impulses to the central nervous system and the efferent division carries motor impulses from the central nervous system to the muscles and glands (effectors). Some, but not all, cranial nerves are sensory; some are motor, and others have both sensory and motor components. All spinal nerves have both sensory and motor components.

12. **C** The autonomic nervous system is the visceral efferent portion of the peripheral nervous system. It comprises sympathetic and parasympathetic divisions and its effectors are cardiac muscle, smooth muscle, and glands.

13. **B** General senses are widely distributed in the body. Proprioception is a general sense of position or orientation and is detected by Golgi tendon organs and muscle spindles. Meissner's and Pacinian corpuscles are receptors that detect the general senses of touch and pressure. Taste and smell are special senses that are localized and closely related.

14. **A** The rods and cones are visual receptors (photoreceptors) located in the retina, which is the innermost layer of the eye. The cornea is the clear portion of the outer fibrous layer. The ciliary body changes the shape of the lens to focus light rays on the visual receptors of the retina.

15. **D** The middle ear contains the malleus, incus, and stapes, the three ossicles that transmit sound waves to the inner ear. The receptors for hearing are located in the organ of Corti, which is a part of the cochlea of the inner ear. The receptors for equilibrium are located in the vestibule and semicircular canals of the inner ear.

16. **D** Aldosterone is a steroid hormone that helps regulate fluid and electrolyte balance and is produced by the adrenal cortex. Steroids are derivatives of cholesterol and react with receptors inside the cell. Protein hormones react with receptors on the cell membrane.

17. **D** Monocytes are a type of leukocytes that do not contain hemoglobin. Thrombocytes, or platelets, are fragments of cells and function in blood clotting. Erythrocytes are red blood cells, which contain hemoglobin and transport oxygen.

18. **B** Blood types are determined by the agglutinogens on the surface of the RBC. Type-A blood has A agglutinogens and anti-B agglutinins. In transfusion reactions, the recipient's agglutinins react with the agglutinogens of the donor. The anti-B agglutinins of the type-A blood (recipient) will react with the type-B agglutinogens found in type-B and type-AB blood; therefore individuals with these two blood types cannot be used as donors. Type O blood, which has no agglutinogens on the RBC surface, may be used.

19. **B** Under normal conditions, no anti-Rh agglutinins are present in either Rh+ or Rh– blood. An Rh– person who comes into contact with Rh+ blood, however, develops these agglutinins. If such a woman becomes pregnant with an Rh+ fetus, some of her anti-Rh

agglutinins may cross the placenta and react with the Rh+ agglutinogens of the fetus. This reaction may cause a breakdown of the fetal RBCs, resulting in hemolytic disease of the newborn, formerly called erythroblastosis fetalis.

20. **A** The descending aorta and left atrium contain blood that has been freshly oxygenated in the lungs. Venous blood, such as that in the hepatic portal vein, has a lower oxygen content. The hepatic portal vein receives blood from the digestive system and has a higher nutrient (glucose) content than other vessels.

21. **B** The right lymphatic duct collects lymph from the upper right quadrant of the body and subsequently drains into the right subclavian vein. Lymph from the remaining three quarters of the body, including the inguinal lymph nodes, enters the thoracic duct, which carries it to the left subclavian vein.

22. **C** The pharynx, trachea, and bronchi are conducting passages for air. The diffusion of gases, oxygen, and carbon dioxide occurs across the simple squamous epithelial walls of the alveoli.

23. **D** The right lung is shorter, wider, and has a greater volume than the left lung. Both lungs are covered by the pleura, a serous membrane. The left lung is divided into two lobes and has an indentation for the apex of the heart. The right lung is divided into three lobes by oblique and horizontal fissures.

24. **A** From the outside inward, the layers of the stomach wall include the serous membrane, muscularis externa (smooth muscle), submucosa (connective tissue with blood vessels and nerves), and the innermost mucosa (simple columnar epithelium).

25. **D** Amylase is an enzyme that hydrolyzes starches into disaccharides. It is produced by the salivary glands and by the pancreas, but not by the stomach. Hydrochloric acid, gastrin, and pepsinogen are all produced by the stomach mucosa.

26. **C** The proximal portion of the small intestine is the short duodenum. This is followed by the jejunum, and then the distal portion, which is the ileum that empties into the large intestine.

27. **C** Cholecystokinin (pancreozymin) stimulates the contraction of the gallbladder and the production of pancreatic enzymes. Gastrin is a hormone that increases stomach activity. Secretin is a hormone produced by the small intestine that stimulates the pancreas to secrete a fluid that is rich in bicarbonate ions. The alkalinity of the bicarbonate ions neutralizes the acid chyme from the stomach so that the pancreatic enzymes can function.

28. **A** Oxygenated blood is transported to the liver by the hepatic artery. The hepatic portal vein delivers nutrient rich blood from the digestive tract to the liver. Venous blood is drained from the liver by the hepatic vein.

29. **C** Urine is produced in the kidney and as it is produced, it flows into the ureter, which transports the urine to the urinary bladder for storage. During micturition, urine flows from the urinary bladder through the urethra to the exterior.

30. **D** Spermatozoa are formed in the seminiferous tubules of the testes and undergo a maturation process in the epididymis. From there, they enter the ductus deferens, and subsequently the ejaculatory duct, which empties into the prostatic urethra.

31. **B** Secretions of the prostate gland contribute approximately 40% of the volume of seminal fluid; the remaining 60% is contributed by the seminal vesicles. Sperm, although numerous, contribute very little to the volume, and there are no glandular cells in the penis that contribute to the seminal fluid.

32. **C** The perimetrium is the outer serous layer of the wall and the myometrium is the middle, thick layer of smooth muscle. The inner layer or lining is the endometrium, which is divided into two layers. The stratum basale is the deeper layer that provides replacement cells for those that are sloughed off from the stratum functionale during menstruation.

33. **B** The basic structure of DNA is a double helix with two strands of DNA running antiparallel to one another. RNA is a single-stranded molecule.

34. **D** Both RNA and DNA are involved in transcription, the process of transferring genetic information from DNA to mRNa. RNA is dissimilar to DNA in that it is single-stranded, contains uridine monophosphate, and is involved in translation of protein.

35. **B** The process of breaking large complex molecules into smaller, simpler units is called catabolism. Anabolism is a process of building large complex molecules from smaller molecules. Electron transport and oxidative phosphorylation is the pathway by which electrons are donated from NADH and $FADH_2$ to a series of proteins, which results in the production of ATP.

36. **C** Lactic acid is a product of aerobic metabolism.

37. **D** "The available surface area is large" is the correct answer. If the concentration gradient were great, the thickness of the membrane were small, the temperature were increased, and the permeability were high, such conditions would facilitate diffusion.

38. **A** Osmosis is associated with H_2O movement across a membrane. The other answers are false. Membrane permeability may affect solute movement, which in turn drags water with it, affecting osmosis.

39. **E** Facilitated diffusion does not require ATP.

40. **C** Action potentials travel down an axon toward the synapse. Action potentials relative to graded potentials are large in amplitude, travel, do not decrement, and are caused by a relatively large flux of positive ions such as Na^+ or Ca^{+2}.

41. **D** A myelinated fiber is large and is insulated by myelin, which allows for saltatory conduction. This fiber's type and size both result in an increased conduction velocity.

42. **C** The absolute refractory period does not allow the production of additional action potentials, which

helps control the number and direction of action potentials.

43. **C** The autonomic nervous system is part of the peripheral nervous system and innervates not only smooth and cardiac muscles, but also glands. It's major neurotransmitters include acetylcholine (parasympathetic) and norepinephrine (sympathetic).

44. **B** No external Ca^{+2} is needed for contraction. All Ca^+ release is regulated by the sarcoplasmic reticulum.

45. **B** Unlike skeletal muscles, which have contraction times of 60 msec, cardiac muscles have contraction times of 200 msec. This length of time ensures that this muscle will not exhibit summation. Cardiac muscles contain a large number of mitochondria and contract in response to norepinephrine but not acetylcholine.

46. **A** The three chemical classes of hormones are amines, peptides, and steroids. (See endocrine section for examples of each.)

47. **B** Parathyroid hormones decrease Ca^{+2} plasma levels in response to hypercalcemia. Parathyroid hormone acts with vitamin D to promote intestinal absorption of Ca^{+2}. It also may influence phosphate handling, but not metabolism, by the kidneys.

48. **C** The pancreas is both an endocrine and an exocrine gland. It produces glucagon, which elevates plasma glucose levels. Its exocrine function results in the secretion of enzymes (not hormones) that break down carbohydrates and proteins.

49. **C** Aldosterone is produced by the adrenal cortex and its secretion is stimulated by low plasma levels of Na^+ and high levels of K^+. Low blood pressure through the renin-angiotensin system also stimulates its production.

50. **D** Glucocorticoids suppress the immune system.

51. **B** Testosterone production is stimulated by luteinizing hormone, stimulates protein production, and increases red blood cell production, resulting in higher hematocrits in men compared with those in women.

52. **B** Estrogen induces the production of progesterone receptors in the uterus, acts as an antioxidant, and increases bone density.

53. **D** Inhibin inhibits production of follicle stimulating hormone.

54. **A** Alveoli perfusion by blood is a major factor associated with normal gas exchange. Because of the differences in solubilities for CO_2 and O_2 (greater for CO_2 than O_2), gas exchange for oxygen is more limited than CO_2 movement. Thus the gradient for O_2 is 60 mm Hg and the gradient for CO_2 is 5 mm Hg. No gas exchange occurs in the bronchi or pulmonary artery.

55. **C** The pleural "space" normally contains only a small amount of fluid. The pressure within the pleural "space" is negative (below atmospheric) because of opposing forces of the lung and chest wall and fluid movements out of the "space." Surfactant is produced by type-II cells in the lungs.

56. **A** Metabolism generally is coupled with ventilation; thus as O_2 demands increase, ventilation increases. Ventilation is depressed by high levels of CO_2 and by anoxia.

57. **A** Bicarbonate ions comprise approximately 72% of the CO_2 that is transported.

58. **D** Increased blood flow to the cells is the only listed condition that would increase O_2 transport or access. Inhalation of carbon monoxide would decrease the amount of O_2 bound to hemoglobin; decreased hemoglobin levels would decrease the amount of hemoglobin available; high altitudes would decrease the alveolar and arterial PO_2; and cyanide poisons enzymes that use O_2 to make ATP.

59. **D** Hyperventilation results in the "blowing off" of CO_2, which also results in a decrease in H^+ and an increased level of O_2.

60. **D** Intrinsic factor is essential to absorption of vitamin B_{12}. The stomach does not produce vitamin B_{12}.

61. **A** The liver produces red blood cells in the embryo and fetus. It synthesizes factors needed for clotting and amino acids. The liver also stores glycogen, iron, copper, and vitamins A and D. Steroid hormones are synthesized primarily in the gonads and in the adrenal cortex.

62. **D** Muscularis externa contains both longitudinal and circular muscle layers. The other layers contain either connective tissue (serosa) and lamina propria or one layer of muscle (muscularis mucosa).

63. **C** Enzymes that digest chyme in the lumen are produced by the pancreas. The small intestine produces only intracellular enzymes.

64. **C** Neither food nor hormones are absorbed by the large intestine. Its major functions include reabsorption of water and electrolytes and movement of fecal material to the rectum for elimination. Intrinsic factor is produced in the stomach.

65. **C** Angiotensin II is produced by endothelial cells in the lung.

66. **D** Blockage of the ureter increases pressures within the kidney and decreases urine excretion.

67. **D** The urethra is a part of the urinary system but is not part of the nephron. All of the other components are parts of the nephron.

68. **A** Efferent arteriole constriction increases GFR. An increase in the leakiness of the Bowman's capsule also increases GFR. Constriction of the afferent arteriole decreases GFR.

69. **C** During respiratory acidosis, the kidneys retain HCO_3^- and excrete H^+.

70. **A** Cardiac output is increased by an increase in the contractility of the heart. Other factors that ↑ cardiac output are increased heart rate, venous return, and stroke volume.

71. **A** Factors that influence total peripheral resistance include the diameter or radius of blood vessels (where R α 1/4) and viscosity (increased viscosity leads to increased resistance). Thus, as the diameter

of blood vessels decrease, total peripheral resistance increases. The radii of blood vessels are increased by the production of metabolites, cytokines, and histamine. Viscosity is increased during dehydration.

72. **C** This is a chemoreceptor for O_2, CO_2, and pH; all others sense pressure or volume changes.

73. **B** Decreased blood pressure causes increased SNS discharge.

74. **A** Hypertension contributes to formation of atherosclerotic plaques. Hypertension also increases the work of the heart and tends to increase with age and obesity.

75. **B** All of these situations, EXCEPT when epinephrine is released rapidly, result in a decrease in blood pressure.

76. **C** Ribosomes that produce protein are located on the rough endoplasmic reticulum or in the cytoplasm, not the plasma membrane.

77. **A** Mitochondria produce ATP. The other organelles are involved in the metabolic handling of internally produced chemicals (Golgi apparatus) and/or externally produced chemicals (peroxisomes and lysosomes), but do not produce ATP.

78. **B** Cl^- is negatively charged and causes the membrane potential to become more negative or hyperpolarized. Depolarization and an excitatory postsynaptic potential occur when negative charges leave the cell or when positive charges enter it. An influx of either Na^+ or Ca^{+2} results in depolarization.

79. **E** Moderate exercise has no effect on synaptic transmission. During hypoxia, less ATP is produced; thus energy-dependent processes, such as the exocytosis of transmitters, are decreased. Administration of tetanus toxin prevents the release of neurotransmitters and results in uncontrolled spasms. When fewer neurotransmitters are released presynaptically, less binding to postsynaptic receptors occurs.

Chapter THREE

Head, Neck, and Dental Anatomy

Margaret J. Fehrenbach, R.D.H., M.S.

 ## Clinical Case STUDY

A *patient is referred to an oral surgeon by a general dentist. Tooth #16 is circled on the referral form, which indicates that extraction is needed for this tooth. After the procedure, a progress report is sent to the patient's general dentist. The report states that the patient had tooth #16 extracted with the use of local anesthesia. After extraction, the patient presented with a fever and swollen lymph nodes, which indicated that a complicating infection had occurred. It was determined that the patient was in excellent health but had not kept the area clean after extraction. Antibiotics were prescribed. The infection healed and the patient is fine.*

Clinical Case QUESTIONS

1. Which tooth was extracted by the oral surgeon?
2. Which nerves should be anesthetized to extract tooth #16 comfortably?
3. Which primary and secondary lymph nodes might be involved in an infection of tooth #16?
4. From which bone and its process did the extraction of #16 take place?
5. Which blood vessels supply the area of the extraction site?
6. What types of roots might an oral surgeon encounter when extracting tooth #16?

Clinical Case RATIONALES

1. Tooth #16, or the permanent maxillary left third molar (wisdom tooth), was extracted.
2. The posterior superior alveolar nerve (for the tooth, associated periodontium, and overlying buccal gingiva) and the greater palatine nerve (for the overlying lingual gingiva) must be anesthetized to extract tooth #16.

3. The primary lymph nodes that directly drain tooth #16 are the superior deep cervical lymph nodes. These subsequently drain into the secondary nodes, which are the inferior deep cervical lymph nodes.
4. Tooth #16 was extracted from the alveolar process of the maxilla.
5. The posterior superior alveolar artery and vein supply tooth #16 and its area.
6. Roots of #16 may be partially or fully fused, poorly developed, and/or curved distally.

Content Review

Anatomy Terminology

Afferent nerve—Sensory nerve that carries information from the periphery of the body to the brain or spinal cord.

Afferent vessel—Type of lymphatic vessel through which lymph flows into the lymph node.

Anastomosis/anastomoses—Communication of one blood vessel with another by a connecting channel.

Arch—Prominent bridgelike bony structure.

Arteriole—Small artery that branches off a larger artery and connects with a capillary.

Artery—Type of blood vessel that carries blood away from the heart.

Articulation—Area where bones are joined to each other.

Aperture—Opening or orifice in bone.

Canal—Opening in bone that is long, narrow, and tube-like.

Capillary—Smaller blood vessel that branches off an arteriole to supply blood directly to tissue.

Condyle—Oval bony prominence typically found at articulations.

Cornu—Small hornlike prominence.

Crest—Roughened border or ridge on surface of bone.

Duct—Passageway that carries a secretion from an exocrine gland to its destination.

Efferent nerve—Motor nerve that carries information away from the brain or spinal cord to the periphery of the body.

Efferent vessel—Type of lymphatic vessel in the area of a node's hilum through which lymph flows out of the lymph node.

Eminence—Tubercle or rounded elevation on a bony surface.

Endocrine gland—Type of gland without a duct; its secretion flows directly into the blood, which carries the secretion to the appropriate region.

Epicondyle—Small prominence that is located on or above a condyle.

Exocrine gland—Type of gland with an associated duct that empties the secretion directly into the location where the secretion will be used.

Fissure—Opening in bone that is narrow and cleftlike.

Foramen/foramina—Short windowlike opening in bone.

Fossa/fossae—Depression on a bony surface.

Ganglion/ganglia—Accumulation of neuron cell bodies outside the central nervous system.

Head—Rounded surface projecting from a bone by a neck.

Hilum—Depression on one side of the lymph node where lymph flows out by way of an efferent lymphatic vessel.

Insertion—End of a muscle that is attached to the more movable structure.

Joint—Site of a junction or union between two or more bones.

Line—Straight small ridge of bone.

Ligament—Band of fibrous tissue that connects bones.

Lymphatic ducts—Larger lymphatic vessels that drain smaller vessels and subsequently empty into the venous system.

Lymphatic vessels—System of channels that drains tissue fluid from surrounding regions.

Lymph nodes—Organized bean-shaped lymphoid tissue that filters lymph by means of lymphocytes to fight disease.

Notch—Indentation at the edge of a bone.

Origin—End of a muscle that is attached to the least movable structure.

Ostium/ostia—Small opening in a bone.

Plexus—Network of blood vessels (typically veins).

Plate—Flat structure of bone.

Process—General term for any prominence on a bony surface.

Spine—Abrupt small prominence of bone.

Sulcus/sulci—Shallow depression or groove, such as on a bony surface.

Suture—Generally immovable articulation in which bones are joined by fibrous tissue.

Tonsillar tissue—Masses of lymphoid tissue located in the oral cavity and pharynx to protect the body against disease processes.

Tubercle—Eminence or small rounded elevation on a bony surface.

Tuberosity—Large, often rough prominence on the surface of a bone.

Venous sinus—Blood-filled space between two layers of tissue.

Vein—Type of blood vessel that carries blood to the heart.

Venule—Smaller vein that drains the capillaries of a tissue area and subsequently joins larger veins.

Surface Anatomy

Knowledge of surface anatomy is essential for performing patient examinations; it is necessary for locating essential landmarks of many deeper anatomical structures, for taking and reading radiographic films, and for proper documentation of anatomical changes.

Regions of the Head (Fig. 3–1)

Include the frontal, parietal, occipital, temporal, orbital, nasal, infraorbital, zygomatic, buccal, oral, and mental regions.

I.   Frontal Region
  A. Includes the supraorbital ridge under each eyebrow.
  B. Frontal eminence forms the prominence of the forehead.
II. Parietal and Occipital Regions
  A. Are covered by the scalp and may be covered by hair.
III. Temporal Region and External Ear
  A. Comprises an auricle and the external acoustic meatus.
  B. Superior and posterior free margin of the auricle is called the helix, which ends inferiorly at the lobule or earlobe.
  C. The tragus is the part of auricle that is anterior to the external acoustic meatus.
  D. The antitragus is the flap of tissue opposite the tragus.
IV. Orbital Region
  A. Includes the eyeball and supporting structures within the orbit or bony socket.
  B. The sclera is the white area of eyeball.
  C. The iris is the circular central area of color.
  D. The pupil is the central opening in iris.
  E. Has movable upper and lower eyelids that cover and protect each eyeball.
  F. The lacrimal gland is located behind each upper eyelid and within orbit; it produces lacrimal fluid or tears.
  G. The conjunctiva is the membrane that lines the inside of eyelids and the front of eyeball.
  H. The lateral canthus is the outer corner where the upper and lower eyelids meet; the inner corner of the eye is called the medial canthus.
V.   Nasal Region and External Nose
  A. Root of the nose is located between the eyes.

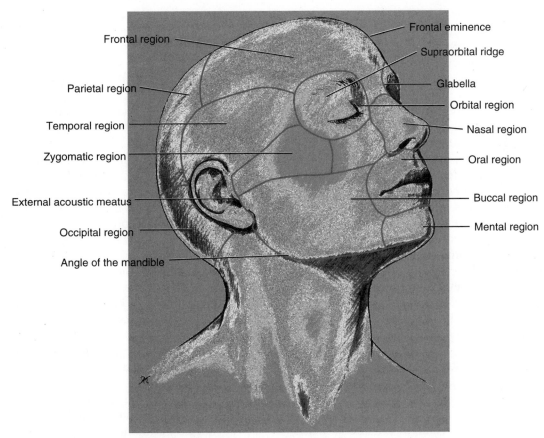

Figure 3.1   Regions of the head.
(From Fehrenbach MJ, Herring SW: Illustrated Anatomy of the Head and Neck. Philadelphia, WB Saunders, 1996, p. 14.)

B. The nasion is a midpoint landmark.
C. The bridge of the nose is inferior to the nasion.
D. The apex of the nose is the tip.
E. The nares or nostrils are separated by the midline nasal septum and bounded laterally by alae.

VI. Infraorbital, Zygomatic, and Buccal Regions
A. Are located on the facial aspect; infraorbital region is inferior to the orbital region and lateral to the nasal region; zygomatic region overlies the cheek bone; buccal region is composed of soft tissues of the cheek.
B. The zygomatic arch extends from just below the lateral margin of the eye to the upper part of the ear.
C. The temporomandibular joint is inferior to the zygomatic arch and just anterior to the ear, where the upper skull forms a joint with the lower jaw.
D. The cheek forms the side of the face between nose, mouth, and ear; is primarily composed of fat and muscles, including the masseter muscle.
E. The angle of the mandible is the sharp angle of the lower jaw that is inferior to the earlobe.

VII. Oral Region
A. Includes lips, oral cavity, palate, tongue, floor of mouth, and parts of the pharynx.
B. Lips are the gateway of the oral region; vermilion zone of lips is darker than surrounding skin; vermilion border that outlines the lips from the surrounding skin is a transition zone.
C. The philtrum is a vertical groove on the midline of the upper lip, extending downward from the nasal septum.
D. The tubercle of the upper lip is the thicker area, where the philtrum terminates.
E. The labial commissure is where the upper and lower lips meet at each corner of mouth.
F. The nasolabial sulcus is the groove running upward between the labial commissure and ala of the nose.
G. The labiomental groove is a horizontal groove to which the lower lip extends and that separates the lower lip from the chin in the mental region.

VIII. Mental Region
A. The chin's mental protuberance or prominence is the region's major feature.
B. Has a midline depression or dimple that marks underlying bony fusion of the lower jaw.

Oral Cavity

The oral cavity is the inside of the mouth and includes the jaws, palate, tongue, floor of the mouth, pharynx, and all associated mucosal tissues.

I. Structures typically are labeled according to their location.
   A. Lingual, if closest to tongue.
   B. Palatal, if closest to palate.
   C. Buccal is closest to inner cheek.
   D. Facial, if closest to facial surface.
   E. Labial, if closest to lips.
II. Mucous Membranes or mucosa line the inner oral cavity. Parts of the lips are lined by labial mucosa; buccal mucosa lines the inner cheek and covers the buccal fat pad, including its parotid papilla, which contains a duct opening from the parotid salivary gland.
III. The Maxillary and Mandibular Vestibules are the upper and lower spaces between the cheeks, lips, and gums. Alveolar mucosa lines each vestibule and meets labial or buccal mucosa at the mucobuccal fold.
IV. The Labial Frenum is the fold of tissue located at the midline between the labial mucosa and alveolar mucosa of the maxilla and mandible.
V. Maxillary and Mandibular Jaws lie beneath the respective lips and contain permanent teeth, including incisors, canines, premolars, and molars.
VI. Gingiva surrounds the maxillary and mandibular teeth.
   A. Attached gingiva tightly adheres to bone around the roots of teeth and may have areas of pigmentation.
   B. The mucogingival junction is a scalloped line of demarcation between attached gingiva and alveolar mucosa.
   C. Marginal gingiva is the nonattached tissue at the gingival margin of each tooth; its inner surface faces a sulcus.
   D. Interdental gingiva is the tissue between the teeth and is an extension of attached gingiva.
VII. Palate
   A. The anterior part is the hard palate and includes the midline ridge, median palatine raphe, and incisive papilla; the palatine rugae, which are irregular ridges of tissue, lie directly posterior to the incisive papilla.
   B. The posterior part is the soft palate and includes the uvula.
   C. The pterygomandibular fold extends from the junction of the hard and soft palates down to mandible, just behind the most distal mandibular tooth, and separates the cheek from the pharynx.
   D. The retromolar pad is located just distal to the last tooth of the mandible.
VIII. Tongue (Fig. 3–2)
   A. The base of the tongue is the posterior one third, which attaches to the floor of the mouth and does not lie within the oral cavity; is located in the oral part of the pharynx.
   B. The body is the anterior two-thirds of the tongue and includes the tip or apex.
   C. Some surfaces have lingual papillae or elevated structures of specialized mucosa, some of which are associated with taste buds.

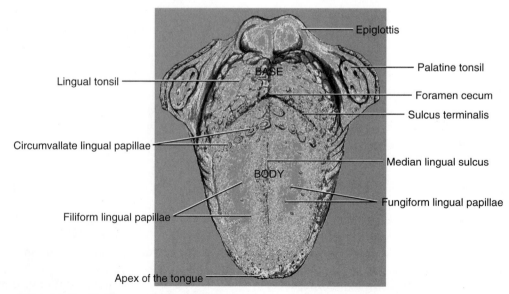

Figure 3.2 Tongue and tonsillar tissues.
(From Fehrenbach MJ, Herring SW: Illustrated Anatomy of the Head and Neck. Philadelphia, WB Saunders, 1996, p. 23.)

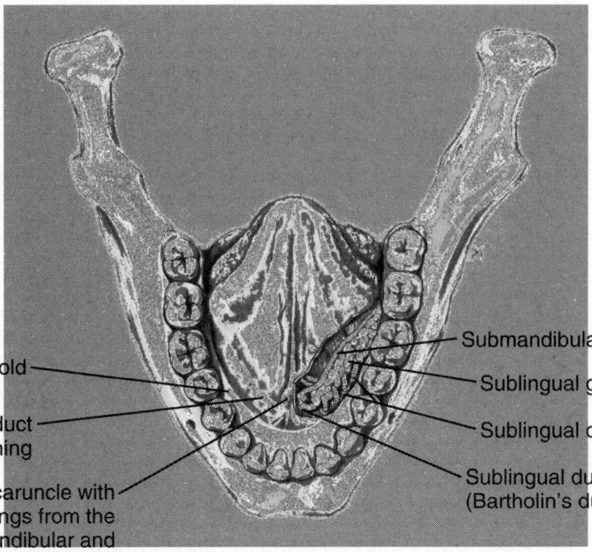

Figure 3.3 Floor of the mouth.
(From Fehrenbach MJ, Herring SW: Illustrated Anatomy of the Head and Neck. Philadelphia, WB Saunders, 1996, p. 150.)

D. The lateral surfaces are located on each side of the tongue.

E. The dorsal surface is located on the top of the tongue; includes the midline depression and median lingual sulcus.

F. The sulcus terminalis is a V-shaped groove located posteriorly on the dorsal surface; separates base from body; has a pit-like depression called the foramen cecum.

G. The lingual tonsil is an irregular mass of tonsillar tissue located more posteriorly than sulcus terminalis on the dorsal surface.

H. The ventral surface of the tongue or underside is noted for its visible deep lingual veins and plica fimbriatae, which have fringe-like projections.

IX. Floor of the Mouth (Fig. 3–3)

A. Is located inferior to ventral surface of tongue.

B. The lingual frenum is a midline fold of tissue between the ventral surface of tongue and floor of mouth.

C. The sublingual fold is a V-shaped ridge of tissue on floor of mouth; contains duct openings from sublingual salivary gland.

D. The sublingual caruncle is a small papilla at the anterior end of each sublingual fold; contains duct openings from both submandibular and sublingual salivary glands.

X. Pharynx

A. Is a muscular tube that serves both respiratory and digestive systems.

B. Is divided into the nasopharynx, oropharynx, and laryngopharynx.

1. The nasopharynx is superior to the level of the soft palate and is continuous with nasal cavity.

2. The oropharynx is located between the soft palate and the larynx opening.

3. The laryngopharynx is inferior to the orophar-

ynx, close to the laryngeal opening, and not visible on intraoral examination.

C. The fauces is the opening from the oral region into the oropharynx and is formed laterally by anterior and posterior tonsillar pillars, which are created by the underlying muscles.

D. Palatine tonsils are located between the pillars.

Regions of the Neck (Fig. 3–4)

The neck regions extend from the skull and mandible down to the clavicles and sternum. They can be divided into different cervical triangles based on large bones and muscles and include the sternocleidomastoid muscle, the thyroid cartilage, and the hyoid bone.

I. The sternocleidomastoid muscle divides each side of the neck diagonally into anterior cervical and posterior cervical triangles.

A. The anterior region of the neck corresponds to the two anterior cervical triangles, which are separated by a midline. The anterior cervical triangle can be subdivided into a submandibular triangle and a midline submental triangle by the digastric muscle.

B. The posterior cervical triangle on each side is considered the lateral region and is posterior to the sternocleidomastoid muscle.

II. The thyroid cartilage at the anterior midline is the prominence of the larynx; vocal cords or ligaments are attached to the posterior surface of the thyroid cartilage.

III. The hyoid bone in the anterior midline is superior to the thyroid cartilage, is attached to many muscles, and controls the position of the base of tongue.

Skeletal System

The skeletal system serves as a base during palpation of soft tissues and as a marker during location of soft tissue

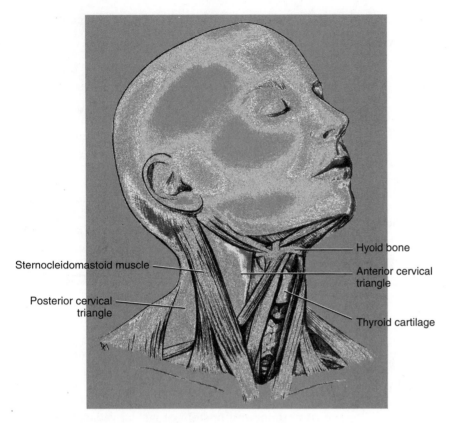

Figure 3.4 Regions of the neck. (From Fehrenbach MJ, Herring SW: Illustrated Anatomy of the Head and Neck. Philadelphia, WB Saunders, 1996, p. 27.)

Sternocleidomastoid muscle

Posterior cervical triangle

Hyoid bone

Anterior cervical triangle

Thyroid cartilage

lesions, administration of local anesthesia, and radiographic procedures. The skeleton may be a factor in the spread of dental infection and may undergo a disease process itself.

Skull Overview

The skull is a series of twenty-two bones, some of which are present in pairs.

I.   Is immovable, with the exception of the mandible and its temporomandibular joint.
II. Has movable articulation with the bony vertebral column in the neck area.
III. Contains bony openings for important nerves and blood vessels (Table 3–1).
IV. Has paranasal sinuses that serve to lighten the bony mass (Fig. 3–5).
V.   Has many associated processes that are involved in important structures.

Views of the Skull

The skull is divided into superior, lateral, inferior, and anterior views.

I.   Superior View of skull has three major sutures.
     A. The coronal suture between the frontal and parietal bones.
     B. The sagittal suture between paired parietal bones.
     C. The lambdoidal suture between the single occipital bone and paired parietal bones.
II. Anterior View of skull includes orbits and nasal cavity (Fig. 3–6).

A. Orbits
   1. Contain and protect the eyeballs.
   2. Orbital walls are composed of orbital plates of the frontal, ethmoid, and lacrimal bones; the orbital surfaces of the maxilla; the zygomatic bone; and the orbital surface of the greater wing of the sphenoid bone.
   3. The orbital apex is composed of the lesser wing of the sphenoid and palatine bones.
   4. The optic canal is the opening in the orbital apex.
   5. The superior orbital fissure is located between the greater and lesser wings of the sphenoid bone and connects the orbit and cranial cavities, carrying the oculomotor, trochlear, abducens, and ophthalmic nerves and veins.
   6. The inferior orbital fissure is between the greater wing of the sphenoid bone and the maxilla; connects orbit with infratemporal and pterygopalatine fossae; carries infraorbital and zygomatic nerves, branches of maxillary nerve, infraorbital artery, and inferior ophthalmic vein.

B. Nasal cavity
   1. The piriform aperture is the anterior opening.
   2. The lateral boundaries are formed by the maxillae.
   3. The nasal conchae are located on each lateral wall.
      a. The superior nasal concha and middle nasal concha are formed from ethmoid bone.

TABLE 3.1	Bony Openings in the Skull and Their Associated Nerves and Blood Vessels	
Bony Opening	**Location**	**Nerves and Vessels**
Carotid canal	Temporal bone	Internal carotid artery
Cribriform plate with foramina	Ethmoid bone	Olfactory nerves
External acoustic meatus	Temporal bone	(Opening to tympanic cavity)
Foramen lacerum	Sphenoid, occipital, and temporal bones	(Cartilage)
Foramen magnum	Occipital bone	Spinal cord, vertebral arteries, and eleventh cranial nerve
Foramen ovale	Sphenoid bone	Mandibular division of the fifth cranial nerve
Foramen rotundum	Sphenoid bone	Fifth cranial nerve
Foramen spinosum	Sphenoid bone	Middle meningeal artery
Greater palatine foramen	Palatine bone	Greater palatine nerve and vessels
Hypoglossal canal	Occipital bone	Twelfth cranial nerve
Incisive foramen	Maxilla	Nasopalatine nerve and branches of the sphenopalatine artery
Inferior orbital fissure	Sphenoid bone and maxilla	Infraorbital and zygomatic nerves, infraorbital artery, and ophthalmic vein
Infraorbital foramen and canal	Maxilla	Infraorbital nerve and vessels
Internal acoustic meatus	Temporal bone	Seventh and eighth cranial nerves
Jugular foramen	Occipital and temporal bones	Internal jugular vein and ninth, tenth, and eleventh cranial nerves
Lesser palatine foramen	Palatine bone	Lesser palatine nerve and vessels
Mandibular foramen	Mandible	Inferior alveolar nerve and vessels
Mental foramen	Mandible	Mental nerve and vessels
Optic canal and foramen	Sphenoid bone	Optic nerve and ophthalmic artery
Petrotympanic fissure	Temporal bone	Chorda tympani nerve
Pterygoid canal	Sphenoid bone	Area nerves and vessels
Stylomastoid foramen	Temporal bone	Seventh cranial nerve
Superior orbital fissure	Sphenoid bone	Third, fourth, and sixth cranial nerves and ophthalmic nerve and vein

From Fehrenbach MJ, Herring SW: Illustrated Anatomy of the Head and Neck. Philadelphia, WB Saunders, 1996, p. 36.

    b. The inferior nasal concha is a separate facial bone.
 4. The nasal meatus are grooves beneath each concha that have openings through which the paranasal sinuses and the nasolacrimal duct communicates with the nasal cavity.

 5. Nasal septum
    a. Divides nasal cavity into two parts.
    b. Is formed by both nasal septal cartilages, a perpendicular plate of ethmoid bone, and the vomer.
III. Lateral View of skull (Fig. 3–5)

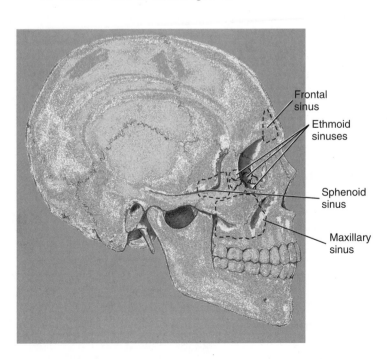

Frontal sinus

Ethmoid sinuses

Sphenoid sinus

Maxillary sinus

Figure 3.5   Lateral view of the skull. (From Fehrenbach MJ, Herring SW: Illustrated Anatomy of the Head and Neck. Philadelphia, WB Saunders, 1996, p. 77.)

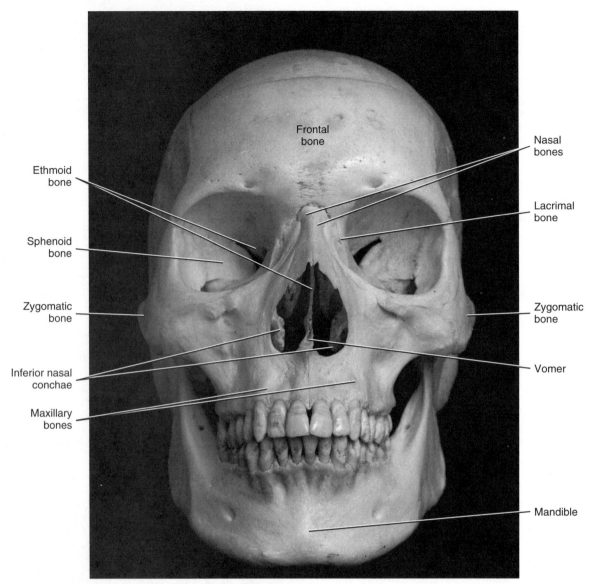

Figure 3.6 Anterior view of the skull.
(From Fehrenbach MJ, Herring SW: Illustrated Anatomy of the Head and Neck.
Philadelphia, WB Saunders, 1996, p. 40.)

A. The superior temporal line is the superior ridge.

B. The inferior temporal line is the superior boundary of the temporal fossa.

C. Has a squamosal suture between the temporal and parietal bones.

D. The temporal fossa is formed by several bones of the skull and contains the body of the temporalis muscle.

E. The infratemporal fossa is inferior to the temporal fossa.

F. The pterygopalatine fossa is deep to the infratemporal fossa.

G. The zygomatic arch is formed by a union of the temporal process of the zygomatic bone and zygomatic process of the temporal bone.

H. The temporomandibular joint is a movable articulation between the temporal bone and the mandible.

IV. Inferior View of the external surface of skull (Fig. 3–7)

A. The hard palate at the anterior section forms the floor of the nasal cavity and roof of the mouth (Fig. 3–8).

1. Is bordered by the alveolar process of the maxilla and its maxillary teeth.

2. Is formed by the palatine processes of the maxilla and horizontal plates of the palatine bones.

3. The median palatine suture is a midline articulation between the palatine processes of the maxillae anteriorly, as well as the horizontal plates of the palatine bones posteriorly.

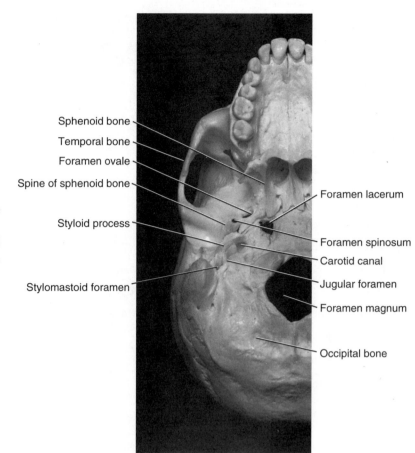

Figure 3.7   Inferior view of the external surface of the skull.
(From Fehrenbach MJ, Herring SW: Illustrated Anatomy of the Head and Neck. Philadelphia, WB Saunders, 1996, p. 51.)

4. The transverse palatine suture articulates the palatine processes of the maxillae and the horizontal plates of the palatine bones.
B. The jugular foramen is the opening through which the internal jugular vein and glossopharyngeal, vagus, and accessory nerves pass.
C. The foramen lacerum is large, irregularly shaped, and filled with cartilage.
V. Superior View of the internal surface of skull (Fig. 3–9)

Bones of the Skull

The skull bones are divided into three categories: cranial, facial, and hyoid.

I. Cranial Bones form the cranium and comprise the occipital, frontal, parietal, temporal, sphenoid, and ethmoid bones.
   A. Occipital bone
      1. Is a single bone located in the most posterior part of the skull.
      2. Articulates with the parietal, temporal, and sphenoid bones.
      3. Is completely formed by the occipital bone.
      4. Has a single foramen magnum on its external surface, which is the largest opening and carries the spinal cord, vertebral arteries, and accessory nerve.

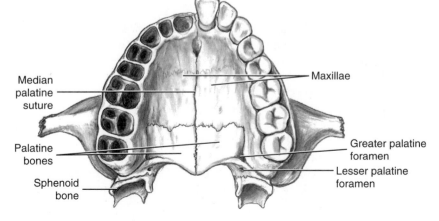

Figure 3.8   Inferior view of the hard palate. (From Fehrenbach MJ, Herring SW: Illustrated Anatomy of the Head and Neck. Philadelphia, WB Saunders, 1996, p. 68.)

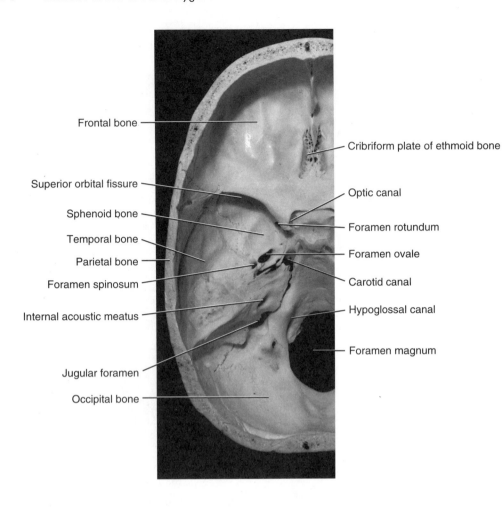

Frontal bone

Superior orbital fissure

Sphenoid bone

Temporal bone

Parietal bone

Foramen spinosum

Internal acoustic meatus

Jugular foramen

Occipital bone

Cribriform plate of ethmoid bone

Optic canal

Foramen rotundum

Foramen ovale

Carotid canal

Hypoglossal canal

Foramen magnum

Figure 3.9 Superior view of the internal surface of the skull. (From Fehrenbach MJ, Herring SW: Illustrated Anatomy of the Head and Neck. Philadelphia, WB Saunders, 1996, p. 52.)

5. Has paired occipital condyles located lateral and anterior to the foramen magnum and has movable articulation with atlas.
6. The basilar part is a four-sided plate.
7. The pharyngeal tubercle is the midline projection anterior to the foramen magnum.
8. Has paired hypoglossal canals that carry the hypoglossal nerve.

B. Frontal bone
1. Is a single bone that forms the forehead and superior part of the orbits.
2. Articulates with the parietal, sphenoid, lacrimal, nasal, ethmoid, and zygomatic bones and maxillae.
3. Contains paired frontal sinuses, superior to the nasal cavity; each sinus communicates with and drains into the nasal cavity by means of the frontonasal duct to the middle nasal meatus (see Fig. 3–5).
4. The supraorbital ridges are elevations over the superior part of the orbit.
5. The supraorbital notch is located on the medial part of the supraorbital ridge.
6. The lacrimal fossa is located just inside the lateral part of the supraorbital ridge and con-

tains a lacrimal gland that produces lacrimal fluid.

C. Parietal bones
1. Are paired bones that articulate with each other at the sagittal suture.
2. Articulate also with the occipital, frontal, temporal, and sphenoid bones.

D. Temporal bones
1. Are paired bones that form the lateral walls of the skull.
2. Articulate with one zygomatic and one parietal bone, the occipital and sphenoid bones, and the mandible.
3. Are composed of squamous, tympanic, and petrous parts.
4. The tympanic part forms most of the external acoustic meatus; the petrous part contains the mastoid process and carotid canal, which carries the internal carotid artery.
5. The mastoid notch is medial to the mastoid process.
6. The styloid process is a bony projection.
7. The stylomastoid foramen carries the facial nerve and is located between the styloid process and the mastoid process.

8. The internal acoustic meatus is on the intracranial surface and carries the vestibulocochlear and facial cranial nerves.

E. Sphenoid bone
   1. Is a single, complex midline bone.
   2. Articulates with the frontal, parietal, ethmoid, temporal, zygomatic, maxillae, palatine, and occipital bones and with the vomer.
   3. The foramen ovale is the oval opening that carries the mandibular division of the trigeminal nerve.
   4. The foramen rotundum is the round opening that carries the maxillary division of the trigeminal nerve.
   5. The foramen spinosum near the spine carries the middle meningeal artery into the cranial cavity.
   6. The body is the middle part; it contains a sphenoid sinus that communicates with and drains into the nasal cavity through an opening superior to each superior nasal concha (see Fig. 3–5).
   7. The lesser wing is anterior and forms the base of the orbital apex.
   8. The greater wing of the sphenoid bone is the posterolateral process with its spine at each corner, divided by the infratemporal crest.
   9. The pterygoid process is inferior and consists of lateral and medial plates, between which is the pterygoid fossa.
   10. The hamulus is the inferior termination of the medial pterygoid plate.

F. Ethmoid bone
   1. Is a single midline bone.
   2. Articulates with the frontal, sphenoid, lacrimal, and maxillary bones and adjoins the vomer.
   3. Has two unpaired plates that cross each other.
   4. Has a perpendicular plate that is midline and vertical.
   5. Has a cribriform plate that is horizontal and perforated by foramina to allow passage of olfactory nerves.
   6. The crista galli is a vertical midline continuation of the perpendicular plate into the cranial cavity.
   7. The ethmoid sinuses in the lateral masses are divided into anterior, middle, and posterior sinuses and open into the superior and middle meatus of the nasal cavity (see Fig. 3–5).
   8. Forms the superior and middle nasal conchae in the nasal cavity.

II. Facial Bones create the facial features and serve as a base for the dentition. They include the vomer, lacrimal, zygomatic, palatine, maxilla, and mandible bones.

A. Vomer
   1. Is a single bone that forms the posterior part of the nasal septum.
   2. Is located in the midsagittal plane, inside the nasal cavity.
   3. Articulates with the ethmoid bone, nasal cartilage, palatine bones and maxillae, and sphenoid bone, and has a free posteroinferior border.

B. Lacrimal bones, nasal bones, and inferior nasal conchae
   1. Paired lacrimal bones form a small part of the anterior medial wall of the orbit and articulate with ethmoid, frontal, and maxilla bones.
   2. The nasolacrimal duct is formed at the junction of the lacrimal and maxillary bones, where lacrimal fluid from the lacrimal gland drains into the inferior nasal meatus.
   3. Paired nasal bones form the bridge of the nose and articulate with each other in the midline above the piriform aperture; also articulate with the frontal bone and maxillae.
   4. Paired inferior nasal conchae project off maxilla to form part of the lateral walls of nasal cavity; articulate with ethmoid, lacrimal, palatine and maxillary bones.

C. Zygomatic bones
   1. Are paired bones that form the cheek bones or malar surfaces.
   2. Articulate with the frontal, temporal, and sphenoid bones and the maxillae.
   3. Are each composed of frontal, temporal, and maxillary processes.
   4. The orbital surface of the frontal process forms the anterior lateral orbital wall.
   5. The temporal process of the zygomatic bone joins the zygomatic process of the temporal bone to form the zygomatic arch.
   6. The orbital surface of the maxillary process forms a part of the lateral orbital wall.

D. Palatine bones
   1. Are paired bones that consist of horizontal and vertical plates.
   2. Articulate with each other and with the maxillae and the sphenoid bone.
   3. Horizontal plates form the posterior part of the hard palate.
   4. Vertical plates form part of the lateral walls of the nasal cavity.
   5. Both plates contribute to the orbital apex.
   6. The posterior part of the median palatine suture is located at the articulation of two horizontal plates.
   7. The greater palatine foramen is located in the posterolateral region of each of the palatine bones, typically distal to the maxillary third

molar; carries greater palatine nerve and blood vessels.

8. The lesser palatine foramen is an opening nearby that carries the lesser palatine nerve and blood vessels to the soft palate and tonsils.

E. Maxilla (Fig. 3–10)

1. Is the upper jaw, which consists of two maxillary bones or maxillae that are fused together.

2. Articulates with the frontal, lacrimal, nasal, inferior nasal conchal, sphenoid, ethmoid, palatine, and zygomatic bones and with the vomer.

3. Each maxilla comprises a body and frontal, zygomatic, palatine, and alveolar processes.

4. The body of the maxilla contains the maxillary sinus, just posterior to the maxillary canine and premolars; this sinus is the largest of the paranasal sinuses; drains into the middle meatus (see Fig. 3–5).

5. The inferior orbital fissure separates each orbital surface from the sphenoid bone, which carries the infraorbital and zygomatic nerves, the infraorbital artery, and the inferior ophthalmic vein (see Fig. 3–6).

6. The infraorbital sulcus is a groove in the floor of the orbital surface, which becomes the infraorbital canal.

7. The infraorbital canal terminates as the infraorbital foramen, which carries the infraorbital nerve and blood vessels.

8. The canine fossa is a depression posterosuperior to the maxillary canine roots; the canine eminence is the facial ridge over the maxillary canine.

9. The anterior part of the median palatine suture is the articulation of two fused maxillae or two palatine processes.

10. The incisive foramen is in the anterior midline part of the palatine process, just posterior to the maxillary central incisors; carries branches of the right and left nasopalatine nerves and blood vessels.

11. The alveolar process typically contains roots of the maxillary teeth.

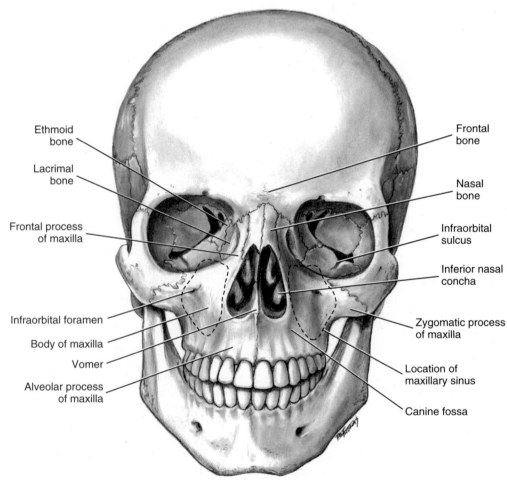

Figure 3.10 Maxilla.
(From Fehrenbach MJ, Herring SW: Illustrated Anatomy of the Head and Neck. Philadelphia, WB Saunders, 1996, p. 69.)

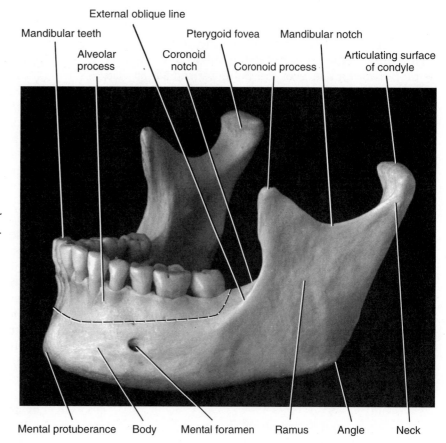

External oblique line
Mandibular teeth
Pterygoid fovea   Mandibular notch
Alveolar process   Coronoid notch   Coronoid process   Articulating surface of condyle

Mental protuberance   Body   Mental foramen   Ramus   Angle   Neck

Figure 3.11 Mandible.
(From Fehrenbach MJ, Herring SW: Illustrated Anatomy of the Head and Neck. Philadelphia, WB Saunders, 1996, p. 73.)

12. The maxillary tuberosity on the posterior part is perforated by the posterior superior alveolar foramina, where the posterior superior alveolar nerve and blood vessel branches enter.

F. Mandible (Fig. 3–11)
1. Is the lower jaw, a single bone that is the only freely movable bone of the skull; articulates with the temporal bones at each temporomandibular joint.
2. The mental protuberance is the prominence of the chin.
3. The mandibular symphysis is the ridge where bone was formed by fusion.
4. The mental foramen is on the lateral surface of the mandible, between the apices of the mandibular premolars; allows entrance of the mental nerve and blood vessels into the mandibular canal.
5. The mandibular foramen is on the internal surface of the ramus, from which the inferior alveolar nerve and blood vessels exit the mandible after traveling in the mandibular canal; overhanging the mandibular foramen is the lingula.
6. The body of the mandible is inferior to the alveolar process.
7. The alveolar process is the part that contains roots of the mandibular teeth.

8. The ramus extends upward and backward from the body on each side and terminates in the coronoid process and its coronoid notch.
9. The external oblique line is a crest where the ramus joins the body.
10. The ramus extends from the angle to the condyle, where it articulates with the temporomandibular joint.
11. The mandibular notch is located between the coronoid process and the condyle.
12. The genial tubercles are at the midline of the medial surface.
13. The retromolar triangle is at the lateral end of each alveolar process.
14. The mylohyoid line extends posteriorly and superiorly on the medial surface.
15. The sublingual fossa contains the sublingual salivary gland; the submandibular fossa contains the submandibular salivary gland.

III. Hyoid Bone
A. Forms the base of the tongue and the larynx; consists of a midline body and two pairs of projections—the greater cornu and lesser cornu.
B. Is suspended in the neck, is mobile, and lacks other bony articulations.
C. Is attached to many muscles.
D. Is superior and anterior to the thyroid cartilage of the larynx.

Muscular System

Knowledge of the location and action of muscles, the relationship of other structures to muscles, and their involvement in the spread of dental infection is essential to proper performance of the patient examination. The muscular system is divided into the cervical muscles, muscles of facial expression, muscles of mastication, hyoid muscles, and muscles of the tongue.

Cervical Muscles

The cervical muscles include the sternocleidomastoid and trapezius muscles.

I. Sternocleidomastoid Muscle (SCM) (see Fig. 3–4)
   A. Is a paired muscle that serves as a primary muscular landmark.
   B. Divides the neck region into anterior and posterior cervical triangles.
   C. Originates from the clavicle and sternum and inserts on the mastoid process of the temporal bone.
   D. If one SCM contracts, the head and neck bend to the same side and the face and front of the neck rotate to the opposite side.
   E. If both SCMs contract, the head flexes at the neck and extends at the junction between the neck and skull.
   F. Is innervated by the accessory nerve.

II. Trapezius Muscle
   A. Is a paired muscle that covers the lateral and posterior surfaces of the neck.
   B. Originates from the occipital bone and the posterior midline of the cervical and thoracic regions; inserts on clavicle's lateral third and parts of the scapula.
   C. Acts to lift the clavicle and scapula.
   D. Is innervated by the accessory nerve and third and fourth cervical nerves.

Muscles of Facial Expression

The facial expression muscles (Fig. 3–12) are innervated by the facial nerve and act in various combinations to alter the appearance of face. The muscles are grouped according to their location in different facial regions. They include the epicranial, orbicularis oculi, corrugator supercilii, orbicularis oris, buccinator, risorius, levator, zygomaticus, depressor, mentalis, and platysma muscles.

I. Epicranial Muscle
   A. Is located in the scalp region and has frontal and occipital bellies, which are separated by a scalp tendon called the epicranial aponeurosis.
   B. Raises the eyebrows and scalp.

II. Orbicularis Oculi Muscle
   A. Encircles the eye.
   B. Closes the eyelid.

III. Corrugator Supercilii Muscle
   A. Is deep to the superior part of the orbicularis oculi muscle.
   B. Originates on the frontal bone and inserts into skin tissue of the eyebrow.
   C. Causes vertical wrinkles in the forehead.

IV. Orbicularis Oris Muscle
   A. Encircles the mouth.
   B. Closes the lips.

V. Buccinator Muscle
   A. Forms the anterior part of the cheek.
   B. Originates from the alveolar processes of the maxilla, mandible, and pterygomandibular raphe; the pterygomandibular raphe is a ligament that extends from hamulus and attaches to the mylohyoid line.
   C. Pulls the angle of mouth laterally and shortens the cheek both vertically and horizontally; keeps food in correct position during chewing.

VI. Risorius Muscle
   A. Originates from the fascia superficial to the masseter muscle and inserts in skin tissue at the angle of the mouth; widens the mouth.

VII. Levator Labii Superioris Muscle
   A. Originates from the infraorbital region of the maxilla and inserts in skin tissue of the upper lip.
   B. Elevates the upper lip.

VIII. Levator Labii Superioris Alaeque Nasi Muscle
   A. Originates from the frontal process of the maxilla and inserts into skin tissue of the ala of nose and upper lip.
   B. Elevates the upper lip and ala of the nose.

IX. Zygomaticus Major Muscle
   A. Originates from the zygomatic bone and inserts in skin tissue at the angle of the mouth.
   B. Elevates the angle of the upper lip and pulls it laterally.

X. Zygomaticus Minor Muscle
   A. Originates on the zygomatic bone and inserts in skin tissue of the upper lip.
   B. Elevates the upper lip.

XI. Levator Anguli Oris Muscle
   A. Originates superior to the root of the maxillary canine teeth and inserts in skin tissues at the angle of mouth.
   B. Elevates the angle of mouth.

XII. Depressor Anguli Oris Muscle
   A. Originates on the mandible and inserts in skin tissue at the angle of mouth.
   B. Depresses the angle of the mouth.

XIII. Depressor Labii Inferioris Muscle
   A. Originates from the mandible and inserts in skin tissues of the lower lip.
   B. Depresses the lower lip.

XIV. Mentalis Muscle
   A. Originates near the mandible midline and inserts in skin tissue of the chin.
   B. Raises the chin, causing lower lip protrusion and narrowing of the oral vestibule.

XV. Platysma Muscle

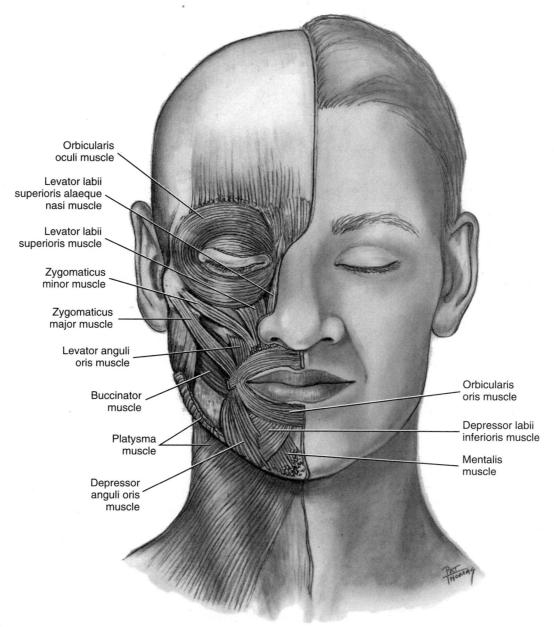

Figure 3.12 Muscles of facial expression.
(From Fehrenbach MJ, Herring SW: Illustrated Anatomy of the Head and Neck.
Philadelphia, WB Saunders, 1996, p. 101.)

A. Runs from the neck to the mouth, covering the anterior cervical triangle.
B. Originates in skin tissue superficial to the clavicle and shoulder and inserts on the mandible and muscles surrounding the mouth.
C. Raises the skin of the neck and pulls down the corner of the mouth.

Muscles of Mastication

Mastication muscles (Figs. 3–13 and 3–14) are paired muscles that attach to the mandible and work with the temporomandibular joint to accomplish the movements of the mandible: depression, elevation, protrusion, re-traction, and lateral deviation. They are innervated by the mandibular division of the trigeminal nerve. These muscles include the masseter, temporalis, medial ptery-goid, and lateral pterygoid muscles.

I. Masseter Muscle
 A. Is the most superficially located and one of the strongest muscles.
 B. Is located anterior to the parotid salivary gland.
 C. Has two heads—superficial and deep—that origi-nate from different areas of the zygomatic arch and insert on the mandible.
  1. The superficial head inserts on the lateral sursface of angle.

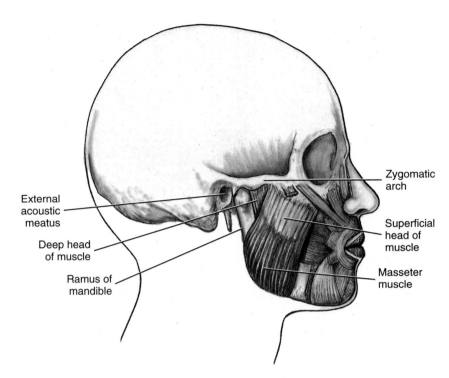

Figure 3.13 Muscles of mastication. (From Fehrenbach MJ, Herring SW: Illustrated Anatomy of the Head and Neck. Philadelphia, WB Saunders, 1996, p. 114.)

2. The deep head inserts on the ramus.
D. When bilateral contraction occurs during closing of the jaws, the mandible elevates, thereby raising the lower jaw.
E. Can become enlarged with clenching or grinding of teeth (bruxism).
II. Temporalis Muscle
A. Originates from the entire temporal fossa and inserts on the coronoid process of mandible.

B. When the entire temporalis muscle contracts during closing of the jaws, the mandible elevates, thereby raising the lower jaw.
C. When only the posterior part of the temporalis muscle contracts, the muscle moves the lower jaw backward, causing retraction of the jaw (usually during closing of the jaws).
III. Medial Pterygoid Muscle
A. Similar to but deeper to the masseter muscle.

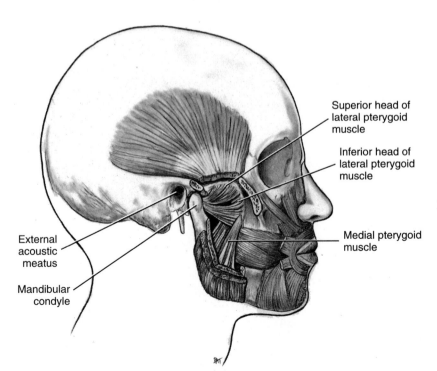

Figure 3.14 Muscles of mastication. (From Fehrenbach MJ, Herring SW: Illustrated Anatomy of the Head and Neck. Philadelphia, WB Saunders, 1996, p. 115.)

B. Originates from the pterygoid fossa, on the medial surface of the lateral pterygoid plate, and inserts on the medial surface of the angle of the mandible.

C. Elevates the mandible during closing of the jaws, thus raising the lower jaw.

IV. Lateral Pterygoid Muscle

A. Has two separate heads of origin, superior and inferior, which are separated by a slight interval anteriorly; these heads fuse posteriorly, within the infratemporal fossa, deep to the temporalis muscle.

  1. Superior head originates from the greater wing of the sphenoid bone.

  2. Inferior head originates from the lateral pterygoid plate.

  3. Both heads of the muscle unite and insert on the mandibular condyle.

B. Has a tendency to depress the mandible during opening of the jaws, thereby lowering the lower jaw.

C. When both muscles contract they serve to bring the lower jaw forward, causing a protrusion of the mandible (typically during opening). When only one lateral pterygoid muscle is contracted, the lower jaw shifts to the opposite side, causing lateral deviation of the mandible.

Hyoid Muscles

The hyoid muscles (Fig. 3–15) are located superficially in the neck tissues and include the suprahyoid and infrahyoid muscle groups. These muscles attach to the hyoid bone and assist in the actions of mastication and swallowing.

I. Suprahyoid Muscles

A. Are located superior to the hyoid and are

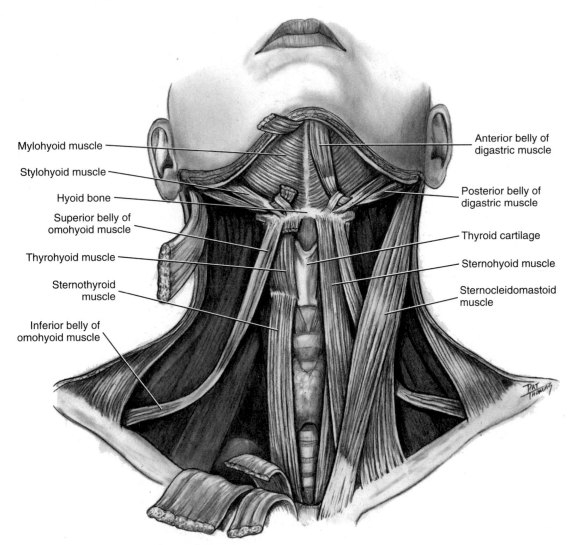

Figure 3.15   Hyoid muscles.
(From Fehrenbach MJ, Herring SW: Illustrated Anatomy of the Head and Neck. Philadelphia, WB Saunders, 1996, p. 117.)

categorized according to their anterior or posterior position relative to the hyoid.

B. Act to elevate the hyoid and larynx by contraction of the muscles of mastication when the mandible is stabilized, which occurs during swallowing.

C. Contraction of the anterior muscles causes the mandible to depress and the jaws to open when the hyoid is stabilized by contraction of the posterior suprahyoid and infrahyoid muscles.

D. Include the digastric, mylohyoid, stylohyoid, and geniohyoid muscles.
1. Digastric muscle
   a. Has anterior and posterior bellies, which are separate.
   b. The anterior belly is part of the anterior suprahyoids and the posterior belly is part of the posterior suprahyoids.
   c. Each muscle demarcates a superior part of the anterior cervical triangle, forming (with the mandible) a submandibular triangle on each side of the neck.
   d. The right and left anterior bellies form a midline submental triangle.
   e. The anterior belly arises from the intermediate tendon and inserts close to the symphysis on the inner surface of the mandible.
   f. The posterior belly arises from the mastoid process and inserts on the intermediate tendon.
   g. The anterior belly is innervated by the mylohyoid nerve.
   h. The posterior belly is innervated by the posterior digastric nerve.
2. Mylohyoid muscle
   a. Is located deep to the digastric muscle; its fibers run transversely between the two sides of the mandible, where it originates from the mylohyoid line (on the inner surface of mandible), and unite medially, forming the floor of the mouth and the most posterior fibers insert on the body of the hyoid bone.
   b. Helps elevate the tongue; also elevates hyoid bone or depresses mandible.
   c. Is innervated by the mylohyoid nerve.
3. Stylohyoid muscle
   a. Is anterior and superficial to the posterior belly of the digastric muscle.
   b. Originates from the styloid process of the temporal bone and inserts on the body of the hyoid bone.
   c. Is innervated by the stylohyoid nerve.
4. Geniohyoid muscle
   a. Originates from the medial surface of the mandible and inserts near the symphysis at the genial tubercles.
   b. Is innervated by the first cervical nerve; innervation is conducted by the hypoglossal nerve.

II. Infrahyoid Muscles
A. Are paired muscles located inferior to the hyoid bone.
B. Are innervated by the second and third cervical nerves and generally act to depress the hyoid bone.
C. Include the sternohyoid, sternothyroid, omohyoid, and thyrohyoid muscles.
1. Sternothyroid muscle
   a. Is superficial to the thyroid gland; deep and medial to the sternohyoid muscle.
   b. Originates from the sternum and inserts on the thyroid cartilage.
   c. Depresses the thyroid cartilage and larynx; does not directly depress hyoid bone.
2. Sternohyoid muscle
   a. Is superficial to the sternothyroid muscle, thyroid gland, and cartilage.
   b. Originates from the sternum and inserts on the hyoid bone.
3. Omohyoid muscle
   a. Is lateral to both the sternothyroid muscle and thyrohyoid muscle.
   b. Has superior and inferior bellies.
   c. The inferior belly originates from the scapula and passes beneath the SCM muscle, where it attaches by a short tendon to the superior belly.
   d. The superior belly originates from a short tendon attached to the inferior belly and inserts on hyoid bone.
4. Thyrohyoid muscle
   a. Is covered by the omohyoid muscle and sternohyoid muscle.
   b. Originates from thyroid cartilage and inserts on hyoid bone; appears as a continuation of sternothyroid muscle.
   c. Raises thyroid cartilage and larynx in addition to depressing hyoid bone.

Muscles of the Tongue

The muscles of the tongue are divided into intrinsic and extrinsic groups. The tongue forms complex movements during mastication, speaking, and swallowing as a result of the combined action of muscles. All tongue muscles are innervated by the hypoglossal nerve.

I. Intrinsic tongue muscles
A. Are located inside the tongue.
B. Change the shape of the tongue.
C. Are named according to their orientation.
D. Include superior longitudinal, transverse, vertical, and inferior longitudinal muscles.

II. Extrinsic Tongue Muscles
A. Originate outside the tongue, yet insert inside tongue.
B. Move the tongue while suspending and anchoring the tongue to the mandible, styloid process, and hyoid bone.

C. Include the genioglossus, styloglossus, and hyoglossus muscles.

Temporomandibular Joint

The temporomandibular joint (TMJ) (Fig. 3–16) is located on each side of the head and allows for movement of the mandible for speech and mastication. It is innervated by the mandibular division of the trigeminal nerve and receives its blood supply from the external carotid artery. Patients may experience a disorder of one or both of these joints.

Bones of the Temporomandibular Joint

The bones of the TMJ are discussed in the section on the skeletal system.

Joint Capsule

The joint capsule completely encloses the TMJ. Membranes that line the inside of the joint capsule secrete synovial fluid, which helps lubricate the joint.

Disc

The disc is located between the temporal bone and the condyle and completely divides the TMJ into two synovial cavities—upper and lower—which are filled with synovial fluid.
I. Is attached to the mandibular condyle anteriorly and not to the temporal bone, except indirectly through the capsule.
II. Is divided posteriorly into two areas where it blends with the capsule.
    A. The upper division is attached to the postglenoid process.
    B. The lower division is attached to the condyle.
III. Nerves and blood vessels enter the joint in the posterior area of attachment to the capsule.

Ligaments Associated with TMJ

Several ligaments are associated with the TMJ. These are the temporomandibular joint, sphenomandibular, and stylomandibular ligaments.
I. Temporomandibular Joint Ligament
    A. Is located on the lateral side of each joint.
    B. Forms a reinforcement of the capsule.
    C. Prevents excessive retraction of the mandible.
II. Sphenomandibular Ligament
    A. Is not a part of the TMJ.
    B. Is located on the medial side of the mandible, some distance from the joint.
    C. Runs from the angular spine of the sphenoid bone to the lingula.
    D. Becomes taut when the mandible protrudes.
III. Stylomandibular Ligament
    A. Is a variable ligament that is formed by thickened cervical fascia.
    B. Runs from the styloid process of the temporal bone to the angle of the mandible.
    C. Becomes taut when the mandible protrudes.

Jaw Movements and Muscle Relationships

Movements of the mandible and TMJ with associated muscles are detailed in Table 3-2.

Vascular System

The vascular system supplies the body's tissues with nutrients. However, it may become compromised by a disease process or during a dental procedure. The system also is capable of spreading infection or cancerous cells in the head and neck area because valveless veins control the direction of blood flow. The vascular system comprises the arterial blood supply, the capillary network, and venous drainage.

Arterial Blood Supply of the Head and Neck

The major arteries that supply the head and neck are the subclavian artery and the common carotid artery. Their

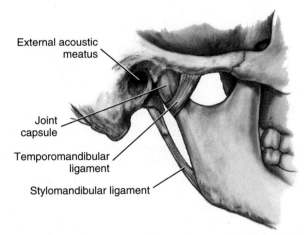

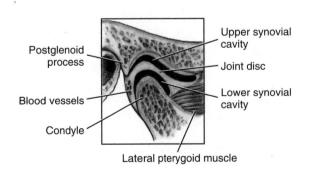

Figure 3.16 Temporomandibular joint.
(From Fehrenbach MJ, Herring SW: Illustrated Anatomy of the Head and Neck. Philadelphia, WB Saunders, 1996, p. 158.)

TABLE 3.2	Movements of the Mandible and TMJ with Associated Muscles	
Mandibular Movements	**TMJ Movements**	**Associated Muscles**
Protrusion of mandible, moving lower jaw forward	Gliding in both upper synovial cavities	Lateral pterygoid, bilateral contraction
Retraction of mandible, moving lower jaw backward	Gliding in both upper synovial cavities	Posterior portion of temporalis, bilateral contraction
Elevation and retraction of mandible, closing jaws	Gliding in both upper synovial cavities and rotation in both lower synovial cavities	Masseter, temporalis, and medial pterygoid, bilateral contraction
Depression and protrusion of mandible, opening jaws	Gliding in both upper synovial cavities and rotation in both lower synovial cavities	Suprahyoids and inferior heads of lateral pterygoid, bilateral contraction
Lateral deviation of mandible, to shift lower jaw to opposite side	Gliding in one upper synovial cavity and rotation in opposite upper synovial cavity	Lateral pterygoid, unilateral contraction

From Fehrenback MJ, Herring SW: Illustrated Anatomy of the Head and Neck. Philadelphia, WB Saunders, 1996, p. 142.

paths from the heart to the head and neck are different, depending on the side of the body; other arteries of the head and neck are symmetrically located on each side of the body.

I. The Subclavian Artery
 A. Is located lateral to the common carotid artery.
 B. Has branches that supply both cranial structures.
II. The Common Carotid Artery
 A. Is branchless and travels up the neck, lateral to the trachea and larynx, to the thyroid cartilage; is contained in a sheath beneath the sternocleidomastoid muscle, along with the internal jugular vein and vagus nerve, until it ends by dividing into internal and external carotid arteries at the level of the larynx.
 B. Bifurcates just past the location of the carotid sinus, a swelling or dilation. The carotid sinus provides the most reliable arterial pulse.
  1. Internal carotid artery
   a. After leaving the common carotid artery, is hidden by the sternocleidomastoid muscle; has no branches in neck, but continues adjacent to the internal jugular vein within the carotid sheath to the skull base, where it enters the cranium to supply the intracranial structures.
   b. Is the source of the ophthalmic artery, which supplies the eye, the orbit, and the lacrimal gland.
  2. External carotid artery
   a. Arises from the common carotid artery.
   b. Supplies the extracranial tissues, including the cavity.
   c. Has anterior, medial, posterior, and terminal branches.
    1) Anterior branches of external carotid artery.
     a) The superior thyroid artery branches into the infrahyoid, sternocleidomastoid, superior laryngeal, and superior and inferior thyroid arteries, which supply tissues inferior to the hyoid bone, including the infrahyoid muscles, the SCM muscle, the muscles of the larynx, and the thyroid gland.
     b) The lingual artery arises above the superior thyroid artery, at the level of the hyoid bone, travels anteriorly to the tongue apex, and supplies tissues superior to the hyoid, including the suprahyoid muscles and the floor of the mouth by the dorsal lingual, deep lingual, sublingual, and suprahyoid branches; also supplies the tongue, including the dorsal lingual branches to the base and body and the terminal part of the deep lingual artery to the terminal part of the apex.
     c) The sublingual artery supplies the mylohyoid muscle, the sublingual salivary gland, and the mucous membranes of the floor of the mouth; the suprahyoid branch supplies the suprahyoid muscles.
     d) The facial artery arises slightly superior to the lingual artery as it branches off anteriorly and has a complicated path; supplies the face in the oral, buccal, zygomatic, nasal, infraorbital, and orbital regions with its major branches, including the ascending palatine, submandibular and submental, inferior labial, superior labial, and angular (which may share common trunk with lingual) arteries.

2) Medial branch of external artery
  a) Includes ascending pharyngeal artery and its pharyngeal and meningeal branches.
3) Posterior branches of external carotid artery
  a) The occipital artery includes the muscular, sternocleidomastoid, auricular, and meningeal branches.
  b) The posterior auricular artery arises superior to the occipital artery and stylohyoid muscle, level with the tip of the styloid process, and has auricular and stylomastoid branches.
4) Terminal branches of external carotid artery
  a) The superficial temporal artery arises within the parotid salivary gland and may be visible in the temporal region; transverse facial branch supplies the parotid; middle temporal branch supplies the temporalis muscle; frontal and parietal branches supply the scalp.
  b) The maxillary artery (Fig. 3–17) gives off many branches within the infratemporal and pterygopalatine fossae, such as the middle meningeal and inferior alveolar arteries, and has branches near

the muscles they supply, including the deep temporal, pterygoid, masseteric artery, and buccal muscles. It branches into the inferior alveolar, posterior superior alveolar, infraorbital, and greater and lesser palatine arteries.
(1) The inferior alveolar artery arises from the maxillary artery in the infratemporal fossa, turns inferiorly to enter the mandibular foramen, and subsequently enters the mandibular canal and the inferior alveolar nerve; it branches into the mylohyoid artery before it enters the canal. In the canal it branches into the mandibular posterior and alveolar (dental) branches to supply the teeth and periodontium of these teeth, and also associated gingiva.
(2) The mylohyoid artery arises before the main artery enters the mandibular canal by way of the mandibular foramen and travels in the mylohyoid groove to supply the floor of the mouth and the mylohyoid muscle.
(3) The mental artery arises from the main artery and subsequently exits

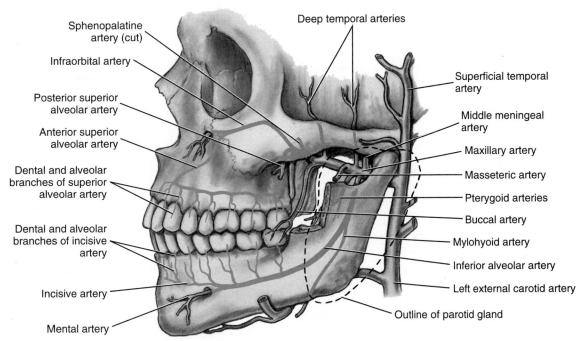

Figure 3.17 Maxillary artery.
(From Fehrenbach MJ, Herring SW: Illustrated Anatomy of the Head and Neck. Philadelphia, WB Saunders, 1996, p. 158.)

the mandibular canal by way of the mental foramen to supply the chin tissues; anastomoses with inferior labial artery.

(4) The incisive artery branches off the main artery and remains in the mandibular canal, where it divides into dental branches to supply the mandibular anterior teeth and alveolar branches to supply the periodontium of these teeth; anastomoses with alveolar branches of incisive artery on other side of the mouth.

(5) The posterior superior alveolar artery is given off just as the maxillary artery leaves the infratemporal fossa and enters the pterygopalatine fossa, where it subsequently enters the posterior superior alveolar foramina and gives off dental branches (to supply the maxillary posterior maxillary teeth) and alveolar branches (to supply the periodontium of those teeth and the maxillary sinus); anastomoses with the anterior superior alveolar artery.

(6) The infraorbital artery branches from the maxillary artery in the pterygopalatine fossa and may share a common trunk with the posterior superior alveolar artery; subsequently it enters the orbit through the inferior orbital fissure and travels through the infraorbital canal, giving off orbital branches to the orbit and gives off anterior superior alveolar artery.

(7) The anterior superior alveolar artery arises from the infraorbital artery and gives off dental branches to supply the anterior maxillary teeth and alveolar branches to supply the periodontium of these teeth; anastomoses with the posterior superior alveolar artery. After giving off these branches in the infraorbital canal orbit, it emerges onto the face—from the infraorbital foramen to the infraorbital region of face; anastomoses with facial artery.

(8) The greater palatine and lesser palatine arteries arise from the maxillary artery in the pterygopalatine fossa, which travels to the palate through the pterygopalatine canal and greater and lesser palatine foramina to supply the hard and soft palate, respectively.

(9) The maxillary artery ends by becoming the sphenopalatine artery, which supplies the nasal cavity and gives rise to the posterior lateral nasal branches and septal branches, including a nasopalatine branch that accompanies the nasopalatine nerve through the incisive foramen.

Venous Drainage of the Head and Neck (Fig. 3–18)

Veins typically are symmetrically located but have greater variability in location than do arteries. They anastomose freely and generally are larger and more numerous than arteries in the same tissue. The internal jugular vein drains the brain and other tissue; the external jugular vein drains only some extracranial tissues, with many anastomoses between them. The internal and external jugular veins are the major venous drainage vessels of the head and neck region. As they leave the head near the base of the neck, they tend to enlarge.

I. Facial Vein
    A. Includes the superior labial, inferior labial, submental, and lingual veins.
    B. Drains into the internal jugular vein.
    C. Begins at the medial canthus, at the junction of the supratrochlear and supraorbital veins, which anastomoses with ophthalmic veins that drain orbit tissues and provides communication with the cavernous venous sinus; may become fatally infected from the spread of a dental infection.
    D. Receives branches from same facial areas supplied by the facial artery and anastomoses with deep veins, such as the pterygoid plexus in the infratemporal fossa and the retromandibular vein, before joining the internal jugular vein at level of hyoid bone.
    E. Has oral tributaries, including:
        1. The superior labial vein, which drains the upper lip.
        2. The inferior labial vein, which drains the lower lip.
        3. The submental vein, which drains the chin tissues and the submandibular region.
        4. The lingual veins, including the dorsal lingual veins, which drain dorsal surface of tongue, the deep lingual veins, which drain the ventral surface, and the sublingual veins, which drain the floor of the mouth and may join to form a single vessel or may empty into larger vessels separately—either indirectly into the facial vein or directly into the internal jugular vein.

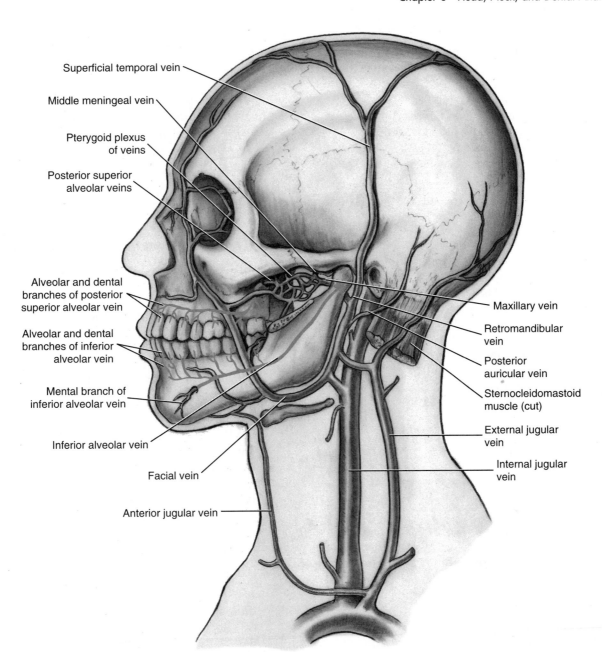

Figure 3.18 Venous drainage of the head and neck.
(From Fehrenbach MJ, Herring SW: Illustrated Anatomy of the Head and Neck. Philadelphia, WB Saunders, 1996, p. 163.)

II. Retromandibular Vein
   A. Is formed by the union of the superficial temporal and maxillary veins; emerges from the parotid salivary gland and drains areas similar to those supplied by the superficial temporal and maxillary arteries.
   B. Divides below the parotid gland; its anterior division joins the facial vein and its posterior division continues and is joined by the posterior auricular vein, which drains the scalp behind the ear and becomes the external jugular vein.
      1. Superficial temporal vein
         a. Drains the lateral scalp; drains into and

   forms the retromandibular vein, along with the maxillary vein.
      2. Maxillary vein
         a. Begins in infratemporal fossa, where it drains the pterygoid plexus near the maxillary artery and receives the middle meningeal vein, posterior superior alveolar vein, inferior alveolar vein, and other veins, such as those from the nose and palate (areas served by maxillary artery).
         b. Subsequently merges with the superficial temporal vein to drain into and form the retromandibular vein.

III. Pterygoid Plexus of Veins
   A. Is a collection of small anastomosing vessels that are located around the pterygoid muscles and surround the maxillary artery, protecting it from compression in the infratemporal fossa.
   B. Drains blood from the maxillary and middle meningeal veins, which drain blood from the meninges and deep facial portions.
   C. Anastomoses with both the facial and retromandibular veins.
   D. May be involved in the spread of infection to the cavernous venous sinus.
   E. Also drains the posterior superior alveolar vein, which is formed by the union of dental branches of the maxillary teeth and alveolar branches of the periodontium of these teeth.
   F. Also drains the inferior alveolar vein, which is formed by the union of the dental branches of the mandibular teeth, the alveolar branches of the periodontium of those teeth, and the mental branches that enter the mental foramen after draining the chin area, where they anastomose with branches of the facial vein.

Glandular Tissue

Glandular tissues include the lacrimal, salivary, thyroid, parathyroid, and thymus tissues. An understanding of their location, innervation, lymphatic drainage, and blood supply is essential to determining the extent of glandular involvement in a disease process.

Lacrimal Glands

These glands are paired exocrine glands that secrete lacrimal fluid or tears for lubrication of the conjunctiva.
I. Secrete lacrimal fluid, which leaves the gland through tubules.
   A. After passing over the eyeball, are drained through a hole in each eyelid, which terminates in the nasolacrimal sac, a structure behind the medial canthus.
   B. Continue from the nasolacrimal sac into the nasolacrimal duct, at the junction of the lacrimal and maxillary bones, and subsequently drain into the inferior nasal meatus.
II. Are located in the lacrimal fossa of the frontal bone, inside the lateral part of the supraorbital ridge, which is inside the orbit.
III. Are innervated by parasympathetic fibers from the greater petrosal nerve, a branch of the facial nerve; synapse occurs at the pterygopalatine ganglion and postganglionic fibers, which reach the gland through branches of the trigeminal nerve.
IV. Drain into the superior parotid lymph nodes.
V. Are supplied by the lacrimal artery, a branch of the ophthalmic artery of the internal carotid artery.

 Clinical Case · STUDY

Sixty-eight-year-old Alice Chin is a new patient. Mrs. Chin has not had a dental examination since her last dentist retired 2 years ago. She frequently experiences a dry mouth and clenches her teeth at night. Further investigation reveals that her jaws ache when she wakes in the morning. An extraoral examination indicates that her cheeks are firm and enlarged. She currently has no pain or discomfort in the jaw area.

Clinical Case QUESTIONS

1. Describe the location and function of the major salivary glands that should be assessed.
2. The patient has dry mouth. What is the medical term for this condition? Does it pose any risk?
3. What caused the firmly enlarged cheeks? Why is there no jaw discomfort except in the morning?
4. Does the condition of cheek firmness and enlargement require treatment? If so, what may be recommended?

Clinical Case RATIONALES

1. The major salivary glands of the mouth that should be assessed for saliva-producing ability are the parotid, submandibular, and sublingual glands. The parotid glands are the largest encapsulated salivary glands located in the cheeks (in the parotid fascial space behind the mandibular ramus) adjacent to the maxillary molars. The parotid glands provide 25% of the total salivary volume, and its secretions are purely serous. The submandibular glands, which are located medial to the mandible in the submandibular fossa, are the second largest encapsulated salivary glands. They produce a mixed secretion that provides 60% to 65% of the total salivary volume. The sublingual glands are the smallest and only unencapsulated salivary glands. They are located beneath the tongue in the sublingual fossa and produce only 10% of total salivary volume in a mixed secretion.
2. Dry mouth, or xerostomia, is caused by inadequate saliva production (often from medication, radiation therapy to the head and neck, or a systemic condition such as Sjögren's syndrome) and can result in difficult swallowing, plaque retention, and an increased risk of caries. Mrs. Chin should be carefully monitored for caries.
3. This patient's firmly enlarged cheeks are caused by an overuse of the masseter muscle during sleep. Jaw discomfort only upon awakening is indicative of a nighttime bruxing or clenching habit. Her teeth should be checked for the presence of occlusal wear or cusp fracture.

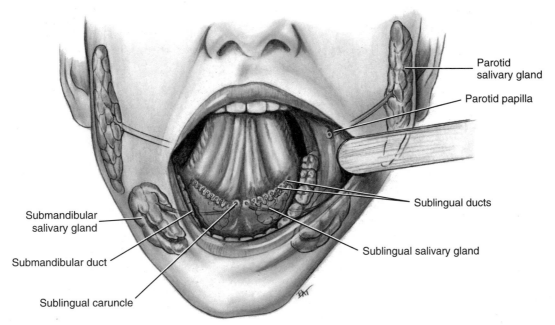

Figure 3.19   Salivary glands.
(From Fehrenbach MJ, Herring SW: Illustrated Anatomy of the Head and Neck. Philadelphia, WB Saunders, 1996, p. 180.)

4. This condition may require treatment with a mouthguard. The mouthguard prevents full closure and allows the masseter muscle to relax. It also helps prevent further wear to the occlusal surfaces of the teeth.

Salivary Glands

Salivary (Fig. 3–19) glands produce saliva, which lubricates and cleanses the oral cavity and aids digestion. The major glands are the parotid, submandibular, and sublingual glands.

I.   Are controlled by the autonomic nervous system.
II. Include both major and minor glands, which are defined by their size.
III. Are exocrine glands with ducts that drain saliva directly into the oral cavity, where saliva is used.
IV. May become enlarged, tender, and possibly firmer in response to various disease processes or blocked with stone (sialolith) formations, which prevents drainage of saliva from the ducts and causes gland enlargement and tenderness.
V.   Production of saliva may decrease or increase in response to certain medications or disease processes.
VI. The major salivary glands are large paired glands whose ducts are named after them; they include the parotid, submandibular, and sublingual glands.

A. Parotid salivary gland
   1. Is the largest, encapsulated salivary gland; provides only 25% of total salivary volume; has a purely serous secretion.
   2. Is divided into two lobes: superficial and deep.
   3. Has parotid duct (Stensen's), which emerges from the anterior border of the gland, pierces the buccinator muscle, and subsequently opens into the oral cavity, at the parotid papilla.
   4. Becomes enlarged and tender with mumps.
   5. Is involved in tumorous growth, which can change the consistency and cause facial paralysis on the involved side (because the facial nerve travels through this gland).
   6. Occupies the parotid fascial space, behind the mandibular ramus, anterior and inferior to the ear; extends irregularly from the zygomatic arch to the angle of mandible.
   7. Is innervated by parasympathetic nerves of the otic ganglion of the glossopharyngeal nerve, as well as afferent nerves from the auriculotemporal branch of the trigeminal nerve.
   8. Drains into the deep parotid lymph nodes.
   9. Is supplied by branches of the external carotid artery.

B. Submandibular salivary gland
   1. Is the second largest encapsulated salivary gland; provides 60% to 65% of the total salivary volume with a mixed secretion.
   2. The submandibular duct (Wharton's):
      a. Arises from the deep lobe and remains inside of the mylohyoid muscle.
      b. Travels along the anterior floor of the mouth and subsequently opens into the oral cavity at the sublingual caruncle.
      c. Its tortuous travel may be the reason that it is the salivary gland most often involved in stone formation.
   3. Occupies the submandibular fossa in the submandibular fascial space, mostly superficial to the mylohyoid muscle—however, the deep lobe wraps around the posterior part and is posterior to the sublingual salivary gland.
   4. Is innervated by parasympathetic fibers of the chorda tympani and submandibular ganglion of the facial nerve.
   5. Drains into the submandibular lymph nodes.
   6. Is supplied by branches of the facial and lingual arteries.
C. Sublingual salivary gland
   1. Is the smallest and only unencapsulated salivary gland; provides only 10% of total salivary volume with a mixed secretion.
   2. Has sublingual ducts (Bartholin's) that open directly into the oral cavity through the sublingual gland.
   3. Has other ducts that open along the sublingual fold.
   4. Is located in the sublingual fossa in the sublingual fascial space at the floor of the mouth.
   5. Is superior to the mylohyoid muscle, medial to the body of the mandible, and anterior to the submandibular gland.
   6. Is innervated by parasympathetic fibers of the chorda tympani and the submandibular ganglion of the facial nerve.
   7. Drains into the submandibular lymph nodes.
   8. Is supplied by the sublingual and submental arteries.
D. Minor salivary glands
   1. Are smaller than the major glands but are more numerous.
   2. Are exocrine glands, with unnamed ducts that are shorter than those of the major glands.
   3. Are scattered in tissues of the buccal, labial, and lingual mucosa, soft palate, lateral parts of the hard palate, and floor of the mouth; include von Ebner's glands (associated with circumvallate lingual papillae).
   4. Secrete primarily mucous saliva, except von Ebner's glands, which secrete only serous secretions.
   5. Are innervated by the facial nerve.
   6. Drain into various lymph nodes.
   7. Are supplied by various arteries.

Thyroid Gland

The thyroid gland (Fig. 3–20) is located in the anterior and lateral regions of the neck, inferior to thyroid cartilage, at the junction between the larynx and trachea. It produces

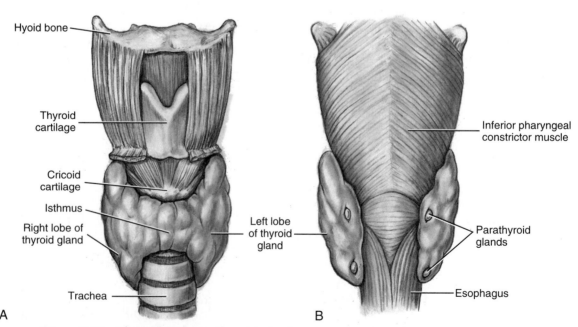

Figure 3.20 Thyroid and parathyroid glands.
(From Fehrenbach MJ, Herring SW: Illustrated Anatomy of the Head and Neck. Philadelphia, WB Saunders, 1996, p. 182.)

thyroxine, which it secretes directly into the blood, stimulating the metabolic rate.

I. Is the largest endocrine gland and is ductless.
II. Consists of two lateral lobes—right and left—which are connected anteriorly by an isthmus.
III. May become enlarged during a disease process; enlargement is called a goiter.
IV. Is innervated by sympathetic nerves through the cervical ganglia.
V. Drains into superior deep cervical lymph nodes.
VI. Is supplied by superior and inferior thyroid arteries.

Parathyroid Glands

The parathyroid glands (see Fig. 3–20) are located close to or inside the thyroid gland on its posterior surface. These ductless glands produce and secrete parathyroid hormone directly into the blood to regulate calcium and phosphorus levels.

I. Consist of four endocrine glands—two on each side.
II. May alter the thyroid gland if involved in a disease process.
III. Are innervated by sympathetic nerves through the cervical ganglia.
IV. Drain into superior deep cervical lymph nodes.
V. Are supplied primarily by inferior thyroid arteries.

Thymus Gland

The thymus gland is a ductless endocrine gland. It is located in the thorax and anterior region of the base of the neck, inferior to the thyroid gland, deep to the sternum and sternohyoid and sternothyroid muscles, and superficial and lateral to the trachea. It is part of the immune system and fights the disease process.

I. As part of immune system, T-cell lymphocytes mature in the gland in response to stimulation by thymus hormones.
II. Grows in size from birth to puberty, when it subsequently stops growing and starts to shrink.
III. Consists of two lateral lobes in close contact at the midline.
IV. May develop thyroid cancer as a result of past radiation therapy.
V. Is innervated by branches of the vagus nerve and the cervical nerves.
VI. Has lymphatics that arise within the substance of the gland and terminate in the internal jugular vein.
VII. Is supplied by the inferior thyroid and internal thoracic arteries.

Nervous System

The nervous system causes muscles to contract and stimulates glands to secrete. It regulates many other systems of the body and allows for sensation perception. Knowledge of the nervous system is important in understanding pain management and nervous system disorders of the head and neck. Head and neck branches include the cranial, trigeminal, and facial nerves.

Cranial Nerves

The cranial nerves (Fig. 3–21) are numbered I through XII and include the olfactory, optic, oculomotor, trochlear, trigeminal, abducens, facial, vestibulocochlear, glossopharyngeal, vagus, accessory, and hypoglossal nerves. They are part of the peripheral nervous system and include twelve pairs that are connected to the brain at its base and pass through the skull by way of fissures or foramina. A cranial nerve may be either afferent or efferent or may have both types of neural processes.

I. Cranial Nerve I (olfactory nerve)
    A. Is afferent for smell from the nasal mucosa to the brain.
    B. Enters the skull through perforations in the cribriform plate of the ethmoid bone to join the olfactory bulb in the brain.
II. Cranial Nerve II (optic nerve)
    A. Is afferent for vision from the retina to the brain.
    B. Enters the skull through the optic canal of the sphenoid bone, where right and left optic nerves join at the optic chasm, and where many fibers cross to the opposite side before continuing into the brain as optic tracts.
III. Cranial Nerve III (oculomotor nerve)
    A. Is efferent to eye muscles.
    B. Carries preganglionic parasympathetic fibers to ciliary ganglion near the eyeball; postganglionic fibers innervate muscles inside the eyeball.
    C. Lies in lateral wall of cavernous sinus and exits the skull through the superior orbital fissure on its way to the orbit.
IV. Cranial Nerve IV (trochlear nerve)
    A. Is efferent to one eye muscle and for proprioception.
    B. Runs in lateral wall of the cavernous sinus and exits the skull through the superior orbital fissure on its way to the orbit.
V. Cranial Nerve V (trigeminal nerve)
    A. Is efferent for muscles of mastication and for other cranial muscles; is afferent for teeth, tongue, and oral cavity and for most of facial skin.
    B. May experience trigeminal neuralgia, a neural lesion involving afferent nerves.
    C. Is the largest cranial nerve; has two roots—sensory and motor.
        1. Sensory root has three divisions: ophthalmic, maxillary, and mandibular; each enters the skull in different locations in the sphenoid bone.
            a. Ophthalmic division provides sensation for upper face and scalp and enters through the superior orbital fissure.

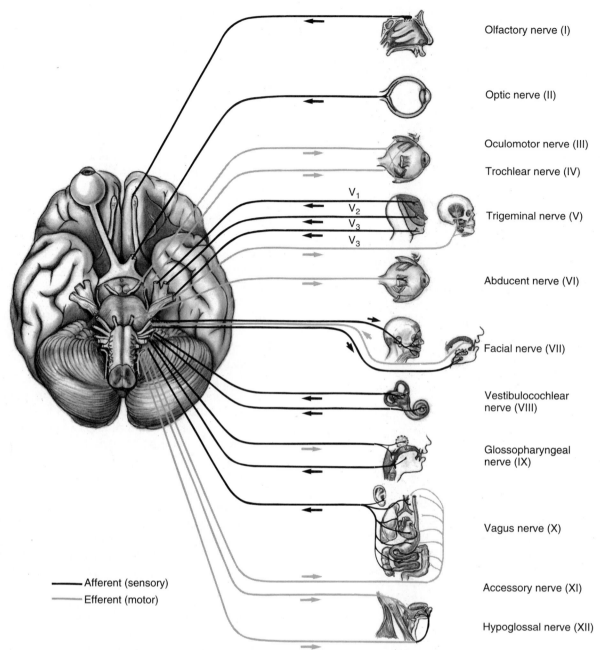

Figure 3.21 Cranial nerves.
(From Fehrenbach MJ, Herring SW: Illustrated Anatomy of the Head and Neck. Philadelphia, WB Saunders, 1996, p. 192.)

b. Maxillary division provides sensation for middle face and enters by way of the foramen rotundum.

c. Mandibular division provides sensation for the lower face and passes through the skull by way of the foramen ovale.

d. Has trigeminal ganglion (semilunar or Gasserian), located on anterior surface of the petrous part of the temporal bone.

2. Motor root accompanies the mandibular division of the sensory root and also exits the skull through the foramen.

VI. Cranial Nerve VI (abducens nerve)

A. Is efferent to one of the eyeball muscles.

B. Exits the skull through the superior orbital fissure on its way to the orbit.

C. Runs through the cavernous sinus and often is the first nerve affected by sinus infection.

VII. Cranial Nerve VII (facial nerve)
  A. Is efferent for the muscles of facial expression, for preganglionic parasympathetic innervation of the lacrimal gland, and for submandibular and sublingual salivary glands; is afferent for skin behind the ear, for taste sensation, and for the body of the tongue.
  B. Leaves the cranial cavity by passing through the internal acoustic meatus, which leads to the facial canal inside the temporal bone.
  C. Exits the skull by way of the stylomastoid foramen.
  D. Lesions of nerves may include facial paralysis—a loss of movement of facial expression muscles caused by injury of the facial nerve, Bell's palsy, or trigeminal neuralgia.
VIII. Cranial Nerve VIII (vestibulocochlear nerve)
  A. Is afferent for hearing and balance.
  B. Enters the cranial cavity through the internal acoustic meatus.
IX. Cranial Nerve IX (glossopharyngeal nerve)
  A. Is efferent for the pharyngeal muscle and preganglionic parasympathetic innervation for the parotid salivary gland; is afferent for the pharynx, for taste, and for general sensation from the base of the tongue.
  B. Passes through the skull by way of the jugular foramen and the tympanic branch; has sensory fibers for the middle ear and preganglionic parasympathetic fibers for the parotid gland; arises here and reenters the skull.
  C. After supplying the ear, the parasympathetic fibers leave the skull through the foramen ovale as the lesser petrosal nerve; these preganglionic fibers subsequently end in the otic ganglion, which is located near the medial surface of the mandibular division of the trigeminal nerve.
X. Cranial Nerve X (vagus nerve)
  A. Is efferent for muscles of the soft palate, pharynx, and larynx, and for parasympathetic fibers to many major body organs, including the thymus gland, heart, and stomach; is afferent for skin around the ear and for taste sensation of the epiglottis.
  B. Passes through the skull by way of the jugular foramen.
XI. Cranial Nerve XI (accessory nerve)
  A. Is efferent for trapezius and sternocleidomastoid muscles, as well as muscles of the soft palate and pharynx.
  B. Is only partly a cranial nerve; consists of two roots—one arising from the brain and one from the spinal cord.
  C. Exits the skull through the jugular foramen.
XII. Cranial Nerve XII (hypoglossal nerve)
  A. Is efferent for intrinsic and extrinsic muscles of the tongue.
  B. Exits the skull through the hypoglossal canal.

Clinical Case STUDY

Twelve-year-old Nick Bartlett complains of a sore mouth from eating pizza. A visual examination reveals a 6-mm burn (diameter) on the roof of the mouth, behind the central incisors. Enlarged tonsils, bilaterally and near the fauces, also are noted.

Clinical Case QUESTIONS

1. Which nerves are involved in the patient's discomfort from the thermal burn?
2. Which bone underlies the tissue in the thermal burn area?
3. Identify the unique intraoral landmark located near or within the burn area.
4. Which tonsils are involved in the enlargement and which primary lymph nodes would one expect to find enlarged during the extraoral examination?

Clinical Case RATIONALE

1. The nasopalatine nerve is involved in the patient's discomfort from the thermal burn.
2. The maxillary bone underlies soft tissues in the burn area.
3. The unique intraoral landmark located near or within the burn area is the incisive papilla.
4. The palatine tonsils are enlarged. Palpation of the neck would reveal enlargement of the superior deep cervical lymph nodes.

Trigeminal Nerve and its Sensory Root

The trigeminal nerve (cranial nerve V) comprises the ophthalmic, maxillary, and mandibular branches.
I. Ophthalmic Division (ophthalmic nerve)
  A. Is the first and smallest division and is carried by way of the superior orbital fissure.
  B. Includes the frontal, lacrimal, and nasociliary nerves.
    1. Frontal nerve
      a. Is afferent and located in the orbit.
      b. Comprises a union of the supraorbital nerve from the forehead and anterior scalp and the supratrochlear nerve from the bridge of the nose and medial parts of the upper eyelid and forehead.
      c. Courses along the roof of the orbit toward the superior orbital fissure, where it is joined by the lacrimal and nasociliary nerves to form the ophthalmic nerve.
    2. Lacrimal nerve
      a. Is afferent for the lateral part of the upper eyelid, conjunctiva, and lacrimal gland and

also delivers the postganglionic parasympathetic to the gland.

    b. Runs posteriorly along the lateral roof of the orbit and subsequently joins the frontal and nasociliary nerves near the superior orbital fissure to form the ophthalmic nerve.

  3. Nasociliary nerve

    a. Formed from afferent branches that converge. These include the infratrochlear nerve from the skin of the medial part of the eyelids and side of the nose; ciliary nerves to and from the eyeball; and the anterior ethmoidal nerve from the nasal cavity and paranasal sinuses.

    b. The anterior ethmoidal nerve is formed by the external nasal nerve from the skin of the ala and apex and the internal nasal nerves from the anterior part of nasal septum and lateral walls of the nasal cavity.

    c. Runs within the orbit, superior to the optic nerve; joins the frontal and lacrimal nerves near the superior orbital fissure to form the ophthalmic nerve.

II. Maxillary Division of Trigeminal Nerve (maxillary nerve) (Fig. 3–22)

  A. Is the second division of the trigeminal nerve and is a nerve trunk formed in the pterygopalatine fossa by the convergence of many nerves.

  B. Enters the skull through the foramen rotundum.

  C. Contains the following branches: zygomatic, infraorbital, anterior superior alveolar, middle superior alveolar, posterior superior alveolar, greater palatine, lesser palatine, and nasopalatine nerves.

    1. Zygomatic nerve

      a. Is afferent and composed of the union of the zygomaticofacial and zygomaticotemporal nerves in the orbit.

      b. Conveys postganglionic parasympathetic fibers from the lacrimal gland to the lacrimal nerve.

      c. Courses posteriorly along the lateral orbit floor, enters the pterygopalatine fossa through the inferior orbital fissure, and subsequently joins the maxillary nerve.

    2. Infraorbital nerve (IO)

      a. Is afferent and is formed by a union of cutaneous branches from the upper lip, medial part of cheek, lower eyelid, and side of the nose.

      b. Passes into the infraorbital foramen and travels through the infraorbital canal, along with infraorbital blood vessels, where it is joined by the anterior superior alveolar nerve.

      c. Passes from the infraorbital canal and groove into the pterygopalatine fossa through the inferior orbital fissure.

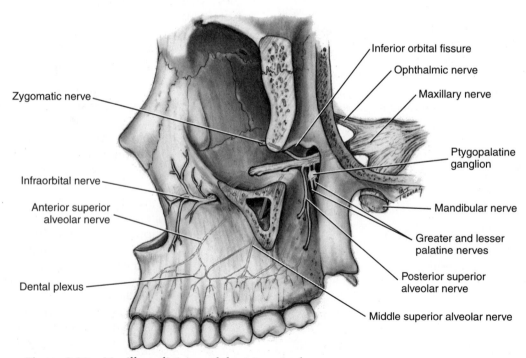

Figure 3.22 Maxillary division of the trigeminal nerve. (From Fehrenbach MJ, Herring SW: Illustrated Anatomy of the Head and Neck. Philadelphia, WB Saunders, 1996, p. 201.)

d. After it leaves the infraorbital groove, and within the pterygopalatine fossa, it receives the posterior superior alveolar nerve.

3. Anterior superior alveolar (ASA) nerve
   a. Is afferent for the maxillary central incisors, lateral incisors, and maxillary canines by way of the dental and interdental branches; forms the dental plexus and innervates overlying facial gingiva.
   b. Ascends along the anterior wall of the maxillary sinus to join the infraorbital nerve in the infraorbital canal.

4. Middle superior alveolar (MSA) nerve
   a. Is afferent for the maxillary premolar teeth and possibly the mesial buccal root of the maxillary first molars.
   b. Originates from the dental, interdental, and interradicular branches and forms the dental plexus.
   c. Ascends to join the infraorbital nerve by running in the lateral wall of the maxillary sinus.
   d. Communicates with both ASA and PSA nerves.
   e. May or may not be present; if not present, area is innervated by both ASA and PSA nerves, but primarily the ASA nerve.

5. Posterior superior alveolar (PSA) nerve
   a. Is afferent for most parts of the maxillary molar teeth (possibly mesiobuccal root of maxillary first molars) and maxillary sinus.
   b. Joins the infraorbital nerve (or maxillary nerve directly) in the pterygopalatine fossa.
   c. Some branches remain external to the posterior surface of the maxilla and provide innervation for the buccal gingiva overlying the maxillary molars.
   d. Other branches originate from the dental, interdental, and interradicular branches, forming a dental plexus.
   e. All internal branches exit from the posterior superior alveolar foramina.
   f. Both external and internal branches ascend along the maxillary tuberosity, which forms in the posterolateral wall of the maxillary sinus, to join the infraorbital or maxillary nerve.

6. Greater palatine nerve (anterior palatine)
   a. Is afferent for the posterior hard palate and posterior lingual gingiva.
   b. Is located between the mucoperiosteum and bone of the anterior hard palate.
   c. Communicates with terminal fibers of the nasopalatine nerve.
   d. Enters the greater palatine foramen in the palatine bone to travel in the pterygopalatine canal, along with the greater palatine blood vessels and lesser palatine nerves and blood vessels.
   e. Ascends through the pterygopalatine canal, toward the maxillary nerve in the pterygopalatine fossa.

7. Lesser palatine nerve (posterior palatine)
   a. Is afferent for the soft palate and palatine tonsillar tissues.
   b. Enters the lesser palatine foramen in the palatine bone, along with the lesser palatine blood vessels.
   c. Joins the greater palatine nerve and blood vessels in the pterygopalatine canal.
   d. Ascends through the pterygopalatine canal, toward the maxillary nerve in the pterygopalatine fossa.

8. Nasopalatine (NP) nerve
   a. Is afferent for the anterior hard palate, lingual gingiva of maxillary anterior teeth, and nasal septal tissues.
   b. Originates in the mucosa of the anterior hard palate.
   c. Communicates with the greater palatine nerve.
   d. Has right and left nerves, which enter the incisive canal by way of the incisive foramen.
   e. Subsequently travels along the nasal septum.

III. Mandibular Division of the Trigeminal Nerve (mandibular nerve) (Fig. 3–23).
   A. Is the largest of the three divisions that form the trigeminal nerve.
   B. Has meningeal and muscular branches, which arise from the trunk before its separation into two trunks. The main trunk is formed by the union of an anterior trunk and posterior trunk in the infratemporal fossa, before it passes through the foramen ovale.
      1. The anterior trunk of the mandibular division is formed by a union of the buccal nerve and muscular branches.
      2. The posterior trunk is formed by a union of the auriculotemporal, lingual, and inferior alveolar nerves.
   C. The mandibular division joins the ophthalmic and maxillary nerves to form the trigeminal ganglion of the trigeminal nerve.
   D. Includes the buccal, muscular, auriculotemporal, lingual, inferior alveolar, mental, incisive, and mylohyoid nerves.
      1. Buccal nerve (long buccal)
         a. Is afferent for the skin of the cheek, buccal mucous membranes, and buccal gingiva of the mandibular posterior teeth.

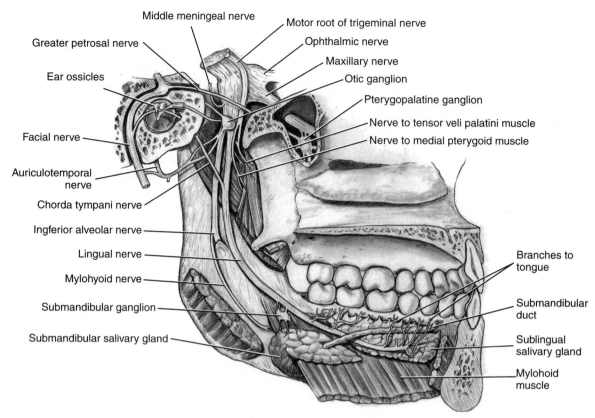

Figure 3.23 Mandibular division of the trigeminal nerve.
(From Fehrenbach MJ, Herring SW: Illustrated Anatomy of the Head and Neck. Philadelphia, WB Saunders, 1996, p. 206.)

b. Is located on the surface of the buccinator muscle and travels posteriorly in the cheek, deep to the masseter muscle.

c. Subsequently crosses in front of the anterior border of the ramus, between the two heads of the lateral pterygoid muscle, to join the anterior trunk.

2. Muscular branches
   a. Arise from the motor root of the trigeminal nerve.
   b. Have deep temporal nerves that are efferent for temporal muscle.
   c. Includes the masseteric nerve, which is efferent for the masseter muscle, and a sensory branch to the temporomandibular joint.
   d. Includes the lateral pterygoid nerve, which is efferent for the lateral pterygoid muscle.

3. Auriculotemporal nerve
   a. Is efferent for the external ear and scalp.
   b. Subsequently joins the posterior trunk of the mandibular nerve.

4. Lingual nerve
   a. Is afferent for the general sensation of body of the tongue, floor of the mouth, and lingual gingiva of the mandibular teeth.
   b. Is formed from afferent branches from the body of the tongue that travel along the lateral surface of the tongue.
   c. Subsequently passes posteriorly from the medial to the lateral side of the submandibular salivary gland.
   d. Communicates with the submandibular ganglion located superior to the deep lobe of the submandibular salivary gland, which is part of the parasympathetic efferent innervation for sublingual and submandibular salivary glands (note: chorda tympani travels along with the lingual nerve).
   e. At the base of the tongue, it ascends and runs between the medial pterygoid muscle and mandible, anterior and slightly medial to the inferior alveolar nerve.
   f. Subsequently continues to travel upward; joins the posterior trunk of the mandibular nerve.

5. Inferior alveolar (IA) nerve
   a. Is efferent for the mandibular posterior teeth and is formed from a union of the mental and incisive nerves.

b. Subsequently continues to travel posteriorly through the mandibular canal, along with the inferior alveolar nerve and the alveolar blood vessels.

c. Is joined by dental, interdental, and inter-radicular branches from the mandibular posterior teeth, forming a dental plexus.

d. Subsequently exits the mandible through the mandibular foramen, where it is joined by the mylohyoid nerve.

e. Subsequently travels lateral to the medial pterygoid muscle, between the sphenomandibular ligament and ramus and within the pterygomandibular space, posterior and slightly lateral to the lingual nerve.

f. Subsequently joins the posterior trunk of the mandibular nerve.

6. Mental nerve
   a. Is composed of external branches that are afferent for the chin, lower lip, and labial mucosa near the mandibular anterior teeth.
   b. Subsequently enters the mental foramen to merge with the incisive nerve to form the inferior alveolar nerve in the mandibular canal.

7. Incisive nerve
   a. Is afferent and composed of dental branches from the anterior mandibular teeth and in-terdental branches, which form a dental plexus.
   b. Subsequently merges with the mental nerve, just posterior to the mental foramen, to form the inferior alveolar nerve in the mandibular canal.

8. Mylohyoid nerve
   a. Is a branch of the inferior alveolar nerve after it exits the mandibular foramen.
   b. Subsequently pierces the sphenomandibular ligament; runs in the mylohyoid groove and subsequently onto the lower surface of the mylohyoid muscle.
   c. Is efferent for the mylohyoid muscle and anterior belly of the digastric muscle.

Facial Nerve

The facial nerve (cranial nerve VII) has the following branches: greater petrosal, chorda tympani, posterior auricular, stylohyoid, and posterior digastric. It also inner-vates the muscles of facial expression.

I. Carries both efferent and afferent nerves.

II. Emerges from the brain and enters the internal acoustic meatus; gives off efferent branches to the middle ear muscle and greater petrosal and chorda tympani nerves, which carry parasympathetic fibers.

III. Main trunk subsequently emerges from the skull through the stylomastoid foramen and gives off the posterior auricular nerve and a branch to the posterior belly of the digastric and stylohyoid muscles.

IV. Subsequently passes into the parotid salivary gland and forms numerous branches to supply the muscles of facial expression, but not the parotid.

A. Greater petrosal nerve
   1. Branches off the facial nerve before it exits the skull.
   2. Has efferent fibers that are preganglionic para-sympathetic fibers to the pterygopalatine gan-glion in the pterygopalatine fossa.
   3. Has postganglionic fibers that arise in the pterygopalatine ganglion, subsequently join with branches of the maxillary division of the trigeminal nerve, and are carried to the lacrimal gland (via zygomatic and lacrimal nerves), nasal cavity, and minor salivary glands of the hard and soft palate.
   4. Is also afferent for taste sensation in the palate.

B. Chorda tympani nerve
   1. Is a branch of the facial nerve and is parasympa-thetic; is efferent for the submandibular and sublingual salivary glands and afferent for taste sensation for the body of the tongue.
   2. After branching off the facial nerve within the petrous part of temporal bone, it crosses the tympanic membrane (eardrum) and exits the skull by the petrotympanic fissure, located immediately posterior to the temporomandibu-lar joint.
   3. Subsequently travels with the lingual nerve along the floor of the mouth in the same nerve bundle.
   4. In the submandibular triangle, appears as part of the lingual nerve and has communication with the submandibular ganglion.

C. Posterior auricular, stylohyoid, and posterior di-gastric nerves
   1. Are given off of the facial nerve after it exits the stylomastoid foramen.
   2. Are all efferent; the posterior auricular nerve supplies the occipital belly of the epicranial muscle and the other two nerves supply the stylohyoid muscle and posterior belly of the digastric muscle, respectively.

D. Branches to the muscles of facial expression
   1. Are efferent branches of the facial nerve, which originate in the parotid salivary gland and pass to the muscles they innervate.
   2. Include the temporal, zygomatic, buccal, (mar-ginal) mandibular, and cervical nerves.
   3. Are rarely seen as five independent nerves and may vary in number and connect irregularly.

Lymphatic System

The lymphatic system is part of the immune system and helps to fight disease. It is a network of lymphatic vessels that link lymph nodes throughout most of body. Examina-tion for and documentation of the presence of palpable nodes is essential to identifying disease, such as cancer or infection, its area of involvement, and the need for referral.

Lymph Nodes of the Head

Lymph nodes of the head are either superficial or deep.

I. Superficial Nodes of the Head (Fig. 3–24)
   A. Occipital nodes
      1. Are located bilaterally in the occipital region.
      2. Drain this part of the scalp.
      3. Empty into the inferior deep cervical nodes.
   B. Retroauricular nodes (mastoid or posterior auricular)
      1. Are located posterior to each ear and drain the surrounding area.
      2. Empty into the superior deep cervical nodes.
   C. Anterior auricular nodes
      1. Are anterior to each ear and drain the surrounding area.
      2. Empty into the superior deep cervical nodes.
   D. Superficial parotid nodes (paraparotid)
      1. Are superficial to each parotid salivary gland and drain the surrounding area.
      2. Empty into the superior deep cervical nodes.
      3. Some group anterior auricular and superficial parotid together.

   E. Facial lymph nodes
      1. Are positioned along the length of the facial vein to drain the area.
      2. Are further categorized into four subgroups: malar (or infraorbital), nasolabial, buccal, and mandibular nodes.
      3. Drain into each other and subsequently into the submandibular nodes.
II. Deep Lymph Nodes of the Head
   A. Deep parotid lymph nodes
      1. Are located deep in the parotid salivary gland.
      2. Drain the middle ear, auditory tube, and parotid.
      3. Drain into the superior deep cervical nodes.
   B. Retropharyngeal lymph nodes
      1. Are located near the deep parotid nodes.
      2. Drain the pharynx, palate, paranasal sinuses, and nasal cavity.
      3. Drain into the superior deep cervical nodes.

Cervical Lymph Nodes

Cervical lymph nodes are located in the neck and are divided into superficial and deep branches. Many clinicians record cervical nodes in relationship to the SCM, placing the nodes into three overlapping categories:

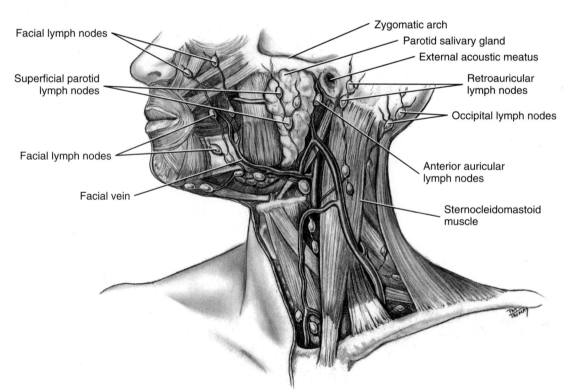

Figure 3.24 Superficial nodes of the head.
(From Fehrenbach MJ, Herring SW: Illustrated Anatomy of the Head and Neck. Philadelphia, WB Saunders, 1996, p. 252.)

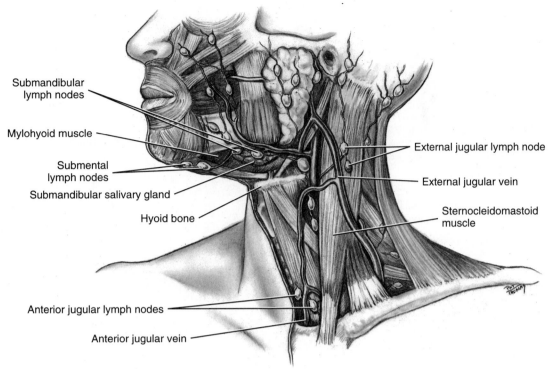

Figure 3.25   Superficial cervical nodes.
(From Fehrenbach MJ, Herring SW: Illustrated Anatomy of the Head and Neck. Philadelphia, WB Saunders, 1996, p. 255.)

superior or inferior, anterior or posterior, and superficial or deep.

I.   Superficial Cervical Nodes (Fig. 3–25)
   A.   Submental nodes
      1.   Are located inferior to the chin in the submental fascial space, superficial to the mylohyoid muscle and near the midline.
      2.   Drain both sides of the chin, lower lip, floor of the mouth, apex of the tongue, and mandibular incisors.
      3.   Subsequently empty into the submandibular nodes or deep cervical nodes.
   B.   Submandibular nodes
      1.   Are located at the inferior border of the ramus, superficial to the submandibular salivary gland and within the submandibular fascial space.
      2.   Drain the cheeks, upper lip, body of tongue, anterior part of hard palate, and all teeth (except the mandibular incisors and maxillary third molars).
      3.   May be secondary nodes for the submental nodes and facial regions because they also drain the sublingual and submandibular salivary glands.
      4.   Subsequently empty into the superior deep cervical nodes.
   C.   External jugular nodes (superficial lateral cervical)

      1.   Are located on each side of the neck along the external jugular vein, superficial to the sterno-cleidomastoid muscle.
      2.   May be secondary nodes for the occipital, retroauricular, anterior auricular, and superficial parotid nodes.
      3.   Subsequently empty into the superior or inferior deep cervical nodes.
   D.   Anterior jugular nodes (superficial anterior cervical)
      1.   Are located on each side of the neck along the length of the anterior jugular vein, anterior to the sternocleidomastoid muscle; drain infrahyoid region of neck.
      2.   Subsequently empty into inferior deep cervical nodes.

II.   Deep Cervical Nodes (Fig. 3–26)
   A.   Superior deep cervical nodes
      1.   Are located deep beneath the sternocleidomastoid muscle, superior to where the omohyoid muscle crosses the internal jugular vein.
      2.   Drain the posterior nasal cavity, posterior part of the hard palate, soft palate, base of tongue, maxillary third molars, esophagus, trachea, and thyroid gland.
      3.   May be secondary nodes for all other nodes of the head and neck (except occipital nodes and inferior deep cervical nodes).

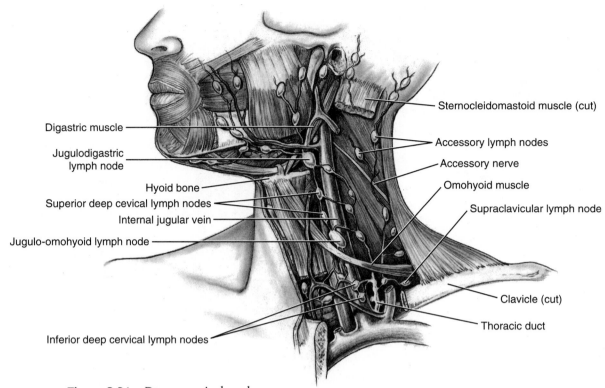

Figure 3.26 Deep cervical nodes.
(From Bath-Balogh M, Fehrenbach MJ: Illustrated Dental Embryology and Anatomy. Philadelphia, WB Saunders, 1997, p. 257.)

4. Empty into the inferior deep cervical nodes or directly into the jugular trunk.
5. The jugulodigastric lymph node (tonsillar node) easily becomes palpable when the palatine tonsils and/or pharynx are inflamed; is located below the posterior belly of the digastric muscle.

B. Inferior deep cervical lymph nodes
1. Are a continuation of the superior deep cervical group.
2. Are located deep to the sternocleidomastoid muscle, at the level where the omohyoid muscle crosses the internal jugular vein or inferior to this point; extend inferiorly into the supraclavicular fossa, superior to each clavicle.
3. Drain the posterior part of the scalp and neck, the superficial pectoral region, and part of the arm.
4. May be secondary nodes for the occipital and superior deep cervical nodes.
5. Efferent vessels form a jugular trunk, which is one of the tributaries of the right lymphatic duct (on right side) and thoracic duct (on the left).
6. Communicate with the axillary lymph nodes that drain the breast region.

7. The jugulo-omohyoid lymph node is located at the crossing of the omohyoid muscle and internal jugular vein and drains the tongue and submental region.

C. Accessory nodes
1. Are located along the accessory nerve.
2. Drain the scalp and neck.
3. Empty into the supraclavicular nodes.

D. Supraclavicular nodes (transverse cervical)
1. Are located along the clavicle.
2. Drain the lateral cervical triangles.
3. May empty into one of the jugular trunks or into the right lymphatic duct or thoracic duct.

Tonsils

Tonsils are masses of lymphoid tissue that drain into the superior deep cervical nodes, especially the jugulodigastric lymph node. They include the palatine, lingual, pharyngeal, and tubal tonsils.

I. Palatine Tonsils (see Fig. 3–2)
A. Are two rounded masses of variable size located between the anterior and posterior tonsillar pillars.

II. Lingual Tonsil (see Fig. 3–2)
A. Is an indistinct layer of lymphoid tissue located on the base of the dorsal surface of tongue.

III. Pharyngeal Tonsils (adenoids)
  A. Are located on the posterior wall of naso-pharynx.
  B. Are normally enlarged in children.
IV. Tubal Tonsils
  A. Are located in the nasopharynx, posterior to openings of the eustachian or auditory tubes.

 Clinical Case **STUDY**

Two-year-old Ethan James, while waiting for his bath, slips and hits his upper front teeth on the edge of the bathtub. He bleeds profusely and his upper lip is severely swollen. His parents rush him to the dental office. An intraoral examination reveals that both primary maxillary central incisors are intruded (pushed up into the sockets).

Clinical Case QUESTIONS

1. How many teeth make up the primary dentition?
2. At 2 years of age, which teeth should be fully erupted?
3. Identify the blood and nerve vessels that are most likely to be injured in this situation.
4. What effect might this trauma have on the child's physical oral development?

Clinical Case RATIONALES

1. There are 20 teeth in the primary dentition.
2. At 2 years of age, the primary maxillary and mandibular central and lateral incisors, canines, and first molars are fully erupted. The primary second molars erupt between the ages of 27 and 29 months, depending on the arch.
3. The infraorbital artery innervates the upper lip and the anterior superior alveolar nerve innervates the maxillary anterior teeth and bone.
4. An intrusion injury occurs when the tooth root is forcibly compressed into the alveolar bone. This severe injury caused damage to the patient's primary maxillary central incisor roots and the alveolar bone. When this injury occurs in a primary dentition, the displacement of the tooth also can cause injury to adjacent developing permanent maxillary teeth. Enamel development of the permanent maxillary central and lateral incisors begins 3 to 4 months after birth and continues to age 5; therefore his permanent maxillary central incisors may possibly exhibit enamel defects.

Content Review

The Dentition

The dentition consists of the natural teeth in the jaw bones and includes both primary and permanent dentitions.

Primary Dentition

The primary dentition (deciduous) (Fig. 3–27) is the first dentition. It consists of twenty teeth (8 incisors, 4 canines, and 8 molars), which are exfoliated or shed and replaced by the permanent dentition.

Permanent Dentition

The permanent dentition (Fig. 3–28) is the second dentition; it replaces the primary dentition. It consists of 32 teeth (8 incisors, 4 canines, 8 premolars and 12 molars). The anterior and premolar teeth are succedaneous and have primary predecessors; the molars are nonsuccedaneous and do not have primary predecessors.

Tooth Types

Tooth types are related to the masticatory function of the tooth and to its role in speech and aesthetics. The form and function of each type is similar for both primary and

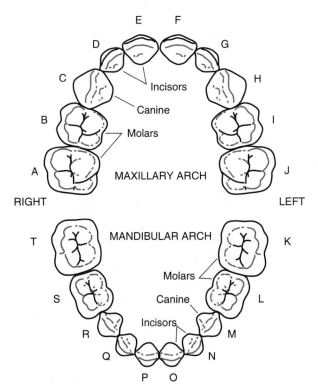

Figure 3.27   Primary dentition. (From Bath-Balogh M, Fehrenbach MJ: Illustrated Dental Embryology and Anatomy. Philadelphia, WB Saunders, 1997, p. 214.)

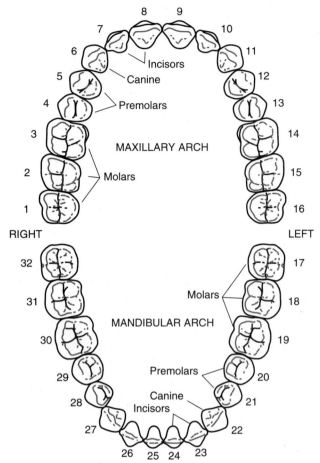

Figure 3.28 Permanent dentition.
(From Bath-Balogh M, Fehrenbach MJ: Illustrated Dental Embryology and Anatomy. Philadelphia, WB Saunders, 1997, p. 214.)

permanent dentitions. The types include incisors, canines, premolars, and molars.

I. Incisors function as instruments for biting and cutting food because of their triangular proximal form.
II. Canines function to pierce or tear food because of their prominent cusp and tapered shape.
III. Premolars, which exist only in the permanent dentition, function to assist molars in grinding food because of their broad occlusal surface and prominent cusps; they also assist canines in piercing and tearing food with their cusps.
IV. Molars function to grind food, assisted by the premolars, because of their broad occlusal surfaces and prominent cusps.

Tooth Designation

Two systems of tooth designation, The Universal Tooth Designation System and the International Standards Organization Designation System (ISO System), are widely used. These systems offer a standardized method of identifying teeth for the purposes of treatment, identification, and documentation.

I. The Universal Tooth Designation System is the most widely used system in the United States and is adaptable to electronic data transfer.
   A. Primary teeth are designated by the capital letters A through T, consecutively, starting with the maxillary right second molar, moving in a clockwise fashion, and ending with the mandibular right second molar.
   B. Permanent teeth are designated by numbers #1 through #32, consecutively, starting with the maxillary right third molar, moving in a clockwise fashion, and ending with the mandibular right third molar.
II. The International Standards Organization Designation System (ISO System) by the World Health Organization is used internationally and is adaptable to electronic data transfer.
   A. Teeth are designated by using a 2-digit code.
   B. The first digit of the code indicates the quadrant and the second indicates the tooth in the quadrant.

Dentition Periods and Eruption Time Table

Dentitions may be in one of three states: the primary, mixed, or permanent period Tables 3-3 and 3-4).

I. The primary dentition period begins with eruption of the primary mandibular central incisor; occurs approximately between 6 months and 6 years of age, and ends when the first permanent tooth, the mandibular first molar, erupts.
II. The mixed dentition period follows the primary dentition period; occurs approximately between 6 and 12 years of age; begins with the eruption of the first permanent tooth (the mandibular first molar) and ends with the shedding of the last primary tooth.

TABLE 3.3	Approximate Eruption Ages for Primary Teeth (in Months)
Maxillary Teeth	**Age (Months)**
Second molar	29
First molar	16
Canine	19
Lateral incisor	11
Central incisor	10
Mandibular Teeth	
Second molar	27
First molar	16
Canine	20
Lateral incisor	13
Central incisor	8

Adapted from Ash MM: Wheeler's Dental Anatomy, Physiology and Occlusion. 7th ed. Philadelphia, WB Saunders, 1993.

TABLE 3.4	Approximate Eruption Ages for Permanent Teeth (in Years)

Maxillary Teeth	Age (Years)
Third molar	17–21
Second molar	12–13
First molar	6
Second premolar	10–12
First premolar	10–11
Canine	11–12
Lateral incisor	8–9
Central incisor	7–8

Mandibular Teeth	
Third molar	17–21
Second molar	11–13
First molar	6–7
Second premolar	11–12
First premolar	10–12
Canine	9–10
Lateral incisor	7–8
Central incisor	6–7

Adapted from Ash MM: Wheeler's Dental Anatomy, Physiology and Occlusion. 7th ed. Philadelphia, WB Saunders, 1993.

III. The permanent dentition period begins with the shedding of the last primary tooth; typically occurs just after 12 years of age and includes the eruption of all permanent teeth.

Dental Anatomy Terminology

Alveolus, alveoli—Bone of tooth socket that surrounds and supports each tooth.

Alveolar process—Tooth-bearing part of jaw bone where each alveolus is located.

Anterior teeth—Incisors and canines; teeth located in the anterior part of the mouth.

Dental arch—Both alveolar processes of the jaw bones—the maxilla and mandible.

ISO System—A tooth identification system that designates areas by a two-digit number, in which at least one of the two digits is zero.

Mandibular teeth—Teeth in the mandibular arch of the lower jaw bone or mandible.

Maxillary teeth—Teeth in the maxillary arch of the upper jaw bones or maxillae.

Midline—An imaginary vertical plane that divides each dental arch into two approximately equal halves (a right and a left half).

Occlusion—The anatomic alignment of teeth and their relationship to the rest of the masticatory system; how the teeth of the mandibular arch contact those of the maxillary arch.

Posterior teeth—Molars and premolars; teeth located in the posterior part of the mouth.

Quadrant—A division of each dental arch into two parts, based on the relationship to the midline; four sections or quadrants make up the oral cavity.

Sextant—A division of each dental arch into three parts, based on the relationship to the midline; six sextants make up the oral cavity.

Tooth Anatomy Terminology (Fig. 3–29)

Anatomical crown—The part of the tooth composed of dentin covered by enamel.

Anatomical root—The part of the tooth composed of dentin covered by cementum.

Cementoenamel junction (CEJ)—The part of the tooth where the enamel of the crown and cementum of the root typically meet.

Clinical crown—The part of the anatomical crown that is visible and not covered by gingiva.

Clinical root—The part of the anatomical root that is visible and not covered by gingiva.

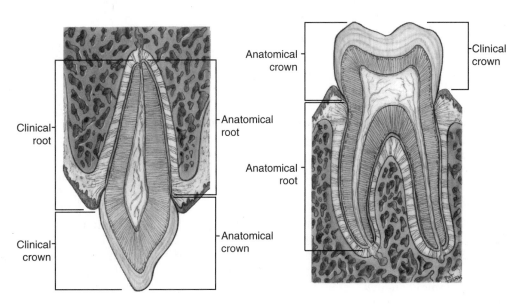

Figure 3.29   Tooth anatomy. (From Bath-Balogh M, Fehrenbach MJ: Illustrated Dental Embryology and Anatomy. Philadelphia, WB Saunders, 1997, p. 222.)

Contact area—Area where adjacent tooth crowns in the same arch physically touch on each proximal surface.

Cusp—A major elevation on the masticatory surface of canines and posterior teeth.

Distal surface—Surface farthest from the midline.

Embrasures—Spaces that occur when two teeth in the same arch contact at the crown curvatures; they are continuous with the interproximal spaces.

Facial surfaces—Surfaces closest to the lips and inner cheeks; termed labial if nearest lips and buccal if nearest cheeks.

Height of contour or crest of curvature—The greatest elevation of the tooth, either incisocervically or occlusocervically, on a specific surface of the crown.

Interproximal space—Area between adjacent tooth surfaces.

Line angle—Is formed by the junction of two crown surfaces.

Linear elevations or ridges—Raised areas on masticatory surfaces that are named according to their location (i.e., lingual, buccal, mesial, distal).

Lingual surfaces—Surfaces closest to the tongue are termed lingual; lingual surfaces closest to the palate are also termed palatal.

Masticatory surface—The chewing surface on the most superior surface of the crown; typically called incisal for anterior teeth and occlusal for posterior teeth.

Mesial surface—Surface closest to the midline.

Point angle—The junction of three crown surfaces.

Proximal surfaces—Include both mesial and distal surfaces between adjacent teeth.

Pulp cavity—Is covered by the inner part of the dentin of both the crown and roots and includes the pulp chamber, pulp canals, apex, apical foramen, and possibly the pulp horns.

Root axis line (RAL)—An imaginary line that represents the long axis of a tooth; drawn through the apex of the root and subsequently through the crown, bisecting the CEJ.

Tooth—Consists of a crown and one or more roots.

Permanent Anterior Teeth

The permanent anterior teeth include the incisors and the canines.

Developmental Considerations of Anterior Teeth

The anterior teeth are composed of four developmental lobes—three labial and one lingual—and two vertical labial developmental depressions. Succedaneous teeth that replace primary teeth are of the same type.

Morphology of Anterior Teeth

An anterior tooth has a long crown and its masticatory surface is incisal. Its outline is trapezoidal from the labial and lingual and triangular from its proximal. Compared with posterior teeth, anterior teeth are wider mesiodistally than labiolingually.

Features of Anterior Teeth

Anterior teeth typically are single-rooted teeth with cingulum on their lingual surfaces.

I. The height of contour for the labial and lingual surfaces of the crown is in the cervical third.

II. Contact areas typically are centered labiolingually on proximal surfaces and have a smaller area than contact areas of posterior teeth.

III. On each proximal surface, there is greater CEJ curvature than in posterior teeth.

IV. Lingual surfaces have a cingulum, which is a raised, rounded area on the cervical third, in varying degrees of development.

V. Ridges are present on lingual surfaces and are bordered mesially and distally by rounded raised borders called marginal ridges.

VI. Some anterior teeth have more complicated lingual surfaces; may have fossa, which are shallow, wide depressions; some have developmental pits located in the deepest part of the fossa.

VII. May have on their lingual surface a developmental groove that marks the junction among developmental lobes.

VIII. The supplemental groove also may be present on the lingual surface, which is more shallow and irregular.

Permanent Incisors

The permanent incisors (Fig. 3–30) comprise two types—the central and the lateral incisors. When newly erupted they may contain three mamelons or rounded enamel extensions on the incisal ridge, which are extensions from labial developmental lobes. Two incisal angles are formed from the incisal ridge on each proximal surface. The incisal ridge is flattened and becomes an incisal edge through attrition. The cingulum, lingual fossa, and marginal ridges are located on the lingual surface at different levels, depending on the type of incisor.

I. Permanent Maxillary Incisors

A. Have crowns that are larger in all dimensions, especially mesiodistally, compared with mandibular incisors; labial surfaces are more rounded from the incisal aspect, with the tooth tapering toward the lingual.

B. Lingual surface features are more prominent than on the mandibular incisors.

C. The incisal edge is just labial to the long axis of the root from either proximal view.

D. The shovel-shaped incisor has greater prominence of lingual marginal ridges and deeper lingua fossa; its lingual pit is susceptible to caries development.

E. Maxillary central and lateral incisors resemble each other more than they resemble the similar type of incisors of the opposing arch; the maxillary central is larger than the lateral incisor, but overall they have a similar form and both are wider mesiodistally than labiolingually.

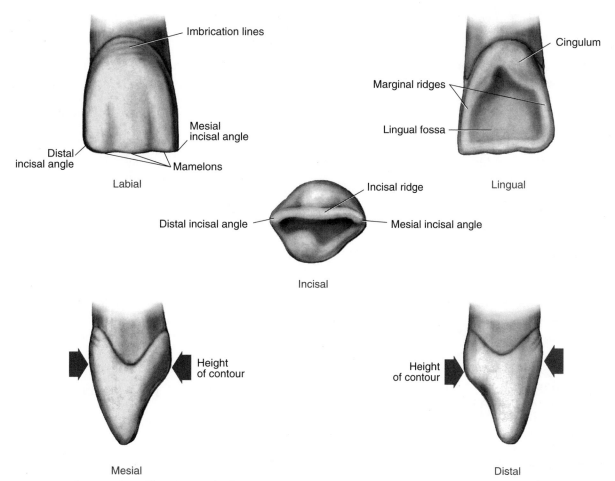

Figure 3.30 Permanent incisors.
(From Bath-Balogh M, Fehrenbach MJ: Illustrated Dental Embryology and Anatomy. Philadelphia, WB Saunders, 1997, p. 232.)

F. Roots are short compared with other maxillary teeth and typically do not have root concavities.
1. Permanent maxillary central incisors (#8 and #9).
  a. Are the largest incisors.
  b. Crown is the widest of any anterior tooth.
    1) Outline when viewed from labial or lingual is trapezoidal.
    2) Lingual surface is narrower overall than the labial.
    3) Has horizontally-placed lingual groove; linguogingival groove or lingual pit may be present.
    4) CEJ curvature on the mesial is deep incisally and has the greatest depth of curvature of any tooth surface in permanent dentition; also has largest height of contour for both labial and lingual surfaces.
  c. Root
    1) Has a conical shape, which is smooth and slightly straight; typically narrows through the middle to blunt the apex.
    2) Is approximately the same length or shorter but wider than the lateral of the same arch.
    3) Is triangular in cervical cross section because it is wider on the labial.
  d. Pulp cavity
    1) Has only one root canal, which is a rather large pulp chamber; has three sharp pulp horns.
2. Permanent maxillary lateral incisor (#7 and #10).
  a. Crown
    1) Has greater variation in form than any other permanent tooth, except for permanent third molars.
    2) Typically resembles the maxillary central incisor in all views of tooth, but has a smaller and slightly more rounded crown.
    3) The horizontal lingual groove is more common and better developed than on the central, with a more common lingual pit.
    4) Outline is more rounded or oval from an incisal view, not triangular as is the central; mesiodistal measurement is wider

than labiolingual measurement and labial surface is more rounded than that of central.

    5) Commonly exhibits partial microdontia (peg lateral) and partial anodontia (congenitally missing).

  b. Root

    1) Is conical in shape, relatively smooth and straight, yet may curve slightly to the distal; same length or longer than central, yet thinner.

    2) Frequently is confused with small mandibular canine, yet typically has no depressions on proximal surface, as is common on mandibular canine.

    3) The apex is not rounded like central, but sharp.

  c. Pulp cavity

    1) Is simple in form, with a single pulp canal and pulp.

II. Permanent Mandibular Incisors

  A. Are the smallest and most symmetrical, uniform teeth.

  B. May experience attrition to the incisal edge, which changes the symmetrical form.

  C. Root is elliptical on the cervical cross section; narrow on the labial and lingual; and wide on both proximal surfaces.

  D. Proximal root concavities also are present and, if deep enough, give the teeth a double-rooted appearance.

1. Permanent mandibular central incisor (#24 and #25)

  a. Crown

    1) Difficult to distinguish between the right and left.

  b. Root

    1) Has pronounced proximal root concavities.

  c. The pulp cavity is simple because it has a single pulp canal and three pulp horns.

2. Permanent mandibular lateral incisor (#23 and #26)

  a. Crown

    1) Is slightly larger than that of central, yet resembles it.

    2) Is not as symmetrical as that of central; from both labial and lingual views, it appears tilted or twisted distally in comparison with the long axis of the tooth.

  b. Root

    1) Has pronounced proximal root concavities, especially on the distal surface, which vary in both length and depth.

  c. Pulp cavity

    1) Is simple; has a single pulp canal and three pulp horns.

Permanent Canines

Permanent maxillary and mandibular canines (cuspids) are similar (Figs. 3–31 and 3–32). They have large cingu-

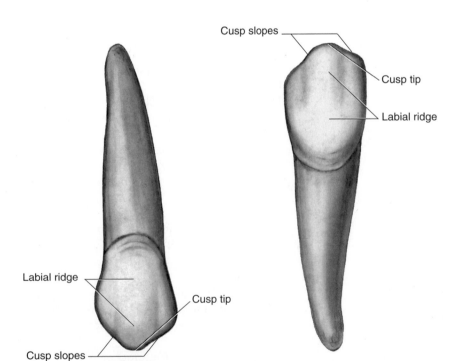

Cusp slopes

Cusp tip

Labial ridge

Labial ridge

Cusp tip

Cusp slopes

Labial View
Permanent Maxillary Right Canine

Labial View
Permanent Mandibular Right Canine

Figure 3.31 Labial view of permanent canines.
(From Bath-Balogh M, Fehrenbach MJ: Illustrated Dental Embryology and Anatomy. Philadelphia, WB Saunders, 1997, p. 246.)

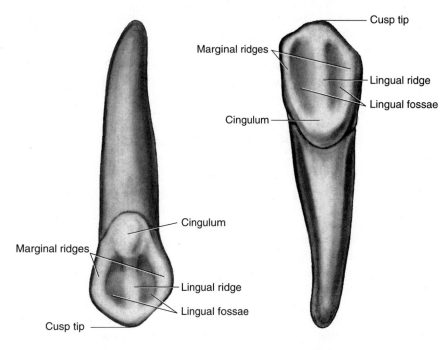

Figure 3.32 Lingual view of permanent canines.
(From Bath-Balogh M, Fehrenbach MJ: Illustrated Dental Embryology and Anatomy. Philadelphia, WB Saunders, 1997, p. 247.)

lum and marginal ridges on their lingual surfaces, which are narrower than the labial surfaces, and crowns that taper lingually. Canines are the longest teeth. Each has a long, thick root, which is externally manifested by the canine eminence. Proximal root concavities are on both proximal root surfaces and are ovoid on cervical cross section, with wide facial and proximal surfaces that show increased convergence to a narrow lingual surface.

I. Permanent Maxillary Canines (#6 and #11)
   A. Crown
      1. Is similar in length or even shorter than that of maxillary central incisor.
      2. Outline is asymmetrical from the incisal view; the distal part appears thinner than the mesial and gives the impression of being 'stretched' to make contact with the first premolar.
      3. The arch space often is partially closed; the tooth may erupt labially or lingually to the surrounding teeth or may fail to erupt and remain impacted.
   B. Root
      1. Is the longest in the maxillary arch.
      2. Has a blunt apex.
      3. Has developmental depressions on both proximal surfaces that are especially pronounced on the distal.
   C. Pulp cavity
      1. Consists of single pulp canal and large pulp chamber, with only one pulp horn.
II. Permanent Mandibular Canines (#22 and #27)
   A. Crown
      1. Can be as long or even longer than the maxillary canine.
      2. Rarely has lingual pits or lingual grooves.
   B. Root
      1. May be as long as maxillary canine, but typically is somewhat shorter; has the longest mandibular root.
      2. Has a slight mesial inclination.
      3. Has more pronounced and often deeper mesial developmental depression than the maxillary canine.
      4. Has a distal developmental depression similar to the mesial one; gives the tooth a double-rooted appearance.
   C. Pulp cavity
      1. Resembles the maxillary canine, with only one pulp horn; may have two separate pulp canals.
      2. One is placed labially and the other lingually; these may join at the apex or have separate apical foramina if the tooth has two canals.

Permanent Posterior Teeth

The permanent posterior teeth include the premolars and molars.

Crowns of Posterior Teeth

The crowns of posterior teeth are trapezoidal when viewed from the buccal and lingual. The height of contour for the buccal surface is in the cervical third and for the lingual surface is in the middle or occlusal third. The posterior teeth are wider labiolingually than mesiodistally, except for the mandibular molars, when compared with anterior teeth. The contact areas of posteriors are wider than those of anteriors, typically are located to the buccal of center, and also are closer to the same level on each proximal surface. On each proximal surface, the CEJ curvature is less pronounced on posterior teeth than on anteriors and may be quite straight.

Occlusal Table of Posterior Teeth

The occlusal tables of posterior teeth (Fig. 3–33) are bordered by raised marginal ridges located on the distal and mesial and have two or more cusps, with four cusp ridges descending from each cusp tip and inclined cuspal planes between them.

I. Has triangular cusp ridges that descend from cusp tips toward central part.

II. May have a transverse ridge that occurs with the joining of two triangular ridges that cross the occlusal table transversely or from the labial to the lingual outline.

III. Has shallow and wide depressions called fossa (plural, fossae); central fossae are located at the converging of cusp ridges in a central point, where there is a junction of grooves and triangular fossa which appears to have a triangular shape at the convergence of cusp ridges and are associated with the termination of the triangular grooves.

IV. Contains developmental pits, where two or more grooves meet; sometimes located in the deepest parts of fossae.

V. Has developmental grooves or primary grooves, which are sharp, deep, and V-shaped linear depressions; the most prominent is the central groove, which generally travels mesiodistally and separates the occlusal table buccolingually.

VI. Has other developmental grooves called marginal grooves, which cross the marginal ridges, and triangular grooves, which separate a marginal ridge from the triangular ridge of a cusp and which at their terminations form the triangular fossae.

VII. Has different levels of supplemental grooves or secondary grooves, which are shallower, more irregular linear depressions.

VIII. Has complex pit and groove patterns, which make these teeth susceptible to caries.

Permanent Premolars: First and Second

Permanent premolars (bicuspids) are succedaneous and replace primary first and second molars. They are sometimes extracted in each quadrant for orthodontic purposes to improve dental arch spacing (typically first premolar). The premolars have a shorter crown than the anterior teeth and their buccal surface is rounded, with a prominent buccal ridge and buccal developmental depressions. The height of contour labially is in the cervical third, similar to anterior teeth, and lingually is in the middle third. Permanent premolars typically have one root, except for the maxillary first premolar, which has two roots. They also have proximal root concavities.

I. Permanent Maxillary Premolars

A. The crown of both types resemble each other more than that of the mandibular premolar. The maxillary first premolar is larger than the maxillary second. The crowns have two cusps of almost equal size, which are centered over the long axis of the tooth from a proximal view. They are shorter occlusocervically than those of maxillary canines, yet slightly longer than those of molars. Unlike those of mandibular premolars, the crowns are centered over the root and show no lingual inclination. The crowns have greater buccolingual than mesiodistal width compared with mandibular premolars.

B. The premolar outline from the proximal is trapezoidal.

C. The occlusal table outline is somewhat hexagonal.

D. The roots on the maxillary premolars are shorter than those of the maxillary canines and the same as those of molars. They show a slight lingual and distal inclination.

E. On cervical cross-section, the root appears elliptical; appearance may be slightly altered by proximal root concavities.

F. The root may penetrate the maxillary sinus during accidental trauma or during tooth extraction because of their proximity. Discomfort from sinusitis may be confused with tooth-related discomfort, or vice-versa.

1. Permanent maxillary first premolars (#5 and #12)
a. Crown
1) Is the widest mesiodistally of all premolars; is wide at the level of contact areas and more narrow at the CEJ.
b. Occlusal table
1) Has a transverse ridge perpendicular to the central groove, and mesial and distal pits.
c. Roots
1) Typically have two root branches or are

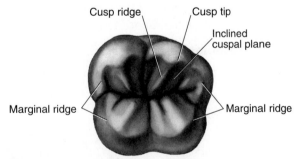

Figure 3.33 Occlusal table of posterior teeth. (From Bath-Balogh M, Fehrenbach MJ: Illustrated Dental Embryology and Anatomy. Philadelphia, WB Saunders, 1997, p. 254.)

bifurcated in apical third; have one buccal root and one lingual or palatal root.

    2) May be fused or laminated.

  d. Pulp cavity shows two pulp horns (one for each cusp) and two pulp canals (one for each root).

2. Permanent maxillary second premolar (#4 and #13)

  a. Crown

    1) Is less angular and more rounded in shape than the maxillary first, with more variations.

  b. Occlusal table

    1) Has numerous supplemental grooves radiating from a central groove; other features are similar to those of the maxillary first premolar.

  c. Roots

    1) Typically are single; these teeth may have two.

    2) Have less pronounced greater root length of the second mesial concavity.

  d. Pulp cavity has two pulp horns and one single pulp canal.

II. Permanent Mandibular Premolars

  A. Crowns do not resemble each other as much as those of maxillary premolars; first premolar is smaller than the second.

  B. Buccal outline shows strong lingual inclination when viewed proximally.

  C. When viewed occlusally, it appears almost round, with a strong buccal ridge.

  D. Contact areas are nearly on the same level and have similar CEJ curvatures.

  E. Proximally, the outlines are rhomboidal, with a lingual incline.

  F. May have more than two cusps; the lingual cusps are always smaller than the buccal.

  G. Root is single, with a slight distal inclination; in cervical cross section is either ovoid or elliptical; may be slightly altered by proximal root concavities, most frequently found on mesial surface.

  1. Permanent mandibular first premolar (#21 and #28)

    a. Crown

      1) Resembles the mandibular canine in many more ways than it does the mandibular second premolar; smaller overall than the canine.

      2) Shows a transition in the dental arch from canine to molar-like second premolar.

    b. Occlusal table

      1) Lingual cusp is very small, typically no more than half the height of the buccal, with four lingual cusp ridges, four lingual inclined cuspal planes, and a lingual triangular ridge.

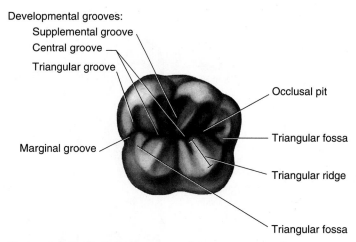

Developmental grooves:
Supplemental groove
Central groove
Triangular groove
Marginal groove
Occlusal pit
Triangular fossa
Triangular ridge
Triangular fossa

Figure 3.34 Occlusal surface of permanent molars. (From Bath-Balogh M, Fehrenbach MJ: Illustrated Dental Embryology and Anatomy. Philadelphia, WB Saunders, 1997, p. 255.)

  c. Root

    1) Is smaller and shorter than the mandibular second premolar.

    2) May have a deep groove on the distal.

    3) Pulp cavity consists of two pulp horns and a single pulp canal; each pulp horn is located within a cusp; the buccal pulp horn more pronounced.

2. Permanent mandibular second premolars (#20 and #29)

  a. Crown

    1) The three-cusp type (tricuspidate form) develops from three lobes; is most common; has one large buccal cusp and two smaller lingual cusps; grooves form a distinctive Y-shaped pattern on the occlusal table; resembles a small molar.

    2) The two-cusp type (bicuspidate form) develops from two lobes; is similar to that of the mandibular first premolars; has a larger buccal cusp and single smaller lingual cusp; the central groove typically is crescent or U-shaped; appears rounded from the occlusal view.

  b. Root

    1) Is larger and longer than that of the first premolar, yet shorter than that of the maxillary premolars.

    2) Has pronounced proximal root concavities.

  c. Pulp cavity

    1) Three-cusp type has three-pointed pulp horns; two-cusp type has two pulp horns.

Permanent Molars: First, Second, and Third

Permanent molars (wisdom teeth) (Figs. 3–34 and 3–35) are nonsuccedaneous and do not replace primary

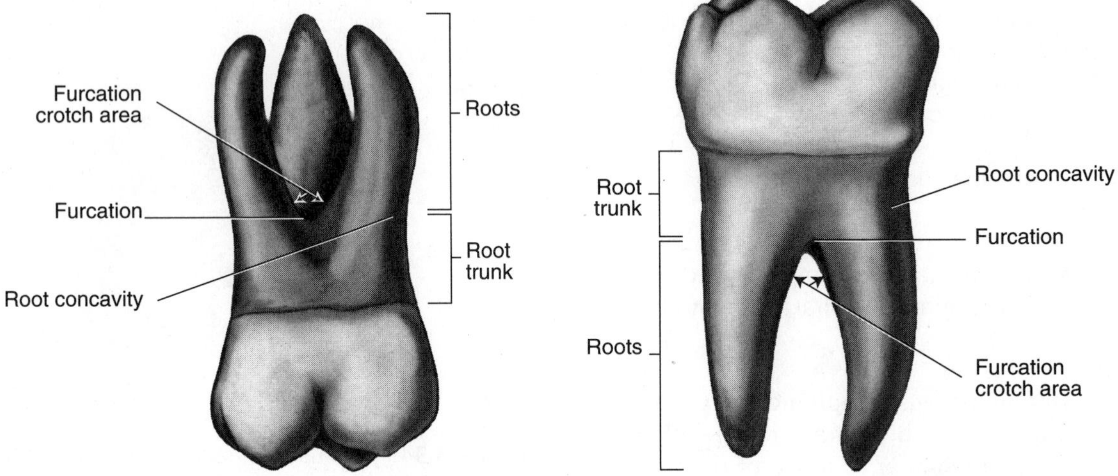

Figure 3.35 Features of permanent molars.
(From Bath-Balogh M, Fehrenbach MJ: Illustrated Dental Embryology and Anatomy. Philadelphia, WB Saunders, 1997, p. 275.)

teeth. They show evidence of developmental lobe separation in the developmental grooves on the occlusal table and do not exhibit buccal developmental depressions. Permanent molars have large crowns in comparison with the rest of the permanent dentition and are shorter occlusocervically than teeth anterior to them. The molar typically has three or more cusps, of which at least two are buccal cusps, and its buccal surface has a prominent cervical ridge running mesiodistally in the cervical one-third. The molar occlusal table is bordered by cusp ridges and marginal ridges that are even more complicated than those of premolars because there are more developmental grooves, supplemental grooves, and occlusal developmental pits. Grooves and pits are located on occlusal and lingual surfaces of the maxillary and on occlusal and buccal surfaces of the mandibular molars. Molars typically are multirooted; the maxillary molars usually have three and the mandibular molars usually have two root branches. A cervical cross-section of the root trunk follows the form of the crown but subsequently divides into the number of root branches. Furcations lie between two or more of these root branches before they divide from the trunk. The furcation crotches are the spaces between the roots at the furcation. Root concavities are found on many root branches and furcal surfaces.

With the loss of periodontal tissue support from advanced periodontal disease, the furcations, furcation crotches, and root concavities of the molars may loose their bony coverage in varying degrees and present a challenge during instrumentation and performance of oral hygiene. Localized enamel hypoplasia from congenital syphilis can result in mulberry molars. When molars have one or more tubercles or accessory cusps, dilaceration also can occur, making extraction and endodontic treatment difficult.

I. Permanent Maxillary Molars
   A. Crowns typically are shorter occlusocervically than the crowns of teeth anterior to them, but are larger in all other measurements than other maxillary teeth. They are wider buccolingually than mesiodistally. From the occlusal, the outline is rhomboidal and from the proximal it is trapezoidal.
   B. The occlusal table (Fig. 3–36) typically has four major cusps, with two cusps on the buccal part and two on the lingual. It has an oblique ridge—a type of transverse ridge formed by the union of the triangular ridge of the DB cusp and the distal cusp ridge of the ML cusp.
   C. The roots typically are trifurcated into three root branches: MB, DB, and lingual (palatal). The lingual branch typically is largest and longest.
   D. When located farther (distally) in the maxillary arch, have shorter and more varied roots in size, shape, and curvature, but are less divergent.

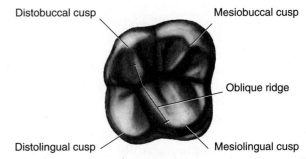

Figure 3.36 Occlusal table of permanent maxillary molars.
(From Bath-Balogh M, Fehrenbach MJ: Illustrated Dental Embryology and Anatomy. Philadelphia, WB Saunders, 1997, p. 278.)

E. The roots show great lingual and moderate distal inclination and have three furcations—typically located on the mesial, buccal, and distal surfaces—that begin near the junction of the cervical and middle thirds.

F. May have root concavities on the mesial surface of the MB root, on the lingual surface of the lingual root, and on all three furcal surfaces.

G. The roots may penetrate the maxillary sinus, from accidental trauma or during tooth extraction, because of their close proximity.

H. Commonly are associated with discomfort from sinusitis.

I. Have a possible lingual pit that is susceptible to carries.

J. Are the teeth most commonly involved in concrescence among those of the permanent dentition.

1. Permanent maxillary first molars (#3 and #14)
   a. Crown
      1) Is the largest among those of the permanent dentition; has much more complex form than that of nearby maxillary premolars.
      2) Is the least variable in form among maxillary molars.
      3) Is composed of five developmental lobes—two buccal and three lingual.
   b. Occlusal table (Fig. 3–37)
      1) ML cusp is the largest cusp; has a rounded cusp tip.
      2) May have the minor cusp of Carabelli, with its groove, which is the smallest cusp.
      3) Has three triangular grooves: MB, ML, and D; also has an oblique ridge.
   c. Roots
      1) Are larger and more divergent than those of the second molar, and more complex in

form than those of the maxillary premolars.
      2) Are twice as long as the crown; thus furcations are well removed from the cervical area.
      3) The pulp cavity typically has one pulp horn for each major cusp; roots typically have three main pulp canals.

2. Permanent maxillary second molars (#2 and #15)
   a. Crown
      1) Is one of two outline types; when viewed occlusally, is either rhomboid or heart-shaped.
   b. Occlusal table
      1) Of rhomboid type has cusps similar to major cusps of the maxillary first molar.
      2) Of heart-shaped type has a DL cusp that is small and sometimes absent.
   c. Roots
      1) Furcation notches are narrower than those of the first molar; have a greater chance of fusion, especially of the buccal roots or all three roots.
   d. Pulp cavity consists of a pulp chamber, three main pulp canals, and four pulp horns.

3. Permanent maxillary third molars (#1 and #16)
   a. Crown
      1) Has no standard form; is the smallest molar and most variable in shape in the permanent dentition.
      2) May exhibit partial microdontia (peg third molar) or partial anodontia (congenitally missing) or may fail to erupt and remain impacted.
   b. Occlusal table
      1) With a heart-shaped occlusal outline is most common; similar to that of the maxillary second molar but with more supplemental grooves; has only three cusps: MB, DB, and ML.
      2) With a rhomboid occlusal outline has four cusps; no oblique ridge is present on small DL cusp.
   c. Roots
      1) Typically are trifurcated and so close together that they are fused, either partially or fully; are poorly developed and shorter than second molar; are curved distally.
      2) May have an accessory root.
   d. Pulp cavity may have a pulp chamber and three pulp canals; the number of pulp horns varies and is dependent on the number of cusps present.

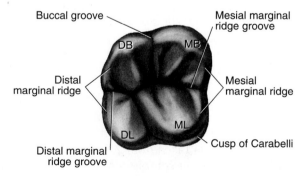

Figure 3.37 Occlusal table of permanent maxillary first molars.
(From Bath-Balogh M, Fehrenbach MJ: Illustrated Dental Embryology and Anatomy. Philadelphia, WB Saunders, 1997, p. 281.)

II. Permanent Mandibular Molars
   A. Have crowns that are wider mesiodistally than buccolingually, similar to anterior teeth.
   B. From an occlusal view, have an outline that is rectangular or pentagonal. The buccal crown outline shows a strong lingual inclination viewed proximally (like nearby premolars), or is rhomboidal.
   C. Have four or five major cusps; always with two lingual cusps of approximately the same width.
   D. Typically have two roots or are bifurcated, with mesial and distal roots; show distal root inclination.
   E. Have two furcations located on the buccal and lingual surfaces, midway between the proximal surfaces.
   F. Have root concavities on the mesial surface of the mesial root and on furcal surfaces of both the mesial and distal roots; concavities on the mesial root are especially prominent if this root also has two root canals.
      1. Permanent mandibular first molars (#19 and #30)
         a. Crown
            1) Is the widest mesiodistally of any permanent tooth because it has a fifth major cusp.
         b. Occlusal table
            1) Has the most complex groove pattern of all mandibular molars: a Y-shaped groove pattern by the cusps and mesiobuccal, distobuccal, and lingual grooves, but no transverse ridges.
         c. Roots
            1) Are widely separated buccally; root trunk is shorter than the second.
            2) Pulp cavity typically has three root canals and five pulp horns.
      2. Permanent mandibular second molars (#18 and #31)
         a. Crown
            1) Is smaller than that of the first molar and rectangular in occlusal view.
         b. Occlusal table (Fig. 3–38)
            1) Has a cross-shaped groove pattern formed by well-defined grooves that divide it into four parts, with nearly equal-sized cusps.
         c. Roots
            1) Are smaller, shorter, less divergent, and closer together than those of the first molar.
         d. Pulp cavity can have two pulp canals (one for each root).
      3. Permanent mandibular third molars (#17 and #32)
         a. Crown
            1) Has no standard form; often has an oval occlusal outline; can be smaller or the same size as that of the first molar of the same arch.

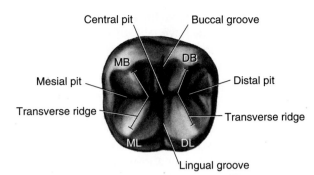

Figure 3.38 Occlusal table of permanent mandibular second molars.
(From Bath-Balogh M, Fehrenbach MJ: Illustrated Dental Embryology and Anatomy. Philadelphia, WB Saunders, 1997, p. 295.)

            2) May fail to erupt and remain impacted or partially erupted; may exhibit partial anodontia (congenitally missing)
         b. Occlusal table
            1) Has two mesial cusps, which are larger than the two distal cusps.
            2) Has an irregular groove pattern, with numerous supplemental grooves and occlusal pits.
         c. Roots
            1) The two roots often are fused, irregularly curved, and shorter than those of the mandibular second molar.
         d. Pulp cavity typically is similar to that of the second molars, with four pulp horns and two or three pulp canals.

Primary Teeth

The primary teeth make up the first dentition.

Developmental Considerations of Primary Teeth

The developmental considerations of primary teeth include patterns of calcification, eruption, and exfoliation.
   I. Are exfoliated or shed and replaced by the permanent dentition.
   II. Begin calcification between 13 and 16 weeks' gestation; by 18 to 20 weeks' gestation have started to calcify.
   III. Eruption of the primary mandibular central incisor occurs first, at an average age of 8 months; thus no primary teeth are visible at birth.
   IV. Root formation takes from 2 to 3 years to be completed, including completion of roots of maxillary second molar; a 6-month delay or acceleration is considered normal.

Features of Primary Teeth

There are 20 primary teeth—10 per dental arch. They include incisors, canines, and molars (Fig. 3–39).

I. Are labeled in the Universal Tooth Designation System by capital letters, A through T.

II. Are smaller and have a whiter enamel than the permanent dentition.

III. Crowns are short relative to the total length and more constricted or narrower at the CEJ, which makes them appear bulbous-shaped.

IV. Masticatory surfaces may show high levels of attrition.

V. Have cervical ridges on both the labial and lingual surfaces of the anteriors and buccal surfaces of the molars.

VI. Roots are narrower and longer when compared with the crown length and also may show partial resorption.

VII. Pulp cavity is relatively large in proportion to the permanent dentition, especially the mesial pulp horns of the molars, which increases the risk of pulpal exposure during cavity preparation.

VIII. Hold eruption space for succedaneous permanent teeth; early assessment for appropriate preventive orthodontic intervention is important; supervising adults and child patients sometimes discount the importance of these teeth.

IX. Have thinner enamel and dentin than the permanent teeth; risk of endodontic complications is greater.

X. May demonstrate extensive extrinsic staining because of Nasmyth membrane.

Primary Incisors

The primary incisors include the primary maxillary and mandibular central and lateral incisors.

I. Primary Maxillary Central Incisor (E and F)
   A. Crown
      1. Is wider mesiodistally than incisocervically (the opposite of its permanent successor); appears thick even at the incisal third (can be altered by attrition); incisal edge is nearly straight.
      2. Has no mamelons and no lingual pits, unlike its permanent successors.
      3. Has cingulum and marginal ridges that are more prominent and lingual fossa that are deeper than in the permanent teeth.
      4. The CEJ curvature curves distinctly toward incisal, but not as much as on its permanent successor.
   B. The root is single and round and tapers evenly to the apex.

II. Primary Maxillary Lateral Incisor (D and G)
   A. Crown
      1. Is similar to that of the central incisor but is much smaller.
      2. Is longer incisocervically than mesiodistally.
      3. Has incisal angles that also are more rounded than those of the central incisor.
   B. The root also is similar to that of the central incisor but the apex is sharper.

III. Primary Mandibular Central Incisor (O and P)
   A. Crown
      1. Looks more like that of primary mandibular lateral incisor than its permanent successor or any other primary maxillary incisor.
      2. Is a symmetrical tooth, similar to its permanent successor; its incisal edge is centered over the root.
      3. Is not as constricted at the CEJ as the primary maxillary central.
      4. Labially, appears wide in comparison with its permanent successor; has mesial and distal outlines that taper evenly from the contact areas.
      5. The lingual surface appears smooth and tapers toward the prominent cingulum, which has less

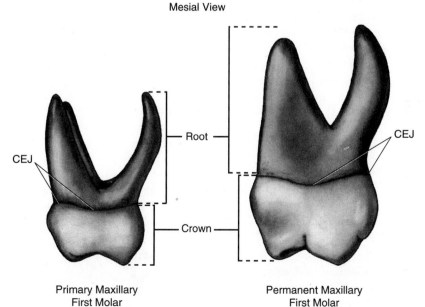

Figure 3.39 Features of primary teeth. (From Bath-Balogh M, Fehrenbach MJ: Illustrated Dental Embryology and Anatomy. Philadelphia, WB Saunders, 1997, p. 301.)

Mesial View

CEJ

Root

CEJ

Crown

Primary Maxillary First Molar

Permanent Maxillary First Molar

pronounced marginal ridges and shallow lingual fossa.

    6. Mesially, is much wider labiolingually than its permanent successor.

  B. The root is single, long, and slender; the labial and lingual surfaces are rounded, yet the proximal surfaces are slightly flattened.

IV. Primary Mandibular Lateral Incisor (Q and N)

  A. Crown

    1. Is similar in form to that of the mandibular central incisor; wider and longer than the central, but not as symmetrical.

    2. Cingulum also is more developed; is offset toward distal, and has a deeper lingual fossa than the central.

    3. Incisal edge slopes distally; its distoincisal angle is more rounded.

  B. Root may have distal curvature in its apical third and distal longitudinal groove.

Primary Canines

The primary canines include the primary maxillary and mandibular canines.

I. Primary Maxillary Canine (C and H)

  A. Crown

    1. Is relatively longer, with a sharper cusp, than that of its permanent successor, when it first erupts; has rounder mesial and distal outlines that greatly overhang the cervical line.

    2. Mesial cusp slope is longer than the distal.

    3. Cingulum, lingual ridge, and marginal ridges are well-developed; tubercle often is present on cingulum.

    4. Lingual ridge divides the lingual surface into shallow mesiolingual and distolingual fossae.

    5. Incisally, is diamond-shaped; the cusp tip is offset distally.

  B. The root is twice as long as the crown, more slender than that of its permanent successor, and is inclined distally.

II. Primary Mandibular Canine (M and R)

  A. Crown

    1. Resembles the primary maxillary canine; is smaller labiolingually; the incisal edge is straight and centered labiolingually.

    2. Distal cusp slope is longer than the mesial.

    3. Lingual surface is smoother than that of the maxillary canine, with a shallow lingual fossa.

  B. The root is long, narrow, and almost twice the crown length; is shorter and more tapered than that of the maxillary canine.

Primary Molars

The primary molars include the primary maxillary and mandibular first and second molars.

I. General Considerations

  A. Crown

    1. Does not resemble any other tooth in either dentition; the primary second in both arches does resemble the permanent first molars that will erupt distal to them.

    2. Is shorter occlusocervically than mesiodistally.

    3. Presence of the newly erupted permanent first molar of either arch may not be noticed.

  B. Occlusal table

    1. Is more constricted buccolingually than the permanent molars, with buccal and lingual surfaces that are flatter occlusal to CEJ.

    2. Anatomy of cusps is not as pronounced as on its permanent successors.

  C. Roots

    1. Are flared beyond the crown outlines; widely separated to create additional space between the roots for developing permanent premolar crowns.

    2. Have a short root trunk, which creates more space for developing permanent premolar crowns.

    3. Have greater root spread of primary molars, along with their narrow shape and lack of root trunk, making primary molars easier to fracture during extraction procedures.

II. Primary Maxillary First Molar (B and I)

  A. Crown

    1. Does not resemble other crowns of either dentition.

    2. From the buccal view, mesial and distal outlines are rounded and constricted at the CEJ.

    3. CEJ on the mesial half of the buccal surface curves around the prominent buccal cervical ridge.

    4. Height of contour on the buccal is at the cervical one third and for the lingual is at the middle one third.

  B. Occlusal table

    1. Can have four cusps: MB, ML, DB, and DL; mesial cusps are largest and distal cusps are very small.

    2. Frequently has only three cusps; DL cusp may be absent.

    3. Has a prominent transverse ridge and oblique ridge running between ML cusp and DB cusp, though not as prominent as on its permanent counterpart.

    4. Has an H-shaped groove pattern and central, mesial triangular, and distal triangular fossae, with the central groove connecting the central, mesial, and distal pits.

    5. Buccal groove separates the MB and DB cusps and the distal triangular fossa contains the disto-occlusal groove.

  C. Roots

    1. Are the same in number and position as those of the permanent dentition.

    2. Have a short root trunk, with three root

branches that are thinner and have greater flare than on the permanent molar.

3. The MB root is wider buccolingually than the DB root; the lingual root is longest and most divergent.

III. Primary Maxillary Second Molar (A and J)
   A. Crown and occlusal table
      1. Most closely resembles the form of the permanent maxillary first molar, yet is smaller in all dimensions.
      2. Typically has a cusp of Carabelli, a minor fifth cusp.

IV. Primary Mandibular First Molar (L and S)
   A. Crown
      1. Is unlike any other tooth of either dentition.
      2. Has a prominent buccal cervical ridge on the mesial half of the buccal surface.
      3. Height of contour on the buccal is at the cervical one third and for the lingual is in the middle one third.
      4. Mesiolingual line angle is rounder than any other.
   B. Occlusal table
      1. Has four cusps; the mesial cusps are larger.
      2. The ML cusp is long, pointed, and angled.
      3. A transverse ridge runs between MB and ML cusps.
   C. The roots are both positioned similarly to those of other primary and permanent mandibular molars.

V. Primary Mandibular Second Molar (K and T)
   A. Crown
      1. Is larger than that of the primary mandibular first molar.
      2. Most closely resembles the form of the permanent mandibular first molar that erupts distal to it.
   B. Occlusal table
      1. Has five cusps.
      2. Has three buccal cusps of nearly equal size.
      3. Has overall oval occlusal shape.
   C. The roots are both positioned similarly to those of other primary and permanent mandibular molars.

Occlusion

Occlusion is the contact relationship between the maxillary and mandibular teeth when the jaws are in a fully closed position. It also refers to the relationship between teeth in the same arch.

Dental Considerations

Dental considerations of occlusion include the effects of eruption and muscle, nerve, and joint function.
   I. Occlusion develops as the primary teeth erupt.
   II. Occlusion involves interrelated factors in development, such as associated musculature, neuromuscular patterns, and temporomandibular joint functioning.

III. Occlusal disharmony may lead to occlusal trauma, which could be an adverse factor in periodontal disease development.
IV. Occlusal disharmonies must be considered during dental treatment; occlusal adjustment involving removal of restorative, prosthetic, or natural tooth material may be needed.

Normal Occlusion

Normal occlusion is ideal occlusion. It rarely exists; thus the concept of normal provides the basis for treatment. The position of the dentition in centric occlusion serves as a basis for reference.
   I. Centric occlusion (CO) or habitual occlusion is a voluntary position of the dentition that allows maximum contact when teeth occlude, serving to equalize the forces of impact.
   II. Overjet occurs when the maxillary dental arch naturally overhangs the mandibular arch facially; overjet is measured in millimeters with a probe.
   III. Overbite occurs as the maxillary incisors overlap the mandibular incisors to allow for maximum contact of the posterior teeth; overbite is measured in millimeters with a probe.
   IV. Contact areas protect the interdental gingiva and stabilize each tooth in the dental arch; open contact allows for food impaction and reduces mesiodistal stability.
   V. Centric stops occur in three places between the two arches where the teeth contact: at the height of cusp contour of supporting cusps, at the marginal ridges, and at the central fossae.
   VI. Centric relation (CR) is the end point of closure of the mandible, when the mandible is in the most retruded position; CR is a base measurement from which to evaluate the patient's occlusion.
   VII. When the mandible is in centric relation, the dentition ideally should be in centric occlusion (CR = CO), with allowance for a 1-mm shift (more is most often caused by premature contacts, which may cause occlusal disharmony).
   VIII. The mandibular rest position is the physiological rest position of the mandible when it is held in a relaxed state; an average of 2 to 3 mm space is between the maxillary and mandibular arch or interocclusal clearance (failure of patient to assume may mean they have parafunctional habits which may be involved in occlusal problems).

Malocclusion

Malocclusion is related to the lack of an overall ideal form of dentition in centric occlusion.
   I. Rarely is directly associated with severe occlusal trauma.
   II. May affect patients by having a negative impact on appearance and may increase difficulty with oral hygiene procedures; may be corrected by an

orthodontist and other specialists when occlusal functioning of dentition is considered.

III. Most commonly includes problems of crowding and excessive overjet of the maxillary incisors.

IV. Often is classified using Angle's Classification of Malocclusion because it gives a starting point for describing a particular case of permanent teeth; does not describe normal or even ideal occlusion.

    A. Classification of malocclusion (Table 3–5)

        1. Primary occlusion

            a. Is similar to that of the permanent dentition; has an ideal form and canine relationship between the arches is the same.

            b. Ideal molar relationship is referred to as the terminal plane, and which facilitates an ideal permanent molar relationship

                1) May involve a flush terminal plane, where the maxillary and mandibular second molars are in an end-to-end relationship.

                2) May involve a mesial step, where the primary mandibular second molar is mesial to the maxillary molar.

                3) May involve distal step, where the mandibular second molar is distal to the maxillary second molar; not an ideal molar relationship and thus not a terminal plane relationship.

            c. Primate spaces between teeth may be present (between maxillary lateral incisor and canine and between mandibular first molar and canine), which allows ideal permanent molar relationship to develop.

TABLE 3.5   Angle's Classification of Malocclusion*

Class	Model	Arch Relationships	Descriptions
Class I		Molar: MB cusp of the maxillary first occludes with the MB groove of the mandibular first. Canines: Maxillary occludes with the distal half of the mandibular canine and the mesial half of the mandibular first premolar.	Dental malalignment(s) present (see text), such as crowding or spacing. Mesognathic profile.
Class II	Division I	Molar: MB cusp of the maxillary first occludes (by more than the width of a premolar) mesial to the MB groove of the mandibular first. Canines: Distal surface of the mandibular canine is distal to the mesial surface of the maxillary canine by at least the width of a premolar.	Division I: Maxillary anteriors protrude facially from the mandibular anterior, with deep overbite. Retrognathic profile.
	Division II		Division II: Maxillary central incisors are either upright or retruded, and lateral incisors are either tipped labially or overlap the central incisors with deep overbite. Mesognathic profile.
Class III		Molar: MB cusp of the maxillary first occludes (by more than the width of a premolar) distal to the MB groove of the mandibular first. Canines: Distal surface of the mandibular is mesial to the mesial surface of the maxillary by at least the width of a premolar.	Mandibular incisors in complete crossbite. Prognathic profile.

*Note that this system deals with the classification of the permanent dentition.
MB, Mesiobuccal.
From Bath-Balogh M, Fehrenbach MJ: Illustrated Dental Embryology, Histology, and Anatomy. Philadelphia, WB Saunders, 1997.

Parafunctional Habits

Movements of the mandible that are not normal motions associated with mastication, speech, or respiratory movements are called parafunctional habits.

I. Often are subconscious.

II. Etiology and treatment are controversial and are not conclusive contributing factors in malocclusion or other dentition problems.

III. Include clenching, in which the teeth are held in centric occlusion for long periods of time without a break (without mandibular rest position or interocclusal clearance).

IV. Include grinding of teeth (bruxism), which is associated with attrition and large areas of hyperkeratinized buccal mucosa.

V. Include thumb/finger sucking, characterized by excessive anterior overjet, lips irreversibly stretched by protruding teeth, deep narrow palate, and callus on thumb/finger.

VI. May enlarge masseter muscles.

Skeletal Considerations with Malocclusion

Skeletal considerations, such as discrepancies between the maxilla and mandible, not only those problems linked with the teeth, may be factors in many malocclusions. Skeletal abnormalities of the jaws can be corrected by an oral surgeon—in conjunction with an orthodontist, or using certain orthodontic appliances to direct bone growth of the jaws.

 CONTENT REVIEW QUESTIONS

1. How many erupted primary teeth does a 4-year-old child typically have?
   A. 10
   B. 12
   C. 16
   D. 18
   E. 20

2. The function of permanent incisors is:
   A. biting and tearing
   B. grinding and cutting
   C. biting and cutting
   D. tearing and grinding

3. Which of the following structures or features are found in numbers of four in the oral cavity only during the permanent dentition period?
   A. molars
   B. dental arches
   C. canine cusp slopes
   D. maxillary premolars
   E. quadrants

4. When viewed proximally, the crown of the permanent mandibular first molar is inclined:
   A. buccally
   B. lingually
   C. mesially
   D. distally

5. Which of the following describes the typical groove pattern on the occlusal table of the permanent mandibular second molar?
   A. linear
   B. snake eyes
   C. crescent
   D. cross

6. Which of the following teeth is succedaneous?
   A. #13
   B. #14
   C. #18
   D. #19

7. Which of the following features is located on the lateral surface of the mandible?
   A. lingula
   B. submandibular fossa
   C. genial tubercles
   D. external oblique line
   E. mental foramen

8. Which of the following bones of the skull is paired?
   A. sphenoid bone
   B. ethmoid bone
   C. occipital bone
   D. vomer
   E. parietal bone

9. Which of the following bones of the skull is a facial bone?
   A. occipital
   B. parietal
   C. sphenoid
   D. zygomatic
   E. frontal

10. Which of the following landmarks of the temporomandibular joint is located on the mandible?
    A. articular eminence
    B. coronoid process
    C. articular fossa
    D. postglenoid process

11. Which of the following lymph nodes are initially affected in a patient who develops an infection in the lower lip after trauma from an accident?
    A. submandibular
    B. deep cervical
    C. submental
    D. buccal
    E. malar

12. Which of the following nerves is also called the trigeminal nerve?
    A. cranial nerve V
    B. cranial nerve VII
    C. cranial nerve X
    D. cranial nerve XII

13. Which of the following nerves to the parotid salivary gland is affected by medication that causes dry mouth?

A. facial nerve
B. trigeminal nerve
C. glossopharyngeal nerve
D. chorda tympani nerve

14. Which of the following provides the most reliable arterial pulse of the body and is located in the head and neck area?
    A. internal carotid artery
    B. common carotid artery
    C. lingual artery
    D. facial artery
    E. superior thyroid artery

15. Which muscle can become enlarged with the parafunctional habit of bruxism?
    A. mentalis
    B. masseter
    C. orbicularis oris
    D. risorius
    E. epicranial

16. Which of the following muscles is palpated during an extraoral examination of the posterior cervical triangle?
    A. suprahyoid muscles
    B. infrahyoid muscles
    C. sternocleidomastoid muscle
    D. temporalis muscle

17. When local anesthesia is used to anesthetize the inferior alveolar nerve, which nerve is secondarily anesthetized?
    A. posterior superior alveolar nerve
    B. anterior superior alveolar nerve
    C. lingual nerve
    D. infraorbital nerve

18. Which teeth may cause sensations that suggest a carious or endodontic situation when only a sinus infection is diagnosed?
    A. maxillary anteriors
    B. maxillary posteriors
    C. mandibular anteriors
    D. mandibular posteriors

19. Which of the following salivary glands is commonly involved in stone formation?
    A. parotid
    B. submandibular
    C. sublingual
    D. submandibular and sublingual

20. Which of the following structures divides the tongue into the body and the base?
    A. circumvallate lingual papilla
    B. sulcus terminalis
    C. foramen cecum
    D. median lingual sulcus
    E. lingual tonsil

21. Which of the following in the primary dentition will *not* allow for the efficient eruption of a normal permanent dentition?
    A. presence of primate spaces
    B. mesial step

C. distal step
D. flush terminal plane

22. Which of the following terms is used to describe the maxillary incisors overlapping the mandibular incisors in centric occlusion?
    A. overbite
    B. cross-bite
    C. overjet
    D. end-to-end

23. Which of the following nerves or branches of a nerve cause discomfort during disorders of the temporomandibular joint?
    A. lingual
    B. auriculotemporal
    C. inferior alveolar
    D. buccal

24. Which pair of bones forms the floor of the nasal cavity?
    A. frontal and ethmoid
    B. ethmoid and lacrimal
    C. lacrimal and maxillary
    D. maxillary and palatine
    E. zygomatic and palatine

25. Which of the following methods is MOST commonly used in America for the designation of teeth?
    A. Universal Tooth Designation System
    B. Palmer Method for Tooth Designation
    C. International Standards Organization Designation System for Teeth

26. Which of the following statements concerning the pterygoid plexus is CORRECT?
    A. located around the infrahyoid muscles
    B. protects the superficial temporal artery
    C. contains valves to prevent the backflow of blood
    D. injury can lead to hematoma

27. Which of the following permanent teeth has an oblique ridge?
    A. mandibular second molar
    B. maxillary first molar
    C. mandibular third molar
    D. maxillary third molar

28. Which permanent tooth has a buccal pit that is susceptible to caries?
    A. mandibular first molar
    B. maxillary first molar
    C. mandibular second molar
    D. maxillary second molar

29. Which of the following structures is located just posterior to the most distal molar of the mandibular dentition?
    A. maxillary tuberosity
    B. median palatine suture
    C. incisive foramen
    D. greater palatine foramen
    E. retromolar triangle

30. The mandibular third molar, compared with the mandibular second molar, is:
    A. larger in the crown

B. less smooth on its occlusal surface
C. less variable in form
D. longer in the roots

31. Which of the following nerves supplies the muscles of mastication?
    A. hypoglossal
    B. vagus
    C. facial
    D. chorda tympani
    E. trigeminal

32. The submandibular duct opens into the oral cavity:
    A. opposite the maxillary second molar
    B. on the sublingual caruncle
    C. on the buccal mucosa
    D. at the base of the mandibular labial frenum

33. Which of the following permanent teeth typically has two roots?
    A. maxillary first molar
    B. maxillary second premolar
    C. maxillary first premolar
    D. maxillary third molar

34. Which of the following permanent teeth has two pulp canals?
    A. maxillary first premolar
    B. mandibular first premolar
    C. maxillary first molar
    D. mandibular first molar

35. Which of the following muscles, when fully contracted, helps close the jaws?
    A. lateral pterygoid
    B. platysma
    C. mentalis
    D. buccinator
    E. temporalis

REVIEW QUESTION RATIONALES

1. **E** All of a 4-year-old child's primary teeth would have erupted in the oral cavity because the average age for primary dentition completion is approximately age 3. There are 20 teeth in the primary dentition.

2. **C** Incisors function as instruments for biting and cutting food during mastication because of their incisal ridge, triangular proximal form, and arch position.

3. **D** It is only during the permanent dentition period that four maxillary premolars are present. Two types of molars are found during the primary dentition period—first and second molars. Three types of molars are found during the permanent dentition period. Only two arches are found in both the primary and permanent dentition periods. Only two canine cusp slopes per tooth are found during both periods. There are four quadrants, but they are present during both the primary and permanent dentition periods.

4. **B** All permanent mandibular molars also show a strong lingual inclination when viewed proximally.

This inclines the crown lingually on the root base, bringing the cusps into proper occlusion with their maxillary antagonists and the distribution of forces along the long axis.

5. **D** A cross-shaped groove pattern is formed when the well-defined central groove is crossed by the buccal groove and lingual groove, dividing the occlusal table into four parts that are nearly equal.

6. **A** Tooth #13 is the permanent second premolar, which is succedaneous for the primary second molar. All of the rest of the teeth listed are permanent molars and all molars are nonsuccedaneous because they do not have primary predecessors and they erupt distal to the primary second molar.

7. **E** The mental foramen is located on the lateral surface of the mandible. All of the other structures listed are located on the internal or medial surface of the mandible.

8. **C** The occipital bone is the only paired bone of the skull. All of the other bones are single bones of the skull.

9. **D** The zygomatic bone is considered a facial bone because it helps create the face. All of the other bones listed are considered cranial bones because they form the cranium.

10. **B** The coronoid process is located on the mandible and is part of the temporomandibular joint. All of the other features listed are part of the joint but are located on the temporal bone.

11. **C** The lower lip drains directly into the submental lymph nodes, which serve as the primary nodes during an infection. The submandibular and cervical lymph nodes would serve as secondary nodes if the infection progressed. The buccal and malar lymph nodes drain the upper and middle cheek.

12. **A** The trigeminal nerve also is considered cranial nerve V. Cranial nerve VII is the facial nerve. Cranial nerve X is the vagus nerve. Cranial nerve XII is the hypoglossal nerve. However, all these nerves innervate important structures of the oral cavity.

13. **C** The parotid salivary gland is supplied by the glossopharyngeal nerve (preganglionic parasympathetic innervation). Even though the facial nerve travels through the parotid gland, it does not supply it. The chorda tympani supplies the submandibular and sublingual salivary glands, which also may be affected by medication. The trigeminal nerve serves many other oral cavity structures but not the parotid.

14. **B** The common carotid artery provides the reliable carotid pulse from the carotid sinus, which is a swelling of the common carotid before it bifurcates into the internal and external carotid arteries. The other arteries listed are branches off of the internal carotid artery after the bifurcation.

15. **B** The masseter muscle can become enlarged or undergo hypertrophy in a patient who habitually grinds his or her teeth (bruxism). The action of the masseter muscle during bilateral contraction of the

entire muscle is to elevate the mandible, thus raising the lower jaw. Elevation of the mandible occurs during closing of the jaws or grinding of the teeth. The rest of the muscles are those of facial expression and not of mastication.

16. **C** The sternocleidomastoid muscle divides each side of the neck into the anterior and posterior cervical triangle. The posterior cervical triangle is located on the side of the neck and the anterior cervical triangle corresponds to the anterior region of the neck that contains the suprahyoid and infrahyoid muscles. The temporal muscle is located in the temporal region on the lateral surface of the skull.

17. **C** At the base of the tongue, the lingual nerve ascends and runs between the medial pterygoid muscle and the mandible, anterior and slightly medial to the inferior alveolar nerve. Thus the lingual nerve is anesthetized by an inferior alveolar anesthetic nerve block. The other nerves listed innervate structures of the maxilla.

18. **B** Discomfort from sinusitis can be confused with tooth-related discomfort from the maxillary posterior teeth because their roots are in close proximity to the maxillary sinus. All of the other teeth listed are not near the maxillary sinus, which is the sinus most commonly involved in sinus infections.

19. **B** The duct for the submandibular gland is the submandibular duct. This long duct travels along the anterior floor of the mouth. Its tortuous upward travel for a considerable distance during its course may be the reason that the submandibular gland is the salivary gland most commonly involved in salivary stone formation.

20. **B** The sulcus terminalis divides the tongue into the posterior base and anterior body. The other structures listed also are on the dorsal surface of the tongue.

21. **C** A distal step will not allow for the efficient eruption of a normal permanent dentition. A distal step occurs when the primary mandibular second molar is distal to the maxillary second molar and thus is not in a terminal plane relationship. Mesial step and flush terminal plane are both types of terminal plane relationships that allow for efficient eruption, along with primate spaces. A flush terminal plane occurs when the primary maxillary and mandibular second molars are in an end-to-end relationship; a mesial step occurs when the primary mandibular second molar is mesial to the maxillary molar. If primate spacing exists in the primary mandibular arch after the eruption of the permanent first molar, the permanent first molar will put pressure on the primary second and first molars, causing forward movement of the primary mandibular canine and first molar.

22. **A** In centric occlusion, the maxillary incisors overlap the mandibular incisors in what is called an overbite. When the maxillary dental arch naturally 'overhangs'

the mandibular arch facially, the placement is called overjet. Crossbite occurs when a mandibular tooth or teeth are placed facially to the maxillary teeth. An end-to-end bite occurs when the teeth occlude without the maxillary teeth overlapping the mandibular teeth.

23. **B** The auriculotemporal nerve serves as an afferent nerve for the external ear and scalp near the temporomandibular joint. The other nerves are afferent for oral structures.

24. **D** The horizontal plates of the palatine bones and maxillary bones together form the floor of the nasal cavity. The other bones listed form the orbital walls.

25. **A** The Universal Tooth Designation System currently is the most widely used system in America for the designation of both dentitions because it is adaptable to electronic data transfer.

26. **D** The pterygoid plexus of veins is located around the pterygoid muscles and surrounds the maxillary artery on each side of the face in the infratemporal fossa. It protects the maxillary artery from being compressed during mastication. It may be involved in the spread of infection to the cavernous venous sinus because it does not have valves. When it is pierced, a small amount of blood escapes and enters the tissues, causing a hematoma.

27. **B** The maxillary first molar has an oblique ridge that is formed by the union of the triangular ridge of the distobuccal cusp and the distal cusp ridge of the mesiolingual cusp, crossing the occlusal table obliquely. The other teeth do not have oblique ridges.

28. **A** The mandibular first molar's mesiobuccal groove almost always ends in the buccal pit. The buccal pit is susceptible to carries from increased plaque retention and because of the thin enamel that forms the walls of the pit. The other teeth listed do not have buccal pits.

29. **E** The retromolar triangle is located just posterior to the most distal molar of the mandibular dentition. The other structures listed are found on the maxilla.

30. **B** In general, the more posterior the tooth, the more supplemental grooves are present—such that the occlusal table appears more 'wrinkled.' Thus the mandibular third molar is less smooth on its occlusal surface than the third molar of the same arch. The other features listed refer to the second molar and not the third molar.

31. **E** The muscles of mastication are four pairs of muscles that are attached to the mandible; they include the masseter, the temporalis, the medial pterygoid, and the lateral pterygoid muscles. The mandibular division of the fifth cranial or trigeminal nerve innervates all the muscles of mastication.

32. **B** The submandibular duct opens up into the oral cavity on the sublingual caruncle, on the floor of the mouth. The parotid duct opens opposite the maxil-

lary second molar on the buccal mucosa. The mandibular labial frenum has only minor salivary gland ducts nearby in the labial mucosa.

33. **C** The maxillary first premolar typically has two roots. All maxillary molars have three roots or are trifurcated; however, sometimes the roots of the third molar are so close together that they are fused roots, either partially or fully, and thus may give the appearance of a single root. The maxillary second premolar has a single root and only occasionally is bifurcated.

34. **A** The pulp cavity for the maxillary first premolar typically shows two pulp canals, even if there is only one undivided root. The mandibular first premolar has a single pulp canal. Both the maxillary and mandibular first molars primarily have three pulp canals.

35. **E** Both the lateral pterygoid and temporalis are muscles of mastication, which affect the movement of the jaws. If the entire temporalis muscle contracts, its main action is to elevate the mandible, thus raising the lower jaw. Elevation of the mandible occurs during the closing of the jaws. The main action when both lateral pterygoid muscles contract is to bring the lower jaw forward, thus causing the protrusion of the mandible. Protrusion of the mandible often occurs during the opening of the jaws. If only one lateral pterygoid muscle is contracted, the lower jaw shifts to the opposite side, causing a lateral deviation of the mandible. The others muscles listed are muscles of facial expression only.

Additional Readings

Ash MM, Ramford S: Occlusion. 4th ed. Philadelphia, WB Saunders Company, 1995.

Ash MM: Wheeler's Dental Anatomy, Physiology and Occlusion. 7th ed. Philadelphia, WB Saunders Company, 1993.

Bath-Balogh M, Fehrenbach MJ: Illustrated Dental Embryology, Histology, and Anatomy. Philadelphia, WB Saunders, 1997.

Clemente CD: Anatomy: A Regional Atlas of the Human Body. 3rd ed. Philadelphia, Lea and Fibiger, 1987.

Darby ML, Walsh MM: Dental Hygiene Theory and Practice. Philadelphia, WB Saunders Company, 1994.

Dorland's Medical Dictionary. 28th ed. Philadelphia, WB Saunders Company, 1994.

Fehrenbach MJ, Herring SW: Illustrated Head and Neck Anatomy. Philadelphia, WB Saunders, 1996.

Gray H: Gray's Anatomy. 38th ed. Edinburgh, Churchill and Livingstone, 1995.

Ibsen AC, Phelan JA: Oral Pathology for Dental Hygienists. 2nd ed. Philadelphia, WB Saunders Company, 1997.

Leeson TS, Leeson CR, Paparo AA: Text/Atlas of Histology. Philadelphia, WB Saunders Company, 1988.

Leonard PC: Medical Terminology. Philadelphia, WB Saunders Company, 1990.

Moore KL, Persaud TVN: The Developing Human. 5th ed. Philadelphia, WB Saunders Company, 1993.

Nominal Anatomica. 6th ed. Edinburgh, Churchill and Livingstone, 1989.

O'Toole M: Miller-Kean: Encyclopedia and Dictionary of Medicine, Nursing and Allied Health. 5th ed. Philadelphia, WB Saunders Company, 1992.

Perry DA, Beemsterboer PL, Taggart EJ: Periodontology for Dental Hygienist. Philadelphia, WB Saunders Company, 1996.

Chapter FOUR

Microbiology and Immunology

William A. Cafruny, Ph.D. • Thomas A. Langworthy, Ph.D.

 Clinical Case **STUDY**

Jane Smith is a 5-year-old who attends day care. Three weeks after starting at her new day care center in September, she abruptly developed fever and general malaise of several days' duration. After obtaining some laboratory data, her family physician diagnoses hepatitis A virus (HAV) infection.

Clinical Case **QUESTIONS**

1. What was the likely source of the HAV infection?
2. What laboratory tests would help in the diagnosis of this infection?
3. What is the likely outcome of this case?
4. Are her family members or other children at risk for developing this infection? If so, what might help prevent infection?

Clinical Case **RATIONALES**

1. Transmission of HAV is primarily fecal-oral. The case history suggests likely exposure in the institutional day care setting, most likely from contaminated food or water.
2. Laboratory determination of elevated blood levels of aminotransferase and increases in antibodies to HAV would confirm the diagnosis.
3. Complications of HAV infection are uncommon; within a few weeks an immunocompetent patient will clear the infection.
4. Her family and other children are at risk for HAV infection. Because contamination occurs through the fecal-oral route, hand washing and septic handling of foods and drink are important. Family members may receive immunoglobulins as a preventive measure.

Content Review

General Terminology

Adjuvant—Substance that stimulates an immune response (typically a vaccine component).

Aerobic—Requiring oxygen for growth and reproduction.

Allergy (hypersensitivity)—Pathologic immune response characterized by harmful inflammatory mechanisms.

Aminoglycosides—Antibiotics that inhibit bacteria by blocking protein synthesis at the level of the 30s ribosome.

Anaerobic—Growth and reproduction only in the absence of oxygen.

Antibiotic—Compound produced by one organism that is capable of inhibiting the growth of another organism.

Antibody—Antigen-specific glycoprotein produced by B cells and plasma cells.

Antibody class (isotype)—Functionally distinct type of antibody.

Antibody titer—Describes the highest dilution of antibody (e.g., serum) that yields a detectable antigen reaction.

Antigen—Reacts with specific B cell (Ab) or T cell (TCR) receptors.

Antigen presenting cell (APC)—Presents antigenic peptides to T cells.

Autoimmunity—Pathologic immune response directed against self-antigens.

B-lymphocyte—Antibody-producing cell that is central in the development of humoral immunity.

Bacteriocidal—Describes an agent that is able to kill a bacterium.

Bacteriophage—Virus that specifically infects bacterial cells.

Bacteriostatic—Describes an agent that is able to stop the growth of a bacterium, but does not kill the cell.

Cephalosporins—Antibiotics that inhibit bacteria by blocking the cross-linking of peptidoglycan in cell wall biosynthesis.

Chemotroph—Cell that derives its energy from chemical compounds.

Conjugation—Transfer of DNA from a donor bacterium to a recipient by attachment of the two cells by means of pili.

Complement—Set of proteins that participates in diverse inflammatory and antimicrobial responses.

Cross-reaction—Chemical similarity between two different antigens.

Cytokine—Hormone-like protein messengers that regulate immune cells.

Delayed-type hypersensitivity—T cell-mediated hypersensitivity characterized by cytokine-induced inflammation.

Dental plaque—Dense masses of bacteria that adhere to teeth by means of the glycocalyx.

Disinfection—Removal of most organisms, which reduces the chance of an infectious agent being present.

ELISA—Immunoassay (enzyme-linked immunosorbent assay) that measures antigen-antibody reactions.

Endospore—Small resistant structure produced by some bacteria as a means of survival.

Endotoxins—Lipopolysaccharides that are components of Gram-negative cell walls. These may cause fever and shock during infection.

Eukaryotic—Cell possessing a true nucleus with a defined nuclear membrane.

Exotoxins—Toxic substances excreted from the bacterial cell.

Exoenzymes—Hydrolytic enzymes excreted by a cell into the external environment.

Facultative anaerobe—Microorganism that grows and reproduces in the presence or absence of oxygen.

Fc receptor—Cell membrane ligand for the antibody Fc domain.

Fermentation—Anaerobic energy-yielding process in which an organic compound serves as the final electron acceptor.

Flagella—Employed for locomotion by some bacteria.

Generation time—Time required for a bacterial cell to undergo cell division.

Genome—Entire genetic make up of a cell.

Gram-negative—Describes bacteria that possess, in addition to peptidoglycan, a lipid-rich outer membrane composed of lipopolysaccharides, lipoproteins, phospholipids, and proteins. This layer is removed during the decolorization step of the Gram stain procedure.

Gram-positive—Describes bacteria that possess primarily a thick peptidoglycan layer with associated teichoic acids; these bacteria are not decolorized during the Gram stain procedure.

Helminths—Flatworms and roundworms capable of parasitizing the tissues, blood, or organs of animals.

Heterotroph—Cell that derives its carbon from organic compounds.

Human leukocyte antigen (HLA) gene locus—Codes for human MHC proteins.

Immunoblot ("western blot")—Immunoassay that reveals the molecular specificity of antibodies.

Immunodeficiency—Defect in some component(s) of the immune system.

Immunoglobulin—All antibodies are immunoglobulins (a class of proteins).

Immunosuppression—Impairment of any component(s) of the immune system.

Latent period—Time it takes for a virus to reproduce itself.

Lysis—Disintegration of a bacterial cell.

Major histocompatibility complex (MHC)—Gene cluster that codes for cell surface molecules; important to immune regulation (known as HLA in humans).

Mast cell—Cell that contains chemical mediators of type-I hypersensitivity.

Mold—Filamentous fungi.

Monoclonal antibodies—Products of a single clone of B cells that react with a single antigenic determinant or epitope.

Mutation—Stable genetic change that is inherited by the population.

Opportunistic infection—Potentially harmful organisms that are typically members of the normal flora. If given the opportunity, they may cause disease.

Oxidative phosphorylation—Cellular energy (ATP) generated by the electron transport chain.

Parasite—Organism that derives its nutrients by living in or on a host.

Pathogen—Microorganism that is capable of causing disease.

Penicillin—Antibiotic that inhibits cell wall biosynthesis in bacteria by blocking the cross-linking of the peptidoglycan chains.

Peptidoglycan—Macromolecular structure of bacteria that encompasses the cell, forming the bacterial cell wall.

Plasmid—Self-replicating DNA elements found in bacteria that are capable of transmission to another bacterial cell.

Pleomorphic—Lacking a defined cellular shape (e.g., the mycoplasmas).

Prokaryotic—Cell that lacks a nuclear membrane, such that the DNA is not separated from the cytoplasm (e.g., bacteria).

Protozoa—Free-living unicellular eukaryotes.

Radioimmunoassay (RIA)—Immunoassay often used to measure hormones or other small antigens that compete with radiolabeled antigens for binding to antibodies.

Resolving power—Ability of a microscope to distinguish the fine detail of a specimen.

Respiration—Aerobic or anaerobic energy-yielding process in which an inorganic compound serves as the final electron acceptor.

Saprophyte—Organism that grows on dead organic material.

Specificity—Describes the ability of antibodies to recognize unique chemical structures known as antigenic determinants or epitopes.

Sterilization—The killing of all life.

Substrate level phosphorylation—Cellular energy (ATP) generated by the glycolytic pathway.

T lymphocyte—Lymphocyte that uses the antigen-specific T cell receptor for interaction with antigens.

Tetracyclines—Antibiotics that inhibit bacteria by blocking protein syntheses at the level of the 30s ribosome.

Tinea—Fungal infections (ring worm) of the scalp, nails, body, or feet.

Transcription—The copying of DNA into messenger RNA by RNA polymerase.

Transduction—Transfer of DNA from a donor bacterium to a recipient by a bacteriophage.

Transformation—Transfer of free "naked" DNA to a recipient bacterium.

Translation—Process by which the message in the messenger RNA directs the biosynthesis of a specific protein.

Vector—Means by which a microorganism is transmitted to the host.

Vegetative—Describes an actively growing bacterial cell.

Virus—Obligate intracellular parasite lacking its own metabolic machinery and composed of either DNA or RNA (never both) surrounded by a protein coat.

Yeast—Free-living single-cell fungi.

Fundamental Microbiology

Microorganisms are life forms that normally cannot be seen with the unaided human eye. They possess characteristics common to all cellular life in terms of their physiology, morphology, and reproduction. They may inhabit most niches of the earth's environment. Microorganisms are normal inhabitants of the human body. Medically important microorganisms include those that inhabit the human host and are pathogenic (disease-causing).

Spectrum of Microorganisms

The spectrum of microorganisms comprises prokaryotes, eukaryotes, and viruses. The classification of prokaryotes and eukaryotes employs the Latin binomial system of genus and species.

I. Prokaryotes (bacteria) possess a relatively simple cellular structure and are more primitive cells.
  A. Bacteria are divided into two major taxa: eubacteria and archaeobacteria.
    1. Eubacteria (true bacteria) comprise bacteria of medical importance.
      a. Mycoplasmas are the smallest free-living bacteria.
      b. Rickettsias and chlamydials are the smallest members of the bacteria and are obligate intracellular parasites.

2. Archaeobacteria are primitive nonpathogenic bacteria normally associated with extreme or unusual environments (e.g., thermophilic, halophilic, and methanogenic bacteria).
3. Prokaryotes are operationally classified into divisions and classes based primarily on morphologic and physiologic characteristics.
  a. Division I: *Gracilicutes* (typical Gram-negative bacteria)
    1) Class I: *Scotobacteria* (non-photosynthetic)
    2) Class II: *Anoxyphotobacteria* (photosynthetic anaerobes)
    3) Class III: *Oxyphotobacteria* (photosynthetic aerobes)
  b. Division II: *Firmicutes* (typical Gram-positive bacteria)
    1) Class I: *Firmibacteria* (simple bacteria)
    2) Class II: *Thallobacteria* (branching or filamentous)
  c. Division III: *Tenericutes* (bacteria lacking a cell wall)
    1) Class I: *Molecutes* (mycoplasmas)
  d. Division IV: *Mendosicutes* (bacteria with defective cell walls or lacking peptidoglycan)
    1) Class I: *Archaeobacteria*

II. Eukaryotes possess a relatively complex cellular structure and are more highly evolved.
  A. Fungi are non-photosynthetic and include a number of human pathogenic molds and yeasts.
  B. Protozoa and helminths are non-photosynthetic and include some human pathogens.
  C. Algae are photosynthetic and do not include human pathogenic representatives.
III. Viruses comprise acellular life forms that are principally composed of proteins and nucleic acid. All are parasitic and require a viable (living) host cell for their replication.
  A. Classification is based on shape (symmetry), type of nucleic acid, type of host cell, type of vector (agent of transmission), and/or the associated disease produced.

Observation

The observation of microorganisms may be either macroscopic or microscopic, depending upon the total number of organisms present.

I. Macroscopic observation is necessary when organisms are present in large numbers.
  A. Turbidity (cloudiness) in liquid cultures.
  B. Colonial morphology occurs when organisms are grown on a solid surface such as an agar Petri dish.
    1. A colony is defined as a mass of cells that arise from a single cell.
    2. A colony may provide the distinguishing characteristics of an organism in terms of color (pigmentation), texture, size, and shape.
II. Microscopic observation of individual cells is required because of their small size; bacteria may range in size

from approximately 10 μm (approximately the size of a red blood cell) to 0.1 μm (micrometer = 10^{-6} of a meter). Viruses are even smaller; they range in size from approximately 0.25 μm to as small as 15 nm (nanometer = 10^{-9} of a meter). Compound microscopes, which have two or more lenses, provide enlargement of the specimen (magnification) and allow the observer to distinguish fine details of the object (resolving power). Resolving power is dependent upon the wavelength of light and is employed with decreasing wave length, resulting in a higher resolving power.

A. Bright field microscopy (via a compound microscope), which uses visible light and oil immersion, is most commonly employed (magnification = approximately 1000X and resolution = approximately 0.25 μm). Specimens must be stained to be observed.

B. Dark field microscopy is used for observing living, unstained specimens. Oblique light increases the contrast such that specimens appear bright against a dark background.

C. Phase-contrast microscopy is used for observing unstained specimens. Contrast is amplified by the detection of small differences in the refractive indices of the specimen and the surrounding medium.

D. Fluorescence microscopy is used to visualize objects that fluoresce or emit light when exposed to light of a different wavelength. It detects florescent objects that are illuminated by ultra violet or near-ultraviolet light. Specimens absorb this light and emit visible light. Fluorescent dyes conjugated with specific antibodies are the basis of immunofluorescence, which is employed in the identification of microorganisms. Is commonly used for the tracking of antigen-antibody complexes.

E. Electron microscopy (EM) takes advantage of the short wavelength of electrons, which greatly increases magnification and resolving power. Is used to observe cellular ultrastructure and viruses.
   1. Transmission EM is used to observe thin sections of specimens.
   2. Scanning EM is used to observe whole cells and cells attached to surfaces.

Specimen Preparation and Staining

Specimens must be prepared and stained in order to be seen under the light microscope because the refractive index of most organisms is clear. Basic dyes (e.g., crystal violet, methylene blue, safranin) are positively charged and combine with negatively charged cell constituents. Acidic dyes (e.g., eosin, nigrosin, basic fuchsin) possess a negative charge and combine with positively charged cell components.

I. Specimens must be heat-fixed to the microscope slide for bright field microscopy so that cells adhere to the slide and are not washed off during staining procedures.

II. Simple staining employs a single stain, such as methylene blue or crystal violet. Is useful only to distinguish cellular morphology.

III. Differential stains employ two different-colored stains to indicate cellular morphology and distinguish between groups of organisms and/or cellular structures.
   A. Gram stain
      1. Separates all bacteria into two groups: Gram-positive (purple-blue) cells or Gram-negative (red-pink) cells.
      2. Is the most important staining procedure in microbiology and is the paramount first step in bacterial identification.
      3. Reflects differences in cell wall structure.
      4. Staining procedure consists of a four-step application.
         a. Crystal violet (purple) is the primary stain.
         b. Iodine is the mordant that helps to "fix" the primary stain to the cells.
         c. Alcohol is the wash that decolorizes only Gram-negative cells.
         d. Safranin (red) is the counter stain that enables observation of the colorless Gram-negative cells.
   B. Acid-fast stain
      1. Is used to differentiate *Mycobacteria*, the causative agents of tuberculosis; *Mycobacteria* appear red and other bacteria appear blue.
      2. Primary stain must be heated into the cell and is not washed out, even with acid alcohol, because of the hydrophobic waxy nature of the cell wall; thus the stain is acid "fast".
      3. Employs three steps.
         a. Carbolfuchsin (red) is the primary stain heated into the cell.
         b. 3% HCl in alcohol is the wash that decolorizes non-acid-fast cells.
         c. Methylene blue is the counter stain that enables observation of the non-acid-fast cells.

Major Differences Between Eukaryotic and Prokaryotic Cells

The ultrastructures of prokaryotic and eukaryotic cells have important primary differences (Table 4–1).

Bacterial (prokaryotic) Structure and Function

Small bacteria possess a variety of shapes and sizes and internal or external structures that aid the survival of the organisms and also assist in the identification of different bacteria.

I. Cellular Shape
   A. Coccus (plural cocci): spherical
      1. Diplococci (pairs): *Streptococcus pneumonia*
      2. Chains of cocci: *Streptococcus mutans*, *Streptococcus pyogenes*

TABLE 4.1	Differences Between Prokaryotic and Eukaryotic Cells	
Cellular Structure	**Prokaryotes**	**Eukaryotes**
Chromosome number	One (haploid)	Two (diploid)
DNA topology	Circular	Linear
Nuclear membrane	No	Yes
Mitotic division	No	Yes
Endoplasmic reticulum	No	Yes
Mitochondria	No	Yes
Chloroplasts	No	Yes
Phagocytosis	No	Yes
Ribosomes	70S	80S

3. Tetrads (groups of four): *Gaffkyia tetragena*
4. Sarcina (groups of eight): *Sarcina lutea*
5. Random clusters: *Staphylococcus aureus*

B. *Bacillus* (plural bacilli): cylindrical rods
1. Large rods: *Bacillus subtilis, Clostridium botulinum*
2. Small rods: *Escherichia coli, Salmonella, Shigella,* enterics
3. Chains aligned end to end: *Streptobacillus moniliformis*
4. Fusiform types are rods with rounded ends.
5. Coccobacillary types are indistinguishable rod or coccal shape

C. *Spirillum* (plural spirilla): cylindrical with an amplitude
1. *Leptospira, Treponema, Borrelia*
2. Vibrios have a comma shape: *Vibrio cholerae*

D. Palisade arrangement (snapping division): *Corynebacterium diphtheriae*

E. Pleomorphic (lack a defined cell shape): *Mycoplasma pneumoniae*

II. Cellular ultrastructure
A. Internal cellular structures
1. Chromosomal DNA is circular and haploid; possesses most cellular genes and genetic information.
2. Plasmids are autonomously self-replicating, small, circular DNA molecules. They may be transferred from cell to cell and may contain genes for resistance to multiple antibiotics. Are not present in all bacteria.
3. Ribosomes are composed of 30S and 50S subunits, which make up the 70S ribosomal RNA required for protein synthesis. Are distributed throughout the cytoplasm.
4. Inclusion bodies may be present in some bacteria; consist of energy storage molecules, such as poly-beta-hydroxybutyrate, that form granules or refractive bodies.

B. The cytoplasmic membrane encompasses the cytoplasm. It comprises lipids, proteins, and ions,

which provide a hydrophobic matrix that typically exists as a bilayer. It provides a permeability barrier and a support for transport proteins and the electron transport system.
1. Mesosomes are invaginations of the cytoplasmic membrane; extend into the cytoplasm of some bacteria. May be related to cell division.

C. The cell wall surrounds the cytoplasmic membrane, which provides cellular shape and rigidity. The cell wall prevents the cell from lysing because of increased internal osmotic pressure.
1. Periplasmic space is a region between the cytoplasmic membrane and the cell wall; contains various enzymes and proteins, many of which are associated with transport.

D. Cell surface structures external to the cell wall
1. The capsule, generally composed of polysaccharides, is a thick tightly-bound structure found in some bacteria. When present, the capsule may be antigenic and may protect against phagocytosis and desiccation.
2. The slime layer, composed of polypeptides, exits as a relatively thin layer over the cell surface of some bacteria and is loosely bound. In some instances it must be present to provide virulence in bacteria.
3. The glycocalyx surrounds the surface of some bacteria and is composed of a macromolecular network of primarily polysaccharide molecules. It provides cellular adhesion to surfaces such as tooth enamel (*Streptococcus mutans*).
4. Flagella are long (as long as 70 µm), thin protein (flagellin) filaments extending from the cell surface; provide bacterial motility by turning in a circular motion. They allow movement toward or away from chemical substances (chemotaxis). Bacteria without flagella must depend upon Brownian motion (random activity by van der Waals forces) for movement.
   a. Monotrichous flagellation involves a single flagellum extending from a bacterium.
   b. Lophotrichous flagellation involves a tuft of flagella extending from one point on a bacterium.
   c. Amphitrichous flagellation involves flagella extending from the opposite end of a bacterium.
   d. Peritrichous flagellation involves the most common arrangement of flagella, which extend randomly over the entire surface of the bacterium.
5. Pili (singular pilus) and fimbriae are short, proteinaceous, hair-like structures that extend from the cell surface; are associated with Gram-negative bacteria.
   a. Pili are involved with the cell-to-cell transfer of genetic material between bacteria.

b. Fimbriae provide cell-to-cell adhesion (e.g., in pellicle formation—the clumping together of cells).

E. Endospores are large, generally spherical structures that form within the cytoplasmic interior of the cell. One spore is formed per cell and one bacterium is produced per spore upon germination.

1. Spores are a means of survival and not reproduction.

2. The spore coat contains large amounts of dipicolinic acid and divalent cations (Ca^{++}).

3. Spores resist high temperatures, desiccation, ultraviolet light, and disinfectants and are the major reason for elaborate and harsh sterilization procedures. They are prevalent throughout the environment and may remain viable for thousands of years.

4. Spore formation is induced by deteriorating growth conditions.

5. *Bacillus* (aerobic) and *Clostridium* (anaerobic) are the two major genera of spore-forming bacteria.

III. Chemical differences in cell wall structure of Gram-positive and Gram-negative bacteria

A. Peptidoglycan (murine) is present in both Gram-positive and Gram-negative cells. It is a three-dimensional macromolecular net that surrounds the cytoplasmic membrane. It is composed of a polysaccharide backbone (repeating *N*-acetyl glucosamine-*N*-acetyl muramic acid subunits) to which amino acid chains are attached (to muramic acid residues). The amino acid chains are further cross-linked to amino acid chains on adjacent peptidoglycan molecules by additional amino acid residues, thus providing the three dimensional structure.

1. Gram-positive bacteria possess thick, highly cross-linked peptidoglycan layers because of high internal osmotic pressures.

2. Gram-negative bacteria possess thin, sparsely cross-linked peptidoglycan layers because of relatively low internal osmotic pressures.

B. Gram-positive wall macromolecules

1. Teichoic acid is composed of polymers of repeating glycerol phosphate or ribitol phosphate residues attached to peptidoglycan; may serve as antigenic determinants or receptor sites for bacterial viruses.

2. Lipoteichoic acids have similar structures to teichnoic acid, but with diglyceride residue(s) on one end that provide an anchor into the cytoplasmic membrane.

3. Various polysaccharides may bind to peptidoglycan.

C. Gram-negative wall macromolecules

1. A lipid-enriched outer membrane is formed externally to the peptidoglycan layer by the presence of lipopolysaccharides and lipoproteins.

2. Lipopolysaccharides (endotoxins) are composed of a complex lipid: a molecule linked to a polysaccharide chain oriented on the outer surface of the peptidoglycan, with polysaccharide chains extending into the environment. Lipopolysaccharides are potent endotoxins, are antigenic, and may serve as receptor sites for bacterial viruses.

3. Lipoproteins are composed of lipid and extended amino acid chains and are oriented in a manner similar to that of lipopolysaccharides.

4. Porins are globular hollow proteins that form pores in the lipid-rich outer membrane.

IV. Mycobacterial (acid-fast) cell walls differ from those of typical Gram-positive or Gram-negative cells; waxes (wax D) and mycolic acids cover the peptidoglycan layer, creating a hydrophobic surface layer that is correlated with the staining reaction of the mycobacteria.

Bacterial Growth and Nutrition

Bacterial growth is the increase in the number of bacterial cells as a result of cell division by binary fission. Growth is influenced by the physical environment and the availability of essential nutrients.

I. Bacterial Growth

A. Generation time is the amount of time it takes a single cell to divide into two cells (approximately 30 minutes for a typical bacterium growing under ideal conditions).

B. Expressed as cell numbers is log to the base 10 (e.g., $1 \times 10^7 = 10$ million cells). This is for convenience because of the large number of bacterial cells that may be attained under ideal growth conditions.

C. Is measured by visually observing the turbidity of a culture, the increase in optical density, and the increase in protein concentration, or by direct cell counts in a Coulter counter.

D. A curve in culture has 4 phases.

1. Lag phase: on inoculation into a new medium, cells do not immediately divide. Cells swell and begin metabolic preparation for growth in the new medium.

2. Exponential (logarithmic) phase: cells divide and generation time is at a minimum. All cells are viable (alive). A Gram stain is most reliable during this phase; antibiotics are most effective.

3. Stationary phase: the number of drying cells equals the number of dividing cells. Endospore formation may begin. Nutrients are being depleted and toxic metabolic products are increasing.

4. Death phase: cells begin dying exponentially.

II. Nutritional Requirements for Bacterial Growth
  A. Include liquid water, inorganic elements, carbon, and an energy source for growth and reproduction.
  B. Bacteria may be physiologically classified based on how they derive their carbon and/or energy.
    1. Heterotrophs obtain carbon from an organic compound (e.g., glucose).
    2. Autotrophs obtain carbon from an inorganic source (e.g., CO_2).
    3. Phototrophs derive energy from light.
    4. Chemotrophs derive energy from the oxidation of chemical compounds.
  C. Bacteria may be further subdivided based on the carbon plus the energy source.
    1. Photolithotrophs obtain energy from light and carbon from CO_2.
    2. Photoorganotrophs obtain energy from light and carbon from organic compounds.
    3. Chemolithotrophs obtain energy from inorganic compounds (e.g., sulfur, iron) and carbon from inorganic CO_2.
    4. Chemoorganotrophs obtain both energy and carbon from organic compounds—often from the same molecule (e.g., glucose).
    5. Saprophytes grow on dead organic matter.
    6. Parasites grow on living organic matter.
III. Media for Bacterial Growth
  A. May be liquid or solidified by the addition of 1.5% agar; agar is obtained from Kelp and is inert to bacterial metabolism.
  B. May be identified as one of several media based on its composition.
    1. A defined medium is one in which the exact concentration and exact composition of all compounds added are known.
    2. A complex medium is one in which the exact concentration of components added is known; however, the exact composition of all constituents is not known.
      a. Contains various digests and extracts of plant and animal products (e.g., yeast extract, trypticase digest of soybeans, beef heart infusion).
      b. Provides the typical base for the isolation and identification of most bacteria.
    3. A selective medium is one to which agents are added that inhibit the growth of one group of bacteria but not another.
      a. Crystal violet inhibits Gram-positive but not Gram-negative bacteria.
      b. Deoxycholate (bile salts) inhibits Gram-positive and non-enteric (intestinal) but not enteric Gram-negative bacteria.
      c. Phenethyl alcohol inhibits Gram-negative but not Gram-positive bacteria.
    4. A differential medium distinguishes between different organisms.
      a. A fermentation medium that contains glucose and a pH indicator distinguishes between a glucose fermenter and a nonfermenter.
      b. Eosin methylene blue (EMB) agar contains a pH indicator (EMB) and lactose to distinguish between lactose fermenters, which produce greenish colonies, and non-lactose fermenters, which do not.
    5. A differential and selective medium contains components of both selective and differential mediums.
    6. Enriched media are employed for fastidious (difficult to culture) organisms and contain such complex components as serum and/or red blood cells.
    7. Reducing media and special techniques are necessary for the cultivation of anaerobic organisms that cannot be grown in the presence of oxygen. Reducing agents such as thioglycollate, hydrogen sulfide, and cysteine are added to remove oxygen from the medium. Air may be replaced with nitrogen, hydrogen, and/or carbon dioxide. Special jars, which use a hydrogen generator and palladium catalyst to remove oxygen from the air, are employed for cultivating organisms on agar plates.
IV. Factors that Influence Microbial Growth
  A. Include temperature, pH, salt concentration, and oxygen
    1. Temperature
      a. Psychrophiles grow only at low temperatures, between approximately 0°C and 20°C.
      b. Mesophiles grow at temperatures between 20°C and 45°C. The common optimal temperature for human pathogens is 37°C.
      c. Thermophiles grow only at high temperatures, between 45°C and 110°C; *Pyrodictium occultum* grows at 110°C and not below 100°C, which is the highest temperature recorded for cellular life.
    2. Hydrogen ion concentration (pH)
      a. Most bacteria grow optimally near neutrality (pH 7.0).
      b. Acidophiles grow only at acidic pH values, between approximately 0 and 4.0.
      c. Alkalophiles grow only in alkaline pH values greater than 9.0.
    3. Osmotic pressure
      a. Most bacteria grow optimally at salt concentrations near salinity (0.9%).
      b. Halophiles grow only in saturated salt concentrations greater than 20% sodium chloride.
    4. Oxygen requirements for growth and reproduction
      a. Aerobes (O_2) require and use oxygen.

b. Microaerophiles (low O_2) require and use oxygen but only in low concentrations.

c. Facultative anaerobes (O_2 or no O_2) may grow by using oxygen or may grow in the absence of oxygen.

d. Aerotolerant anaerobes (no O_2) may grow in the presence of oxygen, but they do not use it.

e. Anaerobes (no O_2) grow only in the absence of oxygen; exposure to oxygen may be toxic to the organism.

V. Microbial Growth Relationships

A. May be beneficial, harmful, or benign metabolic interactions between microorganism and host.

B. Involve growing on or within other organisms (hosts), including humans.

C. Provide a means of obtaining nutritional requirements.

1. Syntrophism: two or more microorganisms degrade a substance that neither can degrade alone.

2. Competition: two or more organisms vie for the same nutrients. Some microorganisms produce antibiotics to inhibit the growth of competitors.

3. Predation: one microorganism feeds upon another.

D. Interactions may be summarized as in Table 4–2.

Microbial Metabolism

Microbial metabolism includes the sum total of all biochemical reactions that occur in the cell.

I. Exoenzymes

A. Are enzymes that are excreted into the external cellular environment.

B. Break down polymers and other molecules into subunits that are small enough to be transported into the cell.

C. May be potent exotoxins (e.g., *Clostridium botulinum* and *Clostridium tetani* produce lipases that affect the central nervous system).

D. Examples:

1. Carbohydrases degrade polysaccharides to individual sugar residues.

2. Proteases degrade proteins to amino acids.

3. Lipases degrade lipid molecules.

4. Hemolysins degrade (lyse) red blood cells.

TABLE 4.2 Microbial Interactions		
Term	**Microorganism**	**Host**
Symbiosis	Benefits	Benefits
Commensalism	Benefits	Benign
Parasitism	Benefits	Benign or Harmed
Pathogenesis	Benefits	Harmed

II. Transport of Molecules for Metabolism

A. Includes transport of individual molecules to the cell and the concentration of these molecules within the cell.

B. Includes four principle transport mechanisms.

1. Passive diffusion is the random movement of molecules into or out of the cell, progressing from a higher to lower concentration gradient. Cellular energy or carrier proteins are not involved; the diffusion of H_2O is an example.

2. Facilitated diffusion involves the transport of molecules, such as sugars, mediated by a carrier protein that follows a concentration gradient; cellular energy is not expended.

3. Active transport is mediated by a carrier protein and the expenditure of cellular energy to move molecules into the cell against a concentration gradient.

4. Group translocation (phosphotransferase system) moves molecules into the cell against a concentration gradient. A carrier protein and energy (in the form of phosphoenol pyruvate) are involved and the substrate (e.g., glucose molecule) becomes phosphorylated in the process. The molecule becomes negatively charged (e.g., glucose-phosphate) and is retained inside the cell. Group translocation is the most efficient and most common form of transport in bacteria.

III. Metabolism

A. Involves metabolic pathways; once inside the cell, a molecule (e.g., glucose) enters metabolic pathways.

B. Includes two major classes of metabolic reactions.

1. Catabolic reactions are degradative reactions that:

a. Produce energy (ATP).

b. Produce carbon skeletons.

c. Produce reducing power.

2. Anabolic reactions are biosynthetic reactions that:

a. Use up energy (ATP).

b. Use up carbon skeletons.

c. Use up reducing power.

IV. Oxidation-Reduction Reactions

A. Are employed in cellular metabolism.

B. A compound is oxidized when it gives up or loses electrons.

C. A compound is reduced when it receives or gains electrons.

D. These reactions are simultaneous; when a molecule is oxidized another is simultaneously reduced.

V. Energy Production (catabolism)

A. Bacteria produce cellular energy, primarily in the

form of ATP, by passing a pair of electrons through the cell.

1. The molecule that gives up the pair of electrons and becomes oxidized is called the electron donor.
2. The molecule that ultimately receives these electrons after they pass through the cell is called the final electron acceptor.
3. Molecules that accept and transfer these electrons (within the cell) from the donor to the final electron acceptor are called electron carriers.
   a. A typical electron carrier involved in energy metabolism is nicotine adenine dinucleotide (NAD).
4. When the electron donor (e.g., glucose) becomes oxidized, NAD receives the pair of electrons (and protons) and becomes reduced to $NADH_2$. However, the cell is limited in number of oxidized NAD molecules; soon all would become reduced to $NADH_2$ and energy metabolism cease.
5. The reduced $NADH_2$ molecule must be able to donate its electrons to an acceptor to regenerate oxidized NAD; *this is from where the definition of fermentation and respiration is derived.*
   a. Fermentation occurs when an organic molecule serves as the final electron acceptor.
   b. Respiration occurs when an inorganic molecule serves as the final electron acceptor.

VI. Fermentation
   A. Is an energy inefficient process that results in the production of two ATPs from the partial oxidation of one glucose molecule.
   B. Is strictly an anaerobic process that results in:
      1. Glucose (electron donor) entering the glycolytic pathway.
      2. Glycolysis, which results in the oxidation of one glucose molecule (C6) into two pyruvate molecules (C3) and the net production of two reduced $NADH_2$ molecules and two molecules of ATP, which is referred to as substrate level phosphorylation.
      3. Pyruvate, an organic compound, which is the central "hub" of fermentation reactions and serves as the final electron acceptor in the simplest fermentation; reduced $NADH_2$ donates its electrons directly to pyruvate, reducing it to lactic acid (C3), which is released into the external environment.
   C. Is accomplished by microorganisms capable of carrying out fermentations that result in a wide variety of metabolic end products, including CO_2, H_2, organic acids, and alcohols.
   D. The ability or inability of an organism to ferment different substrates is one of the key features that enables distinction among bacterial species.

VII. Respiration
   A. Is an energy efficient process that results in the production of 38 ATPs from the complete oxidation of one glucose molecule.
   B. Can be either an aerobic or anaerobic process that results in the following:
      1. Glucose (C6) entering the glycolytic pathway, with the same result as in fermentation: 2 ATP, 2 $NADH_2$, and 2 pyruvate (C3) molecules are formed.
      2. Pyruvate becoming decarboxylated and bound to coenzyme A, resulting in acetyl-CoA, CO_2, and the production of one reduced $NADH_2$ molecule.
      3. Acetyl-CoA feeding into the tricarboxylic acid (TCA) cycle. One turn of the TCA cycle results in the production of 2 CO_2 molecules and 4 reduced $NADH_2$ molecules.
      4. The second pyruvate molecule generated by glycolysis undergoing the same series of reactions. At this point glucose is completely oxidized to 6 molecules of CO_2; 2 ATPs have been produced and a total of 12 reduced $NADH_2$s have been formed. Cells regenerate oxidized NAD and generate more energy by means of the electron transport system.
      5. The electron transport chain being made up of a series of electron transfer molecules called cytochromes that are located in the cytoplasmic membrane.
         a. A reduced $NADH_2$ will donate its electrons and protons to the electron transport chain, becoming reoxidized to NAD.
         b. Passage of the electrons through the electron transport chain results in the production of 3 ATP molecules. This is called oxidative phosphorylation.
         c. At the end of the electron transport chain the electrons and protons combine with O_2, reducing it to H_2O. There are a total of 12 reduced $NADH_2$ molecules, which results in the production of 36 ATPs (3 x 12) in addition to the 2 ATPs produced from glycolysis, for a total production of 38 ATPs from one glucose molecule.

VIII. Differences between Aerobes and Anaerobes
   A. Aerobic respiration
      1. Of bacteria involves the use of O_2 as the final electron acceptor in respiration.
      2. Involves a combination of O_2, electrons, and protons at the terminus of the electron transport chain, resulting in the formation of toxic intermediates, superoxide anions (O_2^-), and hydrogen peroxide (H_2O_2).
      3. Requires bacterium that grow aerobically to possess two enzymes for the removal (conversion) of these toxic products.

a. Superoxide dismutase converts O_2^- into H_2O_2.

b. Catalase (peroxidase) subsequently converts H_2O_2 into H_2O and O_2.

B. Anaerobic respiration

1. Is carried out by bacteria that possess an electron transport chain but lack either or both superoxide dismutase and catalase and are unable to remove toxic byproducts of aerobic respiration.

2. Uses oxidized inorganic compounds other than O_2 as the final electron acceptor; some common inorganic compounds used in anaerobic respiration include sulfate (SO_4), sulfur (S), nitrate (NO_3), and carbon dioxide (CO_2).

C. Anaerobic fermentation enables bacteria that lack components of, or do not have, an electron transport chain to grow anaerobically by means of fermentation.

IX. Biosynthesis (anabolism)

A. Fermentation and respiration produce the energy for driving the biosynthetic (anabolic) reactions of the cell for the necessary synthesis of nucleic acids, proteins, carbohydrates, and lipids (see Chapter 2).

Bacterial Genetics

Bacterial genetics is the study of the variability and inheritance of bacteria. Microorganisms vary in the composition of their DNA and RNA and in the way their genetic codes are expressed.

I. Composition of DNA (deoxyribonucleic acid) and the genetic code

A. DNA is composed of 4 nucleotide bases: the purines, adenine (A) and guanine (G), and the pyrimidines, cytosine (C) and thymine (T).

1. Adenine pairs with thymine via two hydrogen bonds (A = T).

2. Guanine pairs with cytosine via three hydrogen bonds (G≡C).

B. DNA exists as two strands of bases in a double helix.

1. Replication of the double helix is semiconservative (a copy of each of the original strands is made) and occurs by the enzyme DNA polymerase.

C. DNA Genetic Code

1. Is a triplet code because three nucleotide bases (a codon) code for one amino acid.

2. Is a degenerate code because more than one codon codes for the same amino acid.

3. A stop codon occurs with a codon that codes for no amino acid.

II. Composition of RNA (ribonucleic acid)

A. Is the same as for DNA, except that the base uracil replaces the base thymine.

B. Consists of three types of RNA molecules

1. Messenger RNA (mRNA), which are single-stranded molecules.

2. Ribosomal RNA (rRNA), which are composed of a complex of RNA molecules.

a. Prokaryotic rRNA are 70s consisting of 30s and 50s subunits.

b. Eukaryotic rRNA are 80s consisting of 40s and 60s.

3. Transfer RNA (tRNA), which are convoluted molecules that carry an amino acid.

III. Protein Synthesis

A. Transcription of the genetic code occurs when one strand of the DNA is copied (transcribed) as complimentary bases into a single strand of mRNA by the enzyme RNA polymerase.

B. Translation of the genetic code involves the following:

1. Initiation

a. Messenger RNA combines with two individual ribosomal subunits.

b. A complimentary (anticodon) tRNA charged with an amino acid combines with the mRNA-ribosome complex.

c. The ribosomes move one codon down the mRNA and another charged tRNA associates with the mRNA.

d. A peptide bond is formed between the amino acids and the uncharged tRNA is released.

2. Elongation

a. Movement of the ribosomes along mRNA continues, as does the addition and release of charged and uncharged tRNAs.

b. Movement and addition of tRNAs continue, resulting in a growing polypeptide chain.

3. Termination

a. At the end of the mRNA molecule, the ribosomes dissociate into two individual subunits and the completed protein is released.

IV. Mutations in DNA

A. A change in a codon sequence (mutation) results in a translational change in the amino acid sequence of the polypeptide (protein product).

1. Example of the genetic code in protein synthesis:

2. DNA: AAA————CTG——GCA——CTT

3. mRNA: UUU————GAC——CGU——GAA

Amino acid sequence produces phenylalanine-aspartate-arginine-glutamate.

B. Types of mutations (sequence changes) in DNA

1. A point mutation is a change in one nucleotide base, resulting in one changed amino acid.

2. Frameshift mutations are caused by the insertion or deletion of a nucleotide base.

a. An insertion results in a shift in the entire reading frame (codon sequences) in one direction, by one nucleotide base.

b. A deletion results in a shift in the entire reading frame in the other direction, by one nucleotide base.

3. Transition is the replacement of a purine base by a purine base or the replacement of a pyrimidine by a pyrimidine.

4. Transversion is the replacement of a purine base by a pyrimidine or the replacement of a pyrimidine by a purine base.

C. Effect of mutations on transcription and translation

1. Missense mutation occurs when a single amino acid is substituted for another in a polypeptide chain.

2. Nonsense mutation occurs when a stop codon is coded for in place of a codon specifying an amino acid.

3. Suppressor mutation occurs when a second mutation corrects a previous mutation.

D. Spontaneous mutations within DNA occur naturally but infrequently, when adenine or thymine undergo tautomeric shifts (a temporary jump to an unstable high energy state).

1. Adenine shifts from its normal amino form to the imino form, which can form three hydrogen bonds that may pair with cytosine (instead of thymine).

2. Thymine shifts from its normal keto form to the enol form, which can form three hydrogen bonds that may pair with guanine (instead of adenine).

3. Mutagenic agents increase the rate of spontaneous mutations (changes in nucleotide bases).

V. Genetic Transfer between Bacteria

A. Involves the passage of DNA from a donor bacterial cell to a recipient cell.

B. Spontaneous mutations occur infrequently in a population but recipient bacteria may instantly acquire new genes, which changes the genetic constitution and capabilities of the organism.

C. Incoming DNA may be degraded by nucleases of the recipient or may be exchanged and integrated with existing sequences in the recipient DNA by recombination.

1. The exogenote is the donor or incoming DNA.

2. The endogenote is the recipient cell's DNA.

3. During recombination the exogenote contains sequences that are homologous to sequences within the endogenote; the sequences align and the DNA of the endogenote exchange with the sequences of the endogenote and integrate into the recipient cell's DNA.

D. Types of transfer between bacteria

1. Transformation is gene transfer mediated by free "naked" DNA.

2. Transduction is gene transfer mediated by bacteriophages (bacterial viruses).

a. Generalized transduction is host cell DNA transmitted by lytic bacteriophages. Random host DNA segments are mistakenly packed into capsids during bacteriophage replication.

b. Specialized transduction is host cell DNA transmitted by temperate bacteriophages. A specific host DNA gene is always transferred based on the specific integration site of the prophage.

3. Conjugation is plasmid-mediated gene transfer, which requires cell-to-cell contact.

a. Cell contact requires sex pili, which are coded for by the conjugative plasmid F (so called fertility factor).

b. An F^+ donor cell that comes in contact with an F^- cell (possesses no F plasmid or pili) will transfer an F plasmid and the recipient will become F^+.

4. Types of conjugation

a. High frequency recombination (Hfr) is the transfer of many chromosomal genes from the donor to the recipient cell. This occurs infrequently, but occurs when the F plasmid integrates into and resides in the chromosomal DNA of the donor cell.

b. Sexduction (F plasmid) occurs when an F plasmid that is integrated into the chromosome is excised and mistakenly acquires chromosomal gene sequences. When transferred, donor chromosomal DNA sequences reside on the F plasmid within the recipient cell.

5. Significance of conjugation and gene transfer

a. After gene transfer the existing genes of one bacterium can be acquired at any moment by a bacterium that is lacking these genes.

b. Many different plasmids are capable of mediating their own transfer. Of special concern are those that code for multiple antibiotic resistance.

c. Not only can these plasmids be donated and spread like an infection throughout a bacterial population, they also may be transferred between different genera of bacteria and between species of the same genus.

Terminology

Antiseptic—Disinfecting agent that is mild enough to be applied to the surface of the human body.

Aseptic—Refers to manipulations and technical procedures that help minimize the chances of infection or contamination.

Bactericidal—Refers to an agent that kills bacteria. Some agents are specifically viricidal or fungicidal.

Bacteriostatic—Refers to an agent that stops the growth of a bacterium but does not kill it. Some agents are specifically virostatic or fungistatic.

Disinfection—The removal of most organisms from an object, which reduces the chances of infection by a pathogenic agent. Many disinfectants are rather harsh chemical agents.

Sterilization—The killing of all life. Harsh procedures are applied to inanimate objects to sterilize them. Examples include exposure to high temperatures, steam, and toxic chemicals.

Control of Microorganisms by Chemical and Physical Agents

Microbial growth is controlled through the use of chemical and physical agents. These agents range from those that inhibit or slow growth to those that kill microorganisms. The effectiveness of these agents depends on a number of parameters.

I. The effectiveness of controlling agents is modified by the following parameters:
   A. Number of microorganisms present
   B. Concentration of the agent
   C. Temperature during treatment
   D. Duration of exposure to the agent
   E. Environment (e.g., microorganisms trapped in pus or dried blood)

II. Cell Death by Chemical or Physical Agents
   A. Does not occur instantly or simultaneously for members of a microbial population.
   B. Is typically exponential; it may take an extended time to eliminate the last remaining cell or endospore.
   C. Is resisted most by endospores.

III. Physical Agents and Their Effects include:
   A. Moist heat
      1. Pasteurization is a process of disinfection typically applied to dairy products, wines, and beers.
         a. Items are heated to a temperature that is high enough to kill only known pathogenic organisms that might be present.
         b. Milk, for example, is pasteurized when heated at 65°C for 30 minutes, which eliminates the possible presence of *Mycobacterium tuberculosis* (the causative agent of TB), *Brucella abortus* (an agent of abortion), and *Coxiella burnetii* (the agent of Q-fever)—all of which may be transmitted through milk. Many bacteria survive pasteurization, which is why milk eventually sours.
      2. Autoclaving is a process of sterilization that employs steam under pressure.
         a. At 15 lb/in^2, moist steam generates a temperature of 121°C, which is standard.
         b. Any item can be sterilized by autoclaving, and depending on the nature of the materials and the load, an exposure time of 20 minutes or more is employed. Some objects, such as plastics, are destroyed under these conditions.

B. Dry Heat
   1. Is less efficient than moist heat; requires longer exposure and higher temperatures.
   2. By electric dry air oven requires materials to be exposed to a temperature of 180°C for at least 2 hours.
   3. Is the best method of sterilization for materials such as powders, jellies, and sharp instruments.

C. Cold temperatures
   1. Refrigeration only slows microbial growth and metabolism.
   2. Freezing stops microbial growth and kills some but not all cells of a microbial population; deep freezing at -70°C is an excellent means of preserving many microbial cultures.

D. Radiation
   1. Ionizing radiation (gamma rays)
      a. Penetrates cells.
      b. Can react with macromolecules, but reacts primarily with water molecules in the cell; when hit by a gamma ray, a water molecule is converted into a hydroxyl radical (•OH) and a hydride radical (•H), which are potent oxidizing and reducing agents, respectively.
      c. Is useful for sterilizing many items that would be destroyed by high temperatures, such as plastic Petri dishes, sutures, prosthetic devises, and brachioscopes.
   2. Ultraviolet light
      a. Is absorbed by thymine molecules present in the DNA of the cell; subsequently forms thymine dimers that inhibit DNA replication.
      b. Has no effect on bacterial endospores, which are resistant.
      c. Does not penetrate glass, plastic, or other materials.
      d. Is used primarily for disinfecting surfaces and sometimes air.

E. Filtration
   1. Employs membrane filters with pore sizes in the approximate range of 0.25 µm to 0.01 µm, which retain bacteria and viruses.
   2. Is used to sterilize sensitive material that would be destroyed by other means, such as antibiotics solutions, vitamins, serum, and biological fluids.

IV. Chemical Agents and Their Effects
   A. Most chemical agents are disinfectants because endospores may not be killed by these agents.
   B. Many are mild enough to be used as topical skin antiseptics.
   C. Types include:
      1. Detergents
         a. Act by disrupting the cellular membrane.
         b. When cationic, posses a net positive charge; examples are cetylpyridinium chloride and benzalkonium chloride, representatives of the quaternary amine compounds.

c. When anionic, posses a net negative charge; examples are soap and sodium lauryl sulfate.

d. When nonionic, lack a charge; examples are Triton-X and Tween compounds, which are fairly ineffective disinfectants.

2. Phenolic compounds

   a. Are based on the phenol nucleus, which by itself is caustic.

   b. Work by disrupting membranes and ultimately precipitating proteins.

   c. Examples include:

   1) Cresols, which are methylated phenol derivatives; in mixture form, Lysol is an example.

   2) Halogenated diphenyls, which are two phenol molecules linked together and which also contain additional chlorine molecules, such as hexachlorophene (pHisoHex) and hexylresorcinol (ST-37 in mouth wash).

   3) Alcohols, which disrupt cellular membranes and precipitate cellular proteins.

      a) 100% alcohol is not effective because it only serves to dehydrate the cell.

      b) 70% isopropyl alcohol is most commonly used and is made by dilution with water.

   4) Heavy metal compounds

      a) Are those that contain a mercury or silver molecule.

      b) Include mercurochrome, merthiolate Metaphen, and silver nitrate.

      c) React reversibly with sulfhydryl groups of proteins to form mercaptide bonds.

      d) Are bacteriostatic.

   5) Oxidizing agents

      a) Include iodine, chlorine, hypochlorous acid (bleach), and hydrogen peroxide.

      b) React irreversibly with active hydrogen molecules of proteins, such as sulfhydryl groups, to form covalently-linked disulfide bonds.

      c) Are bactericidal.

   6) Alkylating agents

      a) Include formaldehyde (solution), glutaraldehyde (solution), and ethylene oxide (gas).

      b) React with reactive hydrogen molecules in the cell, such as sulfhydryl groups, by adding (alkylating) hydroxy methyl or hydroxy ethyl groups to these residues.

      c) Are bactericidal.

   7) Ethylene oxide

      a) Is the major gaseous sterilant for sterilizing nonbiological materials at room temperature.

Control of Microorganisms by Antibiotics and Other Chemotherapeutic Agents

Antibiotics are natural chemotherapeutic compounds that typically are produced by a bacterium or mold. They inhibit the growth of other bacteria or molds and may be taken internally.

I. Antibiotics

   A. Ideal antibiotic

   1. Is broad spectrum; has the ability to inhibit a wide range of microorganisms.

   2. Prevents the development and spread of organisms resistant to the antibiotic.

   3. Is selective for the pathogenic organism and not detrimental to the human host (e.g., does not cause allergy or toxicity).

   4. Does not eliminate the normal flora of the human host.

   5. Has not been found.

   B. Sites of action

   1. Cell wall biosynthesis

      a. Includes an important group of agents because bacteria possess peptidoglycan but eukaryotic (human) cells do not; without a complete peptidoglycan, bacterial growth will stop or cells will lyse.

      b. Inhibitors of earlier stages of peptidoglycan biosynthesis include:

      1) Cycloserine

      2) Vancomycin and Ristocetin

      3) Bacitracin

      c. Beta lactam antibiotics inhibit peptidoglycan cross-linking, the last stage of peptidoglycan biosynthesis. The active site of all of these antibiotics is the lactam ring, which is an internal amide bond; are effective primarily on Gram-positive bacteria.

      1) Penicillin

         a) Was the first antibiotic discovered.

         b) Can be rendered ineffective by penicillinase, an enzyme produced by resistant bacteria that opens the lactam ring on the penicillin molecule.

         c) Causes allergy in some people.

         d) Original molecule was chemically modified in an attempt to overcome resistance and allergy problems, resulting in derivatives such as ampicillin, nafcillin, methicillin, and cloxacillin.

      2) Cephalosporins, monobactams, and carbapenams

         a) Are other classes of lactam antibiotics, some of which have a broader spectrum and some of which are used to treat individuals who are allergic to penicillin.

2. Cell membranes
   a. Agents are few in number, because bacterial and eukaryotic membranes are very similar, which makes targeting the cell membrane difficult.
   b. Include these topically applied agents:
      1) Polyene antibiotics
         a) Are molecules that contain many double bonds.
         b) Complex with sterols in the membrane, causing disruption.
         c) Are useful for fungal infections because bacteria do not contain sterols in the membrane.
         d) Include amphotericin and nystatin.
      2) Polymyxins
         a) Are small polypeptides that disrupt membranes by a detergent-like action.
         b) Are useful for stopping infection in individuals who have suffered severe burns.

3. DNA synthesis; inhibitors of DNA gyrase
   a. Are typically toxic to both bacteria and the human host because of the universal structure of DNA and its biosynthesis; bacteria do differ from eukaryotes in that the DNA is circular and the enzyme DNA gyrase is required for supercoiling and DNA stability.
   b. Antibiotics include:
      1) Nalidixic acid, which is the basis for the class of antibiotics called quinolones.
      2) Novobiocin.

4. Protein synthesis
   a. An important class of useful antibiotics work at this site to inhibit bacteria at the level of protein synthesis.
   b. Antibiotic action consists of two major stages:
      1) Transcription
         a) In which the genetic code is copied (transcribed) from DNA into mRNA and translation, wherein information in the mRNA molecule (in combination with ribosomes and tRNA) is translated into amino acid sequences of a protein.
            (1) Bacteria and eukaryotic cells differ in the structure of their ribosomal RNA.
                (a) Bacteria possess 70S ribosomes made up of 30S and 50S subunits.
                (b) Eukaryotes posses 80S ribosomes made up of 40S and 60S subunits.
            (2) Prolonged use of these antibiotics typically has detrimental side effects because the mitochondria of eukaryotic cells possess 70S ribosomes.
      b) Inhibitor, which produces few clinically-useful antibiotics because of the universal nature of the transcription process.
            (1) Rifampin inhibits the initiation of mRNA synthesis by inhibiting RNA polymerase. Rifampin is a primary agent in the treatment of mycobacterial infections.
      2) Translation
         a) By binding to the 30S ribosome
            (1) Aminoglycosides (e.g., streptomycin, neomycin kanamycin, gentamycin, tobramycin) contain unusual amino sugars in their structures and are bactericidal because they bind irreversibly to the 30S ribosomal subunit.
            (2) Tetracyclines (e.g., Aureomycin, Terramycin, Declomycin) are broad spectrum antibiotics that contain a series of cyclohexyl rings in their structure and are bacteriostatic because they bind reversibly to the 30S ribosomal subunit.
         b) By binding to the 50S ribosome
            (1) Inhibits by blocking transpeptidation or translocation; agents generally are bacteriostatic.
            (2) Examples include:
                (a) Chloramphenicol, which is quite toxic; reserved for typhoid fever and infectious agents that are resistant to less toxic antibiotics.
                (b) Macrolides (e.g., erythromycin, oleandomycin, spiramycin), which are effective on Gram-positive bacteria. The antibiotic of choice for mycoplasma infections and Legionnaires disease.
                (c) Clindamycin and lincomycin, which have a spectrum similar to the macrolides; are used in dental medicine as a substitute for penicillin and for *Bacteroides* infections. May cause pseudomembranous colitis.

5. Antimetabolites
   a. Are not antibiotics but are chemically derived chemotherapeutic agents that stereochemically resemble metabolic intermediates that block important biosynthetic pathways in bacteria.

b. Examples include:
   1) Sulfonamides and Trimethoprim, which resemble paraaminobenzoic acid (PABA), an intermediate; reversibly block (bacteriostatic) folic acid biosynthesis in bacteria.
   2) Isoniazid, which stereochemically resembles niacin and nicotinamide; appears to block synthesis of these two coenzymes.

II. Chemotherapeutic Drug Resistance
   A. Mechanisms include:
      1. Enzymatic inactivation (e.g., penicillinase).
      2. Modification of the agent's binding site.
      3. Decreased cell permeability or loss of ability to transport the agent into the cell.
      4. Overproduction of biosynthetic intermediates that are inhibited by the agent.
   B. Reasons for judicial use of antibiotics
      1. Include potentially harmful side effects (e.g., allergy, liver damage, bone deposition, nerve damage).
      2. Viruses are not affected by antibiotics.
      3. Indiscriminate use of antibiotics and their unnecessary placement into the environment ultimately selects for organisms that become resistant to the antibiotic, thereby reducing its usefulness.
   C. Origins of antibiotic resistance
      1. Random natural genetic mutations followed by selection.
      2. Gene transfer. Multiple antibiotic resistance genes are carried on plasmids, which may be transferred from an antibiotic resistant donor bacterium to an antibiotic sensitive bacterium, rendering the recipient immediately resistant to antibiotics.

Terminology

Latent period—The time between uncoating and production of mature virions.

Lytic infection—Immediate replication of some bacteriophages, as well as destructive release of some viruses from animal cells.

Latent infection—Delayed viral replication; for example, when viral nucleic acid integrates into bacterial (prophage) or animal (provirus) host cells. Subsequent replication along with the host chromosome occurs; eventually the viral nucleic acid may be excised, which leads to viral replication (a lytic cycle).

Temperate bacteriophages—Bacteriophages capable of both integration ("lysogeny") and lytic replication; "virulent" bacteriophages only cause lytic infections.

Persistent (chronic) virus infections—May involve latency or some other mechanism that promotes continuous internal infection.

Viruses

Viruses are the smallest (approximately 0.2 μm to 0.02 μm) and simplest infectious agents. The genome of a virus consists of RNA or DNA (not both). Structurally, viruses are composed of protein molecules and some viral proteins are glycosylated or associated with lipids. Viruses are obligate intracellular parasites, which require a host cell's metabolic apparatus for their reproduction. There are two major groups of viruses: those that infect prokaryotic (bacterial) cells and are called bacteriophages, and those that infect only eukaryotic cells.

I. Composition and Morphology of Virions (complete infectious virus particles):
   A. Nucleic acid may be single-stranded (ss) or double-stranded (ds) forms of either DNA or RNA.
   B. The viral capsid is protein that surrounds the nucleic acid; capsid subunits are called capsomers.
   C. Some viruses have an envelope that surrounds the capsid. The envelope contains lipid acquired from the membrane of the host cell. Viral proteins and glycoproteins typically are embedded in the lipid envelope and serve as antigens and virulence factors.
   D. Viral symmetry (shape) is one of three basic types:
      1. Icosahedral (cubic) symmetry
      2. Helical (rod shape) symmetry
      3. Complex symmetry also may occur (e.g., the combination of icosahedral and cubic symmetry found in bacteriophages).

II. Classification of Viruses
   A. Is increasingly based on nucleic acid sequence homology. Traditional classification has been based on size, symmetry, type of nucleic acid, and virus-host interactions such as cellular location of replication (nucleus or cytoplasm), type of disease associated with the virus (e.g., hepatitis), and tissue site from which the virus was isolated.
   B. Is periodically updated, as new molecular data become available.
   C. Includes different families of viruses, which are classified according to the criteria above.
      1. Virus classification and clinically important examples:
         a. Bacteriophages—9 separate families
         b. Plant viruses—20 separate families
         c. Animal viruses—20 separate families
            1) Picornaviruses (small "RNA" viruses); include polio and a common cold virus (rhinovirus).
            2) Reoviruses (dsRNA); include rotavirus, which causes diarrheal illness.
            3) Orthomyxoviruses (ssRNA); include influenza virus.
            4) Rhabdoviruses (ssRNA); include rabies virus.
            5) Retroviruses (ssRNA); include human immunodeficiency virus (HIV).

6) Herpesviruses (dsDNA); include herpes simplex virus (HSV).

7) Hepadnaviruses (dsDNA); include hepatitis B virus (HBV).

III. Replication within a Host Cell
   A. Requires several basic steps:
      1. Attachment (or adsorption), which is the process of virus attachment to the host cell surface. Is mediated by interaction between viral proteins and host cell surface receptor molecules.
      2. Penetration, which occurs when the virus enters the cell, typically through endocytosis or direct passage through the cell membrane.
      3. Uncoating, which occurs when the virus disassembles and releases its nucleic acid inside the cell.
      4. Multiplication, which refers to viral nucleic acid replication and the production of viral proteins, which happens as the virus takes over some of the host cell biochemical machinery.
      5. Maturation of virus particles, which occurs as viral nucleic acid and proteins are packaged into mature virions and are released from the cell through rupture or budding of the cell membranes.

IV. Pathogenesis
   A. Can be divided into the following categories:
      1. Harmful effects of virus replication on host cells (structural and biochemical damage).
      2. Genetic effects on the host (e.g., carcinogenesis).
      3. Induction of harmful host immune responses (immunopathology) as the infected host attempts to fight the virus.

V. Detection
   A. By culture of viruses in appropriate host cells (bacterial, plant, or animal) grown in the laboratory.
      1. Is one important tool for the detection of viruses and determination of their concentration by virus titration.
      2. Viruses that infect cultured cells often (but not always) cause microscopically visible damage or cytopathic effects.
   B. By structural analysis; electron microscopy is used for the definitive identification of viruses.
   C. By genetic technology; allows specific identification of viral nucleic acid sequences in cells or tissues (e.g., by polymerase chain reaction [PCR], using viral-specific probes to amplify and detect viral nucleic acid).
   D. By presumptive identification of specific virus infection; may be carried out by determining the specific host immune response that occurs during infection (e.g., determination of HIV infection by identifying HIV-specific antibodies in the blood of an infected individual).

VI. Antiviral Therapy
   A. Agents are under intense study and development.
   B. Agents generally are designed to interfere with a biochemical stage that is specific for viral replication (e.g., a viral-coded enzyme or receptor molecule).
   C. Examples of currently available antivirals are included later in this chapter (see Infectious Diseases section).

Molds and Yeasts (fungi)

Molds and yeasts are eukaryotic cells that may reproduce either asexually or sexually. Most are saprophytes (grow on dead organic matter), but many are parasites (grow on living material), which are pathogenic for plants and animals. Some produce potent mycotoxins or aflatoxins that may cause liver tumors. Others are responsible for such afflictions as ringworm, athlete's foot, trench mouth, and thrush. They are metabolically versatile and grow on typical media as well as on cork, hair, paint, and even polyvinyl plastics. Their spores are everywhere and are primarily responsible for the contamination of bacterial cultures and media. Mold and yeast isolation and culture generally employ techniques similar to those used for bacteria.

I. Molds (mycelium)
   A. Typically grow by the production of hyphae, which form a characteristic cotton-like tangled mass called mycelia.
   B. Types of mycelia include:
      1. Non-septate mycelia, which are long, string-like cells that do not contain cross-walls.
      2. Septate mycelia, which are similar but contain perforated cross-walls.
   C. Identification
      1. Is based primarily on morphology and modes of reproduction (e.g., the types of asexual and sexual spores produced).
      2. Four major classes are:
         a. Zygomycetes
            1) Are represented by water molds (*Mucor*) and bread molds (*Rhizopus*).
            2) Are non-septate mycelia.
            3) Include:
               a) Sporangiospores—asexual spores enclosed in a sporangium.
               b) Zygospores—sexual spores freely suspended as a "naked spore" between mycelia of two mating types.
         b. Basidiomycetes
            1) Are represented by the mushrooms.
            2) Are septate mycelia.
            3) Typically do not produce asexual spores.
            4) Include basidiospores—sexual spores produced by the fruiting body (mushroom) above ground.

c. Ascomycetes
1) Are represented by the true yeasts and *Neurospora.*
2) Are septate mycelium.
3) Include:
a) Conidia—asexual spores that are "naked," not enclosed in a structure.
b) Ascospores—sexual spores enclosed in a structure called the ascus.
d. Deuteromycetes (*fungi imperfecti*)
1) Are molds and yeasts that reproduce asexually; no sexual form of reproduction has been found.
2) Examples include *Penicillium*, *Aspergillus*, and *Candida.*
3) Are septate mycelium.
4) Include conidia—asexual spores.
5) Sexual spores not found.

II. Yeasts
A. Are a special class of molds that are egg-shaped, elliptical, single-celled, and larger than bacteria; do not produce mycelia.
B. Reproduce asexually by cell division called budding; asexual spores are not produced. Sexual spores (ascospores) may be produced by some yeasts upon the mating of two cells.
C. Can grow anaerobically by fermentation, with the production of alcohol (ethanol) and CO_2.
D. Examples include:
1. *Saccharomyces*—important in bread, wine, and beer production.
2. *Candida albicans*—the causative agent of thrush or oral candida.

Parasites (Protozoa and Helminths)

Human parasites are eukaryotic animals that are found in two subkingdoms, protozoa and metazoa. Protozoa are unicellular organisms. Metazoa are all parasites other than protozoa. An important group of the metazoa are the helminths, which are worms, including flatworms (*Platyhelminthes*) and roundworms (*Aschelminthes*). The classification of parasites is based on morphology, cytoplasmic structure, locomotion, organelles, life cycles, and means of reproduction.

I. Protozoa
A. General characteristics
1. Are unicellular but may be found in groups as colonies.
2. Range in size from approximately 10 μm to 200 μm in length.
3. Are nutritionally holozoic; ingest solid food particles through a mouth or opening.
4. Cyst formation may occur, which is useful in the transmission of parasitic forms.
5. Reproduce asexually or sexually.

6. Are classified based primarily on mode of locomotion.
7. Typically are transmitted by ingestion but sometimes by penetration of the skin.
B. Protozoa Classes
1. *Mastigophora* (flagellates) move by means of flagella. Major pathogens include:
a. *Giardia lamblia.* Causes giardiasis, an intestinal infection with cramps and diarrhea; fecal-oral transmission.
b. *Trichomonas vaginalis.* Causes trichomoniasis, a genitourinary infection; sexual transmission.
c. *Trypanosoma gambiense.* Causes African sleeping sickness; tsetse fly transmission.
d. *Leishmania tropica.* Causes leishmaniasis, a skin eruption with scaring; sand fly transmission.
2. *Sarcodina* are flexible amoebas. Major pathogen:
a. *Entamoeba histolytica.* Causes amebic dysentery; fecal-oral or venereal transmission.
3. *Sporozoa* are nonmotile. Major pathogens:
a. *Plasmodium malariae.* Causes malaria; mosquito transmission to the blood stream.
b. *Toxoplasma gondii.* Causes toxoplasmosis, a fatigue syndrome; transmission by cat feces or undercooked meat.
4. *Ciliata* (ciliates) move by means of cilia. Major pathogen:
a. *Balantidium coli.* Causes severe dysentery; fecal-oral transmission.

II. Helminths
A. General characteristics
1. Are multicellular complex organisms; elongated and bilaterally symmetrical worms.
2. Are macroscopic in size; range from less than 1 mm to more than 1 mm.
3. Receive nutrition from the host by attachment of suckers, hooks, plates, or teeth. If lacking these structures, nutrients are absorbed by the organism.
4. Life cycles are complex, with intermediate stages and infectious forms. Eggs may develop into larvae in an intermediate host and the larvae may develop into adult worms in the final or definitive host (the definitive host often is human).
5. Reproduce sexually; many are hermaphroditic (male and female organs in the same body).
6. Are classified primarily based on morphologic forms, intermediate stages, eggs, and attachment apparatus.
7. Typically are transmitted by ingestion or skin penetration.
B. Helminth classes
1. Cestodes (tape worms) are flatworms with a ribbon-like structure. They lack an alimentary canal and are hermaphroditic. Some life cycles are simple and others involve one or more intermediate hosts. Major pathogens include:
a. *Taenia saginata.* Beef tapeworm. Larvae are ingested with infected beef.

b. *Taenia solium*. Pork tapeworm. Larvae are ingested with infected pork.

c. *Diphyllobothrium latum*. Fish tapeworm. Larvae are ingested with infected fish.

2. Trematodes (flukes) are flatworms with a leaf-like structure. They have a partial digestive system and are hermaphroditic. Life cycles are complex with first (snails) and secondary (aquatic plants and animals) intermediate hosts. Major pathogens include:

a. *Fasciolopsis buski*. Intestinal fluke; transmitted by ingestion of larvae.

b. *Fasciola hepatica*. Liver fluke; transmitted by ingestion of larvae.

c. *Paragonimus westermani*. Lung fluke; transmitted by ingestion of larvae.

d. *Schistosoma mansoni*. Blood fluke; transmitted by penetration of the skin.

3. Nematodes (roundworms) are round and cylindrical. They have a complete digestive system and the sexes are separate. Nematodes that infect the intestine and muscle are transmitted by ingestion; those that infect blood and tissue are transmitted by the bites of insects (arthropods). Pathogens include:

a. *Trichinella spiralis*. Causes trichinosis in the intestine and muscles; transmitted by ingestion of larvae in meat, especially pork.

b. *Ascaris lumbricoides*. Causes ascariasis in the small intestine; transmitted by ingestion of eggs in food and soil.

c. *Enterobius vermicularis*. Pinworms that infect the large intestine; transmitted by ingestion of eggs.

d. *Necator americanus*. Hookworms in the small intestine; transmitted by penetration of larvae through the skin.

e. *Wuchereria bancrofti*. Causes filariasis, infection of the blood and lymphatic system; transmitted by mosquito.

f. *Onchocerca volvulus*. Causes river blindness; transmitted to the blood by black flies.

Transmission and Pathogenesis

Microorganisms generally must breach host barriers in order to initiate disease-causing reactions. An exception is transmission by ingestion of a preformed microbial toxin.

I. Nonspecific Host Defenses

A. Constitute first-line barriers and reactions against invading microorganisms.

B. Physical defenses include skin cells and hair.

C. Chemical defenses include:

1. Acidic pH present in stomach (acid secretion), vagina (microbial flora), and skin (lipids).

2. Microbe-digesting enzymes at mucosal sites (e.g., lysozyme).

3. Blood proteins termed "acute phase" proteins, which harm microbes by depositing on their surface and facilitating clearance by phagocytosis.

D. Biological defenses include:

1. Phagocytic cells, which internalize and degrade potential pathogens.

2. Complement proteins, which damage microbial membranes and facilitate clearance by phagocytosis.

II. Specific Host Defenses occur when the body's immune system recognizes and responds to microbes or microbial toxins.

 Clinical Case **STUDY**

When 68-year-old Bob Bates visits his dentist for an oral prophylaxis of his mandibular teeth, examination of the oral cavity reveals several white patchy lesions that adhere to the buccal mucosal surfaces and erythematous mucosa underlying his upper denture. Microscopic examination of a small specimen mixed with saline and placed on a slide reveals ovoid cells, some of which appear singly and some of which are budding. When some of the specimen is cultured in the laboratory, irregular cream-colored colonies rapidly appear. Further investigations by Bob's family physician reveal a fasting blood sugar concentration of 200 mg/dL (normal = 70 to 110 mg/dL).

Clinical Case QUESTIONS

1. Bob is diagnosed with a fungal infection. Which of the data mentioned are important to the diagnosis? What organism is the likely cause of the infection?

2. What is the likely source of Bob's fungal infection?

3. What is the most important factor in Bob's susceptibility to this oral infection?

4. What strategies for treating Bob would be appropriate?

Clinical Case RATIONALES

1. The gross appearance of the lesion, the microscopic appearance of the lesion material, and the growth in culture are all consistent with oral *C. albicans* infection, also known as "thrush" or candida.

2. *C. albicans* is ubiquitous (environmental exposure is common) and the likely source of Bob's infection was endogenous (from candida harbored in or on his body). *C. albicans* thus represents an opportunistic pathogen, which causes clinical disease during a breakdown in host defenses.

3. Bob's fasting blood glucose level of 200 mg/dL suggests a diagnosis of diabetes mellitus type II. Diabetes

is known to increase susceptibility to some infections, including opportunistic *C. albicans.*

4. Several antifungal agents may be useful in helping to clear the oral infection, including amphotericin B, nystatin, and clotrimazole. Bob's diabetes must be evaluated and treated by appropriate insulin and/or nutritional therapy.

Immunology

The immune system protects the body from harmful infections and most likely also attacks the development of some tumors. Bone marrow stem cells generate the body's immune cells on a continuous basis throughout life. The body produces both specific and nonspecific immune factors. Immunosuppression or immunodeficiency predisposes the individual to infections and some types of cancers.

Antigens

Antigens are molecules that are recognized as foreign and potentially harmful by the immune system. They are present on all invading microorganisms, are constituents of bacterial toxins, and are targets for specific protective immune reactions.

Lymphocytes

Lymphocytes are the key antigen-specific cells of our immune system. They use antigen receptors on their surface to recognize the presence of foreign microbial invaders, which trigger their responses.

I. Lymphocytes produce antigen-specific molecules that focus immune responses on foreign microorganisms that have entered the body.

II. Lymphocytes also help activate antigen-nonspecific inflammatory responses produced by macrophages, neutrophils, and other cells.

III. These combined immune responses neutralize or destroy agents of pathogenic infections as well as some tumors.

A. B lymphocytes produce antibodies (or "immunoglobulins", the class of blood proteins that contains antibodies).

1. Antibodies chemically bind to specific antigenic determinants known as epitopes (Fig. 4–1).

2. Humoral immunity is mediated by antibodies.

   a. IgG is the major blood antibody; crosses the placenta to protect the newborn.

   b. IgA protects mucosal sites (e.g., GI and GU tracts); is present in tears and saliva and is secreted in breast milk.

   c. IgM is the first antibody produced during an immune response.

   d. IgE attacks parasites and also may harm humans by causing allergies.

   e. IgD is a class of antibodies that participates in immune regulation.

3. Antibodies may bind to the surface of microbes and thereby trigger:

   a. Neutralization.

   b. Destruction via complement activation or phagocytosis by macrophages and neutrophils.

B. T lymphocytes specifically recognize microbial antigens and carry out cell-mediated reactions. T lymphocytes also:

1. Help B cells respond by secreting cytokines (regulatory protein molecules), which stimulate B cells.

2. Kill virus-infected cells by recognizing the presence of viral antigen on the surface of the infected target cells; kill tumor cells by a similar mechanism.

3. Stimulate phagocytosis of microbes by macrophages and neutrophils through the release of activating cytokines.

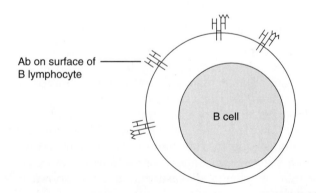

Antigenic determinant (epitope) ⋁⋀

Ab on surface of B lymphocyte

B cell

Figure 4.1 B lymphocyte.

B cell surface antibody (Ab) is shown reacting with specific antigenic determinants. This helps trigger B cell activation and subsequent Ab secretion.

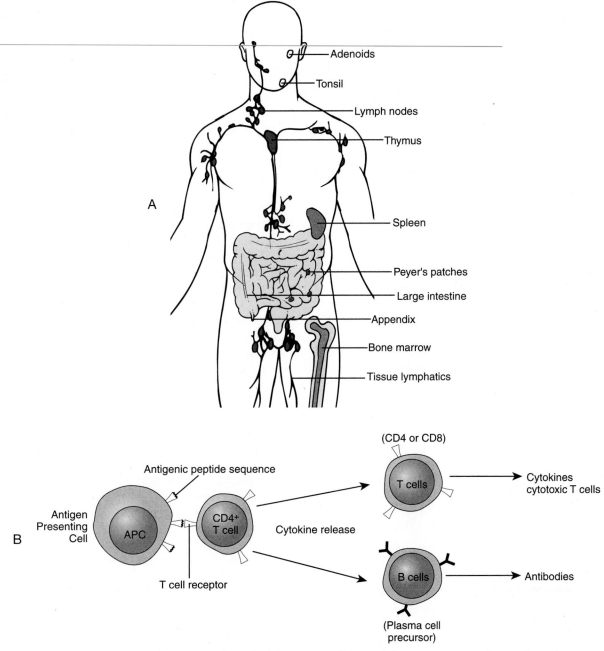

Figure 4.2 *A*, Human lymphoid system. Primary (bone marrow, thymus) and secondary lymphoid tissues are shown. Note interconnections via tissue lymphatics (shown), as well as blood vessels (not shown). *B*, cellular interactions of the immune system.

Development of Immunity

Immune responses occur when antigens are recognized by lymphocytes.

I. Primary immunization describes the first contact with an antigen; may occur by natural infection or by vaccination. It takes time (varies: several days to weeks) for immunity to develop after primary immunization.

II. Secondary immunization is the subsequent rapid, highly vigorous immune response to a second contact with the same antigen, via reexposure or booster vaccination.

Lymphoid Tissue and Cell Interactions

I. All cells of the immune system (Fig. 4–2, *A*) originate from bone marrow stem cells.

II. B lymphocytes are highly dependent on bone marrow because much of their maturation occurs there.

III. T lymphocytes mature in the thymus.

IV. B and T lymphocytes migrate to secondary lymphoid tissue (e.g., lymph node, spleen).

V. Secondary lymphoid tissues are sites of interaction (Fig. 4–2, B) with trapped antigen and also sites of initiation of immune responses.

VI. Accessory cells (e.g., macrophages, dendritic cells) present antigen to lymphocytes, thereby facilitating immune responsiveness.

Autoimmunity

Some individuals' immune systems develop a breakdown in the normal control mechanisms that prevent immune reactions against "self" antigens. There is a spectrum of autoimmune disease that ranges from mild, transient responses to potentially fatal responses. Autoimmune reactions may be organ-specific (e.g., directed against a particular endocrine gland, such as the thyroid) or more generalized (e.g., directed against DNA). Some autoimmune disorders may be successfully treated with immunosuppressive or antiinflammatory drugs, such as corticosteroids or aspirin.

I. Normally, we are self-tolerant:
  A. When lymphocytes that are reactive for self-antigens develop in the body, they are automatically eliminated, which provides us with protection from internal immune attack.
  B. If the mechanisms that normally eliminate self-reactive lymphocytes break down, surviving self-reactive lymphocytes may lead to autoimmune disease (i.e., a clinically apparent immune reaction to self-antigen).
  C. The reasons for breakdown in self-tolerance are not clear; there may be a genetic basis for some autoimmune disease because the major histocompatibility complex (MHC, a gene locus present in all mammals that codes for immunologically important cell-surface proteins; also known as "HLA" in humans) governs immune recognition and regulation. Viral or bacterial infection may trigger some autoimmune disease.
  D. Examples of autoimmune disease:
    1. Hashimoto thyroiditis—Characterized by anti-thyroid autoantibodies.
    2. Insulin-dependent diabetes mellitus—Characterized by autoantibodies against pancreatic beta cells.
    3. Myasthenia gravis—Characterized by muscle weakness and the presence of autoantibodies that disrupt nerve connections to muscle.
    4. Rheumatoid arthritis—Pathogenesis is unknown, but autoantibodies directed against immunoglobulins ("rheumatoid factors") may play a role.
    5. Systemic lupus erythematosus (SLE)—Anti-DNA antibodies are present.
    6. Multiple sclerosis (MS)—Cause is unknown, but autoimmune responses have been implicated in this disease, which is characterized by demyelination of the central nervous system.

Immunodeficiencies

Immunodeficiencies are characterized by a breakdown of one or more immune system components, which leads to the inability to fend off infection or cancer. Some immunodeficiencies may be clinically inapparent (detected only by a laboratory test); others may be mild and treatable with drugs. Some may be severe enough to cause death.

I. The severity of a given immunodeficiency often is related to the location of the cellular defect.
  A. The failure of lymphocyte stem cells to develop properly leads to a wide-ranging immunodeficiency.
  B. A defect late in the developmental pathway of lymphocytes may lead to a selective immunodeficiency (e.g., the inability to produce only a single immunoglobulin isotype, such as IgA).

II. Immunodeficiencies may involve any of the molecules, cells, tissues, or organs that comprise our complex immune defenses, including B and T lymphocytes, phagocytic cells, and complement molecules.
  A. Primary immunodeficiencies are intrinsic (genetic) defects in immunity; are caused by inheritance or mutation. Examples of primary immunodeficiencies include severe combined immunodeficiencies (no functional B or T lymphocytes) and a variety of disorders linked to the X chromosome (generally B cell disorders).
  B. Secondary immunodeficiencies are the result of an insult to the immune system, such as:
    1. Virus infection (e.g., AIDS).
    2. Radiation.
    3. Trauma from burns or toxin exposure.
    4. Malnutrition.

III. Clinical features associated with immunodeficiencies (Table 4–3):
  A. Opportunistic infection—Infection with microbes of normally low virulence.
  B. Reactivated infection—One that the patient had previous exposure to (which normally would stimulate life-long protective immunity).
  C. The incidence of some cancers is higher in patients with an immunodeficiency.

IV. Treatment of Immunodeficiencies
  A. Replacement of antibodies, by injecting the patient with immunoglobulins (passive immunization), may be effective for some B cell disorders, such as X-linked hypogammaglobulinemia.
  B. Transplantation with bone marrow, cord blood, or fetal thymus may provide functioning tissue to patients with T cell or T and B cell disorders.
  C. Treatment with cytokines, to stimulate immune cells, is under development.
  D. Gene therapy, in which missing or defective genes are replaced, is a potentially promising treatment.

TABLE 4.3	Immunodeficiency Types and Clinical Associations

Name/Type	Clinical Associations
Selective IgA deficiency	Mild-to-severe infections at mucosal sites (respiratory, gastrointestinal, genitourinary) because of low levels of IgA.
X-linked hypogamma-globulinemia	Reduced levels of circulating anti-bodies lead to chronic bacterial infections.
DiGeorge syndrome	Absence of the thymus leads to T-cell deficiency, viral infections, and increased susceptibility to some cancers.
Severe combined immunodeficiency (SCID)	Absence of functional T- and B-lymphocytes is potentially fatal.

 Clinical Case STUDY

George Scott, a previously healthy 12 year old, recently experienced trouble breathing after eating a peanut butter sandwich. His symptoms included wheezing and a swollen face. His parents took him to the local emergency room, where his blood pressure was 60/40 mmHg and his breathing was labored. He received an injection of epinephrine (adrenaline), and minutes later his blood pressure normalized and his breathing difficulty abated.

Clinical Case QUESTIONS

1. Describe the pathogenesis and cause of George's illness.
2. What laboratory tests would help confirm the diagnosis?
3. What role did epinephrine play in facilitating George's recovery?
4. What preventive measures should George take in the future?

Clinical Case RATIONALES

1. George appears to have developed an allergic response to peanuts, based on his symptoms and the case history. Therefore the presumptive diagnosis is an anaphylactic response. The pathogenesis is that of a type I (immediate) hypersensitivity response: after becoming sensitized to peanut antigens, George produced an IgE response that triggered his anaphylaxis after a subsequent exposure.
2. Tests to confirm and further explore this diagnosis would include a skin test with peanut antigens (to see

whether George responds with a wheal and erythema), and a RAST (radioallergosorbent test), which specifically seeks out blood IgE antibodies that are reactive with particular antigens.

3. Epinephrine was the solution to George's emergency because this drug causes an increase in mast cell cAMP, which results in rapid inhibition of the type I response. Other drugs that could be administered as a second line of treatment include the corticosteroid, prednisone, and bronchodilators.
4. Future medical precautions would include avoiding peanuts and carrying an emergency epinephrine injection kit, because peanuts may be a hidden component of some foods and thus difficult to avoid entirely.

Allergies

Allergies are immune reactions with pathologic inflammatory side effects.

I. IgE-mediated immune reactions induce basophils and mast cells to release chemical mediators of inflammation.
   A. Asthma/hay fever is a common category.
   B. Anaphylaxis is an emergency that requires immediate treatment with epinephrine.
   C. Drugs (e.g., penicillin) may cause anaphylaxis.
   D. Stings and bites also are causes of anaphylaxis.
   E. Rubber/latex allergy
      1. Apparently occurs with increasing incidence. Latex allergy may occur in anyone, but at-risk groups include health care workers, people who work with latex, food service workers, police, janitors, and firefighters.
      2. Contact with hospital gloves, catheters, tourniquets, dental dams, balloons, baby bottle nipples, condoms, or other latex items may sensitize an individual to latex molecules.
      3. Powdered latex gloves may facilitate inhalation of latex molecules bound to cornstarch powder, which become airborne, setting the stage for an allergic (hypersensitivity) response to inhaled latex molecules. Occasionally, severe or life-threatening hypersensitivity reactions may occur, which require emergency medical treatment (use of epinephrine or other drugs).
II. IgG antibodies may cause allergic reactions.
   A. By attaching to cell-surface antigens and activating complement to injure or kill cells.
   B. By forming circulating immune complexes, which lodge in capillaries to incite inflammatory damage.
III. T cells
   A. Release inflammatory cytokines, which stimulate tissue damage.
IV. Treatment includes:
   A. Drugs that suppress inflammation.
      1. Antihistamines
      2. Corticosteroids

B. Avoidance of the allergen (e.g., food allergy).
C. Desensitization; exposure to an allergen by a different route, which alters the immune response (e.g., modulating it from IgE to IgG).

Immunologic Diagnosis

Immunologic diagnosis uses antibodies or other immune factors to detect immune responses or the presence of antigens.

I. Serodiagnosis detects antibodies to specific antigens, providing evidence of exposure to the antigen (e.g., HIV testing [termed "seroconversion"]).
II. Genetic testing is used to determine MHC genes; has predictive value for some diseases.

Immunotherapy

Immunotherapy may be employed to counter the effects of immunodeficiency or autoimmunity. The immune system may be manipulated by the administration of antibodies, the administration of various drugs (e.g., cytokines, antiinflammatory and immunosuppressive drugs), and by transplantation of immune cells.

I. Passive administration of antibodies (e.g., pooled human immunoglobulins) is a treatment for immunodeficiencies or is a form of prophylaxis for some viruses (e.g., hepatitis A or B).
II. Transplantation of human stem cells (e.g., from bone marrow) is used in the treatment of some immunodeficiencies, such as SCID.
III. Immune stimulators (e.g., cytokines) are used for treatment of immunodeficiencies and some cancers.
IV. Immunosuppression, with drugs or antibodies directed against immune cells, may help treat autoimmunity or graft rejection.

Vaccination

Vaccination (active immunization) is exposure to antigens in a manner that is designed to stimulate protective immunity.

I. Killed vaccines use heat or chemical-treated microorganisms or toxins. They are safe but in some cases may be less effective than live-attenuated vaccines.
II. Live-attenuated vaccines are genetically-altered microorganisms that have lost virulence but still undergo limited replication in the body.
III. Molecular vaccines are composed of critical antigenic determinants, derived as recombinant (from cloned bacteria or yeast) or synthetic peptides. Recently, DNA has been used to vaccinate experimental animals.
IV. Adjuvants may be used to stimulate immune responses to I and III.

Passive Immunization

Passive immunization is the transfer of protective antibodies into an individual. Protection is immediately established but short-lived because of antibody catabolism.

I. Passive immunization is a common form of postexposure prophylaxis after:
A. Possible exposure to infection (e.g., hepatitis viruses A and B).
B. Toxin exposure (e.g., snakebite).
II. Passive immunization occurs naturally during pregnancy, when maternal antibodies are transported into the fetus, and during nursing, when breast milk antibodies are ingested.

 ## Clinical Case STUDY

John Brown is a 40-year-old homeless man living in the streets of New York City. He presents at a walk-in clinic with a cough of several weeks duration, weight loss, and fever. A sputum smear shows the presence of acid-fast bacilli, a chest x-ray film shows evidence of pulmonary lesions, and two days later his tuberculin (TB) test is determined to be positive.

Clinical Case QUESTIONS

1. Does this patient pose a risk to allied health personnel, and if so, what precautions could be taken?
2. What is the significance of the positive TB test?
3. How should therapy of this patient's tuberculosis be handled?

Clinical Case RATIONALES

1. Close contact and heavy exposure enhance tuberculosis transmission by respiratory droplets, so medical personnel are at risk. Limiting droplet exposure by wearing face masks helps reduce the risk of acquiring tuberculosis.
2. The positive TB test indicates active immunity (T cell-mediated hypersensitivity) to the tubercle bacillus. In the context of the symptoms and other lab tests, active infection is likely.
3. Therapy should consist of immediate antibiotic therapy and monitoring of patient compliance with drug therapy.

Infectious Diseases

Examples of the myriad infectious diseases of humans are organized here according to major modes of transmission (respiratory, mucosal, food-borne or vector-borne, sexual, or by exposure to blood or body fluids, toxins, or parasitic infection). These examples have a practical association with major risks for exposure.

Common Respiratory/Mucosal Infections (Oral/Nasopharynx/Tonsils/Lungs/Eyes)

The most common routes for infection transmission are the respiratory system, the eyes, and oral mucosa. These routes of transmission are facilitated by the absence of protective skin cells and also by potential access to various body cells (e.g., epithelial, lymphocytes, macrophages).

I.   Influenza (RNA [orthomyxo-] virus)
  A. Virus is transmitted in aerosols of respiration secretions.
  B. Pathogenesis
    1. Includes virus replication in airway cells.
    2. The inflammatory immune response contributes to tissue damage.
  C. Diagnosis
    1. Symptoms include fever, malaise, headache, and cough.
    2. Is by specific detection of virus antigens in cells from nasopharynx.
  D. Prevention occurs through vaccination.
    1. Protects some but not all individuals.
    2. Vaccine preparation is complicated by mutations and new antigenic strains that arise.
  E. Treatment includes amantadine and rimantadine, antivirals that hasten recovery from some cases if started early.
  F. Epidemiology includes yearly epidemics and occasional world-wide pandemics.
II. Rubeola (RNA [paramyxo-] virus; "measles")
  A. Is transmitted through the respiratory route; involves local infection followed by viremia and systemic spread.
  B. Pathogenesis is by replication of the virus in various body cells, including those of the skin (rash), respiratory tract, and conjunctiva.
    1. The virus may persist for years; rarely causes a fatal brain infection.
  C. Diagnosis can be made
    1. By symptoms, which include fever, sneezing, cough, Koplik spots (small, blue-white ulcerations on buccal mucosa, opposite lower molars), and skin rash (head-to-chest).
    2. By virus isolation or seroconversion.
  D. Prevention includes:
    1. Immune protection after natural infection is life-long.
    2. Vaccination is highly effective.
    3. Passive prophylaxis with measles immunoglobulin.
  E. No specific treatment is available.
  F. Epidemiology
    1. By age 12, most unvaccinated children have had measles and are immune.

  2. Vaccination has greatly reduced the incidence of disease in developed countries.
III. Rubella (RNA [toga-] virus; "German measles")
  A. Virus is transmitted by contact with respiratory secretions or is transmitted directly to a fetus.
  B. Pathogenesis is by virus replication in respiratory and other body cells; congenital rubella may cause fetal/infant damage.
  C. Diagnosis is by presence of typical rash and lymphadenopathy and specifically by virus isolation or seroconversion.
  D. Prevention includes:
    1. Protective immunity occurs after infection or vaccination.
    2. A live-attenuated rubella virus vaccine; not for use during pregnancy.
    3. No specific treatment is available.
  E. Epidemiology
    1. Rubella occurs sporadically in the United States.
    2. Vaccine use has greatly reduced the incidence of the disease.
IV. Mumps (RNA [paramyxo-] virus)
  A. Transmission is by respiratory route (droplets), local virus replication, viremia, and systemic dissemination.
  B. Pathogenesis is by virus replication in parotid gland, testes (after puberty), ovaries, brain, kidneys, and other organs.
  C. Diagnosis made by:
    1. Symptoms, which include malaise and parotid/salivary gland enlargement.
    2. Specifically, by isolation of virus or seroconversion.
  D. Prevention
    1. By immunization is effective; typically is a combination vaccine for measles-mumps-rubella or "MMR."
    2. No specific treatment therapy is currently available.
  E. Epidemiology includes:
    1. World-wide epidemics (primarily children).
    2. Vaccine use has greatly reduced mumps and complications of mumps.
V.   Infectious Mononucleosis ("mono")
  A. Is caused by the Epstein-Barr virus (EBV), a DNA herpes virus.
  B. Is transmitted by saliva to the pharynx and salivary glands.
  C. Pathogenesis of infectious mononucleosis includes:
    1. A 30- to 50-day incubation period, during which the virus replicates in epithelial and B-lymphoid cells.
    2. Development of enlarged lymph nodes and spleen.
    3. Persistence of the virus in B lymphocytes.

4. Suppression of the EBV in the body by immunity.

D. Diagnosis involves:
   1. Symptoms, which include headache, malaise, fatigue, sore throat, and enlarged spleen/lymph nodes.
   2. Specifically, virus isolation and seroconversion.

E. Prevention in the form of a vaccine is not available.

F. No specific treatment therapy for EBV infection is known.

G. Epidemiology
   1. EBV is a common infection that establishes life-long persistence.
   2. EBV infection is associated with two types of cancers—Burkitt's lymphoma and nasopharyngeal carcinoma.

VI. Cytomegalovirus (CMV)
A. Is a DNA herpes virus.
B. Is transmitted by close oral and respiratory contact (saliva and urine shedding) and also by sexual contact.
C. Pathogenesis
   1. Is normally subclinical.
   2. Includes a 4- to 8-week incubation period, followed by an infectious mononucleosis-like syndrome.
   3. Involves congenital and perinatal infections, which may result in severe fetal and newborn infections.
   4. Causes severe infection in immunosuppressed hosts, such as transplant recipients and AIDS and cancer patients.
D. Diagnosis is by:
   1. Symptoms, such as malaise, myalgia, and fever.
   2. Lymphocytosis and atypical lymphocytes.
   3. Virus isolation and seroconversion.
E. Prevention is unavailable, although a vaccine currently is under development.
F. Treatment includes administration of ganciclovir and foscarnet, which may be used to treat CMV retinitis.
G. Epidemiology
   1. Prevalence, determined by antibody (demonstration of immune response to infection), is between approximately 50% and 100%.
   2. Life-long latent infection occurs, with intermittent shedding.
   3. A vaccine currently is under development.

VII. Tuberculosis (TB)
A. Is a bacterial infection caused by *Mycobacterium tuberculosis*.
B. Transmission is by the respiratory route.
C. Pathogenesis is by:
   1. Spread throughout the body via lymphatics and blood.

2. The growth of bacteria in monocytes.
3. Intracellular growth, which stimulates the T-lymphocyte response and results in cell-mediated hypersensitivity and associated tissue damage.

D. Diagnosis is by:
   1. Symptoms, which depend on the organ site.
      a. Typically include fever and fatigue.
      b. With lung involvement, include coughing and spitting blood.
      c. May include meningitis.
   2. Specific diagnosis is by examination of smears and culture; tuberculin ("TB") skin testing reveals a positive cell-mediated response to antigens.

E. Prevention is by:
   1. BCG vaccination, which is sometimes used but has questionable efficacy.
   2. Avoidance of close contact with infectious persons.

F. Treatment includes:
   1. Antibiotics (isoniazid, rifampin, pyrazinamide, or ethambutol)
   2. A required 6- to 9-month course of treatment.
   3. Additional drugs if antibiotic resistance to those given occurs.

G. Epidemiology includes:
   1. Close contact and massive exposure, which enhances transmission rate.
   2. Immunosuppression (e.g., AIDS), which leads to enhanced susceptibility.
   3. Emergence of multi drug-resistant strains.

VIII. Group A Streptococcus
A. Is a common bacterial infection (e.g., "strep throat") caused by S. pyogenes.
B. Is transmitted by any route, but typically is from an infected person (or carrier) via respiratory droplets or skin; nasal discharge is a prominent source of infection.
C. Pathogenesis is site-dependent, with:
   1. Rapid spreading.
   2. Attachment to pharyngeal epithelium in the case of streptococcal sore throat.
   3. Disease ranging from local skin infections to fatal bacteremia or streptococcal toxic shock syndrome.
D. Diagnosis includes:
   1. Presence of strep throat.
   2. Symptoms, which include acute pharyngitis, tonsillitis, redness and edema of mucous membranes, purulent exudate, fever, and enlarged cervical lymph nodes. Symptoms of rheumatic fever (see below) include carditis, polyarthritis, and subcutaneous nodules.
   3. Specific isolation of streptococci in smears or cultures; rapid detection of group A streptococcal antigen from throat swabs is available.

E. Prevention is unavailable, although vaccines are under development.

F. Treatment includes penicillin, which is given for 10 days.

G. Epidemiology of rheumatic fever
   1. Untreated strep throat may progress to rheumatic fever; the incidence is approximately 3%.
   2. Mechanism responsible is antigenic cross-reaction with heart tissue; the immune response becomes directed against heart antigens.

IX. Hepatitis A Virus (HAV)
   A. Is an RNA (hepato-) virus.
   B. Is transmitted via fecal-oral route; commonly caused by contamination of food or water.
   C. Pathogenesis involves the liver, which is the target organ; necrosis of liver cells and inflammatory changes occur.
   D. Diagnosis occurs by detection of elevated liver enzymes (aminotransferase) and anti-HAV antibodies.
   E. Prevention includes prophylaxis by passive administration of immune globulins; no vaccine is available. No specific antiviral therapy currently is available for treatment.
   F. Epidemiology includes:
      1. Common occurrence in families, institutions, camps, and the armed forces.
      2. A short incubation period of 15 to 45 days; the onset is abrupt.
      3. Recovery by means of the immune response.

X. Whooping Cough (pertussis)
   A. Is caused by *Bordetella pertussis*, a Gram-negative bacterium.
   B. The bacterium is transmitted in respiratory droplets.
   C. Pathogenesis involves the colonization of ciliated cells in the respiratory mucosa, followed by the production of bacterial toxins (see below), which most likely play a role in cell damage.
   D. Diagnosis is by laboratory culture, demonstration of specific IgA antibodies, or by molecular detection of *Bordetella* DNA.
   E. Prevention is by vaccination with whole-cell vaccines, which are effective but occasionally toxic. Less toxic acellular vaccines recently have been introduced.
   F. Treatment with erythromycin reduces the infectious period to 5 to 10 days but has little effect on the disease.
   G. Epidemiology
      1. Transmission is direct, from person to person.
      2. The period of highest infectivity occurs soon after infection, when the levels of bacteria are highest, but patients remain infectious for as many as 5 weeks.
      3. In addition to paroxysmal cough, encephalopathy and bronchopneumonia occasionally may develop.
      4. Has been stemmed by vaccination in developed countries but large numbers of humans (primarily infants and children) continue to die from this highly infectious disease in underdeveloped countries.
      5. Recovery is associated with immune protection.

XI. Legionnaire's Disease
   A. Is a bacterial infection of *Legionella*, a Gram-negative bacillus; *L. pneumophila* is the primary species associated with Legionnaire's disease.
   B. Is transmitted to humans via *Legionella* from an infected water supply, primarily in the form of an aerosol.
   C. Pathogenesis is by infection of the lower respiratory tract, which results in toxic effects on lung cells and stimulation of inflammatory responses, which exacerbate tissue damage.
   D. Diagnosis is by laboratory culture of *Legionella*, detection of bacterial antigen in body tissues, or demonstration of seroconversion.
   E. Prevention is by:
      1. Decontamination of contaminated water supplies, by heating or chlorination.
      2. Vaccination has not been attempted in humans.
      3. Erythromycin is the antibiotic of choice for symptomatic infections.
   F. Epidemiology
      1. The bacterium is common in aquatic systems.
      2. Dissemination by aerosols plays an important role in outbreaks (e.g., from evaporative condensers, cooling towers, and nebulizers).
      3. Patient susceptibility appears to play a role; risk factors are greater for health care facilities.

XII. Histoplasmosis
   A. Is a fungal infection; the fungal agent is *Histoplasma capsulatum*.
   B. Pulmonary infection results from inhalation of Histoplasma capsulatum.
   C. Is characterized by intracellular growth of the fungus, which may disseminate to lymph nodes, liver, bone marrow, or brain, causing a life-threatening infection in immunocompromised patients or infants.
   D. Diagnosis is by culture from blood, sputum, bone marrow, or CSF, or by biopsy and histologic examination of tissues.
   E. Treatment of progressive disease is with amphotericin; only 50% success is achieved in immunocompromised patients.
   F. Epidemiology
      1. The fungus is endemic in tropical areas of the world and also in the central U.S.; resides in

soil, from which it may be transported to the air and inhaled.

   2. Fungal spores may spread from alveoli to lymph nodes, resulting in disseminated disease, which may appear years after an initial infection in immunocompromised hosts.

Bacterial toxins

Some bacteria may cause disease in humans because of toxic properties present in protein molecules (toxins), which they carry or release. Disease from toxin exposure may not require bacterial replication in the body, because in some cases exposure to the toxin alone is sufficient to cause disease.

I. Enterohemorrhagic *E. coli*
   A. Is a toxin-producing, enteric Gram-negative rod.
   B. Is commonly transmitted via contaminated food; fecal-oral transmission may occur.
   C. Pathogenesis is by production of toxins, which cause hemorrhagic colitis and hemolytic uremic syndrome (kidney failure, hemolytic anemia, and thrombocytopenia).
   D. Diagnosis is by strain-specific immunological detection and growth in culture.
   E. Prevention is achieved by thoroughly cooking ground beef, which is the most common source of this infection.
   F. Therapy consists of rapid administration of antibiotics, reconstitution of fluid and electrolyte imbalances, and treatment of disseminated intravascular coagulation.
   G. Epidemiology: this infection recently has gained prominence in the news media. Fatal cases may occur; children and debilitated patients seem particularly susceptible.

II. Staphylococcal Enterotoxin
   A. Is a soluble toxin produced by approximately 50% of *S. aureus* strains.
   B. Causes food poisoning; may be present in contaminated foods that support the growth of *S. aureus*.
   C. Pathogenesis is by toxin action on gut nerves, which stimulates vomiting and diarrhea.
   D. Diagnosis typically is based on symptoms and epidemiology but enterotoxins may be assayed immunologically in the laboratory.
   E. Prevention is complicated by the presence of *S. aureus* on the skin and mucous membranes of most humans. Use of antiseptics and good personal hygiene may help control spread to food. Antibiotic therapy for carriers has limited use because of the emergence of drug resistance and the need for long-term therapy.
   F. Treatment of the symptoms of food poisoning is primarily symptomatic because of the short incubation period after exposure to the toxin (1 to 8 hours).
   G. Epidemiology: staphylococcal enterotoxin is a significant cause of food poisoning. The heating of contaminated food may be sufficient to destroy the bacteria, although the toxin remains active.

III. Toxic Shock Syndrome (TSS)
   A. Toxic shock syndrome toxin (TSST) is produced by some strains of *S. aureus*.
   B. TSS is a tampon-associated disease; TSST is absorbed into the blood after growth of the bacteria in a tampon. However, any staphylococcal infection that produces enterotoxin or TSST may cause TSS.
   C. The pathogenesis of TSS is by activation of large numbers of T lymphocytes. by TSST, which is a superantigen; TSST causes activation of T lymphocytes and the release of inflammatory cytokines.
   D. Diagnosis is symptomatic (fever, shock, rash) and by laboratory detection of *S. aureus* and/or enterotoxin; also is indicated by shock and organ system failure.
   E. Prevention of TSS is facilitated by the use of less absorbent tampons.
   F. Therapy for TSS includes administration of antibiotics and supportive measures.
   G. Epidemiology of TSS: recognition of the relationship between TSS and the use of highly absorbent tampons has lead to a reduced incidence; sporadic cases continue to occur and require rapid recognition to reduce mortality and morbidity.

Vector-Borne Infections

Many infections are transmitted from insects or other living carriers. Such carriers acquire an infectious agent from an infected individual or waste and pass it to a susceptible individual, either directly (e.g., bite) or indirectly (e.g., food or environment).

I. Dengue
   A. Is a tropical disease caused by a mosquito-borne RNA (flavi-) virus.
   B. Is transmitted in a cycle, from mosquito to human (mosquitoes pick up the virus from an infected person and inject it into an uninfected person).
   C. Pathogenesis involves:
      1. Virus replication in macrophages throughout the body.
      2. Systemic toxicity.
      3. Immunopathology, which occurs in dengue hemorrhagic fever and dengue shock syndrome, with potentially severe outcomes.
   D. Prevention includes experimental vaccines, which currently are in use, and avoidance of the mosquito vector.
   E. Treatment includes supportive therapy for symptoms.
   F. Epidemiology has a geographic distribution, which includes the Caribbean; there are occasional reports of infection in the southern United States.
   G. Diagnosis is by:
      1. Serology.
      2. Virus detection in the blood.

3. Symptoms, such as fever, chills, malaise, and headache, followed by recovery that lasts from days to weeks.

II. Malaria

A. Is a tropical disease caused by mosquito-borne transmission of a parasite (genus is *Plasmodium*).

B. Transmission occurs in a cycle, from mosquito to human.

C. Pathogenesis involves internal growth of the parasite through its life cycle, resulting in chronic infection and damage to red blood cells and other body sites.

D. Diagnosis is by examination of stained blood specimens, which reveal the parasite; hematologic and liver function tests may be useful.

E. Prevention is through avoidance of mosquito bites, eradication of mosquitoes, prophylactic use of antimalarial drugs, and treatment of infected individuals. Vaccines are under development.

F. Treatment includes chloroquine, the drug of choice for acute attacks of malaria; resistance to chloroquine may occur, necessitating the use of other drugs for therapy or prophylaxis.

G. Epidemiology: malaria has been resistant to eradication in tropical areas. Malaria may be transmitted via contaminated needles, blood transfusions, and from mother to fetus.

Infections Transmitted Sexually or by Blood and Body Fluids

A variety of microorganisms have adapted to a sexual mode of transmission, whereby the protection afforded by intact skin is bypassed and the exchange of body fluids that contain infectious agents or infected cells may occur. Microbial exposure of fragile mucous membranes in body cavities allows for direct infection of target cells near the site of exposure, and also facilitates access to the blood, particularly in the case of concurrent infection or trauma. Blood transfusions and the sharing of contaminated needles during drug injection also facilitate cross-infection between individuals.

I. AIDS (acquired immunodeficiency syndrome)

A. Results from infection with human immunodeficiency virus (HIV), a retrovirus (contains a reverse transcriptase that mediates transcription of viral RNA into DNA). Various strains of HIV exist; most AIDS patients in North America are HIV-1 infected.

B. Transmission occurs via sexual contact, intravenous injection, and from mother to baby.

C. Key features of pathogenesis include:

1. HIV replication in CD4+ T cells, macrophages, and other body cells.

2. A prolonged asymptomatic period (approximately 10 years on average) for most HIV-infected people, during which the body's immune system becomes progressively impaired, apparently from a reduction in CD4+ cells.

3. Development of AIDS-defining infections and/or cancer follows the asymptomatic period, resulting in the death of untreated patients, generally within a few years.

D. Diagnosis of AIDS is by:

1. Case-defining infections (e.g., cytomegalovirus, *Pneumocystis carinii*, candidiasis, histoplasmosis, tuberculosis, toxoplasmosis, cryptococcosis). Patients typically present with one or more of these opportunistic infections.

2. Laboratory findings of HIV RNA in the blood and reduced blood CD4+ cells.

3. Positive ELISA screen for anti-HIV antibodies in blood (i.e., seroconversion).

4. Confirmation of anti-HIV antibodies in blood by immunoblot (a more specific antibody test).

5. History of exposure to HIV; acute HIV disease typically occurs 2 to 4 weeks after infection, and is characterized by fever, adenopathy, pharyngitis, and rash.

E. Prevention includes:

1. Avoidance of contact with blood and other body fluids (tears, saliva, semen, vaginal secretions, amniotic fluid, urine, and cerebrospinal fluid) of HIV-infected individuals.

2. Screening of blood used for transfusion.

F. Management of HIV infection

1. According to current CDC guidelines (www.healthcg.com), the following are methods for monitoring the severity of the infection:

a. Frequent assaying of the HIV RNA level in blood.

b. Frequent determination of blood CD4+ cell counts.

2. Currently recommended treatment options include combination drug therapy (reverse transcriptase inhibitors, such as AZT, D4T, ddI, or ddC, and one or more viral protease inhibitors), which holds promise for extending the length of the disease-free period of infection by:

a. Suppressing viral replication (as determined by blood HIV RNA analysis).

b. Encouraging blood CD4+ count increases.

G. Epidemiology

1. Is a world-wide epidemic; the World Health Organization estimates that approximately 40 million people will be HIV-infected by the year 2000.

2. High risk transmission groups in North America include homosexual males and IV drug users who share needles. In Africa, greatest risk is heterosexual transmission.

3. Fatality rate is very high—greater than 50%.

II. Hepatitis B Virus (HBV)

A. Is a DNA virus.

B. Transmission is intravenous, sexual, by oral exposure to the virus, or from mother to baby; HBV is present in blood, saliva, semen, and other body fluids.

C. Pathogenesis includes chronic infection of the liver, which leads to liver dysfunction and liver cancer.

D. Diagnosis is by:
1. Symptoms, which may vary and include jaundice, rash, and arthritis.
2. Specific immunological tests for viral antigens or antivirus antibodies.
3. Detection of elevated blood levels of some liver enzymes.

E. Vaccination with HBV vaccine is available and involves postexposure prophylaxis with passive injection of hepatitis B-immune globulin in combination with the HBV vaccination. Recombivax is the currently used HBsAg; is derived from expression in yeast cells.

F. Prevention is by avoidance of exposure to body fluids, and HBV vaccination.

G. Treatment: specific therapy is not yet available.

H. Epidemiology: most patients recover completely, but 5% to 10% become chronic carriers of HBV. The 300 million chronic carriers worldwide are at high risk for developing liver cancer.

III. Hepatitis C Virus (HCV)

A. Is a ssRNA virus.

B. Is transmitted much like HBV: by blood transfusion, by IV drug abuse, mother to infant, and sexually.

C. HCV apparently replicates in humans over a long period of time, causing a mild disease in approximately 10% of recipients. Little is known about the pathogenesis.

D. Diagnosis is by demonstration of viral nucleic acid, using a virus-specific cDNA probe, or by seroconversion.

E. Management of HCV infection is by treatment with interferon-alpha and ribavirin. There is no vaccine for HCV.

F. Epidemiology
1. HCV is the most common cause of transfusion-associated hepatitis.
2. Blood donor screening currently is performed to eliminate antibody-positive donors.
3. Chronic active hepatitis develops in approximately 50% of patients.
4. Disease sometimes progresses to cirrhosis and liver cancer.

IV. Herpes Simplex Virus (HSV)

A. Includes the two subtypes of this DNA-virus family, which are HSV type 1 (HSV-1) and HSV type 2 (HSV-2).

B. Is transmitted both nonsexually (primarily HSV-1) and sexually (primarily HSV-2), through breaks in the skin or mucosal contact.

C. Pathogenesis includes a virus-induced cell death and inflammation.

1. The primary infection involves the skin and mucous membranes.
2. The virus maintains latency in the nerve ganglia.
3. Reactivation from the latent site occurs because of stress or immunosuppression; results in recurring secondary infection.

D. Diagnosis is by:
1. Symptoms, which include cold sores on the lips, palate, gingiva, nasal septum, or genitalia.
2. Specific virus isolation or seroconversion.

E. Vaccines are in the experimental stages of development.

F. Treatment includes use of acyclovir, valacyclovir, and famciclovir, which are potentially effective antivirals.

G. Epidemiology
1. HSV is widespread (HSV-1 incidence is greater than 80%).
2. HSV-1 most commonly infects the oropharynx and typically is spread by respiratory droplets or contact with saliva.
3. HSV-2 typically is spread by sexual contact; HSV-2 infection exhibits both symptomatic and asymptomatic shedding of the virus.
4. Other potentially severe but less common herpes infections include encephalitis, meningitis, and neonatal herpes.

V. Human Papillomaviruses (HPVs)

A. Are tumor-associated DNA viruses.

B. Infect epithelial cells of the skin and mucous membranes.

C. Transmission is by intimate contact.

D. Pathogenesis includes:
1. A range of clinical lesions, which depend on HPV type, including skin warts, plantar warts, flat warts, genital condylomas, and laryngeal papillomas. These tumors result from virus infection of epithelial cells.
2. HPV is linked with premalignant and malignant genital lesions.

E. Diagnosis is by clinical appearance and/or viral type detection.

F. Prevention includes:
1. Avoidance of sexual contact, which is effective for genital HPV infection.
2. Vaccines, which are under development but not yet available.

G. Treatment involves removal or destruction of the warts.

H. Epidemiology includes:
1. A wide distribution in humans.
2. Approximately 70 different types of HPV that may infect humans.
3. A majority of genital cancers are associated with types 16 and 18.

VI. Gonorrhea
- A. Is an infection with *Neisseria gonorrhea*, a Gram-negative coccus.
- B. Is transmitted by sexual contact; commonly infects the mucous membranes of the urethra in males and the cervix in females.
- C. Pathogenesis is related to the invasion of epithelial cells and cell damage associated with an inflammatory response. Dissemination to various body sites (e.g., brain, heart, joints, and peritoneal cavity) may occur.
- D. Laboratory diagnosis of a suspected case involves identification of Gram-negative diplococci, culture of oxidase-positive colonies, and specific confirmation by immunologic studies (fluorescent antibody staining; agglutination) or reaction with DNA probes.
- E. Prevention
  - 1. No vaccine is available.
  - 2. Condoms are effective in preventing transmission.
- F. Treatment of gonorrhea is with antibiotics such as ceftriaxone or doxycycline.
- G. Epidemiology of gonorrhea: this STD often is acquired from an asymptomatic sex partner. Hundreds of thousands of new cases occur each year in the United States.

VII. Syphilis
- A. Is infection with *Treponema pallidum* (subspecies pallidum); is sexually transmitted.
- B. Is a complex disease that may involve almost any tissue in the body.
- C. Has a complex pathogenesis, which includes:
  - 1. Primary disease, which occurs at the site of entry (typically a mucous membrane); is characterized by an ulcer ("chancre") that is highly contagious but eventually heals.
  - 2. Secondary disease, which follows weeks to months later and is caused by the dissemination of bacteria to various tissues; results in the development of new contagious lesions. These lesions typically heal within several weeks after their appearance; are caused by host immunological defenses.
  - 3. Tertiary disease, which may occur years later, when treponemes reemerge in body tissues. Tertiary syphilis in cardiovascular or central nervous system tissues is particularly serious and may be fatal.
- D. Diagnosis is by physical symptoms, microscopic identification of treponemes, and positive serology (detection of anti-syphilis antibodies).
- E. Prevention
  - 1. Vaccines are not yet effective.
  - 2. Includes tracing of contacts and prophylactic treatment with penicillin.
  - 3. Condoms are effective in preventing transmission.
- F. Treatment is effective with penicillin.
- G. Epidemiology
  - 1. Sexually-transmitted syphilis is a world-wide problem.
  - 2. Even with improved surveillance, syphilis remains an important public health problem in underdeveloped countries and in some drug-abusing populations of developed countries.

Parasites

Medical parasitology involves study of parasitic protozoa, helminths, and anthropoids. Examples of some medically important parasites, other than the vector-borne plasmodium infection previously described, include:

I. *Giardia lamblia*
- A. Is a protozoan found in the small intestine of humans.
- B. Transmission occurs by ingestion of fecally contaminated food or water that contains *Giardia* cysts; *Giardia* cysts may survive for weeks or months.
- C. Pathogenesis involves:
  - 1. Attachment of the parasite to the wall of the small bowel.
  - 2. Occurrence of persistent infections.
  - 3. Symptoms, which vary; may include weakness, abdominal pain, and weight loss. Patients may be asymptomatic.
- D. Diagnosis is by microscopic examination of stool specimens.
- E. Prevention includes personal hygiene and disinfection of water through filtration, boiling, and chlorination.
- F. Treatment is with quinacrine hydrochloride and/or metronidazole.
- G. Epidemiology of giardiasis includes epidemics in institutional settings and outbreaks in wilderness areas (which suggest transmission from animal sources [zoonosis]).

II. *Toxoplasma gondii*
- A. Is a protozoan that infects a wide range of animals, including the cat family.
- B. Transmission to humans is by exposure to cat feces (which carry an oocyst), eating undercooked meat that contains tissue oocysts, or from mother to fetus.
- C. Pathogenesis includes:
  - 1. A lack of symptoms in most humans (asymptomatic infection).
  - 2. Development of congenital toxoplasmosis when non-immune mothers are infected during pregnancy.
  - 3. Immunosuppression, which is associated with toxoplasmosis.
  - 4. Damage to macrophages and other body cells in which *T. gondii* replicates.
- D. Diagnosis includes:
  - 1. Prenatal toxoplasmosis in a pregnant woman, which is associated with blindness and other

defects, including neurologic damage, occurring in her newborn.
  2. Laboratory tests involving microscopic examination, animal inoculation, and seroconversion.
E. Prevention includes avoidance of cat feces and proper cooking of meats.
F. Treatment is with sulfonamides and pyrimethamine.
G. Epidemiology: most natural infections occur from eating undercooked meat, which contains tissue cysts, or from eating food contaminated with cat feces.

Infections with Neurological Sequelae

Some microorganisms may damage nerve cells, either by direct infection or by toxin production.
I. Poliovirus
  A. Is an RNA (picorna-) virus.
  B. Transmission is by the oral route, from virus present in water or from close contact with carriers who shed the virus in pharyngeal secretions or feces.
  C. Pathogenesis includes:
    1. Infection of the tonsils and small intestine cells.
    2. Invasion of the central nervous system.
    3. Damage of nerve cells, which leads to muscle paralysis.
    4. Primarily self-limiting infections; subsequent immunity to the same strain of virus occurs after recovery.
  D. Diagnosis is by:
    1. Symptoms that range from minor to major, including paralysis.
    2. Laboratory isolation of the virus or demonstration of seroconversion.
  E. Prevention includes vaccination with both live-attenuated and killed vaccines.
  F. Epidemiology includes a world-wide occurrence and susceptibility of children.
II. Meningitis
  A. Is a general term that describes inflammation of the membranes of the brain and spinal cord (meninges).
  B. May be triggered by infection with a variety of microorganisms.
    1. Common bacterial causes are group B streptococci, E. coli, Neisseria meningitidis, H. influenzae, and Streptococcus pneumoniae.
    2. Common viral causes include enteroviruses and the mumps virus.
    3. Some fungi and parasites may cause meningitis.
  C. Transmission is by:
    1. Infection acquired by contact with another individual or other outside source.
    2. Infection as a result of invasion by microorganisms normally carried by patient.
  D. Pathogenesis:
    1. Occurs after microbial invasion of the central nervous system (CNS).

  2. Generally involves the host inflammatory response to local CNS infection (e.g., infiltration by inflammatory cells, immune responses to microbial antigens and toxins, and cytokine release by immune cells).
  3. Some viruses directly infect neural cells.
E. Diagnosis involves:
  1. Clinical appearance, including fever, irritation, headache, and neurological signs.
  2. Laboratory analyses of cerebral spinal fluid (CSF) for cells, elevated protein, and depressed glucose.
  3. Laboratory identification of bacteria present in CSF is critical for rapid institution of antibiotic therapy.
F. Prevention includes:
  1. Vaccines, which are available for several causes of bacterial meningitis (e.g., H. influenzae, Streptococcus pneumoniae, Neisseria meningitidis).
  2. Prophylactic use of antibiotics for close contacts.
G. Treatment involves:
  1. Prompt use of appropriate antibiotics or antifungal/antiparasitic agents.
  2. Antiviral therapy for meningitis caused by HSV.
H. Epidemiology
  1. Meningitis occurs in all age groups.
  2. Neonatal meningitis (typically from group B streptococci or E. coli) has a high fatality rate (approximately 35%).
  3. Use of the H. influenzae vaccine has greatly reduced the incidence of childhood meningitis caused by H. influenzae.
  4. AIDS patients are susceptible to meningitis caused by Cryptococcus neoformans.

CONTENT REVIEW QUESTIONS

1. *Candida albicans* is all of the following, EXCEPT:
   A. reproduced by budding
   B. a yeast
   C. the causative agent of thrush
   D. inhibited by penicillin
2. The rigidity and shape of the bacterial cell is caused by the:
   A. capsule
   B. peptidoglycan layer
   C. lipopolysaccharide layer
   D. teichoic acid layer
3. Which of the following sequences is correct for staining a bacterial smear with the Gram stain?
   A. crystal violet, alcohol, iodine, safranin
   B. crystal violet, iodine, alcohol, safranin
   C. safranin, iodine, alcohol, crystal violet
   D. safranin, alcohol, iodine, crystal violet
4. Which of the following is an INCORRECT characteristic of *Mycobacteria*?
   A. acid fast
   B. lacks cell wall

C. possesses mycolic acids and waxes in the wall structure

D. causes tuberculosis

5. The term sterilization means the killing of _____ .
A. spores
B. microbes that cause disease
C. all life
D. fungus

6. Multiple antibiotic resistance may be rapidly spread through bacterial populations by:
A. transformation
B. transduction
C. Hfr recombination
D. plasmids

7. Penicillin is an effective inhibitor of:
A. cell wall synthesis
B. cytoplasmic membrane
C. nucleic acid
D. transcription

8. A bacteriocidal agent is recognized by the fact that it/its:
A. action is irreversible
B. does not kill bacteria and only stops bacterial growth
C. is effective only on dead cells
D. action is reversible

9. The central intermediate that leads to the production of different fermentation products by bacteria is:
A. pyruvate
B. ATP
C. lactate
D. NADH

10. Which of the following is INCORRECT regarding bacterial respiration?
A. may occur anaerobically
B. an organic compound serves as the final electron acceptor
C. may occur aerobically
D. produces more energy in the form of ATP than does fermentation

11. A facultative anaerobe grows in the presence of:
A. oxygen
B. no oxygen
C. oxygen or no oxygen
D. low concentrations of oxygen

12. The antibiotic of choice in the treatment of a topical yeast or fungal infection would be:
A. nystatin
B. hexachlorophene
C. tetracycline
D. penicillin

13. The principal agent currently used for gaseous sterilization is:
A. formaldehyde
B. isopropyl alcohol
C. gamma rays
D. ethylene oxide

14. Identification of bacterial species depends on all of the following, EXCEPT:
A. presence of plasmids
B. nutritional requirements
C. biochemical characteristics
D. staining and morphology

15. Transduction is a means of gene transfer between bacteria that is mediated by:
A. bacteriophages
B. cell to cell contact
C. free DNA
D. yeasts

16. The enzymes needed for the breakdown of hydrogen peroxide to H_2O and O_2 are:
A. autotrophs
B. heterotrophs
C. aerobes
D. anaerobes

17. Viruses can be distinguished from all other microorganisms by virtue of their:
A. ability to be isolated from the blood
B. need to replicate intracellularly
C. resistance to antibodies
D. possession of only one type of nucleic acid

18. Prokaryotic cells differ in structure from eukaryotic cells in that prokaryotes possess:
A. a nuclear membrane
B. mitochondria
C. 70S ribosomes
D. 80S ribosomes

19. Which of the following statements regarding the control of microorganisms is INCORRECT?
A. widespread and indiscriminate use of antibiotics may select for bacteria that are resistant to antibiotics
B. an antibiotic that inhibits a large variety of different organisms is said to possess a broad spectrum
C. tetracyclines are inhibitors of bacterial cell wall biosynthesis
D. viruses are not affected by antibiotics

20. Bacteria typically reproduce by means of:
A. endospores
B. mitosis
C. binary fission
D. budding

21. The source of carbon for an heterotrophic bacterium is:
A. glucose
B. hydrogen gas
C. carbon dioxide
D. hydrogen sulfide

22. In which phase of bacterial growth is the number of newly formed cells equal to the number of dying cells?
A. lag
B. exponential
C. stationary
D. death

23. The aminoglycoside antibiotics, such as streptomycin, are inhibitors of:
    A. transcription
    B. cell wall biosynthesis
    C. translation
    D. DNA replication

24. Elaborate and harsh procedures are required for sterilization because of the possible presence of:
    A. viruses
    B. endospores
    C. capsules
    D. flagella

25. Which of the following antibiotics is different from all of the others in its mode of action?
    A. erythromycin
    B. tetracycline
    C. cephalosporin
    D. streptomycin

26. Yeasts posses all of the following characteristics, EXCEPT:
    A. reproduce asexually
    B. reproduce sexually
    C. are unicellular
    D. produce mycelia

27. Which type of microorganism may be found growing deep inside a wound and on its surface?
    A. aerobe
    B. anaerobe
    C. facultative anaerobe
    D. microerophile

28. Biologically active solutions such as antibiotics and vitamins are best sterilized by:
    A. autoclaving
    B. ethylene oxide
    C. filtration
    D. gamma radiation

29. Penicillin would NOT be an antibiotic of choice for treatment of an infection by:
    A. *Streptococcus pneumoniae*
    B. *Mycoplasma pneumoniae*
    C. *Staphylococcus aureus*
    D. *Bacillus subtilis*

30. Tuberculosis is characterized by all of the following, EXCEPT:
    A. rapidly cured by antibiotic therapy
    B. emergence of drug-resistant *M. tuberculosis*
    C. susceptibility is enhanced by HIV infection
    D. efficient airborne transmission

31. Antibodies are best characterized by which of the following?
    A. lack of antigen specificity
    B. production of T lymphocytes
    C. specific interaction with antigenic determinants
    D. absence from blood

32. B lymphocytes have which important characteristic?
    A. absence of cell-wall cytokine receptors
    B. inability to produce antibodies
    C. maturation centered in the thymus
    D. clonal expansion after immunization or infection

33. All of the following are true about Immunoglobulin G (IgG), EXCEPT:
    A. is the predominant antibody class found in blood plasma
    B. mediates specific antibacterial and antiviral immunity
    C. is produced by plasma cells
    D. cannot bind to Fc receptors

34. Phagocytic cells:
    A. have no role in the generation of specific immunity
    B. are capable of ingesting foreign molecules in the absence of antibodies
    C. are capable of synthesizing antibodies
    D. do not bear surface Fc receptors

35. All of these are true about the complement system, EXCEPT:
    A. consists of many blood proteins
    B. helps defend the body against infection
    C. facilitates attachment and clearance of foreign molecules by the body
    D. genetic deficiencies do not occur

36. Allergic reactions are BEST characterized by which of the following?
    A. subclinical symptoms
    B. susceptibility that excludes genetic inheritance
    C. lack of T-lymphocyte participation
    D. mediation by IgE

37. The spectrum of antigens recognized by the mammalian immune system (i.e., the antigenic repertoire) is:
    A. restricted to immune recognition of membrane lipid molecules
    B. highly diverse; caused by genetic mechanisms that regulate antigen receptor molecules
    C. very narrow because most B and T cells carry the same antigen receptor molecules
    D. unaffected by B and T cell antigen receptor molecules

38. Immune mechanisms of host defense against infections include all of the following, EXCEPT:
    A. IgG-mediated neutralization of viruses
    B. stimulation of bacterial phagocytosis by antibodies and/or complement (opsonization)
    C. IgD-mediated neutralization of bacteria
    D. complement-mediated degradation of bacteria

39. Graft rejection is characterized by:
    A. immunological tolerance to the grafted tissue
    B. immune recognition of powerful transplantation antigens on the graft
    C. failure of B and T cells to become activated
    D. failure of the complement system to become activated

40. The human major histocompatibility complex (MHC) is a DNA region that:
    A. is a human leukocyte antigen (HLA) complex
    B. encodes antibody molecules

C. is identical among all humans

D. encodes T cell receptor molecules

41. Genetic typing of a person's HLA genes:
    A. has no role in controlling the likelihood of graft rejection
    B. has no role in the diagnosis of certain autoimmune diseases
    C. can be performed using cellular, serological, or genetic technology
    D. cannot yet be performed because HLA alleles are uncharacterized

42. CD4+ T cells are characteristically:
    A. greater in number in individuals with AIDS
    B. known as "helper" T cells
    C. nonresponsive to vaccine injections
    D. unable to produce interleukin-2 (IL-2)

43. Cytokines are:
    A. protein molecules produced by lymphocytes, macrophages, and other cells
    B. normally not involved in regulating immune responses
    C. not involved in the inflammatory process
    D. only produced during humoral immune responses

44. Cytotoxic T cells:
    A. recognize and kill virus-infected and tumor cells
    B. release killer antibody molecules
    C. are not antigen-specific
    D. bear the CD4 cell surface marker

45. Immunological protection of a newborn baby is:
    A. unnecessary because of vigorous nonspecific and innate protection
    B. transferred to the baby only after birth, by contact with foreign antigens
    C. passively transferred to the baby in utero by maternal IgG antibodies
    D. unaffected by nursing

46. Systemic lupus erythematosus (SLE) is characterized by all of the following, EXCEPT:
    A. autoimmunity
    B. circulating anti-DNA antibodies of unknown origin
    C. lack of affect by sex hormones
    D. immune complex-mediated damage to the kidneys

47. All of the following describe immune complexes, EXCEPT:
    A. are found during infections
    B. are formed in response to virus infections
    C. are associated with complement activation
    D. result in tissue repair when deposited in blood vessels

48. Hemolytic disease of the newborn occurs in babies born to Rh-negative mothers and is characterized by all of the following, EXCEPT:
    A. a father whose erythrocytes bear the Rh+ phenotype
    B. a mother whose erythrocytes bear the Rh+ phenotype
    C. maternal antibodies stimulated by paternal erythrocyte antigens, which are recognized as foreign by the mother
    D. antibody-mediated attack against red cells made by the newborn

49. Determination of which of the following characterizes specific serological diagnosis of an infection?
    A. seroconversion after vaccination
    B. blood B cell counts
    C. specific blood antibody response to antigens
    D. elevated total blood IgG levels

50. The ELISA test used to screen for HIV infection detects _____ in the blood.
    A. HIV RNA
    B. CD4+ T cells
    C. cytotoxic T cells
    D. anti-HIV antibodies elicited by HIV infection

51. Bone marrow transplantation:
    A. replaces body stem cells, leading to regeneration of the immune system
    B. is effective only for B cell regeneration; T cells and phagocytes are not affected
    C. is the treatment of choice for anaphylactic reactions
    D. cannot introduce infections into the recipient

52. Important oral signs of HIV infection include all of the following, EXCEPT:
    A. aphthous (oral) ulcers
    B. dental caries
    C. acute necrotizing ulcerative gingivitis (ANUG)
    D. oral hairy leukoplakia

53. Current therapy for HIV infection is based on all of the following, EXCEPT:
    A. treatment with viral reverse-transcriptase inhibitors
    B. management with viral protease inhibitors
    C. reduction of viral load
    D. human bone marrow transplant

54. The secondary immune response is characterized by:
    A. a predominance of IgM
    B. high affinity IgG
    C. absence of IgA
    D. unrelated to booster vaccination

55. The process of antigen presentation to CD4+ T cells:
    A. is not necessary for helper T cell activation, because CD4+ T cells recognize soluble antigen
    B. occurs only in the thymus
    C. is necessary for the immune response to T-dependent antigens
    D. does not depend on recognition of MHC molecules

56. All of the following are B cell-dependent mechanisms of cytotoxicity, EXCEPT:
    A. complement activation caused by IgM
    B. ADCC
    C. CTL activity
    D. K cells

57. Monoclonal antibodies may have all of the following properties, EXCEPT:
    A. are obtained from the serum of immunized animals
    B. are useful in diagnostic testing
    C. have antitumor activity
    D. are specific for one antigenic determinant
58. The hemagglutination test of blood erythrocytes from the following individuals would be positive in all cases, EXCEPT:
    A. a blood group A-positive person tested with anti-A antibody
    B. a blood group A-negative person tested with anti-A antibody
    C. a baby born with hemolytic disease of the newborn
    D. a person with autoimmune hemolytic anemia
59. Select the BEST treatment for a patient with severe combined immunodeficiency (SCID):
    A. transplantation with purified donor T cells
    B. transplantation with purified donor stem cells
    C. passive immunization with pooled human gamma globulins
    D. periodic injections of interleukin-2 (IL-2)
60. Secretory component is:
    A. produced by T cells; stabilizes the T-cell receptor
    B. required for IgE binding to mast cells
    C. required for cross-linking of IgM monomers
    D. produced by epithelial cells; protects IgA
61. The serum protein electrophoresis pattern of a patient with a history of recent infections contains abnormally elevated gamma globulins. Subsequent serum immunoelectrophoresis shows an elevation of the IgM band. The MOST likely diagnosis of this patient is:
    A. hypogammaglobulinemia
    B. DiGeorge syndrome
    C. Waldenstrom's macroglobulinemia
    D. T cell lymphoma

REVIEW QUESTION RATIONALES

1. **D** Penicillin is not effective in the treatment of Candida infections because this organism is a yeast, which is a eukaryotic cell. Thrush is a candida infection that is common in infants. Penicillin inhibits peptidoglycan biosynthesis in bacterial cell walls and peptidoglycan is found only in prokaryotic cells.
2. **B** Peptidoglycan is the three dimensional macromolecular structure of the cell wall that surrounds the cytoplasmic membrane and provides shape and rigidity to bacterial cells. Because of high internal osmotic pressure within the cell, bacteria normally would lyse without this structure.
3. **B** The correct order of reagents used in the Gram stain is crystal violet (the primary stain), iodine (a mordant), alcohol (which decolorizes Gram-negative cells), and safranin (the counter stain). Gram-positive bacteria retain the primary stain and appear purple-blue in color. Gram-negative bacteria are decolorized and take up the counter stain; they appear red-pink in color.
4. **B** Mycobacteria posses a peptidoglycan cell wall that is covered with mycolic acids and waxes. The hydrophobic surface is responsible for the positive acid-fast staining reaction that is characteristic of this causative agent of tuberculosis. Mycoplasmas are organisms that lack a cell wall and are the smallest free-living bacteria.
5. **C** Sterilization is the killing of all life, including bacterial endospores. Major sterilization agents include high temperatures (use of an autoclave or dry air oven), gamma radiation, and ethylene oxide. Disinfectants typically are harsh agents, including chemical agents and ultraviolet light, that kill most but not all organisms.
6. **D** Plasmids are small, circular, self-replicating DNA molecules that may contain multiple genes that code for resistance to different antibiotics. Plasmids may be transmitted from a donor bacterium to a recipient by conjugation. Thus a bacterium that is sensitive to antibiotics may receive a plasmid from a donor cell and become immediately resistant to antibiotics. Transformation, transduction, and Hfr recombination are mechanisms for the transfer of chromosomal genes.
7. **A** Penicillin specifically inhibits the biosynthesis of bacterial cell wall peptidoglycan. It inhibits the cross-linking of peptidoglycan chains, thus disrupting the integrity of the three dimensional structure. Penicillin is effective only on actively growing cells.
8. **A** A bacteriocidal agent is one that binds irreversibly with a microorganism, resulting in the death of the bacterium. A bacteriostatic agent binds reversibly to a bacterium, stopping its growth, but does not kill the organism.
9. **A** Pyruvate is the end product of the glycolytic pathway in which a sugar such as glucose (C6) is broken down into two molecules of pyruvate (C3), resulting in the net production of two ATP molecules and two reduced $NADH_2$ molecules. In perhaps the simplest fermentation, pyruvate itself is the organic compound that serves as the final electron acceptor and is thus reduced to the fermentation product, lactate. Pyruvate is the central "hub" in fermentation reactions.
10. **B** By definition, an inorganic compound serves as the final electron acceptor in respiration, whereas an organic compound serves this function in fermentation. Bacterial respiration may occur aerobically, employing oxygen, or may occur anaerobically, using other inorganic compounds (e.g., sulfate, nitrate); it produces more energy from one glucose molecule in the form of ATP (38 net) than fermentation (2 net).
11. **C** A facultative anaerobe is a bacterium that may grow either aerobically, in the presence of oxygen, or

anaerobically, in the absence of oxygen. An aerobe grows only in the presence of oxygen and an anaerobe grows only in the absence of oxygen; a microaerophile requires limited amounts of oxygen for growth.

12. **A** Nystatin (and amphotericin) are polyene antibiotics that complex with sterol, thereby disrupting membranes of eukaryotic cells such as yeast. Bacterial cells are not affected by these antibiotics because sterol is absent. Tetracycline and penicillin act only on prokaryotic cells. Hexachlorophene is not an antibiotic but a disinfectant.

13. **D** Ethylene oxide is a useful room-temperature gaseous sterilant for materials that may be destroyed by other means.

14. **A** Plasmids are not present in all microorganisms and are not routinely useful for the purposes of identification. Typically identification depends on the Gram stain and morphology (e.g., rods, cocci), biochemical characteristics (such as the ability to grow on different substrates), metabolic end products, requirement for oxygen, and specific nutritional requirements.

15. **A** Transduction occurs upon replication within the host bacterium when a piece of host cell chromosomal DNA is mistakenly incorporated into a phage capsid instead of phage DNA. Upon infection of a new host cell, this piece of DNA is injected and thus transferred to the new bacterial cell. Conjugation is the process of gene transfer that is mediated by cell-to-cell contact and transformation is the incorporation of free "naked" DNA into a recipient cell.

16. **C** In order for bacteria to grow aerobically, using oxygen as the final electron acceptor (respiration), the enzymes catalase and superoxide dismutase are required to break down toxic intermediates that form at the end of the electron transport chain. Superoxide dismutase converts superoxide anions (toxic) to hydrogen peroxide (toxic) and the peroxide is converted to water and oxygen. Without these enzymes, bacteria grow anaerobically. Autotrophs are bacteria that use carbon dioxide as their carbon source; heterotrophs derive their carbon from organic compounds.

17. **D** A distinguishing feature of viruses is that they contain either DNA or RNA but not both as do cellular lifeforms. They are able to replicate themselves from information contained in the DNA or information in their RNA.

18. **C** Prokaryotes (bacteria) possess 70S ribosomes. All of the other features listed are characteristic of the more complex eukaryotic cells. Many useful antibiotics specifically inhibit bacterial protein synthesis because they specifically bind to 70S ribosomes, but not to the 80S ribosomes of eukaryotic cells.

19. **C** Tetracyclines inhibit bacterial protein synthesis. Penicillins, and other beta-lactam antibiotics, inhibit cell wall biosynthesis. The other choices are all true and should be remembered when administering antibiotics.

20. **C** Bacteria reproduce by binary fission. Eukaryotic cells reproduce by mitosis and yeast do so by budding. Endospores are not a mode of reproduction in bacteria but are a means of survival.

21. **A** Organic compounds serve as the carbon source for heterotrophic bacteria. Carbon dioxide is the carbon source for autotrophic bacteria. Although hydrogen and hydrogen sulfide may serve as an energy source for chemolithotrophic bacteria, they do not contain carbon.

22. **C** Dividing and dying bacteria are in balance during the stationary phase of growth. There is no growth during the lag phase. Rapid growth and division of the cell occur during the exponential phase, and cells die exponentially during the death phase.

23. **C** The aminoglycoside antibiotics specifically inhibit protein synthesis at the level of translation by binding to the 30S ribosomal subunit. Antibiotics such as rifampicin inhibit protein synthesis at the level of transcription. Nalidixic acid is an inhibitor of DNA synthesis and the beta- lactam antibiotics (e.g., penicillin) inhibit cell wall biosynthesis.

24. **B** Bacterial endospores are the most resistant form of life known. They are a means of survival and resist heat, ultraviolet light, and desiccation. Viruses are killed by much milder conditions; capsules and flagella are bacterial structures that are easily destroyed by physical and chemical procedures.

25. **C** Cephalosporins are beta-lactam antibiotics that inhibit cross-linking in peptidoglycan biosynthesis. Erythromycin, tetracyclines, and streptomycin are all inhibitors of bacterial protein synthesis.

26. **D** Yeasts do not produce mycelia; they are unicellular fungi. Yeasts may reproduce asexually, by budding, or sexually, by the production of ascospores.

27. **C** Facultative anaerobes may grow on the surface of a wound, in the presence of air, or deep in a wound, where anaerobic conditions exist. Anaerobes grow only deep in a wound and aerobes grow only on the surface. A microerophile might be expected to grow just below the surface.

28. **C** Sterilization by filtration is necessary for biologically active solutions. Alternative methods—autoclaving, ethylene oxide, or gamma radiation—would be too severe and would destroy biological activity.

29. **B** Penicillin inhibits cell wall biosynthesis. Mycoplasmas are bacteria that lack a cell wall and are therefore not affected by any of the cell wall antibiotics. The other organisms possess typical cells walls and are inhibited by penicillin.

30. **A** Drug resistance is a significant problem in treating tuberculosis, as is patient medication compliance, because patients may feel better soon after initiating therapy; however, eradication of *M. tuberculosis* from the body may take many months of treatment. Tuber-

culosis is a growing problem in immunocompromised patients, including those with HIV infection. Infected people may cough up large numbers of the organisms and these may survive for long periods of time because of the outer waxy coat of this bacterium, which makes airborne transmission relatively efficient.

31. **C**   A key property of antibodies (which are produced only by B cells and plasma cells) is specific reactivity with antigens, which allows them to target specific pathogens while avoiding autoimmune responses. Antibodies are soluble proteins that circulate in the blood, facilitating contact with pathogens that invade the body.

32. **D**   The production of antibodies by B lymphocytes is greatly influenced by cytokines (e.g., cytokines such as IL-2, produced by T cells). B lymphocytes are generated by the bone marrow and mature there and in secondary sites such as lymph nodes. Contact with antigens, either naturally or by immunization, selects specific clones of B lymphocytes for expansion.

33. **D**   Plasma cells represent the terminal stage of B-cell differentiation. They secrete antibodies that find their way into the blood (IgG has the highest blood concentration) and other body sites (e.g., mucosal sites where IgA predominates), where they may mediate immune reactions against bacteria, viruses, and other pathogens. Fc receptor binding is a major mechanism by which IgG helps phagocytic cells clear pathogens.

34. **B**   Phagocytic cells (e.g., macrophages, neutrophils) help in the generation of specific (B and/or T cell) immunity by processing antigen molecules, presenting antigen fragments to B/T cells, and releasing cytokines. However, phagocytic cells do not synthesize antibodies, although they are generally rich in surface Fc receptors, which helps them interact with antibodies and immune complexes.

35. **D**   The complement system is a complex biochemical system that comprises more than 30 protein molecules. When activated by contact with antigens and/or antibodies, complement helps stimulate inflammation and magnify immune reactions; it also attaches to and helps clear foreign molecules and pathogens from the body. Various complement proteins may be adversely affected by genetic mutations.

36. **D**   The clinical spectrum of allergy is broad and includes potentially fatal allergic reactions (e.g., anaphylaxis caused by food allergy or drug allergy). Genetic factors that affect susceptibility to allergy include HLA genes. Although T cells may participate in some types of allergies (e.g., delayed-type hypersensitivity), some of the most severe allergies are caused by antibodies.

37. **B**   Diversity is the hallmark of mammalian immunity, being generated by recombination at V(D)J genes which encode for antibodies and T cell receptors. This results in the generation of antibodies that specifically recognize antigens of virtually any molecular structure.

38. **C**   Immune mechanisms of host defense are multifactorial. They include antibody reactions (e.g., direct neutralization and compliment activation) as well as opsonization, which is the term used to describe the facilitation of clearance of bacteria and other foreign invaders by phagocytic cells. IgG is a major mediator of virus neutralization. Although bacteria in some cases may be inhibited by IgG, IgA, or IgA antibodies, which bind to critical receptors, IgD has no known direct antimicrobial function. IgD is involved in the developmental regulation of immune responses.

39. **B**   Tolerance is the lack of immune reactivity to specific antigens (e.g., self antigens). Graft rejection is characterized by active immunity against antigens carried by the graft, the most potent of which appear to be transplantation (MHC) antigens, which activate T/B cells to react against the graft. Complement may play an important role in graft rejection, either through direct activation by graft cells or through antibodies that react against the graft.

40. **A**   MHC is the generic term for the gene complex known as HLA in humans. It carries alleles (specific DNA coding sequences), which are highly diverse within the species. Antibodies and T-cell receptors are encoded on separate and distinct gene regions outside the HLA complex.

41. **C**   HLA typing is an important method that is used to match graft donors and recipients and to help diagnose autoimmune diseases (and some cancers) that have been linked to certain MHC alleles. Classical cellular and serological typing techniques are being replaced with the molecular detection of HLA gene sequences.

42. **B**   CD4 denotes the "helper" T-cell phenotype. CD4+ T cells are destroyed in AIDS (most likely because HIV replicates within these cells). Because CD4+ T cells are important for immune responses and in the production of cytokines such as IL-2, their destruction leads to susceptibility to infections.

43. **A**   Many cell types, including B/T lymphocytes and macrophages, produce cytokines. Cytokines are critical regulators of immunity, and participate in all phases of immune responses.

44. **A**   Cytotoxic (CD8+) T cells are capable of killing other cells by a specific protein-killing mechanism unrelated to antibodies, which are not produced by T cells. Antigen-specific T-cell killing allows these cells to be directed against virus-infected or tumor cells.

45. **C**   The immune system of a newborn is not fully mature. Without passive maternal protection, acquired in utero (maternal IgG crosses the placenta) and during nursing (from breast milk antibodies and cells), the newborn would not be able to cope effectively with exposures to infections. By approximately 6 months of age, the immune system has

reached the stage in which it is likely to respond well to contact with most foreign antigens.

46. **C**   Anti-DNA antibodies are found in the blood of SLE patients, who are predominantly female; thus sex hormones exert an influence on development of SLE, although it is not known why anti-DNA antibodies develop. The clinical spectrum of this autoimmune disease is broad. In more severe cases, kidney failure may occur from the deposition of immune complexes in the kidney and the stimulation of inflammatory responses.

47. **D**   As in the example of SLE, immune complexes may precipitate tissue damage, and the activation of complement is a major pathway for this occurrence. Nonpathogenic immune complexes typically circulate at low levels—for example, as a result of immune responses to microorganisms and their antigens—and are cleared in healthy individuals without causing dangerous immune reactions.

48. **B**   When an Rh-negative mother is exposed to paternal Rh+ antigen during pregnancy (typically because of expression of RhD antigen by erythrocytes of the developing fetus, which leak into the maternal circulation before or during birth), the mother may become sensitized to the RhD antigen. During subsequent pregnancies, maternal IgG anti-RhD antibodies may enter the fetus and damage fetal red blood cells, resulting in hemolytic disease of the newborn. Prophylactic treatment consists of injecting the mother with anti-RhD antibodies at approximately the time of birth; these passively administered antibodies bind to paternal antigen and inhibit the development of maternal anti-RhD antibodies. Reactions to blood group antigens other than RhD also may occur.

49. **C**   Determination of specific antibody responses to pathogens (e.g., anti-HIV detection by ELISA) is a powerful tool for detecting human exposure and infection. However, a specific antibody response that occurs as a result of vaccination would not necessarily indicate infection, because the immunization itself could be responsible for seroconversion. Blood B-cell counts and IgG levels are nonspecific measures of immunity and do not reveal specific exposures.

50. **D**   ELISA screening for HIV infection detects specific immunity that occurs during HIV infection, as represented by circulating IgG or IgM anti-HIV antibodies. False-positive ELISA reactions may occur, because of blood antibodies that cross-react with HIV antigens, even in the absence of HIV infection. Blood HIV RNA detection by molecular techniques, and measurement of CD4+ T cells in the blood by cytochemistry, both provide important correlates of disease progression but are not carried out by ELISA.

51. **A**   By providing a new source of functional stem cells, bone marrow transplantation may effectively treat a variety of immune system disorders, including those that affect B/T cells and phagocytes. The transmission of infection—particularly but not exclusively virus infection—from the donor to the recipient is one of the risks of this procedure.

52. **B**   Dental caries are not indicative of HIV infection, although they may occur when oral hygiene is inadequate or may be caused by xerostomia from medication use. Aphthous ulcers are common in HIV infection. Less common but still prevalent in HIV infection are ANUG (an anaerobic infection that resembles periodontitis and is treatable with systemic metronidazole) and oral hairy leukoplakia (white fuzzy lesions on the bottom and sides of the tongue).

53. **D**   Bone marrow transplant from a human donor has not been developed as an HIV treatment because the donor cells would likely be infected with HIV. The central goal of current HIV therapy is to reduce the viral load present in the body (typically measured by the HIV RNA copy number in the blood). Combination therapy with HIV reverse transcriptase inhibitors such as zidovudine (AZT; a nucleoside reverse-transcriptase inhibitor) or nevirapine (a non-nucleoside reverse-transcriptase inhibitor), and protease inhibitors such as saquinavir, has proven most effective.

54. **B**   High affinity IgG predominates during the secondary immune response. IgM predominates during a primary immune response but the affinity of all antibody isotypes, including IgA, increases during the secondary immune response, which for some vaccinations requires a "booster shot."

55. **C**   Antigen presentation to CD4+ T cells occurs at many lymphoid sites. It is necessary for the generation of immunity to T-dependent antigens and the activation of T-helper activity because CD4+ T cells cannot recognize soluble antigen. CD4+ T cells recognize antigen in combination with MHC molecules that are present on the antigen-presenting cell surface.

56. **C**   CTL (cytotoxic T lymphocyte) activity is independent of antibody, but IgM activation of complement, ADCC, and K cells all require antibody for their role in cytotoxicity.

57. **A**   Monoclonal antibodies are obtained from cultures of cloned cells or in vivo from the ascites fluid of animals injected with cloned cells. Immunization of an animal stimulates polyclonal antibodies, which are not as useful diagnostically or as anti-tumor antibodies because they react against multiple antigenic determinants.

58. **B**   For the cases listed in A, C, and D, erythrocytes will carry either an antigen (the A antigen for A) or antibodies (maternal anti-RhD for C; an autoantibody for D), which results in a positive hemagglutination test.

59. **B**   Transplantation with stem cells (or stem cell-containing tissue) provides the only mechanism for reconstituting the immune system in a patient with SCID; administration of T cells only puts the patient at risk for graft-versus-host disease. Passive immuniza-

tions or cytokine injections have too limited an effect to provide significant benefit to a patient with SCID because all functional B and T cells are absent in these patients.

60. **D**   Secretory component is produced by epithelial cells located near mucosal sites. It becomes attached to IgA and provides protection from degradation at mucous membranes.

61. **C**   Waldenstrom's macroglobulinemia is a B-cell tumor that is characterized by an overproduction of IgM, which in this case was observed on protein electrophoresis and isoelectric focusing. Hypogammaglobulinemia is a B-cell deficiency and DiGeorge syndrome is the absence of the thymus, neither of which would result in elevated serum IgM.

Additional Readings

Brooks GF, Butel JS, Ornston LN, editors: Medical Microbiology. Norwalk, CT, Appleton and Lange, 1995.

Baron S, editor: Medical Microbiology. Galveston, TX, University of Texas Medical Branch at Galveston, University of Texas, 1996.

Mahon CR, Manuselis G, editors: Diagnostic Microbiology. Philadelphia, WB Saunders, 1995.

Murray PR, Rosenthal KS, Kobayashi GS, et al, editors: Medical Microbiology. St. Louis, Mosby, 1998.

Roitt I, Brostoff J, Male D, editors: Immunology. Philadelphia, Mosby, 1988.

Lim D, editor: Microbiology. Boston, WCB/McGraw-Hill, 1998.

Stites DP, Terr AI, Parslow TG, editors: Medical Immunology. Stamford, CT, Appleton and Lange, 1997.

Schuster GS: Oral Microbiology and Infectious Disease. Philadelphia, BC Decker, 1990.

Mims C, Playfair J, Roitt I, et al, editors: Medical Microbiology. London, Mosby, 1998.

Chapter FIVE

General and Oral Pathology

Susan Swanson, D.D.S • Kevin Gyolai, M.S.

 ## Clinical Case STUDY

Willard Quill, a 71-year-old male, presents in the dental office complaining of sores on his lower lip. He is semi-retired and owns a landscaping business; he frequently helps his employees mow lawns and plant shrubbery. He indicates that he had a slight fever two days ago. The extra-oral exam reveals a cluster of vesicles on his lower lip and lymphadenopathy also is noted.

Clinical Case QUESTIONS

1. What is the most likely diagnosis and cause of Mr. Quill's condition?
2. What common signs of inflammation are associated with this condition? Is this an acute or chronic inflammation?
3. Identify the major functions of inflammation. During the healing process for this condition, are tissues restored by regeneration or by repair?
4. What other locations might exhibit this condition? How long does this condition typically last?
5. Are prodromal conditions present? Is his job a factor in this condition?

Clinical Case RATIONALES

1. Recurrent herpes simplex, also known as herpes labialis, cold sore, or fever blister, is caused by a herpes simplex virus. The virus exists in a latent or quiescent state in the trigeminal ganglion and infection follows a stimulus.
2. Common signs of inflammation associated with this condition include fever, pain, and swelling. Functioning of the lip often is limited because of discomfort. This is an acute inflammation because it is an immediate response to viral attack and results in redness, vesicle formation (increased vessel permeability), and the movement of leukocytes to the area.
3. The major functions of inflammation are neutralization or destruction of the injurious agent, cleaning of

necrotic debris, and initiation of repair and regeneration. During the healing process the epithelial tissues are restored by regeneration.

4. Herpes labialis occurs on the vermilion border of the lips; however, recurrent herpes may occur on keratinized mucosa that is fixed to bone, such as the hard palate and gingiva. In contrast, aphthous ulcers generally appear on the lining mucosa. The herpes condition generally lasts for 1 to 2 weeks.
5. Yes, prodromal conditions, such as pain, burning, or tingling occur before vesicle development. The landscaping job is a factor in the condition because exposure to sunlight is one of several stimuli that are known to trigger the viral activity.

Content Review

General Pathology

General pathology includes the study of the destruction and repair of bodily tissues.

Inflammation and Repair

Inflammation is the body's normal response to injury. It is a dynamic and protective process. Repair occurs in response to inflammation and involves both regenerative and reparative processes.

I. Injury
   A. Causes include:
      1. Hypoxia (lack of oxygen) from chemical, physical, and/or microbial agents.
      2. Immunologic factors such as anaphylactic reactions and reactions to self-antigens.
      3. Genetic defects that result in pathologic changes, such as those that result in sickle cell anemia.
      4. Nutritional imbalances, including the lack of sufficient proteins or other nutrients and di-

etary excesses such as a high intake of animal fats.

  B. Mechanisms of injury
   1. Are dependent on multiple factors, including:
      a. The type, duration, and severity of the injury.
      b. The type of cell injured; different types of cells have variable responses to injury.
      c. Biochemical considerations, including the integrity of cell membranes, ATP production systems, protein synthesis mechanisms, and genetic apparatus.

II. Inflammation
  A. Signs of inflammation include heat, redness, swelling, pain, and loss of function.
  B. The pathogenesis of inflammation typically involves circulatory changes, alterations in blood vessel permeability, leukocyte response, and chemical mediators.
  C. Types of Inflammation
   1. Acute—an immediate response to injury; is characterized by increased blood flow, increased vessel permeability, and the movement of leukocytes—primarily neutrophils—into the tissue.
   2. Chronic—typically is a low-grade inflammation that lasts weeks to years, during which inflammation, injury, and healing occur simultaneously. Is characterized by the migration of macrophages, plasma cells, and lymphocytes; repair with new vessel formations; and fibrous connective tissue repair.
  D. Inflammation functions to:
   1. Neutralize, destroy, isolate, and remove the injurious agent.
   2. Clean up necrotic debris.
   3. Initiate repair and regeneration.

III. Regeneration and Repair
  A. Regeneration is the replacement of injured cells with parenchymal cells of the same type and is primarily dependent on cell type, whether labile, stable, or permanent.
  B. Repair is the restoration of cell function and/or morphology after injury.
   1. In response to severe or persistent injury, repair can not be accomplished by regeneration alone.
   2. Repair is accomplished by connective tissue scar.
   3. Factors involved in tissue repair include:
   4. Angiogenesis—the proliferation of new blood vessels.
   5. Remodeling—the secretion of collagen-degrading enzymes.
   6. Fibrosis—repair by fibrous connective tissue.

Immune System Disorders

Immune system disorders are conditions related to the suppression, dysfunction, or destruction of the immune system. They include disorders such as acquired immune deficiency syndrome and systemic lupus erythematosus.

I. Acquired Immune Deficiency Syndrome (AIDS)
  A. Is a fatal syndrome that develops as a consequence of severe immunosuppression after infection by the human immunodeficiency virus (HIV).
  B. Is caused by contact with HIV via contaminated body fluids (e.g., semen, blood), contaminated needles or surgical implements that penetrate the skin, or in utero exposure; has an incubation period of 2 to 8 years.
  C. Early-stage symptoms include weight loss, fever, diarrhea, enlarged lymph nodes, night sweats, and nausea; symptoms during later stages include encephalopathy, dementia, neoplasia, an increase in opportunistic infections, and gastrointestinal disorders.
  D. Common oral lesions include: Kaposi sarcoma of the tongue, candidiasis, herpes ulcers, and acute progressive periodontitis.
  E. Treatment includes vigorous care of opportunistic infections and palliative support.

II. Systemic Lupus Erythematosus
  A. Is an autoimmune disease that affects the skin and collagenous connective tissue.
  B. Is believed to be caused by hypersensitivity to an external or internal antigen.
  C. Signs, symptoms, and manifestations include a butterfly rash on the face, arthritis, dermatitis, glomerulonephritis, anemia, and inflamed spleen and or lymph nodes.
  D. Treatment is nonspecific and may include the use of corticosteroids to control inflammation.

Inflammatory Skin Disease

Inflammatory skin diseases include several common forms of dermatitis.

I. Dermatitis
  A. Is a generic term that refers to acute or chronic inflammation of the skin.
  B. Is caused by stimuli such as chemicals, drugs, radiation, and trauma; has metabolic and immunologic factors.
  C. The most common types of dermatitis include:
   1. Eczema—characterized by nonspecific lesions and itching.
   2. Seborrheic dermatitis—presents with inflammation of sebaceous glands, redness, itching, and scaling.
   3. Psoriasis—characterized by raised papules or patches with silvery scales and thickened skin on extremities.

Infectious Skin Diseases

Skin diseases can be caused by infection with a variety of bacterial or viral organisms.

I. Bacterial Infections (include common diseases and infective agents)
- A. Acne—multiple facial lesions because of plugged sebaceous glands and hair follicles; is most common during adolescence; involves heredity and hormonal factors; is aggravated by stress and/or drugs.
- B. Abscess—raised pocket of necrotic tissue and purulent exudate; is most common around trauma sites or associated with obstructed skin appendage; also called boil or furuncle.
- C. Impetigo—infectious pustules that appear as itchy, honey-colored scabs; is most common around the face; is highly contagious.

II. Viral Infections (include common diseases and infective agents)
- A. Localized viral diseases—include warts, which are caused by strains of human papilloma virus; involve discrete proliferation of squamous epithelium; may disappear spontaneously.

Metabolic Disorders

Metabolic disorders often manifest themselves as either an overproduction or underproduction of secretions. Hypersecretion most often occurs because of a tumor of the secretory cells of a gland; hyposecretion most often occurs because of the agenesis, atrophy, or destruction of secretory cells. Treatment for hypersecretion is removal or destruction of part or all of the gland. Hormone supplementation is prescribed for hyposecretion.

I. Endocrine Gland Disorders
- A. Pituitary gland disorders
  1. Pituitary hyperfunction (hyperpituitarism)—causes gigantism and acromegaly because of the overproduction of growth hormone.
     - a. Oral signs of acromegaly include macroglossia and mandibular prognathism.
  2. Pituitary hypofunction (hypopituitarism and panhypopituitarism)—is associated with diabetes insipidus. Urine production is copious because of the lack of ADH.
- B. Thyroid gland disorders
  1. Hyperthyroidism—is associated with Grave's disease. Involves autoimmune hypertrophy of the thyroid gland; patient presents with hypersecretion of thyroxine, which causes exophthalmos, tachycardia, and severe weight loss.
  2. Hypothyroidism—is associated with cretinism, a congenital lack of thyroxine that leads to dwarfism with stocky stature, protruding abdomen, underdeveloped sex organs, and a typically misshapen face.
- C. Adrenal gland disorders
  1. Hyperadrenalism—is associated with Cushing's syndrome, the hypersecretion of glucocorticoid hormones; patient presents with obesity, striae, easy bruising, red face, pathological fractures, hyperglycemia, and hypertension.
  2. Hypoadrenalism—the hyposecretion of adrenal cortex hormones; patient presents with dehydration, electrolyte imbalances, low blood pressure, weight loss, and altered skin color.

II. Liver Disorders
- A. Cirrhosis of the liver—chronic destruction of liver cells with fibrous, nodular regeneration.
  1. Causative factors include drugs, alcohol, and viral infections; cause may be unknown.
  2. Manifestations include jaundice, hepatic encephalopathy, ascites, splenomegaly, and bleeding.
  3. Treatment for alcoholic patients includes abstinence from alcohol; occasionally involves surgical operations to relieve portal circulatory disruptions.
- B. Viral hepatitis—a liver disease caused by several viruses known as hepatitis A, B, C, D, and E.
  1. Significance
     - a. Is the most prevalent liver disease in the world.
       1) Affects 2 per 1000 individuals every year in the United States.
       2) 40% of Americans have antibodies to hepatitis A and 5% to 10% have antibodies to hepatitis B.
       3) Vaccines exist for hepatitis A and B.
  2. Manifestations include anorexia, malaise, jaundice, enlarged liver, high levels of aspartate aminotransferase (AST—an enzyme released into the blood after liver injury), and dark urine that contains bilirubin.
  3. Types include:
     - a. Hepatitis A
       1) Is transmitted by fecal-oral route from sources such as contaminated food and water and sewage.
       2) Has an incubation period of 15 to 50 days, typically with short-lived, mild symptoms, a rapid recovery, and no long-term consequences.
     - b. Hepatitis B
       1) Is transmitted by exposure to contaminated blood or blood products or by sexual contact.
       2) Has an incubation period of 40 to 180 days; two thirds of all patients have clinically unrecognizable symptoms; 90% of all infected persons recover fully.
     - c. Hepatitis C
       1) Is transmitted by exposure to contami-

nated blood or blood products or by sexual contact.

   2) Has an incubation period of 15 to 150 days; symptoms are identical to Hepatitis B but typically less severe.

   3) Progresses to chronic hepatitis in half of all infected persons.

d. Hepatitis D

   1) Is transmitted by exposure to contaminated blood or blood products or by sexual contact.

   2) Has an incubation period of 30 to 50 days; hepatitis D virus depends on hepatitis B virus for its replication, so infection with both viruses typically occurs simultaneously.

e. Hepatitis E

   1) Is transmitted by fecal-oral route from sources such as contaminated food and water and sewage; often causes waterborne epidemics during the rainy season in parts of Asia, Africa, South America, and Mexico.

   2) Has an incubation period of 14 to 60 days and a mild or asymptomatic course; in most cases there are no long-term consequences (except in 20% of acutely infected pregnant women, who develop liver necrosis).

4. Treatment for viral hepatitis is palliative.

III. Pancreatic Disorders

A. Diabetes mellitus (hyperglycemia) is a multifactorial disease in which the pancreas fails to secrete adequate insulin or target cells fail to respond to insulin.

   1. Types include:

      a. Type I (insulin-dependent diabetes mellitus [IDDM])—juvenile onset; is the more serious type; requires daily insulin injections.

      b. Type II (non-insulin-dependent diabetes mellitus [NIDDM])—mature onset; may be controlled by diet; is more common in females than in males; often accompanies obesity.

   2. Symptoms include polyuria, glycosuria, polyphagia, polydipsia, a large amount of ketone bodies in the blood, acidosis, weight loss, poor wound healing, and an increased susceptibility to infections.

B. Pancreatitis is an inflammation of the pancreas caused by protein- and lipid-digesting enzymes in the pancreas that digest the organ itself. Most severe cases are associated with alcoholism; the disease can be either acute or chronic.

   1. Symptoms

      a. Acute pancreatitis is characterized by severe abdominal pain with sudden onset, nausea and vomiting, elevated serum levels of amy-

lase and lipase, rapidly developing shock, and pancreatic enzymes in the urine.

      b. Chronic pancreatitis is characterized by severe pain, malabsorption, and diabetes.

   2. Treatment of acute pancreatitis centers on controlling the systemic consequences of shock; treatment for chronic pancreatitis centers on treating its symptoms.

Blood Disorders

The basic categories of blood disorders include the clotting disorders and the red and white blood cell disorders. These diseases are related to abnormal levels, function, or structure of some blood components.

I. Red Blood Cell Disorders

A. Anemias

   1. Are caused by low hemoglobin and oxygen concentration in the blood.

   2. Include multiple forms.

   3. Are caused by bleeding, hemolysis, iron or other nutrient deficiency, or improper formation of new red blood cells.

   4. Classifications include:

      a. Pernicious anemia—too few erythrocytes; factor for erythrocyte formation is missing; is treated with injections of missing factor.

      b. Hypochromic anemia—(also called iron-deficiency anemia) too little hemoglobin per erythrocyte; is treated with iron supplementation.

      c. Hemolytic anemia—rupture of erythrocytes; may be environmental or genetic; generally, no effective treatment for genetic forms; treatment for environmentally induced forms centers on the control of environmental factors.

         1) Sickle-cell anemia is an example of a genetically caused hemolytic anemia; generally is confined to African Americans; red blood cells are sickle- or crescent-shaped and cannot function properly.

      d. Aplastic anemia—faulty bone marrow; is treated with transfusion or marrow transplantation.

      e. Secondary anemia—results from another disease; cell numbers are normal but hemoglobin is low.

   5. Oral signs of anemia include:

      a. Angular cheilitis.

      b. Pale skin and mucosa.

      c. Erythematous, burning tongue and/or loss of filiform and fungiform papillae.

      d. Erythematous oral tissues.

B. Other diseases of erythrocytes (other than anemias).

   1. Polycythemia is a disease associated with the overproduction of erythrocytes.

a. Primary polycythemia involves hyperactive bone marrow and elevated hematocrit, blood viscosity, blood pressure, and cardiac workload; treatment involves bloodletting and/or radiation therapy to reduce erythrocyte number.

b. Secondary polycythemia is associated with the need to compensate for inadequate blood oxygen levels caused by heart disease, emphysema, living at high altitude, or increased oxygen demand by muscles (in athletes). Treatment involves controlling the symptoms.

II. Clotting Disorders

A. Hemophilia

1. Is characterized by the improper clotting of blood; is manifested by prolonged, severe bleeding after minor injury.

2. Is a genetic disorder that typically affects only males; females are carriers; bleeding is caused by a lack of the plasma proteins required for clotting.

3. Oral manifestations include spontaneous gingival bleeding, ecchymoses, and petechiae.

4. Treatment includes blood transfusion and administration of clotting protein concentrates before dental/dental hygiene therapy.

III. White Blood Cell Disorders

A. Diseases of leukocytes and bone marrow

1. Leukemia is a cancer of red bone marrow, lymphatic tissue, and/or leukocytes.

a. Causes are largely unknown, although radiation, genetics, and viruses are implicated.

b. Signs and symptoms include pallor, bone and joint pain, abnormal bleeding that leads to bruising, enlarged lymph nodes, hepatomegaly, splenomegaly, and anemia.

c. Oral manifestations include red, tender gingiva, which may exhibit spontaneous sulcular bleeding. Petechial lesions and ecchymosis often are evident on the mucosal membrane.

d. Treatment primarily consists of chemotherapy to kill cancer cells.

2. Agranulocytosis is a severe reduction in the number of granulocytes (basophils, eosinophils, or neutrophils) and results in a greatly reduced immune system. Leukopenia is abnormally low levels of white blood cells. Neutropenia is abnormally low levels of neutrophils (a type of granulocyte or white blood cell).

a. Causes may be immunologic or may involve chemicals (such as medications) or radiation therapy that suppresses bone marrow; acute disease most often is an adverse reaction to toxic levels of medication or to bone marrow suppressing radiation therapy.

b. Signs and symptoms include lymphadenopathy, fever and chills, prostration, jaundice, and bleeding ulcers of the rectum, mouth, and vagina.

c. Oral manifestations include infections, painful ulcerations, and gingival lesions that bleed and can quickly cause periodontal destruction.

d. Treatment includes proper identification of the disease by blood test. White blood cell counts drop to between one fifth and one tenth (1000 to 2500 mm^3) of normal. Transfusions to restore blood cell counts and antibiotics to control infections are prescribed. Infections can be fatal, so they must be treated quickly. Invasive oral procedures, including oral prophylaxis, should not be performed.

Clinical Case STUDY

Jane is a 50-year-old school teacher. She spends many hours sunbathing every summer and uses tanning booths in the winter to maintain her tan. During a routine dental visit a lesion on Jane's neck is noted. The lesion appears to be a preexisting nevi but has a raised, irregular, and reddened border on its most anterior surface that is 1 cm in diameter. The patient states that the nevus becomes irritated and bleeds occasionally. She also believes that the lesion has enlarged recently.

Clinical Case QUESTIONS

1. What is a likely diagnosis of Jane's condition?
2. Which of the usual signs and predisposing factors for this condition does Jane present?
3. How is this condition treated?
4. What could Jane have done to prevent this condition?

Clinical Case RATIONALES

1. Malignant melanoma.
2. Asymmetry of the lesion (flat and raised portions); irregular borders; variation in color; relatively large diameter; preexisting nevus; prolonged, frequent exposure to the sun.
3. Treatment is surgical.
4. Prevention includes reducing exposure to sun, using sun block, and routine examination of existing lesions.

Neoplasia

A neoplasm is uncontrolled cellular growth. A tumor is a mass of neoplastic cells. Carcinogens are causative agents involved in neoplastic development.

I. Causes of Neoplastic Development
  A. Exposure to adequate concentrations of carcinogens (cancer-causing agents).
    1. Carcinogens alter cellular DNA and/or proteins.
    2. There are two general groups of carcinogens:
      a. Exogenous carcinogens, which include chemicals, radiation, viruses, and other environmental factors.
      b. Endogenous carcinogens, which include genetic factors (in genome of cells), hormonal factors, immune systems factors, nutritional factors, and aging.
  B. Susceptible host tissues
    1. The tendency for cells to undergo neoplasia is roughly related to their involvement in physiologic replacement.
  C. Adequate time for initiation, transformation, and growth of mass.
II. Classification of Neoplasms
  A. Benign neoplasia
    1. The suffix *-oma* is added after the name of the tissue (e.g., osteoma).
    2. Criteria for classification as benign.
      a. Single, discrete mass.
      b. In solid organs or connective tissue, formation of a capsule around mass.
      c. Close resemblance to tissue of origin.
      d. Mature cells with minimal to moderate cellular atypia.
      e. Significance—two principal factors influence the effects of benign tumors.
        1) As a benign tumor grows, it may compress adjacent tissue (brain or spinal cord) or cause blockage of a lumen (trachea or intestines).
        2) If a benign tumor has an endocrine function, it may cause uncontrolled hormone secretion.
    3. Common examples of benign neoplasms
      a. Angioma—tumor composed of blood vessels (birth mark).
      b. Lipoma—soft, fatty tumor that develops in adipose tissue.
      c. Nevus—common mole.
      d. Papilloma (polyp)—epithelial tumor that grows from the skin or mucous membrane, such as a wart.
      e. Adenoma—tumor of glandular tissue.
    4. Common treatment options include surgical removal and radiation therapy.
  B. Malignant neoplasia
    1. The term *carcinoma* is added to the tissue name for epithelial tissue (e.g., squamous cell carcinoma), and the term *sarcoma* is added to the tissue name for nonepithelial tissue (e.g., osteosarcoma).
    2. Criteria for classification as malignant
      a. Cells are neoplastic (new growth).
      b. Capacity exists for invasion or metastasis.
      c. Frequency and significance:
        1) In both sexes, malignancies are most common in the lungs, digestive organs (including the pancreas), and sex organs.
        2) In females, breast cancer is most common.
        3) In males, prostate cancer is most common.
    3. Common malignant neoplasms
      a. Malignant melanoma—a malignant tumor involving melanocytes.
      b. Squamous cell carcinoma—a malignant tumor involving squamous epithelium.
      c. Basal cell carcinoma—a malignant tumor involving cells of the epidermis.
    4. Treatment options include surgical incision, chemotherapy, radiation therapy, and bone marrow transplantation. If treatment is ineffective in eliminating the cancer, the disease typically is fatal.

Diseases of the Heart and Blood Vessels

Coronary heart disease, hypertension, and cerebrovascular disease are three significant diseases.

I. Coronary Artery Atherosclerosis (coronary heart disease)
  A. Primary injury to the endothelium of the artery leads to the deposition of platelets and serum lipoproteins and to the proliferation of smooth muscle cells in the wall of the artery.
  B. This plaque formation may lead to occlusion of the coronary arteries, which may cause a myocardial infarction.
  C. Risk factors include age, sex, heredity, diet, hypertension, smoking, obesity, and diabetes mellitus.
  D. Treatments include drugs to lower serum lipid levels and blood pressure, reducing risk factors, bypass surgery, and heart transplant in younger patients.
II. Hypertension
  A. In most hypertensive patients (as many as 90%), no specific cause for elevated blood pressure can be found; this form is called essential or idiopathic hypertension.
  B. Is a multifactorial disease that involves heredity and environment.
  C. May have significant effects on many organs, including the heart, kidneys, blood vessels, and brain.
  D. Treatment includes drug therapy and environmental manipulation.
III. Cerebrovascular Disease
  A. Atherosclerosis of blood vessels in the brain may lead to cerebrovascular accidents (strokes).

I. Strokes typically are caused by one of three principal factors:
   a. Emboli from a larger artery—generally the carotid artery.
   b. Rupture of brain blood vessels because of hypertension, which leads to brain hemorrhage.
   c. Aneurysm of brain blood vessels.

Terminology

Clinical Descriptive Terminology

Bulla—Large fluid-filled vesicle, typically more than 5 mm in diameter.

Erythema—Abnormal redness of tissue.

Lobule—Lobe or well-defined part of a whole.

Macule—Flat area whose color is different from adjacent tissue.

Nodule—Small palpable aggregate of tissue, typically less than 1 cm in diameter. May be subcutaneous, even with tissue, or may protrude above tissue surface.

Pallor—Lack of color.

Papillary—Resembling a small, nipple-like, elevated protuberance.

Papule—Small, elevated, circumscribed lesion, typically less than 1 cm in diameter.

Pedunculated—Possessing a stalk or stem.

Pustule—Elevated pus-containing lesion.

Sessile—Having no peduncle or attached directly by a broad base.

Vesicle—Blister-like elevation containing serous fluid.

Radiographic Descriptive Terminology

Coalescence—Fusion.

Diffuse—Lacking definition; difficult to determine borders.

Multilocular—Having many compartments.

Radiolucent—Appears dark or black on a radiograph.

Radiopaque—Appears light or white on a radiograph.

Unilocular—Area that appears to have one well-defined compartment or unit.

Oral Pathology

Oral pathology includes the study of conditions associated with the mouth, neck, and head.

Dental Diagnostic Process

The foundation of dental treatment is the diagnostic process. A preliminary diagnosis may be made with one or more components of the diagnostic process. The use of differential diagnosis requires the use of diagnostic components to rule out other disease possibilities.

I. Diagnostic Components
   A. Patient history includes medical, dental, and lesion histories.
   B. Clinical assessment requires identification of lesion color, size, shape, or location.
   C. Radiographic assessment is especially useful in osseous and periapical pathology.
   D. Laboratory assessment includes microscopic analysis and blood tests.
   E. Surgical assessment is a visual examination of the surgical site.
   F. Therapeutic trial uses an effective treatment to assist in the diagnostic process.

Variations of Normal

Variants of normal are conditions that are not evident in all patients but are so frequently noted that they are not considered pathologic.

I. Fordyce granules
   A. Are an asymptomatic cluster of yellow lobules of sebaceous origin.
   B. Have an incidence of 75% in adults older than 20 years of age.
   C. Common locations include the buccal mucosa and lower lip.
   D. Require no treatment.

II. Tori
   A. Are an exophytic nodular osseous growth typically found on the palate or bilaterally on the lingual surface of the mandible; typically are asymptomatic; also are called bony exostosis.
   B. Appear on radiographs as radiopaque areas in the mandibular premolar region.
   C. Palatal tori occur twice as often in women compared with men.
   D. Generally require no treatment unless a dental prosthesis is necessary or growth interferes with speech.

III. Pigmentation (physiologic)
   A. Is an asymptomatic, symmetric, brown-colored area located on intraoral tissues—commonly on gingiva.
   B. Appears more often in dark-skinned individuals; nonphysiologic pigmentation is associated with Addison's disease, Peutz-Jeghers' syndrome, smoking, and melanomas.
   C. Requires no treatment, although diagnostic tests for the aforementioned associated diseases and syndromes may be appropriate.

IV. Linea Alba
   A. Is an asymptomatic, bilateral band of white tissue at the level of the occlusal plane on the buccal mucosa.
   B. Is caused by cheek biting.
   C. Requires no treatment.

V. Leukoedema
   A. Is a generalized, opalescent white film located bilaterally on the buccal mucosa caused by cellular edema in the buccal spinous cells.
   B. Has a higher incidence among some ethnic groups (e.g., African-Americans).

C. Requires no treatment.

VI. Lingual Thyroid Nodule
   A. Is a small, nodular mass located slightly posterior to circumvallate papillae.
   B. Is caused by entrapped thyroid tissue.
   C. Treatment may require surgery.

VII. Fissured Tongue
   A. Is characterized by deep grooves or fissures on the dorsal surface of the tongue.
   B. Treatment involves patient instruction on cleaning the tongue.

VIII. Geographic Tongue (benign migratory glossitis)
   A. Is a map-like appearance of erythematous tissue surrounded by a white or yellow border on the dorsal or lateral surface of the tongue.
   B. Histology reveals a desquammation of filiform papillae.
   C. Most likely is caused by stress, heredity, or nutritional factors.
   D. Requires no treatment.

IX. Hairy Tongue
   A. Is characterized by hypertrophy of filiform papillae.
   B. May be caused by the use of mouth rinses or broad spectrum antibiotics.
   C. Color change may be attributed to bacteria, chemicals, tobacco use, foods, or the use of some drugs.
   D. Treatment involves brushing the tongue to remove debris and removal of the cause.

X. Lingual Varices
   A. Are vascularities that appear as red or purple areas on the ventral or lateral surface of the tongue.
   B. Incidence increases among older adults.
   C. Treatment is not required.

 Clinical Case STUDY

Marcus Swenson, a 65-year-old farmer, presents in the office complaining of a painful sore in his mouth. The patient indicates that he noticed the sore several months ago. The medical history reveals that the patient smokes a pack of cigarettes a day and started smoking when he was approximately 15 years old. Mr. Swenson indicates that he consumes alcoholic beverages on the weekends. Examination reveals a 10-mm ulcerated red lesion located on the left lateral border of the tongue.

Clinical Case QUESTIONS

1. What additional information is required for a proper diagnosis?
2. What is the most likely diagnosis of this lesion?
3. Describe the histologic features of this type of lesion.
4. Is this lesion likely to spread to other areas?

5. What risk factors are important in the formation of this type of lesion?

Clinical Case RATIONALES

1. A tissue biopsy is required for proper diagnosis.
2. A biopsy should confirm a squamous cell carcinoma.
3. Histologically, this lesion is an invasion of neoplastic squamous cells through the epithelial basement membrane.
4. Yes, squamous cell carcinomas of the oral cavity are most likely to metastasize to the lymph nodes of the neck.
5. Tobacco and alcohol use are two key risk factors associated with this case.

Injury-Associated Oral Lesions

Traumatic injury, by either chemical or physical means, can result in the development of oral lesions. Typical injury-associated lesions include attrition, abrasion, erosion, burns, tobacco-associated lesions, salivary gland obstruction, connective tissue hyperplasias, and ulcerations.

I. Attrition
   A. Is a physiologic wear of dentition that is accelerated by abnormal grinding or clenching of the teeth (bruxism).
   B. Bruxism may involve incisal or occlusal wear, gingival recession, TMJ disorders, or hypertrophy of the masseter muscle.
   C. Treatment may require fabrication of an occlusal splint or nightguard.

II. Abrasion
   A. Is a wear of dentition associated with the use of an abrasive substance or an abnormal habit.
   B. Is caused by the improper use of a toothbrush or an abrasive dentifrice, which causes a notch at the CEJ, particularly at the canine or premolar area.
   C. Also may be caused by a repetitive habit.
   D. Requires patient education and restorative treatment if indicated.

III. Erosion
   A. Is a loss of tooth structure because of a chemical action.
      1. In bulimia, is a result of the emesis of stomach acids, which typically causes loss of enamel on the lingual surfaces of teeth (called perimolysis).
      2. Also is influenced by diet.
   B. Treatment involves removing the cause and fluoride application.

IV. Burns
   A. Are initiated by heat or chemical exposure, which causes surface tissue necrosis of the oral mucosa.

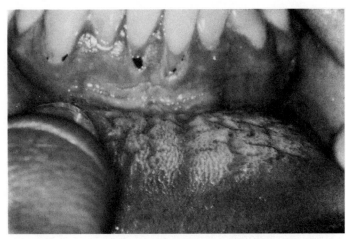

Figure 5.1   Tobacco chewer's lesion located in the area of the labial mucobuccal fold.

B. Are visible as white or ulcerated lesions of the mucous membrane; thermal burns on the palate generally are red.

C. Treatment primarily involves analgesics, topical anesthetics, and in severe cases surgery.

V. Tobacco-Related Lesions (Fig. 5–1)

A. Tobacco chewer's lesions are symptomatic, wrinkled, white lesions located in the mucobuccal fold at the site of tobacco placement.

B. Nicotine stomatitis is red or white lesions with raised red centers (minor salivary glands) on the palatal tissue; is caused by smoking.

C. Treatment involves removal of the cause and possible biopsy to assess for squamous cell carcinoma.

VI. Salivary Gland Obstruction

A. Is an obstruction of a salivary gland (salivary stone or sialolith).

B. Lesions are named according to location (mucocele—typically lower lip; ranula—sublingual or submandibular gland).

C. May appear as a translucent or bluish superficial swelling in the floor of the mouth or as a submental swelling located below the mylohyoid muscle.

D. Is treated by removal of the obstruction.

VII. Connective Tissue Hyperplasia

A. Pyogenic granuloma

1. Is a proliferation of connective and vascular tissue and is most often found on the gingiva; also may be located on the lip, tongue, or buccal mucosa.

2. Formation may be related to hormonal changes (increased incidence occurs during pregnancy) combined with chronic irritants such as plaque.

3. If not spontaneously reduced, is treated by surgical excision.

4. Is similar in clinical appearance to the periph-

eral giant cell granuloma; however, the peripheral giant cell granuloma contains multinucleated giant cells and may lead to bone destruction.

B. Denture-induced hyperplasia

1. Is a proliferation of connective tissue associated with a removable prosthesis.

2. Is indicated by folds of tissue near the denture flange (epulis fissuratum) or fibrous papillary projections of tissue located on the palate (papillary hyperplasia).

3. Is treated by surgical removal of the tissue and a prosthesis reline or redo, if necessary.

C. Gingival hyperplasia

1. Is a proliferation of free or attached gingival tissue, typically in response to local irritants (e.g., plaque, calculus).

2. Is caused by hormonal changes, drugs (e.g., phenytoin, nifedipine, cyclosporin), or heredity and is exacerbated by poor oral hygiene.

3. Appearance varies from soft to fibrous gingiva and color also may vary from pink to red because of increased vascularity.

4. Is referred to as pericoronitis when associated with third molars.

5. May be treated by gingivoplasty, gingivectomy, and oral hygiene instruction.

D. Irritation fibroma (Fig. 5–2)

1. Is a dense connective tissue growth related to chronic irritation.

2. Is an asymptomatic, exophytic growth with color similar to that of adjacent tissues.

3. Appears on the buccal or labial mucosa, gingiva, or tongue.

4. May be treated by excision and possibly biopsy.

VIII. Ulcerations

A. Aphthous ulcers

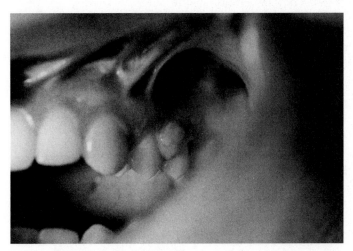

Figure 5.2   Irritation fibroma of the gingiva.

1. Are painful oral lesions also known as canker sores; occur on the unattached mucosa.
2. Often recur and may be associated with a history of trauma or emotional stress.
3. Occur in three forms:
    a. A minor aphthous ulcer is a single lesion 1 cm or less in diameter; is the most common form.
    b. A major aphthous ulcer is a single lesion greater than 1 cm in diameter; generally is more destructive.
    c. A herpetiform aphthous ulcer consists of small clusters of aphthous lesions.
4. Typically heal within 7 to 10 days.
5. Are best treated by an application of topical steroids during the prodromal or preulcerative period.

B. Traumatic ulcers
1. May form as a result of occlusal trauma (biting), irritation from orthodontic or removable appliances, or trauma from food.
2. Often are diagnosed using patient history; heal within 2 weeks.
3. Typically are treated by removing the cause.

Periapical Inflammation and Pathology

Inflammation and pathology of the periapical tissues are found in periapical abscesses, cysts, and granulomas; condensing and alveolar osteitis; and chronic hyperplastic pulpitis.

I. Periapical Abscess
   A. Is an acute, inflammatory condition that develops in the pulp or surrounding periapical tissues.
   B. May cause severe pain, exudate, and radiographic changes ranging from a slight to a distinct periapical radiolucency.
   C. Is treated by endodontic therapy or tooth removal.

II. Peripheral Cemental Dysplasia (cementoma)
   A. Is a lesion associated with a disordered production of cementum and bone.
   B. Radiographic appearance is similar to periapical disease but the tooth is vital and asymptomatic.
   C. Incidence is greater in anterior teeth; in adults older than 30 years of age, requires no treatment.

III. Periapical Cyst (radicular cyst)
   A. Is an epithelial-lined tissue associated with a periapical granuloma.
   B. Often is asymptomatic; radiograph indicates a distinct periapical radiolucency.
   C. May be differentiated from a periapical granuloma only by biopsy.
   D. Is treated by endodontic therapy or tooth removal.

IV. Periapical granuloma
   A. Involves chronic growth of granulation tissue located in the periapical region.
   B. Generally is asymptomatic; radiographic changes range from a slight to a distinct periapical radiolucency.
   C. Is treated by endodontic therapy or tooth removal.

V. Condensing Osteitis (focal sclerosing osteomyelitis)
   A. Is indicated by a formation of dense periapical bone, often in response to a dental infection.
   B. Generally is asymptomatic; is characterized by a radiopaque radiolucency in the periapical region.
   C. Is most commonly associated with the mandibular first molar.
   D. Generally requires no treatment.

VI. Alveolar Osteitis (dry socket)
   A. Is a lack of proper blood clot formation after an extraction.
   B. Causes pain a few days after extraction; patient also may note a foul odor and taste.
   C. Is treated by irrigation and placement of medicated dressing.

VII. Chronic Hyperplastic Pulpitis (pulp polyp)
   A. Is an asymptomatic hyperplasia of the pulp tissue.
   B. Often is associated with a large carious lesion in children or young adults.
   C. Is treated by pulpotomy or extraction.

Clinical Case STUDY

Sixty-five-year-old Virginia Sway complains of a burning mouth, bleeding gums, and soreness when eating. This condition has occurred several times during the past few years. Visual examination of the oral cavity reveals several erythematous areas surrounding grayish-white lesions on the gingiva. A positive Nikolsky's sign also is noted during the exam. Mrs. Sway states that she gets blisters that rupture just before the soreness develops.

Clinical Case QUESTIONS

1. What is the most likely diagnosis of Mrs. Sway's condition? Why?
2. Identify the common signs and symptoms associated with this condition.
3. Describe the treatment for this condition.
4. Does the positive Nikolsky's sign distinguish this condition from pemphigus vulgaris?
5. What other indicators assist in the differential diagnosis?

Clinical Case RATIONALES

1. The condition most likely is benign mucous membrane pemphigoid (BMMP), an autoimmune disorder that results in the development of vesiculobulbous lesions on the gingiva, floor of the mouth, and hard palate. The lesions rupture, giving the appearance of desquamative gingivitis, and cause soreness. These lesions eventually heal, sometimes causing scarring. This dis-

ease tends to occur in older adults and is a chronic condition that is characterized by periods of exacerbation and remission.

2. Common signs and symptoms of the disorder include vesicles that rupture, reddened and ulcerated gingiva, burning, mouth soreness, recurrence of the condition after remission, and scarring.

3. Treatment for this condition is palliative. During active stages, toothbrushing may be impossible; thus the use of a 0.2% chlorhexidine rinse is recommended. Topical anesthetics may be needed to encourage proper nutrition. Topical or systemic corticosteroids are prescribed based on the severity of the condition.

4. No, both BMMP and pemphigus vulgaris may exhibit a positive Nikolsky's sign. A positive Nikolsky's sign appears histologically as a separation of the surface epithelium from the underlying connective tissue.

5. Although a biopsy would confirm the diagnosis of BMMP rather than pemphigus vulgaris, the fact that the patient has had previous oral lesions with no mention of skin lesions indicates that BMMP is the most likely diagnosis. Other autoimmune disorders such as Sjögren's syndrome and lupus erythematosus may occur in association with pemphigus vulgaris.

Immunologic Disorders

Immunologic disorders include hypersensitivity, immunologic pathogenic lesions, and autoimmune diseases.

I. Hypersensitivity
    A. Is an allergic response that varies from a mild cell-mediated response to anaphylaxis.
    B. Is referred to as a mucositis or dermatitis when associated with the oral mucous membrane or skin.
    C. Reaction from latex contact may occur in patients or health care providers.
    D. Treatment varies from none to epinephrine administration and medical assistance.

II. Immunologic Pathogenic Lesions
    A. Erythema multiforme
        1. Lesions may affect both the skin and mucous membrane and resemble a target.
        2. Intraorally, may exhibit red macules and ulcerations on the mucosa or tongue; often characterized by a hemorrhagic crusting of the lips.
        3. Has a greater incidence among young adults and males.
        4. In its severe form is referred to as Stevens-Johnson syndrome.
        5. Is treated with topical corticosteroids.
    B. Lichen planus (Fig. 5–3)
        1. Is a benign, chronic disease that affects the skin and mucosa.
        2. May have one of four forms: atrophic, erosive, reticular, or plaque-like.

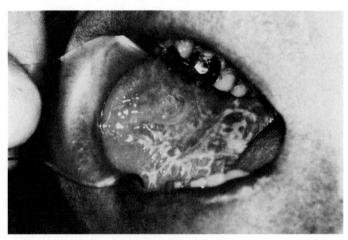

Figure 5.3 Lichen planus exhibiting Wickham's striae on the buccal mucosa.
(Courtesy John L. Hicks, M.D.)

3. In the reticular form is indicated by thin white lines called Wickham's striae and white papules on the buccal mucosa.
        4. Biopsy reveals that the epithelial layer separates from the connective tissue in the erosive and bullous form.

III. Autoimmune Diseases
    A. Lupus erythematosus
        1. Is a chronic and progressive disease that affects the skin and organs; is more common among females.
        2. Displays the classic sign of a butterfly rash over the bridge of the nose.
        3. Is treated with steroids or aspirin.
    B. Pemphigus vulgaris
        1. Occurs most often during middle age and is an autoimmune disease that affects the skin and mucous membranes.
        2. Is a desquammation of tissue that occurs with gentle pressure (Nikolsky's sign).
        3. Is treated with corticosteroids.
    C. Benign mucous membrane pemphigoid (Fig. 5–4).
        1. Also is known as cicatricial (scarring) pemphigoid or mucosal pemphigoid.
        2. Generally affects older adults—women more than men.
        3. Affects the oral mucosa; occurs when the oral epithelium separates from the underlying connective tissue.
        4. Is a chronic, blistering disease of the mouth that causes discomfort; most often is seen on the gingiva (desquamative gingivitis) and may produce the Nikolsky's sign as well as areas of ulceration.

Infectious Diseases

Infectious diseases may be bacterial, viral, or fungal in origin.

I. Tuberculosis

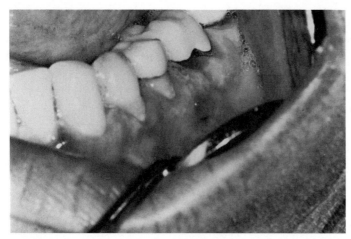

Figure 5.4 Benign mucous membrane pemphigoid with blistering of the gingiva.

A. Is a mycobacterial disease caused by inhaling airborne droplets that contain mycobacterium tuberculosis.
B. Is indicated by fever, malaise, cough, sputum production, pleuritic chest, and occasionally ulcerative oral lesions (typically on the tongue).
C. Is treated with medication and temporary isolation during the infectious state.

II. Acute Necrotizing Ulcerative Gingivitis (ANUG)
A. Is a bacterial disease most likely caused by a fusiform bacillus and *Borrelia vincentii*.
B. Causes red, painful gingiva and necrosis of interdental papilla; patient may note a foul taste and odor.
C. Treatment involves debridement and antibiotics.

III. Candidiasis
A. Is a fungal disease caused by an overgrowth of *Candida albicans*, which may be related to the use of antibiotics or corticosteroids or to an immune deficiency.
B. Most common oral location is the oral mucosa or labial commissures.
C. Presents in a variety of forms:
1. Acute pseudomembranous candidiasis (thrush) is a curdlike superficial plaque that is easily removed.
2. Angular cheilitis is the form associated with a labial commissure.
3. Chronic hyperplastic candidiasis is a more penetrating and hyperplastic form.
4. Acute atrophic candidiasis is the form associated with antibiotic use.
5. Chronic atrophic candidiasis is the form associated with denture use.
6. Is treated with antifungal topical (e.g., Nystatin) or systemic medications.

IV. Verruca Vulgaris
A. Also is known as the common wart; is caused by the papillomavirus.

B. Is a white papillary lesion whose most common site is on the lip.
C. Treatment is by surgical excision.

V. Herpes Simplex (Fig. 5–5)
A. Is a viral disease that presents as one of the following:
1. Type 1—oral herpes; also described as primary herpetic gingivostomatitis or recurrent herpes simplex; also is known as a "cold sore."
a. In its primary form is indicated by edematous, red, painful gingiva with multiple vesicle formation on the oral mucosa.
b. Incidence is greatest in children from 6 months to 6 years.
c. When recurrent, lesions appear most often on the lip (herpes labialis) or perioral tissues; however, lesions also may be noted on keratinized mucosa; recurrent lesions may be multiple vesicles or a single ulcer.
2. Type 2—genital herpes; is a sexually-transmitted disease.
3. Herpetic whitlow—occurs on the fingers.
B. Condition often heals spontaneously in 1 to 2 weeks or may be treated with antiviral drugs such as acyclovir.

VI. Varicella (chicken pox) and Herpes Zoster (shingles)
A. Are caused by the varicella zoster virus. Chicken Pox is caused by an acute infection with the virus; shingles is caused by a reactivation of the virus.
B. As chickenpox, typically presents as skin lesions; oral lesions may occur, which often are associated with the trigeminal nerve.
C. As shingles, may present as unilateral painful vesicles or ulcers that occur on the skin or mucosa; the ophthalmic division of the trigeminal nerve is the area of the face most commonly affected.
D. May be associated with immunodeficiency.

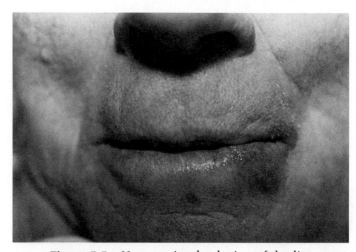

Figure 5.5 Herpes simplex lesion of the lip.

E. May require supportive treatment with antiviral drugs such as acyclovir.

VII. HIV Infection

A. Is caused by the human immunodeficiency virus, which impairs T helper cell function; virus is spread by contact with body fluids, especially blood.

B. In its severe form is known as acquired immunodeficiency syndrome (AIDS).

C. Manifestation ranges from asymptomatic to acute illness.

D. Exhibits numerous oral lesions, which may include:

1. Candidiasis.
2. Herpes simplex or zoster.
3. Hairy leukoplakia (corrugated white lesion often located on the lateral surface of the tongue).
4. HIV gingivitis or linear gingival erythema (chronic red linear band associated with the marginal gingiva—despite minimal plaque—and spontaneous bleeding).
5. Kaposi's sarcoma (an oral malignancy that appears as a red-to-purple lesion; most often seen on the hard palate).
6. Aphthous ulcers.
7. Non-Hodgkin's lymphoma (appears as a large, rapidly growing purple mass in the palate or retromolar area).
8. Other opportunistic infections.

E. Many of the conditions noted with HIV infection may be treated individually as they occur.

F. Is treated, not cured, by a number of drugs; when treated by a combination of drugs, such as AZT, DDI, and nevirapine, the quality and length of life are improved.

 ## Clinical Case STUDY

Twenty-two-year-old Adam Zawada complains of discomfort in the region of the mandibular third molars. Upon visual examination, acute inflammation is noted in the gingival tissues surrounding his newly erupting terminal molars. A panoramic radiograph is taken and development of the third molars is assessed. In addition, a nickel-sized radiolucency is located between the roots of the maxillary right lateral incisor and canine. The roots of the teeth are spread apart from each other.

Clinical Case QUESTIONS

1. Name the condition Adam is experiencing in the molar regions of his mouth. What has caused the condition?
2. What can be done to alleviate Adam's discomfort?
3. What is indicated by the radiolucency located between the roots of the maxillary lateral incisor and canine?
4. What caused the radiolucency and how is it treated?

Clinical Case RATIONALES

1. Adam is experiencing pericoronitis in the molar regions of his mouth. This condition occurs when bacteria collects beneath the flap of gingival tissue (operculum) that commonly covers the most distal surface of newly erupting molars and causes an acute infection. The result is pain and inflammation.

2. Adam's discomfort can be relieved by gently irrigating the sulcus with saline solution, warm water, or hydrogen peroxide. Debridement of the area at the initial appointment, using a topical anesthetic, is recommended if the patient can tolerate it. If not, debridement should occur during the second visit, when the inflammation has subsided somewhat. The use of systemic antibiotics also may be indicated. Surgical removal of the tooth or the operculum may be necessary to prevent a recurrence.

3. The radiolucency located between the roots of the maxillary right lateral and canine most likely is a globulomaxillary cyst. This type of cyst typically is asymptomatic; thus the teeth remain vital. The roots of the adjacent teeth often diverge because of pressure from the cyst. The cyst, because it is non-calcified, appears radiolucent.

4. The radiolucency is "caused by" a developmental disorder, a cyst, that is treated by surgical excision.

Developmental Disorders

A developmental disorder is a disturbance or lack of development of a structure; such disorders include odontogenic and nonodontogenic cysts and other abnormalities. These may occur in a variety of oral structures, including the teeth, soft tissues, and supportive structures of the teeth.

I. Odontogenic Cysts (cysts related to tooth development)

A. Dentigerous (follicular) cyst

1. Is a disturbance associated with reduced enamel epithelium; leads to a cyst that forms around the crown of an unerupted tooth.
2. Appears as a well-defined, unilocular radiolucency associated with a tooth—most commonly a third molar.
3. Is treated by removal of both the cyst and the tooth.

B. Eruption cyst

1. Is a soft-tissue swelling around a newly erupting crown.
2. Requires no treatment because the lesion dissipates during the eruption process.

C. Primordial cyst

1. Develops in place of a tooth and is caused by a disturbance of the enamel organ.
2. Is a well-defined, unilocular or multilocular

radiolucency; is noted most often in the third molar region.

    3. Is treated by cyst removal.

D. Odontogenic keratocyst

    1. Is a cyst lined by both epithelium and parakeratin; is capable of moving or resorbing teeth.

    2. Is a well-defined, multilocular, radiolucent lesion; is noted most commonly in the mandibular third molar region.

    3. Is treated by excision but has a high rate of recurrence.

E. Lateral periodontal cyst

    1. Is an asymptomatic soft-tissue or osseous cyst indicated by a swelling in the interdental papillae.

    2. Exhibits a radiolucent lesion; is noted most commonly in the mandibular canine or premolar area.

    3. Is treated by excision.

II. Nonodontogenic cysts (cysts in the oral cavity not related to tooth development)

A. Nasopalatine cyst

    1. Occurs within the incisive papilla or duct.

    2. Is noted as an asymptomatic, heart-shaped radiolucency.

    3. Frequency is greatest in adults between 40 and 60 years of age.

    4. Is treated by excision.

B. Median palatine cyst

    1. Is located slightly posterior to the incisive papilla.

    2. Is similar to the median mandibular cyst in that the cyst is located between the central incisors.

    3. Is visible as a well-defined, unilocular, radiolucent lesion.

    4. Is treated by excision.

C. Globulomaxillary cyst

    1. Is visible as a pear-shaped radiolucency between the maxillary lateral and canine; may cause root divergence.

    2. Is asymptomatic; the teeth test vital, indicating that periapical pathology is not likely.

    3. Is treated by excision.

D. Nasolabial cyst

    1. Is a soft-tissue cyst located in the mucolabial fold.

    2. Incidence is greatest among 40- to 50-year-old adults.

    3. Is treated by excision.

E. Epidermoid and dermoid cysts

    1. Consist of epithelial cells (epidermoid cyst) or involve the epithelium, mesoderm, and endoderm (dermoid cyst).

    2. Both occur in the mandible and are more common among young adults.

    3. Are treated by excision.

F. Static bone cyst (lingual mandibular bone concavity)

    1. Is not considered a true cyst because it has no epithelial lining and is caused by a depression in the medial side of the mandible, where a portion of the sublingual salivary gland lies.

    2. Is visible as a radiolucency in the posterior mandible.

    3. Requires no treatment.

G. Simple bone cyst (traumatic bone cyst)

    1. Is a well defined, unilocular or multilocular radiolucency; is noted most often between the mandibular molar roots.

    2. Has a greater incidence among young adults.

    3. Is treated by excision.

H. Aneurysmal bone cyst

    1. Has a soap-bubble appearance on a radiograph and may cause bone expansion.

    2. May follow a history of a previous lesion and is more common among young adults.

    3. Is treated by excision (bleeding noted).

III. Developmental Abnormalities Associated With Teeth

A. Hypodontia

    1. Is a fairly common condition that is indicated by a lack of one or more teeth; anodontia (a complete lack of tooth formation) is rare.

    2. Occurs with greater incidence in third molars, maxillary laterals, and mandibular premolars of the permanent dentition; in lateral incisors of the primary dentition.

    3. Is treated by placement of fixed or removable prostheses (e.g., implants, bridges, or partial dentures).

B. Supernumerary teeth

    1. Refers to the formation of extra teeth.

    2. Often are smaller (a microdont) and remain unerupted.

    3. Occur most often in the maxillary arch (90%) and are termed:

       a. Mesiodens, when located between the maxillary centrals.

       b. Distomolars or fourth molars, when located distal to the third molar.

       c. Paramolars, when located buccally or lingually.

    4. Are treated by removal.

C. Germination

    1. Occurs when a single tooth bud forms two teeth (one root and two crowns).

    2. Is more common in the primary mandibular incisors.

D. Fusion (Fig. 5–6)

    1. Is the joining of two tooth germs (a joining of cementum only is referred to as concrescence) to form a single tooth.

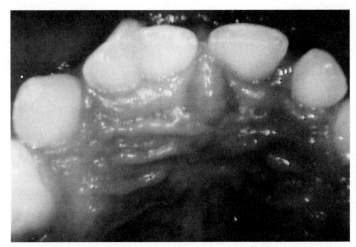

Figure 5.6   Fusion of a primary central and lateral incisor.

    2. Is more common in the primary than in the permanent dentition; typically is associated with anterior teeth.

E. Dilaceration
    1. Is indicated by a curvature of the root and may be caused by trauma during tooth development.
    2. Is more common in third molars.
    3. Requires no treatment; however, does present a challenge during tooth removal or endodontic therapy.

F. Enamel pearl
    1. Is an exophytic area of enamel on a root surface caused by displaced ameloblasts during root formation.
    2. Typically is located near the CEJ, with a greater incidence in the maxillary molars.
    3. May be mistaken for calculus.
    4. May be treated by removal.

G. Taurodontism
    1. Is the formation of an elongated pulp and short root, which result from the improper invagination of the Hertwig sheath.
    2. Appears on a radiograph as teeth with elongated pulps and short roots.
    3. Incidence is greater in molars of Native Americans and Eskimos.
    4. Requires no treatment.

H. Enamel hypoplasia
    1. Is incomplete enamel formation that is caused by disturbances or damage to ameloblasts during enamel formation.
    2. Enamel formation may vary from pits to complete hypoplasia; color varies from white to brown.
    3. Is noted radiographically as thin or absent enamel.
    4. Is seen in Turner's tooth (a single affected tooth), fluorosis, congenital syphilis, tetracycline stain, and amelogenesis imperfecta.

Neoplasia

A neoplasm is an uncontrolled new growth of abnormal cells. This growth may be slow-growing, well differentiated, and not characterized by metastasis (benign neoplasia). It also may vary from well differentiated to anaplastic, with slow or rapid growth, and may be invasive and likely to metastasize (malignant neoplasia). Three possible causes of neoplasms include chemical, viral, and/or radiation exposure.

I. Vascular Neoplasias
  A. Hemangioma
    1. Is a benign vascular lesion that develops at birth or during early childhood.
    2. Is a vascular, exophytic lesion that often occurs on the skin (50%); rarely occurs in the mucous membrane of the head and neck region.
    3. Those that are located intraorally most often are found on the tongue or buccal mucosa.
    4. May require surgical removal.
  B. Kaposi's sarcoma
    1. Is a malignant vascular lesion often associated with HIV infection.
    2. Presents as a dark purple, flat, or exophytic lesion; occurs in a variety of intraoral and extraoral sites.
    3. Is treated by surgery, radiation, or chemotherapy.
  C. Melanocytic nevi
    1. Is a blue- or black-pigmented, generally benign lesion that is commonly referred to as a mole.
    2. May require a biopsy.
  D. Malignant melanoma
    1. Is a malignancy found on the skin; occasionally occurs on fixed mucous membranes.
    2. Grows aggressively and is dark in color; 20% of these lesions are found on the skin of the head and neck.
    3. Often exhibits changes in symmetry, border, color, or diameter.
    4. Appears to be caused by excessive exposure to sunlight.
    5. Is treated by surgery, radiation, or chemotherapy.

II. Osseous Neoplasias
  A. Osteosarcoma
    1. Is a malignant, osseous neoplasia.
    2. Appears as a poorly defined radiolucency in the maxilla or mandible.
    3. Is noted most often in adults who are 30 to 40 years of age; may cause pain, swelling, and paresthesia.

III. Soft Tissue Neoplasias
  A. Are most often benign.
  B. Occur in a variety of tissues, including adipose, muscle, blood, and lymphatic tissues.
    1. Fibroma
      a. Is a mesenchymal tumor associated with an excessive growth of connective tissues.

  b. Is an exophytic lesion whose tissue color matches that of surrounding tissues.
  c. May occur on any oral tissue but often is found on buccal or labial tissues.
  d. When associated with gingiva and cells of the periodontal ligament (PDL), the lesion is referred to as a peripheral odontogenic fibroma.
IV. Odontogenic Neoplasias
  A. Ameloblastoma
    1. Is an epithelial tumor associated with cells of the enamel organ; most often found in the posterior mandible.
    2. Radiographic evidence may reveal multilocular bone destruction; ameloblast-like cells may be noted in biopsy.
    3. Is treated by surgical removal.
V. Epithelial Squamous Cell Neoplasias
  A. Papilloma
    1. Is a benign, pedunculated or sessile, white lesion associated with squamous cells.
    2. Incidence is greater on the palate.
    3. Is treated by excision.
  B. Squamous Cell Carcinoma (Fig. 5–7)
    1. Is a malignancy associated with squamous cells that invades through the basement membrane.
    2. Appearance may vary; color may be red and/or white.
    3. Of the head and neck region is most commonly found on the lower lip; the lateral border of the tongue is the second most common location.
    4. Incidence is greater among males; also is more common in adults aged 40 or older; is associated with chronic tobacco and alcohol use.
    5. May metastasize to lymph nodes of the neck.
    6. Verruca carcinoma.
      a. Is a type of squamous cell carcinoma that is slow growing.
      b. Does not invade the basement membrane, and is unlikely to metastasize; the prognosis

for verruca carcinoma is better than for most squamous cell carcinomas.
      c. Is treated by excision, radiation, or chemotherapy.
  C. Basal cell carcinoma
    1. Is a malignancy that is characterized by an increase in basal epithelial cells; often is associated with sun exposure.
    2. Appears as a small lesion on the skin with rolled borders.
    3. Incidence is greatest among older adults.
    4. Is treated by excision, radiation, or chemotherapy.
VI. Salivary Gland Neoplasms
  A. Pleomorphic adenoma
    1. Is generally a benign salivary gland tumor that consists of a mixture of epithelial and connective tissue cells.
    2. Is the most common benign salivary gland tumor.
    3. Is an asymptomatic mass often associated with the parotid gland or palate.
    4. Is more common among adults older than age 40.
    5. Is treated by excision.
  B. Adenoid cystic carcinoma
    1. Is a slow-growing malignancy associated with a major or minor salivary gland.
    2. Microscopically, has a Swiss-cheese-like appearance.
    3. Is treated by excision.
  C. Mucoepidermoid carcinoma
    1. Is a malignancy associated with epithelial and mucous cells.
    2. Is a slow-growing mass associated with the palate or parotid gland.
    3. Is treated by excision.

Inherited Disorders

Several inherited disorders have an effect on the oral cavity. These include disorders that affect the gingival and periodontal tissues, bone, and teeth.
I. Gingival and Periodontal Disorders
  A. Cyclic neutropenia
    1. Is an autosomal dominant disorder that results in decreased neutrophil production.
    2. May be indicated by severe ulcerative gingivitis, ulcers on the tongue and mucosa, and an increased incidence of periodontal disease.
  B. Papillon-Lefevre syndrome
    1. Is an autosomal recessive disorder that results in early periodontal disease.
    2. Is by indicated by early-onset advanced bone destruction and tooth loss.
  C. Hemophilia
    1. Type A, which is the most common form, is x-linked; thus the disease is transmitted from

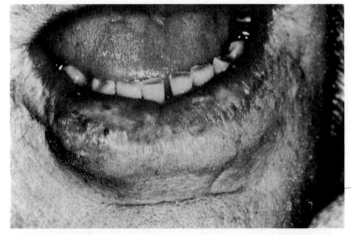

Figure 5.7 Squamous cell carcinoma of the lip.

unaffected daughters to grandsons and affects only males.

2. Exhibits a deficiency in blood clotting factors (type A: factor VIII deficiency; type B: factor IV deficiency; and type C: factor IX deficiency).

3. Is indicated orally by spontaneous gingival bleeding, petechiae, and ecchymoses.

D. Hereditary fibromatosis

1. Is a condition associated with several inherited disorders, such as Laband's syndrome, which causes gingival fibromatosis, nail dysplasia, and joint hypermobility.

2. Develops soon after tooth eruption.

3. May be seen as a generalized enlargement of the gingival tissue, which eventually may cover the dentition completely.

   a. Tissue generally is firm and slightly lighter in color than surrounding gingiva.

   b. Is treated by oral hygiene instruction and surgical excision of excess tissue.

II. Osseous Disorders

A. Cherubism

1. Is an autosomal dominant disorder that develops early in life.

2. Is distinguished by bilateral facial swelling.

3. Is seen radiographically as a multilocular, soap-bubble appearance of the mandible.

4. Is associated with abnormal tooth development and eruption.

B. Cleidocranial dysplasia

1. Is an autosomal dominant disorder.

2. Is indicated by hypoplasia of the clavicles, an underdeveloped premaxilla, supernumerary teeth, malformed teeth, and an abnormal eruption sequence.

C. Osteogenesis imperfecta

1. Is an autosomal dominant disorder.

2. Is indicated by multiple bone fractures and loss of enamel because of abnormal dentin formation.

III. Teeth Disorders

A. Amelogenesis imperfecta

1. This malformation of enamel has a number of causes, including heredity, childhood illness, nutritional deficiency, and medication.

2. Appears as thin, pitted, mottled, snow-capped or yellowish, and poorly calcified enamel.

3. Treatment often requires the placement of esthetic veneers.

B. Dentinogenesis imperfecta

1. Is an autosomal dominant disorder caused by a defect in the odontoblasts.

2. Type I is associated with osteogenesis imperfecta and type II is indicated by opalescent, blue-to-brown colored dentition.

3. May be noted in primary or permanent dentitions.

4. May cause enamel to fracture easily because of unsupportive dentin.

5. Is indicated radiographically by a lack of pulp chamber and root canal formation, bell-shaped crowns, and severe incisal or occlusal wear.

C. Ectodermal dysplasia

1. Is an x-linked recessive disorder.

2. Is indicated by conical or missing incisors and a lack of body hair and sweat glands.

D. Dentin dysplasia

1. Is an autosomal dominant condition described as type I or type II.

2. Type I is indicated by short roots with nearly complete obliteration of the pulp.

3. Type II is similar to type I radiographically; however type II is characterized by large coronal pulps filled with abnormal dentin.

4. Of either type may cause tooth loss because of short roots and periapical lesions.

Systemic Diseases

Systemic diseases that affect the oral tissues include hyperpituitarism, hyperthyroidism, hyperparathyroidism, diabetes mellitus, Paget's disease, anemia, and leukemia.

I. Hyperpituitarism

A. Is caused primarily by a pituitary adenoma.

B. May be associated with the secretion of growth hormone during adulthood, which is demonstrated by acromegaly (enlarged skull, hands, feet) and an enlarged tongue (macroglossia).

II. Hyperthyroidism

A. May cause premature primary exfoliation and early eruption of permanent teeth.

B. May cause osteoporosis of the maxilla and mandible.

III. Hyperparathyroidism

A. Is indicated by radiolucencies in the mandible and by mobile teeth.

IV. Diabetes Mellitus

A. Non-insulin-dependent diabetes mellitus (NIDDM) accounts for the majority of cases of diabetes mellitus.

B. Clinical manifestations are greatest when associated with poorly controlled blood sugar.

C. May be indicated by *Candida albicans*, xerostomia, increased periodontal disease, slow wound healing, and tooth loss and mobility.

D. Is treated by controlling glucose levels and minimizing infections by effective plaque and calculus removal during home care.

V. Paget's Disease

A. Is a chronic bone disease characterized by bilateral bone resorption and replacement; typically is seen in the maxilla.

B. Exhibits a classic cotton-wool appearance on lateral head radiograph.

C. May be associated with hypercementosis, loss of lamina dura, and PDL obliteration.

D. Is noted more often in adults older than 40 years of age.

VI. Anemia
  A. Is a reduction in the number of red blood cells or concentration of hemoglobin; has a variety of causes including heredity, inability to absorb Vitamin B_{12}, and iron deficiency.
  B. Is indicated by a loss of filiform and fungiform papillae, red and atrophic oral mucosa, angular cheilitis, and a painful tongue.
  C. Treatment focuses on treatment of the specific anemia.

VII. Leukemia
  A. Is a malignant neoplasm of cells of the bone marrow and may be acute or chronic; laboratory tests indicate elevated white blood cell counts (100,000 to 500,000 mm^3).
  B. Is indicated orally by enlargement, infection and bleeding of the gingiva, petechiae, ecchymoses, and enlarged lymph nodes.

Temporomandibular and Facial Disorders

Disorders of the temporomandibular joint (TMJ) include dysfunctions and trigeminal neuralgia.

I. Temporomandibular Dysfunction
  A. Is a masticatory muscular disorder that may be accompanied by joint dysfunction.
  B. Is caused by a disorder of the muscles of mastication or TMJ damage.
  C. May exhibit joint or muscle pain, restrictive movement of the mandible, and occlusal disorder.
  D. Is diagnosed using TMJ arthrography and MRI and TMJ arthroscopy.
  E. Is treated by drugs, physical therapy, occlusal splint fabrication, or surgery.

II. Trigeminal Neuralgia
  A. Is a unilateral pain associated with the maxillary or mandibular branch of the trigeminal nerve.
  B. Is found most commonly in women older than age 50.
  C. Is generally treated with medication; surgery typically is reserved for severe conditions.

Dental Implant Pathology

Pathology of the dental implant often results in implant failure.

I. Dental Implant Failure
  A. Is caused by a bacterial infection or mechanical overload.
  B. May be characterized by increased mobility of the implant, bleeding, swelling, suppuration, and erythema.
  C. Is identified on radiograph by minimal bone support and peri-implant radiolucency.
  D. Is treated with surgery, prosthesis modification, debridement, antibiotics, and home care instruction.

 CONTENT REVIEW QUESTIONS

1. Which of the following is TRUE regarding the cellular response to injury?
   A. the duration of an injury has little impact on the cellular response to injury
   B. the response to injury is the same in all cell types
   C. cell necrosis will occur if cell membrane integrity is compromised
   D. cell necrosis will occur only if the genetic apparatus of the cell is damaged

2. Which of the following causes an irreversible injury that leads to cell death?
   A. swelling of the cytoplasm
   B. fragmentation of the nucleus
   C. condensation of the cytoplasm
   D. brief hypoxia

3. The cardinal signs of inflammation include all of the following, EXCEPT:
   A. pain
   B. heat
   C. redness
   D. swelling
   E. odor

4. Which one of the following factors involved in tissue repair is correctly defined?
   A. angiogenesis is the formation of new blood vessels
   B. fibrosis is the formation of a new epithelial layer
   C. remodeling is the formation of a fibrous collagen patch
   D. chemotaxis is the secretion of collagen-degrading enzymes

5. What circulatory system changes take place during inflammation?
   A. a decrease in blood vessel permeability
   B. a release of chemical mediators such as histamine
   C. the constriction of arterioles
   D. an inhibition of diapedesis of leukocytes

6. Which of the following statements about tissue regeneration is CORRECT?
   A. regeneration is accomplished by the formation of a fibrous connective tissue scar
   B. in terms of tissue function, repair is more desirable than regeneration
   C. regeneration is the replacement of damaged cells with parenchymal cells of the same type
   D. the type of cell injured has little impact on whether the tissue heals by regeneration or repair

7. Which of the following is NOT a necessary condition for neoplasia formation?
   A. exposure to adequate concentrations of carcinogens
   B. susceptible host tissue
   C. adequate time for establishment
   D. existence of a genetic defect

8. Which of the following statements is CORRECT regarding the name of a neoplasia?

A. for a benign neoplasia, the suffix *-oma* is added to the tissue name —

B. for a malignant neoplasia, the suffix *-oma* is added to the tissue name

C. a benign neoplasia of squamous epithelium is called a squamous cell carcinoma

D. a malignant neoplasia of bone tissue is called an osteoma

9. Endogenous carcinogens include which one of the following?

A. radiation

B. viruses

C. chemicals (such as benzene)

D. genetic anomalies —

10. The process by which cells with cancer potential establish themselves and give rise to cancer is called:

A. initiation

B. transformation —

C. metastasis

D. promotion

11. The MOST common site for malignant cancers in females is the:

A. lungs

B. uterus

C. breast —

D. colon

12. A 14-year-old boy died of an osteosarcoma that metastasized to the lungs. Which one of the following statements regarding this case is CORRECT?

A. the cancer in the lungs most likely originated in the liver

B. osteosarcoma is a benign tumor

C. metastasis of the osteosarcoma most likely was by blood —

D. metastasis is the best criteria for classifying a tumor as benign

13. Psoriasis:

A. is a generic term that refers to many acute or chronic inflammations of the skin

B. presents as raised papules or patches with silvery scales and thickened skin —

C. is a bacterial infection characterized by multiple facial lesions from plugged sebaceous glands

D. is most commonly found on the trunk and neck

14. A 16-year-old male presents with numerous pus-containing pimples on his face and neck. Which of the following statements is INCORRECT regarding this condition?

A. the condition most likely is acne

B. the condition most likely is caused by a viral infection of the sebaceous glands —

C. a clear relationship exists between hormonal factors and this patient's condition

D. the condition most likely is caused by a bacterial infection of the sebaceous glands

15. Which of the following statements BEST describes the relationship between acne and seborrheic dermatitis?

A. both acne and seborrheic dermatitis are skin diseases that affect the sebaceous glands and hair follicles —

B. both acne and seborrheic dermatitis are bacterial skin infections

C. acne is a bacterial skin infection and seborrheic dermatitis is a viral skin infection

D. both acne and seborrheic dermatitis are autoimmune disorders

16. Many honey-colored, itchy, raised pustules are noted on the skin around the face and neck of a 3 year old. They are signs of which of the following diseases?

A. acne

B. seborrheic dermatitis

C. impetigo —

D. psoriasis

17. Pituitary hyperfunction is a characteristic of which of the following diseases?

A. acromegaly —

B. diabetes insipidus

C. Graves' disease

D. Cushing's syndrome

18. Which of the following is a manifestation of hypopituitarism?

A. oversecretion of growth hormone

B. acromegaly

C. hyperactive thyroid gland

D. copious urine production —

19. Grave's disease is associated with which of the following glands?

A. pituitary gland

B. thyroid gland —

C. pancreas

D. adrenal glands

20. A cause of Cushing's syndrome could be:

A. administration of glucocorticoid steroids by a physician —

B. destruction of the thyroid gland as treatment for disease

C. atrophy of the adrenal glands

D. autoimmune hypertrophy of the parathyroid glands

21. The most common cause of hyperparathyroidism is:

A. pituitary adenoma

B. parathyroid adenoma —

C. thyroid adenoma

D. medullary carcinoma of the adrenal gland

22. Which of the following is NOT a complication of cirrhosis of the liver?

A. hyperglycemia —

B. ascites

C. splenomegaly

D. jaundice

23. Characteristics of type I diabetes mellitus include all of the following, EXCEPT:

A. insulin dependence

B. mature onset —

C. juvenile onset

D. more serious than type II

24. Chronic pancreatitis often causes an inadequate secretion of pancreatic juices. Which of the following might be a manifestation of this?

    A. nutrient malabsorption—

    B. chronic constipation

    C. severe jaundice

    D. diverticula of the intestine

25. Hypochromic anemia also might be called:

    A. secondary anemia

    B. hemolytic anemia

    C. iron-deficiency anemia —

    D. aplastic anemia

26. Which type of anemia is characterized by the rupturing of erythrocytes?

    A. pernicious anemia

    B. hypochromic anemia

    C. aplastic anemia

    D. hemolytic anemia —

27. Which of the following statements is INCORRECT regarding hemophilia?

    A. hemophilia is characterized by low blood hemoglobin concentration —

    B. hemophilia is a genetic blood disease

    C. hemophilia is a blood disease characterized by improper blood clotting

    D. treatment for hemophilia includes transfusion and administration of clotting proteins

28. All of the following are correct regarding primary polycythemia, EXCEPT:

    A. primary polycythemia is an increase in the number of erythrocytes in circulation

    B. hyperviscosity of the blood is a manifestation of primary polycythemia

    C. emphysema is a cause of primary polycythemia

    D. treatment for primary polycythemia includes bloodletting

29. Bone marrow infiltrated by malignant cells, an increased number of immature leukocytes in the blood, and treatment by chemotherapy are characteristic of:

    A. leukemia

    B. primary polycythemia

    C. secondary polycythemia

    D. hemophilia

30. Which of the following is NOT correct regarding AIDS?

    A. AIDS is a fatal syndrome that develops after infection by HIV

    B. AIDS is best classified as an autoimmune disease

    C. AIDS is contracted by contact with HIV-contaminated blood

    D. late-stage symptoms of AIDS include increased opportunistic infections

31. For which condition would radiographic diagnosis be conclusive?

    A. alveolar osteitis

    B. periapical abscess

    C. periapical granuloma

    D. condensing osteitis

32. Which of the following closely resembles or is slightly lighter in color than the tissue on which it is located?

    A. pyogenic granuloma

    B. fibroma

    C. papillary hyperplasia

    D. peripheral giant cell granuloma

33. A bilateral, lobulated, exophytic bone located in the lingual mandibular premolar area most likely is:

    A. condensing osteitis

    B. genial tubercles

    C. mandibular tori

    D. ranula

34. Which of the following is observed as a radiopaque area at the tooth apex and often is associated with a restored or carious tooth?

    A. periapical granuloma

    B. focal sclerosing osteomyelitis

    C. periapical abscess

    D. compound odontoma

35. A target-like lesion is a clinical manifestation of:

    A. lichen planus

    B. ectodermal dysplasia

    C. erythema multiforme

    D. lupus erythematosus

36. Loss of lingual tooth structure associated with bulimia is described as:

    A. attrition

    B. erosion

    C. bruxism

    D. abrasion

37. A cluster of sebaceous glands observed on the buccal mucosa most likely is:

    A. lipomas

    B. linea alba

    C. mucoceles

    D. Fordyce granules

38. Which of the following could NOT occur in response to a hypersensitivity to latex?

    A. contact mucositis

    B. angioedema

    C. contact dermatitis

    D. lichen planus

39. Which term best describes a freckle?

    A. pedunculated

    B. sessile

    C. macule

    D. papule

40. Which of the following presents as a painful, erythematous necrosis of the interdental papilla?

    A. pericoronitis

    B. acute necrotizing ulcerative gingivitis

    C. pemphigus vulgaris

    D. pyogenic granuloma

41. Geographic tongue is associated with the desquammation of _____ papillae.

A. fungiform
B. filiform
C. circumvallate
D. foliate

42. Acantholysis and Nikolsky's sign are associated with which one of the following conditions?
    A. lupus erythematosus
    B. pemphigus vulgaris
    C. tuberculosis
    D. pemphigoid

43. Which cyst is MOST commonly found between the maxillary canine and lateral incisor teeth?
    A. dentigerous cyst
    B. radicular cyst
    C. globulomaxillary cyst
    D. lateral periodontal cyst

44. The union of two teeth by cementum is referred to as:
    A. gemination
    B. fusion
    C. dilaceration
    D. concrescence
    E. dens in dente

45. The most likely etiology for basal cell carcinoma is:
    A. heredity
    B. tobacco
    C. alcohol
    D. sunlight

46. Hutchinson's incisors and mulberry molars are associated with which condition?
    A. congenital syphilis
    B. amelogenesis imperfecta
    C. ectodermal dysplasia
    D. tuberculosis

47. A supernumerary tooth mesial to teeth #8 and #9 is termed a:
    A. Turner tooth
    B. dens in dente
    C. microdont
    D. mesiodens

48. Improper invagination of the Hertwig's sheath may cause:
    A. an enamel pearl
    B. a peg lateral
    C. a talon cusp
    D. taurodontism

49. The MOST common microdont is the:
    A. maxillary central incisor
    B. mandibular lateral incisor
    C. maxillary lateral incisor
    D. mandibular third molar

50. A pseudocyst that forms in the mandibular premolar or molar region and is caused by a bone depression adjacent to a salivary gland is a:
    A. simple bone cyst
    B. static bone cyst
    C. salivary cyst
    D. traumatic bone cyst

51. All of the following may cause gingival hypertrophy, EXCEPT:
    A. cyclosporine
    B. tetracycline
    C. Procardia
    D. Dilantin

52. Patients with this x-linked recessive disorder lack body hair and sweat glands and may have missing or cone-shaped incisors:
    A. dentin dysplasia
    B. dentinogenesis imperfecta
    C. amelogenesis imperfecta
    D. hypohidrotic ectodermal dysplasia

53. The loss of lamina dura and a cotton-wool radiographic appearance of bone are associated with:
    A. fibrous dysplasia
    B. insulin-dependent diabetes mellitus
    C. osteogenesis imperfecta
    D. Paget's disease

54. An autosomal dominant disorder that is characterized by opalescent blue or brown crowns is:
    A. amelogenesis imperfecta
    B. ectodermal dysplasia
    C. dentin dysplasia
    D. dentinogenesis imperfecta

55. Which of the following does not meet the criteria for a diagnosis of AIDS?
    A. Kaposi's sarcoma
    B. histoplasmosis
    C. herpes simplex
    D. candidiasis of the respiratory system
    E. lymphoma of the brain

REVIEW QUESTION RATIONALES

1. **C** The cellular response to injury depends on multiple factors, including the type, duration, and severity of the injury; the cell type; and biochemical considerations such as cell membrane, genetic apparatus, and protein integrity.

2. **B** Damage to the nucleus of the cell and therefore to the genetic apparatus of the cell is considered an irreversible cell injury. Cytoplasmic changes that occur without the loss of cell membrane integrity are normal signs of reversible cell injury. Prolonged hypoxia may cause irreversible cell damage. Brief hypoxia most often is manifested by cytoplasmic swelling without damage to the cell membrane.

3. **E** Odor is not a cardinal sign of inflammation. The cardinal signs of inflammation include heat, redness, pain, swelling, and loss of function.

4. **A** Angiogenesis is the proliferation of local blood vessels into the site of tissue damage. Fibrosis is the formation of a fibrous collagen patch in and around the damaged tissue. Remodeling is the generation of collagen-degrading enzymes. Chemotaxis is the

movement of white blood cells toward a chemical substance that attracts it.

5. **B** The pathogenesis of inflammation is characterized by circulatory and cellular changes. Circulatory changes include increases in blood flow and blood vessel permeability because of the release of chemical mediators. Cellular changes include the emigration or diapedesis of leukocytes and phagocytosis.

6. **C** Injured tissues heal by regeneration or repair. Regeneration is the replacement of injured cells with parenchymal cells of the same type. Repair is healing with the formation of a connective tissue scar. The type of cell injured is the primary factor that determines whether tissue healing is by regeneration or repair. Some tissues, such as epithelial tissues, have a high capacity for regeneration. Other tissues, such as cardiac muscle and nervous tissue, have a very limited capacity for regeneration and heal by repair.

7. **D** Neoplasia formation occurs only if certain conditions are met. These conditions include: exposure to adequate concentrations of carcinogens; susceptible host tissue; and adequate time for neoplasia initiation, transformation, and growth. The existence of a genetic defect is not a necessary condition.

8. **A** Several general guidelines are followed in naming a neoplasia. For a benign neoplasia, the suffix *-oma* is added to the name of the tissue (with the exception of malignant melanoma, which is always cancerous). For a malignant neoplasia in nonepithelial tissue, the term *sarcoma* is added to the tissue name. For a malignant neoplasia in epithelial tissue, the term *carcinoma* is added to the tissue name. A malignant neoplasia of bone is an osteosarcoma.

9. **D** Endogenous carcinogens include genetic factors, hormonal imbalances, immunologic and nutritional factors, and aging. Radiation, viruses, and chemicals are considered exogenous carcinogens.

10. **B** Transformation occurs when cells with cancer potential establish themselves and give rise to cancer. Initiation occurs when cells undergo an alteration or series of alterations to acquire autonomous growth potential. Metastasis is the spread of cancerous cells to a new site. Promotion is not a part of the process of cancer development.

11. **C** The most common site for malignant cancers in females is the breast. In males the most common site for malignant cancers is the prostate gland. The second most common site in both males and females is the lungs.

12. **C** An osteosarcoma is a malignant tumor of bone tissue. Metastasis is the primary criteria for classifying a tumor as malignant. Osteosarcomas metastasize by blood and secondary tumors often develop in the lungs.

13. **B** Psoriasis is a type of dermatitis that is characterized by raised papules or patches with silver-colored scales. Its cause is unknown, although it tends to run

in families. Lesions most commonly are found on the extremities and lead to thickened skin.

14. **B** The condition most likely is acne, a bacterial infection of the sebaceous glands. This condition is most common during adolescence, has hormonal and hereditary components, and may be aggravated by stress and/or drugs. Viruses do not cause acne.

15. **A** Acne and seborrheic dermatitis are both skin diseases that affect the sebaceous gland and hair follicles. Acne is caused by bacteria and is thus considered an infectious disease. Seborrheic dermatitis is a multifactorial disorder and is not an infectious disease.

16. **C** Impetigo is a highly contagious infectious disease that is common in children. The key signs are honey-colored, itchy, raised pustules around the head and neck. Acne lesions are raised but typically are not honey-colored or itchy. Seborrheic dermatitis exhibits redness, itching, and scaling, and psoriasis lesions are raised, scaly patches on the extremities.

17. **A** Gigantism and acromegaly occur when the pituitary gland oversecretes growth hormone. Diabetes insipidus is caused by pituitary hyposecretion. Graves' disease is caused by hypersecretion of the thyroid gland. Cushing's syndrome is caused by hypersecretion of the adrenal glands.

18. **D** Hypopituitarism is characterized by a hypoactive pituitary gland. The condition is caused by agenesis, atrophy, and/or destruction of secretory cells in the pituitary gland. A lack of the pituitary hormone antidiuretic hormone (ADH) leads to copious urine production. Oversecretion of growth hormone, acromegaly, and hyperactive thyroid gland are all characteristics of hyperpituitarism.

19. **B** Graves' disease is associated with hyperthyroidism and is characterized by an autoimmune hypertrophy of the thyroid gland. Manifestations include the hypersecretion of thyroxine, which leads to exophthalmos, tachycardia, and severe weight loss.

20. **A** Cushing's syndrome is characterized by the hypersecretion of adrenal gland hormones, such as glucocorticoids. The administration of glucocorticoid steroids by a physician in inappropriate amounts could lead to elevated blood levels of glucocorticoids and Cushing syndrome.

21. **B** Parathyroid adenoma is the primary cause of hyperparathyroidism. Remember, an adenoma is a tumor in secretory epithelium that often leads to hypersecretion by the affected epithelial cells.

22. **A** Hyperglycemia is not a complication of cirrhosis of the liver. The most common complications include jaundice, hepatic encephalopathy, ascites (accumulation of fluid in the abdominal cavity), splenomegaly, and bleeding.

23. **B** Characteristics of type I diabetes mellitus include insulin dependency and juvenile onset. Type I diabetes mellitus is more serious than type II. Mature onset is typical of type II diabetes mellitus.

24. **A** Pancreatitis may lead to an inadequate secretion of pancreatic juices, which are necessary for the digestion of nutrients in the intestine. Malabsorption is a key manifestation of chronic pancreatitis.

25. **C** Anemia is a blood disorder that is characterized by low blood oxygen and hemoglobin levels. There are several types of anemia. Hypochromic anemia is characterized by too little hemoglobin per erythrocyte and often is caused by iron deficiency. Hemolytic anemia is characterized by erythrocytes that rupture too easily. Pernicious anemia is a disease in which too few erythrocytes are present. In aplastic anemia the red bone marrow is faulty. Secondary anemia occurs as a consequence of another condition.

26. **D** Hemolytic anemia is characterized by erythrocytes that rupture too easily.

27. **A** Hemophilia is the improper clotting of blood. It is a genetic disease characterized by prolonged bleeding after even minor injuries. Treatment for hemophilia includes blood transfusion and administration of blood clotting proteins. Low blood hemoglobin concentration is a characteristic of anemia.

28. **C** Primary polycythemia is the oversecretion of erythrocytes by hyperactive bone marrow. Factors such as emphysema, heart disease, and living at high altitude may lead to secondary polycythemia.

29. **A** Leukemia is a cancer of bone marrow. The most common manifestations of leukemia are malignant cells in the bone marrow, an increased number of immature leukocytes in the blood, and complications such as joint pain, unusual bleeding, hepatomegaly, and splenomegaly. Polycythemias involve red blood cells and hemophilia involves blood clotting factors.

30. **B** Acquired immune deficiency syndrome is not considered an autoimmune disease because the body's immune system is not attacking its own tissues. Rather, AIDS is a syndrome that develops as a result of infection by HIV.

31. **D** Condensing osteitis or focal sclerosing osteitis has a characteristic radiopaque appearance. A dry socket or alveolar osteitis would not indicate a periapical change. A periapical abscess and a periapical granuloma may exhibit a similar radiographic appearance, ranging from a slight radiolucency to a very distinct periapical radiolucency.

32. **B** A fibroma typically is similar in color to adjacent tissues. Because of an increase in vascularity, the pyogenic granuloma, papillary hyperplasia, and peripheral giant cell granuloma typically are more erythematous than the surrounding tissue.

33. **C** The mandibular tori is a lobulated overgrowth of dense bone found in the mandibular premolar region. Condensing osteitis is not exophytic; a ranula is associated with a blocked salivary gland and would be located in the floor of the mouth; and genial tubercles are located inferior to the mandibular central incisors.

34. **B** Focal sclerosing osteomyelitis is observed as an apical radiopacity. The periapical granuloma and abscess both would be observed as a radiolucency, and a compound odontoma would exhibit a collection of tooth-like radiopacities between two teeth.

35. **C** Only erythema multiforme exhibits a target-like lesion, typically on the skin but occasionally on the oral mucosa.

36. **B** A client who exhibits chronic bulimia will have erosion of the lingual tooth structure, which is caused by the emesis of gastric acids (chemical wearing of the tooth). Tooth loss associated with attrition and bruxism is caused by physiological wear of the incisal edge or occlusal surface and is not associated with tooth loss because of acid exposure. Tooth loss associated with abrasion occurs at the location of the repetitive habit (e.g., buccal CEJ from toothbrush abrasion).

37. **D** Fordyce granules or spots appear as a yellow cluster on the buccal mucosa. Linea alba appears as a white line on the buccal mucosa corresponding to the occlusal plane. A mucocele appears as a clear vesicle and a lipoma is a single neoplasia composed of mature fat cells.

38. **D** Lichen planus is an autoimmune disease. Contact mucositis, dermatitis, and angioedema are all examples of a hypersensitivity response and may occur after latex exposure in a sensitive individual.

39. **C** A macule is a flat lesion. A pedunculated lesion has a stalk, a sessile lesion is a broad-based lesion, and a papule is an elevated lesion.

40. **B** Acute necrotizing ulcerative gingivitis is a painful, red lesion that often involves necrosis of the interdental papilla. Pericoronitis may be red and painful, however, it is associated with the distal surface of the last erupted molar. Although the other lesions may be associated with the gingival tissue, they do not cause necrosis of the interdental papilla.

41. **B** A migratory, reversible desquammation of the filiform papillae is noted with geographic tongue (benign migratory glossitis). A change in the fungiform, foliate, and circumvallate papillae is not noted with this condition.

42. **B** Pemphigus vulgaris is a separation of the epithelial tissue; the removal of epithelium may be noted when gauze is rubbed across the lesion (Nikolsky's sign). Lesions associated with lupus erythematosus, tuberculosis, and pemphigoid do not exhibit acantholysis (a separation of epithelial cells) and the Nikolsky's sign.

43. **C** A globulomaxillary cyst is most often found between the maxillary canine and lateral incisors. Dentigerous and radicular cysts may be found in a variety of locations and a lateral periodontal cyst typically is located in the mandibular canine and premolar area.

44. **D** A condition in which two neighboring teeth are joined only by cementum is concrescence. Germina-

tion involves the incomplete formation of two teeth from one; fusion involves the confluence of both cementum and dentin; dilaceration refers to an abnormal root curvature; and dens in dente involves the invagination of the enamel organ during tooth development.

45. **D** Basal cell carcinoma is associated with sun exposure. Heredity, alcohol, and tobacco are associated with squamous cell carcinoma rather than basal cell carcinoma.

46. **A** Irregularly shaped mandibular incisors and mandibular first molars may develop as a result of congenital syphilis. Ectodermal dysplasia and amelogenesis imperfecta may cause defects in enamel but are not confined to incisors and first molars. Lesions associated with tuberculosis do not affect the hard tissue.

47. **D** A supernumerary or extra tooth located between the maxillary incisors is referred to as a mesiodens. A microdont is a small tooth that could be found in a variety of locations in the oral cavity. A dens in dente would not be located between central incisors.

48. **D** Taurodontism is caused by a decrease in the normal invagination of Hertwig's root sheath and is found only in multirooted teeth. A peg lateral is a small lateral incisor; a talon cusp is a tooth with an accessory cusp; and an enamel pearl is a small formation of enamel on the root surface caused by misplaced ameloblast activity.

49. **C** The maxillary lateral incisor is the most common microdont and the maxillary third molar also is a common microdont. The mandibular third molar and lateral incisor are seldom associated with microdontia.

50. **B** A static bone cyst is identified on a radiograph as a small well-defined radiolucency in the lower posterior region of the mandible. It is not a true cyst because it is a bone depression caused by the adjacent salivary gland. Simple and traumatic bone cysts are true cysts. Salivary gland cysts do occur in the molar and premolar areas, however, they are not specific to these areas. The blockage of a salivary gland duct also may be noted with salivary gland cysts.

51. **B** Tetracycline taken during tooth formation may cause tooth discoloration but does not cause hyperplasia of gingival tissues. Procardia, cyclosporine, and Dilantin have been shown to cause gingival hypertrophy.

52. **D** Missing or cone-shaped incisors are associated with the hereditary disorder ectodermal dysplasia. Lack of or thin body hair and a lack of sweat glands also are characteristic of this disorder. A dysplasia of tooth structure is noted in dentin dysplasia, amelogenesis imperfecta, and dentinogenesis imperfecta; however, cone-shaped incisors and ectodermal changes are not characteristics of these disorders.

53. **D** Radiographic evidence reveals a cotton-wool appearance and a loss of lamina dura in patients with Paget's disease. Patients with IDDM may show evidence of bone loss associated with periodontal disease and patients with fibrous dysplasia may show a diffuse radiopacity. Patients with osteogenesis imperfecta present with abnormally formed bones that fracture easily and abnormal dentin formation.

54. **D** Dentinogenesis imperfecta type II, also known as hereditary opalescent dentin, exhibits crowns that appear opalescent brown to blue. Anodontia, not opalescent teeth, is characteristic of ectodermal dysplasia. Dentin dysplasia (radicular type) exhibits normal tooth color. Coronal dentin dysplasia exhibits amber translucent teeth in the primary dentition and normal color in the permanent dentition. Amelogenesis imperfecta is characterized by poorly calcified, mottled, or thin enamel that may appear yellowish-brown.

55. **C** Herpes simplex infection would not typically be considered an indicator of AIDS, unless the herpes simplex infection persisted longer than one month. The other diseases or conditions are important in AIDS diagnosis.

Additional Readings

Damjanov I: Pathology for the Health-Related Professions. 1st ed. Philadelphia, WB Saunders Company, 1996.

Crowley LV: Introduction to Human Disease. 4th ed. Sudbury, MA, Jones and Bartlett, 1997.

Ibsen OA, Phelen JA: Oral Pathology for the Dental Hygienist. 2nd ed. Philadelphia, WB Saunders Company, 1996.

Kumar V, Cotran R, Robbins S: Basic Pathology. 6th ed. Philadelphia, WB Saunders Company, 1997.

Langlais RP, Miller C: Color Atlas of Common Oral Diseases. 2nd ed. Baltimore, Williams and Wilkins, 1998.

Laskin D, Damm D: Benign Ulcerative Lesions of the Mouth, AAOMS Surgical Update, Fall 1997.

Mulvihill ML: Human Diseases: A Systemic Approach. 4th ed. Norwalk, Appleton and Lange, 1995.

Regezi JA, Sciubba JJ: Oral Pathology: Clinical-Pathologic Correlations. 2nd ed. Philadelphia, WB Saunders, 1993.

Shafer W, Hine M, Levy B: A Textbook of Oral Pathology. 4th ed. Philadelphia, WB Saunders Company, 1983.

Taber's Cyclopedic Medical Dictionary. 17th ed. Philadelphia, FA Davis, 1993.

Chapter SIX

Nutrition

Mary Danusis Cooper, R.D.H., M.S.Ed

Clinical Case STUDY

Lisa, who is 8 years old, is in the dental office for a six-month oral prophylaxis maintenance appointment. Upon reviewing her medical history with her mother, the dental hygienist asks whether there have been any changes in her health status since her last visit. Lisa's mother shares that Lisa had a severe chest cold 2 months ago and that she recently has been waking up frequently during the night to urinate. In fact, Lisa wet her bed a couple of nights ago and her mother is truly concerned. She also notes that Lisa recently has had an increased appetite yet has lost weight.

Clinical Case QUESTIONS

1. What is the most likely diagnosis of Lisa's condition?
2. Identify the usual causes and predisposing factors for this condition.
3. What is the best treatment for this condition?
4. Is this condition preventable? And if so, how?

Clinical Case RATIONALES

1. Insulin-dependent diabetes mellitus (Type 1).
2. The onset of type 1 diabetes typically occurs in individuals who are under the age of 20. An associated condition that may trigger the onset of insulin-dependent diabetes is a viral infection. The infection may effect an immune response that attacks the pancreas, leading to an inability to make insulin. Symptoms include polyuria (frequent urination), increased appetite, and weight loss.
3. This condition must be treated by insulin therapy, regular blood glucose monitoring, and careful nutritional assessment.

4. This disease cannot be prevented, but it can be controlled. Although a viral infection can play a part in the development of insulin-dependent diabetes, its determination as a cause cannot always be made.

Content Review

Nutrients

Nutrients are substances that are obtained from food and are used by the body to promote growth, maintenance, or repair. There are six classes of nutrients, including proteins, carbohydrates, lipids, vitamins, minerals, and water.

Proteins

Proteins are organic compounds that are composed of amino acids, which are the building blocks of proteins. They contain carbon, hydrogen, oxygen, and nitrogen.

I. Types
   A. Amino acids are held together by peptides; a carboxyl (COOH) group of one amino acid is linked to an amino (NH_2) group of another; there are 22 amino acids.
      1. Essential (indispensable) amino acids cannot be synthesized by the body; must be obtained from the diet. There are nine essential amino acids; nitrogen balance can be achieved from proper proportions and adequate amounts of these.
      2. Nonessential (dispensable) amino acids can be synthesized by the body as long as nitrogen is present. There are 11 nonessential amino acids.
   B. Complete proteins (high-quality) are foods that consist of *all* the essential amino acids in sufficient amounts; completely supply the needs of the

body for maintenance, repair, and growth; are found in meat, fish, poultry, eggs, cheese, and milk.

C. Incomplete proteins (low-quality) lack one or more essential amino acids; include plant proteins; can support life but not normal growth.

D. Complementary proteins are two or more proteins that combine to compensate for deficiencies in amino acid content; use of whole grains important.

II. Physiology

A. Digestion/absorption—no digestion begins in mouth, mechanical breakdown of food only.

1. Digestion begins in the stomach.
   a. The hormone gastrin releases the enzyme pepsin, which breaks down protein into smaller amino acid units called peptones.
   b. Hydrochloric acid is essential for protein digestion.

2. Digestion continues in the small intestine.
   a. Peptones stimulate the release of the hormone cholecystokinin (CCK) from intestinal walls.
   b. CCK travels via the bloodstream to the pancreas and gallbladder.
      1) CCK releases bile from the gallbladder.
      2) In the pancreas, the enzymes trypsin and chymotrypsin break down peptones into short peptides and amino acids.
   c. The final digestion of all peptides into amino acids occurs inside the absorptive cells of the small intestine.
   d. Amino acids travel via the portal vein to the liver, where they convert to glucose or fat, are used for energy, or released in the bloodstream.

B. Metabolism

1. Liver is the primary site of catabolism (breakdown into simpler compounds).
2. Food protein provides amino acids, which are absorbed from the small intestine.
   a. Synthesized into tissue proteins, enzymes, or hormones.
   b. Protein synthesis is controlled by deoxyribonucleic acid (DNA).
3. Nitrogen balance is the balance between the input and output of nitrogen.
   a. Negative nitrogen balance: output exceeds intake as a result of fever, anorexia nervosa, surgery, blood loss, infection, or use of protein for energy.
   b. Positive nitrogen balance: input exceeds output as a result of growth, pregnancy, or recovery from surgery.

III. Functions

A. Role in overall body needs.
   1. Assist in growth and maintenance—construction and repair of body tissue.

2. Provide essential components of hormones and enzymes.
3. Provide precursors of antibodies.
4. Provide an energy source when carbohydrate and fat intake are inadequate—4 kilocalories (kcal) per gram (g).
5. Regulate acid-base balance.

B. Role in oral health

1. Important in the growth and development of the oral cavity.
2. If absent, results in crowded and/or rotated teeth because of inadequate growth of the jawbone.
3. If deficient, can cause Kwashiorkor, which results in delayed eruption and hypoplasia of deciduous teeth.
4. Can help neutralize acids produced by plaque bacteria.

C. Role in periodontal disease

1. Important in maintaining the health of the periodontium.
2. Essential for cellular defenses against subgingival plaque bacteria.
3. Essential for healing and repair of tissue after periodontal surgery.

IV. Dietary Requirements and Nutrient Sources

A. Requirements

1. Recommended daily allowance (RDA) is 0.8 g/kg (2.2 lb) of body weight.
2. Increase during periods of growth, pregnancy, and lactation.

B. Sources

1. Complete proteins—meat, fish, poultry, eggs, and milk.
2. Incomplete proteins—legumes, grains, vegetables, and soybeans.

V. Nutritional Deficiency and Disease

A. Phenylketonuria (PKU)—disease in which the liver cannot metabolize the essential amino acid phenylalanine into the nonessential amino acid tyrosine. Phenylalanine accumulates in the liver and blood and reaches the kidneys in high concentrations. Toxic by-products build up in the body and damage the developing nervous system. An enzyme in the kidneys converts phenylalanine to the ketone phenylpyruvic acid, which empties into the urine. Diet: restrict phenylalanine, enough to support normal growth; supplement tyrosine; avoid aspartame (Nutrasweet/Equal).

B. Protein-energy (calorie) malnutrition (PCM)

1. Marasmus—inadequate food intake. Is common in children between 6 and 18 months of age in impoverished nations; impairs brain development and learning; causes wasting and weakening of muscles; no edema.
2. Kwashiorkor—severe protein deficiency. Begins at approximately 2 years of age; without severe wasting of body fat; symptoms include

apathy, failure to grow and gain weight, listlessness, changes in hair color, and edema in the
abdomen and legs.
3. Adult PCM occurs in alcoholics (with nutritional
liver disease) and in patients who are hospitalized for long periods.
C. Protein needs increase during episodes of trauma,
fear, anxiety, surgery, and fever.

Carbohydrates

Carbohydrates are organic compounds (contain carbon)
that also contain the elements hydrogen and oxygen.
They provide energy during metabolism.
I. Types
   A. Simple carbohydrates
      1. Monosaccharides (single sugars)
         a. Pentoses (C_5) act as coenzymes in energy
            production (e.g., ribose, deoxyribose).
         b. Hexoses (C_6) have major nutritional impor-
            tance.
            1) Glucose (blood sugar or dextrose) is the
               form that is used most efficiently by the
               body. Can be obtained from all plant
               carbohydrates; serves as primary fuel for
               the brain; is found in honey, fruits, and
               corn syrup.
            2) Fructose (levulose or fruit sugar) is the
               sweetest of all sugars. Is closely related
               to glucose structurally; is found in honey,
               fruits, and corn syrup.
            3) Galactose is derived from the hydrolysis
               of lactose. Is a constituent of many plant
               polysaccharides. During lactation, the
               body converts glucose to galactose in
               mammary tissue to synthesize lactose in
               breast milk.
      2. Disaccharides (double sugars; two mono-
         saccharides)
         a. Lactose (milk sugar) is composed of glucose
            and galactose and is obtained from milk
            products.
         b. Sucrose (table sugar; cane and beet sugar) is
            composed of glucose and fructose; is ob-
            tained from sugar beets, sugarcane, or ma-
            ple syrup.
         c. Maltose (plant sugar) is composed of two
            molecules of glucose; forms as starch in
            grains and breaks down during germination;
            is used in the fermentation of alcohol.
   B. Complex carbohydrates (long chains of sugars)
      1. Polysaccharides
         a. Starch (mixture of amylose and amylopec-
            tin): nutritionally is the most important car-
            bohydrate. Is digestible by humans; stores
            energy; breaks down at a slower rate than
            mono- and disaccharides; is found in rice,
            wheat, corn, rye, potatoes, and legumes.
         b. Glycogen is the animal equivalent of starch.

Provides a food storage system for all forms
of animal life; is stored in liver, where it
regulates blood sugar, and in muscle, where
it serves as an energy source for muscle
contraction.
         c. Insulin is produced by the pancreas; is used
            for storing energy.
         d. Dextran forms a substrate for dental plaque;
            serves as an energy source for dental caries-
            producing bacteria such as *Streptococcus
            mutans*.
         e. Fibers
            1) Cellulose: provides a fibrous framework
               for plants. Is a good source of fiber; is not
               digestible and therefore provides rough-
               age and bulk to aid in peristalsis and the
               elimination of water; is found in fruits,
               legumes, and all vegetables.
            2) Hemicellulose: group of insoluble fibers
               (do not easily dissolve in water); is a
               primary constituent of cereal fibers.
            3) Pectin: responsible for the thickening of
               jams and fruit preserves and keeps salad
               dressing from separating; is found in
               vegetables and fruits, especially citrus
               fruits and apples.
II. Physiology
   A. Digestion: digestive enzymes are released (se-
      creted) from pancreas and cells of intestinal walls.
      1. Polysaccharides: The initial breakdown of starch
         begins in the mouth during chewing; is assisted
         by the enzyme salivary amylase (which breaks
         starch down into disaccharides such as malt-
         ose). Pancreatic amylase completes the process
         in the small intestine (breaks down remaining
         disaccharides into monosaccharides).
      2. Disaccharides are digested in the walls of the
         small intestine.
         a. Lactose is hydrolyzed to glucose and galac-
            tose by the enzyme lactase.
         b. Sucrose is hydrolyzed to glucose and fruc-
            tose by the enzyme sucrase.
         c. Maltose is hydrolyzed to two molecules of
            glucose by the enzyme maltase.
      3. Monosaccharides enter the capillaries; glucose
         enters the blood directly.
   B. Absorption: single sugars (from food or as by-
      products) are taken up by the absorptive cells in
      the small intestine.
         a. Monosaccharides enter the villi and are
            transported to the liver via the portal vein.
         b. The liver transforms monosaccharides to:
            1) Glucose and releases them directly into
               bloodstream or
            2) Stores carbohydrates as glycogen or
            3) Produces fat
   C. Metabolism: glucose is the primary source of
      energy for the body.

1. Sources of blood glucose
   a. Dietary carbohydrates (sugars, starches)
   b. Glycogenolysis is the process by which stored liver glycogen is converted to glucose by a liver enzyme
   c. Gluconeogenesis is the process by which the liver makes glycogen from amino acids derived from the body's protein and/or from fatty acids.
2. Blood glucose reactions (production of energy)
   D. Glycolysis is the process by which cells oxidize glucose to pyruvic acid and subsequently pyruvic acid oxidizes to CO_2 and water, yielding usable energy in the form of adenosine triphosphate (ATP).
3. Storage
   a. Glycogenesis is the conversion of glucose to glycogen (storage form for excess glucose in liver and muscle).
   b. Lipogenesis occurs when more glucose is available than the body can use for energy; glycogen needs of the liver and muscle are filled and excess is deposited as fat in adipose cells.

III. Functions of Carbohydrates
   A. Provide energy (4 kcal/g).
   B. Spare proteins: protein can supply energy when necessary but its primary function is to build tissue and replace cells.
   C. Aid in oxidation (burning) of fats to prevent ketosis (a partial breakdown of fats, which leads to high levels of ketones in the bloodstream).
   D. Furnish fiber for normal peristalsis. Also provide bulk, reduce risk of heart and artery disease, and prevent constipation and diverticular disease.

IV. Dietary Requirements and Nutrient Sources
   A. Requirements
      1. Minimum adult requirement is 60 to 100 g/day. Infants and children require more carbohydrates to prevent the use of protein for energy.
      2. Dietary fiber: minimum requirement is 20 to 30 g/day for adults.
   B. Sources
      1. Cereals and breads provide starch.
      2. Some vegetables (leafy) provide cellulose and hemicellulose.
      3. Some vegetables (root tuber and seed: potatoes, beans, beets, squash) provide starch and sucrose.
      4. Fruits provide primarily glucose and fructose.
      5. Sugar, honey, and corn syrups provide monosaccharides and disaccharides.
      6. Sweeteners
         a. Sucrose is a disaccharide found in table sugar, beet sugar, and cane sugar.
         b. High-fructose corn syrup contains 40% to 90% fructose; is made by treating corn starch with acid and enzymes; is broken down into glucose and changed into fructose.

   c. Turbinado sugar is a partially refined version of raw sugar; has a slight molasses flavor.
   d. Brown sugar is white sugar that contains some molasses; the molasses is either added or not totally removed.
   e. Maple syrup is made by boiling down sap obtained from sugar maple trees.
      7. Alternative sweeteners
         a. Sugar alcohols are sugarlike compounds (nutritive sweeteners) that, like carbohydrates, yield 4 kcal/g of energy. Metabolized more slowly than sucrose by bacteria in the mouth and therefore do not promote tooth decay.
            1) Sorbitol is made from glucose by hydrogenation; is used in foods, especially diabetic foods and sugarless chewing gums; is not readily absorbed by the small intestine and therefore can cause diarrhea.
            2) Mannitol is made from mannose and galactose by hydrogenation; is used in sugarless chewing gum and candies; also is not readily absorbed by the small intestine and may cause diarrhea.
            3) Xylitol is derived from cellulose products such as wood straw and pulp cane; may produce diarrhea when taken in excess; is equivalent to sucrose in sweetness.
         b. Artificial sweeteners include noncarbohydrate, noncaloric sweeteners.
            1) Saccharin is derived from coal-tar compounds; is 500 times sweeter than sucrose; is widely used in soft drinks and table sweeteners; may cause cancer and therefore products must contain a warning label.
            2) Aspartame is the active ingredient in Nutrasweet and Equal; is composed of amino acids (phenylalanine and aspartic acid) and methanol; is used in beverages, gelatin desserts, and chewing gum; cannot be used in baking (low calorie sweetener yields 4 kcal/g).
            3) Acesulfame-K is 200 times sweeter than sucrose; is used in chewing gum, powdered drink mixes, gelatin puddings, and nondairy creamers; can be used in baking.

V. Nutritional Management of Deficiency and Disease
   A. Diabetes mellitus is a metabolic disorder characterized by a high blood glucose level due to insufficient or ineffective insulin function. High levels of glucose in the blood and cells subsequently result in tissue damage.
      1. Types
         a. Insulin-dependent diabetes mellitus (IDDM) is type 1, juvenile onset diabetes

that typically begins during late childhood. The islets of Langerhans in the pancreas cannot synthesize insulin and therefore glucose is unable to enter cells; individual must inject insulin to assist cells in taking up needed glucose; cells break down protein and fat for energy; as fatty acids are released, liver responds by making ketone bodies (which accumulate in blood and urine); onset has been associated with viral infection.

   b. Noninsulin–dependent diabetes mellitus (NIDDM) is type 2, adult-onset diabetes that characterizes the majority of cases of diabetes; usually develops in adulthood; has a genetic component and is associated with obesity. The body lacks the ability to make sufficient insulin or improperly uses that which it does make; cells in the body resist the action of insulin at receptor sites (entryways of cells).

2. Role of insulin (hormone produced in beta cells of islets of Langerhans in pancreas)
   a. Normal function
      1) Is a protein hormone secreted in response to a high level of glucose.
      2) Stimulates the liver to make glycogen (storage form of glucose) through the process of glycogenesis.
      3) Allows fat cells to increase glucose absorption; in muscle, glucose is transformed into glycogen.
   b. Abnormal function: without insulin, ketoacidosis results.
      1) An acidic state is caused by a rapid breakdown of body fat.
      2) The liver normally breaks down small amounts of fatty acids to form ketones.
      3) Ketones subsequently are metabolized for energy.
      4) In uncontrolled diabetes, ketone production exceeds use and the excess is excreted in urine (ketonuria).

3. Symptoms
   a. Acetone breath: fruity odor on the breath of a person who is experiencing ketosis (ketone acetone).
   b. Hyperglycemia is an abnormally high blood glucose concentration.
   c. Ketonemia is ketones in blood.
   d. Ketonuria is ketones in urine.
   e. Polydipsia is increased thirst caused by frequent urination.
   f. Polyuria is frequent urination to remove excess ketones and glucose.
   g. Polyphagia is increased appetite because of a need for energy.
   h. IDDM is characterized by weight loss and increased appetite.
   i. NIDDM is characterized by weight gain and increased appetite.

4. Chronic complications
   a. Blood vessel and nerve damage
   b. Poor circulation
   c. Increased infections
   d. Blindness (diabetic retinopathy)
   e. Cardiovascular disease
   f. Atherosclerosis
   g. Loss of kidney function

5. Treatment
   a. Obese patients
      1) Restrict calories and reduce weight.
      2) Engage in regular exercise (assists muscles in taking up more glucose).
      3) Space meals evenly throughout the day.
      4) Discourage alcohol consumption.
   b. Insulin-dependent patients
      1) Require careful nutritional assessment; should eat regular meals with a precise carbohydrate-to-protein-to-fat ratio.
      2) Insulin delivery—a mixture of two or more types two or more times daily.
      3) Intensive therapy, including regular blood glucose monitoring.
      4) Regular exercise.

6. Oral manifestations
   a. Periodontal disease involves an increased incidence of gingival inflammation, bleeding, and advanced periodontal pocket formation.
   b. Xerostomia (dry mouth) involves an increased incidence of caries.

7. Dental treatment
   a. Update and review medical histories.
   b. Emphasize plaque control.
   c. Schedule regular prophylaxis maintenance appointments (every 3 to 4 months).
   d. Recommend fluoride treatments to help prevent root caries.

B. Hypoglycemia is a disorder characterized by low blood glucose levels.
1. Reactive hypoglycemia occurs in reaction to the ingestion of food; typically occurs 1 to 4 hours after meals.
   a. Symptoms include weakness, rapid heartbeat, sweating, anxiety, and hunger; are caused by the release of epinephrine (hormone), which is triggered by falling blood glucose.
   b. Treatment: eating regular meals with protein, fat, and complex carbohydrates that contain soluble fiber; avoiding concentrated sweets.
2. Fasting sets in gradually and affects the brain and central nervous system (CNS).

a. Symptoms include headaches, fatigue, blurred vision, and confusion; are not related to epinephrine release.
b. Treatment is eating balanced meals at regular intervals.

C. Lactose intolerance is an intestinal condition in which lactose digestion may be reduced because of a deficiency of the digestive enzyme lactase. Lactase hydrolyzes lactose to glucose and galactose in the intestine. When lactase is absent in the small intestine, lactose travels to the large intestine, where bacteria breaks it down into gas and acids.
1. Symptoms include cramps, abdominal distention, gas symptoms, and diarrhea after the consumption of dairy products.
2. Treatment includes:
a. Eating smaller servings of milk products.
b. Including fat in meals, which slows digestion and leaves more time for lactase action.
c. Eating cheese; lactose is lost when milk is processed into cheese.
d. Consuming yogurt with active bacteria cultures; lactose is digested by yogurt.

D. Dental caries—five oral and dental factors contribute to the initiation and progression of dental caries, including tooth structure, bacteria, types of fermentable carbohydrates eaten, salivary flow, and frequency of food intake.
1. Tooth chemistry—the following are susceptible to caries:
a. Pits and fissures of posterior surfaces
b. Buccal pits and grooves of mandibular molars
c. Cingulum of maxillary incisors
d. Crowded or overlapped teeth
2. Dental plaque bacteria types—sucrose and glucose are broken down into lactic acid as a result of the enzymatic activity of streptococci and lactobacilli.
a. *Streptococcus mutans* initiates the caries process; synthesizes polysaccharides (glycogen, dextran, levan) for future fermentation.
1) Polysaccharides are used for energy when they are needed.
2) Dextrans form a substrate for dental plaque and serve as an energy source for dental caries.
3) Demineralization begins at a pH of 5.5.
b. *Lactobacillus acidophilus* extends the caries process.
3. Fermentable carbohydrates ingestion: the concentration of sugars in food is a key factor in the development of dental caries.
a. Starch-rich foods: if left on teeth for long periods of time, will degrade to organic acids and can contribute to dental caries.
b. Sugar-rich foods: the cariogenic activity of sucrose, glucose, and fructose is similar; physical form of food affects cariogenic activity (oral clearance time of liquids is faster than that of solids or retentive sweets, thus liquids are less cariogenic).
c. A concentration of 0.8 M must be present for sugar to pass through 1 mm of dental plaque and undergo harmful fermentation. A 1-M solution of sugar contains 342.3 g of sugar in water.
4. Salivary flow rate: an inadequate salivary flow interferes with the oral clearance time of cariogenic foods and decreases natural salivary buffers, subsequently initiating caries development.
5. Daily food intake frequency: the development of caries is related to between-meal snacking; eating sweets with a meal makes them less cariogenic.

Lipids (Fats)

Lipids are organic compounds that are composed of carbon, hydrogen, and oxygen. They include triglycerides (fats and oils), phospholipids, and sterols (cholesterol).

I. Types
A. True fats are composed of glycerol (a trihydroxy alcohol) that is attached to one, two, or three fatty acids to form monoglycerides, diglycerides, or triglycerides, respectively.
1. Saturated fatty acid carries the maximum number of hydrogen atoms; remains solid at room temperature; increases serum cholesterol.
a. Stearic acid sources include beef and lard.
b. Palmitic acid sources include animal fat and palm oil.
c. Myristic acid is found in coconut.
d. Lauric acid is found in coconut oil.
2. Monounsaturated fatty acid contains a point of unsaturated linkage (with no hydrogen atom); is viscous in form; has no effect on serum cholesterol.
a. Oleic acid sources include olive oil, shortening, lamb, and canola oils.
3. Polyunsaturated fatty acid contains two or more points of unsaturation; is liquid in consistency (includes oils); decreases serum cholesterol.
a. Omega-6 fatty acids are linoleic; found in corn, cottonseed, safflower, and sunflower oils.
b. Omega-3 fatty acids are linolenic; are found in fatty fish oils, green leafy vegetables, and soybean products (tofu).
4. Essential fatty acids must be obtained from diet (i.e., linoleic and linolenic acids); regulate blood pressure, assist in clot formation, maintain cell membranes, make hormone-like sub-

stances, and support the functioning of the retina.

B. Compound lipids are compounds that are added to glycerol and fatty acids.
1. Phospholipids are built on the backbone of glycerol, with one fatty acid replaced by a compound that contains phosphorus.
   a. Lecithin is found in cells and participates in fat digestion in the intestine; acts as an emulsifier by mixing oil with water (e.g., in salad dressings, mayonnaise); is most commonly found in egg yolk.
2. Lipoproteins are produced in the liver and allow cholesterol, triglycerides, and phospholipids to be transported in the bloodstream.
   a. Chylomicrons are made in the intestine after fat absorption; contain triglycerides and a small amount of protein.
      1) Transport newly absorbed lipids from intestinal cells to the bloodstream via the lymphatic system.
      2) During circulation, cells remove lipid content and therefore become smaller.
      3) The liver picks up and breaks down chylomicrons and assembles new lipoproteins known as very low-density lipoproteins (VLDL).
   b. VLDL: liver coats cholesterol and triglycerides with a shell of protein and lipids.
      1) VLDLs leave the liver and triglycerides are broken down into fatty acids and glycerol by the enzyme lipase.
      2) VLDLs become much heavier as triglycerides are released.
      3) VLDLs gather cholesterol from other lipoproteins and become low-density lipoproteins (LDL).
   c. Low-density lipoproteins (LDLs) are primarily composed of cholesterol; contain a few triglycerides; are larger, lighter, and more lipid-filled than VLDLs.
      1) Cells absorb LDLs from the bloodstream and break them down.
      2) Most LDLs are taken up by liver cells when a diet is low in saturated fats and cholesterol.
      3) Scavenger cells in blood vessels engulf LDLs that are not taken up.
      4) Over time, cholesterol builds on inner blood vessel walls and plaque develops.
      5) The blood supply to organs subsequently is cut off and may result in a heart attack.
   d. High-density lipoproteins (HDLs)—are produced by the liver and intestine; are smaller, denser, and contains a high amount of protein
      1) HDLs travel in the bloodstream and pick up cholesterol.
      2) Cholesterol is transported, via other lipoproteins, back to liver for excretion.
      3) High HDLs slow the development of heart disease.
C. Cholesterol (Sterol) is capable of forming esters with fatty acids; makes important hormones (estrogen, testosterone); makes bile, an emulsifier needed for digestion; is found in animal foods only. The liver can make what the body needs; high levels raise total plasma cholesterol level.
D. Fat replacements
1. Olestra is made by adding fatty acids to sugar; yields no energy to the body; may lower blood serum cholesterol levels; reduces the absorption of vitamin E; has no kilocalories.
2. Simplesse is a protein; feels like fat in the mouth but contains no fatty acids; cannot be used in cooking; contains 1.3 kcal/g.
3. Hydrogenation is a process that is used to reduce the amount of fat per serving (e.g., in diet margarine).
4. Gums are derived from plant sources and are added to thicken products such as diet salad dressings.

II. Physiology
A. Digestion
1. Tongue secretes the enzyme lingual lipase; acts primarily on the short- and medium-chain fatty acids of triglycerides.
2. Stomach—actual digestion occurs with enzyme, gastric lipase.
3. Small intestine
   a. Pancreatic lipase
      1) Hormone cholecystokinin (CCK) acts to release lipase from the pancreas after food is eaten.
      2) Digests triglycerides and other lipids with long-chain fatty acids into monoglycerides and fatty acids.
   b. Stored bile from the gallbladder emulsifies fats.
B. Absorption
1. If the chain length of a fatty acid is less than 12 carbon atoms, it is water-soluble and travels through the portal vein.
2. If the chain length is long, it must become a triglyceride molecule and enter circulation through the lymphatic system.
   a. Covered with a protein coat, triglycerides combine with cholesterol and other substances.
   b. The end result is a lipoprotein that enters the lymphatic system at the villus and eventually enters the bloodstream to carry absorbed fats.

III. Functions
   A. Provide energy (9 kcal/g).
   B. Store energy.
   C. Insulate to maintain body temperature and protect organs.
   D. Transport fat-soluble vitamins to the small intestine and aid in absorption.
   E. Provide satiety (fullness).
   F. Provide flavor and texture to foods.

IV. Dietary Requirements and Nutrient Sources
   A. Requirements—less than or equal to 30% of total kilocalories.
      1. Saturated—less than 10% of total kilocalories.
      2. Monounsaturated—approximately 10% of total kilocalories.
      3. Polyunsaturated—approximately 10% of total kilocalories.
      4. Cholesterol—less than or equal to 300 mg/day.
      5. Essential fatty acids—1% to 3% of total kilocalories.
   B. Sources
      1. Saturated—animal fat and palm oil.
      2. Monounsaturated—olive oil, shortenings, and lamb.
      3. Polyunsaturated—soybean, cottonseed, and vegetable oils.
      4. Cholesterol—animal foods.
      5. Essential fatty acids—vegetable oils; recommendation is 1 tablespoon per day.

V. Nutritional Management of Deficiency and Disease
   A. Atherosclerosis—is a degenerative disease that produces a hardening of large and medium arteries.
      1. Formation of plaques
         a. Includes the formation of atheromata, which are deposits of lipids on the inner walls of arteries.
         b. With age, plaque becomes fibrotic and narrows blood vessels.
         c. Eventually ischemia occurs (decreased blood supply).
      2. Risk Factors include:
         a. Total blood cholesterol greater than 240 mg/100 mL.
         b. LDL cholesterol greater than 160 mg/100 mL.
         c. HDL cholesterol less than 35 mg/100 mL.
         d. Men older than age 45; women older than age 55.
         e. Smoking
         f. Family history
         g. Hypertension
      3. Treatment
         a. Reduce saturated fat from diet (less than 10% of total kilocalories lowers LDL cholesterol level); maintain polyunsaturated and monounsaturated fat intake at approximately 10% of total kilocalories.
         b. Eat less than 300 mg of cholesterol per day.
         c. Substitute foods rich in animal fat, butter, coconut oil, and hydrogenated (solid) fats with less hydrogenated forms.
         d. Increase consumption of dietary fiber (20–35 g per day).
         e. Lose weight or maintain desirable body weight.
         f. Avoid smoking.
      4. Low-fat food recommendations
         a. Meat, fish, poultry—lean cuts; trim fat; grill, roast, or bake; tuna packed in water.
         b. Dairy—low-fat or nonfat milk, cheese, and yogurt; nonfat frozen yogurt.
         c. Fruits and vegetables—nonfat salad dressing; steam vegetables; eat fruit for dessert.
         d. Breads and cereals—use jellies on bread instead of butter/margarine; avoid croissants, coffee cakes, and sweet rolls.
   B. Obesity—decrease fat and calorie intake. (See weight control section.)

 Clinical Case **STUDY**

Carol, a 21-year-old woman, is in the dental office for an oral prophylaxis appointment. The dental hygienist reviews Carol's medical history and Carol notes that she may be 2 weeks pregnant. Carol has not seen her physician yet but shares her concern regarding the pregnancy. There is a history of spina bifida in her family.

Clinical Case QUESTIONS

1. Identify the typical causes of and predisposing factors for spina bifida.
2. How can this condition be prevented?
3. What food sources are essential in preventing spina bifida?

Clinical Case RATIONALES

1. Folic acid (folate, folacin) deficiency during pregnancy is associated with an increased risk of spina bifida. Because folate is necessary for nucleic acid synthesis, a deficiency may impair cell growth—thus causing anomalies of the fetus. Defects typically occur within the first 6 weeks of inception.
2. The patient must see a physician as soon as possible. Most women are encouraged to increase folate consumption even before they conceive. An adequate intake of foods containing folate is important. The patient also may be given prenatal vitamins.
3. Food sources high in folate include fruits and vegetables—especially green leafy vegetables. Raw vegetables are better than cooked vegetables because

cooking easily destroys folate. Orange juice also is a good source of folate.

Vitamins

Vitamins are organic nutrients that are needed by the body in small quantities. They do not contribute energy to the body but are needed as facilitators of body processes. Fat-soluble vitamins include A, D, E, and K. Water-soluble vitamins include the Bs and C.

I. Fat-Soluble Vitamins (soluble in fats and fat solvents; are not readily excreted and therefore can build up to toxic levels; are stored in the liver and in fatty tissues)
   A. Vitamin A
      1. Function
         a. Is important for night vision; retinal forms rhodopsin
         b. Assists in maintenance of epithelial cells and mucous membranes.
         c. Is necessary for immune defenses.
         d. Promotes normal growth and development.
         e. Assists in formation of ameloblasts and odontoblasts.
      2. Dietary requirements—1000 retinol equivalent (RE)/day for men; 800 RE/day for women
      3. Nutrient sources
         a. Preformed vitamin A (retinoids; animal form) is found in liver, body fat of fish, egg yolk, and vitamin A-fortified milk.
         b. Provitamin A (carotenoids; from plant-derived precursor carotene) is converted in the body to vitamin A; most potent form is beta-carotene (an antioxidant); is found in orange-yellow and dark green fruits and vegetables (e.g., carrots, spinach, apricots, and broccoli).
      4. Nutritional deficiency and disease—may cause night blindness (nyctalopia); dry, rough skin; or dry mucous membranes.
      5. Toxicity may cause irritability; enlarged liver and spleen; dry skin; and bone and joint pain.
   B. Vitamin D
      1. Functions as a hormone. Assists in:
         a. Regulating proper serum levels of calcium and phosphorus.
         b. Absorbing calcium and phosphorus.
         c. Promoting the mineralization of teeth and bones.
      2. Dietary requirements—5 to 10 g (200 to 400 IU)/day
      3. Nutrient sources
         a. Sunlight—the liver makes a vitamin D precursor (7-dehydrocholesterol) that surfaces on the skin, is activated by sunlight, and is converted into vitamin D_3 (cholecalciferol).
         b. Fortified milk and fatty fish.
      c. Vitamin D_2 (ergocalciferol)—is derived from plants, especially yeasts and fungi.
      4. Nutritional deficiency and disease
         a. Rickets—in children, manifests as a softening of the bones (because of failure to calcify normally); symptoms include bowed legs, enlarged head, joints, and rib cage, and deformed pelvis.
         b. Osteomalacia—occurs in adults; calcium is taken from bones to make up for insufficient absorption by the intestine; symptoms include bowed legs, bent posture, and pain in ribs, pelvis, and legs.
         c. Toxicity—occurs with high blood calcium levels; symptoms include loss of appetite and mental confusion.
   C. Vitamin E (tocopherol)
      1. Functions
         a. Is an antioxidant—prevents the oxidation of vitamin A and polyunsaturated fatty acids.
         b. Protects red blood cells (RBCs) from damage.
      2. Dietary requirements—8 to 10 mg/day
      3. Nutrient sources
         a. Plant (vegetable) oils—including safflower, cottonseed, and peanut.
         b. Green leafy vegetables.
         c. Legumes, nuts, whole grains.
      4. Nutritional deficiency and disease—deficiency may lead to erythrocyte hemolysis (breakdown of RBCs).
      5. Toxicity—interferes with blood coagulation.
   D. Vitamin K
      1. Function—synthesizes blood-clotting factor prothrombin.
      2. Dietary requirements—60 to 80 µ/day
      3. Nutrient sources—green leafy vegetables; also is synthesized by the intestine.
      4. Nutritional deficiency may lead to hemorrhage.
      5. Toxicity—in infants, manifests as jaundice; also reduces effectiveness of anticoagulant drugs.
II. Water-Soluble Vitamins—because water-soluble vitamins (Bs and C) are easily excreted, they are less likely to reach toxic levels.
   A. Thiamin (B_1)
      1. Functions
         a. Aids in the metabolism of carbohydrates, fats, and proteins.
         b. Assists in proper functioning of nervous system, heart, and muscles.
         c. Promotes proper functioning of the digestive tract.
      2. Properties—is sensitive to heat; avoid overcooking.
      3. Dietary requirements—1.1 to 1.5 mg/day
      4. Nutrient sources—include pork, whole grains (wheat germ), sunflower seeds, and organ meats.
      5. Nutritional deficiency and disease

a. Beri beri (I can't, I can't)
   1) Wet—symptoms include rapid pulse, enlarged heart, and severe edema.
   2) Dry—symptoms include paresthesia, numbness of feet, and cramps in legs; edema is not a symptom.
   3) Infantile—symptoms include dyspnea (shortness of breath) and cardiac failure.

B. Riboflavin (B_2)
   1. Functions—aids in the metabolism of carbohydrates, fats, and proteins; assists in the formation of ATP.
   2. Properties—is sensitive to light; milk should be stored in cardboard/opaque containers.
   3. Dietary requirements—1.2 to 1.7 mg/day.
   4. Nutrient sources—milk products, organ meats, and green vegetables (broccoli, turnip greens, asparagus).
   5. Nutritional deficiency and disease—deficiency may lead to glossitis, cheilosis, dermatitis, and eye disorders.

C. Niacin (B_3)
   1. Functions
      a. Is a coenzyme that assists in energy metabolism.
      b. Aids normal functioning of the CNS.
      c. Maintains healthy skin and mucous membranes.
   2. Properties—amino acid tryptophan can be converted to niacin; is one of the most stable vitamins.
   3. Dietary requirements—15 to 19 mg/day
   4. Nutrient sources
      a. Meat, poultry, and fish
      b. Enriched breads and cereals
      c. Green leafy vegetables, mushrooms, and asparagus
   5. Nutritional deficiency and disease
      a. Pellagra (rough, painful skin)—symptoms include the 4 Ds: dementia, diarrhea, dermatitis, and death.
      b. Gastrointestinal disturbances
      c. Glossitis
   6. Toxicity—leads to blood vessel dilation (flushing) caused by increased blood flow, headaches, nausea, and vomiting.

D. Pantothenic acid
   1. Functions
      a. Aids in the metabolism of carbohydrates, fats, and proteins for energy.
      b. As coenzyme A, assists in fatty acid metabolism and initiates fatty acid synthesis.
      c. Aids in the formation of hormones and nerve-regulating substances.
   2. Properties—is easily destroyed by heat.
   3. Dietary requirements—4 to 7 mg/day.

4. Nutrient sources include liver, eggs, whole grains, legumes, and potatoes (white and sweet).
5. Nutritional deficiency and disease
   a. Poor muscle coordination
   b. Fatigue, headaches, and nausea
   c. Paresthesia of the hands and feet

E. Biotin
   1. Functions—in coenzyme form assists in energy metabolism and serves as a carrier of carbon dioxide, thus promoting the synthesis of glucose and fatty acids.
   2. Properties—avidin, a protein that is present in raw egg whites, can bind to biotin and interfere with its absorption.
   3. Dietary requirements—30 to 100 µ/day
   4. Nutrient sources—include egg yolk, liver, and meats; also is synthesized by intestinal bacteria.
   5. Nutritional deficiency and disease
      a. Patients who are fed intravenously for long periods are at risk.
      b. Deficiency may lead to nausea, muscle pain, and loss of appetite and sleep.

F. Pyridoxine (B_6)
   1. Functions
      a. Is involved in carbohydrate, protein, and fat metabolism.
      b. Aids in the synthesis of hemoglobin and neurotransmitters.
      c. Regulates blood glucose.
   2. Properties—is stable to heat.
   3. Dietary requirements—1.8 to 2 mg/day.
   4. Nutrient sources
      a. Animal sources—meat, fish, and poultry
      b. Fruits and vegetables—bananas, cantaloupe, and broccoli
   5. Nutritional deficiency and disease—deficiency leads to a weakened immune system, weakness, irritability, insomnia, dermatitis, anemia, and glossitis.
   6. Toxicity—sensory nerve damage, numbness in extremities, and walking difficulties.

G. Folate (folacin, folic acid)
   1. Functions
      a. Assists in forming DNA and protein.
      b. Manufactures RBCs.
   2. Properties—is easily destroyed by processing and heating.
   3. Dietary requirements—180 to 200 µ/day
   4. Nutrient sources—include liver, dark green leafy vegetables, and fruits (oranges, orange juice, cantaloupe).
   5. Nutritional deficiency and disease
      a. Megaloblastic anemia
      b. Impaired cell division
      c. Gastrointestinal (GI) tract deterioration
      d. Glossitis

e. Diarrhea

f. Birth defects (spinal; spina bifida)

H. Cobalamin (B$_{12}$)

1. Functions

a. Assists folate metabolism.

b. Maintains myelin sheaths that insulate nerve endings.

c. Is essential for the proper functioning of *all* cells.

2. Properties

a. Intrinsic factor (protein)—is made in stomach; is needed for absorption of B$_{12}$; prevents pernicious anemia.

b. Extrinsic factor—must be obtained through foods; prevents pernicious anemia.

3. Dietary requirements—2 μ/day

4. Nutrient sources—found exclusively in foods of animal origin (meat, liver, eggs, cheese).

5. Nutritional deficiency and disease

a. Occur in strict vegetarians.

b. Deficiency may lead to pernicious anemia—symptoms include weakness, sore tongue, and apathy.

I. Vitamin C (ascorbic acid)

1. Functions

a. Promotes the synthesis of protein collagen, which is found in connective tissue, bone, teeth, and blood vessels; assists in wound healing.

b. Is an antioxidant—reduces the formation of cancer-causing nitrosamines in the stomach; keeps folate coenzymes intact.

c. Promotes iron absorption.

d. Protects the body from infections.

2. Properties—cannot be stored in the body for long periods.

3. Dietary requirement—60 mg/day

4. Nutrient sources—include citrus fruits, cantaloupe, strawberries, broccoli, and organ meats (liver and kidneys).

5. Nutritional deficiency and disease

a. Scurvy—is characterized by ruptured blood vessels, swollen and bleeding gingiva, delayed wound healing, and rough skin.

6. Toxicity

a. Symptoms include nausea, abdominal cramps, and diarrhea.

b. May lead to iron toxicity.

c. Obscures test results used to detect diabetes.

 Clinical Case **STUDY**

Emma, who is 60 years old, is in the dental office complaining that her denture does not fit well. She also notes that she fractured her arm 3 months ago when she slipped and fell while walking up the stairs in her home.

After an initial examination, a panoramic radiograph is taken and thinning of the mandible is noted. Emma is questioned regarding her diet. She states that she has never been a milk drinker. She also mentions she still smokes cigarettes.

Clinical Case QUESTIONS

1. What is the most likely diagnosis of Emma's condition?

2. Identify the most common causes of and predisposing factors for this condition.

3. What is the best treatment for this condition?

4. Is this condition preventable? And if so, how?

Clinical Case RATIONALES

1. Osteoporosis.

2. Genetics are a factor in the development of osteoporosis and in the attainment of bone mass. Early menopause is a predictor for the development of osteoporosis. Other contributing factors include deficiencies in calcium and vitamin D, lack of physical activity, cigarette smoking, and excessive intake of protein or caffeine.

3. Traditional treatment includes the use of estrogen, calcium and vitamin D supplements, and regular exercise. Exercise may increase bone mass.

4. Adequate calcium intake is necessary throughout an individual's life. Consuming caffeine in moderation is vital because an increase in caffeine increases the excretion of calcium; decaffeinated teas and coffee can be substituted.

Minerals

Minerals are inorganic nutrients that are used in the body for building and regulating functions. Minerals yield no energy to the body but assist in regulating the release of energy.

Macrominerals

The major minerals (macrominerals) are present in the body in amounts that are greater than 5 grams.

I. Calcium is the most abundant mineral in the body.

A. Functions

1. Forms and maintains bones and teeth.

2. Aids in blood coagulation.

3. Assists in muscle contraction/relaxation.

4. Maintains normal functioning of the nervous system.

5. Regulates cellular metabolism.

B. Properties

1. Vitamin D is required for its proper absorption.

2. Parathyroid hormone (PTH) maintains a normal level of serum calcium.

C. Dietary Requirement—800 mg/day

D. Nutrient sources

1. Dairy products—milk, yogurt, and cheese
2. Calcium-fortified orange and fruit drinks
3. Calcium supplements

E. Nutritional deficiency and disease—women are most likely to be at risk.
  1. Calcium tetany—is characterized by a failure of the muscles to relax after contraction.
  2. Deficiency may lead to stunted growth in children; rickets.
  3. Hypertension
  4. Osteoporosis—is a bone disease that develops primarily in women and is characterized by decreased bone density.
    a. Type I—postmenopausal (occurs directly after menopause)
    b. Type II—senile (occurs during advanced years)
    c. Prevention includes:
      1) Hormone replacement therapy with estrogen
      2) Use of active vitamin D hormone or hormone calcitonin
      3) Meeting RDA requirements
      4) Exercising regularly
      5) Avoiding alcohol and smoking
      6) Decreasing caffeine consumption

II. Phosphorus—is the second most abundant mineral in body.
  A. Functions
    1. Assists in the formation of bones and teeth.
    2. Is involved in the production and transfer of high-energy phosphates.
    3. Regulates acid-base balance.
    4. Releases energy from carbohydrates, protein, and fat metabolism.
    5. Plays an active role in cell protein synthesis.
  B. Properties—its absorption is affected by vitamin D and PTH.
  C. Dietary Requirements—800 mg/day
  D. Nutrient sources—include milk, cheese, bakery products, and meats.
  E. Nutritional deficiency and disease—are uncommon; risk is greater among elderly individuals, strict vegetarians, and alcoholics.

III. Magnesium
  A. Functions
    1. Acts in *all* cells of soft tissues.
    2. Relaxes muscles after contraction.
    3. Assists in the mineralization of bones and teeth.
    4. Aids transmission of nerve impulses.
    5. Facilitates the operation of enzymes.
    6. Assists in the production of energy.
  B. Properties—vitamin D enhances its absorption.
  C. Dietary requirements—350 mg/day for men; 280 mg/day for women.
  D. Nutrient sources—include nuts, legumes, whole grains, and dark green leafy vegetables.

E. Nutritional deficiency and disease—risk is greater among women; symptoms include vomiting, diarrhea, tetany, weakness, and convulsions.

IV. Potassium
  A. Functions
    1. Assists in the transmission of nerve impulses.
    2. Maintains fluid/electrolyte balance.
    3. Maintains cell integrity.
    4. Assists in carbohydrate and protein metabolism.
    5. Aids in muscle contraction (including heart muscle).
  B. Nutrient sources
    1. Is inside *all* living cells, both plant and animal.
    2. Fresh fruits and vegetables.
    3. Milk, meat, whole grains, dried beans, and legumes.
  C. Nutritional deficiency and disease
    1. Are caused by dehydration, diabetic acidosis, vomiting, diarrhea, diuretics, and steroids.
    2. Symptoms include muscle weakness, cramps, loss of appetite, constipation, mental confusion, and apathy.
  D. Toxicity may lead to muscle weakness and cardiac arrest.

V. Sodium
  A. Functions
    1. Retains body water.
    2. With chloride and potassium, aids in the maintenance of acid-base and fluid balance.
    3. Facilitates the transmission of nerve impulses and muscle contraction.
  B. Properties—contributes to high blood pressure, which can lead to heart disease and stroke. High blood pressure may be controlled by:
    1. Limiting the intake of processed foods.
    2. Restricting the intake of sodium to 3 g/day.
    3. Exercising.
  C. Dietary requirements—500 mg/day
  D. Nutrient sources include table salt and processed foods.
  E. Nutritional deficiency and disease occurs in individuals who restrict sodium intake; symptoms include muscle cramps, mental apathy, dizziness, decreased appetite, and nausea.

VI. Chloride
  A. Functions
    1. Aids in maintaining normal acid-base and fluid balance.
    2. Is a component of hydrochloric acid in the stomach and is necessary for digestion.
    3. Assists in the maintenance of nerve functions.
  B. Properties—is a negative ion of extracellular fluid.
  C. Dietary requirement—700 mg/day
  D. Nutrient sources include table salt and processed foods.

E. Nutritional deficiency and disease
   1. Are caused by starvation, fever, diarrhea, and vomiting.
   2. Symptoms include muscle cramps, mental apathy, and decreased appetite.

VII. Sulfur
   A. Functions
      1. Aids in maintaining normal acid-base balance.
      2. Stabilizes the shape of proteins by forming bridges between sulfur molecules (creates rigid proteins in hair, nails, skin).
      3. Is used to preserve foods.
   B. Properties—is a component of amino acids and vitamins biotin and thiamin.
   C. Dietary requirements—none
   D. Nutrient sources—include all protein-containing sources.
   E. Nutritional deficiency and disease—protein deficiency occurs before sulfur deficiency.

Water

Water, the main constituent of the body, comprises 50% to 60% of total body weight. Most of the water in the body is located in the cells. Water is required on a daily basis.

I. Intracellular/Extracellular Fluid
   A. Water flows in and out of cells through cell membranes.
      1. Intracellular fluid
         a. Refers to water inside cells.
         b. Is composed primarily of intracellular potassium and phosphate concentration.
      2. Extracellular fluid
         a. Refers to water outside of cells or in the bloodstream.
         b. Is composed primarily of extracellular sodium and chloride.
   B. The body controls the amount of water in cells by controlling ion concentration.
      1. Ions have electrical charges.
      2. Water follows ions such as sodium, chloride, and potassium.

II. Osmosis is the process that regulates water in cells and in the bloodstream.
   A. Water balance
      1. Refers to an osmotic equilibrium between body fluid compartments.
      2. Water intake equals output.
   B. Semipermeable membrane
      1. Separates extracellular fluid from intracellular fluid.
      2. Allows water to pass into cells when dissimilar ion concentrations exist; equalizes particle concentrations in compartments.

III. Functions
   A. Removes waste products, including urea (by-product of protein metabolism, which contains nitrogen).
   B. Maintains body temperature.
   C. Serves as a solvent for minerals, vitamins, glucose, and amino acids.
   D. Acts as a lubricant around joints.
   E. Participates in chemical reactions.
   F. Transports inorganic nutrients.
   G. Maintains normal kidney function and electrolyte balance.

IV. Dietary Requirements—approximately 1 mL/kcal of energy expended.

V. Nutrient Sources are primarily water and beverages.

VI. Nutritional Deficiency and Disease—survival without water is limited to 2 to 3 days.
   A. Dehydration is caused by:
      1. Blood loss.
      2. Malfunctioning kidneys.
      3. Vomiting/diarrhea.
      4. Lack of water intake.
   B. Toxicity is characterized by:
      1. Sodium retention.
      2. Hypertension.

Effects of Nutrients on Cells of Oral Tissues

Nutrients significantly affect the function and health of oral tissues by providing components for synthesis, repair, and immunity.

Epithelial Barrier

Several nutrients are needed for the formation, maintenance, and repair of the epithelial barrier.

I. Iron, Vitamin C, and Zinc are needed for collagen synthesis and wound healing.
   A. The basement membrane, which acts as a barrier against toxins, is composed of collagen.
   B. Sources include:
      1. Iron—beef, liver, and beans.
      2. Vitamin C—citrus fruits, broccoli, and peppers.
      3. Zinc—red meats and shellfish.

II. Folate and Protein are needed for cell formation.
   A. The sulcular epithelium has a rapid turnover of cells.
   B. Sources include:
      1. Folate—asparagus, broccoli, and liver.
      2. Protein—meat, fish, and poultry.

III. Vitamin A maintains the integrity of epithelium.
   A. Synthesizes the protein matrix for enamel and dentin.
   B. Sources include carrots and squash.

Repair Process

The speed and effectiveness of the repair process is greatly influenced by nutrients such as proteins, vitamins, and minerals.

I. Zinc speeds wound healing and the repair process; sources include oysters, shrimp, crab, bran cereal, lean pork, lamb, ham, and hamburger.

II. Calcium, Phosphorus, and Vitamin D promote bone density and calcify the protein matrix of cementoblasts, ameloblasts, and odontoblasts; sources include milk and hard cheeses.

III. Protein and Vitamin C are involved in connective tissue formation; sources for protein include animal sources and water-packed tuna; sources for vitamin C include citrus fruits and green vegetables.

Immune Mechanisms

Proteins are needed for the body's immune system and aid in controlling infection.

Weight Control

Weight control is achieved when the calories gained from food equal the energy needs of body.

Measurement of Energy

One kilocalorie is the amount of heat produced to raise the temperature of 1 kg of water 1°C.

I. Energy Needs of the Body
   A. The basal metabolism rate (BMR) is a measure of the energy that is needed to maintain life at rest.
      1. Includes the energy needed for breathing, beating of the heart, circulation, muscle tone, and body temperature.
      2. Is influenced by factors such as age, gender, body size, infection, injury, surgery, and thyroid hormone level.
   B. The degree of physical activity is the voluntary component of energy.
      1. Varies from sedentary to strenuous activity.
      2. Is influenced by factors such as the intensity and length of activity and the size of the individual.
   C. Specific dynamic activity (SDA) is the energy required to digest and absorb food.
      1. Contributes approximately 10% of total kilocalories consumed.

Obesity

Obesity is characterized by excess body fat; the weight of an obese individual exceeds the standard weight for height by 20% or more.

I. Causes include:
   A. A positive energy balance (kilocalorie intake exceeds expenditure).
   B. Genetics: A child with one obese parent has a 40% risk of becoming obese, whereas a child with two obese parents has an 80% risk.
   C. The development of excess fat cells during childhood.
      1. During childhood an increased number of fat cells develops in response to excess kilocalorie intake (hyperplasty).
      2. After puberty, fat cells enlarge (hypertrophy).
   D. The set-point theory: the body chooses a weight and defends its set-point by internal factors.
   E. Psychological factors (e.g., finding comfort in eating).
   F. Physical activity (i.e., lack of energy expenditure).

II. Prevention and Weight Control
   A. Diet involves:
      1. Controlling energy intake.
      2. Eating low-fat, carbohydrate foods such as fresh fruits, vegetables, and whole grains.
      3. Drinking adequate water to satisfy thirst and fill the stomach.
      4. Meeting RDA nutritional needs.
   B. Behavior modification (changing eating behavior) involves:
      1. Becoming aware of current behaviors.
      2. Stimulus control; changing the environment to minimize the stimuli for eating (e.g., shopping after eating to avoid poor choices).
      3. Cognitive restructuring; altering one's state of mind regarding eating (e.g., avoiding excuses for overeating such as having a difficult day).
      4. Self-monitoring; (i.e., keeping a diary of foods and eating patterns).
      5. Contingency management; developing a plan for responding in an environment where overeating is most likely to occur (e.g., at a party where snacks are served).
   C. Physical activity
      1. Increases energy output.
      2. Controls appetite.
      3. Aids in stress reduction.
      4. Increases basal metabolism.
      5. Increases self-esteem.

Eating Disorders

Anorexia nervosa, bulimia, and compulsive overeating are common eating disorders in today's society.

I. Anorexia Nervosa
   A. Is self-starvation; individual has a distorted body image (i.e., belief that one is overweight).
   B. Behavior profile includes:
      1. Female gender, typically; middle to upper socioeconomic class.
      2. Competitiveness and obsessive behavior.
      3. Conflict within the family; an overbearing parent.
      4. Control over eating by the affected individual.
   C. Characteristics include:
      1. Dramatic weight loss; weight that is 20% to 40% below desirable body weight.
      2. Excessive exercising.
      3. Aversion to food and altered eating habits.
      4. Amenorrhea—the absence of a menstrual cycle in response to hormonal changes.
      5. Low self-esteem.
      6. Lanugo—downy hair that appears on the body to help insulate against heat loss.
      7. Iron-deficiency anemia because of a lack of nutrient intake.

8. Decreased heart rate caused by slowing of the metabolism.
9. Electrolyte imbalance.
10. Constipation and/or diarrhea.

D. Treatment is:
   1. Dietary
      a. Food intake is increased to raise metabolic rate to normal.
      b. Regular eating habits and proper food intake are restored.
   2. Psychological; a therapist works with the patient to determine underlying issues associated with the eating disorder.

II. Bulimia
   A. Involves episodes of binge eating followed by purging (vomiting or laxative/diuretic abuse) to prevent weight gain.
   B. Behavior profile includes:
      1. Female gender, typically.
      2. Weight at or slightly above normal.
      3. Turning to food for comfort.
      4. Awareness that behavior is abnormal.
      5. Low self-esteem and impulsiveness.
   C. Characteristics include:
      1. A general lack of physical signs because of normal body weight; calluses on knuckles may be present from digital purging (vomiting).
      2. Clinical depression (often).
   D. Oral manifestations include:
      1. Dental erosion (perimolysis)—especially on the lingual surfaces of the maxillary teeth from constant exposure to acid.
      2. Erosion from restorations; restorations appears 'raised' from adjacent teeth.
      3. Thermal sensitivity.
      4. Enlarged parotid glands.
      5. Cheilosis.
      6. Enlarged interdental papillae as a result of constant irritation from acidic vomitus.
   E. Treatment is:
      1. Dietary; to establish regular eating patterns.
         a. Sodium fluoride rinses aid remineralization.
         b. Sodium bicarbonate rinses help neutralize acids from vomiting.
      2. Psychological
         a. Involves a team approach.
         b. Is easier to treat than anorexia because a bulimic person is aware of engaging in abnormal behavior.

III. Compulsive Overeating
   A. Is uncontrolled chronic episodes of overeating without other signs of an eating disorder.
   B. Behavior profile includes:
      1. Overeating in response to stress or feelings of anxiety or depression.
      2. Bingeing on foods that are easy to eat in large portions (e.g., noodles, rice).

3. Eating foods categorized as 'junk' foods, such as ice cream and chips (typically).
   C. Characteristics include:
      1. Eating large quantities in isolation to induce a sense of well-being.
      2. Grazing, in some individuals.
      3. Lack of preoccupation with weight, typically.
      4. A difficulty expressing and dealing with feelings.
   D. Treatment is:
      1. Dietary
         a. Eating until full (a must).
         b. Avoiding diets that may encourage more binge eating.
      2. Psychological
         a. Focusing on responding to hunger rather than emotions.
         b. Identifying personal needs and expressing them.

Nutritional Counseling

Counseling for weight control and proper health and nutrition involves diet counseling, diet management, and nutritional counseling.

I. Diet Counseling
   A. Patient selection
      1. Patient must be willing to improve and/or change eating habits.
      2. Patient has a need for dietary improvement.
   B. Communication techniques are necessary to create motivation in patient.
      1. Maintain good eye contact.
      2. Use effective verbal and nonverbal methods of communication—tone of voice, gestures, and facial expressions can communicate sincerity and concern to patient.
      3. Adapt education to patient's needs and understanding.
   C. Patient interview
      1. Purpose:
         a. Understand the problem.
         b. Determine factors that contribute to the problem.
         c. Understand the personality and motivation of the patient.
   D. Counseling approaches
      1. Directive—decisions are made by counselor; patient is passive.
      2. Nondirective—counselor assists in understanding needs and recommends changes; patient is involved in planning, implementing, and evaluating diet.

II. Principles of Diet Management
   A. Food diary
      1. Patient keeps a 5-day food diary (including a weekend).
      2. Patient records all meals and between-meal snacking.

B. Interview
  1. Assess patient's primary problem/complaint.
  2. Ascertain patient's routine and habits.
  3. Review medical history for any changes or problems—may reveal systemic conditions that can influence medical health, including the ability to digest and/or metabolize food.
  4. Evaluate diet.
    a. Review adequacy of food intake.
    b. Determine amount of foods that contain sugar and frequency of intake.
  5. Assess clinical signs of deficiencies/diseases.
    a. Cheilosis, glossitis
    b. Dry skin
    c. Dental caries
  6. Diagnosis—try to determine possible causes for clinical signs.
C. Follow-up
  1. Review a second 5-day diet plan.
  2. Compare second plan with first.
  3. Stress good changes patient has made.
III. Nutritional Management
  A. Dental caries
    1. Cariogenic factors associated with diet
      a. Frequency of between-meal snacking—the more frequent the exposure to sugar, the more cariogenic the diet (best to eat sugar-rich foods at mealtime).
      b. Physical form of food—solid and retentive forms have a slower oral clearance time and therefore are more cariogenic than liquid forms.
      c. Amount of sugar added to foods and beverages (e.g., to cereals, coffee)
    2. Dietary prescription
      a. Eat nutritionally balanced diet.
      b. Eliminate sugary snacks.
      c. Restrict sugar to mealtimes.
      d. Eat hard cheeses to help neutralize pH.
      e. Use fluoride rinses to promote remineralization process.
    3. Dietary modifications
      a. Use USDA Food Guide Pyramid to determine recommended servings.
      b. Establish needs to meet body's requirements for essential nutrients.
  B. Acute necrotizing ulcerative gingivitis (ANUG) is an acute bacterial infection of the gingiva associated with poor oral hygiene.
    1. Diet consists of empty-calories and sugar-rich foods because of patient's decreased ability to chew.
    2. Dietary prescription
      a. Recommend food sources that contain protein, calcium, folate, iron, zinc, and vitamins A and C.
      b. Patient should eat 6 to 8 small meals per day (1 or 2 foods at each meal).

  3. Dietary modification
    a. Use USDA Food Guide Pyramid for serving recommendations.
    b. Choose good food sources high in nutrients.
    c. Initially, menus should consist of liquids or soft foods.
    d. Avoid spicy foods.
C. Chronic periodontal disease
  1. Dietary prescription
    a. Considerations
      1) Evaluate information obtained for any factors that may interfere with nutritional status.
      2) Determine patient's eating patterns and food habits.
      3) Patient should assist in determining revised diet.
    b. Procedure
      1) Patient determines deficiencies and makes appropriate choices to improve diet.
      2) Direct patient to choices that can benefit the periodontium.
      3) Stress the importance of decreasing sugar-rich foods in diet.
      4) Instruct patient to add variety to meal planning and to focus on nutritionally sound foods that the patient likes.
  2. Dietary modifications
    a. Goals
      1) Assist patient in meeting stress of surgery.
      2) Aid wound healing and recovery time.
      3) Increase resistance to infections.
    b. Preoperative diet
      1) Recommend an increased intake of vitamin C one week before surgery, which conditions tissues to heal; sources include orange juice, green pepper, and broccoli.
      2) Recommend adequate amounts of carbohydrates to spare protein.
    c. Postoperative diet
      1) First postoperative day—include fluids such as water, juices, and broths; recommend more frequent feedings.
      2) Second postoperative day—include blended fruits and vegetables, oatmeal, ice cream, milk, milk shakes, eggs, and/or meat broths.

 CONTENT REVIEW QUESTIONS

1. A complete protein is:
  A. adequate in *all* the essential amino acids
  B. synthesized by the body
  C. provided through plant foods
  D. a dispensable amino acid

2. All of the following conditions are examples of negative nitrogen balance, EXCEPT:
   A. infection
   B. anorexia nervosa
   C. blood loss
   D. pregnancy
3. Phenylketonuria is a condition that:
   A. involves protein-energy malnutrition
   B. restricts the consumption of aspartame
   C. ineffectively metabolizes phenylalanine to threonine
   D. involves a disorder in carbohydrate metabolism
4. Kwashiorkor is a disease that:
   A. occurs most commonly in children in underdeveloped countries
   B. occurs most commonly in children in underdeveloped countries and presents without severe wasting of body fat
   C. occurs most commonly in children 6 to 12 months of age in underdeveloped countries
   D. is common in children 6 to 12 months of age and is not characterized by edema
5. The main function of carbohydrates is to:
   A. repair body tissues
   B. neutralize acid—base
   C. provide energy
   D. regulate metabolism
6. The primary form of carbohydrate storage in humans is:
   A. glucose
   B. sucrose
   C. glycogen
   D. starch
7. Starch digestion initiates in the:
   A. mouth
   B. stomach
   C. small intestine
   D. large intestine
8. One gram of carbohydrate yields:
   A. 9 kcal
   B. 7 kcal
   C. 5 kcal
   D. 4 kcal
9. Sorbitol, which is a sugar alcohol used in diabetic foods and sugarless gum, is made from:
   A. fructose
   B. glucose
   C. galactose
   D. mannitol
10. The majority of cases of diabetes are in this category:
    A. juvenile-onset
    B. adult-onset
    C. infantile
    D. all types are equally common
11. All of the following are symptoms of diabetes mellitus, EXCEPT:
    A. acetone breath
    B. hyperglycemia
    C. ketonuria
    D. decreased appetite
12. All of the following are chronic complications that may result from diabetes, EXCEPT:
    A. poor circulation
    B. blindness
    C. atherosclerosis
    D. increased infections
    E. obesity
13. Oral manifestations associated with diabetes include a higher incidence of which of the following?
    A. periodontal disease
    B. cheilosis
    C. glossitis
    D. lichen planus
14. Which of the following foods would be MOST cariogenic?
    A. dried apricots
    B. soda pop
    C. cake
    D. milk
15. Lipids are transported in the blood by means of:
    A. bile
    B. phospholipids
    C. lipoproteins
    D. water
16. A high level of this lipoprotein actually slows down the development of cardiovascular disease:
    A. chylomicron
    B. very low-density lipoprotein
    C. low-density lipoprotein
    D. high-density lipoprotein
17. All of the following are characteristics of cholesterol, EXCEPT which of the following?
    A. is a phospholipid
    B. can be made by the body
    C. acts as an emulsifier
    D. increases the risk of heart disease
18. Important functions of dietary lipids include:
    A. providing essential fatty acids and aiding in absorption of B vitamins
    B. aiding in absorption of B vitamins and providing satiety
    C. providing essential fatty acids, aiding in absorption of B vitamins, and providing satiety
    D. providing essential fatty acids, providing satiety, and aiding in absorption of vitamins A, D, E, and K
    E. providing essential fatty acids, preventing night blindness, and aiding in absorption of B vitamins
19. Overconsumption of these foods can increase the risk of atherosclerosis, EXCEPT for which of the following?
    A. butter
    B. coconut oil
    C. beef
    D. skim milk

20. Risk factors associated with atherosclerosis include all of the following, EXCEPT:
    A. hypertension
    B. LDL cholesterol of 120 mg/100 mL
    C. total blood cholesterol greater than 240 mg/100 mL
    D. smoking

21. Fat-soluble vitamins include all of the following, EXCEPT:
    A. A
    B. E
    C. C
    D. K
    E. D

22. Preformed vitamin A is found in which of the following food sources?
    A. carrots
    B. body fat of fish
    C. broccoli
    D. cauliflower

23. Rickets is a disease associated with which vitamin deficiency?
    A. A
    B. D
    C. E
    D. C

24. The function of vitamin E is to:
    A. aid in the prevention of night blindness
    B. promote the mineralization of teeth
    C. act as an antioxidant
    D. synthesize prothrombin

25. A function of water-soluble vitamins is to:
    A. aid in the metabolism of energy-producing nutrients
    B. assist with immune defenses
    C. regulate serum levels of calcium and phosphorus
    D. absorb calcium and phosphorus

26. The amino acid tryptophan can be converted into this water-soluble vitamin:
    A. riboflavin
    B. pantothenic acid
    C. thiamin
    D. niacin

27. Interference with the intrinsic-extrinsic factor leads to a deficiency in this vitamin:
    A. cobalamin
    B. folate
    C. biotin
    D. pantothenic acid

28. A 'pure' vegetarian diet most likely will be deficient in this vitamin:
    A. cobalamin
    B. folate
    C. biotin
    D. thiamin

29. A disease caused by vitamin C deficiency is:
    A. beri beri
    B. pernicious anemia
    C. scurvy
    D. pellagra

30. Which of the following characteristics is NOT true concerning calcium?
    A. aids coagulation
    B. assists in muscle contraction and relaxation
    C. 400 mg/day is recommended
    D. vitamin D assists in its absorption

31. The most abundant mineral in the body is:
    A. calcium
    B. phosphorus
    C. copper
    D. fluorine
    E. magnesium

32. The best food sources of magnesium include:
    A. citrus fruits
    B. dairy products
    C. dark yellow vegetables
    D. whole grains and nuts

33. The functions of sodium include all of the following, EXCEPT:
    A. nerve impulse conduction
    B. maintenance of acid-base balance
    C. retention of body water
    D. use as an immune response

34. This mineral is used to preserve foods:
    A. sodium
    B. chloride
    C. sulfur
    D. phosphorus

35. Body water possesses all of the following characteristics, EXCEPT which of the following?
    A. is found extracellularly as well as intracellularly
    B. makes up 85% of total body weight
    C. assists in maintaining body temperature
    D. acts as a lubricant around joints

36. Several nutrients have an effect on the cells of the oral tissues. Which of the following nutrients assist in speeding up wound healing?
    A. zinc
    B. folate
    C. calcium
    D. phosphorus

37. With regard to energy measurement, 1 kcal is the amount of heat produced to raise the temperature of:
    A. 1 g of water 1°C
    B. 1 kg of water 1°F
    C. 1 kg of water 1°C
    D. 1 g of water 1°F

38. Which of the following activities is NOT included in the measurement of the BMR?
    A. breathing
    B. maintaining body temperature
    C. beating of the heart
    D. digesting food

39. Which of the following is the major gland that affects the BMR?
    A. thyroid

B. endocrine

C. hypothalamus

D. sebaceous

40. In order for an individual to lose weight, a reduction in energy intake must take place. The individual also should decrease physical activity.

    A. both statements are true

    B. both statements are false

    C. the first statement is true; the second is false

    D. the first statement is false; the second is true

41. The individual with anorexia nervosa is:

    A. typically female

    B. typically female and exercises excessively

    C. typically female and aware that her behavior is abnormal

    D. typically female and often is difficult to diagnose because of a lack of physical signs

42. Bulimia is an eating disorder that involves:

    A. weight loss 40% to 60% below desirable body weight

    B. mostly males

    C. episodes of binge eating followed by purging

    D. a decreased heart rate in response to a decreased metabolism

43. Compulsive overeating is associated with:

    A. eating large quantities of food and purging

    B. eating large quantities of food in response to stress or an emotional outlet

    C. an aversion to food

    D. a fear of becoming overweight

44. The best counseling technique for increasing patient involvement and responsibility in making his/her own decisions:

    A. is directive

    B. is nondirective

    C. involves motivation

    D. involves listening

45. Which of the following is the BEST example of a nondirective approach?

    A. the counselor makes all recommendations for a diet modification program and the patient accepts

    B. the patient is involved in the diet analysis and evaluation and the counselor makes recommendations for diet modification

    C. the patient is involved in the diet analysis, evaluation, and diet modification program and the counselor explains each process to the patient

    D. the counselor provides information regarding the diet analysis, evaluation, and diet modification and the patient accepts all recommendations

46. The recommended number of days for recording a diet diary is:

    A. 2 to 3 days

    B. 4 to 7 days

    C. 7 to 10 days

    D. 14 days

47. The basic postsurgery diet for patients recovering from periodontal surgery is a:

A. diet that is nutritionally adequate and modified for the patient's chewing ability

B. clear liquid diet with supplements of vitamins A and E

C. diet high in fiber with 6 to 8 glasses of water

D. diet that consists of foods recommended in the Food Guide Pyramid and high in vitamin C and cobalamin

CONTENT REVIEW RATIONALES

1. **A** Animal proteins are considered complete (high-quality) proteins. The composition of human tissue more closely resembles that of animal tissue than that of plant tissue. These tissue similarities enable the human body to use animal proteins more effectively for its primary functions—body maintenance, repair, and growth. Animal proteins contain *all* the essential amino acids in amounts that are sufficient for the body.

2. **D** Nitrogen balance refers to a balance between the input and output of nitrogen. If the body is not growing or in need of extra protein to recover from an illness or infection, only enough protein is needed to equal the input to output. Negative protein balance exists when the output is greater than the input (as occurs with semistarvation, infection, fever, and blood loss). However, if the body is growing, as during childhood or pregnancy, or recovering from an illness, more protein will be necessary to supply the body with the needs for tissue repair. This increased need for protein intake is defined as a positive protein balance.

3. **B** Phenylketonuria (PKU) is a disease in which the liver is not able to metabolize the essential amino acid phenylalanine into the nonessential amino acid tyrosine. By-products of phenylalanine build up in the body, damaging the nervous system and therefore causing mental retardation. It is recommended that individuals with PKU not consume aspartame because it contains high levels of phenylalanine.

4. **B** Kwashiorkor is a disease caused by protein-energy malnutrition and characterized by a severe protein deficiency. Affected children who are approximately two years old and raised in underdeveloped countries show evidence of edema in the abdomen and legs but no severe wasting of body fat. Other signs of the disease include listlessness, failure to grow and gain weight, and changes in hair color.

5. **C** The main function of carbohydrates is to provide energy. Although proteins can provide energy, the use of carbohydrate energy spares proteins for their primary function—to repair body tissues. Carbohydrates also aid in the oxidation of lipids to prevent ketosis. The polysaccharides, fibers, provide for normal peristalsis. One of the main functions of the water-soluble B vitamins is to regulate the metabo-

lism of carbohydrates. Minerals such as phosphorus help regulate the body's acid-base balance.

6. **C** Glycogen provides a food storage system for all forms of animal life. One area of storage is in the liver, which assists in regulating blood sugar. Glycogen storage also occurs in the muscle, where glycogen serves as an energy source for muscle contraction.

7. **A** The initiation of starch digestion begins in the mouth during chewing. The enzyme salivary amylase begins to break starch into disaccharides such as maltose. Stomach acids hydrolyze maltose and sucrose, but only to a small extent. Digestion continues in the small intestine; there, the enzyme pancreatic amylase (from the pancreas) breaks down the remaining disaccharides into monosaccharides.

8. **D** The energy yield for carbohydrates is 4 kcal/g (the same as for proteins). However, fats, which can be broken down and used as an energy source, yield 9 kcal/g.

9. **B** Sorbitol is a sugar alcohol made from glucose through hydrogenation. Sugar alcohols are carbohydrates, yield approximately the same energy as sucrose (4 kcal/g), and are also referred to as nutritive sweeteners. An advantage that sugar alcohols have over sucrose is that they do not promote caries because they are not easily metabolized by bacteria in the mouth. Fructose is a monosaccharide and the sweetest of all sugars. It is found in honey, fruits, and corn syrup. Mannitol is another sugar alcohol made from mannose and galactose.

10. **B** The majority of cases of diabetes (90% to 95%) are adult-onset or noninsulin-dependent types. The onset typically occurs in individuals older than 40 years of age and is associated with obesity. Although the individual is able to produce some insulin, the body is unable to use it properly.

11. **D** Diabetes mellitus has several symptoms. An individual with diabetes may experience acetone breath—a fruity odor that is caused by ketosis. Ketonuria (ketones in the urine) is a result of an incomplete breakdown of fat when carbohydrates are not available. Diabetics experience an abnormally high blood glucose level in response to ineffective or insufficient insulin. However, individuals with either type 1 or type 2 diabetes mellitus show an increase in appetite.

12. **E** Several complications are associated with diabetes mellitus. Circulation becomes poor and structures of the blood vessels and nerves weaken. Infections increase because of poor circulation. Blindness and kidney failure may result from disorders of the capillaries. Atherosclerosis and cardiovascular disease also are prevalent among diabetics. Obesity is not a result of diabetes but instead is related to its development and is associated with complications of the disease.

13. **A** Oral manifestations associated with diabetes mellitus include periodontal involvement and xerostomia. Cheilosis and glossitis are generally seen with vitamin B deficiencies. Lichen planus is a chronic, benign skin lesion of unknown etiology and is not associated with diabetes mellitus.

14. **A** The consistency of food plays a major role in caries development. Food with a sticky consistency will remain on the teeth longer and have a slower clearance time. Dried apricots, like raisins, are a dried fruit and remain on the teeth longer than other foods. Retention is a contributing factor to the initiation and progression of dental decay. Although soda pop, cake, and milk contain moderate to large amounts of sugar, they are cleared from the oral cavity more quickly.

15. **C** Lipoproteins are a means of transportation through the bloodstream for cholesterol, triglycerides, and phospholipids. The lipoproteins include chylomicrons, very low-density lipoproteins, low-density lipoproteins, and high-density lipoproteins.

16. **D** High-density lipoproteins (HDLs) are capable of transporting cholesterol back to the liver, where it can be disposed. They contain a higher level of protein, making them smaller and denser than very low-density and low-density lipoproteins. HDLs often are referred to as 'good' cholesterol because elevated levels of HDLs are associated with a low risk of heart and vessel disease.

17. **A** Cholesterol is a sterol—one of the three main types of lipids. It can be synthesized by the body (in the liver) and makes bile to aid in the digestion (emulsification) of fats. Because dietary cholesterol elevates blood cholesterol, it may increase the risk of coronary disease.

18. **D** Dietary lipids have essential functions in the body. They provide a concentrated source of energy—9 kcal/g. In addition, they assist with the absorption of fat-soluble vitamins and provide insulation, essential fatty acids, flavor and texture to foods, and a sense of satiety. A deficiency in fat-soluble vitamin A may cause night blindness.

19. **D** Skim milk is considered a nonfat food source. Butter, coconut oil, and beef contain high levels of saturated fat. A high intake of saturated fats (more than 30% of daily intake) is associated with the development of atherosclerosis, a disease characterized by plaque build-up on arterial walls. To reduce the amount of fat from one's diet, it is essential to reduce the amount of saturated fats. This can be accomplished by eating foods such as fish, skinless poultry, and low-fat or nonfat dairy products.

20. **B** Atherosclerosis obstructs blood flow along the arterial walls. High blood pressure is evidence that the heart is applying more pressure to circulate the blood because of narrowing of the walls of arteries from plaque buildup. Smoking also is a risk factor for cardiovascular disease, as is a low-density lipoprotein cholesterol (LDL) reading at or above 160 mg/100 mL and a total blood cholesterol greater than 240

mg/100 mL. Men who are older than 45 and women who are older than 55 also are at greater risk for this disease.

21. **C** Fat-soluble vitamins include A, D, E, and K. These vitamins are soluble in fat and are not readily excreted. All B vitamins and vitamin C are water-soluble.

22. **B** Preformed vitamin A (retinoid) is found in animal sources. Provitamin A (carotenoid) is found in plant foods, especially deep green and yellow fruits and vegetables.

23. **B** Rickets is a bone disease that affects children as a result of a vitamin D deficiency. The bones soften because they fail to calcify normally. Signs of rickets characteristically include bowed legs.

24. **C** Vitamin E is a fat-soluble antioxidant; it protects other substances from oxidation. It also serves to protect red blood cell membranes.

25. **A** Water-soluble vitamins must be consumed regularly because they are easily excreted or lost in cooking and therefore readily dissolved. Although vitamins do not provide energy, they play an active role in the metabolism of energy. Carbohydrates, lipids, and proteins require vitamin input for their energy metabolism.

26. **D** Niacin is found in protein foods such as fish, beef, turkey, and chicken. However, 1 mg of niacin can be converted from 60 mg of the amino acid tryptophan.

27. **A** The intrinsic factor is made in the stomach and is needed for the absorption of cobalamin. If the intrinsic factor becomes inadequate or halts due to the surgical removal of the stomach, absorption will be affected. This results in a deficiency is known as pernicious anemia. A deficiency in the extrinsic factor, which must be obtained from food, also causes pernicious anemia but can be prevented by altering the diet to include animal foods.

28. **A** A 'pure' vegetarian will be deficient in cobalamin because the major source is almost exclusively animal-derived foods.

29. **C** Scurvy is a disease caused by vitamin C deficiency. A deficiency in vitamin C is not uncommon because this water-soluble vitamin is not stored for long periods. The first sign of a deficiency is bleeding gingiva. Subsequently the muscles begin to degenerate and the skin takes on a dry and scaly appearance. It takes approximately 10 mg of vitamin C per day to prevent overt scurvy; however, the RDA for adults is 60 mg per day.

30. **C** Although the major function of calcium is to form and maintain bones, it also has other important functions. Calcium aids in the contraction of muscles and in the blood coagulation process. It also may reduce the risk of colon cancer. Most of its absorption is in the upper intestine, with the assistance of active vitamin D hormone. The recommended daily allowance for both calcium and phosphorus is 800 mg/day.

31. **A** Calcium is the most abundant mineral found in the body (followed by phosphorus). Ninety-nine percent of the body's calcium is stored in the bones and teeth. It plays a vital role in keeping bones healthy and in preventing bone disease, such as osteoporosis, in later life.

32. **D** Magnesium facilitates the operation of enzymes and assists with the relaxation of muscles after contraction. Foods rich in magnesium include dark green leafy vegetables, whole grain breads and cereals, nuts, legumes, and seafood.

33. **D** Sodium, a major mineral, is active in maintaining the acid-base balance in the body. Along with calcium, potassium, and magnesium, it plays a vital role in nerve conduction. Sodium also helps retain water by triggering a thirst reaction when it is consumed. A thirsty individual will drink more water to help balance the sodium-water ratio.

34. **C** Sulfur is present in all proteins and in the vitamins biotin and thiamin. It aids in maintaining a normal acid-base balance in the body. In addition, sulfur compounds are used to preserve foods.

35. **B** Water is the main constituent of the body and comprises 50% to 60% of total body weight. Water is required on a daily basis and flows in and out of cells through cell membranes. Its roles include removal of waste products, maintenance of body temperature, transport of inorganic nutrients, lubrication around joints, and maintenance of normal kidney function.

36. **A** Adequate zinc intake is essential for the proper development of sexual organs and bone. Zinc also is needed for DNA and protein metabolism and it assists with wound healing.

37. **C** Energy is measured by heat expenditure. One kilocalorie is the amount of heat produced to raise the temperature of 1 kilogram of water 1°C.

38. **D** Basal metabolism requires approximately 60% to 70% of the total energy used by the body. It is the minimal amount of energy necessary to maintain life at rest. The BMR involves circulation, beating of the heart, breathing, and maintaining body temperature. It does not include specific dynamic activity, which is the energy required for the digestion of food.

39. **A** The major gland that affects the basal metabolism rate is the thyroid gland. Higher thyroid hormone levels increase the metabolic rate.

40. **C** A reduction in weight can be accomplished by a reduction in energy input together with an increase in physical activity (energy output). An increase in physical activity controls the appetite, aids in stress reduction, increases the basal metabolism rate, and raises one's self-esteem.

41. **B** Anorexia nervosa is an eating disorder that is characterized by self-starvation. The individual, typically female, has a distorted body image (believes that she is overweight). She has a tendency to exercise excessively and her weight typically is 20% to 40% below desirable body weight. The individual,

who has a low self-esteem, is competitive in nature and is not aware of her problem.

42. **C** Bulimia is an eating disorder that involves episodes of binge eating followed by purging—by means of vomiting and/or the use of diuretics. The individual typically is female, maintains a normal body weight, and is aware that her behavior is abnormal.

43. **B** Compulsive overeating is characterized by uncontrolled episodes of overeating without other signs of an eating disorder. Typically the individual eats foods that are easy to eat in large portions, such as noodles or rice and foods that are categorized as 'junk' foods. Most who compulsively overeat do so in response to stress or feelings of depression.

44. **B** The most effective counseling approach when decisions need to be made is nondirective. The counselor assists the patient in understanding the needs and changes that are recommended and subsequently the patient is an active participant in planning, implementing, and evaluating the changes.

45. **C** A directive approach in diet counseling involves a passive participant and decisions are made by the counselor. In a nondirective counseling approach, the counselor assists with the process but the patient is an active participant in the analysis, evaluation, and modifications of the diet.

46. **B** A diet diary should be recorded for 5 days and should include a weekend. This gives the reviewer sufficient data to review the adequacy of food intake and determine both the foods that contain sugar and the frequency of their consumption.

47. **A** A diet after surgery for a patient recovering from periodontal surgery should include more frequent feedings and mostly fluids on the first day. On the first day after surgery, the patient typically consumes plenty of water, juices, and broths. The diet on the second day can include blended fruits and vegetables, oatmeal, and dairy products such as milk shakes and ice cream. For protein, the patient may have meat broths or eggs. The patient's comfort in chewing will determine what the patient is able to consume.

Additional Readings

Cataldo CB, DeBruyne LK, Whitney EN: Nutrition and Diet Therapy, 4th ed. St Paul, West, 1995.

Nizel AE, Papas AS: Nutrition in Clinical Dentistry, 3rd ed. Philadelphia, WB Saunders, 1989.

Peckenpaugh NJ, Poleman CM: Nutrition: Essentials and Diet Therapy, 7th ed. Philadelphia, WB Saunders, 1995.

Wardlaw GM, Insel PM, Seyler MF: Contemporary Nutrition: Issues and Insights, 2nd ed. St Louis, Mosby, 1994.

Chapter SEVEN

Radiology

Jacqueline N. Brian, R.D.H., M.S.Ed

Clinical Case STUDY

Molly Hagan, a 42-year-old certified public accountant, states that she has had a bad cold for the past couple of weeks. On her medical history, she also states that she had a mammogram last week. The reason for today's visit is the sensitivity of her maxillary posterior teeth. Her clinical exam reveals suspicious areas and several fractured restorations on the maxillary arch. She states that her fillings feel as if they are moving when she bites down. It has been at least 6 or 7 years since she has had radiographs taken. The dental hygienist recommends a full mouth series of radiographs. Ms. Hagan is reluctant to have radiographs taken because of what she has read in recent articles in the newspaper and heard on television about the dangers and misuse of radiation.

Clinical Case QUESTIONS

1. What is the most probable diagnosis of Ms. Hagan's condition? Identify all possible causes for her symptoms. What other information should be gathered to determine the cause of Ms. Hagan's sensitivity?
2. What issue must be addressed to provide this patient with the best treatment?
3. What procedures are used to protect the patient from unnecessary radiation?

Clinical Case RATIONALES

1. Carious lesions. The sensitivity of the maxillary teeth could be related to the closeness of the maxillary teeth roots to enlarged, inflamed sinuses; such sensitivity should dissipate as the sinusitis clears up. The movement of the restorations is more serious in nature and is indicative of fractured restorations. Ill-fitting restorations often exhibit marginal leakage and/or recurrent decay. Other information can be gained by asking: "What are the teeth sensitive to (e.g., temperature,

pressure, sweets)?", "How long have they been sensitive?", and "Does anything seem to exacerbate or alleviate the discomfort?"
2. The benefit versus the risk of having radiographs taken should be discussed with the patient. The medical and clinical exams warrant radiographs to confirm the exact diagnosis and direction of proper treatment. Although a minimal amount of radiation exposure occurs, the benefit of the diagnosis far outweighs the risk.
3. Devices on the x-ray machine such as the filter, collimator, and lead-lined position-indicating device reduce radiation exposure to the patient. In addition, using a lead apron with a thyroid collar and film-holding devices with fast-speed film keep patient exposure to a minimum while providing good quality diagnostic radiographs.

Content Review

Historical Contributions

The contributions of early discoverers have profoundly impacted the status that radiology enjoys today. In order to appreciate the value of radiology, it is necessary to be aware of events that led to our current technology.

Innovators

Several individuals are responsible for discovering radiation and developing the uses that we are familiar with today.

I. Wilhelm Roentgen
   A. Discovered x-rays on November 8, 1895.
   B. Used a cathode tube and an electrical current, which caused permanent images to appear on photographic plates.
   C. Was honored when the unknown rays were named "Roentgen rays."

II. Otto Walkoff
   A. Was a German dentist who, in January, 1896, made the first dental x-rays using a photographic plate, his own mouth, and 25 minutes of exposure time.
III. William Rollins
   A. Was a Boston dentist and physician who first alerted the profession to the importance of radiation hygiene and protection.
   B. Is known as the Father of the Science of Radiation Protection.

Equipment

Dental x-ray equipment historically has consisted of a cathode tube and the pre-set controls on the x-ray machine.
I. Hot Cathode Tube
   A. Was invented by William Coolidge in 1913.
   B. Provided an electron source, rather than gas, for ionization in the x-ray tube.
II. X-Ray Machine
   A. Was first created in 1923 by the Victor X-Ray Corporation.
   B. In 1957 was greatly improved by General Electric, which created the first dental x-ray machine with variable kilovoltage.

Techniques

Several individuals are responsible for developing the radiographic techniques that are used today.
I. Howard Raper
   A. Was an Indiana University professor who introduced the bitewing technique in 1925.
   B. Wrote the first dental radiography textbook.
   C. Established the first full-time radiography course in a dental college in 1910.
II. Edmund Kells
   A. First introduced the paralleling technique in 1896.
   B. Was the first in the United States to expose an intraoral radiograph on a live patient.

Fundamental Radiation Physics

Understanding radiation physics requires a basic knowledge of atomic structure, radiation types, and properties of radiation.

Atomic Structure

The nucleus and electrons in the orbiting shells of an atom function in a state of equilibrium until ionization occurs (Fig. 7–1).
I. The Nucleus
   A. Contains protons, which are positively charged, and neutrons, which have no charge.
II. Orbiting Shells
   A. Contain electrons, which are negatively charged, and circle the nucleus in shells.
   B. Have binding energy, which keeps the electrons in their shells as a result of centripetal force and the attraction of opposites.

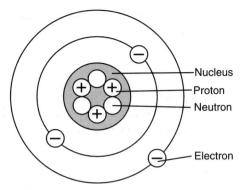

Figure 7.1 Atomic structure.

III. Ionization
   A. Occurs when an atom loses an electron from one of its shells and becomes part of an ion pair.
   B. An ion pair is created when an x-ray photon ejects a negative electron from its shell and the neutral atom becomes positive.
   C. Ionizing radiation is any radiation that is capable of producing ions.

Types of Radiation

Particulate and electromagnetic radiation are two types of ionizing radiation that are common in dentistry.
I. Particulate or Corpuscular Radiation
   A. Involves mass and particles that travel at high speeds.
   B. Four types are recognized:
      1. Electrons, which originate from radioactive atoms, are called beta particles.
      2. Protons, which are heavily charged particles (namely hydrogen nuclei).
      3. Neutrons, which have mass but no electrical charge.
      4. Alpha particles, which are large and are emitted from the nucleus of heavy metals; typically are unable to penetrate tissue.
II. Electromagnetic Radiation
   A. Comprises electric and magnetic fields of energy that move through space in a wave-like motion.
   B. Some forms are ionizing and others are not, depending on their energy (wavelengths); for example, x-rays have short wavelengths and are ionizing.
   C. Is arranged in a spectrum according to its energies, which is demonstrated by its wavelengths and frequencies.
      1. The wave concept suggests that electromagnetic radiation is much like waves or ripples of water and involves wave frequency and length.
         a. Wavelength
            1) Is the distance between the peaks or crests of a wave.
            2) Determines the energy of radiation; the longer the distance, the less energetic the radiation and the less ability it has to penetrate objects.

3) Is measured according to the distance between peaks. Longer wavelengths are measured in meters; shorter wavelengths are measured in nanometers (0.01 nm to 0.05 nm).

b. Frequency
1) Is the number of peaks or crests that occur in a given amount of time.
2) The frequency of the peaks determines the energy of the wavelength; the more frequent the peaks, the shorter and more energetic the radiation.

Properties of X-Rays

X-rays are ionizing forms of radiation that have unique properties.

I. Are bundles of pure energy (short wavelengths) that have no electrical charge but travel at the speed of light (3×10^8 m/sec).
II. Are invisible, weightless, and undetectable by any of the senses.
III. Are absorbed by matter according to the atomic structure of the material that is exposed.
IV. Cause ionization, which produces biologic change in interaction with matter.

The X-Ray Machine and its Components

The x-ray machine has basic operable components and internal components that are important in the safe operation and functioning of the machine.

Basic Operable Components

The control panel, tube head, and position-indicating device make up the major operable parts of the x-ray machine.

I. Control Panel
   A. Is operated by visible on-off switches, an exposure button, and indicator light.
   B. Controls milliamperage, time, and kilovoltage settings by dials on the panel.
II. Tubehead (Figure 7–2)
   A. Is a heavy, metal housing for the transformers and x-ray tube that serves as an attachment for the position-indicating device (PID), filter, and collimator.
   B. Contains insulating oil, which surrounds the x-ray tube and the transformers to prevent overheating.
III. Position-Indicating Device
   A. Attaches to the tubehead.
   B. Is a lead-lined, open-ended cylinder or rectangle that directs the x-ray beam to the object and the film.

Internal Components

Internal components of the x-ray machine include the x-ray tube, power supply, circuit, and transformer.

I. X-Ray Tube
   A. Is a lead glass vacuum tube that is 1 inch by several inches long. Contains two types of electrodes:
      1. Cathode-negative electrode
         a. Has a tungsten filament, which is a wire that is the source of electrons when heated.
         b. Has a molybdenum cup, which is semicircular in shape, to focus the direction of the electrons toward the anode.
      2. Anode-positive electrode
         a. Has a tungsten plate or target that electrons hit (when they leave the cathode) to produce x-rays and heat.
         b. Has a copper stem with an anode embedded in it to dissipate the excessive amount of heat produced.
         c. Has a focal spot, which is hit by the electrons leaving the cathode.
II. Power Supply
   A. Is the electricity that provides energy to the unit to produce x-rays and is described by its current, amperage, and voltage.
   B. Is an electric current, or the flow of electrons through a wire in a given point of time.
      1. When a direct current (DC), electrons flow in one direction.
      2. When an alternating current (AC), electrons flow in one direction and then change to flow in another direction.
   C. Is measured in amperes; in dentistry we use the milliampere, which is 1/1000 of an ampere.
   D. Uses voltage as the unit of force between two points; is measured in kilovolts (1000 volts).
III. Circuit
   A. Is a route that the electrical current takes.
   B. Filament and high-voltage are two types of circuits.
      1. Filament circuit
         a. Adjusts the flow through a low-voltage circuit.
         b. Controls the heating of a filament and the quantity of available electrons.
         c. Is controlled by the milliamperage (mA) setting.

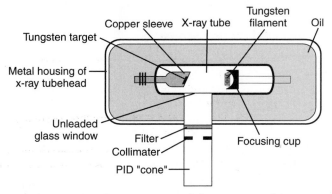

Copper sleeve   X-ray tube   Tungsten filament   Oil
Tungsten target
Metal housing of x-ray tubehead
Unleaded glass window
Filter
Collimater
Focusing cup
PID "cone"

Figure 7.2   Components of the x-ray machine.

2. High-voltage circuit
   a. Uses 65,000 to 100,000 volts to provide the high voltage necessary to propel electrons and produce x-rays.

IV. Transformer
   A. Is a mechanism used in an electrical circuit to increase or decrease the voltage.
   B. May be a step-up, step-down, or autotransformer type.
      1. Step-down transformer
         a. Is needed to produce electrons by heating the tungsten filament in a cathode.
         b. Decreases the incoming line voltage (110 to 220) to the required 3 to 5 volts.
         c. Has more wires in the primary coil (input coil) than in the secondary coil (output coil).
      2. Step-up transformer
         a. Provides the energy needed to propel electrons from the negative pole to the positive pole to produce x-rays.
         b. Increases the incoming line voltage (110 to 220) to the required 65,000 to 100,000 volts.
         c. Has more wires in the secondary coil than in the primary coil.
      3. Autotransformer
         a. Changes the voltage input into the primary coil of the step-up transformer.

Generation of X-Rays

X-rays are produced in the x-ray tube through a complex process that involves negative and positive poles.

Process

The x-ray process involves the use of both a cathode and an anode.

I. Cathode
   A. Is the negative pole in the x-ray tube.
   B. Contains a tungsten filament that is heated by the filament circuit and that generates electrons.
      1. The heating temperature is controlled by milliamperage.
      2. The available electrons are "boiled off" from the filament by a process called thermionic emission.
   C. Includes the focusing cup, which is made of molybdenum; the cup surrounds the filament and directs the electrons to the focal spot on the anode.

II. Anode
   A. Is the positive pole in the x-ray tube.
   B. Has a copper stem that serves as a good thermal conductor and dissipates heat away from the anode.
   C. Includes a target made of tungsten, which is imbedded in the copper stem.
      1. The target's purpose is to convert the electrons from the cathode into x-rays.
      2. This process results in the generation of x-rays (1%) and heat (99%).

Types of X-Rays Produced

X-rays are produced in an x-ray tube when kinetic energy from electrons hits the target in the anode. Types include Bremsstrahlung and characteristic radiation.

I. Bremsstrahlung Radiation
   A. Means "braking action" in German; it is the major source of x-rays produced in dentistry.
   B. Results when high energy electrons come close to the nuclei of tungsten atoms but are slowed down by the positive pull of the nuclei.
   C. X-ray production results from the slowing down of the electrons, which releases energy.

II. Characteristic Radiation
   A. Is not generated frequently.
   B. Involves electrons dislodging electrons from the K or L shell of the tungsten atom.
   C. Requires the filling of a vacancy by a lower energy shell electron, which results in an x-ray that comprises the binding energy between these two different shell electrons.

Interaction of X-Rays With Matter

An x-ray weakens whenever it reacts with matter. When x-rays pass through the atoms of tissue but do not react with the tissue, no interaction occurs.

Photoelectric Effect

Photoelectric effect is ionization that occurs when an x-ray photon interacts with an inner shell electron.

I. When photons are absorbed and electrons are ejected, the effect ceases to exist (no penetrating power).
II. The photoelectric effect is responsible for approximately 30% of all interactions in dental x-rays.

Compton Scatter

Compton scatter is ionization that occurs when an x-ray photon interacts with an outer shell electron.

I. Occurs when an electron is ejected and the x-ray photon scatters in a different direction.
II. Is responsible for approximately 62% of all scatter in dental x-rays.

Coherent or Thompson Scatter

Coherent scatter results without the occurrence of ionization.

I. Occurs when a low-energy photon reacts with an outer shell electron and no loss of energy occurs.
II. The x-ray photon scatters in a different direction.

Mechanisms of Radiation Injury of Living Tissue

Two theories attempt to explain the biologic effects of radiation that result in injury to living tissues.

Direct Theory

According to the direct theory, radiation damage to tissues is caused by a direct hit on the DNA molecule of a cell, which causes cell death.

I.   Seldom causes radiation injury.

Indirect Theory

According to the indirect theory, radiation damage to tissues involves the formation of free radicals.

I.   Applies when an x-ray photon is absorbed in a cell, which creates toxins (free radicals) and damages the cell.
II. States that indirect injuries are common because of the reaction with water (70% to 80%) in cells (i.e., formation of hydrogen peroxide).

Dose Response Curve

The dose response curve is a graphic means of plotting the biologic response (damage) to radiation exposure (dose) to determine acceptable levels of radiation exposure.

I.   For low doses of radiation, very little information is available about the dose response curve.
II. Graphically, a linear nonthreshold curve occurs, which indicates that a response is seen at any dose.
III. Results indicate that there is no safe level of radiation exposure.

Units of Radiation Measurement

Units of radiation were established to measure exposure, dose, and dose equivalent by the International Commission on Radiation Units and Measurements. Two systems are used for each unit: Standard and Systeme International (SI).

Exposure

Exposure is a radiation quantity that measures ionization in air; it is described in roentgens or SI units.

I.   Intensity is measured by the roentgen (R).
II. In other SI units, is equivalent to coulombs per kilogram (C/kg).

Dose

Dose is the amount of radiation energy absorbed by tissue.

I.   Rate is the amount of radiation absorbed per unit of time.
II. Often is identified with the radiation absorbed dose (RAD).
   A. Is the traditional unit of dose.
   B. The SI equivalent is the gray (Gy).
   C. Conversion is:

$$1 \text{ Gy} = 100 \text{ rad}$$

$$1 \text{ rad} = 0.01 \text{ Gy}$$

Dose Equivalent

Dose equivalents have different biologic effects when compared with different types of radiation.

I.   The quality factor is a specific number, according to exposure effect, that is given to each type of radiation.
II. Roentgen-equivalent-man (REM).
   A. Is the traditional unit of absorbed dose.
   B. The SI equivalent is the sievert (Sv).
   C. Conversion:

$$1 \text{ Sv} = 100 \text{ rem}$$

$$1 \text{ rem} = 0.01 \text{ Sv}$$

Factors That Determine Radiation Injury

Several factors determine the amount of injury that occurs from radiation. These include total dose, amount of area exposed, types of cells exposed, and cell sensitivity.

Total Dose

Total dose is the amount of radiation absorbed in the tissue that determines the effect.

I.   Acute exposure refers to an ionizing radiation given in a short amount of time; results in more dramatic biologic effects.
II. Chronic exposure refers to small amounts of ionizing radiation given over a longer period of time; results in less effect on tissue.
III. The latent period is the time (hours, days, or months) between radiation exposure and its observed clinical effect.

Exposure Area

The amount of the body that is exposed to radiation also determines the biologic effect of radiation on the tissues.

I.   Whole-body exposure is exposure of the entire body to radiation, which results in more severe biologic effects; can be either acute or chronic.
   A. Acute exposure, such as occurs in nuclear warfare or occupational hazards, can result in the symptoms of nausea, vomiting, bleeding, and diarrhea.
   B. Chronic exposure involves exposure to natural background radiation; the largest single cause is cosmic rays.
II. Limited-area exposure involves irradiation to a specific body area; can be either acute or chronic.
   A. Acute exposure involves high doses of radiation directed at a specific area, such as occurs during radiation therapy.
   B. Chronic exposure is exposure to low doses of radiation, such as occurs during dental radiography.

Cell Types

Effects of radiation are determined by cell maturity and cell type.

I.   The Law of Bergonie and Tribondeau states that the greatest radiation effects occur in cells that are immature, not highly specialized, and that frequently divide.

II. Cell Maturity
   A. Immature cells are nonspecialized and experience rapid cell division.
   B. Mature cells are specialized in their function; divide at a slow rate, or do not divide at all.

III. Basic Tissue Cell Types
   A. Somatic tissue cells are not inherited and are not involved in reproduction (e.g., skin, kidney cells).
   B. Genetic tissue cells are reproductive tissue cells (e.g., ovaries in female/testes in the male).

Cell Sensitivity

Human tissue cells have different sensitivities to radiation.

I. Radiosensitivity applies to tissues and cells that are highly sensitive to radiation (e.g., bone marrow, reproductive, small lymphocyte).

II. Radioresistant tissues and cells are those that are more resistant to radiation (e.g., salivary glands, lungs, kidneys, muscle).

Radiation Exposure and Risks

Exposure and risks associated with radiation include those from the environment (background) and those associated with direct irradiation of organs.

Background Radiation

The greatest contribution to radiation is from naturally occurring sources in the environment.

I. External radiation is from cosmic and terrestrial sources and comprises approximately 15% of the radiation exposure to the population.

II. Internal radiation occurs from exposure to radionuclides through inhalation and ingestion; comprises approximately 67% of radiation exposure. Radon is the largest single contributor to natural radiation.

III. Artificial radiation comprises approximately 17% of radiation exposure and includes sources such as medical and dental radiation.

Critical Organs

When sensitive organs and tissues are exposed to radiation during dental irradiation, a significant decrease in the quality of a person's life may occur. These critical organs include the skin, eye lens, thyroid, and bone marrow (hematopoietic).

I. Skin irradiation may lead to erythema—the first clinical sign of overexposure (250 rad in a 14-day period).

II. Eye irradiation can lead to cataract formation if exposure to the eyes is 200,000 mrad.

III. Thyroid irradiation can result in cancer, particularly when radiation exposure of 6,000 mrads or more occurs.

IV. Bone marrow irradiation poses a cancer risk (particularly leukemia) at exposures of 5,000 mrads or more of radiation.

Radiation Protection

Proper use of equipment, patient and operator positioning, and technique can provide acceptable limits to radiation exposure.

Patient

Patient exposure to radiation can be reduced through the proper use of filtration, collimation, positioning, and shielding.

I. Filtration involves the filtering-out of nonproductive x-rays; inherent filtration plus added filtration equals the total filtration for the machine.
   A. Inherent filtration is inside the tubehead (i.e., the oil, glass window, and tubehead seal).
   B. Added filtration includes the aluminum disk placed around the seal of the machine.
      1. Is used to filter out longer, nonproductive wavelengths, resulting in a primary beam with more energy.
      2. Federal and state laws dictate the thickness of the total filtration according to the kilovolt peak (kVp) setting of the machine (at or below 70 kVp = 1.5 mm thickness of aluminum; 70 kVp and above = 2.5 mm thickness).

II. Collimation restricts the size and shape of the x-ray beam and therefore restricts patient exposure.
   A. The collimator is a lead diaphragm placed over the opening of the tubehead.
   B. Exposure reduction is possible by limiting the size of the x-ray beam at the end of the PID to no more than 2.75 inches in diameter.

III. The PID is the aiming device that is used to direct the x-ray beam; also is called the beam-indicating device (BID).
   A. A cone-shaped PID is a closed, pointed, plastic device that increases scatter radiation and should not be used.
   B. A round PID is open-ended, circular in shape, and lead-lined. Standard lengths are 8 inches and 16 inches; 16 inches is preferable because it provides more parallel rays.
   C. A rectangular lead-lined PID is highly recommended because it offers the most reduction in radiation exposure to the patient; standard lengths are 8 inches and 16 inches.

IV. Lead aprons are shields that patients wear to protect their tissues from scatter radiation. Use of these aprons is mandated by law in many states; should be used in conjunction with a thyroid collar for intraoral films.

V. Fast film is one of the most effective means of reducing patient exposure; E-speed film is the fastest and is twice as fast as D-speed film.

VI. Film-holding devices are necessary to stabilize film and ultimately reduce additional exposure to the patient.

Operator

Measures must be taken to protect the operator from unnecessary radiation. These include proper positioning, the use of monitors, and attention to proper methods.

I. Positioning
  A. Involves an awareness of distance; remaining at least 6 feet from the source of radiation and in a safe quadrant (at right angles to the primary beam) is one of the most effective ways to eliminate unnecessary operator exposure.
  B. The operator should never hold the tubehead or film in the patient's mouth during exposure.
  C. Involves standing behind a lead shield or barrier whenever possible (cinderblock or 2½ inches of dry wall provides adequate protection).

II. Monitoring
  A. Involves personnel monitoring and following national guidelines when measuring occupational radiation exposure.
  B. Requires the use of film badges that measure exposure to low doses of radiation; should be worn at waist level.
    1. Metal filters inside the badge measure the amount of radiation that reaches the badge.
    2. Hard radiation shows a faint shadow; soft radiation casts a pronounced shadow.
  C. Maximum permissible dose (MPD)
    1. Relates to the amount of radiation exposure that is permissible through occupational exposure.
    2. Is considered the maximum dose that does not produce significant injury in a lifetime.
    3. Formula represents the whole body dose equivalent of ionizing and electromagnetic radiations and is expressed in sieverts.
    4. Was developed by the National Council on Radiation Protection (NCRP) in 1957. MPD for occupationally exposed persons:

    = 50 mSv (5000 mrem) per year

    = 4 mSv (400 mrem) per month

    = 1 mSv (100 mrem) per week

  D. ALARA concept
    1. Is the philosophy of radiation protection that currently is practiced by all radiation workers.
    2. Means *As Low As Reasonably Achievable.*
    3. Implies that every effort will be made to keep the radiation exposure to occupational and non-occupational workers as low as possible.

Radiographic Examination

The radiographic examination involves the use of intraoral, extraoral, and special imaging techniques to produce quality radiographs for use in the examination, interpretation, and diagnosis of dental conditions.

Intraoral Techniques and Errors

Intraoral radiography includes bisecting, paralleling, and occlusal techniques. The proper recognition of errors can help the operator correct a technique problem before it is repeated.

I. Bisecting Technique (Fig. 7–3)
  A. Also called the angle technique.
  B. Is based on the rule of isometry, which states that two triangles are equal if they have equal angles and share a common side.
  C. Requires bisection of the angle, which forms two equal triangles. The angle is formed by the plane of the film and the plane of the long axis of the tooth.
  D. If technique is strictly followed, directs the primary beam of radiation 90 degrees to the bisected line, resulting in an accurate image of the tooth.

II. Paralleling Technique
  A. Is based on the geometric figures of parallelism.
  B. Requires that the film be placed parallel to the long axis of the tooth.
  C. Requires a film holder for proper film placement.
  D. Directs the primary beam perpendicular to the film and the long axis of the tooth.

III. Occlusal Technique
  A. Is used for the detection of salivary stones and foreign bodies in the jaw and to locate supernumerary, unerupted, and impacted teeth.
    1. For anterior topographical mandibular occlusal
      a. Type-4 film is placed with the pebble side on the mandibular occlusals.
      b. The head is tilted backward, using a negative 55-degree vertical angulation, and the central ray is directed through the point of the chin.

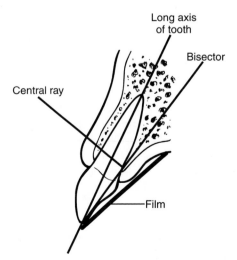

Figure 7.3   Bisection technique.

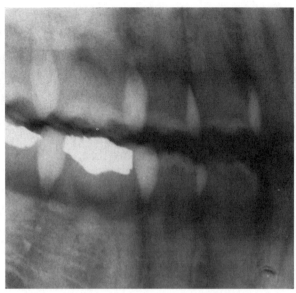

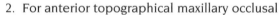

Figure 7.4 Overlapping of tooth structures caused by faulty horizontal angulation.

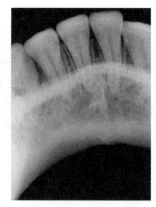

Figure 7.5 Foreshortening from excessive vertical angulation.

    2. For anterior topographical maxillary occlusal
       a. The patient is positioned with the sagittal plane perpendicular to the floor and the occlusal plane parallel to the floor.
       b. A positive vertical angulation of 65 degrees is used and the central ray is directed just above the tip of the nose.
    3. For cross-sectional maxillary occlusal
       a. The patient is positioned with the sagittal plane perpendicular to the floor and the occlusal plane parallel to the floor.
       b. The central ray is directed to the film at 90 degrees, with the PID centered between the eyebrows.
    4. For cross-sectional mandibular occlusal
       a. The patient's head is tilted backward until the ala-tragus line is almost perpendicular to the floor.
       a. A 90-degree vertical angulation is used, and the central ray is directed 3 cm below the chin.
IV. Intraoral Technique Errors
   A. Overlap (Fig. 7–4)
     1. Appears as adjacent tooth structures superimposed on each other.
     2. Can be corrected by redirecting the primary beam through the contacts.
   B. Foreshortening (Fig. 7–5)
     1. Teeth appear shorter than their actual size because of excessive vertical angulation.
     2. Can be corrected by decreasing the vertical angulation.
   C. Elongation (Fig. 7–6)
     1. Teeth appear distorted and larger than their actual size because of insufficient vertical angulation.

     2. Can be corrected by increasing the vertical angulation.
   D. Bent film (Fig. 7–7)
     1. Appears as a radiolucent mark across the film; is caused by creasing or improperly placing film.
     2. Can be corrected by not creasing the film corners and by positioning the film to keep the surface of the film in the same plane.
   E. Cone cut (Fig. 7–8)
     1. Appears as a radiopaque area with a circular border; is caused by failure of the PID to cover the entire surface of the film.
     2. Can be corrected by redirecting the PID to completely cover the surface of the film.
   F. Backward placement (Fig. 7–9)
     1. Film appears much lighter, with a herringbone or waffle patterned effect on both sides; is caused by backward placement of the film in

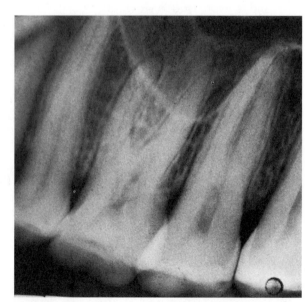

Figure 7.6 Elongation from inadequate vertical angulation.

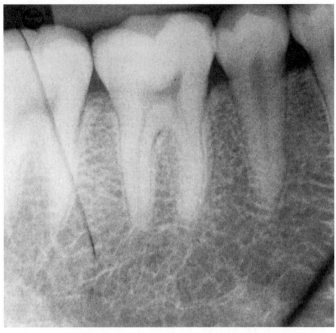

Figure 7.7   Radiolucent mark associated with a creased or bent film.

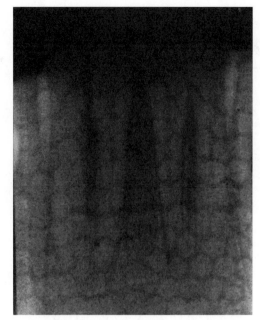

Figure 7.9   A film placed backward in the mouth has a waffle or herringbone appearance.

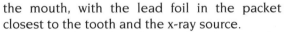

the mouth, with the lead foil in the packet closest to the tooth and the x-ray source.
  2. Can be corrected by placing the film with the smooth side next to the tooth.
G. Movement (Fig. 7–10)
  1. Appears as a blurred or unclear image; is caused by movement of the patient or the tubehead during exposure of the film.
  2. Can be corrected by giving the patient more specific directions about not moving and by

checking to be sure the tubehead is stabilized before exposing the film.
H. Double exposure (Fig. 7–11)
  1. Appears as a darker film, with distinct outlines of many teeth; is caused by a film order mix-up during exposure or by exposing a single film twice.
  2. Can be corrected by keeping the film in order of exposure and by keeping the film in a different place after exposure.

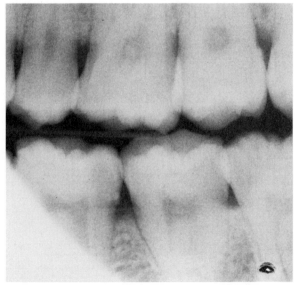

Figure 7.8   Cone cut caused by inadequate PID coverage of the film.

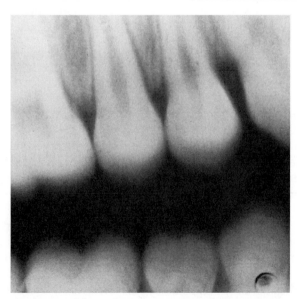

Figure 7.10   A blurred image is caused by movement of either the patient or the tubehead during film exposure.

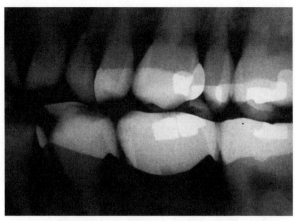

Figure 7.11 A double exposure occurs when a single film is exposed to radiation twice.

~ Clinical Case STUDY ~

Eight-year-old Shawn is visiting the dental office for the first time. He has fetal alcohol syndrome (FAS) and an IQ of 70. His medical history does not indicate any health problems or medications. At his appointment, Shawn demonstrates nervousness and a short attention span. His guardian states that Shawn often has bad breath and wonders whether he has any cavities.

Clinical Case QUESTIONS

1. What is fetal alcohol syndrome and what are the oral manifestations of this disorder?
2. What radiographs are recommended and why?
3. What could cause Shawn's bad breath and what recommendations should be made to Shawn and his guardian?
4. A double image appeared on one of the two films. What caused this?

Clinical Case RATIONALES

1. FAS is caused by maternal ingestion of alcohol during pregnancy. Alcohol ingestion during the early stages of pregnancy often leads to mental retardation and other developmental disabilities in the child. Hyperactivity and attention deficit disorder (ADD) often accompany the syndrome. Oral manifestations may include cleft lip, with or without palate, underdeveloped maxilla, and micrognathia.
2. A panoramic radiograph with accompanying bitewings is recommended because of Shawn's FAS and lack of medication for ADD or hyperactivity. In addition, his small jaw size would make numerous intraoral films difficult to obtain.
3. Shawn's bad breath most likely is caused by bacteria and should improve after he receives a complete prophylaxis. Oral hygiene instructions are crucial and

must be given to Shawn and his guardian, who most likely will supervise this activity. If the halitosis has not disappeared by his 6-month recall appointment, referral to a physician for a possible medical disorder might be in order.

4. A blurred image on a film is caused by movement of either the tubehead or the patient during exposure. In this situation, it most likely is caused by patient movement because hyperactivity accompanies FAS and this patient is not taking any medication.

Extraoral Techniques

During the performance of extraoral techniques, the film is placed outside of the mouth during exposure; most of these require the use of screen film. These techniques include panoramic imaging, lateral jaw exposures, and cephalometric and Waters projection techniques.

I. Panoramic Imaging
   A. Requires rotational movement of the film and radiation source around the head; also is called tomography (Fig. 7–12).
   B. Uses a focal trough or plane of acceptable focus in the shape of the dental arches.
   C. Any images in this trough are clear; the images outside the trough are blurred, thus correct patient positioning is crucial.
   D. Is used to evaluate impacted teeth, eruption patterns, and growth and to detect diseases, conditions of the jaw, and trauma.
   E. Errors in technique are common.
      1. Lip and tongue placement
         a. Lips must be closed to prevent the appearance of a dark shadow on the anterior teeth.

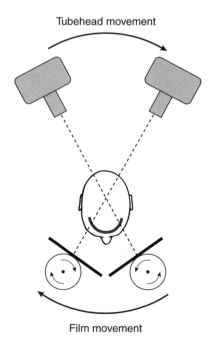

Tubehead movement

Film movement

Figure 7.12 Focal trough used in panoramic imaging.

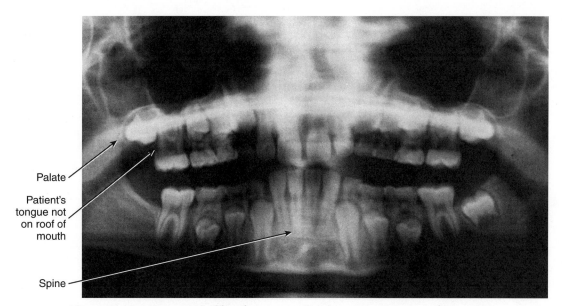

Palate

Patient's
tongue not
on roof of
mouth

Spine

Figure 7.13   Panoramic film demonstrating improper tongue placement.

b. The tongue must be placed on the palate to prevent the appearance of radiolucent areas over the apices of the maxillary teeth (Fig. 7–13).
2. Chin placement
   a. If the chin is tipped up, a "frown" results, with blurring and magnification of the maxillary teeth.
   b. If the chin is tipped down, an "exaggerated smile" results, with blurring and magnification of the mandibular incisors.
3. Placement of the anterior teeth
   a. If the anterior teeth are placed forward to the focal trough (notch in the bite-block), they will appear "thin."
   b. If the anterior teeth are placed behind the focal trough (notch in the bite-block), they will appear thick and wide.

II. Lateral jaw exposure (Fig. 7–14)
   A. Requires that film be placed laterally to the jaw during exposure.
   B. Is used to examine the posterior portion of the mandible or for patients who are unable to open the mouth because of swelling or possible fractures.
III. Lateral cephalometric projection (Fig. 7–15)
   A. Requires that a cassette be placed on the side of the head to image the outline of the face.
   B. Is used to evaluate trauma, facial growth and development, and any developmental abnormalities.
IV. Posteroanterior projection (Fig. 7–16)
   A. Requires that film be placed on the face, with the forehead and nose touching the film.
   B. Is used to show frontal and ethmoid sinuses, orbits, and the nasal cavity.

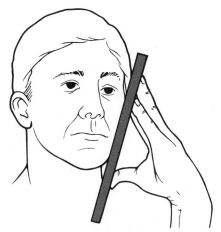

Figure 7.14   Lateral jaw exposure is useful for examining traumatic injury to the posterior jaw.

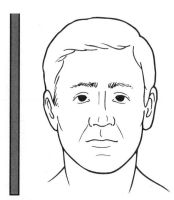

Figure 7.15   Lateral cephalometric projection often is used to detect developmental or traumatic disturbances.

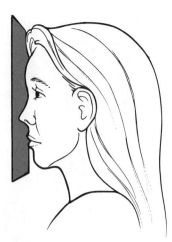

Figure 7.16 Posteroanterior projection is used to evaluate the frontal and ethmoid sinuses, the eye orbits, and the nasal cavity.

V. Waters projection (Fig. 7–17)
   A. Requires that film be placed on the patient's face, with the chin touching the film and the head tipped back so that the tip of the nose is 1 inch from the film.
   B. Is used specifically to evaluate the maxillary sinus area.

Special Imaging Techniques

Digital imaging, magnetic resonance imaging, and computed tomography are three types of specialized imaging techniques that currently are in use.
   I. Digital Imaging
   A. Requires that a nonfilm sensor be placed inside the mouth; the sensor is electronically attached to a computer, which immediately produces an image on the monitor.

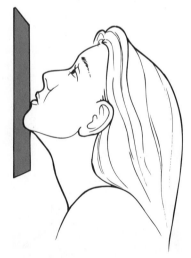

Figure 7.17 Waters projection is useful for examining maxillary sinuses.

   B. Images can be stored, retained as a hard copy, or sent to a different site.
   C. Images can be displayed immediately, which eliminates darkroom procedures.
   D. Provides less radiation exposure to the patient.
   II. Magnetic Resonance Imaging (MRI)
   A. Derives energy from a magnetic field 10,000 times more powerful than the earth's magnetic field and is superior for imaging soft tissue.
   B. Hydrogen nuclei in the body are realigned by radiofrequency pulses.
   C. Realignment of the nuclei is received by a sensor and transmitted to a computer to generate an image.
   III. Computed Tomography (CT scanning)
   A. Is computer generated; uses ionizing radiation as the energy source.
   B. Must be performed in a special CT unit in the hospital.
   C. Allows multiple images of the patient to be fed into a computer, resulting in an image on the monitor or film.
   D. Is useful in dentistry for implant planning; special software is required.

Characteristics of Radiation Images

Radiation images are characterized by their quantity, quality, intensity, and clarity.

Quantity

Image quantity refers to the number of x-rays that are produced and is measured in amperes, milliampere-seconds, and the density of the radiographs.
   I. Ampere
   A. Is the number of electrons that flow through a filament.
   B. A milliampere (mA) is equal to 1/1000 of an ampere.
   C. Milliamperage controls the temperature of the cathode filament.
   II. Milliampere-seconds (mA-s)
   A. Are a combination of milliamperes and seconds.
      1. Milliamperes have a direct effect on the number of electrons produced.
      2. Seconds have the same effect on the quantity of electrons produced.
   B. To maintain similar density:
      1. If the seconds are increased, milliamperage must be decreased.
      2. If the seconds are decreased, milliamperage must be increased.
   III. Density
   A. Is the overall darkness of a radiograph.
   B. Is affected by milliamperage and by the quantity of electrons produced.
      1. If the mA is increased, the film will be darker.
      2. If the mA is decreased, the film will be lighter.

Quality

Quality is the energy or penetrating power of the beam. It is measured in kilovolts and affects image contrasts.

I. Kilovolt (kV)
  A. Is equal to 1000 volts and is the measurement used to determine the energy in a tubehead.
  B. The kilovoltage peak represents the peak or maximum voltage; determines the speed and ultimately the energy of the electrons.
    1. If kVp is increased, the primary beam will have more energy and density will increase.
II. Contrast
  A. Is the difference between the light and dark colors on a radiograph.
  B. An increase in kVp (90 or higher) results in many shades of gray on the film (long scale contrast).
  C. A decrease in kVp (65 to 70) results in more black and white areas on a radiograph (short-scale contrast).

Beam Intensity

Beam intensity is affected by mA, kVp, time, and distance.

I. Milliamperage affects the intensity by controlling the number of electrons produced; the higher the mA, the more intense the beam.
II. The kilovoltage peak controls the energy of the electrons traveling from the cathode to the anode; higher the kVp, the more the intense beam.
III. Exposure time affects the intensity in the same manner as the mA; increase in time = more intense beam
IV. Distance also affects beam intensity; as the beam travels a longer distance to the film or tooth, it becomes less intense.
  A. Inverse square law states that "the intensity of radiation is inversely proportional to the square of the distance from the source of radiation"; explains how the beam loses its intensity as it travels farther from the source.
  B. Half-value layer is a term used to describe the reduction in beam intensity by one half with the use of aluminum filters; the filters remove the less penetrating, longer wavelengths in the beam.

Accurate Image Formation

Accurate image (geometric) formation is best produced by controlling image sharpness, magnification, and distortion.

I. Sharpness (umbra)
  A. Is the clarity or distinctness of the outlines of an object; penumbra is the fuzziness or lack of sharpness in an image.
  B. Is influenced by the focal spot size; the tungsten target of the anode should be small to increase sharpness.
  C. Is associated with film composition. The size of the crystals on the film determines sharpness; the larger the crystals, the less sharp the image.
  D. Is influenced by movement of the patient or the tubehead; movement of either will reduce image sharpness.
II. Magnification
  A. Is the enlargement of an actual image.
  B. Is influenced by the target-film distance; an increased distance from the target in the x-ray tube to the film allows more parallel rays to hit the film, which produces less magnification.
  C. Is affected by the object-film distance; the closer the tooth is to the film, the less the magnification.
III. Distortion
  A. Is the disfigurement of the shape and size of an image.
  B. Is affected by the object-film alignment; the film and long axis of the tooth must be parallel to each other (so that rays will hit at a right angle) to decrease distortion.
  C. Is influenced by beam direction; the beam must be directed perpendicular to both the film and the tooth to record an accurate, distortion-free image.

Image Production

Producing a good image requires knowledge of proper film processing and darkroom techniques, processing problems and solutions, film reproduction methods, and infection control practices.

Film Processing

Film processing, whether manual or automatic, is the transformation of a latent image into a visible image by means of chemical processing.

I. Manual processing is also called the time-temperature method and involves manual developing, washing, fixing, washing, and drying steps.
  A. Optimum developing takes approximately 5 minutes at 68°F; reduces exposed silver halide crystals into black metallic silver through the use of four ingredients in the solution:
    1. Hydroquinone or elon is a developing agent that converts energized crystals into metallic silver.
    2. Sodium sulfite is a preservative that prevents rapid oxidation of the developer.
    3. Sodium carbonate softens film emulsion and speeds up the action of the developing agents.
    4. Potassium bromide is a restrainer that inhibits the development of unexposed silver halide crystals.
  B. Fixing takes approximately 10 minutes, or twice the developing time; it clears all unexposed silver halide crystals from the film emulsion by means of four ingredients in the solution:
    1. Sodium thiosulfate clears the unexposed silver halide crystals from the emulsion.

2. Sodium sulfite prevents the break down of the sodium thiosulfate.
3. Potassium alum shrinks and hardens the emulsion.
4. Acetic acid is an acidifier that keeps the medium acetic and stops additional development.

II. Automatic processing is a procedure that automatically processes the film.
  A. A roller transport system moves the film through the solutions in the following order: developer, fixer, water, and drying chamber.
  B. The developing and fixing solutions are different from those used in manual processing.
    1. The developing solution works at a higher temperature and more rapidly.
    2. The fixing solution has a hardening agent to keep the film sturdy as it continues through the rollers.

Darkroom

The darkroom environment is important in the production of good quality radiographs. Attention to lighting is particularly significant.
I. Room Lighting
  A. The darkroom should be without any light leaks to prevent fogging of the film.
  B. Safelighting requires the use of a low-wattage bulb (7½ or 15 watts) with a filter that removes blue-green wavelengths; safelights must be spaced at least 4 feet from the working surface.

Film Duplication

Film duplication is the process of copying or reproducing a second film or set of films without re-exposing the patient to radiation.
I. Requires special duplicating film that must be used under safelight conditions.
  A. The duplicating film is coated only on one side.
  B. The duplicating film is a direct positive film. A darker film requires less exposure time; conversely, a lighter film requires more exposure time.
II. The procedure requires placing the original film next to the light source, placing the duplicate film on top of it, and exposing the films to the light source for a specified amount of time.

Film Mounting

Film mounting is the process whereby processed radiographs are organized and placed in a frame for ease of reading, to protect the films from wear, and to reduce interpretation errors.
I. Depending on the teaching method, radiographs are either mounted "dot-in" or "dot-out."
  A. The dots-in method or lingual method (as if inside the mouth looking out)—films are mounted with the patient's left side films on the left side of the mount and right side films on the right side of the mount; is the least common method.

B. The dots-out method or labial method (as if outside the mouth looking in)—films are mounted with the patient's right side films on the left side of the mount and the left side films on the right side of the mount; is the most common method.

II. Procedure
  A. The appropriate mount for the type and quantity of exposed film is selected.
  B. Once the films are dry, they are placed on a clean viewbox surface with dots up; the use of a magnifying viewer is helpful.
  C. The films are separated into maxillary, mandibular, and bitewing. For each of the three groups:
    1. Bitewing radiographs are mounted first, "with curve of Spee" directed up and distally, to guide the placement of posterior periapical films. Maxillary molars are three-rooted and mandibular molars are double-rooted.
    2. Posterior films with the most posterior structures are placed in the molar areas of the mount; subsequently posterior films with the least posterior structures are placed in the premolar areas of the mount.
    3. Anterior films exhibiting both central incisors are placed in the appropriate maxillary and mandibular central anterior sections of the mount.
    4. Remaining right and left-of-central anterior films are placed in their appropriate sections to either side of the central films.
  D. Films are arranged by the anatomic landmarks as they logically appear in the dental arches: maxillary posterior right, posterior left, and anterior; mandibular posterior right, posterior left, and anterior.

Quality Assurance Program

Quality assurance is a systematic procedure used to guarantee that quality radiographs are produced with minimal exposure to the patient.
I. Quality Control
  A. X-ray equipment
    1. Is evaluated annually as recommended by the American Academy of Oral and Maxillofacial Radiology.
    2. Is inspected by specifically trained inspectors who check kVp, mA output, half-value layer, timer, collimation, beam alignment, and tube head stability.
  B. Radiographer expertise
    1. Only individuals skilled in radiographic procedures and techniques should expose patients to x-rays.
  C. Processing solutions (manual and automatic)
    1. Are mixed and replenished according to the manufacturer's recommendations.
    2. Are changed as needed, according to degree of use.
    3. Can be evaluated by:
      a. Stepwedge (constructed of aluminum layers)

to provide a standard radiograph for evaluating density on a daily basis.

b. A dental radiographic normalizing device (DRND) to compare the density of film and monitor the strength of the solution.

D. Darkroom
   1. The safelight is evaluated every 6 months.
   2. Is evaluated for light leaks around doors and vents by means of the coin test.
E. Cassette intensifying screens
   1. Are inspected and cleaned monthly.

II. Administration
   A. Assign duties to appropriate personnel.
   B. Write descriptions of the plan and its expectations.
   C. Maintain records for equipment.
   D. Create forms to keep records of monitoring procedures.
   E. Document all monitoring procedures.

 ## Clinical Case STUDY

Eighty-five-year-old Marvin presents to the dental office complaining of a sore jaw and difficulty opening his mouth. He fell while getting dressed yesterday and hit his head on the headboard of his bed. Visual examination reveals a large bruise on the right side of his face along the lower jaw line. Teeth #30 and #31 are missing their anatomic crowns.

Clinical Case QUESTIONS

1. Which type of radiograph would provide the best assessment of this patient's jaw and teeth? What information should be obtained from the radiograph? Describe the appearance of such information.
2. After the film is processed, a 9-mm semicircular radiopaque mark is found on the lower right corner of the radiographs. What is the mark and what caused it?
3. During examination of the processed film, a pyramid-shaped radiopacity is observed in the center of the panoramic image. What is it and how was it caused?
4. "Branch-out" radiolucent marks appear on several areas of the film. What are they and what caused them?

Clinical Case RATIONALES

1. A panoramic radiograph should be taken to allow assessment of a larger area of the jaws and teeth; it also is easier for the patient, given that he has difficulty opening his mouth. One would look for indications of a jaw fracture (vertical radiolucent line) on the right side, possible tooth discoloration, noncontinuous lamina dura, and infected retained root tips on the right side.
2. The 9-mm semicircular radiopaque mark located on the lower edge of the film most likely is a fingernail scratch mark caused by improper handling of the film during processing. Scratching of the emulsion causes a radiopaque artifact on the processed film.

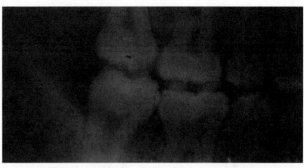

Figure 7.18 Overdeveloped film appears too dark.

3. The pyramid-shaped opacity is a ghost image of the spine caused by a slumped position of the patient during the exposure. The patient should be required to stand erect so that the spinal column is not superimposed on the film.
4. These "tree-like" marks are artifacts caused by static electricity. They typically occur because of low humidity.

Processing Problems and Solutions

Many problems occur when processing technique and procedure errors are made. The following are some of the most common problems.

I. Overdeveloped Film (Fig. 7–18)
   A. Appears too dark.
   B. May be caused by overdevelopment (excessive development time).
   C. May be caused by developing solution at a temperature that is too high.
   D. May be caused by developing solution that was incorrectly mixed or too concentrated.
II. Underdeveloped Film (Fig. 7–19)
   A. Appears too light.
   B. May be caused by underdevelopment (inadequate development time).
   C. May be caused by developing solution at a temperature that is too low.

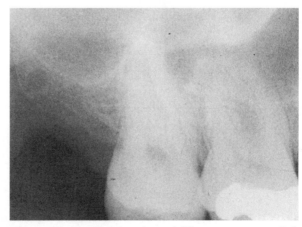

Figure 7.19 Underdeveloped film appears too light.

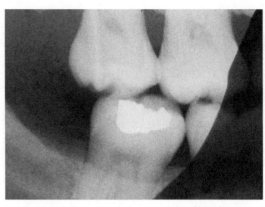

Figure 7.20 Developer contamination.

D. May be caused by exhausted (over-used) developing solution.
III. Reticulation
  A. Appears as cracked emulsion; is caused by a sudden temperature change between the developer and the fixer solution.
IV. Contamination From Chemicals
  A. Developer contamination appears as dark areas and occur when the developing solution comes into contact with the film before the processing procedure (Fig. 7–20).
  B. Fixer contamination appears as white areas and occur when the fixer solution comes into contact with the film before the processing procedure.
  C. Yellow-brown stains are caused by exhausted solutions or insufficient time in the solutions.
  D. Developer cut-off is a straight white border caused by a low level of solution (Fig. 7–21).
  E. Fixer cut-off is a straight black border caused by incomplete immersion of the film into the fixer solution (Fig. 7–22).
  F. Overlapped films exhibit white or darks areas in the shape of the outline border of another film and result from contact with each other in the solutions (Fig. 7–23).
  G. Air bubbles appear as white spots and are caused by air that is trapped on the surface of the film during processing.
  H. Static electricity exhibits thin, black, branch-like lines, which are caused by low humidity and opening the film packet too quickly (Fig. 7–24).
  I. Scratched films demonstrate white lines that are caused by the removal of emulsion during the processing process.
  J. Fogged films exhibit a gray hue that is caused by improper safelighting, outdated film, or light leaking into the darkroom.

Infection Control

The disinfection and sterilization of equipment and clinical areas involves proper attention to infection control procedures and standards.
I. Equipment and Supplies
  A. The chair, headrest, tubehead, and PID should be covered with a disposable barrier material such as a plastic bag.

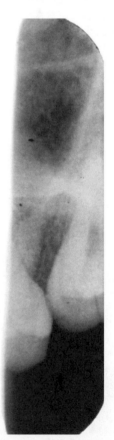

Figure 7.21 Developer cut-off exhibits a straight white border.

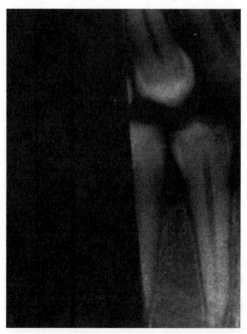

Figure 7.22 Fixer cut-off exhibits a straight black border.

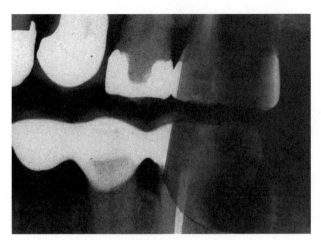

Figure 7.23 Overlapped films carry the outline shape of a second film.

B. Controls on the machine, including the activating switch, should be covered with a clear wrap or disposable item.

C. The lead apron should be sanitized by misting with a disinfectant and wiping the apron's surface.

D. The surface of the work area should be covered with a disposable barrier material.

E. Film holders should be sterilized and film should have protective coverings or should be contained in a disposable cup to prevent contamination of other surfaces.

F. If a lead barrier is used, the barrier should have protective coverings on all handled areas.

II. Operator Preparation

A. Hands should be washed and gloved; mask and eyewear are optional.

B. Operator should wear a gown or some protective outer wear.

III. Exposure Procedures

A. Contaminated items (e.g., paper cups, bite-wing tabs, cotton rolls) should be carefully discarded.

B. All uncovered surfaces (e.g., arm rests, chair, countertops) that might be contaminated should be disinfected with an EPA-registered disinfectant; operator should wear utility gloves.

Normal Anatomic Landmarks

Familiarity with normal anatomic landmarks of the oral cavity is essential to the development of proper radiographic technique, assessment, and diagnosis.

General Considerations

The proper identification of pathology involves familiarity with basic oral landmarks and principles of assessing radiographs.

I. The radiopaque or radiolucent appearance of an image helps determine specific landmarks.

II. Not all landmarks are seen on every full mouth series.

III. When a lesion is suspect, the appropriate landmarks for that site should be ruled out.

Maxillary Arch

Approximately 11 commonly identified intraoral landmarks are evident on maxillary films.

I. Nasopalatine (incisive) Foramen (Fig. 7–25)

A. Is the passageway for the nasopalatine nerves and vessels and is located in the middle of the palate, behind the central incisors.

B. Is an oval-shaped object located between the roots of the maxillary central incisors.

C. Is radiolucent in appearance.

II. Median Palatal Suture (intermaxillary suture) (see Fig. 7–25)

A. Appears as a thin line between the roots of the maxillary central incisors.

B. Runs vertically from the alveolar crest to the hard palate.

C. Is radiolucent in appearance and exhibits thin lines of cortical bone on each side.

III. Nasal Fossa (see Fig. 7–25)

A. Are air-filled spaces.

B. Appear as radiolucent oval shapes above the maxillary central incisors and are outlined by radiopaque bone.

IV. Nasal Septum (see Fig. 7–25)

A. Is a thin wall that divides two spaces.

B. Is formed by the ethmoid, vomer bones, and cartilage.

C. Appears as a radiopaque, vertical strip that separates the nasal fossae.

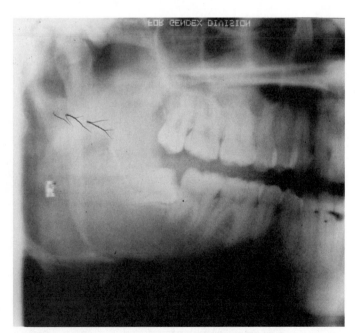

Figure 7.24 Static electricity on this half of a panoramic film caused a black, branch-like image.

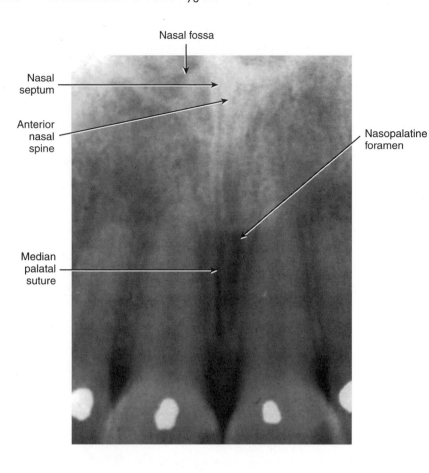

Nasal fossa

Nasal septum

Anterior nasal spine

Median palatal suture

Nasopalatine foramen

Figure 7.25 Anatomic structures commonly seen on maxillary anterior radiographs.

V. Anterior Nasal Spine (see Fig. 7–25)
   A. Is a pointed projection of bone located anterior and inferior to the nasal cavity, between the maxillary central incisors.
   B. Appears as a radiopaque, triangular shape at the intermaxillary suture (where the nasal septum and fossa meet).

VI. Maxillary Sinus (Fig. 7–26)
   A. Are hollow spaces in bone above the apices of the molars and premolars.
   B. Appear as large, oval, radiolucent areas outlined with thin lines of cortical bone.

VII. Inverted Y-Junction of Two Anatomic Landmarks (Fig. 7–27)

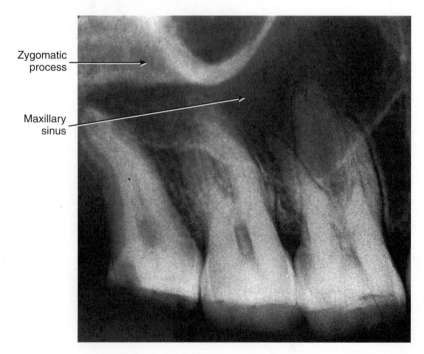

Zygomatic process

Maxillary sinus

Figure 7.26 The maxillary sinus and zygomatic process commonly appear on maxillary posterior radiographs.

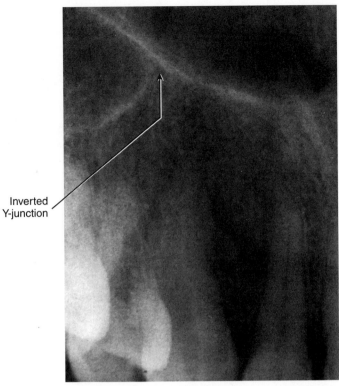

Figure 7.27   The inverted y-junction is the meeting point of the nasal fossa and maxillary sinus.

A. Is the point where the nasal fossa and the maxillary sinus meet and is located above the maxillary canine apices.
B. Appears as two oval, radiolucent areas outlined by a thin line of cortical bone.

VIII. Maxillary Tuberosity (Fig. 7–28)
A. Is a rounded, radiopaque elevation distal to the third molar region.

IX. Hamulus (Fig. 7–29)
A. Is a radiopaque, hooklike protrusion located posterior to the maxillary tuberosity.

X. Zygomatic Process (see Fig. 7–26)
A. Together with the zygoma make up the zygomatic arch.

B. Starts as a U-shaped band above the apices of the maxillary molars and extends posteriorly, where it continues as a radiopaque band.

XI. Coronoid Process of Mandible (Fig. 7–28)
A. Is the anterior portion of the ramus.
B. Appears as a radiopaque triangular projection, typically superimposed over the maxillary tuberosity.

Mandibular Arch

Approximately eight commonly identified intraoral landmarks are evident on mandibular films.

I. Genial Tubercles (Fig. 7–30)
A. Are four bony spines that are used for muscle attachment.
B. Appear as circular radiopacities below the apices of the mandibular central incisors.

II. Lingual Foramen (see Fig. 7–30)
A. Is the opening and exit for the incisive vessel branches.
B. Appears as a radiolucent circle inside the genial tubercles.

III. Mental Process (Fig. 7–31)
A. Is a bulge or ridge of bone located on the labial surface of the mandible.
B. Appears as bilateral radiopaque lines, starting below the apices of the premolars and extending forward toward the midline.

IV. Mental Foramen (Fig. 7–32)
A. Is the opening for nerves and blood vessels located below the apices of the premolars.
B. Appears as a round radiolucent area that can be mistaken for periapical pathology.

V. External Oblique Line/Ridge (Fig. 7–33)
A. Is a linear raised area of bone on the external surface of the mandible.
B. Appears as a radiopaque line that runs anterior from the ramus across the molar region.

VI. Internal Oblique Line/Ridge (mylohyoid) (see Fig. 7–33)
A. Is a linear raised area of bone on the internal surface of the mandible.

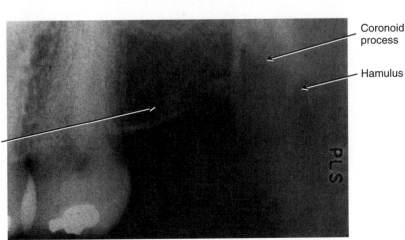
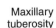

Figure 7.28   The coronoid process appears superimposed over the maxillary tuberosity.

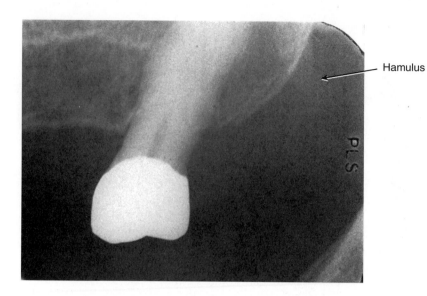

Hamulus

Figure 7.29   The hamulus is a radiopaque protrusion posterior to the maxillary tuberosity.

B. Appears as a radiopaque line that runs anterior along the apices of the molars and premolars, from the anterior part of the ramus to the anterior part of the mandible.

VII. Mandibular Canal (Fig. 7–34)
  A. Serves as a nutrient canal for blood supply and nerves; its posterior opening is the mandibular foramen and its anterior opening is the mental foramen.

B. Appears as a radiolucent band; is outlined with a thin line of cortical bone below the apices of the molars and premolars.

VIII. Submandibular Fossa (see Fig. 7–34)
  A. Is a thin, depressed area of bone on the internal surface of the mandible.
  B. Appears as a radiolucent band below the mylohyoid and the apices of the molars and premolars.

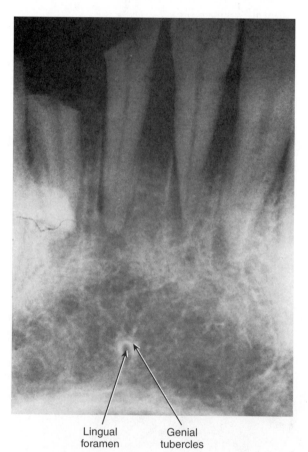

Lingual
foramen   Genial
                 tubercles

Figure 7.30   The lingual foramen (radiolucent) is surrounded by the genial tubercles (radiopaque).

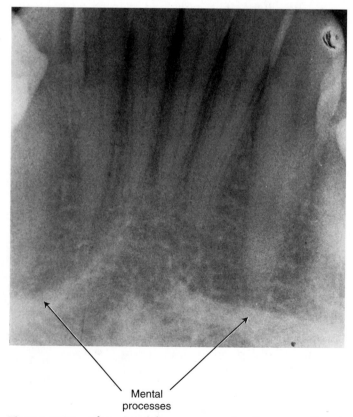

Mental
processes

Figure 7.31   The mental processes (radiopaque lines) extend from the apices of the mandibular premolars to the central incisors.

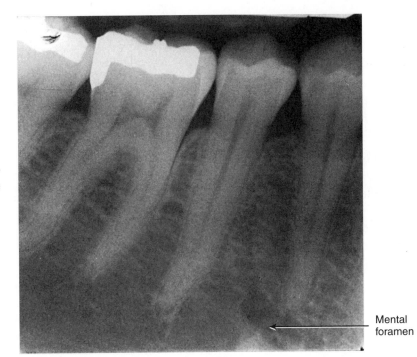

Figure 7.32   The mental foramen, located beneath the mandibular premolar apices, may be mistaken for periapical pathology.

Mental foramen

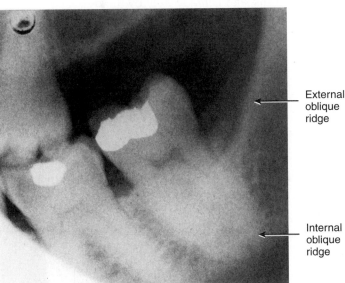

External oblique ridge

Internal oblique ridge

Figure 7.33   The internal and external oblique ridges are radiopaque structures that run from the ramus through the molar region (external) or to the anterior region (internal).

Figure 7.34   The mandibular canal and submandibular fossa are located beneath the root apices of the mandibular molars and premolars.

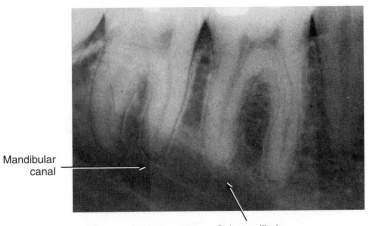

Mandibular canal

Submandibular fossa

Clinical Case STUDY

While updating her health history, 32-year-old Debra indicates that she is in her second month of pregnancy. She recently had her orthodontic bands removed. Visually, her clinical examination reveals a large restoration on tooth #30 and recession on the right side of her mouth. Her examination reveals no apparent caries. She made this appointment because she is experiencing sensitivity when she eats.

Clinical Case QUESTIONS

1. What is (are) the most likely reason(s) for Debra's sensitive teeth? What home care recommendations can be made?
2. Given Debra's history, what types of radiographs are recommended?
3. During examination of the radiographs, a well-defined radiopacity is seen apical to tooth #30. What is this and how does it relate to her sensitivity?
4. Radiographically, the apices of teeth #27 and #28 appear blunted and the roots appear shorter than normal. What condition does this most likely indicate?

Clinical Case RATIONALES

1. Debra's sensitivity may be caused by gingival recession, the recent removal of her orthodontic bands, or erosion associated with morning sickness. To determine the cause, further information must be gathered from Debra. Because she did not present clinically with caries and has only one restoration, providing oral hygiene instructions on toothbrushing technique (to reduce the incidence of recession) and encouraging the use of fluoride rinses (for sensitivity) is the best approach. Debra should be examined in 1 month to evaluate the effectiveness of the home care procedures in reducing her sensitivity.
2. Because Debra is pregnant and has no obvious signs of decay, radiographs can be postponed until after the pregnancy, unless the sensitivity does not abate after the practice of home care recommendations. Although the use of a lead apron (covering both front and back) with a thyroid collar eliminates the chance of radiation reaching the developing fetus, most dental practitioners prefer to take only those x-rays that are absolutely necessary to the safety and health of the patient. If the tooth discomfort continues at the 1-month visit, specific areas of sensitivity must be identified and appropriate radiographs must be exposed.
3. The radiopaque area most likely indicates condensing osteitis (also known as chronic focal sclerosing osteomyelitis), which results from a low-grade infection or mild irritation. The tooth most likely is nonvital; most frequently the affected teeth contain large restorations. Condensing osteitis most commonly occurs in

mandibular first molars in adults. Because this condition is asymptomatic, no treatment is necessary.

4. This most likely indicates external resorption of the apices of teeth #27 and #28 from mechanical forces placed on them by orthodontic movement. This type of resorption does not have any signs or symptoms and cannot be detected clinically. There is no treatment for external resorption.

Radiographic Interpretation

Radiographic interpretation involves the explanation or clarification of what is seen on a dental radiograph.

Ethical Considerations

Interpretation and diagnosis differ in both definition and use.

I. Interpretation is the means of explaining or clarifying what is seen on a dental radiograph.
II. Diagnosis is the specific identification of a condition or disease by examination, or a conclusion drawn from symptoms, and is made only by the dentist.
III. Commonly identified lesions
  A. Caries
    1. The loss of tooth structure caused by microorganisms; are radiolucent in appearance.
    2. Include:
      a. Interproximal caries (Fig. 7–35)
        1) Are located on the mesial or distal surfaces of a tooth.
        2) May progress from incipient to advanced, depending on the length of time involved.
        3) Appear as radiolucencies that advance as the caries get larger.
      b. Occlusal caries
        1) Occur on the biting surfaces of posterior teeth.

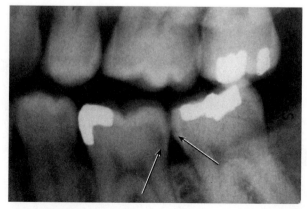

Figure 7.35 Interproximal caries (*arrows*) commonly appear as radiolucencies at the contact areas between adjacent teeth.

2) Appear as radiolucent shadows under the enamel as they progress.
   c. Root surface caries (Fig. 7–36)
      1) Occur only on the root surface.
      2) Are preceded by bone loss and gingival recession.
      3) Appear as a ditched-out, radiolucent area on the root.
B. Periodontal disease (Fig. 7–37)
   1. Is a group of diseases that affect supporting structures of the teeth.
   2. Includes:
      a. Gingivitis
         1) Affects the marginal gingiva and is a continuation of infection that is not apparent on radiographs.
      b. Periodontitis
         1) Is an infection that involves alveolar bone loss.
         2) Appears radiographically:
            a) Initially as a fuzzy or ditched-out area where destruction of the cortical crest of bone occurs.
            b) In more advanced stages, as horizontal or vertical bone loss (Fig. 7–38).
               (1) Horizontal bone loss appears radiographically in a plane parallel to the CEJ of adjacent teeth.
               (2) Vertical bone loss appears along one side of a tooth in an angular form; is not parallel to the CEJ of adjacent teeth.
   3. Assessment of periodontal disease requires the use of radiographs; bone loss, calculus, overhanging margins of restorations, caries, root resorption, and periapical lesions are assessed by appearance.
C. Trauma changes
   1. Are caused by injuries resulting from external forces.

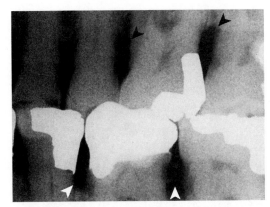

Figure 7.37   Periodontal disease is typified on radiographs by a fuzzy appearance of alveolar crest bone. Arrows indicate areas of advanced bone loss.

   2. Include:
      a. Tooth fractures
         1) A crown fracture typically involves anterior teeth and results from blows to the face or mouth or falls; the space from the missing structure appears radiolucent on a radiograph.
         2) A root fracture occurs most frequently in the anterior portion of the mouth and appears as a radiolucent horizontal line on the root.
      b. Avulsion, which is complete removal of the tooth from the bone; appears radiographically as a radiolucent space in the bone.
D. Resorption
   1. Is the loss of tooth structure with no resultant clinical recognition; can be either internal or external.
   2. Includes:
      a. External resorption, which starts on the root surface with a loss or flat rather than conical

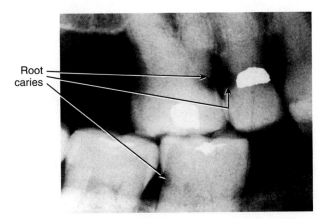

Root caries

Figure 7.36   Root caries appear as ditched-out radiolucent areas located at the cervical third of the exposed root surface.

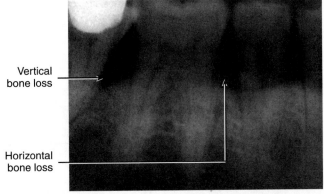

Vertical bone loss

Horizontal bone loss

Figure 7.38   Vertical or horizontal bone loss is assessed by determining whether the bone level maintains parallelism with the CEJs of associated teeth; parallelism is maintained with horizontal bone loss but not with vertical bone loss (often appears angular).

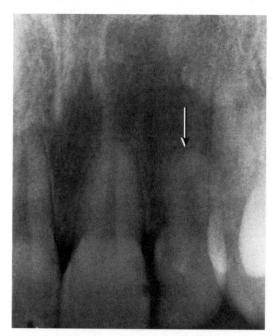

Figure 7.39 External resorption appears as a blunted or flat appearance of the apices.

shape appearance radiographically; bone and lamina dura appear normal (Fig. 7–39).

b. Internal resorption, which appears as an asymptomatic radiolucency; results from trauma or pulp capping; begins in the pulp and travels into the dentin.

E. Pulpal lesions
  1. Are commonly seen on radiographs.
  2. Include:
    a. Pulp stones, which are round, radiopaque calcifications most commonly seen in the pulp of molars (Fig. 7–40).

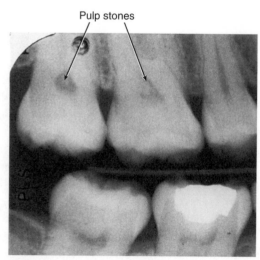

Pulp stones

Figure 7.40 Pulp stone calcifications in the pulps of molars.

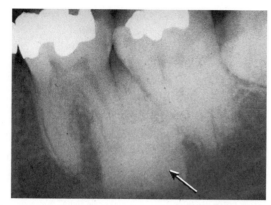

Figure 7.41 Condensing osteitis at the root apex of a nonvital tooth.

b. Pulp erasure, which is the disappearance of the radiolucent pulp canal because of pulp cavity trauma caused by caries, abrasion, or abnormal forces; the canal appears radiopaque because secondary dentin forms in the pulp chamber or canals.

F. Periapical lesions
  1. Are located around the apex of a tooth.
  2. Include:
    a. Periapical abscess, which is a radiolucent area located at the end of the apex of a symptomatic tooth with an infected pulp; appears as a widening of the PDL and an obliteration of the lamina dura.
    b. Periapical granuloma, which is a radiolucent area at the apex of a nonvital, typically asymptomatic tooth (caused by pulp death or necrosis).

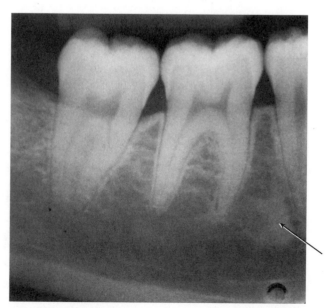

Figure 7.42 Sclerotic bone near the root apex of an asymptomatic vital tooth.

c. Condensing osteitis (chronic focal sclerosing osteomyelitis), which is a radiopaque area (attached to the apex of a nonvital tooth) associated with a low-grade infection (Fig. 7–41).

d. Sclerotic bone (osteosclerosis), which is a radiopaque, defined area around the apices of an asymptomatic, noncarious, nonvital tooth; most likely is associated with inflammation (Fig. 7–42).

 CONTENT REVIEW QUESTIONS

1. Which radiology innovator is known as the father of the science of radiation protection?
   A. Wilhelm Roentgen
   B. Howard Raper
   C. Edmund Kells
   D. William Rollins –

2. Which one of the following energies in the electromagnetic spectrum is considered ionizing radiation?
   A. radar rays
   B. radio waves
   C. infrared rays
   D. gamma rays –

3. What is the source of electrons used for x-ray production?
   A. tungsten filament –
   B. molybdenum cup
   C. tungsten target
   D. copper stem

4. What part of the circuit provides the energy to propel the electrons and produce x-rays?
   A. filament circuit
   B. high-voltage circuit –
   C. step-down transformer
   D. milliampere

5. Where does the generation of x-rays in the x-ray tube actually occur?
   A. tungsten filament
   B. focusing cup
   C. copper stem
   D. tungsten target –

6. When x-rays interact with an outer shell electron of an atom, causing ionization and scattering in a different direction, it is called:
   A. the photoelectric effect
   B. coherent/Thompson scatter
   C. Compton scatter –
   D. no interaction

7. Which theory best describes the free radical formation that is so injurious to living tissue?
   A. direct theory
   B. indirect theory –
   C. dose response curve

8. What unit of radiation represents the amount of radiation energy absorbed by the tissue?
   A. roentgen
   B. sievert
   C. dose rate
   D. gray –

9. What factor is most important when considering the biologic effects of radiation used in dentistry?
   A. whole body exposure
   B. limited area exposure –
   C. acute exposure (limited area)
   D. latent period

10. Which one of the following cell types is most sensitive to radiation?
    A. highly specialized cells
    B. mature cells
    C. slowly dividing cells
    D. immature cells –

11. All of the following reduce patient exposure to radiation, EXCEPT:
    A. filtration
    B. collimation
    C. positioning –
    D. lead apron

12. Which one of the following reduces operator exposure to radiation?
    A. fast film
    B. distance –
    C. PID
    D. film-holding device

13. Which radiographic technique has less distortion and magnification and creates a more accurate image on film?
    A. bisecting-angle
    B. occlusal
    C. paralleling –
    D. panoramic

14. Which one of these extraoral techniques is used specifically to evaluate the maxillary sinuses?
    A. Waters –
    B. lateral cephalometric
    C. panoramic
    D. lateral jaw

15. Which one of the following is used to restrict the size of the x-ray beam?
    A. filtration
    B. collimation –
    C. film-holding device
    D. fast film

16. If the source-to-film distance is changed from 8 to 24 inches, the intensity of the beam becomes:
    A. three times as intense
    B. nine times as intense
    C. one ninth as intense –
    D. one third as intense

17. Magnification occurs when there is a:
    A. long object-film distance
    B. small focal spot
    C. parallel object and film
    D. short target-film distance

18. Which one of these film processing ingredients converts energized crystals into metallic silver?
    A. sodium carbonate
    B. sodium thiosulfate
    C. potassium alum
    D. hydroquinone/elon

19. What is the processing order that films undergo in an automatic film processor?
    A. water, developer, water, fixer, dry
    B. developer, water, fixer, dry
    C. developer, fixer, water, dry
    D. developer, water, fixer, water, dry

20. Which of the following is LEAST likely to cause fogged film?
    A. improper safelighting
    B. developer spots
    C. outdated film
    D. light leakage

21. Which radiopaque maxillary anatomic landmark is MOST likely to be seen on a maxillary incisor periapical radiograph?
    A. nasal septum
    B. median palatal suture
    C. zygomatic process
    D. genial tubercles

22. Which radiolucent mandibular anatomic landmark is MOST likely to be seen on a mandibular molar periapical radiograph?
    A. lingual foramen
    B. external oblique line
    C. submandibular fossa
    D. mental foramen

23. The arrow in picture A indicates which condition?U
    A. root surface caries
    B. vertical bone loss
    C. horizontal bone loss
    D. gingivitis

24. The arrow in picture B, which points to a radiopaque area, indicates which condition?

A. external resorption
B. periapical abscess
C. sclerotic bone
D. condensing osteitis

25. Which of the following steps in the radiograph mounting process is first?
    A. organizing films by anatomic area
    B. separating maxillary from mandibular films
    C. placing films dot-side up
    D. mounting premolar films first

26. Root caries are:
    A. typically located at the middle third of the root
    B. identified as well-circumscribed radiopacities
    C. associated with bone loss and gingival recession
    D. found more often in adolescents

27. Partially formed third molars on a panoramic radiograph indicate that the patient is MOST likely _____.
    A. 6 to 10 years of age
    B. 11 to 15 years of age
    C. 16 to 20 years of age
    D. 21 to 25 years of age

28. Overlap on a left molar bitewing radiograph is caused by improper:
    A. exposure time
    B. horizontal angulation
    C. film placement
    D. patient movement

29. When placed backwards, a film exposed in the mouth will exhibit:
    A. fogginess
    B. no image
    C. a waffle pattern
    D. a cone cut

30. A patient of record complains of temperature sensitivity in the maxillary right second molar region of the mouth. A full-mouth series of radiographs was taken 2 years previously. Which radiographs should be prescribed?
    A. panoramic
    B. horizontal bitewings
    C. vertical bitewing
    D. periapical

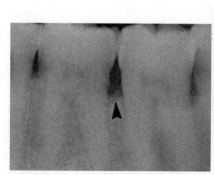

A

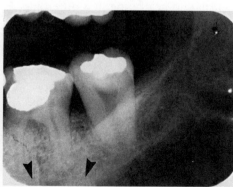

B

31. The "coin test" is a method of assessing:
    A. film freshness
    B. proper kVp settings
    C. contamination by developer
    D. proper safelighting

32. If films are properly exposed at 6 mA for 4 seconds, films exposed for 3 seconds would have an mA of _____?
    A. 2
    B. 8
    C. 16
    D. 24

33. A radiolucent shadow that obscures the apices of the maxillary dentition on a panoramic film indicates that the following error occurred:
    A. the lips were not closed
    B. the midsagittal plane was not perpendicular to the floor
    C. the tongue was not touching the palate
    D. the teeth were not in the focal trough

34. If the x-ray machine is operating at 70 kVp, the following thickness of filtration is necessary:
    A. 1.5 mm
    B. 2.0 mm
    C. 2.5 mm
    D. 3.0 mm

35. The lead diaphragm in the tube head is referred to as the _____.
    A. target
    B. filament
    C. filter
    D. collimator

36. Developing solution splashed on the film prior to processing will result in:
    A. white spots
    B. dark spots
    C. brown stain
    D. yellow stain

37. Which of the following increases penumbra?
    A. increased object-to-film distance
    B. reduced focal spot size
    C. faster-speed film
    D. movement of film

38. The lingual foramen should be evident on the:
    A. maxillary posterior film
    B. maxillary anterior film
    C. mandibular posterior film
    D. mandibular anterior film

39. On a mandibular molar film the most superior radiopaque anatomic landmark is the:
    A. external oblique ridge
    B. coronoid process
    C. internal oblique line
    D. mental process

40. Exposure of a radiograph for ⅗ of a second is equal to _____ impulses?
    A. 3
    B. 15

C. 22
D. 36

41. A white area with a right-angle-shaped border on a film is caused by:
    A. rectangular PID
    B. cylindrical PID
    C. fixer cut off
    D. developer cut off

REVIEW QUESTION RATIONALES

1. **D** William Rollins first alerted the profession to the importance of radiation hygiene and protection and is considered the father of the science of radiation protection. Wilhelm Roentgen discovered x-rays in November of 1895, Howard Raper introduced the bitewing technique in 1925, and C. Edmund Kells introduced the paralleling technique in 1896.

2. **D** Gamma rays are ionizing forms of radiation in the electromagnetic spectrum. Radar rays and infrared rays are not high-energy forms of radiation, thus they do not cause ionization. Radio waves have long wavelengths and therefore cannot cause ionization.

3. **A** Heating the tungsten filament is necessary to provide a source of electrons for the generation of x-rays. The molybdenum cup directs the electrons to the tungsten target in the anode. The tungsten target is the spot in the anode that the electrons hit to produce x-rays. The copper stem in the anode dissipates the heat that is produced.

4. **B** The high voltage circuit provides the voltage necessary to propel the electrons to the anode. The filament circuit controls the heating of the filament and the quantity of available electrons. A step-down transformer is necessary to decrease the incoming voltage to heat the filament. A milliampere is 1/1000 of an ampere and determines the quantity of electrons produced.

5. **D** Electrons hit the tungsten target and convert kinetic energy into heat and x-rays. The tungsten filament has to be heated to provide electrons for x-ray production. The focusing cup in the cathode surrounds the filament and directs the electrons to the target. The target is imbedded in the copper stem, which helps to keep the target cool.

6. **C** Compton scatter occurs when an outer shell electron is removed and scatters in a different direction. The photoelectric effect occurs when an inner shell electron is removed and is absorbed so that it ceases to exist. Coherent/Thompson scatter occurs when an outer shell electron scatters in a different direction but no ionization takes place. No interaction occurs when x-rays pass through the atoms of tissue but never react with them.

7. **B** The indirect theory explains tissue damage by theorizing that x-ray photons are absorbed into cells, causing the production of free radicals (toxins); this damage is believed to be caused by the water

content in cells. The direct theory explains damage as occurring from a direct hit to the target within a cell; this damage seldom occurs. The dose response curve graphically demonstrates that any level of radiation exposure causes a response from the tissue.

8. **D** Gray is the (SI) unit that represents the amount of energy absorbed by the tissue. Roentgen is the standard unit for measuring the quantity of ionization in air. Sievert is the (SI) unit for dose equivalent and is used to compare different types of radiation. Dose rate is the amount of radiation absorbed per unit of time.

9. **B** Limited area exposure refers to radiation in a small area, such as occurs in dental radiation. Whole body exposure is more extensive but is not used in dentistry. Acute exposure-limited area refers to exposure to high doses of radiation in a specific area. The latent period is the time between exposure and the observable effect.

10. **D** Immature cells divide rapidly and therefore are the most sensitive to radiation. Highly specialized cells are more radioresistant to radiation. Mature cells do not change; because they are more specialized in function, they are less sensitive to radiation. Cells that divide at a slow rate have less cell activity and less reaction to radiation.

11. **C** Positioning the patient reduces the risk of exposure to the operator but not to the patient. Filtration reduces radiation by filtering out the nonproductive x-rays. Collimation reduces radiation exposure by restricting the size of the beam directed at the patient's face. A lead apron shields the patient from unnecessary nonproductive scatter radiation.

12. **B** A distance of at least 6 feet from the primary beam is essential for reducing operator exposure. Faster film reduces exposure to the patient. A PID (position-indicating device) should be lead-lined and rectangular to reduce patient exposure. Film-holding devices reduce exposure to the patient's hand.

13. **C** The paralleling technique is superior and provides a more accurate image because the primary beam is at right angles to the tooth and the film. The bisecting-angle technique is not as accurate because the use of a bisecting line allows for more errors. The occlusal technique results in a large amount of distortion, which is caused by the dramatic angles used and the need for greater coverage. The panoramic technique leads to greater distortion because of the blurred images outside the focal trough due to the need for a larger survey.

14. **A** Waters projection is specifically designed to show the maxillary sinus area. The lateral cephalometric technique is designed to show trauma, facial growth, and development. Panoramic projection is used to evaluate impactions, diseases, and growths of the jaw. Lateral jaw exposure is designed to show the posterior part of the mandible and is used for patients who are unable to open their mouths.

15. **B** Collimation is a lead diaphragm that restricts the size of the x-ray beam directed at the patient's face to 2.75 inches. Filtration uses an aluminum disc to filter out the nonproductive, longer wavelengths from the primary beam. A film-holding device is used to hold the film in place but does not restrict the size of the primary beam. Fast film reduces radiation exposure to the patient but does not restrict the size of the beam.

16. **C** According to the inverse square law, the intensity decreases as the distance from the source increases; this would be adding the same amount of distance each time when it really should be squared. The intensity of the beam does not increase as this suggests, but decreases; because the distance is three times the original, it cannot be one third the original intensity.

17. **A** An increased target-film distance allows more parallel rays to hit the film, thus less magnification occurs. A small focal spot size in the x-ray tube increases sharpness. If the object and film are parallel to each other, distortion is decreased. A short target-film distance increases magnification because less parallel rays hit the film.

18. **D** Hydroquinone in the developing solution converts the energized crystals into metallic silver. Sodium carbonate softens the emulsion and speeds up the action of the developing agents. Sodium thiosulfate, in the fixer solution, clears the unexposed silver halide crystals from the emulsion. Potassium alum, in the fixer, shrinks and hardens the emulsion.

19. **C** The processing order that films go through in the automatic processor is "developer-fixer-water-dry." In automatic processing, a reduced number of water baths and the addition of hardeners in the developer and fixer solutions allow film emulsion to remain firm throughout the automated procedure. Film exposed to too much moisture will become soft and prone to stick to the machine roller. In manual processing, water baths between developing and fixing are necessary and film softness is not an issue because the chemical concentrations and temperatures used are not as high as those used in automatic processing.

20. **B** Developer spots occur when the developing solution contacts the film before the processing procedures begin. Proper safelighting (with a bulb of no more than 15 watts, a red filter, and a minimum distance of 4 feet from the working surface) is necessary. The expiration date on the film should be checked and the film should be stored in a cool, dry environment. Because film is sensitive to white light, the darkroom should be "white-light tight."

21. **A** The nasal septum is a vertical radiopaque strip that separates the nasal fossa. The median palatal suture is a thin radiolucent line between the maxillary central incisors. The zygomatic process is a radiopaque u-shaped band located above the apices of the maxillary molars. Genial tubercles are four radi-

opaque bony spines located below the apices of the mandibular central incisors.

22. **C** The submandibular fossa is a radiolucent band that runs below the mylohyoid and the apices of the molars. The lingual foramen is a radiolucent circle inside the genial tubercles, below the apices of the mandibular central incisors. The external oblique line is a radiopaque line that runs anterior from the ramus across the mandibular molars. The mental foramen is a radiolucent oval below the apices of the premolars.

23. **C** Horizontal bone loss appears as a fuzziness of the lamina dura and is located more than 1.5 to 2.0 mm below the CEJ. Root surface caries are indicated by a radiolucent ditched-out area on the root of the tooth. Vertical bone loss appears as a fuzziness of the lamina dura and is angular along one side of the tooth. Gingivitis is inflammation of the marginal gingiva but is not apparent on dental radiographs.

24. **D** Condensing osteitis is a radiopaque area at the apex of a nonvital tooth, typically in mandibular first molars with large carious lesions or restorations. External resorption is a loss or blunting of the apex of a tooth. A periapical abscess is a radiolucent area at the apex of a tooth. Sclerotic bone is a defined area below, but not attached to, the apex of a tooth.

25. **C** Films should be placed dot-side up on a lighted viewbox first. Next, films should be organized by anatomic area, separated into maxillary and mandibular groups, and subsequently mounted in the appropriate area. Premolar films typically are mounted after the molar films are in place.

26. **A** Root caries are associated with bone loss and gingival recession, are located on exposed root surfaces (often in cervical areas), are identified as a ditched-out radiolucency, and are found more often in elderly persons (who experience more root exposure and are at risk of medication-induced xerostomia).

27. **B** Partially formed third molars on a panoramic radiograph indicate that the patient is most likely 11 to 15 years of age. The roots of third molars develop approximately 6 years before their expected eruption at age 18 to 21. Third molars may not be present in individuals 6 to 10 years of age. Individuals 16 years of age and older should exhibit well formed third molars.

28. **B** Overlap on a left molar bitewing radiograph is caused by improper horizontal angulation. Improper exposure time affects the darkness or lightness of a film, poor film placement affects which teeth get exposed or how well the film is centered, and patient movement results in blurring.

29. **C** A film that is exposed when placed backward in the mouth will exhibit a waffle or herringbone pattern. Fogginess is associated with old film, no image indicates a lack of exposure, and a cone cut is associated with cone placement.

30. **D** For a patient of record with a specific complaint (temperature sensitivity in the maxillary right second molar region of the mouth) and a fairly recent full-mouth series of radiographs, a periapical radiograph is the best choice. Temperature sensitivity often is associated with pulpal pathology, and periapical film provides coverage of the entire tooth structure and the bone surrounding the apex of the specific site. A panoramic film is not recommended because it may not provide the clarity required to detect pulpal pathology or other site-specific conditions and it requires exposure to greater amounts of radiation than a periapical film. Horizontal and vertical bitewing films do not provide coverage of the root apex and surrounding bone and thus are not as helpful.

31. **D** The "coin test" is a method of assessing improper safelighting caused by excessive bulb wattage, improper distance, or inadequate filtration. Film freshness is confirmed by the expiration date and by the absence of film fogginess. Proper kVp settings affect film quality as determined by the gray, black, and white tones of a film. Contamination by developer solution is identified by dark spots on the film.

32. **B** Multiplying milliamperage and time gives the total number of x-rays produced (mA X seconds = mAs). The total number of x-rays produced affects the film density; therefore, an increase in one (mA or time) requires a decrease in the other (time or mA) to maintain a similar density.

33. **C** The patient's tongue must be touching the palate or the resulting air space will appear as a radiolucent line, obscuring the apices of the anterior teeth. Open lips result in a radiolucent shadow that obscures the anterior teeth. Improper midsagittal alignment results in unequal magnification of the ramus and the posterior teeth. Distortion of the anterior teeth (a wide or thin appearance) occurs if the teeth are outside of the focal trough.

34. **C** According to federal and state regulations, the filtration (thickness of aluminum) for machines operating below 70 kVp is 1.5 mm. Machines operating at 70 kVp and above are required to have a filtration thickness of 2.5 mm.

35. **D** The collimator, which is located in the tube head, is a lead doughnut or diaphragm. The target refers to the tungsten target in the anode. The filament is the tungsten filament in the cathode. The filter refers to the aluminum filter that is used to eliminate longer wavelengths from the beam.

36. **B** Precontamination of the film with developing solution results in an overdevelopment of the affected areas and causes dark spots. Precontamination with fixer solution clears the film of silver halide in the emulsion, resulting in white spots. Insufficient washing of films after fixing results in brown or yellow stains.

37. **B** Reducing the focal spot size increases penumbra; film movement and increasing the object-to-film distance or film speed decreases penumbra (sharpness).

38. **D** Because the lingual foramen is located below the apices of the mandibular anterior incisors at the midline, it can be seen only on mandibular anterior film.

39. **A** The external oblique ridge is the most superior radiopaque anatomic landmark on mandibular molar film. The coronoid process appears only on maxillary molar films. The internal oblique line is the inferior radiopaque landmark on a mandibular film, and the mental process is a radiopaque landmark located below the mandibular incisors.

40. **D** Converting seconds to impulses requires cross-multiplication. It is necessary to know that each impulse equals 1/60 of a second (3/5 = x/60; 5x = 180; x = 36). Therefore, 3/5 of a second equals 36 impulses.

41. **A** The right-angle shape is the border of a rectangular PID. A circular border is caused by a cylindrical PID. Fixer cut-off has a straight black border, and a developer cut-off has a straight white border.

Suggested Readings

Brian J: Radiology Flash Cards. Anaheim, California, Bryan Edwards Publishing, 1999.

Haring JI, Lind LJ: Dental Radiography: Principles and Techniques. Philadelphia, WB Saunders, 1996.

Langland OE, Langlais RP: Principles of Dental Imaging. Baltimore, Williams and Wilkins, 1997.

Goaz PW, White SC: Oral Radiology, 3rd ed. St Louis, Mosby, 1994.

Quality Assurance in Dental Radiography. Rochester, New York, Eastman Kodak Company, 1998.

Miles DA, Vandis ML, Jensen CW, Ferretti AB: Radiographic Imaging for Dental Auxiliaries. Philadelphia, WB Saunders, 1999.

Chapter EIGHT

Infection Control

Donal Scheidel, DDS

 ## Clinical Case STUDY

Maureen is a new dental assistant in the office. She has had no education or experience in dental assisting but has held a dental office receptionist position for 3 months. Between patients, Maureen carefully washes her gloves. She wears the same mask throughout the day, even though it appears moist and has a small bloodstain on it. At the end of the day, Maureen walks out of the office without changing her clothes.

Clinical Case QUESTIONS

1. What training should Maureen have had before participating in patient treatment?
2. What immunization issues must be addressed if Maureen is to continue employment at Dr. Jones' office?
3. Identify mistakes that Maureen made on her first day of work.
4. What implications do these mistakes have regarding Maureen's health and the health of the patients?

Clinical Case RATIONALES

1. Maureen should have had comprehensive training in office infection control policy and procedures before she began seeing patients. Maureen does not understand the concepts of cross contamination, chain of infection, or how to use personal protective equipment.
2. Maureen must review her personal immunization record to verify her present status. She must be up to date with immunizations against measles, mumps, rubella, and tetanus. In addition, she must begin the hepatitis B vaccination series (or sign a waiver of refusal) within 10 days of employment in order to maintain employment in Dr. Jones' office. She can continue employment while she receives the three-dose regimen. She also would be well advised to receive the influenza vaccine to help prevent future sickness and missed workdays.
3. Maureen was washing and reusing her latex gloves. She was not changing her mask between patients or when it became soiled or damp. She also wore her office uniform home after work. Because Maureen was violating these infection control rules, she may have been violating others and contaminating the office with infectious agents.
4. Maureen's health was in danger because of her lack of knowledge of infection control practices. She had been endangering the health and well-being of her staff members and patients since her employment began. In addition, her family and friends also were at risk for infection from contaminated items (including her uniform and her skin) that Maureen carried outside of the dental office.

Content Review

General Terminology

Bioburden—Build-up of organic debris on instruments and occupational surfaces during the course of care delivery.

CDC—The Centers for Disease Control and Prevention, an agency of the Department of Health and Human Services. The mission of CDC is to promote health and quality of life by preventing and controlling disease, injury, and disability.

Disinfection—Inhibition or destruction of pathogens on inanimate surfaces. Spores are not killed during disinfection.

Infective agents—Bacteria, viruses, protozoa, and fungi that have the capacity to cause infectious diseases in humans.

Oral health care worker (OHCW)—Anyone who is involved in patient care or who comes in contact with items contaminated with blood or saliva. Included in this category would be the dentist, dental assistant, dental hygienist, sterilization technician, and laboratory technician. Occasionally, clerical personnel fall into this category when they are called on to assist in patient care, clean patient treatment rooms, or clean and sterilize instruments.

OSHA—The Occupational Safety and Health Administration, a division of the Department of Labor. OSHA's mission is to protect workers in America from physical, chemical, or infectious hazards in the workplace.

Personal protective equipment—Protective barriers that OHCWs are required to wear; are designed to eliminate OHCW exposure to bloodborne pathogens and infectious agents.

Sanitation—A process of cleaning inanimate objects that is designed to reduce the microbial count to levels that are considered safe by the public health community.

Sterilization—Destroys or removes all forms of life, including bacteria and mycotic spores.

Infective Agents

The successful practice of infection control in the dental office requires a defined program that is designed to prevent the transmission of communicable disease from patient to patient, from patient to dental professional, and from dental professional to patient.

Infections of Bacterial Origin

The many types of bacteria are involved in different disease processes in the mouth and body and are of great importance to dental professionals.

I. *Mycobacterium tuberculosis* (TB)
   A. Negatively impacts the patient's overall health; has significant implications in the delivery of dental care.
   B. Affects the patient's oral health as a result of poor systemic health.
   C. Infection typically requires a long antibiotic treatment regimen for elimination of the disease.
      1. Some patients have multi-drug resistant tuberculosis.
         a. Multi-drug resistant tuberculosis typically is associated with HIV infection.
         b. HIV-positive patients with undiagnosed pulmonary infection should be suspected of having tuberculosis.
   D. Mode of transmission is through water droplets produced by coughing.
      1. Dental professionals can contract tuberculosis from infected patients if barrier techniques are not used.
      2. Tuberculosis can be transmitted from patient to patient if infection control procedures are not followed.

3. Performance of elective dental care on patients with active TB should be avoided when possible.

II. Upper Respiratory Tract Infections of Bacterial Origin
   A. Are easily transmitted in the dental office because of the close proximity of patient and dental professional.
   B. Are transmitted through coughing, sneezing, and aerosolization of the bacteria.
   C. Can involve the sinuses, larynx, pharynx, and the lungs.
   D. Infective agents include *Haemophilus influenzae*, *Klebsiella pneumoniae*, and *Mycoplasma pneumoniae*.
   E. Preventing transmission involves breaking the chain of infection by frequent hand washings, changing of masks, sterilization of instruments, and disinfection of environmental surfaces.

Infections of Viral Origin

The transmission of viral infections has long been a concern for dental professionals. Viruses such as hepatitis, herpes, measles, and influenza are particularly important. During the past 15 years, the human immunodeficiency virus has refocused the concerns of those in the dental profession on the importance of infection control in the dental office.

I. Several viral infections that have been long-standing occupational hazards for dental professionals include:
   A. Viral hepatitis infection
      1. Results in inflammation of the liver, cirrhosis, and carcinoma of the liver.
      2. Is caused by several specific causative agents: hepatitis A virus (HAV), hepatitis B virus (HBV), hepatitis C virus (HCV), and hepatitis D virus (HDV or delta virus).
         a. Hepatitis A (HAV) infection
            1) Causes an illness characterized by an abrupt onset and fever, malaise, abdominal discomfort, and jaundice.
            2) Is transmitted by person-to-person contact (fecal-oral contamination) or by food or water contamination.[1]
            3) Is a low risk for dental professionals; no recommendation for hepatitis A vaccination for dental professionals exists at this time.
         b. Hepatitis B (HBV) infection
            1) Is a major health problem in the United States and has a direct impact on the practice of dental hygiene.
            2) Affects approximately 1 to 1.25 million HBV carriers in the United States.[2]
            3) Approximately 5,000 to 6,000 deaths in the United States occur annually from the infection or its complications.[2]
            4) Has a long onset with symptoms similar to hepatitis A.

5) Is transmitted in the dental office, typically from patient to dental professional, through:
   a) Injuries from contaminated sharps.
   b) Splatter of contaminated blood and saliva onto open mucous membranes or open areas of the skin.
   c) Spread of contaminated blood to open lesions on ungloved hands or through torn gloves.
   c. Hepatitis C (HCV) infection
      1) Accounts for approximately 30% of all cases of acute viral hepatitis in the United States.
      2) Is transmitted via IV drug use, transfusions, and occupational exposure (in health care workers).
      3) 75%–85% of infected persons become chronically infected carriers of HCV.[3]
   d. Hepatitis D (HDV) infection
      1) Is infective only in the presence of HBV; is considered a complication of HBV and is not common in the United States, except among populations with a high incidence of percutaneous exposures (i.e., drug abusers).
B. Herpes simplex (HSV-1 or HSV-2) infection
   1. Is transmitted by direct mucocutaneous contact with infected lesions.
   2. Initially may be asymptomatic or may present with fever, malaise, gingival inflammation, and eruption of small clusters of vesicles throughout the mouth.
   3. Recurrent forms produce clusters of vesicles that ulcerate.
      a. Vesicles follow the distribution of the infected nerve.
      b. Vesicles form on extraoral sites (e.g., the lip in recurrent herpes labialis) or on intra-oral tissues overlying bone (e.g., the palate or the gingiva).
      c. Weeping of the lesions may easily spread the infection to other sites (intraoral or extraoral) or other persons.
C. Colds and upper respiratory tract viral infections
   1. Are caused by influenza A and B, *Rhinovirus, adenovirus, and Coronavirus.*
   2. Are easily transmitted by aerosolization (direct contact between patient and dental health professional) and by contact with contaminated surfaces (indirect contact).
D. Human immunodeficiency virus (HIV) infection
   1. Is caused by the HIV virus, which was discovered in 1981 and changed the way dental hygiene is practiced; several mutations of the original virus are known to exist.

2. Involves an HIV attack on T4 lymphocytes, which results in a significant decrease in the T4 cell count as the disease progresses.
   a. Once the cell-mediated immune system is depleted, the patient experiences infections not normally seen in healthy individuals or infections that have a greater severity than those typically seen.
3. Is caused by transmission of HIV through intimate sexual contact (involving the exchange of semen or vaginal secretions); exposure to contaminated blood or blood products, or blood-contaminated bodily fluids; or from infected mother to child.
   a. HIV is easily killed outside the body (more easily than HBV or *Mycobacterium tuberculosis*).

Infection Control Rationale

A planned system of preventing disease transmission is an important element of dental office protocol. Most diseases that are transmissible in the dental office are difficult or impossible to cure; consequently, preventing transmission is of the utmost importance.

Elements of Infection Control Protocol

The Centers for Disease Control (CDC) Bloodborne Pathogens Standard Recommendations, which were adopted by the Occupational Health and Safety Administration (OSHA), focus on taking and reviewing detailed patient medical histories, appropriate immunization of dental professionals, sterilization and disinfection of multiple use instruments and environmental surfaces, use of barrier techniques in the care of all patients, and appropriate disposal of dental sharps and waste generated during care delivery to prevent the transmission of disease.

I. Sources of Contamination in the Dental Office
   A. Aerosols created by:
      1. Coughing, sneezing, or breathing.
      2. Prophylaxis angles, brushes, or cups.
      3. Air-water syringes used to rinse the oral cavity; air water syringes also pick up contaminants through capillary action and act as a possible source of contamination for the next patient.
      4. Ultrasonic and sonic scalers.
      5. High-speed handpieces and air-polishing devices.
   B. Suction tips and lines:
      1. May contain residues of infectious material from previous procedures.
      2. May harbor permanent colonies of bacteria if not regularly cleaned.
   C. Dental unit water lines:
      1. May serve as a source of bacterial contamination.
      2. Serve as a safe harbor for bacteria that naturally occur in the water supply.

3. Also harbor patient bacteria by drawing back (sucking back) contaminated oral fluids.
   a. Waterlines that contain bacteria have not yet been identified as a major threat regarding the spread of infection to dental patients; current studies are attempting to determine patient risk. Immunocompromised patients may be at greatest risk.
   b. Self-contained water units, antiretraction valves, and backflow preventive devices are commercially available and were developed to help eliminate the risk of a patient drawing back contaminated water.

II. Possible Modes of Disease Transmission (patient to patient, patient to OHCW, OHCW to patient) in the dental office involve:
   A. A chain of infection that relies on the presence of an infectious agent, an area for the infectious agent to grow, and a way to move from the growth niche to the host.
      1. The chain of infection must be broken to prevent disease transmission in the dental office.
      2. Methods used to break the chain of infection include OHCWs washing their hands between patients and when gloves tear; wearing gloves; using protective barriers for mouth, nose, and eyes; wearing protective clothing; and laundering clinic attire and street clothing separately.
      3. Additional methods used to break the chain of infection include:
         a. Sterilization (destruction of all forms of life) of reusable dental instruments; is recommended for all dental instruments; is a must for instruments in the critical category (e.g., scalers, burs, bone chisels, scalpels) and in the semicritical category (if heat-stable).[4,5]
         b. Disinfection (destruction of pathogens but not of spores) of instruments unable to withstand the heat of sterilization; must be high-level disinfection for heat-unstable instruments in the semicritical category; can be used for noncritical surfaces.[4,5]
         c. Disinfection of environmental surfaces in the operatory
         d. Reducing the oral microflora population with an antimicrobial rinse before treatment.
         e. Minimizing the aerosolization of microorganisms with a high-volume suction and avoiding the use of a combined air-water spray.
   B. Occupational exposure to infected blood, saliva, or serum (direct contact) by:
      1. Needlestick/sharps injuries.
      2. Transfer of an open skin wound or mucous membrane.
      3. Airborne transfer of infectious agents.
      4. Splatter involved in the delivery of oral health care (rinsing the patient's mouth, using the prophy angle to polish, debridement with sonic and ultrasonic scalers).
      5. Failure to use high-volume suction.
      6. Depressing the air and water buttons on the air-water syringe at the same time.

III. Immunizations
   A. OHCWs must be up to date on their vaccinations for many vaccine-preventable diseases.
      1. Hepatitis B (HBV)
         a. Full-time, part-time, temporary, and probationary employees must begin the series of vaccine injections during the first 10 working days of employment.
         b. New employees can continue to provide patient care during the 6 months needed to complete the series of vaccinations; new employees may refuse the vaccination, but must read and sign the "Refusal for Hepatitis B Vaccination" form.
         c. Vaccinations must be made available to the employee free of charge and at a reasonable time and location.
         d. A licensed physician or appropriate health care professional must supervise the administration of the vaccine.
         e. Employees who receive the vaccination must have appropriate documentation in their medical records.
         f. Employees who are vaccinated against hepatitis B (HBV) also are considered protected against Hepatitis D.
         g. Primary immunization with hepatitis B vaccine consists of three intramuscular doses; the second and third doses should be given 1 and 6 months after the first, respectively.
         h. The vaccine is administered unless the individual has antibodies to HBV antigens or has HBV antigens in his or her blood.
         i. Vaccinated individuals should be tested after the last of the three injections to verify a positive response to the vaccine.
   B. Recommended vaccination for influenza virus, rubella, measles, mumps, tetanus, and polio (Table 8–1).

IV. Complete, updated patient medical histories are important for the protection of all parties involved in providing and receiving dental care.
   A. Medical histories identify prescription and over-the-counter (OTC) medications that the patient is taking.
      1. Medications give clues to the patient's medical condition and enable dental care professionals to explain the possible impact on oral health that the condition or the medications may have.
      2. A combination of written and oral questions gives a patient the opportunity to explain his or her condition.

TABLE 8.1	Recommended Vaccination Schedule for OHCWs	
Generic Name of Vaccine	**Primay Schedule/Boosters**	**Precautions/Contraindications**
Hepatitis B recombinant DNA	Two doses IM 4 weeks apart; third dose 5 months after second.	Pregnancy not a contraindication if patient is otherwise eligible; history of anaphylactic reaction to baker's yeast.
Rubella live virus	One dose SC; no booster.	Pregnancy; immunocompromised condition; history of anaphylactic reaction after taking neomycin.
Measles live virus	One dose SC; 2nd dose in 1 month; no routine boosters.	Pregnancy; immunocompromised condition; history of anaphylactic reaction after taking neomycin, eating gelatin, or eating eggs; recent administration of immune globulin.
Mumps live virus	One dose SC; no booster.	Pregnancy; immunocompromised condition; history of anaphylactic reaction after taking neomycin, eating gelatin, or eating eggs.
Influenza (inactivated whole-virus and split-virus vaccine)	Annual vaccination with current vaccine; use either whole- or split-virus vaccine.	History of anaphylactic reaction after egg ingestion.
Tetanus-diphtheria toxoid	Two doses IM 4 weeks apart; third dose 6–12 months after second dose; booster every 10 years after previous dose.	Pregnancy (first trimester); immunocompromised history of neurologic reaction or immediate hypersensitivity reaction.
Enhanced-potency inactivated poliovirus (E-IPV) or live oral poliovirus (OPV)	E-IPV is preferred for primary vaccination of adults; two doses SC 4–8 weeks apart, a third dose 6–12 months after the second. For adults with a completed primary series and for whom a booster is indicated, either OPV or E-IPV can be given.	OPV should not be given to immunocompromised individuals or to patients with known or possibly immunocompromised family members; E-IPV is recommended in such situations.

IM, intramuscularly; SC, subcutaneously.

3. Noting the specialties of listed physicians gives clues as to medical conditions that the patient is monitoring.
4. Increased trust between the patient and the provider promotes patient honesty in divulging his or her medical history.

B. A dental office must maintain the confidentiality of patients' medical records.

 ## Clinical Case STUDY

Randy Johnson has returned for his 6-month recall appointment. Randy says that he is very faithful about keeping his recall appointments because "I don't want to wear dentures like my dad." A review of Randy's medical history reveals allergies to milk, eggs, and bee stings. He has no known allergies to any medications. Because Randy has not had dental radiographs taken during the past 18 months, four bitewing radiographs are taken. Upon returning from developing the radiograph films, the dental hygienist observes that Randy's lips appear swollen. Randy complains that he is having difficulty breathing. His breathing appears labored and is noisy (wheezing).

Clinical Case QUESTIONS

1. What is the most likely cause of Randy's symptoms?
2. What should be done immediately?
3. What office preparations are necessary to ensure that Randy does not have the same experience during his next dental appointment?
4. OHCWs also can develop this response. What precautions can minimize the risk of developing this response?

Clinical Case RATIONALES

1. Randy appears to be having an anaphylactic reaction. The swelling of his lips indicates that he has had contact with an allergen. Because latex is a common allergen, exposure to the powders on latex gloves is a likely cause of this response.
2. Activate the office emergency plan. Inform the dentist, call 911, and provide oxygen if necessary. The dentist must determine whether appropriate medications from the emergency kit should be administered.
3. The office must identify all instruments, equipment, and protective devices (anything that contacts the patient) that contain latex. The office should order replacement devices that do not contain latex to ensure safe patient care.

4. Powder free, hypoallergenic gloves help prevent latex allergies. Residual latex proteins are the allergens responsible for the latex allergic response. These proteins bind to the powder that is used to facilitate glove application and are transmitted to the wearer. Hypoallergenic gloves are specially treated to remove most of the residual latex proteins responsible for the allergic response. Oral health care professionals must wash their hands after wearing latex gloves. Oil-based lotions (e.g., petroleum, mineral oil, lanolin, coconut oil) should not be worn because these oils break down the glove barrier and cause the release of more allergens.

Universal Precautions

Whenever there is a potential for contacting blood, blood-contaminated saliva, mucous membranes, or respiratory secretions, Universal Precautions must be instituted to ensure that care is taken to prevent exposure to the body fluids of others. All body fluids have the potential to be contaminated and these precautions should be applied equally to all patients.[6]

I. Protective Barriers
   A. Include gloves, mask, protective clothing, and protective eyewear that must be changed between patients and when visible contamination is present.

BOX 8.1 Recommendations for Latex Allergy

1. Oral health care providers should be familiar with both immediate and delayed latex hypersensitivity and the risks involved.
2. Hand washing after glove use may reduce the likelihood of developing latex hypersensitivity.
3. All people with immediate-type allergy symptoms (eye itching and watering, coughing, sneezing, runny nose, decreased blood pressure, shortness of breath, and dizziness that develop within minutes of latex exposure) should avoid all contact with latex products.
4. Latex allergens in the air can cause respiratory and/or anaphylactic symptoms in susceptible individuals.
5. Exposure to latex may cause reactions (allergic, anaphylactic) that should be treated aggressively.
6. Oral health care providers with hand dermatitis are advised to use hypoallergenic gloves.
7. Dental patients may be at risk for developing latex allergies to latex gloves, rubber dams, prophy cups, or orthodontic elastics during a dental procedure.
8. Patients with spina bifida should be treated in a latex-free environment because of the high incidence of reactions to latex among this population.
9. People with latex allergies should wear an allergy alert label as a precautionary measure.
10. Latex allergies must be documented in the dental record and given the same importance as other drug allergies the patient may have.
11. Dental offices should identify all latex-containing devices in their office and have backup devices that are latex-free for the hypersensitive patient.

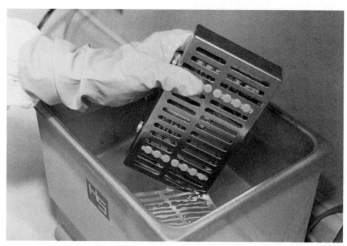

Figure 8.1 Sturdy utility gloves are used when handling contaminated instruments.

I. Gloves
   a. Types of gloves include:
      1) Single-use examination gloves (nonsterile). Can be made of latex, vinyl, or non-vinyl materials (Box 8–1).
      2) Single-use sterile gloves (typically used in conjunction with surgical procedures). Can be either latex or vinyl.
      3) Single-use plastic overgloves; are worn over treatment gloves to prevent cross-contamination (e.g., of charts, drawers, writing instruments).
      4) Multiple-use utility gloves made of heavy latex, rubber, or neoprene and used during handling of contaminated instruments, cleaning of operatories, or handling of chemicals (Fig. 8–1).
   b. Protocols for glove use
      1) Gloves must be used whenever contact with blood, saliva, mucous membranes, or blood-contaminated objects is a possibility.
      2) Hands must be washed before and after wearing gloves.
      3) Gloves should extend over the cuffs of long-sleeved treatment gowns.
      4) Defective gloves must be changed immediately (accompanied by appropriate hand washing).
      5) Gloves must be changed between patients or during long appointments (approximately one third of all gloves allow bacteria leakage during 40 to 50 minutes of use).[9]
      6) When OHCWs decide to double-glove, they must double-glove for every patient; double-gloving increases costs, decreases manual dexterity, and is not recommended by the CDC, ADA, or OSHA.

2. Masks
   a. Types of masks include:
      1) Glass fiber mat and synthetic fiber mat are the most effective types.
      2) Dome masks with elastic bands provide space between the mask and mouth and reduce moistening of the mask (which increases its effectiveness).
      3) Surgical masks (ear-loop or tie-on type) filter smaller particles better but become moist quicker, thus compromising operator protection.
   b. Mask wearing recommendations include:
      1) Changing masks between patients.
      2) Placing and adjusting the mask before hand washing.
      3) Avoiding touching of the mask during an appointment.
      4) Continuing to wear mask after completion of procedures for protection against particulate matter/microorganisms in the ambient air.
      5) Avoiding contamination of the mask with disinfectants or other chemicals.
      6) Removing the mask over the head by the elastic or ties; avoiding touching of the mask proper and dangling mask around the neck.
3. Protective eyewear
   a. Types of protective eyewear:
      1) Prescription eyewear offers limited protection because of open top, sides, and bottom.
      2) Safety glasses or goggles cover all areas around the eye, offer excellent protection from splatter, and are shatter resistance.
      3) Face shields ensure maximum coverage but a mask also must be worn for protection from inhalation of contaminants (Fig. 8–2).

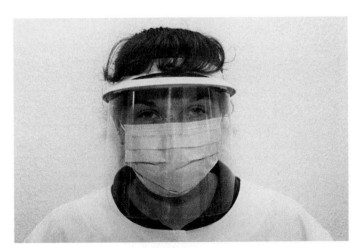

Figure 8.2 Face shields worn with a mask provide protection during aerosol-producing procedures.

   b. Reasons for wearing protective eyewear include:
      1) Prevention of disease transmission (e.g., conjunctivitis, ocular herpes, hepatitis B).
      2) Protection against a penetrating eye injury.
      3) Protection against chemical splatter (e.g., disinfectants, chemicals with a low pH).
      4) Patient protection (e.g., against chemical splatter, oral debris, dropped instruments).
   c. Eyewear protocols include:
      1) Cleaning and disinfecting eyewear between patients.
      2) Avoiding touching of protective eyewear during care delivery to reduce the possibility of contamination.
      3) Wearing eyewear for every clinical appointment (to prevent loss of or forgetting to use eyewear).
4. Protective clothing
   a. Protocols for wearing protective clothing include:
      1) Wearing protective wear whenever contamination with blood or bodily secretions is likely (e.g., from aerosolization of blood, saliva, respiratory secretions, and microorganisms during ultra-sonic scaling or polishing of teeth).
      2) Changing protective clothing daily or when visibly soiled.
      3) Avoiding wearing of protective clothing outside of the health care facility.
      4) Limiting handling of protective clothing as much as possible after wearing; placing clothing in bags for transportation to laundering facility.
      5) Thoroughly laundering protective clothing between wearings; must be washed separately using commercial laundry detergent, high water temperature (60 to 70°C), and normal bleach concentration. Protective clothing should be machine dried at temperatures above 110°C.
   b. Types of protective clothing include:
      1) Reusable or disposable gowns or uniforms.
      2) Surgical gowns (which are the best choice).
      3) Laboratory coats.
   c. Selection of protective clothing:
      1) Any protective clothing must cover street clothing, fit closely around the neck and wrists, and cover the arms.
      2) Protective clothing made from synthetic material is more protective (more fluid resistant).

II. Environmental Surfaces should be covered to prevent contamination during patient care and should be re-covered between patients to break the chain of infection.
   A. Disinfection of surfaces in the treatment area
      1. Involves identifying the surfaces that must be disinfected after patient treatment (e.g., patient chair, operator chair, dental light, countertops, tray tables, handpiece/air-water syringe supports, all tubing in treatment area, knobs, drawers used during treatment). Some of these surfaces can be isolated using plastic wrap or bags to reduce the time and effort needed to prepare a treatment area for the next patient.
      2. Disinfection technique (Table 8–2)
         a. Dental personnel must wear heavy rubber, nitrile, or neoprene gloves, personal protective clothing, a mask, and protective eyewear when disinfecting treatment areas.
         b. Plastic coverings should be removed and disposed of properly.
         c. Uncovered or contaminated surfaces should be precleaned using a cleaner (detergent) or a cleaner/disinfectant. It is best to use an EPA-registered, tuberculocidal disinfectant for both the cleaning step and the disinfecting step. Surfaces should be sprayed and wiped to dislodge accumulations. Surfaces subsequently should be sprayed again with the disinfectant and should remain wet for the recommended amount of time (10 minutes or less depending on the manufacturer).
            1) Criteria for agent(s) used for disinfection
               a) Must be a water-based disinfectant.
               b) Must be an EPA-registered hospital disinfectant that is labeled viricidal and fungicidal.
               c) Must kill *Mycobacterium tuberculosis* (an organism that is very resistant to disinfection because of its tough cell wall).
               d) Must be compatible with treatment area surfaces.
               e) Must remain active in the presence of organic matter.
               f) Must be compatible with pump spray delivery.
               g) Must be accepted by the ADA Council on Scientific Affairs as an effective disinfectant for use in the dental environment.
            2) Acceptable disinfection agents
               a) Iodophors kill a broad spectrum of microorganisms with minimal allergic reactions; can stain light-colored vinyl and corrode metals.
               b) Sodium hypochlorite (1:10 solution) is viricidal, bactericidal, tuberculocidal, and inexpensive to use; has a strong odor, is unstable, corrodes metals, and is irritating to skin and eyes.
               c) Complex phenols (water-based are better than alcohol-based) are bactericidal and tuberculocidal; most are viricidal (check specific product); are economical; are irritating to skin, eyes, and epithelial tissue; corrode some plastics.
               d) Chlorine dioxide is viricidal only; works rapidly (2 minutes); is corrosive; use should be limited to well-ventilated areas.
   B. Care and disinfection of dental unit water lines
      1. All retraction valves should be replaced with anti-retraction valves; retraction valves were installed before 1981 to prevent the dripping of water from dental handpieces.
      2. Anti-retraction valves should be checked to ensure proper function; they may become stuck (open) over time.
      3. Water lines should be flushed at the beginning of each day for 3 to 5 minutes to reduce

---

TABLE 8.2 Levels of Disinfection		
Level of Disinfection	**Action**	**Use**
High	Kills some but not all bacterial spores and is tuberculocidal. EPA registered disinfectant/sterilizant agents are high-level disinfectants.	Instruments that have touched mucous membranes, have penetrated soft tissue but not touched bone, or those that will not withstand sterilization.
Intermediate	Kills HBV, HIV, *Mycobacterium tuberculosis* (var. bovis); does not kill spores.	Instruments that have contact with intact skin.
Low	Kills most bacteria, some fungi, some viruses; does not kill spores or *Mycobacterium tuberculosis* (var. bovis).	General cleaning.

bacterial counts (e.g., for handpieces, ultrasonic scalers, and air-water syringes).

4. Water lines should be flushed for 20 to 30 seconds between patients to eliminate bacterial accumulation (if unit has been idle for some time, it should be flushed for 3 to 5 minutes).

III. Personal hygiene, including hand washing, is an effective defense against spreading diseases from patient to patient or from patient to dental professional.

A. Hands must be washed between patients, both before placing and after removing gloves. Washing with an antimicrobial liquid soap provides additional protection by leaving a protective layer on the skin.

1. Short hand-washing method: wash hands twice (rinsing in between) for 15 seconds, using an antimicrobial soap, at the beginning of each day. Between patients, wash for 15 seconds using antimicrobial soap.

2. Surgical hand scrub: before surgical procedures, scrub hands and forearms for 5 minutes, repeatedly washing with antimicrobial soap and a soft brush and rinsing off debris. Dry with a sterile towel.

B. Whenever gloves are punctured or torn, hands must be washed and covered with new gloves. (The FDA tests gloves for two minutes. If 2.5% of a particular manufacturer's gloves fail the test, they cannot be sold in the United States. Independent tests show that after 40 to 50 minutes, 33% of tested latex gloves fail.[9])

C. Gloves must not be reused between patients (health care workers must not wash gloves and reuse or attempt to sterilize gloves and reuse).

IV. Care must be taken during instrument processing.

A. To ensure that reusable instruments are safely cleaned and sterilized.

1. Instruments should be presoaked, by an individual wearing heavy rubber, nitrile, or neoprene gloves, to soften dried blood and debris.

2. Instruments should be cleaned by:

a. Hand scrubbing only those instruments that would be damaged if exposed to the ultrasonic cleaner (i.e., some handpieces); extra care should be used in hand scrubbing instruments; heavy rubber/neoprene gloves and personal protective equipment also should be used.

b. Transferring instruments to an ultrasonic cleaner and sonicating for the time recommended by the solution manufacturer (typically 1 to 10 minutes); sonication for cassettes should last longer (15 minutes).

1) Ultrasonic cleaning acts by physical agitation (tiny bubbles form and collapse in the solution) and chemical action (ultrasonic solution helps dissolve organic residue on instruments).

2) Overloading should be prevented; the ultrasonic solution must contact all surfaces.

3) Instruments with detachable parts should be disassembled. Hinged instruments must be opened.

4) Observe the manufacturer's recommended cleaning time.

3. Instruments should be removed, rinsed, and allowed to air dry (if towel drying, carefully pat dry).

4. Instruments must be dry if they are to be packaged in paper sterilizer bags or placed in a dry heat, ethylene oxide, or chemical vapor sterilizer.

5. Instruments must be packaged in appropriate sterilizer bags (or in cassettes).

6. Instruments should be sterilized if they can withstand the heat (otherwise disposable instruments should be used).

7. Instruments should be cooled before being stored.

8. Instruments should be stored to preserve their sterility for future procedures.

B. To prevent the transmission of microorganisms between patients or between patients and dental personnel.

C. To avoid damaging expensive instruments.

D. To disinfect according to the categories of critical surfaces (see Table 8–2).

1. Critical surfaces are items that are used to penetrate soft tissue or bone; they must be sterilized.

2. Semicritical surfaces touch intact mucous membranes or oral fluids but do not penetrate tissues; they require sterilization or high-level disinfection.

3. Noncritical surfaces contact only the skin (do not contact mucous membranes); they require intermediate disinfection.

E. To adequately sterilize reusable instruments (Table 8–3).

1. Types of sterilizers

a. Moist heat (standard)

1) Uses steam under pressure.

2) Is useful for all instruments able to withstand high temperatures.

3) Uses pressure to achieve the high temperatures needed to kill spores, tubercle bacillus, and other contaminants.

4) Requires that instruments have space around them to enable steam to reach all instrument surfaces.

TABLE 8.3 Methods of Sterilization

Method	Time (minutes)	Temperature	Pressure (psi)
Moist heat (Steam autoclave)			
Standard	20	250°F 121°C	15
Quick	12	270°F 130°C	30
Dry heat (Oven)			
Standard	60–120	320°F 160°C	
Quick	12	375°F 190°C	
Unsaturated chemical vapor	20	270°F 130°C	20–40

5) Requires a tight seal against the outside to provide necessary pressure and temperature.

6) Disadvantages include: possibility of corroding instruments, inability to penetrate oils or powders, inability of some instruments to withstand the heat generated in the steam autoclave.

b. Dry heat (standard)
1) Sterilizes by oxidation.
2) Is used for instruments that cannot be sterilized safely by steam autoclave.
3) Is effective for oils and powders if stable at temperatures reached during sterilization.
4) Depends on rapid heat transfer from circulating air to instruments (similar to cooking oven).
5) Advantages include: maintenance of sharp edges on instruments, noncorrosiveness, and usefulness on materials unable to withstand steam under pressure.
6) Disadvantages include: longer sterilization cycle, requirement of careful loading to ensure sterilization, and inability of unwrapped instruments to stay sterile for long.

c. Chemical vapor
1) Uses chemical combinations (e.g., alcohol, formaldehyde, ketone, acetone, and water) that are heated to a gas to effectively sterilize instruments.
2) Requires purchasing the manufacturer's chemical solution, which increases sterilization costs.

3) Gas vapors must penetrate the instrument packaging.
4) Advantages include: corrosion- and rust-free operation, shorter sterilization cycle time, ease of operation, and quick drying of instruments.
5) Disadvantages include: use of hazardous chemicals and need for adequate ventilation because of chemical odor.

d. Ethylene oxide
1) Works by producing a gas that is toxic to all microorganisms at a low temperature.
2) Is used primarily in hospitals and larger clinics; is not used in dental offices.
3) Advantages include: effectiveness without damaging most instruments, use of low temperatures for effective sterilization, and ability to penetrate different wrapping materials.
4) Disadvantages include: very long processing times, high cost of equipment, use of hazardous chemicals, and need for aeration of non-metal items for 24 to 48 hours.

e. Quick turn-around sterilization
1) Dry heat sterilization (e.g., Cox sterilizer)
   a) Maintains internal heat at 375°F.
   b) Sterilizes wrapped instruments in 12 minutes, dental handpieces in 8 minutes.
   c) Is continuously ready; requires no warm-up time.
2) Steam sterilization (e.g., Statim, Kwikclave sterilizer)
   a) Sterilizes wrapped instruments in 12 minutes.
   b) Uses greater pressure and heat than traditional steam sterilizers.

f. Chemical sterilants/disinfectants[4]
1) Must be EPA approved as a high-level disinfectant to be used for semi-critical items.
2) Are reserved only for items (non-critical, semi-critical) that cannot withstand heat sterilization (called cold sterilization); are not a substitute for sterilization by steam, dry heat, chemical vapor, or ethylene oxide.
3) May be reused for 28 to 30 days.
4) Require following manufacturer's directions for use; to achieve high-level disinfection, items must be immersed for long periods of time (6 to 10 hours at 200 to 250°C)[10]
5) Are limited in use because of an inability to verify sterilization of instruments.
6) Cannot be used on packaged instruments; consequently, maintaining a

"sterile" state is difficult; after immersion, instruments must be rinsed with sterile water, dried, and stored in sterile containers.[4]

    7) Contain chemicals that are toxic to patients and OHCWs.

F. Instruments must be appropriately packaged to ensure maximal effectiveness of the sterilization process.

G. Most dental offices use steam autoclave sterilization and use packaging appropriate to the selected autoclave.

    1. Heat-stable autoclave pouches, plastic tubing, and cassettes are effective in steam autoclaves. These types of packaging also maintain the sterility of instruments until their use.

    2. Instruments must be packaged loosely to promote adequate sterilization.

    3. Instruments must be allowed to cool down before their use.

    4. Instruments can be safely stored in autoclave packaging for as long as 30 days; such packaging maintains the sterility of the instruments inside.

    5. Instruments must be stored in a clean, dry drawer or shelf, with a door to promote instrument sterility.

Care and Disposal of Infectious and Biomedical Waste

Infectious waste, according to the Environmental Protection Agency (EPA), consists of sharps, tissue, extracted teeth, blood, and blood-soaked items. The ADA has further categorized waste that is generated in the dental office into two types—biohazardous waste and biomedical waste.

I. Types of Waste

A. Biohazardous waste includes:

    1. Sharps (used and unused syringe needles, broken instruments, scalpel blades, burs, disposable syringes, local anesthetic cartridges, broken glass, and suture needles).

    2. Teeth and other body tissues.

    3. Blood, blood-soaked items, blood-caked items, and items soaked or caked with other potentially infectious material.

B. Biomedical waste

    1. Is waste generated during the course of care delivery that does not qualify as biohazardous.

    2. Includes gloves, masks, patient napkins, surface barriers, and paper towels.

II. Disposal of Infectious (biohazardous) Waste

A. Involves separating this waste from biomedical waste.

B. Involves determining which disposal options (incineration, burial, sterilization) are available and which is the most cost effective.

C. Involves labeling the infectious waste with a biohazard label to alert those who will handle the waste container and inform them of its contents.

D. Involves discarding sharps in a puncture-resistant container for disposal.

III. Disposal of Biomedical Waste

A. Involves the same procedures as disposal of regular trash unless state or local regulations stipulate different handling procedures.

Biological Monitoring of Sterilization Process

Weekly biological monitoring of the sterilization process must be performed to ensure that the process is effective. The Centers for Disease Control require dental offices to verify the proper functioning of sterilization cycles weekly, using biologic indicators.

I. Indicator Types

A. Heat-sensitive indicators verify only that sterilizing conditions have been reached, not that sterilization has been achieved.

B. Biologic indicators:

    1. Contain specific organisms, depending on the type of sterilizer that is tested.

      a. *Bacillus stearothermaphilus* spores are used for autoclave and chemiclave sterilizers.

      b. *Bacillus subtilis* spores are used for dry heat and ethylene oxide sterilizers.

    2. Verify that sterilization of the chamber contents has been achieved when spores contained in the biologic indicator are destroyed.

    3. Test packaging procedures and materials and the loading, use, and function of the sterilizer.

II. Spore Testing

A. Is indicated

    1. Once a week.

    2. Whenever a new packaging material is tried.

    3. Whenever a new sterilizer is used.

    4. During the training of new instrument processing staff.

    5. After a sterilizer has been repaired.

    6. When a different method of loading the sterilizer is employed.

B. Records of the process and results of biologic monitoring must be kept to comply with federal regulations and to provide documentation in case of a liability suit.

Handling Sharps and Care of Equipment

Every sharp dental instrument and all dental equipment should be considered potentially infectious and should be handled with safety and injury-prevention in mind.

I. Sharps

A. Include used and unused syringe needles, scalpels, burs, broken instruments, suture needles, local anesthetic cartridges, broken glass, and sharp wires.

B. Must be disposed of in a puncture-resistant container.

C. Are considered biohazardous (infectious) waste and therefore must be disposed of in a puncture-proof, leak-resistant container according to local, state, or federal regulations (whichever take precedence).

D. Must be handled carefully to avoid an occupational exposure (puncture of skin with contaminated sharps).

1. Occupational exposure incident
   a. Consists of eye, mouth, mucous membrane, nonintact skin, or parenteral contact with blood or other potentially infectious materials during the performance of an employee's duties.
   b. Requires that the affected OHCW have a confidential medical evaluation and follow-up as soon as possible.[12]
      1) Both the OHCW and the source individual are tested.
      2) The OHCW is notified of the results of the evaluation.
      3) The OHCW is provided counseling regarding the occupational exposure.
         a) The OHCW is told that the average risk for HIV transmission after a percutaneous exposure to HIV-infected blood is 0.3%, after a mucous membrane exposure is 0.09%, and after skin exposure is estimated to be less than the risk for mucous membrane exposure (no HCW's enrolled in Post-Exposure studies have seroconverted after an isolated skin exposure).[11]
         b) The OHCW also is asked to alter behaviors, especially during the first 6 to 12 weeks Post-Exposure; changes may involve sexual abstinence or the use of condoms to prevent sexual transmission of disease or pregnancy; the OHCW also may be asked to refrain from donating blood, plasma, organs, tissue, or semen.
         c) If the OHCW is breast feeding, the risk of HIV transmission through breast milk is discussed.
         d) Exposed OHCWs are advised to seek medical evaluation for any acute illness that occurs during the follow-up period, including fever, rash, myalgia, fatigue, malaise, or lymphadenopathy.
      4) HIV Post-Exposure prophylaxis (PEP) is discussed with the OHCW.
         a) The PEP is recommended to the OHCW after the need for the protocol is established (Figs. 8–3).
         b) The prophylaxis regimen is recommended for OHCWs who have had an exposure to a source person with HIV or when information suggests that the source person may be HIV positive.
         c) If the need for PEP has been established, the exposed OHCW must be told that the knowledge about the effectiveness and toxicity of PEP drugs is limited.
         d) Zidovudine (ZDV) is the only antiretroviral drug that has been shown to prevent HIV transmission in humans.
         e) No data indicates that adding other antiretroviral drugs increases PEP efficacy, but a two or three drug regimen is recommended to increase potency and to address concerns about drug-resistant viruses.
         f) Toxicity data for persons without HIV or for pregnant women is available only for AZT, and not for the other antiretroviral drugs.
         g) Any and all drugs can be declined by the OHCW.
      5) All activities are documented in the OHCW's medical records.
      6) The employer is provided with a copy of the health care professional's evaluation of the incident.

2. Needle recapping
   a. Requires use of the scoop technique (one-handed) or a mechanical cap-holding device.
      1) Occupational exposures often happen during handling of the syringe after anesthesia administration.
      2) Avoid recapping needles using the two-handed technique.
      3) Do not bend, break, or manipulate needles by hand after the anesthesia administration is complete.

II. Dental Equipment
   A. Handpieces
      1. Must be appropriately sterilized for patient protection.
         a. Newer handpieces can be heat sterilized. These handpieces should be a priority when purchasing new handpieces.
         b. Older handpieces cannot be adequately sterilized and require a compromise in the office infection control plan.
      2. May be damaged by disinfectants used in the dental office (i.e., fiber optic handpieces).
      3. Must be maintained and sterilized according to the manufacturer's instructions to maximize the life of the handpiece.
   B. Prophy angles, contraangles, and air-water syringes
      1. Must be sterilized to prevent the transmission of infectious agents from patient to patient.

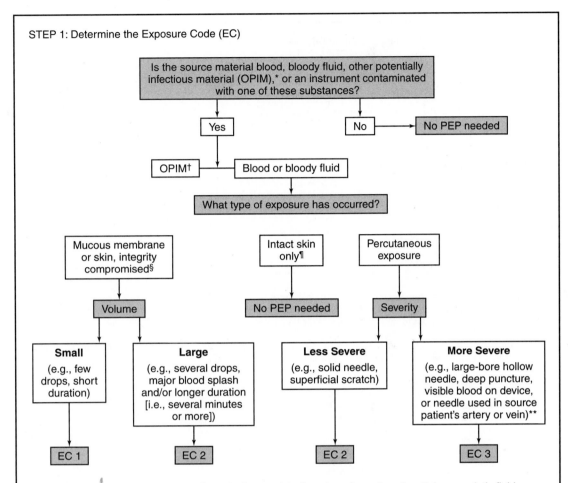

STEP 1: Determine the Exposure Code (EC)

Is the source material blood, bloody fluid, other potentially infectious material (OPIM),* or an instrument contaminated with one of these substances?

Yes → No → No PEP needed

OPIM† → Blood or bloody fluid

What type of exposure has occurred?

Mucous membrane or skin, integrity compromised§ | Intact skin only¶ | Percutaneous exposure

Volume | No PEP needed | Severity

Small (e.g., few drops, short duration) | **Large** (e.g., several drops, major blood splash and/or longer duration [i.e., several minutes or more]) | **Less Severe** (e.g., solid needle, superficial scratch) | **More Severe** (e.g., large-bore hollow needle, deep puncture, visible blood on device, or needle used in source patient's artery or vein)**

EC 1 | EC 2 | EC 2 | EC 3

* Semen or vaginal secretions; cerebrospinal, synovial, pleural, peritoneal, pericardial, or amniotic fluids; or tissue.

† Exposures to OPIM must be evaluated on a case-by-case basis. In general, these body substances are considered a low risk for transmission in health-care settings. Any unprotected contact to concentrated HIV in a research laboratory or production facility is considered an occupational exposure that requires clinical evaluation to determine the need for PEP.

§ Skin integrity is considered compromised if there is evidence of chapped skin, dermatitis, abrasion, or open wound.

¶ Contact with intact skin is not normally considered a risk for HIV transmission. However, if the exposure was to blood, and the circumstance suggests a higher volume exposure (e.g., an extensive area of skin was exposed or there was prolonged contact with blood), the risk for HIV transmission should be considered.

** The combination of these severity factors (e.g., large-bore hollow needle *and* deep puncture) contribute to an elevated risk for transmission if the source person is HIV-positive.

Continued.

Figure 8.3 Determining the need for HIV postexposure prophylaxis (PEP) after an occupational exposure. This algorithm is intended to guide initial decisions about PEP and should be used in conjunction with other guidance provided in this report.
(From Centers for Disease Control and Prevention: Public Health Service Guidelines for the Management of Health Care Worker Exposures to HIV and Recommendations for Postexposure Prophylaxis. MMWR 47:RR-7:14–15, May 15, 1998.)

STEP 2: Determine the HIV Status Code (HIV SC)

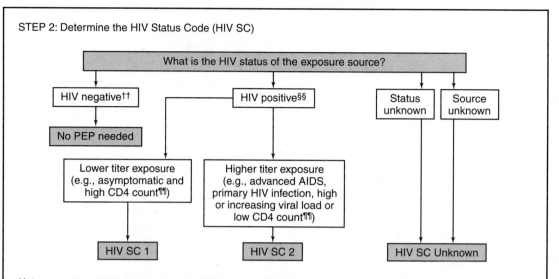

†† A source is considered negative for HIV infection if there is laboratory documentation of a negative HIV antibody, HIV polymerase chain reaction (PCR), or HIV p24 antigen test result from a specimen collected at or near the time of exposure and there is no clinical evidence of recent retroviral-like illness.

§§ A source is considered infected with HIV (HIV positive) if there has been a positive laboratory result for HIV antibody, HIV PCR, or HIV p24 antigen or physician-diagnosed AIDS.

¶¶ Examples are used as surrogates to estimate the HIV titer in an exposure source for purposes of considering PEP regimens and do not reflect all clinical situations that may be observed. Although a high HIV titer (HIV SC 2) in an exposure source has been associated with an increased risk for transmission, the possibility of transmission from a source with a low HIV titer also must be considered.

STEP 3: Determine the PEP Recommendation

EC	HIV SC	PEP recommendation
1	1	**PEP may not be warranted.** Exposure type does not pose a known risk for HIV transmission. Whether the risk for drug toxicity outweighs the benefit of PEP should be decided by the exposed HCW and treating clinician.
1	2	**Consider basic regimen.***** Exposure type poses a negligible risk for HIV transmission. A high HIV titer in the source may justify consideration of PEP. Whether the risk for drug toxicity outweighs the benefit of PEP should be decided by the exposed HCW and treating clinician.
2	1	**Recommend basic regimen.** Most HIV exposures are in this category; no increased risk for HIV transmission has been observed but use of PEP is appropriate.
2	2	**Recommend expanded regimen.**††† Exposure type represents an increased HIV transmission risk.
3	1 or 2	**Recommend expanded regimen.** Exposure type represents an increased HIV transmission risk.
Unknown		If the source or, in the case of an unknown source, the setting where the exposure occurred suggests a possible risk for HIV exposure and the EC is 2 or 3, consider PEP basic regimen.

*** Basic regimen is four weeks of zidovudine, 600 mg per day in two or three divided doses, *and* lamivudine, 150 mg twice daily.

††† Expanded regimen is the basic regimen plus *either* indinavir, 800 mg every 8 hours, *or* nelfinavir, 750 mg three times a day.

Figure 8.3 *Continued*

2. Should be kept in sufficient supply; treatment areas should contain several replacement pieces to facilitate the sterilization of contaminated handpieces/air-water syringes.
3. Must be maintained and sterilized according to the manufacturer's instructions to maximize the life of the equipment.
    a. Prophy angles
        1) Must be taken apart before sterilization.
        2) Are lubricated according to manufacturer's recommendations, typically before and after sterilization.
    b. Air-water syringes
        1) Must be thoroughly flushed before sterilization.
        2) Some types are autoclavable (both the syringe and tips).
        3) May have interchangeable tips that can be sterilized.
        4) If not autoclavable, must be scrubbed with an EPA-registered disinfectant and subsequently allowed to dry for the recommended time for tuberculocidal effect.

 ## Clinical Case STUDY

Misty has been employed as a dental hygienist for 9 months. She is nearly an hour behind schedule because of unforeseen scheduling problems. Her final appointment of the day is with Mrs. Palmer, who is scheduled to receive two quadrants of non-surgical scaling and root planing. Misty administers an inferior alveolar nerve block, a long buccal nerve block, and a lingual infiltration on the mandibular right side. While recapping the needle, the cap she is holding in her left hand slips and she accidentally sticks herself in her left index finger. A pool of blood the size of a dime forms under her glove. Misty proceeds with completion of the appointment and subsequently dismisses the patient.

Clinical Case QUESTIONS

1. What is the primary cause of this needlestick injury?
2. How should Misty have handled the situation immediately after the injury occurred?
3. What is the protocol that must be followed after a needlestick injury?
4. Is any follow up required after a needlestick injury?
5. When do most needlestick injuries occur?

Clinical Case RATIONALES

1. This needlestick injury was a direct result of using a two-handed recapping technique.
2. After the injury occurred, Misty should have stopped treating the patient, carefully removed and disposed of her gloves, washed the needlestick area thoroughly with soap and water (making sure to express blood from the wound to help flush it out), and applied a bandage to the injury. She subsequently should have asked the patient to immediately accompany her to a medical office where both could have blood drawn to test for infectious agents.
3. Within a few hours of exposure, Misty must complete an exposure incident form, have the patient tested for HBV and HIV, be evaluated by a health care professional, and have herself tested for HIV and HBV. Her dentist employer must send Misty's job description, a report of the incident, relevant medical information for both Misty and the patient, and a copy of the blood-borne pathogens standard to the health care provider. Misty should be counseled on her test results, her infectious status, and associated risks. She should be given recommendations for Post-Exposure prophylaxis and for preventing accidental exposure to her family and others.
4. Misty must be provided with a report containing her health care provider's written opinion regarding the incident. Depending on the circumstances surrounding the incident, Misty may need to take prophylactic medication and be medically reexamined in 6 months.
5. Most needlestick injuries occur during the recapping of used needles.

Maintaining Asepsis

Maintaining asepsis during radiologic, clinical, and laboratory procedures is essential in preventing the spread of infective agents to other office areas.

I. Dental Radiography Asepsis
    A. Preparing the operatory
        1. Surfaces that must be disinfected before seating the patient include the tube head and extension device, the chair and chair controls, the exposure controls and panel, any surfaces that exposed film has contacted, and the lead shield.
        2. The OHCW must use personal protective equipment when disinfecting the treatment area.
        3. Barriers
            a. Non-barrier technique
                1) Is totally aseptic only for taking dental radiographs without barriers, using the two-person technique.
                2) Involves one person placing and removing the film from the patient's mouth and another person adjusting the x-ray cone, chair, and headrest and operating the exposure controls.
                3) Is impractical for most dental offices.

b. Barrier technique
1) The operatory must be prepared to prevent the spread of infectious agents.
2) Most areas can be covered with plastic wrap or a bag to isolate the contaminants from the equipment.
3) A bag must be placed over the x-ray cone (Fig. 8–4).
4) Chair, headrest, and chair controls should be covered.
5) Exposure controls must be covered.
6) Film holders need special attention.
   a) Must disinfect/sterilize between patients.
   b) Use disposable film holders whenever possible.
   c) After use, keep film holder in contaminated area of treatment room.
7) Handling of radiographic film
   a) Store unexposed film in an uncontaminated drawer or container.
   b) Once exposed, the plastic-covered film must be cleaned and disinfected.
   c) Film can be placed in plastic pouches before exposure; subsequently remove the film from plastic pouches before developing, taking great care to avoid contaminating the film.
8) Precautions during film exposure.
   a) Place plastic covering on as many environmental surfaces as possible to minimize post-treatment clean-up time. OHCWs must wear personal protective equipment during x-ray exposure.
   b) Drape patient with lead apron and thyroid shield.

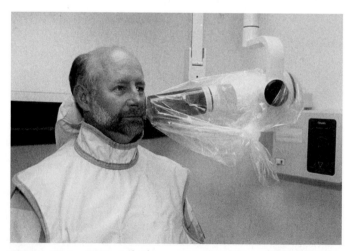

Figure 8.4 Parts of the x-ray machine that may be exposed to contaminants should be covered with disposable wraps and bags.

c) Wipe excess saliva from exposed x-ray films before placing them in a paper cup. Avoid contaminating the outside of the paper cup.
d) After the radiographs have been exposed, place overgloves or remove contaminated gloves, wash hands, and reglove before proceeding to the radiograph developing station.
9) Precautions during film developing
   a) Darkroom film developing
      (1) Designate two zones in the darkroom—contaminated and non-contaminated—and place paper towels over each zone. Place the contaminated radiographs in the contaminated area.
      (2) Remove overgloves, or place powder-free gloves, before opening the film packets.
      (3) Open each film packet, avoiding contact with the film inside, and place the exposed film on the uncontaminated paper towel.
      (4) After all of the film packets have been opened and the film has been carefully placed on the non-contaminated paper towel, remove gloves, wash hands, place new examination gloves, and develop the radiograph films.
      (5) Carefully discard all trash by wrapping the paper towel around the waste and disposing of it in the trash receptacle. Remove gloves, wash hands, and exit the darkroom.
   b) Developing film in a daylight loader
      (1) With clean hands, line the bottom surface of the daylight loader with a barrier. Place the cup containing the exposed film on the barrier, along with a pair of examination gloves and a second empty cup.
      (2) Place clean hands through the sleeves of the daylight loader and place examination gloves.
      (3) Open exposed film and carefully allow film to drop on the barrier, avoiding contamination; place contaminated film packets in the second cup.
      (4) Remove gloves, place film in the developer, and remove hands from the daylight loader.
      (5) Open the top of the daylight loader and carefully wrap the contaminated trash in the barrier,

avoiding contamination; dispose in a trash receptacle.

(6) Wash hands.

(7) Place a plastic cover over the panoramic bite pieces to maintain asepsis.

(8) After the panoramic radiograph has been taken, have patient remove the plastic cover and dispose it in a nearby trash receptacle.

(9) If plastic covers are not used, the bite pieces must be sterilized to maintain aseptic technique.

II. Dental Laboratory Asepsis

A. Items that ultimately will come in contact with mucous membranes must be sterilized.

B. Laboratory items that can withstand the heat of sterilization should be sterilized to increase the overall level of infection control in the dental laboratory.

C. High-level disinfection of laboratory products (prostheses) that contact mucous membranes often is sufficient if laboratory infection control protocols prevent cross-contamination.

D. Routine cleaning and disinfection of laboratory equipment and environmental surfaces should be accomplished with the same regularity as in the dental office.

E. Dental impressions

1. Carry saliva, blood, and many microorganisms and must be decontaminated.

2. Must be rinsed with tap water after an impression is taken.

3. Are soaked in a disinfectant that is recommended for the impression material, for the period of time recommended by the manufacturer; different disinfectants may be needed for different impression materials.

4. Are rinsed again with tap water to remove the disinfectant before an impression is poured.

5. The laboratory area used for pouring an impression must be organized for aseptic operation.

a. Paper should be placed on countertops.

b. Plastic coverings should be placed over areas that are likely to be touched.

c. A shielding device and high-volume suction are used during polishing or grinding to minimize the aerosolization of microorganisms and grinding products.

d. Personal protective equipment is worn during work with contaminated laboratory materials.

e. Complete, fixed, and removable partial dentures are disinfected.

6. Fixed and removable prosthetic devices are disinfected after they are returned from the laboratory, after placement in the mouth, and after in-office adjustment.

a. The disinfectant is checked for compatibility with the materials used in the prosthetic device.

b. The prosthetic device is rinsed with tap water.

c. The prosthetic device is disinfected for the time recommended for tuberculocidal disinfection.

d. The device is rinsed again with tap water and allowed to dry.

7. Cleaning removable prosthetic devices in the dental office

a. Always wear personal protective equipment when handling orally contaminated devices.

b. Place the removable prosthetic device in a zippered plastic bag that contains the disinfectant appropriate for the materials contained in the prosthesis.

c. Place the zippered bag in an ultrasonic cleaner to promote disinfection and removal of "loose" concretions.

d. Place the prosthesis in another zippered bag that contains a single-unit dose of stain, plaque, and calculus remover; subsequently place in ultrasonic cleaner for the recommended time.

e. Wearing gloves, remove the prosthesis from the bag after pouring off the cleaning solution.

f. Thoroughly rinse the prosthesis (e.g., to remove cleaning solution, remaining stain). If necessary, brush the remaining stain and calculus off the appliance. Rinse again.

g. Store in a sealed bag that contains diluted mouthwash to promote a fresh taste for the patient.

h. Rinse before returning the prosthesis to the patient.

III. Dental Operatory Asepsis

A. Preparing the treatment area for an appointment involves the coordination of all of the information discussed in this chapter. Every OHCW must participate in the mission of maintaining general office asepsis.

B. Objectives include:

1. Control of disease transmission from patient to patient, patient to OHCW, OHCW to patient, and OHCW to OHCW (breaking the chain of infection).

2. Efficient use of office facilities and staff to effectively serve as many patients as possible while maintaining aseptic technique.

3. Demonstrating a high standard of cleanliness to patients and for their benefit.

4. Prolonging the life and efficiency of costly dental equipment.

C. Procedure:

1. Before patient arrival:

   a. Disinfect and/or sterilize all environmental surfaces, sinks, faucets, dental equipment, dental instruments, dental chair, operator's chair, and handpieces using the appropriate sterilizing agent or disinfecting agent, flush all water lines to reduce the microorganism count in the delivery system, clean the vacuum system, and follow an office asepsis plan designed to prevent cross-contamination between patients.

   b. Cover as many environmental surfaces as possible with plastic barriers to prevent contamination and promote efficient clean up of the treatment area.

   c. Wear personal protective equipment, including heavy-duty utility gloves, while disinfecting the treatment area. Personal protective equipment also should be worn during operatory set up.

   d. Bring the armamentarium needed for the next patient from the instrument processing area and cover the instrument tray with an imperviously backed patient napkin to prevent contamination from ambient air.

   e. Ensure that there is a plentiful supply of sterile gauzes, cotton rolls, and other necessary paper goods during care delivery.

2. During care delivery

   a. Have the patient rinse with chlorhexidine gluconate or an antibacterial mouthwash to reduce the oral microorganism count by as much as 90%.

   b. Wear personal protective equipment, including protective eyewear, face mask, approved clinic attire, and examination gloves (Fig. 8–5).

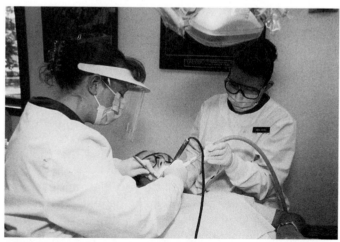

Figure 8.5 Personal protective equipment is worn during all dental procedures where blood or saliva contamination is possible.

   c. Focus on the reduction of splatter, droplet formation, and the aerosolization of microorganisms during care delivery.

   d. Maintain contaminated and non-contaminated zones. The operator must avoid the non-contaminated zones to contain the spread of infectious microorganisms.

   e. Avoid touching switches, drawer handles, pens, pencils, patient charts, and other objects outside the contaminated area.

      1) If the operator needs something in the non-contaminated zone, ask for assistance from another member of the office staff.

      2) If no assistance is available, wear over-gloves to isolate the microorganisms on the treatment gloves from the non-contaminated zone.

   f. Avoid touching mask, protective glasses, or shield to minimize the spread of microorganisms.

   g. Take special precautions if local anesthesia is administered during patient treatment.

   h. Avoid pointing the needle at the patient or self to avoid an unintended needlestick injury.

   i. Recap needles using the one-handed technique (scoop technique) or a mechanical needle recapper.

   j. Take special care when disassembling the syringe after patient care is completed; many sharps injuries occur during disassembly.

   k. Follow office asepsis policy during the exposure of radiographic films to prevent contamination between patients.

   l. Follow the appropriate infection control procedures for handling dental impressions whenever impressions are taken or poured.

3. After care delivery is completed:

   a. Wear personal protective equipment, including heavy nitrile or neoprene gloves, while cleaning the treatment area.

   b. All sharps and blood-caked or soaked gauzes must be removed from the treatment tray and placed in an approved puncture-resistant container.

   c. All water lines are flushed for 20 seconds between patients.

   d. Treatment trays/cassettes are transported to the decontamination area; any contamination on the tray or in the cassette must be contained during transport.

   e. All single-use items (disposable syringes, instruments, paper goods, barrier plastics) must be discarded and disposed of according to local, state, or federal regulations.

   f. All reusable instruments should be rinsed

with water and placed in an ultrasonic cleaner to remove accumulated bioburden. The instruments must be covered with the ultrasonic solution and allowed to remain in the ultrasonic cleaner for the manufacturer's recommended length of time.

g. The vacuum system (both high- and low-volume) is cleaned and flushed with a commercially prepared cleansing/disinfecting solution.

h. All instruments are inspected upon removal from the ultrasonic cleaner; any remaining bioburden must be carefully removed to maximize the sterilant effect of the autoclave.

i. Instruments are thoroughly rinsed with water and packaged in an appropriate autoclave bag.

j. Any contaminated surfaces in the treatment area are disinfected with the appropriate solution for the recommended time.

k. All environmental surfaces are newly recovered with a plastic barrier to ready the treatment area for the next patient.

Minimum Standards for Office Safety

Today's dental office must have a written, comprehensive safety plan to protect patients and staff from infectious disease. This plan should include the following:

I.   Information and training for employees who are at reasonable risk for occupational exposure.

II. Use of Universal Precautions when exposure to bodily fluids is a possibility.

III. Study of the office to determine which job descriptions involve the risk of an occupational exposure to bloodborne pathogens.

IV. HBV should be available at no charge for all employees at risk for occupational exposure to bloodborne pathogens.

V.   Provision of personal protective equipment to all employees at risk for occupational exposure.

VI. Periodic office cleaning and decontamination for patient and staff protection.

VII. Evaluation and follow up of occupational exposures to monitor the health of affected employees.

VIII. Maintenance of accurate medical records after occupational exposures.

IX. Labeling of all containers of regulated waste with a biohazard label.

 CONTENT REVIEW QUESTIONS

1. What condition is associated with multi-drug resistant tuberculosis?
   A. lupus erythematosus
   B. acquired immunodeficiency disease syndrome
   C. trisomy 21
   D. bullous pemphigoid

2. Select from the following the route that is NOT involved in HIV transmission
   A. exposure to contaminated blood, blood products, or blood-contaminated body fluids
   B. infected mother to unborn child
   C. intimate sexual contact involving the exchange of semen or vaginal secretions
   D. casual contact with a recently seroconverted HIV-positive individual

3. An important deterrent against the transmission of disease in the dental office is:
   A. requiring that patients undergo HIV testing
   B. refusing to treat patients from high-risk groups
   C. vaccinating office staff who are exposed to blood-borne pathogens for HBV
   D. asking whether patients have AIDS during the medical history

4. Identify the first step in the process of sterilizing instruments:
   A. storing instruments to preserve their sterility for future procedures
   B. packaging instruments in appropriate sterilizer bags
   C. steam-sterilizing instruments to kill bacteria, fungi, and viruses
   D. soaking instruments to solubilize dried blood and debris

5. Biological testing during the sterilization process must be accomplished on a _____ basis to ensure the effectiveness of the process.
   A. daily
   B. weekly
   C. biweekly
   D. monthly

6. Identify the FALSE statement regarding infection control procedures:
   A. gloves must be worn by dental professionals whenever they are at risk for contacting blood, blood-contaminated saliva, mucous membranes, or respiratory secretions
   B. gloves should be washed between patients to prevent the spread of disease
   C. protective clothing should be changed daily or when visibly soiled
   D. hand washing, when combined with barrier techniques, is an effective defense against spreading disease between patients

7. Select the TRUE statement regarding hepatitis B vaccinations:
   A. new employees must receive all doses of the hepatitis B vaccination before they begin working in the dental office
   B. new employees are required to pay only one third of the cost of their hepatitis B vaccinations
   C. hepatitis B vaccinations typically are administered in dental offices by dentists to control costs
   D. new employees must begin the hepatitis B vaccination series within 10 days of employment,

unless contraindicated by medical reasons or declined by the employee

8. Which of the following statements regarding OSHA regulations is FALSE?
   A. advocate recapping needles using the scoop technique
   B. advocate recapping needles using the two-handed technique
   C. advocate recapping needles using the one-handed technique
   D. advocate recapping needles using a mechanical cap-holding device

9. Select the statement that best describes OSHA requirements regarding occupational exposures:
   A. the dental office must have a plan for documenting and evaluating employee occupational exposures
   B. employees are responsible for the documentation and evaluation of occupational exposures
   C. OSHA directly monitors and evaluates employee occupational exposures
   D. the CDC directly monitors and evaluates employee occupational exposures

10. Employers must provide employees at risk for exposure to bloodborne pathogens all of the following, EXCEPT:
    A. information and training regarding occupational exposures and how to avoid them
    B. HIV immunization at no charge
    C. personal protective equipment
    D. hepatitis B vaccination at no charge

11. HIV causes significant health changes in infected individuals by:
    A. attacking the T4-lymphocytes, thus causing an increase in opportunistic infections
    B. attacking plasma cells, thus interrupting the production of antibodies and reducing the host's resistance to disease
    C. increasing capillary permeability, thus causing redness, itching, and swelling in affected areas
    D. attacking plasma cells, thus altering antibodies so that they do not recognize the person's own tissues as friendly

12. Identify the safest and most effective utilization of face masks as personal protective equipment:
    A. change on a daily basis for maximum operator protection
    B. change at the end of morning and afternoon schedules for maximum operator protection
    C. change after every other patient for maximum operator protection
    D. change after every patient, or when visibly contaminated, for maximum operator protection

13. After prophylaxis of an HIV-positive individual has been completed, the instruments should be:
    A. soaked in household bleach
    B. sterilized for 10 minutes longer than the standard sterilization time

C. sterilized using the same techniques as for all other sterilizable instruments
D. placed in double sterilizer bags to avoid the cross contamination of other instruments

14. Identify the method of sterilization most commonly employed by dental offices:
    A. steam sterilization
    B. dry heat sterilization
    C. ethylene oxide sterilization
    D. chemical vapor sterilization

15. Levels of disinfection are based upon:
    A. the desires of the practitioner
    B. the needs of the patient
    C. the guidelines of the practice
    D. the type of procedure performed

16. During ultrasonic scaling, the operator should wear:
    A. eye protection and a facial mask
    B. eye protection and a facial shield
    C. a facial shield and a facial mask
    D. a facial shield, eye protection, and a facial mask

17. Blood-saturated gauze should be disposed of by:
    A. packaging for incineration
    B. carefully placing in the trash
    C. thoroughly rinsing with water
    D. soaking in cold sterilant

18. Dental handpieces used for coronal polishing procedures should be:
    A. heat sterilized
    B. disinfected with chemical agents
    C. sonicated in general purpose cleaner
    D. wiped with alcohol

19. Dry heat sterilization is NOT suitable for:
    A. paper
    B. plastics
    C. metals
    D. rubber
    E. glass

20. Chemical sterilization is best suited for:
    A. paper
    B. plastics
    C. metals
    D. rubber
    E. liquids

21. Cold sterilization/disinfection is best suited for:
    A. paper
    B. plastics
    C. metals
    D. rubber
    E. liquids

22. When moving instruments from the ultrasonic bath to the sink for rinsing, one should wear:
    A. multiple-use utility gloves
    B. sterile examination gloves
    C. non-sterile examination gloves
    D. plastic overgloves

23. To retrieve additional gauze from a drawer during an oral prophylaxis appointment, one should do which of the following?

A. use rinsed examination gloves

B. wear overgloves

C. ask the patient to assist

D. use a paper towel

24. Latex hypersensitivity is most commonly a symptom of which of the following medical conditions?

   A. pregnancy

   B. spina bifida

   C. cardiovascular disease

   D. diabetes

25. To be classified as a hospital-grade disinfectant, a disinfectant must be able to kill _____ .

   A. hepatitis B virus

   B. human immunodeficiency virus

   C. *Mycobacterium tuberculosis*

   D. *Staphylococcus aureus*

26. All of the following are standard agents used in disinfection, EXCEPT:

   A. alcohols

   B. iodophors

   C. sodium hypochlorite

   D. complex phenols

27. Which one of the following statements is FALSE?

   A. high-level disinfection is used for instruments that have penetrated soft tissues and is capable of killing bacterial spores and *Mycobacterium tuberculosis*

   B. intermediate-level disinfection is used for instruments that have contacted intact skin and is capable of killing *Mycobacterium tuberculosis* but not bacterial spores

   C. low-level disinfection is used for the general cleaning of instruments and is capable of killing bacteria and some fungi and viruses but not *Mycobacterium tuberculosis*

   D. all disinfection procedures kill bacterial spores and *Mycobacterium tuberculosis*

28. Which of the following is NOT a method of reducing airborne transmission of infectious agents?

   A. having the patient rinse with antimicrobial mouth rinse

   B. using high-volume suction during ultrasonic scaling procedures

   C. wearing protective clothing, gloves, and mask

   D. rinsing the mouth with an air/water spray

29. Laundering of contaminated protective clothing requires:

   A. cool water temperatures, a commercial laundry detergent, and a cool dryer

   B. tepid water temperatures, bleach, a commercial laundry detergent, and a warm dryer

   C. warm water temperatures, bleach, a commercial laundry detergent, and a warm dryer

   D. hot water temperatures, bleach, a commercial laundry detergent, and a hot dryer

 30. Waterlines are best disinfected by:

   A. flushing for 1 to 3 minutes at the beginning of the day and for 10 to 15 seconds between patients

   B. flushing for 3 to 5 minutes at the beginning of the day and for 20 to 30 seconds between patients

   C. flushing for 5 to 10 minutes at the beginning of the day and for 35 to 45 seconds between patients

   D. flushing for 10 to 15 minutes at the beginning of the day and for 50 to 60 seconds between patients

31. Moist heat sterilization:

   A. uses steam under pressure

   B. is safe for all instruments

   C. prevents corrosion of instruments

   D. penetrates oils and powders

32. Of the following methods of sterilization, which one requires the longest cycle?

   A. moist heat

   B. dry heat

   C. chemical vapor

   D. ethylene oxide

33. Biomedical waste includes all of the following, EXCEPT:

   A. extracted teeth

   B. gloves

   C. patient napkins

   D. facial masks

34. Biohazardous waste:

   A. is disposed of with regular trash

   B. is incinerated, buried, or sterilized

   C. is placed in plain packaging

   D. is disposed of with biomedical waste

35. The biological indicator *Bacillus stearothermaphilus* is used to determine effective sterilization by _____ sterilizers.

   A. moist heat and chemical vapor

   B. chemical vapor and dry heat

   C. ethylene oxide and moist heat

   D. dry heat and ethylene oxide

REVIEW QUESTION RATIONALES

1. **B**   Multi-drug resistant tuberculosis is always associated with AIDS. In 1997, a total of 19,855 cases of tuberculosis were reported to the CDC. Of these, 171 were considered multi-drug resistant (resistant to rifampin and isoniazid).[13] Trisomy 21 is Down syndrome, a genetic disorder that is characterized by an extra chromosome 21. Affected patients have slanted eyes, shorter stature, heart abnormalities, variations in intelligence levels, and a greater tendency to develop periodontal disease. Lupus erythematosus is a chronic autoimmune disease of unknown cause. Skin lesions are the most common sign of the disease (butterfly rash over the nose, erythematous lesions on the fingertips) and oral lesions include bleeding gingiva and reddened lesions with white striae radiating from the center.

2. **D**   HIV is commonly transmitted through contact with blood, from infected mother to fetus, and through secretions of intimate sexual contact. HIV is

transmitted only through the exchange of body fluids (e.g., saliva, semen, blood). Casual contact with an HIV-infected individual (carrying on a conversation, standing nearby, riding in an elevator) is not a risk factor for transmission of the HIV virus.

3. **C** Staff immunizations against hepatitis B are an effective way to deter the transmission of communicable disease in the dental office. HIV testing of patients provides the professional with only a momentary view of a patient's HIV status because detection of seroconversion takes several weeks to months and because the test does not detect any other disease the patient may have. Testing has no impact on the spread of communicable disease in the dental office. Discriminating against patients from perceived "high-risk" groups is illegal and unethical. One cannot tell whether a person is infected with HIV by appearance. Although knowing whether a patient has AIDS may be important when considering treatment choices and regimens, knowing a patient's HIV status has no effect on the transmission of communicable disease in the dental office. Universal Precautions protect patients and professional staff from infectious diseases that are transmissible in the dental office.

4. **D** The first step in the sterilization of instruments is to loosen dried blood and debris by soaking them and running them through an ultrasonic cleaner. The instruments are subsequently packaged in appropriate sterilization bags, sterilized, allowed to cool, and stored to preserve their sterility.

5. **B** Biological testing should occur on a weekly basis to monitor the effectiveness of the sterilization process.

6. **B** Gloves should never be washed and reused. Gloves must be changed between patients or when they are torn.

7. **D** New employees must begin the hepatitis B vaccination regimen within 10 days of hiring. The dentist must pay the cost of the vaccinations, they must be administered by appropriate medical personnel, and new employees can work while they are receiving the vaccinations.

8. **B** The two-handed needle recapping technique is dangerous and can lead to occupational exposures. The one-handed (scoop) technique or mechanical needle holders are recommended.

9. **A** The dental office must have a plan for documenting and evaluating employee occupational exposures. OSHA and the CDC do not directly monitor such exposures. OSHA monitors dental offices to see whether they have an appropriate plan for handling occupational exposures.

10. **B** Employers must have a plan for providing employees with information and training regarding occupational exposures and their avoidance. Employers also must provide personal protective equipment and hepatitis B vaccination at no charge to the employee. No effective HIV immunization has been developed.

11. **A** HIV attacks T-4 cells, thereby decreasing an individual's cell-mediated immunity. Answer B refers to the humoral immune system. Answer C describes the effects of histamine release in tissues. Answer D describes an autoimmune disease process.

12. **D** Face masks should be changed after every patient or when visibly soiled. Face masks slowly lose their effectiveness as a barrier against infective agents. Moreover, if face masks become damp they lose their effectiveness. Consequently, changing face masks only once or twice daily or after every other patient compromises the effectiveness of the face mask as a barrier against infective agents.

13. **C** Universal Precautions, including autoclaving instruments, are designed to protect OHCWs and patients from bloodborne pathogens and infective agents. The instruments used for an HIV-infected individual should be handled as all other autoclavable instruments are handled. No extra time is needed and double bagging is not necessary. Soaking instruments in bleach will corrode them and not significantly improve sterilization results.

14. **A** Steam sterilization is the most efficient method of sterilization used for the dental office (it is relatively quick, involves no dangerous chemicals, and can sterilize most instruments with a minimum of degradation). Dry heat takes 3 to 6 times as long. Chemical vapor sterilization uses toxic chemicals as the sterilant. Ethylene oxide sterilization requires overnight sterilization.

15. **D** The type of procedure performed dictates the level of disinfection that is necessary. For example, instruments that have penetrated mucosa or gingiva (critical items) must have a higher level of disinfection (sterilization) than a radiographic holding device (semicritical item) or an x-ray head (noncritical item).

16. **C** Ultrasonic scaling, even with high-speed suction, produces tiny, contaminated droplets in the air around the patient's mouth. The operator must use barrier techniques for protection. A facial shield provides the best eye protection but has an opening in the chin and neck area that allows aerosols access to the operator's respiratory system. Consequently, the facial mask is needed to complete the barrier protection for an operator.

17. **A** Blood-stained or blood-soaked gauze is considered infectious waste (EPA) or biohazardous waste (ADA) and must be disposed of according to established guidelines. Management of blood-contaminated gauze by placement in the trash, rinsing in water, or soaking in cold sterilant is not in compliance with infectious waste disposal guidelines.

18. **A** All dental handpieces must be heat sterilized between patients to prevent the spread of infectious disease.

19. **B**   Most plastics cannot withstand dry heat sterilization.
20. **C**   Chemical sterilization is best suited for metals because it does not cause metal instruments to corrode or lose their edge (sharpness). Chemical sterilization may damage plastic instruments, may contaminate paper and liquid products, and may degrade rubber items.
21. **B**   Cold sterilization should be used only for plastics that cannot withstand steam sterilization.
22. **A**   Multiple-use utility gloves provide maximum operator protection against inadvertent occupation exposures. Examination gloves and overgloves do not provide adequate protection for handling contaminated instruments during sonication and sterilization procedures.
23. **B**   If the dental hygienist does not have an assistant to retrieve extra gauze from a drawer, overgloves should be worn to prevent the spread of contamination outside the localized treatment area. Rinsed examination gloves will carry contamination into noncontaminated areas.
24. **B**   Patients with spina bifida commonly have latex allergy as a side effect. The other medical conditions do not predispose patients to latex allergy.
25. **C**   The *Mycobacterium* bacillus is extremely virulent and difficult to eliminate. Consequently *M. tuberculosis* is used as the standard for hospital-grade surface disinfectants.
26. **A**   Alcohols are not effective against *Mycobacterium tuberculosis* and are not recommended by the ADA or the CDC.
27. **D**   Not all disinfection procedures kill *M. tuberculosis* and provide a high level of disinfection. The three levels of disinfection are appropriate depending on the exposure level of the instruments.
28. **D**   Rinsing with the air/water spray increases the aerosolization of the infectious agents in the treatment area. All of the other choices help to reduce the airborne transmission of infectious agents.
29. **D**   Contaminated protective clothing should be washed with the hottest water temperatures available, bleached, and dried at the highest temperature the garment can withstand.
30. **B**   Recommended flushing times are 3 to 5 minutes at the beginning of the day (or if the unit has not been used for a few hours) and 20 to 30 seconds between patients. These times have been shown to be effective for rinsing dental unit water lines. Longer rinse times are not harmful but are not an efficient use of time.
31. **A**   Moist heat sterilization uses steam under pressure. Not all instruments can withstand the conditions in a steam autoclave (e.g., metal instruments can corrode). Steam sterilization does not penetrate oils or powders.
32. **D**   Ethylene oxide requires 10 to 16 hours to be effective. A dry heat cycle must last 1 to 2 hours and a moist heat cycle must last 15 to 20 minutes (flash sterilization occurs in 3.4 to 12 minutes). Chemical vapor cycles require 20 minutes for effective sterilization.
33. **A**   Extracted teeth, blood-soaked sponges and gauze, sharps, and tissue removed from patients are considered biohazardous wastes. All other choices fall into the category of biomedical waste.
34. **B**   Biohazardous waste is treated differently than biomedical waste. Biohazardous waste must be incinerated, buried, or sterilized but biomedical waste can be disposed of with regular trash.
35. **A**   Moist heat and chemical vapor sterilizers use spores of *B. stearothermaphilus*. Ethylene oxide and dry heat sterilizers use spores of *B. subtilis*.

References

1. Centers for Disease Control and Prevention: Hepatitis A Fact Sheet. Department of Health and Human Services, October 1998.
2. Centers for Disease Control and Prevention: Hepatitis B Fact Sheet. Department of Health and Human Services, October 1998.
3. Centers for Disease Control and Prevention: Hepatitis C Fact Sheet. Department of Health and Human Services, October 1998.
4. Centers for Disease Control and Prevention, DHHS: Recommended Infection-Control Practices for Dentistry. MMWR 41:RR-8:1–12, May 18, 1993.
5. Centers for Disease Control and Prevention, DHHS: Immunization of Health-Care Workers: Recommendations of the Advisory Committee on Immunization Practices (ACIP) and the Hospital Infection Control Practices Advisory Committee (HICPAC). MMWR 46:RR-18:1–42; December 26, 1997.
6. American Dental Association: Infection Control Recommendations for the Dental Office and Dental Laboratory. ADA Council on Scientific Affairs and ADA Council on Dental Practice, 1996.
7. National Institute for Occupational Safety and Health: NIOSH Facts: Latex Allergy. Department of Health and Human Services, June 1997.
8. National Institute for Occupational Safety and Health: NIOSH Alert: Preventing Allergic Reactions to Natural Rubber Latex in the Workplace (Pub. No. 97–135). Department of Health and Human Services, July 1997.
9. Cornell S: Is there a hole in your safety net? Examining the permeability of latex. Advance for Nurse Practitioners, November 1997.
10. Miner N: Chemical Disinfectants in Central Service Departments (IAHCSMM Self-Study Series, Lesson 31). CEA/CIS Information Services, Purdue University, February 1997.
11. Gluck GM, Morganstein WM: Jong's Community Dental Health, 4th ed. St. Louis, Mosby, 1998.
12. American Dental Association: Occupational Exposure to Bloodborne Pathogens: A Step-by-Step Guide to Compliance. December 1997.
13. Centers for Disease Control and Prevention, DHHS: Tuberculosis Morbidity—United States, 1997. MMWR 47:RR-13:253–57, April 10, 1998.

Additional Readings

Cottone JA, Terezhalmy GT, Molinari JA: Practical Infection Control in Dentistry, 2nd ed. Media, Pa, Williams and Wilkins, 1996.
Gluck GM, Morganstein WM: Jong's Community Dental Health, 4th ed. St. Louis, Mosby, 1998.
Miller CH, Palenik CJ: Infection Control and Management of Hazardous Materials for the Dental Team. St. Louis, Mosby-Year Book, 1994.
Wilkins EM: Clinical Practice of the Dental Hygienist, 7th ed. Malvern, Pa, Williams and Wilkins, 1994.

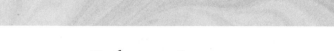

Chapter NINE

Pharmacology

Kimberly A. Stabbe, R.D.H., M.S.

 ## Clinical Case STUDY

Mr. Carroll is a 45-year-old recall patient with a history of myasthenia gravis and rheumatoid arthritis. For the past 2 years he has taken 15 mg of prednisone and neostigmine daily. He also takes diazepam before all dental treatment. He is scheduled for an oral prophylaxis today and mentions his dislike of visiting the dental office.

Clinical Case QUESTIONS

1. Mr. Carroll takes prednisone and neostigmine daily. What types of drugs are these and why is he taking them?
2. Mr. Carroll takes diazepam before all dental appointments. What type of drug is diazepam? Identify its common uses.

Clinical Case RATIONALES

1. Prednisone is a corticosteroid, which is an antiinflammatory agent. It is used to treat various diseases of allergic, inflammatory, and autoimmune origin. Mr. Carroll takes prednisone to treat his rheumatoid arthritis, which is an inflammatory disease of the joints. Neostigmine is an anticholinesterase muscle stimulant that markedly improves muscle strength by improving muscle contraction. Mr. Carroll takes neostigmine to treat his myasthenia gravis, a disease of muscular weakness.
2. Diazepam (Valium) is a benzodiazepine, which is an antianxiety agent. Mr. Carroll takes the drug to help him cope with his dental anxiety.

Content Review

General Terminology

Adverse effects are undesirable side effects and/or toxicities that occur with therapeutic drug doses.

Agonist is a drug that causes an effect by interacting with a receptor.

Antagonist is a drug that counteracts another drug's effect on a receptor.

Chemical name is a drug name that is determined by chemical structure.

Drug allergy is an immunologic response to a drug that ranges from rash to anaphylaxis and results in an antibody-antigen reaction.

Efficacy is the ability to produce a desired effect.

Generic name is drug name given to a drug before marketing.

Pharmacokinetics is the study of the metabolism and actions of drugs, including their absorption, duration, distribution, and excretion.

Pharmacology is the study of drugs, their origins, and their effects on the body.

Potency is the strength of a drug in terms of its ability to achieve a particular result.

Spectrum is the range of organisms that a drug is effective against.

Superinfection (suprainfection) is a new infection caused by an organism other than that which caused the initial infection.

Therapeutic effects are a drug's desirable effects.

Tolerance is the decreased susceptibility to a drug's effects because of repeated use.

Toxicology is the study of toxic and harmful effects of drugs and chemicals.

Trade name is the proprietary or brand name given to a drug by a pharmaceutical company; the name by which a drug is marketed.

Abbreviations/Acronyms

ACh: Acetylcholine
AHA: America Heart Association
AIDS: Acquired immunodeficiency syndrome
ANS: Autonomic nervous system
CHF: Congestive heart failure
CNS: Central nervous system
COPD: Chronic obstructive pulmonary disease
CVS: Cardiovascular system
GI: Gastrointestinal
IDDM: Insulin-dependent diabetes mellitus
IM: Intramuscular
IV: Intravenous
LJP: Localized juvenile periodontitis
MAO: Monoamine oxidase
MI: Myocardial infarction
NIDDM: Noninsulin-dependent diabetes mellitus
NSAIA: Nonsteroidal antiinflammatory agents
OTC: Over the counter
PO: Oral
PANS: Parasympathetic autonomic nervous sytem
RAP: Rapidly advancing periodontitis
SANS: Sympathetic autonomic nervous system
TCA: Tricyclic antidepressant

Basic Principles and Concepts

The successful provision of dental hygiene services involves an understanding of pharmacology. The hygienist continually strives to provide care to patients in the safest manner possible.

I. Understanding a drug's pharmacology, its effect on the patient, and its interaction with other drugs is essential to the safe provision of care.
II. A thorough health history helps the clinician identify potential drug interactions with current medications, dental medications, and OTC medications.
III. Dental medications often are needed for patient comfort and are commonly used.

Administration

Drugs have two basic routes of administration—enteral and parenteral.

I. Enteral includes PO and rectal administration.
II. Parenteral includes topical, intradermal, IV, subcutaneous, IM, intrathecal, and intraperitoneal administration and administration of drugs by inhalation.

Distribution

The distribution of a drug results in the unbound drug reaching (1) the specific site of action and (2) the nonspecific area where it is stored so it becomes a bound site.

I. Plasma proteins (albumin and globulin) bind drugs reversibly to the storage site.

II. A bound drug may become unbound by another drug competing for the same protein binding site.

Metabolism

Metabolism, or biotransformation, is the process of chemical changes in a drug by means of enzymes in the body (e.g., in the liver and blood). It changes the drug into a more polar and water-soluble particle, which aids in excretion.

Excretion

Most drugs are excreted by means of the renal (kidney) route; extrarenal excretion routes include the lungs, the GI tract, saliva, and breast milk.

Reactions

The administration of a drug produces both desired and adverse effects on the body.

I. Desired Effects
   A. Dose-related, predictable, pharmacologic effects that act on target organs to achieve a therapeutic response.
II. Adverse Effects
   A. Side effects typically are predictable and dose-related and act on nontarget organs. An example is nausea and vomiting from the use of erythromycin as an antibiotic.
   B. Toxic reactions, like side effects, are predictable and dose-related but they act on target organs and involve extended pharmacologic effects. An example is hepatotoxicity when methotrexate is used as an antineoplastic agent.
   C. Allergic reactions are not predictable or dose-related; they are the body's immunologic response to a drug. There are four basic types:
      1. Type I (immediate hypersensitivity) is an allergic reaction that occurs immediately (within minutes) after exposure to a previously encountered antigen (e.g., penicillin). It can be life threatening if it produces anaphylaxis, which requires immediate medical attention.
      2. Type II (cytolytic/cytotoxic) is an allergic reaction that inhibits or prevents cell function and results in cell destruction; may be a result of blood transfusion reactions.
      3. Type III (Arthus) is an allergic reaction that occurs within 6 to 8 hours after exposure; is similar to serum sickness. Penicillins and sulfonamides can cause such a reaction; symptoms include urticaria (wheals), lymphadenopathy, and fever.
      4. Type IV is a cell-mediated delayed hypersensitivity (occurs within 48 hours) that results in an inflammatory reaction such as contact dermatitis; often is seen with penicillin allergy or poison ivy.
   D. Idiosyncratic reactions are abnormal and have genetic causes.

Drug Effects on the ANS

Many drugs exert their effects on the ANS. These medications include adrenergic agents, adrenergic blocking agents, cholinergic agents, and anticholinergic agents.

The Autonomic Nervous System

The ANS includes two systems that maintain the body's functions: the sympathetic autonomic nervous system (SANS) and the parasympathetic autonomic nervous system (PANS).

I. Functions of the ANS
   A. The SANS enables the body to function during emergencies (engage in fight or flight) or respond to stressful situations by means of the release of its neurotransmitters, which include norepinephrine and epinephrine.
      1. These neurotransmitters subsequently stimulate the SANS receptors, which include alpha and beta receptors.
      2. Stimulation of alpha receptors causes vasoconstriction of the skin and skeletal muscles.
      3. Excitation of beta$_1$ receptors causes stimulation of the heart muscle and glycogenolysis.
      4. Stimulation of beta$_2$ receptors causes smooth muscle relaxation, which results in bronchodilation of the lungs.
   B. The PANS enables the body to maintain bodily functions during normal, daily activities by means of the release of the neurotransmitter ACh. This neurotransmitter subsequently stimulates its receptor sites (muscarinic and nicotinic) to enhance bodily function.

Effects of Adrenergic Agents

Adrenergic agents stimulate alpha and beta receptors. Common adrenergic agents include epinephrine, isoproterenol, levonordefrin, ephedrine, and dopamine III.

I. Therapeutic Uses
   A. Vasoconstriction, which increases the duration of local anesthetic actions and decreases their systemic location and toxicity; also control bleeding through hemostasis and act as nasal decongestants (via alpha receptors).
   B. Treatment of cardiac arrest by epinephrine (via beta$_1$ stimulation).
   C. Bronchodilation (via beta$_2$ receptors) for the treatment of respiratory diseases such as asthma and emphysema.
   D. Stimulation of the CNS by Ritalin (methylphenidate) or pemoline (Cylert) for the treatment of attention deficit-hyperactivity disorder (ADHD).
II. Contraindications
   A. Narrow-angle glaucoma from an increase in intraocular pressure
   B. Cardiac dysrhythmias.

III. Pharmacologic Effects
   A. Excitation of CNS.
   B. Effects on CVS include hypertension, dysrhythmias, tachycardia, blood vessel vasodilation with beta$_2$ receptors, and vasoconstriction with alpha$_1$ receptors.
   C. Bronchodilation of the bronchioles.
   D. Hyperglycemia from beta$_1$ stimulation, which increases glycogenolysis and decreases the release of insulin.
   E. Mydriasis (dilation of the pupil).
   F. Xerostomia from a decreased flow of saliva.
IV. Adverse Reactions
   A. CNS stimulation, resulting in anxiety and tremors.
   B. Increased blood pressure (if drug affects alpha receptors).
   C. Palpitations of the heart and dysrhythmias.
V. Drug Interactions
   A. A decreased pressor effect with the use of haloperidol, phenothiazines, thioxanthenes, and diuretics.
   B. Cardiac dysrhythmias when halogenated general anesthetics, cardiac glycosides, and TCAs are used.
   C. Hypertension with the administration of beta blockers, which block the beta-adrenergic effects of epinephrine.

Effects of Adrenergic Blocking Agents

Adrenergic blocking agents inhibit alpha and beta receptors and include three types: alpha-adrenergic blocking agents such as tolazoline (Priscoline) and phentolamine (Regitine); beta-adrenergic blocking agents, including nonspecific blocking agents such as propranolol (Inderal) and nadolol (Corgard) and specific blocking agents such as metoprolol (Lopressor); and alpha and beta-adrenergic blocking agents such as labetalol (Normodyne, Trandate).

I. Therapeutic Uses
   A. Alpha blocking agents are used in the treatment of peripheral vascular disease or Raynaud's disease; also are used in the treatment of pheochromocytoma, a catecholamine-secreting tumor of the adrenal medulla.
   B. Beta blocking agents and alpha$_1$-selective blocking agents are used in the treatment of hypertension, angina pectoris, dysrhythmias, and migraine headaches; also are used for MI prophylaxis.
II. Contraindications
   A. Hypersensitivity to adrenergic blocking agents
   B. CHF
   C. Bronchial asthma
III. Pharmacologic Effects
   A. Alpha blocking agents inhibit vasoconstriction in blood vessels (alpha receptor effects).

B. Beta blocking agents competitively block the effects of adrenergic agents on beta receptors and may inhibit specific beta receptors or be a nonspecific receptor site inhibitor.

IV. Adverse Reactions and Drug Interactions
  A. Few occur because the effects of these drugs on receptors is more site specific.
  B. Common reactions include:
    1. Xerostomia (dry mouth) (Table 9–1)
    2. Hypotension (low blood pressure)
    3. Nausea and vomiting

V. Drug Interactions (see also antiadrenergic agents under antihypertensives)
  A. The effects of beta blockers are decreased by sympathomimetics, NSAIA, and rifampin.
  B. The effects of beta blockers are increased by calcium channel blockers.

Effects of Cholinergic Agents

Cholinergic agents stimulate bodily functions by direct action (choline esters) or indirect action (inhibition of acetylcholinesterase). Common agents in this category include pilocarpine and bethanechol (Urecholine).

I. Therapeutic Uses
  A. Xerostomia (dry mouth), by increasing salivation.
  B. Glaucoma, by decreasing intraocular pressure.
  C. Urinary retention after surgery, by increasing secretions and activity of GI tract.
  D. Myasthenia gravis, by decreasing muscle weakness.

II. Contraindications
  A. Severe cardiac disease (because of CVS effects).
  B. Peptic ulcer (because of an increase in secretions).
  C. Asthma (because of an increase in mucous secretion).
  D. Obstruction of GI tract (GIT) or urinary tract (because of an increase in secretions).
  E. Uncontrolled hyperthyroidism that causes impaired drug metabolism.
  F. Patients with myasthenia gravis who take cholinesterase inhibitors (neostigmine).

III. Pharmacologic Effects
  A. Effects on the CVS, such as bradycardia and hypotension (direct effect on heart) and tachycardia and hypertension (indirect effect on blood vessels).
  B. Nausea, diarrhea, and dyspepsia (indigestion).
  C. Miosis (pupil constriction) and decreased intraocular pressure.

IV. Adverse Reactions
  A. An increase in salivation, lacrimation, urination, and defecation.

V. Drug Interactions
  A. Reduced effects with anticholinergics.
  B. Enhanced effects with cholinergics.

TABLE 9.1 Drugs Implicated in Xerostomia

>10%	1% to 10%
Alprazolam	Acrivastine and Pseudoephedrine
Amitriptyline hydrochloride	Albuterol
Amoxapine	Amantadine hydrochloride
Anisotropine methylbromide	Amphetamine sulfate
Atropine sulfate	Astemizole
Belladonna and opium	Azatadine maleate
Benztropine mesylate	Beclomethasone dipropionate
Bupropion	Bepridil hydrochloride
Chlordiazepoxide	Bitolterol mesylate
Clomipramine hydrochloride	Brompheniramine maleate
Clonazepam	Carbinoxamine and pseudoephedrine
Clonidine	Chlorpheniramine maleate
Clorazepate dipotassium	Clemastine fumarate
Cyclobenzaprine	Clozapine
Desipramine hydrochloride	Cromolyn sodium
Diazepam	Cyprohepatidine hydrochloride
Dicyclomine hydrochloride	Dexchlorpheniramine maleate
Diphenoxylate and Atropine	Dextroamphetamine sulfate
Doxepin hydrochloride	Dimenhydrinate
Ergotamine	Diphenhydramine hydrochloride
Estazolam	Disopyramide phosphate
Flavoxate	Doxazosin
Flurazepam hydrochloride	Dronabinol
Glycopyrrolate	Ephedrine sulfate
Guanabenz acetate	Flumazenil
Guanfacine hydrochloride	Fluvoxamine
Hyoscyamine sulfate	Gabapentin
Interferon Alfa-2a	Guaifenesin and Codeine
Interferon Alfa-2b	Guanadrel sulfate
Interferon Alfa-N3	Guanethidine sulfate
Ipratropium bromide	Hydroxyzine
Isoproterenol	Hyoscyamine, Atropine, Scopolamine, and Phenobarbital
Isotretinoin	Imipramine
Loratadine	Isoetharine
Lorazepam	Levocabastine hydrochloride
Loxapine	Levodopa
Maprotiline hydrochloride	Levodopa and carbidopa
Methscopolamine bromide	Levorphanol tartrate
Molindone hydrochloride	Meclizine hydrochloride
Nabilone	Meperidine hydrochloride
Nefazodone	Methadone hydrochloride
Oxybutynin chloride	Methamphetamine hydrochloride
Oxazepam	Methyldopa
Paroxetine	Metoclopramide
Phenelzine sulfate	Morphine sulfate
Prochlorperazine	Nortriptyline hydrochloride
Propafenone hydrochloride	Ondansetron
Protriptyline hydrochloride	Oxycodone and Acetaminophen
Quazepam	Oxycodone and Aspirin
Reserpine	Pentazocine
Selegiline hydrochloride	Phenylpropanolamine hydrochloride
Temazepam	Prazosin hydrochloride
Thiethylperazine maleate	Promethazine hydrochloride
Trihexyphenidyl hydrochloride	Propoxyphene
Trimipramine maleate	Pseudophedrine
Venlafaxine	Risperidone
	Sertraline hydrochloride
	Terazosin
	Terbutaline sulfate

From Wynn RL, Meiller TF, Crossley HL: Drug Information Handbook for Dentistry, 4th ed. Hudson, New York, Lexi-Comp, 1998–1999.

Effects of Anticholinergic Agents

Anticholinergic agents inhibit bodily functions by blocking muscarinic cholinergic receptors. Common agents in this category include atropine and propantheline bromide (Pro-Banthine).

I. Therapeutic Uses
   A. Preoperative medication to inhibit salivary and bronchial secretions (to produce a dry field) and to block vagal slowing of the heart in response to general anesthetics.
   B. Treatment of Parkinson-like tremors caused by smooth muscle relaxation from antipsychotic agents.
   C. Treatment of motion sickness; also aid sleep by depressing the CNS.
   D. Treatment of GI disorders (e.g., gastric ulcers) by decreasing secretions and hypermotility.
   E. Eye examinations; produce relaxation of the lens and mydriasis.
II. Contraindications
   A. Prostatic hypertrophy or intestinal or urinary obstruction or retention (because of increased urinary retention).
   B. Cardiovascular disease (because of tachycardia [vagal blockade]).
   C. Glaucoma (narrow-angle) (because of an increase in intraocular pressure).
III. Pharmacologic Effects
   A. On the CNS are dose dependent; high doses result in stimulation and therapeutic doses result in depression.
   B. On the CVS are dose dependent; high doses result in tachycardia (vagal blockade) and small doses result in bradycardia.
   C. Smooth muscle relaxation results in bronchodilation and constipation.
   D. The exocrine gland reduces secretions in the respiratory, genitourinary, and GI tracts.
   E. Include mydriasis (pupil dilation) and cycloplegia (blurred vision).
IV. Adverse Reactions
   A. Xerostomia, photophobia, blurred vision, signs of CNS stimulation, tachycardia, and hyperpyrexia (high fever).
   B. Urinary and GI stasis.
V. Drug Interactions
   A. Increased anticholinergic effects with TCAs, antihistamines, antidepressants, opioids and antipsychotics.
   B. Decreased absorption of ketoconazole.

Anxiety and Pain Management

The management of pain and anxiety during dental treatment involves the use of a variety of agents, including antianxiety agents, analgesics, anesthetics, and sedatives.

Effects of Antianxiety Agents

The main purpose of antianxiety agents is to decrease anxiety through depression of the CNS. Common agents in this category include benzodiazepines, barbiturates, chloral hydrate, and meprobamate.

I. Benzodiazepines
   A. Therapeutic uses
      1. Treatment of anxiety with diazepam (Valium), alprazolam (Xanax), temazepam (Restoril), and triazolam (Halcion).
      2. Treatment of insomnia by means of CNS depression with flurazepam (Dalmane).
      3. Treatment of alcohol withdrawal (agitation or tremors) with chlordiazepoxide (Librium), lorazepam (Ativan), and oxazepam (Serax).
      4. Treatment of seizures/epilepsy with clonazepam (Klonopin) and diazepam (Valium).
   B. Contraindications include hypersensitivity to benzodiazepines, pregnancy, psychosis (these patients experience CNS stimulation with benzodiazepines), and chronic pain (because of possible abuse and addiction).
   C. Pharmacologic effects include antianxiety and anticonvulsant effects and muscle relaxation.
   D. Adverse reactions generally include:
      1. Depression of the CNS, which results in sedation and fatigue.
      2. Thrombophlebitis, if given intravenously.
      3. Possible teratogenicity, especially if taken during the first trimester of pregnancy.
      4. Xerostomia.
      5. Possible addiction; occurs less often than with barbiturates.
   E. Drug interactions include increased effects with alcohol and CNS depressants.
II. Barbiturates (among the first antianxiety medications)
   A. Are classified by length of action and include:
      1. Ultrashort acting—methohexital (Brevital) and thiopental sodium (Pentothal).
      2. Short acting—pentobarbital (Nembutal) and secobarbital (Seconal).
      3. Intermediate acting—amobarbital (Amytal) and butabarbital (Butisol).
      4. Long acting—phenobarbital (Luminal).
   B. Therapeutic uses are determined by duration of action.
      1. Ultrashort-acting barbiturates are used for short-term general anesthesia.
      2. Short-acting and intermediate-acting barbiturates typically are replaced by benzodiazepines for antianxiety and insomnia.
      3. Long-acting barbiturates are used for the treatment of seizures/epilepsy.
   C. Contraindications

1. Hypersensitivity.
2. Addiction.
3. Porphyria (excess amount of porphyrins)—barbiturates can stimulate and increase the production of porphyrins.
4. Chronic pain (because of abuse and addiction).

D. Pharmacologic effects include depression of the CNS, which results in sedation (higher doses of these agents result in greater CNS depression, including respiratory and CV depression), and an anticonvulsant effect. Barbiturates stimulate microsomal enzymes in the liver to stimulate the metabolism of other drugs that are metabolized by liver.

E. Drug interactions
   1. Decreased effects of acetaminophen, beta-blockers, oral contraceptives, doxycycline, phenytoin, steroids, TCA, and warfarin.
   2. Enhanced effects with the use of disulfiram, MAO inhibitors, and propoxyphene.
   3. Enhanced CNS depression with the use of alcohol and other CNS depressants.

III. Chloral hydrate is given orally and used for the sedation of children.

IV. Meprobamate is used for dental anxiety disorders and as a muscle relaxant for acute TMJ muscle spasm.

Effects of Analgesic Agents

Analgesic agents, which include both opioid and nonopioid types, inhibit the perception of pain. Opioid agents depress pain perception in the CNS by binding with opioid receptors. Nonopioid agents reduce pain perception by inhibiting prostaglandin synthesis; they are more effective if they are taken before the onset of pain. Common agents in this category include salicylates, nonsteroidal antiinflammatory agents (NSAIA), and acetaminophen.

I. Nonopioid agents (Tables 9–2 and 9–3)
   A. Salicylates include aspirin and diflunisal (Dolobid), a long-acting salicylate.
      1. Therapeutic uses include:
         a. Analgesia for mild-to-moderate pain.
         b. Reduction of fever (antipyretic effect).
         c. Reduction of pain and swelling (antiinflammatory effect); also are used to treat inflammatory conditions such as arthritis.
         d. Prevention of post-MI (antiplatelet effect).
      2. Contraindications
         a. Hypersensitivity to salicylates.
         b. GI bleeding or bleeding disorders (because of GI irritation and antiplatelet effect).
         c. Children with flu-like symptoms (Reye syndrome can occur with the use of salicylates during some viral infections).
         d. Peptic ulcers (because of GI irritation).
      3. Pharmacologic effects
         a. Analgesia for mild-to-moderate pain relief.
         b. Antipyretic effect (reduces fever).
         c. Antiinflammatory effect via inhibition of prostaglandin synthesis, which decreases vasodilation and swelling.
         d. Antiplatelet effect via reduction of platelet aggregation, which results in reduced clotting.
         e. Uricosuric effect; high doses of aspirin (more than 5 g/24 hours) cause an increase in uric acid secretion in urine.
      4. Adverse reactions
         a. GI irritation, which is most common and is caused by direct irritation of the stomach mucosa
         b. Increased bleeding also can occur because of an increase in prothrombin time (bleeding time) via the drug's antiplatelet effect.
      5. Drug interactions
         a. An increased risk of bleeding with the use of anticoagulants.
         b. An increased risk of GI complaints with the use of NSAIAs, corticosteroids, and alcohol.
         c. An increased risk of hypoglycemia with the use of oral antidiabetic agents.
         d. Decreased effects of gout medications such as probenecid and sulfinpyrazone.
         e. An increased risk of toxicity with the use of methotrexate, lithium, and zidovudine.
   B. NSAIAs include naproxen (Naprosyn, Anaprox, OTC—Aleve), ibuprofen (Motrin, OTC—Advil,

TABLE 9.2 Nonopioids: Comparison of Analgesic Efficacy			
Drug	**Dose (mg)**	**Dosing Interval (hr)**	**Peak (hr)**
Ibuprofen (Nuprin, IB, Motrin, Pamprin)	400	4–6	1–2
Acetaminophen (Tylenol)	325–650	4–6	0.5–2
Naproxen sodium (Aleve)	250–500	6–8	1–2
Aspirin (Empirin, Genuine Bayer)	650	4–6	1–2
Diflunisal (Dolobid)	Loading dose: 1000; subsequent doses: 500	8–12	2–3

TABLE 9.3 Drug Interactions with Commonly Used Analgesics

NSAIA	Increase effects of anticoagulants
	Decrease antihypertensive effects of ACE inhibitors (captopril), beta blockers, loop diuretics, and thiazide diuretics
	Nephrotoxicity with cyclosporine
	Increase effects of digoxin
	Increase effects of phenytoin
	Increase effects of lithium
	Increase methotrexate toxicity
	Increase effects of sympathomimetics
	Probenecid increases NSAIA concentrations
	Salicylates decrease NSAIA concentrations
Salicylates (aspirin)	Corticosteroids decrease salicylate concentrations
	Nizatidine increases salicylate concentrations
	Alcohol increases GI ulceration and bleeding time
	Increase effects of anticoagulants
	Decrease antihypertensive effects of ACE inhibitors (captopril), beta blockers, loop diuretics, and thiazide diuretics
	Decrease NSAIA concentrations
	Decrease uricosuric effect of probenecid and sulfinpyrazone
	Increase effect of sulfonylureas and exogenous insulin, thereby increasing hypoglycemic effect
	Dose >2 g per day displaces valproic acid (VA) from binding site, thereby increasing VA effect
Acetaminophen (Tylenol)	Alcohol increases hepatotoxicity
	Beta blocker (propranolol) increases effects of acetaminophen
	Oral contraceptives decrease half-life

Pamprin), etodolac (Lodine), ketorolac (Toradol), and indomethacin (Indocin).

1. Therapeutic uses include the control of mild-to-moderate pain, fever, and inflammatory conditions such as rheumatoid arthritis.
2. Contraindications include:
   a. Hypersensitivity to any antiinflammatory agents.
   b. Any blood clotting problems (because of antiplatelet effect).
   c. Renal disease (because of higher risk of adverse renal reactions).
   d. GI disorders such as peptic ulcer.
   e. Asthma.
3. Pharmacologic effects include analgesic, antipyretic, and antiinflammatory effects similar to those of aspirin.
4. Adverse reactions
   a. Stomach mucosa irritation similar to aspirin's effect on the GI tract; xerostomia also may occur.
   b. Inhibition of platelets; occur only for drug's duration.
   c. Depression of the CNS, including sedation, dizziness, and depression.
5. Drug interactions
   a. Decreased effects of antihypertensive agents.
   b. Increased effects of oral anticoagulants, lithium, digoxin, phenytoin, and sympathomimetics.

   c. Increased risk of toxicity with the use of methotrexate.

II. Acetaminophen (para-aminophenols)
   A. Tylenol, Datril, and Tempra
   B. Therapeutic uses include reduction of mild to moderate pain and fever.
   C. Contraindications include hypersensitivity to acetaminophen and hepatic or renal disease.
   D. Pharmacologic effects include analgesic and antipyretic effects similar to those of aspirin and NSAIA; little or no antiinflammatory effect occurs.
   E. Adverse reactions include hepatotoxicity and nephrotoxicity and are associated with long-term use or excessively high doses.
      1. The minimum toxic dose is 10 g (140 mg/kg) but liver damage occurs with one 5.85-g dose.
      2. Chronic excessive use (of more than 4 g/day) can cause transient hepatotoxicity.
      3. The safe dose for chronic alcoholics should not exceed 4 g/day; should be 2 g/day or less if hepatotoxicity has occurred (occurs in some chronic alcoholics who take the therapeutic dose).
   F. Drug interactions are relatively rare at therapeutic doses.

III. Opioid Agents (Tables 9–4 and 9–5)
   A. Depress the CNS by interacting with opioid receptors.
   B. Common agents include morphine, hydromorphine (Dilaudid), meperidine (Demerol), propoxyphene (Darvon), and codeine; can be addicting.

C. Therapeutic uses include analgesia for moderate to severe pain, cough suppression, sedation, and anxiety relief.
D. Contraindications
  1. Hypersensitivity to opioids.
  2. Respiratory problems, including asthma and emphysema (because of respiratory center depression).
  3. Chronic pain (because addiction may occur).
  4. Head injury (because of an increase in intracranial pressure).
E. Pharmacologic effects
  1. Analgesic effect for relief of moderate to severe pain.
  2. Sedative effect for relief of mild anxiety.
  3. Antitussive effect, which aids cough suppression.
  4. Antidiarrheal effect (via increase in smooth muscle tone in GI tract).
F. Adverse reactions are related to the drug's potency (a drug with greater potency is more likely to have adverse reactions) and include:
  1. Decreased rate and depth of respiration.
  2. Increased intracranial pressure (because of cranial vasodilation).
  3. Bradycardia and orthostatic hypotension.
  4. Drowsiness, sedation, and (occasionally) stimulation.
  5. Nausea, emesis (vomiting), and constipation.
  6. Miosis (pupil constriction); may be used to determine abuse of opioids or overdose
  7. Urinary retention.
G. Drug interactions include increased sedation and respiratory depression in conjunction with the use of other CNS depressants or alcohol.
IV. Opioid Antagonists
  A. Short-acting naloxone (Narcan), which is used to reverse respiratory depression caused by opioids
  B. Long-acting naltrexone (ReVia, Trexan), which is used for the treatment of opioid addiction after detoxification.

Effects of Anesthetic Agents

Anesthetic agents include local and general anesthetics that are used for the control of pain. This section also addresses the use of vasoconstrictors.
I. Local Anesthetic Agents
  A. Amides
    1. Shorter-acting amides include lidocaine, mepivacaine, prilocaine.
    2. Longer-acting amides include bupivacaine and etidocaine.
  B. Esters
    1. Include procaine/propoxycaine.
    2. Esters were withdrawn from the US market in January 1996.
II. Pharmacologic Effects
  A. Reversibly blocked peripheral nerve conduction.

TABLE 9.4   Analgesic Drug Combinations and Uses

Drug Name	Opioid Component	Nonopioid Component	Dental Use
Hydrocodone w/APAP Bancap HC Dolacet Vicodin	Hydrocodone	Acetaminophen	Mild-to-moderate pain; posttreatment pain control
Acetaminophen w/codeine Capital w/codeine Phenaphen w/codeine Tylenol w/codeine	Codeine	Acetaminophen	Mild-to-moderate pain; posttreatment pain control
Propoxyphene N/APAP Darvocet-N 100 Propacet 100 Wygesic	Propoxyphene napsylate	Acetaminophen	Mild-to-moderate pain; posttreatment pain control
Roxicet Percocet Tylox	Oxycodone	Acetaminophen	Moderate-to-severe pain; treatment of postoperative pain
Hydrocodone w/aspirin Lortab ASA Alora 5/500 Azdone	Hydrocodone	Aspirin	Mild-to-moderate pain; posttreatment pain control
Oxycodone w/aspirin Percodan Codoxy Percodan-Demi Roxiprin	Oxycodone	Aspirin	Moderate-to-severe pain; treatment of postoperative pain

TABLE 9.5	DEA Controlled Substances (DEA Controlled Substance Act of 1970)			
Schedule	**Abuse Potential**	**Medical Use**	**Examples**
I	High	None, except research	Heroin, hallucinogens, opium derivatives
II Requires prescription; nonrefillable	High (severe dependence possible)	Legal medical uses	Oxycodone, amphetamines, morphine
III Requires prescription; five refills in 6 months	Lower than Schedule I or II drugs (moderate dependence possible)	Legal medical uses	Codeine, anabolic steroids
IV Requires prescription; five refills in 6 months	Low (limited dependence possible)	Legal medical uses	Benzodiazepines, barbiturates
V Requires prescription; five refills in 6 months	Lower than Schedule IV drugs	Legal medical uses	Codeine cough syrups

B. Depressed cardiac conduction and excitability that results in hypotension.

C. Adverse reactions
1. Talkativeness, apprehension, tremors, and seizures (sometimes followed by CNS depression, respiratory and CV depression, and coma).
2. A hematoma at the site of injection.
3. Allergy, ranging from a rash to anaphylaxis; allergic reaction to esters occur more often than allergic reactions to amide local anesthetics; if there is an allergy to both esters and amides the antihistamine Benadryl can be used for a local anesthetic effect.

D. Metabolism (biotransformation) of amides occurs primarily in the liver; pseudocholinesterase, an enzyme found in plasma, hydrolyzes esters.

E. The excretion of both amides and esters occurs by means of the kidneys.

F. Drug interactions include an additive effect with the use of CNS depressants.

III. Vasoconstrictors
A. Are agents that vasoconstrict blood vessels via stimulation of alpha$_1$ receptors.
B. Common agents include epinephrine and levonordefrin (Neo-cobefrin).
C. Clinical applications of vasoconstrictors found in local anesthetics
1. Hemostasis (decreased bleeding) by means of blood vessel constriction.
2. Decreased absorption of local anesthetics into CVS because of blood vessel constriction.
3. Increased duration of local anesthetics because of decreased absorption into CVS.
D. Pharmacologic effects
1. Vasoconstriction of blood vessels in response to alpha$_1$ receptor stimulation.

2. Cardiac stimulation and lipolysis in response to beta$_1$ receptor stimulation.
3. Bronchodilation in response to beta$_2$ receptor stimulation.

E. Adverse reactions include tremors, anxiety, palpitations, and hypertension.

F. Drug interactions
1. Vasoconstriction; is enhanced with TCA when epinephrine is given intravenously.
2. Hypertension, when used in conjunction with nonselective beta blockers.
3. An increase in blood glucose with the use of oral antidiabetic agents.
4. Cardiovascular patients who undergo elective dental treatment should:
   a. Receive a local anesthetic with a vasoconstrictor to increase pain control and its duration, which lowers patient stress level.
   b. Receive no more than the maximum epinephrine dose of .04 mg.

IV. General Anesthetic Agents
A. Are agents that depress the CNS.
B. Stages of anesthesia
1. Guedel's four stages of ether anesthesia
   a. Stage I: analgesia (reduced pain sensation)
   b. Stage II: delirium or excitement (unconsciousness and involuntary movement)
   c. Stage III: surgical anesthesia
   d. Stage IV: respiratory or medullary paralysis (death occurs if stage IV is not reversed)
2. Flagg's stages provide a more modern description of anesthesia levels (because of the more rapidly acting agents currently in use).
   a. The induction phase occurs before surgery.
   b. The maintenance phase begins when the depth of anesthesia that is necessary for

the operation is achieved; continues until the procedure is completed.

   c. The recovery phase occurs at the end of the operation and continues through the postoperative period until the patient is fully responsive.

C. Adverse reactions

   a. Dysrhythmias, cardiac arrest, hypertension, and hypotension.

   b. Respiratory depression and arrest.

   c. Teratogenicity, with chronic exposure.

   d. Hepatotoxicity, with chronic exposure.

D. Common agents

1. Nitrous oxide, an inhalation gas (relatively odorless and colorless); is used in dentistry for conscious sedation.

   a. Contraindications

     1) Respiratory obstruction or stuffy nose (because no exchange of gas is possible through nasal passages).

     2) COPD—The patient cannot tolerate receiving additional oxygen outside the room O_2 they breathe.

     3) Emotional instability or mental illness (altered sense or euphoria may occur).

     4) Pregnancy (spontaneous abortion or miscarriage may occur; chronic exposure reduces fertility in women).

     5) Contagious disease, such as tuberculosis or hepatitis, if nonautoclavable tubes are used.

   b. Pharmacologic effects include analgesia and amnesia, with no significant effect on the respiratory system.

   c. Adverse reactions

     1) Peripheral vasodilation.

     2) Nausea and vomiting, especially if patient consumes a large meal before nitrous oxide is administered.

     3) Diffusion hypoxia may result in headache or other adverse reactions if patient does not receive 5 minutes of 100% oxygen when nitrous oxide administration is terminated.

     4) Neuropathy and paresthesia result with abuse; symptoms include numbness of hands and legs and liver and kidney problems.

2. Inhalation volatile liquids

   a. Halogenated ether, including enflurane (Ethrane).

     1) Produces greater skeletal muscle relaxation than halothane.

     2) Adverse reactions

       a) Respiratory depression.

       b) Myocardial contractility depression.

       c) Hypotension.

       d) Dysrhythmias (occur less often than with halothane).

       e) Depressed renal function.

       f) Possible seizure activity.

   b. Halogenated hydrocarbon, including halothane (Fluothane).

     1) Characteristics include a fruity odor; is nonflammable/nonexplosive; is safe for asthmatics because it does not irritate bronchioles.

     2) Adverse reactions

       a) Incomplete muscle relaxation.

       b) Depression of renal function.

       c) Uterine muscle relaxation.

       d) Possible bradycardia, hypotension, and dysrhythmias.

   c. Halogenated ether, including isoflurane (Forane).

     1) Is a commonly used general anesthetic.

     2) Adverse reactions encompass respiratory depression, hypotension, and muscle relaxation; does not cause liver toxicity. Deeper levels of anesthesia result in respiratory acidosis.

     3) Intravenous agents

       a) Ultrashort-acting barbiturates such as thiopental (Pentothal), methohexital (Brevital), and thiamylal (Surital); IV administration results in a rapid onset of action; are not analgesics—local anesthetics are required for pain control.

     4) Contraindications include porphyria and status asthmaticus.

     5) Adverse reactions encompass bronchospasm, laryngospasm, hiccups, increased muscle activity, and delirium on recovery.

   d. Ketamine (Ketalar) is chemically related to phencyclidine (PCP) and produces dissociative anesthesia (patient fails to respond to environment but is not asleep.)

     1) Contraindications include hypertension and cerebrovascular disease.

     2) Adverse reactions encompass elevated blood pressure and pulse, nausea, and excessive salivation (atropine may be required for dry field); causes hallucinations and delirium during recovery.

   e. Opioids include sufentanil (Sufenta), fentanyl (Sublimaze), alfentanil (Alfenta), and morphine.

     1) Do not cause significant peripheral vascular resistance or CV changes.

     2) Primary adverse reaction is respiratory depression, which is reversible with the use of naloxone, an opioid antagonist.

f. Innovar is a neuroleptic agent combination of the antipsychotic agent (droperidol) with the opioid analgesic (fentanyl). Droperidol causes sedation and catatonia, and this drug combination produces a wakeful anesthetic state.
1) Contraindications include Parkinson's disease and pulmonary insufficiency.
2) Adverse reactions
   a) A boardlike chest, which requires ventilatory assistance.
   b) Respiratory depression.
   c) Tremors.

 ## Clinical Case STUDY

Ms. Hancock, a 29-year-old recall patient, apologizes for missing her last 6-month recall appointment. Although she currently takes no medications, she reveals that she took Redux last year for 3 months. Her mandibular anterior gingiva is visibly hemorrhagic, and Ms. Hancock confirms that her gums bleed when she brushes. Her blood pressure reading is 148/98. Her previous blood pressure reading was 120/76.

Clinical Case QUESTIONS

1. What type of drug is Redux and why is it prescribed?
2. What might explain the change in Ms. Hancock's blood pressure readings?
3. Should Ms. Hancock receive dental treatment at this recall appointment?

Clinical Case RATIONALES

1. Redux (dexfenfluramine) is an anorexiant agent. It suppresses appetite and is prescribed as an aid to weight loss.
2. Although one adverse effect of Redux is hypertension, this effect typically disappears after the drug is discontinued. A moderate weight gain after discontinuing the medication might be a cause of Ms. Hancock's high blood pressure. A more serious cause might be primary pulmonary hypertension, which is a side effect of the drug and is associated with dyspnea, angina, syncope, edema of the lower extremities, and possible congestive heart failure. Her diastolic reading is considered stage-1 (mild) hypertension according to the Fifth Report of the Joint Medical Committee on Detection, Evaluation, and Treatment of High Blood Pressure, 1993. Redux (dexfenfluramine) and Pondimin (fenfluramine), once commonly prescribed diet drugs, were both removed from the market in 1997 because of their adverse effects on the heart and lungs. The effects of these drugs currently are being studied. It is possible that as many as one third of the individuals who took these drugs have permanent damage to their heart valves, which puts them at risk for bacterial endocarditis.
3. She should not receive invasive dental treatment (including oral prophylaxis) at this time. The USDHHS recommends a medical consultation for patients who have taken Redux or Pondimin when there is a possibility of significant oral bleeding or before any invasive procedure (oral prophylaxis) is performed. This patient should be referred to her physician because of her blood pressure reading and history of Redux use. The physician most likely will recommend that the patient have an echocardiogram to determine whether heart valve damage has occurred. If the echocardiogram reveals heart valve damage, the patient must be premedicated (according to the AHA recommendations for the prevention of bacterial endocarditis) before any invasive dental procedure. Invasive procedures that must be performed before a thorough medical evaluation require preventive coverage with the recommended antibiotic.

Infection Management

Agents that are used for infection management include medications in the antibiotic, antifungal, antiviral, and antituberculosis categories. The AHA Recommendations for the Prevention of Infectious Endocarditis are in Boxes 9–1 and 9–2 and Table 9–6.

Oral Antimicrobial Agents

Oral antimicrobial agents destroy microorganisms or prevent their growth. Common agents in this category include chlorhexidine, essential oils, triclosan, and sanguinarine.

I. Chlorhexidine (Peridex, Perioguard)
   A. Requires a prescription.
   B. Contains 0.12% alcohol.
   C. Has high substantivity.
   D. Reduces plaque and gingivitis.
   E. Is used for the treatment of ANUG, candidiasis, and herpetic stomatitis; also is used postsurgically.
II. Essential Oils (Listerine)
   A. Contains thymol, menthol, eucalyptol, methylsalicylate, and 25% alcohol.
   B. Has low substantivity.
   C. Is nonprescription.
   D. Reduces gingivitis.
III. Triclosan (Colgate's Total toothpaste)
   A. Is second-generation to Listerine.
   B. Reduces plaque and gingivitis.
IV. Sanguinarine (Viadent)
   A. Originates from the blood root of the sanguinaria canadensis plant.

BOX 9.1 Cardiac Conditions Associated with Endocarditis

Endocarditis Prophylaxis Recommended

High-risk category
Prosthetic cardiac valves, including bioprosthetic and homograft valves
Previous bacterial endocarditis
Complex cyanotic congenital heart disease (e.g., single ventricle states, transposition of the great arteries, tetralogy of Fallot)
Surgically constructed systemic pulmonary shunts or conduits

Moderate-risk category
Most other congenital cardiac malformations (other than mentioned here)
Acquired valvar dysfunction (e.g., rheumatic heart disease)
Hypertrophic cardiomyopathy
Mitral valve prolapse with valvar regurgitation and/or thickened leaflets

Endocarditis Prophylaxis Not Recommended

Negligible-risk category (no greater risk than the general population)
Isolated secundum atrial septal defect
Surgical repair of atrial septal defect, ventricular septal defect, or patent ductus arteriosus (without residua beyond 6 months)
Previous coronary artery bypass graft surgery
Mitral valve prolapse without valvar regurgitation
Physiologic, functional, or innocent heart murmurs
Previous Kawasaki disease without valvar dysfunction
Previous rheumatic fever without valvar dysfunction
Cardiac pacemakers (intravascular and epicardial) and implanted defibrillators

From Dajani AS, Taubert KA, Wilson W, et al: Prevention of Bacterial Endocarditis: Recommendations by the American Heart Association. JAMA 277(22):1794–1801, 1997.

B. Has minimal substantivity.
C. Is nonprescription.
D. Reduces plaque and gingivitis.
E. Is found in tooth pastes and mouth rinses.

Effects of Antibacterial Agents

Antibacterial agents stop the growth of bacteria and include penicillins, tetracyclines, cephalosporins, clindamycin, macrolides, aminoglycosides, vancomycin, metronidazole, and trimethoprim-sulfamethoxazole.

I. Penicillins
  A. Include three subgroups: narrow-spectrum, penicillinase-resistant, and broad-spectrum/wide-spectrum/extended-spectrum penicillins.
    1. Narrow-spectrum penicillins include Penicillin G and Penicillin V (Pen-Vee K); Penicillin V is used more often in dentistry because of its better oral absorption.
    2. The therapeutic uses of Penicillin V include treatment of ANUG, periodontal abscesses, soft tissue infections, and osteomyelitis.
    3. Penicillinase-resistant penicillins include cloxacillin and dicloxacillin, which are narrow spectrum; therapeutic uses include treatment of infections caused by penicillinase-producing cocci.
    4. Broad-/extended-/wide-spectrum penicillins include ampicillin and amoxicillin; amoxicillin is used more often in dentistry. The therapeutic uses of amoxicillin are similar to those of Penicillin V; it is the first drug of choice for the AHA prophylactic antibiotic regimen (adults 2.0 g, children 50 mg/kg PO 1 hour before procedure).
  B. Contraindications include hypersensitivity to penicillin.

BOX 9.2 Dental Procedures and Endocarditis Prophylaxis

Endocarditis Prophylaxis Recommended*

Dental extractions
Periodontal procedures including surgery, scaling and root planing, probing, and recall maintenance
Dental implant placement and reimplantation of avulsed teeth
Endodontic (root canal) instrumentation or surgery only beyond the apex
Subgingival placement of antibiotic fibers or strips
Initial placement of orthodontic bands but not brackets
Intraligamentary local anesthetic injections
Prophylactic cleaning of teeth or implants when bleeding is anticipated

Endocarditis Prophylaxis Not Recommended

Restorative dentistry† (operative and prosthodontic) with or without retraction cord‡
Local anesthetic injections (nonintraligamentary)
Intracanal endodontic treatment; post placement and buildup
Placement of rubber dams
Postoperative suture removal
Placement of removable prosthodontic or orthodontic appliances
Taking of oral impressions
Fluoride treatments
Taking of oral radiographs
Orthodontic appliance adjustment
Shedding of primary teeth

From Dajani AS, Taubert KA, Wilson W, et al: Prevention of Bacterial Endocarditis: Recommendations by the American Heart Association. JAMA 277(22):1794–1801, 1997.
*Prophylaxis is recommended for patients with high- and moderate-risk cardiac conditions.
†This includes restoration of decayed teeth (filling cavities) and replacement of missing teeth.
‡Clinical judgment may indicate antibiotic use in selected circumstances that may create significant bleeding.

TABLE 9.6 Prophylactic Regimens for Dental, Oral, Respiratory Tract, or Esophageal Procedures

Situation	Agent	Regimen*
Standard general prophylaxis	Amoxicillin	Adults: 2.0 g; children: 50 mg/kg orally 1 hr before procedure
Unable to take oral medications	Ampicillin	Adults: 2.0 g IM or IV; children: 50 mg/kg IM or IV within 30 min before procedure
Allergic to penicillin	Clindamycin or	Adults: 600 mg; children: 20 mg/kg orally 1 hr before procedure
	Cephalexin† or cefadroxil† or	Adults: 2.0 g; children: 50 mg/kg orally 1 hr before procedure
	Azithromycin or clarithromycin	Adults: 500 mg; children: 15 mg/kg orally 1 hr before procedure
Allergic to penicillin and unable to take oral medications	Clindamycin or	Adults: 600 mg; children: 20 mg/kg IV within 30 min before procedure
	Cefazolin†	Adults: 1.0 g; children: 25 mg/kg IM or IV within 30 min before procedure

From Dajani AS, Taubert KA, Wilson W, et al: Prevention of Bacterial Endocarditis: Recommendations by the American Heart Association. JAMA 277(22):1794–1801, 1997.
*Total children's dose should not exceed adult dose.
†Cephalosporins should not be used in individuals with immediate-type hypersensitivity reaction (urticaria, angioedema, or anaphylaxis) to penicillins.

C. Adverse reactions are similar to those of other antiinfective agents and include superinfection, allergic reaction, and GI irritation.
D. Drug interactions
1. Decreased effectiveness of oral contraceptives.
2. Increased anticoagulant effect.
3. Decreased antimicrobial effectiveness with tetracyclines and erythromycins.
II. Tetracyclines
A. Include tetracycline, doxycycline, and minocycline.
B. Therapeutic uses include treatment of syphilis, gonorrhea, acne, LJP, and RAP.
C. Contraindications include hypersensitivity to tetracycline and patients who are younger than 8 years of age (because of effects on developing teeth).
D. Adverse reactions
1. Allergic reactions (allergenicity rate is low).
2. Permanent discoloration of teeth (if taken during developmental period involving enamel calcification).
3. GI irritation, including nausea, vomiting, diarrhea, and xerostomia.
4. Superinfection.
5. Increased risk of hepatotoxicity (liver damage) when tetracycline is given intravenously.
6. Nephrotoxicity (with the use of old tetracycline).
7. Photosensitivity as result of sunburn (because of an exaggerated response of skin to sun exposure).

E. Drug interactions
1. Decreased effectiveness of oral contraceptives.
2. Decreased tetracycline effect in response to chelation, when concomitantly administered with dairy products (Ca), mineral supplements (Fe, Ca, fortified foods), or antacids (Ca, Mg, Al).
3. Enhanced effect of oral sulfonylureas, which results in hypoglycemia.
4. Increased effect of anticoagulants.
III. Cephalosporins
A. Include cephalexin (Keflex), cefadroxil (Duricef), cefazolin (Ancef), and cefaclor (Ceclor).
B. Therapeutic uses
1. Treatment of most infections caused by Gram-positive cocci and penicillinase-producing staphylococci and some Gram-negative bacteria; salmonella and E. coli; respiratory and urinary tract infections; and otitis media.
2. Is the drug of choice for the AHA prophylactic antibiotic regimen for penicillin-allergic patients (cephalexin—adult 2.0 g, children 50 mg/kg PO 1 hour before procedure).
C. Contraindications include hypersensitivity to cephalosporins.
D. Adverse reactions
1. Allergic reactions ranging from rash to anaphylaxis.
2. GI irritation, which commonly includes diarrhea, nausea, and vomiting.
3. Superinfections.
4. Nephrotoxicity.
5. Hemostasis impairment.

6. Local reactions include localized pain and swelling in response to IM administration.

E. Drug interactions include decreased effectiveness of oral contraceptives and decreased effectiveness of cephalosporins with the use of tetracyclines and erythromycins.

IV. Clindamycin
   A. Therapeutic uses
      1. Treatment of infections caused by *Bacteriodes fragilis* and Gram-positive organisms.
      2. Is the drug of choice for the AHA prophylactic antibiotic regimen for penicillin-allergic patients (adult 600 mg, children 20 mg/kg PO 1 hour before procedure).
   B. Contraindications include hypersensitivity to clindamycin and lincomycin and ulcerative colitis/enteritis (because of GI irritation).
   C. Adverse reactions encompass superinfections, allergic reactions, and GI irritation.
   D. Drug interactions
      1. Decreased effectiveness when given with erythromycin.
      2. Increased effects of nondepolarizing muscle relaxants.

V. Macrolides
   A. Include erythromycin stearate, erythromycin ethylsuccinate (EES), azithromycin (Zithromax), and clarithromycin (Biaxin).
   B. Therapeutic uses
      1. Treatment of mild to moderate respiratory tract infections, otitis media, syphilis, and Legionnaire's disease.
      2. Is the drug of choice for the AHA prophylactic antibiotic regimen for penicillin-allergic patients (azithromycin—adult 500 mg, children 15 mg/kg PO 1 hour before procedure).
   C. Contraindications include hypersensitivity to erythromycin.
   D. Adverse reactions include GI irritation with standard therapeutic doses; allergic reactions are uncommon.
   E. Drug interactions
      1. Increased cardiac toxicity with use of terfenadine (Seldane) or astemizole (Hismanal).
      2. Increased serum concentration with the use of digoxin, warfarin, carbamazepine (Tegretol), or cyclosporine.
      3. Decreased effectiveness of oral contraceptives.

VI. Aminoglycosides
   A. Gentamicin is used for the treatment of Gram-negative infections that require hospitalization (e.g., bone, respiratory tract, and urinary tract infections); is combined with ampicillin for the AHA regimen for patients with prosthetic heart valves (who cannot use the oral prophylaxis regimen).
   B. Neomycin is a topical agent used in the treatment of skin infections.

VII. Vancomycin
   A. In combination with gentamicin is the drug of choice in the AHA regimen for patients in high-risk categories (e.g., with prosthetic heart valves or history of previous bacterial endocarditis) who are allergic to penicillin.

VIII. Metronidazole (Flagyl)
   A. Therapeutic uses in dentistry include the treatment of infections caused by anaerobes such as *Bacteroides* organisms and treatment of RAP. Medical uses include the treatment of intestinal amebiasis, trichomoniasis, and giardiasis.
   B. Contraindications include:
      1. Hypersensitivity to metronidazole.
      2. CNS disorders (because of CNS effects).
      3. Renal disease (because of renal toxicity).
   C. Adverse reactions
      1. Metallic taste, black hairy tongue, and xerostomia.
      2. Effects on the CNS, including dizziness, headache, and vertigo.
      3. Nausea, vomiting, and diarrhea.
      4. Renal toxicity.
   D. Drug interactions
      1. Disulfiram (Antabuse) reactions occur with the use of alcohol and alcohol-containing products; antimicrobial rinses (e.g., chlorhexidine and Listerine) that contain alcohol are contraindicated.
      2. Decreased effect with the use of phenobarbital.

IX. Trimethoprim-Sulfamethoxazole (TMP-SMX) (Bactrim)
   A. Is the drug of choice for the treatment of *Pneumocystis carinii* pneumonia (in patients with AIDS), urinary tract infections (UTI), and otitis media.
   B. Adverse reactions include skin rash and hematologic reactions (e.g., leukopenia, thrombocytopenia).

Effects of Antifungal Agents

Antifungal agents inhibit or destroy fungal growth. Common agents in this category include nystatin, clotrimazole, ketoconazole, and fluconazole.

I. Nystatin (Mycostatin) is used for the treatment and prevention of candidiasis.
II. Clotrimazole (Mycelex) is used to treat candidiasis.
   A. Drug interaction with terfenadine (Seldane) or astemizole (Hismanal) can produce cardiac dysrhythmia.
III. Ketoconazole (Nizoral)
   A. Is used therapeutically to treat candidiasis.
   B. Contraindications include hypersensitivity to ketoconazole.

C. Adverse reactions occur more often than with the use of other antifungal agents.
  1. GI irritation is most common (including nausea and vomiting).
  2. Hepatotoxicity is the most serious reaction.
  3. Other effects include headache, photophobia, and allergic reactions.
D. Drug interactions include decreased effect with the use of anticholinergics, H_2 blockers, antacids, and rifampin; cardiac toxicity occurs with the use of terfenadine and astemizole.
IV. Fluconazole (Diflucan) is a candidiasis prophylactic agent for immunocompromised patients; also is used for the treatment of nonresponsive candidal infections.

Effects of Antituberculosis Agents

Antituberculosis agents inhibit the spread of tuberculosis in patients and include such common agents as isoniazid, rifampin, and pyrazinamide.

I. Isoniazid (INH) is used in the treatment and prevention of tuberculosis (TB); can be used alone or in combination with rifampin and pyrazinamide.
  A. Contraindications include hypersensitivity to the agent(s).
  B. Adverse reactions
    1. Effects on the CNS that include peripheral neuropathy, toxic encephalopathy, and convulsions.
    2. Hepatotoxicity.
    3. Vitamin B_6 deficiency.
    4. Xerostomia.
    5. Hematologic effects that include hemolytic anemia, thrombocytopenia, and agranulocytosis.
  C. Drug interactions
    1. Increased hepatotoxicity with the use of alcohol or acetaminophen.
    2. Decreased effect of ketoconazole.
II. Rifampin (Rifadin, Rimactane)
  A. When administered with another antituberculosis agent, reduces the development of antituberculosis drug resistance.
  B. Contraindications include hypersensitivity to rifampin.
  C. Adverse reactions encompass stomatitis, discolored (red-orange) saliva, nausea, vomiting, diarrhea, and thrombocytopenia.
  D. Drug interactions
    1. Increased hepatotoxicity with the use of alcohol and acetaminophen.
    2. Decreased effect of ketoconazole.
III. Pyrazinamide
  A. Combined with INH and rifampin to treat tuberculosis.

Effects of Antiviral Agents

Antiviral agents oppose a virus by weakening its action or inhibiting its DNA synthesis. Common agents in this category include acyclovir and other agents used in the treatment of AIDS.

I. Acyclovir (Zovirax)
  A. Used topically, orally, and parenterally for various herpetic viruses.
II. Antiviral agents (used in the treatment of AIDS)
  A. Zidovudine (AZT; Retrovir)—acetaminophen and aspirin inhibit AZT's glucuronidation or excretion, which increases the toxicity of both drugs.
  B. Didanosine (ddI; Videx) is used when AZT is ineffective; absorption is decreased when coadministered with tetracycline.
  C. Zalcitabine or dideoxycytidine (ddC; HIVID) is combined with AZT when AZT alone does not work.
  D. Stavudine (d4T; Zerit) is used for patients who are intolerant to other therapies.
  E. Lamivudine (3TC; Epivir) works synergistically with AZT.
  F. Saquinavir mesylate (SAQ; Invirase) is a protease inhibitor used in combination with AZT or ddC.
  G. Indinavir (Crixivan) is a protease inhibitor used in triple drug therapy with AZT and 3TC (or other nucleoside medications used to treat AIDS).
  H. Ritonavir (Norvir) is a protease inhibitor used in monotherapy or in triple drug therapy.
  I. Nelfinavir mesylate (Viracept) is a protease inhibitor used in monotherapy or in combination drug therapy.
III. Adverse Reactions
  A. Headache, nausea, diarrhea, anemia, peripheral neuropathy, and oral ulcers.

 Clinical Case **STUDY**

Mrs. Jones, who is 60 years old, is due to return for a recall examination and oral prophylaxis appointment. To facilitate the appointment, her chart is reviewed before scheduling. Her health history reveals an allergy to penicillin and a history of infective endocarditis. When she is scheduled for the recall appointment her health history is reviewed and updated. Mrs. Jones reconfirms that she takes Lanoxin daily. Upon further questioning, she indicates that she began taking Seldane this spring.

Clinical Case QUESTIONS

1. Does Mrs. Jones require prophylactic antibiotic treatment before her appointment? If so, what antiinfective agent should be prescribed and why?
2. Why is Mrs. Jones taking Seldane?
3. Mrs. Jones takes Lanoxin for the treatment of which condition?
4. What types of drugs are Seldane and Lanoxin?

Clinical Case RATIONALES

1. Yes; the AHA prophylactic antibiotic regimen that was updated in 1997[1] should be followed. Amoxicillin should not be used because of her history of penicillin allergy. Erythromycin is no longer a recommended drug for the penicillin-allergic patient because of the high incidence of GI upset and the variability of the pharmacokinetics of the various erythromycin preparations. Azithromycin (Zithromax) or clarithromycin (Biaxin) most likely should be avoided in this particular patient because of potential drug interactions. Azithromycin and clarithromycin belong to the same family (macrolides) of antibiotics as erythromycin. Erythromycin may cause cardiac dysrhythmias when combined with Seldane, and Lanoxin in combination with erythromycin tends to increase Lanoxin availability, thereby increasing the risk of digoxin toxicity. Therefore the drug of choice in the AHA regimen, clindamycin (600 mg 1 hour before procedure), should be used. Postoperative dosage is unnecessary because sufficiently high plasma levels of antibiotic are present long enough to prevent endocarditis.
2. Terfenadine (Seldane) is used to treat rhinitis and seasonal allergies.
3. Digoxin (Lanoxin) is used to treat CHF.
4. Seldane is an H_1 receptor antagonist and Lanoxin is a cardiac glycoside.

Management of Special Patients

The Cardiovascular Patient

The cardiovascular patient has damage or disease of the heart and/or the blood vessels. Many of these patients take medications that have systemic and/or oral effects. Medications are used to treat a variety of cardiovascular disorders, including hypertension, congestive heart failure, dysrhythmias, and angina pectoris. Common therapeutic agents in this category include antihypertensives, digitalis glycosides, antidysrhythmics, antianginals, antihyperlipidemics, and anticoagulants.

I. Effects of Antihypertensive Agents
  A. These agents are used in the treatment of hypertension, the most common cardiovascular disease.
  B. Common agents
    1. Diuretics, such as:
      a. Thiazide-type diuretics, including hydrochlorothiazide (HCTZ).
        1) Adverse reactions include hypokalemia (low blood potassium), hyperglycemia (high blood glucose), and hyperuricemia (excessive uric acid in the body).
        2) Drug interactions include a decrease in hypotensive effect with the use of NSAIA.
      b. Loop diuretics, including furosemide (Lasix)—adverse reactions and drug interactions are the same as those for thiazides.
      c. Potassium-sparing diuretics, including spironolactone (Aldactone).
        1) Adverse reactions include hyperkalemia.
        2) Drug interactions are the same as those for thiazides.
      d. Thiazides combined with potassium-sparing diuretics, including Maxzide and Dyazide, which reduce the incidence of hypokalemia.
    2. Angiotensin-converting enzyme (ACE) inhibitors, including captopril (Capoten), enalapril (Vasotec), and lisinopril (Zestril).
      a. Adverse reactions include neutropenia (abnormal decrease in neutrophils in the blood), cough, dysgeusia (altered taste), xerostomia, and hypotension.
      b. Drug interactions include a decreased effect with the use of indomethacin and possibly other NSAIA.
    3. Calcium channel blockers, including verapamil (Isoptin, Calan), diltiazem (Cardizem), and nifedipine (Procardia).
      a. These agents also are used in the treatment of angina pectoris and dysrhythmias.
      b. Adverse reactions include hypotension, dizziness, lightheadedness, nausea, xerostomia, and gingival hyperplasia (Table 9–7).
      c. Drug interactions include a decreased effect with the use of indomethacin and possibly other NSAIA.
    4. Adrenergic blocking agents
      a. Nonselective beta agents block both beta receptors and include propranolol (Inderal).
        1) Other therapeutic uses include treatment of angina pectoris and migraine headaches and MI prophylaxis.
        2) Adverse reactions include bronchospasm, xerostomia, and bradycardia.
        3) Drug interactions
          a) NSAIA decrease antihypertensive effects.

TABLE 9.7	Drugs That Cause Gingival Hyperplasia	
Generic Name	**Brand Name**	**Drug Classification**
Diltiazem	Cardizem; Dilacor	Calcium channel blocker
Felodipine	Plendil	Calcium channel blocker
Nifedipine	Adalat; Procardia	Calcium channel blocker
Verapamil	Calan; Isoptin; Verelan	Calcium channel blocker
Phenytoin	Dilantin	Hydantoin

b) Hypertension and bradycardia occur with epinephrine use.

b. Selective beta-blocking agents block more beta$_1$ receptors and include atenolol (Tenormin) and metoprolol (Lopressor).

1) Other therapeutic uses include the treatment of angina pectoris.

2) Adverse reactions and drug interactions are the same as for nonselective beta-blocking agents.

c. Centrally acting antiadrenergic agents stimulate central alpha-adrenergic receptors and include clonidine (Catapres) and methyldopa (Aldomet).

1) Adverse reactions include xerostomia and sedation.

2) Drug interactions include:

a) Increase in CNS depression with the use of CNS depressant agents.

b) Decrease in hypotensive effect with the use of NSAIA and sympathomimetics.

d. Alpha$_1$ selective blockers include prazosin (Minipress).

5. Vasodilators include minoxidil (Loniten).

C. Pharmacologic effect—antihypertensive drugs lower blood pressure.

D. Adverse reactions include CNS depression, xerostomia, and orthostatic hypotension.

II. Effects of Digitalis Glycoside Agents

A. These agents are used in the treatment of congestive heart failure, which results from an inability of the heart to pump efficiently.

B. Digoxin (Lanoxin), a commonly prescribed agent, increases cardiac contractility and output.

C. Contraindications include hypersensitivity, ventricular fibrillation, and tachycardia.

D. Adverse reactions include:

1. Sensitive gag reflex.

2. Nausea and vomiting.

3. Effects on the CNS, including headache, drowsiness, and fatigue.

4. Muscular weakness.

5. Blurred vision and photophobia.

6. Dysrhythmias and hypotension.

E. Drug interactions include:

1. Possible dysrhythmias when used in conjunction with epinephrine or levonordefrin.

2. Digoxin toxicity when used in conjunction with erythromycin or tetracycline.

III. Effects of Antiarrhythmic Agents

A. These agents are used to treat cardiac dysrhythmias, which are altered rhythmic contractions of cardiac muscle.

B. Common agents include disopyramide (Norpace), lidocaine (Xylocaine; used parenterally), and propranolol (Inderal).

C. The pharmacologic effect is the suppression of dysrhythmias by various mechanisms, depending on the drug classification.

IV. Effects of Antianginal Agents

A. These agents are used to treat angina pectoris, which is caused by an insufficient oxygen supply to the myocardium and results in pain in the chest.

B. Common agents include nitroglycerin (Nitro-Bid, Nitrostat), isosorbide dinitrate (Isordil), beta blockers (see antihypertensives), and calcium channel blockers (see antihypertensives).

C. Contraindications include hypersensitivity to nitroglycerin or nitrites.

D. Pharmacologic effects include the reduction of oxygen consumption, which decreases the work of the heart and relieves anginal pain.

E. Adverse reactions of nitroglycerin include xerostomia, headache, and postural hypotension.

F. Drug interactions include increased hypotensive effects with the use of alcohol, opioids, benzodiazepines, and phenothiazines.

V. Effects of Antihyperlipidemic Agents

A. These agents treat hyperlipidemia (excess lipids in the plasma), which can result in arteriosclerosis.

B. Common agents include lovastatin (Mevacor) and simvastatin (Zocor).

C. Adverse reactions include flatulence (excess air or gas in the GI tract), abdominal pain, constipation, diarrhea, and headaches.

D. Drug interactions include myalgia (diffuse muscle pain) and myositis (inflammation of muscle tissue) with the use of erythromycin or cyclosporine.

VI. Effects of Anticoagulant Agents

A. These agents decrease the risk of embolism formation by interfering with blood clotting.

B. Common agents include warfarin (Coumadin).

C. Therapeutic uses include:

1. Post-MI treatment.

2. Treatment of pulmonary emboli (blood clots in the lung).

3. Treatment of thrombophlebitis (inflammation of a vein).

4. Treatment of atrial dysrhythmias.

D. Contraindications include blood disorders.

E. Adverse reactions include gingival bleeding and hemorrhage.

F. Drug interactions include:

1. Increased action with the use of diflunisal, salicylates, metronidazole, erythromycin, and NSAIA.

2. Decreased action with the use of barbiturates and vitamin K.

The Psychiatric Patient

Psychiatric patients include those who are treated for mental disorders or psychoses that affect one's ability to recognize reality. Treatment often involves the use of antipsychotic agents or antidepressants.

I. Antipsychotic Agents
  A. Types
    1. Phenothiazines such as chlorpromazine (Thorazine), prochlorperazine (Compazine), and thioridazine (Mellaril).
    2. Butyrophenones such as haloperidol (Haldol).
  B. Therapeutic uses
    1. Treatment of psychoses (e.g., schizophrenia, obsessive compulsive disorder).
    2. Preoperative relaxation.
    3. Treatment of nausea and vomiting.
  C. Contraindications include hypersensitivity; adverse reactions may include blood dyscrasias.
  D. Pharmacologic effects:
    1. Antipsychotic agents calm patient's emotions and slow down psychomotor responses.
    2. Also increase the effects of CNS depressant agents (opioids), and reduce the amount of opioids required.
    3. Act as antiemetics (antivomiting agents) by depressing the chemoreceptor zone.
  E. Adverse reactions
    1. Orthostatic hypotension and tachycardia.
    2. Sedation (tolerance develops).
    3. Xerostomia.
    4. Extrapyramidal effects (movements of the body) include:
      a. Parkinson-like symptoms: tremors, rigidity, and akathisia (increased motor restlessness).
      b. Acute dystonia: muscle spasms of the face, tongue, back, and neck.
      c. Tardive dyskinesia: involuntary, abnormal movement of the tongue, lips, face, and neck.
      d. Seizures: occur as a result of a lower seizure threshold.
  F. Drug interactions
    1. An additive effect with the use of CNS depressant agents, including barbiturates, alcohol, general anesthetics, and opioid analgesics.
    2. Hypotension and tachycardia with epinephrine given intravenously; epinephrine can be safely administered as a vasoconstrictor in a local anesthetic.
    3. Increased anticholinergic effects (xerostomia) with the use of anticholinergic agents.
    4. Increased photosensitivity with the use of tetracycline.

II. Antidepressant Agents
  A. Common agents
    1. TCAs
      a. Include amitriptyline (Elavil) and nortriptyline (Pamelor, Aventyl).
      b. Effective onset of action make take as long as several weeks.
      c. Therapeutic uses include the treatment of depression; may be used in combination with phenothiazines. Nortriptyline (Pamelor, Aventyl) is prescribed if less sedation is desired.
      d. Pharmacologic effects
        1) Mild sedation and fatigue in normal patients.
        2) Elevation of mood and decreased depression in depressed patients.
      e. Adverse reactions include:
        1) Drowsiness (tolerance may develop), confusion, and sometimes tremors.
        2) Hypertension, dysrhythmias, and MI.
        3) Xerostomia, blurred vision, and constipation (tolerance does develop).
      f. Drug interactions include:
        1) Increased anticholinergic effects with the use of antihistamines and phenothiazines.
        2) Increased effects of epinephrine and CNS depressant agents.
        3) Hypertension, tachycardia, seizures, and death may occur with the use of monoamine oxidase inhibitor agents (MAOIA).
    2. Second-generation antidepressants
      a. Common agents include:
        1) Fluoxetine (Prozac) does not have adverse interactions with vasoconstrictors; produces xerostomia.
        2) Trazodone (Desyrel) produces CNS stimulation, not depression; may cause nausea, diarrhea, xerostomia, and aphthous stomatitis.
        3) Bupropion (Wellbutrin) increases the occurrence of seizures; is a last resort for treatment of depression.
        4) Sertraline (Zoloft): most common side effects are dizziness and nausea.
        5) Paroxetine (Paxil): prolonged use may inhibit salivary flow during use of drug.
      b. Adverse reactions include anticholinergic effects; cause fewer CVS/CNS side effects than TCAs.
    3. Other psychotherapeutic agents
      a. Monoamine oxidase inhibitors (MAOI) react with many foods containing tyramine (e.g., cheeses, fish, and wines) and drugs (e.g., TCAs, disulfiram, beta-blockers) to create possible life-threatening reactions. Avoidance of these combinations is critical.
      b. Lithium is used to treat manic depression. Lithium toxicity can be avoided if blood levels are monitored; NSAIAs increase lithium toxicity.
    4. Other antidepressants
      a. Venlafaxine (Effexor) is a bicyclic antidepressant; has no adverse interactions with vasoconstrictors; xerostomia occurs during drug therapy.
      b. Nefazodone (Serzone) has no adverse interactions with vasoconstrictors; serious and

possibly fatal reactions occur in conjunction with the use of monoamine oxidase inhibitors; xerostomia occurs during drug therapy.

The Patient with a Seizure Disorder

Patients who suffer from seizure disorders such as epilepsy are treated with anticonvulsant agents. Agents in this category include phenytoin, carbamazepine, valproic acid, phenobarbital, and benzodiazepines. Anticonvulsant agents depress the CNS and thus prevent seizures. Adverse reactions to these agents include CNS depression and stimulation (in young and elderly individuals), xerostomia, gingival hypertrophy, nausea and vomiting, and teratogenicity (see Table 9–7).

I. Phenytoin (Dilantin)
   A. Adverse reactions
     1. Gingival hyperplasia; good oral hygiene helps to control growth.
     2. Nausea and vomiting.
     3. Drowsiness, mental confusion, blurred vision, and insomnia.
     4. Vitamin D and folate deficiencies.
     5. Rashes; can cause Stevens-Johnson syndrome.
   B. Drug interactions include:
     1. Decreased effect when taken with barbiturates and carbamazepine.
     2. Decreases effects of steroids and doxycycline.

II. Carbamazepine (Tegretol)
   A. Is used to treat seizures and trigeminal neuralgia (tic douloureux).
   B. Has other pharmacologic effects: is an anticholinergic, antiarrhythmic, antineuralgic, antidiuretic, and muscle relaxant.
   C. Adverse reactions
     1. Xerostomia, glossitis, nausea, and constipation.
     2. Aplastic anemia, thrombocytopenia, and leukocytosis; lab monitoring of blood is necessary.
     3. Rashes, photosensitivity, and erythema multiforme.
     4. Abnormal liver function.
   D. Drug interactions
     1. Decreased effect of phenobarbital, benzodiazepines, doxycycline, warfarin, and oral contraceptives.
     2. Increased effect with the use of erythromycin, isoniazid, propoxyphene, calcium channel blockers, and cimetidine.

III. Valproic Acid (Depakene/Depakote)
   A. Adverse reactions include hepatotoxicity, increased bleeding (PT) time, nausea, vomiting, constipation, and sedation.
   B. Drug interactions include:
     1. Additive effect when used in conjunction with CNS depressants.
     2. Increased bleeding when taken with salicylates and NSAIA.

IV. Phenobarbital (Luminal)

   A. Is used as an anticonvulsant agent by itself or in combination with other anticonvulsants (e.g., phenytoin).
V. Benzodiazepines
   A. Agents include clonazepam (Klonopin) and diazepam (Valium).
   B. Diazepam is used in the treatment of recurrent tonic-clonic seizures.

Clinical Case STUDY

Thirty-four-year-old Craig Booth is scheduled for four appointments for quadrant scaling and root planing. These procedures will require the administration of local anesthesia. Mr. Booth's medical history reveals a history of Graves' disease, seasonal allergies, and GI distress. He currently takes methimazole and Pepcid daily.

Clinical Case QUESTIONS

1. What gland in the body does Graves' disease involve and what are some common symptoms of the disease?
2. Why does Mr. Booth take methimazole and Pepcid?
3. Are there any contraindications to the use of local anesthetics for Mr. Booth?

Clinical Case RATIONALES

1. Graves' disease is a thyroid disorder that causes hyperthyroidism. It is more common in females and typically is diagnosed between the ages of 30 and 40. Common symptoms include an enlarged thyroid gland (goiter), exophthalmos, hyperactivity, weight loss, and tachycardia.
2. Methimazole is an antithyroid agent that is used to suppress hyperactivity of the thyroid gland. Pepcid is an H_2-receptor antagonist that is used to treat patients with GI disorders such as heartburn and acid indigestion; it acts by decreasing gastric secretions.
3. Contraindications to treatment for Mr. Booth include the use of epinephrine in the local anesthetic, which may cause a thyroid storm. A thyroid storm can be fatal and is associated with fever, tachycardia, arrhythmia, hypermetabolism, and other serious complications.

The Patient With an Endocrine Disorder

Patients with endocrine disorders such as diabetes and hypothyroidism take endocrine agents (e.g., undergo hormone replacement therapy) to control the disorder. These agents include adrenocorticosteroids, diabetic agents, thyroid gland agents, and female hormones.

I. Adrenocorticosteroids
   A. Common agents
     1. Glucocorticoids, which affect carbohydrate metabolism, and mineralocorticoids, which affect water and electrolyte balance.

2. Glucocorticoids are used more often than mineralocorticoids; they include hydrocortisone, prednisone (Deltasone), triamcinolone (Kenalog), and dexamethasone (Decadron).

B. Therapeutic uses
1. Antiinflammatory effects are used to treat acute bronchial asthma, systemic lupus erythematosus, scleroderma, rheumatoid arthritis, and severe and acute allergic reactions.
2. Are used in replacement therapy for adrenal gland insufficiency (Addison's disease).
3. Treatment of emergencies such as shock or adrenal crisis.
4. Treatment of aphthous stomatitis and noninfectious inflammatory oral lesions (e.g., erythema multiforme, lichen planus, pemphigus).

C. Contraindications
1. Psychosis (because of effects on behavior during either presence or withdrawal of the drug).
2. Infection (because antiinflammatory effects may mask symptoms of infection; also may decrease resistance to infection).
3. Ulcers (because of stimulation of stomach acid secretions).
4. CV disease (because an increase in blood pressure is associated with the use of mineralocorticoids)

D. Pharmacologic effects include a decrease in inflammatory response, allergic reactions, and immunosuppression.

E. Adverse reactions
1. Decreased resistance to infections.
2. Delayed wound healing and development of osteoporosis.
3. Adrenal crisis (including hypertension, circulatory collapse, and death) as a result of abrupt drug withdrawal or stress; may be avoided by premedication with additional steroids.
4. Weight gain and hyperglycemia.
5. Behavioral changes, including agitation, euphoria, and depression.
6. Increased stomach acid.

F. Drug interactions include:
1. Decreased effect with the use of barbiturates and rifampin.
2. Increased adverse reactions with the use of alcohol, salicylates, and NSAIA.

II. Agents for the Treatment of Diabetes Mellitus
A. Classifications of diabetes
1. Insulin-dependent diabetes mellitus (IDDM) type-I, juvenile-onset results from an absence of insulin secretion.
2. Noninsulin-dependent diabetes mellitus (NIDDM) type-II, adult-onset occurs when insulin secretion is insufficient for daily needs.

B. Common agents
1. For IDDM
   a. Rapid acting—Humulin R.
   b. Intermediate acting—Humulin L and Humulin N (NPH).
   c. Long acting—Humulin U
   d. Mixed—Humulin 70/30; the most common combination is Humulin R and NPH.
2. For NIDDM—oral hypoglycemic agents (sulfonylureas) include tolbutamide (Orinase), tolazamide (Tolinase), chlorpropamide (Diabinese), glyburide (DiaBeta, Micronase), and glipizide (Glucotrol).

C. Adverse reactions include hypoglycemia (when insulin overdose results in insulin shock) and hyperglycemia (insufficent insulin). Hyperglycemia is less common and is treated in the hospital.

D. Drug interactions include:
1. Increased hypoglycemia with the use of salicylates, NSAIA, or alcohol.
2. Hyperglycemia with the use of corticosteroids or epinephrine.

III. Thyroid Gland Agents
A. Thyroid hormones maintain the function of organ systems, regulate metabolism, and control energy use.

B. Thyroid disorders
1. Hypothyroidism (cretinism) is thyroid hypofunction that requires thyroid replacement therapy for treatment.
   a. Thyroid agents include levothyroxine sodium (Synthroid) and liotrix (Euthroid, Thyrolar).
   b. Drug interactions include increased sensitivity to opioids and sedatives.
2. Hyperthyroidism (Graves' disease)[25] is excess thyroid hormones circulating in the body (thyrotoxicosis).
   a. Treatment involves the use of antithyroid drugs (e.g., iodide, radioactive iodine) or thyroidectomy.
   b. The use of antithyroid medications with epinephrine must be avoided; may cause life-threatening thyroid storm.

IV. Female Sex Hormones
A. Are responsible for female sex characteristics, reproductive development, and preparation for conception.

B. Common agents include estrogens and progesterones.
1. Estrogen and synthetic formulations of estrogen (include Premarin and Estraderm)
   a. Estrogen is responsible for puberty changes, increased fat deposition, salt and water retention, and bone cell activity (osteoblasts).
   b. Therapeutic uses
      1) Contraception occurs by inhibition of ovulation.

2) Treatment of menstrual disturbances (e.g., dysmenorrhea, dysfunctional uterine bleeding).
3) Treatment of osteoporosis increases osteoblastic activity.
4) Treatment of symptoms of menopause that are caused by a depletion of estrogen.
5) Treatment of cancer (e.g., prostate cancer, breast cancer, and endometrial cancer).

  c. Adverse reactions include:
1) Nausea and vomiting (tolerance does develop).
2) Edema and weight gain.
3) Uterine bleeding.
4) Hypertension.
5) Thrombophlebitis (inflammation of vein).

  d. Drug interactions increases the action of corticosteroids.

2. Progesterones, which include medroxyprogesterone (Provera, Depo-Provera) and levonorgestrel (Norplant) implants.
  a. Prepare uterus for fertilization.
  b. Therapeutic uses include:
1) Contraception.
2) Treatment of endometriosis, dysmenorrhea, dysfunctional uterine bleeding, and premenstrual tension.
3) Treatment of postmenopausal symptoms (in combination with estrogen).
4) Treatment of cancer.

  c. Adverse reactions are similar to those for estrogens.

The Allergic Patient

Patients who suffer from allergies often are medicated with H_1-receptor antagonists or antihistamines. Common agents in this category are classified as either first-generation or second-generation.

I. First-Generation H_1-Receptor Antagonists
  A. Include diphenhydramine (Benadryl), clemastine (Tavist), dimenhydrinate (Dramamine), doxylamine (Unisom), chlorpheniramine (Chlor-Trimeton), and hydroxyzine hydrochloride (Atarax).
  B. Therapeutic uses include:
    1. Control of symptoms of allergic reactions; if anaphylaxis occurs, epinephrine rather than antihistamine should be used for bronchodilation.
    2. OTC sleep aids (e.g., diphenhydramine in Nytol and Compoz).
    3. Preoperative sedation; also may be used as antiemetics.
  C. Contraindications include hypersensitivity and an acute asthma attack (epinephrine is more effective for the latter).
  D. Pharmacologic effects include:

1. Decreased vasodilation, bronchodilation, pain, and itching (antihistamine effects).
2. Antiemesis.
3. Xerostomia.
4. Sedation (stimulation can occur).
5. Benadryl provides a local anesthetic effect.

  E. Adverse reactions include drowsiness, xerostomia, nausea, and constipation.
  F. Drug interactions include:
    1. Effect of CNS depressants, including alcohol, is increased.
    2. Increased anticholinergic effect occurs with the use of anticholinergics, phenothiazines, and TCAs.

II. Second-generation H_1-receptor antagonists include terfenadine (Seldane), astemizole (Hismanal), and loratadine (Claritin).
  A. Therapeutic uses include the treatment of rhinitis and seasonal allergy symptoms.
  B. Pharmacologic effects include antihistaminic and anticholinergic actions similar to those of first-generation agents but without sedation.
  C. Adverse reactions include:
    1. Xerostomia and constipation.
    2. Seldane may have cardiotoxic effects; CV effects of Hismanal include hypotension, bradycardia, and tachycardia (may be cardiotoxic); Claritin does not have CV effects.
    3. Drug interactions include:
      a. All of those listed for first generation H_1-antagonists.
      b. Increased risk of cardiac dysrhythmias when Seldane or Hismanal are used in conjunction with ketoconazole or macrolides antibiotics.

The Patient with a GI Disorder

Patients with GI disorders often are medicated with H_2-receptor antagonists or antihistamines.
  I. Common H_2-Receptor Antagonist Agents (antihistamines)
    A. Include cimetidine (Tagamet), ranitidine (Zantac), famotidine (Pepcid), and nizatidine (Axid).
    B. Therapeutic uses include the treatment of ulcers.
    C. Pharmacologic effects include decreased gastric secretions.
    D. Adverse reactions include nausea, diarrhea, and constipation; Tagamet and Zantac may cause tachycardia and bradycardia.
    E. Drug interactions
      1. Decreased absorption with ketoconazole.
      2. Tagamet results in increased blood levels of metronidazole, alcohol, lidocaine, and opioids.

The Patient with Cancer

Cancer patients undergo a variety of treatments to attempt to eradicate neoplastic growth from their bodies. Common treatments include surgery, radiation therapy, and chemotherapy. Cancer chemotherapeutic agents also are called antineoplastic agents.

I. Classification of Chemotherapeutic Agents (antineoplastics)
  A. Alkylating agents include Mustargen, Leukeran, Ifex, carmustine (BCNU, BiCNU), and Myleran.
  B. Antimetabolites include methotrexate (Amethopterin), floxuridine (FUDR), and mercaptopurine (6-MP, Purinethol).
  C. Miscellaneous antineoplastics include Velban, Actinomycin-D, medroxyprogesterone, Nolvadex, and Alferon N.
II. Pharmacologic Effects
  A. Chemotherapeutic agents destroy and suppress the growth and spread of malignant cells.
III. General Adverse Reactions (Table 9–8)
  A. Bone marrow suppression (BMS) symptoms include thrombocytopenia, leukopenia, and anemia, which result in susceptibility to infection, bleeding, and fatigue.
  B. Hepatotoxicity, which occurs most often with the use of methotrexate.
  C. Dermatologic effects, which vary from mild erythema to exfoliative dermatitis and alopecia (hair loss).
  D. Nephrotoxicity.
  E. Nausea, vomiting, stomatitis, and oral ulcerations.
  F. Mucosal pain and ulceration, gingival hemorrhage, and xerostomia.
  G. Inhibition of spermatogenesis and oogenesis.
  H. Peripheral neuropathy and convulsions.

The Patient with Respiratory Disease

Asthma and COPD are common types of respiratory disease that are encountered in dental patients.

TABLE 9.8	Primary Drugs for Treatment of Oral Infections and Disease
Infection	**Drug**
Recurrent aphthous stomatitis	Tetracycline (if severe may use systemic steroid)
Lichen planus	Topical steroids; if severe, systemic steroids (e.g., Decadron, dexamethasone)
Primary herpes	Orabase, acyclovir, lidocaine
Oral candidiasis	Nystatin or clotrimazole troches, systemic ketoconazole or fluconazole
Cellulitis; periapical abscess; acute necrotizing ulcerative gingivitis (ANUG); pericoronitis osteomyelitis	Penicillin VK, amoxicillin
Periodontal abscess	Penicillin VK
Localized juvenile periodontitis	Doxycycline, tetracycline

These patients are treated with adrenergic agonists, xanthines, corticosteroid inhalers, and anticholinergic agents.

I. Respiratory Diseases
  A. Asthma is severe bronchoconstriction that results in airway obstruction.
    1. Drugs used for treatment include adrenergic agonists (beta$_2$ agonists), corticosteroid inhalers, xanthines, anticholinergics, and cromolyn.
      a. Local anesthetics that contain sulfite preservatives (vasoconstrictor antioxidants) should not be administered to patients with asthma because the vasonconstrictor's "sulfite preservatives" are likely to cause allergic reactions in these patients.
  B. COPD is chronic irreversible airway obstruction.
    1. Occurs with either chronic bronchitis or emphysema.
      a. Chronic bronchitis is chronic inflammation of the airways and excess sputum.
      b. Emphysema is caused by the destruction of alveoli; is characterized by air space enlargement and airway collapse.
    2. Drugs used for treatment include adrenergic agonists, xanthines, corticosteroids, and anticholinergics.
II. Common Respiratory Agents
  A. Sympathomimetic agents (adrenergic agonists) include albuterol (Proventil, Ventolin) and metaproterenol (Alupent).
    1. Pharmacologic effects include bronchodilation by means of beta$_2$ receptor stimulation in the lungs.
    2. Adverse reactions include:
      a. Tachycardia with the use of nonselective adrenergic agonists (epinephrine and isoproterenol).
      b. Nervousness, insomnia, and tachycardia with the use of selective adrenergic beta$_2$ agonists; however, fewer adverse reactions occur with these selective agents than with the use of nonselective adrenergic agonists.
  B. Corticosteroid inhalers include triamcinolone (Azmacort) and beclomethasone (Beclovent, Vanceril).
    1. The aerosolized form provides significant improvement of pulmonary function.
    2. Adverse reactions include candidiasis.
  C. Cromolyn (Intal) is effective only for the prevention of acute bronchospasm; is not a treatment.
  D. Xanthines
    1. Are used to treat acute and chronic asthma; also are used for maintenance treatment of emphysema.
    2. Pharmacologic effects include bronchodilation.
    3. Adverse reactions include nausea, vomiting, anxiety, cardiac palpitations, and increased respirations.

4. Drug interactions include increased action with the use of erythromycin; increased dysrhythmias with CNS stimulants; and a decreased effect with barbiturates, carbamazepine, and ketoconazole.

E. Anticholinergics include atropine (an old asthma drug) and Atrovent (a newer drug with fewer adverse reactions than atropine).

 Clinical Case **STUDY**

Dawn Gates is a 16-year-old high school student. She presents for her oral prophylaxis appointment in an agitated state and demands "laughing gas." Her behavior is in direct contrast to her behavior at previous oral prophylaxis appointments. Her pulse and blood pressure readings are somewhat elevated compared with earlier readings.

Clinical Case QUESTIONS

1. What might be the cause of Dawn's unusual behavior?
2. What is "laughing gas?" Identify its drug classification and common uses. Should it be used at this appointment?
3. What is the significance of the higher-than-normal vital signs at this appointment?

Clinical Case RATIONALES

1. Dawn's unusual behavior could have several possible causes, including anxiety, emotional disturbance, illness, fatigue, and substance abuse.
2. Laughing gas is a slang term for nitrous oxide/oxygen analgesia. It is classified as a CNS depressant, along with opioids, barbiturates, benzodiazepines, and alcohol. In dentistry, it is used to relax anxious patients during dental therapy. Before the gas is administered, a careful medical and dental history interview and physical assessment must be conducted to determine whether Ms. Gates is using any drugs or medications; this is necessary to avoid potential problems such as drug-drug interactions (e.g., with phenothiazines, lithium, and TCA) and CNS suppression.
3. The significance of the higher-than-normal vital signs at this appointment is that they may be one indicator of substance abuse, emotional distress, or a similar problem. Alone, the vital signs offer little information; however, when combined with other information, they may lead to an explanation of the patient's behavior.

General Terminology

Addiction is a physical or psychological dependence on a substance (or both); is a primary, chronic, and progressive disease process.

Drug/substance abuse is the use of chemicals despite adverse consequences to self and others.

Drug dependence is a physical or psychological need to administer a chemical to prevent the body's reaction to an absence of the chemical.

Physical dependence is a physical need for a chemical to maintain certain body functions.

Tolerance is the need to increase the dose of a drug to produce the same effect.

The Substance Abuse Patient

Substance abuse can be described as the use of chemicals despite their adverse effects on the user or others. Dental patients with substance addiction or dependence may be problematic for two reasons: (1) they may seek dental care in order to obtain legal but addictive drugs; and (2) patients with drugs in their bloodstream may be at risk for experiencing an adverse drug interaction with a dentally prescribed drug.

I. Oral Manifestations Observed in Drug Abusers
    A. Rampant caries and/or tooth loss
    B. Halitosis and xerostomia
    C. Gingival recession and/or periodontal disease
    D. Tissue ulceration
    E. Oral cancer
    F. Leukoplakia
    G. Trauma to the mouth and tissues
    H. Bruxism
II. Commonly Abused Drugs
    A. CNS stimulants include the following agents: nicotine, caffeine, amphetamines, and cocaine.
        1. Nicotine is found in tobacco products.
            a. Serious diseases can result from its use (e.g., coronary artery disease, oral cancer, and lung cancer).
            b. Withdrawal symptoms may be different for each person; nicotine chewing gum (Nicorette) or nicotine patches (Nicoderm, Nicotrol, Prostep, Habitrol) may be used to reduce symptoms.
        2. Caffeine
            a. Physical dependence can occur with the consumption of 2 to 3 cups of caffeine daily.
            b. Tolerance can develop.
            c. Withdrawal can occur 24 hours after last cup; symptoms include headache, lethargy, irritability, anxiety, and constipation.
        3. Amphetamines include dextroamphetamine (Dexedrine), methylphenidate (Ritalin), and methamphetamine (Desoxyn).
            a. These drugs provide a sense of euphoria and increased energy.
            b. Tolerance to the euphoria develops.
            c. Toxic symptoms include anxiety, hallucinations, paranoia, and aggressiveness.
            d. Symptoms of acute overdose include mydri-

asis, elevated blood pressure and pulse rate, and cardiac dysrhythmias.

  e. Withdrawal symptoms can include psychological depression and suicidal tendencies.

 4. Cocaine (also known as crack or rock)

  a. Creates a sense of euphoria.

  b. Has a short duration of action (only a few minutes).

  c. Tolerance to the drug does not occur; withdrawal symptoms also do not occur.

  d. Elevated blood pressure, MI, stroke, seizure, or dysrhythmias may occur with use.

B. CNS depressants comprise a wide variety of substances, including opioids, barbiturates, benzodiazepines, volatile solvents (glue and gasoline), nitrous oxide, and alcohol.

 1. Opioid analgesics include heroin, hydromorphone (Dilaudid), morphine, methadone (Dolophine), oxycodone (Percodan), and meperidine (Demerol).

  a. Pharmacologic effects include elevated mood, euphoria, suppressed hunger, reduced sexual drive, slowed respirations, constipation, urinary retention, and peripheral vasodilation.

  b. Physical dependence and tolerance develop; more drug is needed to achieve "high" feeling.

  c. Symptoms of opioid overdose include respiratory depression, miosis, and coma; overdose is treated by administration of short-acting naloxone (Narcan).

  d. Withdrawal effects include lacrimation, rhinorrhea, chills, diaphoresis, tremors, and increased heart rate and blood pressure.

  e. Treatments include methadone maintenance programs, counseling, and Narcotics Anonymous (NA).

 2. Sedative-hypnotics include benzodiazepines (Valium), barbiturates, meprobamate (Miltown), Quaalude, and Librium.

  a. Symptoms of abuse resemble those of alcohol intoxication, with more respiratory depression, and decreased GI, urinary, and cardiac output.

  b. Prolonged abuse causes paranoia and suicidal tendencies.

  c. Withdrawal symptoms are similar to those of opioids but can be life threatening (withdrawal replacement drugs may include benzodiazepines).

 3. Effects of nitrous oxide abuse include hallucinations, paresthesias of the extremities, and mood swings; chronic abuse can cause death.

 4. Alcohol

  a. Alcoholism is a chronic disease characterized by excessive use of alcohol that results in mental and/or physical impairment.

  b. Genetics is considered a contributing factor.

  c. Impaired judgment, mydriasis, slurred speech, ataxia, seizures, coma, and even death may occur from abuse.

  d. Chronic consumption during pregnancy causes fetal alcohol syndrome, which results in mild to severe developmental disturbances in the fetus.

  e. Disulfiram (Antabuse) may be used during the treatment of alcoholism; ingestion of alcohol while taking disulfiram causes the patient to get sick (i.e., to vomit).

C. Psychedelics (hallucinogens) include marijuana (marihuana, cannabis), lysergic acid diethylamide (LSD), and phencyclidine (PCP or angel dust).

 1. The effects of psychedelics are psychological—they disturb reality perception; tolerance develops quickly.

 2. Abuse can cause lasting psychological disturbances that range from panic attacks to schizophrenic episodes to life-threatening depression.

 3. Marijuana (Marihuana, cannabis)

  a. Increases pulse rate; causes reddening of eyes and euphoria.

  b. Active ingredient has an antiemetic effect; can be used to treat nausea that occurs during cancer chemotherapy.

 4. Lysergic acid diethylamide (LSD)

  a. Overdose symptoms include mydriasis, increased blood pressure, visual distortions, hallucinations, and paranoia.

  b. Flashbacks can occur years after using LSD.

 5. Phencyclidine (PCP, peep, or angel dust)

  a. Users exhibit bizarre behavior and elevated blood pressure and pulse.

  b. Is abused alone or with other street drugs; is associated with a high incidence of "bad trips."

III. Dental Concerns Regarding Substance Abuse

A. Drug abusers seek drugs through dental offices (by requesting drugs for pain relief); they request specific drugs, therefore suspicions of drug abuse should be aroused when specific drugs are requested.

B. Eliminating the source of a patient's pain and prescribing NSAIA if pain control is necessary are preferable to prescribing habit-forming medications.

C. Drug abusers are at increased risk for contracting disease, including HIV and hepatitis.

IV. See Table 9–9 for the top 100 drugs prescribed in the United States in 1999.

TABLE 9.9 Top 100 Drugs Prescribed in the United States, 1999*

Rank	Brand Name	Generic Name	Common Uses	Pharmacologic Class
1	Premarin	Conjugated estrogens	Hormone replacement (menopause)	Estrogen
2	Synthroid	Levothyroxine	Hypothyroidism	Thyroid hormone
3	Trimox	Amoxicillin	Infection	Antibiotic
4	Hydrocodone w/APAP	Hydrocodone w/acetaminophen	Analgesic	Opioid and nonopioid analgesics
5	Prozac	Fluoxetine	Major depressive disorders	Antidepressant
6	Prilosec	Omeprazole	Gastroesophageal reflux disorder	Antiulcer
7	Zithromax	Azithromycin	Upper/lower respiratory infection	Macrolide antibiotic
8	Lipitor	Atorvastatin	Hypercholesterolemia	Antihyperlipidemic
9	Norvasc	Amlodipine	Hypertension; chronic, stable angina	Calcium channel blocker
10	Claritin	Loratadine	Allergies	H_1 antihistimine
11	Lanozin	Digoxin	Congestive heart failure	Cardiac glycoside
12	Zoloft	Sertraline	Major depression	Antidepressant
13	Albuterol aerosol	Albuterol	Asthma; bronchospasm	Beta$_2$-adrenergic (bronchodilator)
14	Paxil	Paroxetine	Depression	Antidepressant
15	Amoxicillin (Biocraft)	Amoxicillin	Infections	Antibiotic
16	Prempro	Conjugated estrogens/ medroxyprogesterone	Hormone replacement (menopause)	Conjugated estrogen; progestogen
17	Zestril	Lisinopril	Hypertension	Ace inhibitor
18	Vasotec	Enalapril	Hypertension	ACE inhibitor
19	Augmentin	Amoxicillin/clavulanate	Sinus infection; pneumonia; otitis media	Antibiotic/Beta-lactamase inhibitor
20	Cephalexin (Biocraft)	Cephalexin	Gram-negative bacilli	Antibiotic (cephalosporin)
21	Zocor	Simvastatin	Hypercholesterolemia	Antihyperlipidemic
22	Glucophage	Metformin	Type-II diabetes mellitus (NIDDM)	Oral hypoglycemic
23	Coumadin	Warfarin	Pulmonary embolism; myocardial infarction	Anticoagulant
24	Acetaminophen/Codeine	Acetaminophen/codeine	Analgesic	Nonopioid analgesic; opioid analgesic
25	Ibuprofen	Ibuprofen	Arthritis; fever; analgesic	NSAIA
26	Furosemide	Furosemide	Pulmonary edema; edema in congestive heart failure	Diuretic (loop)
27	Cipro	Ciprofloxacin	Adult upper respiratory tract infection	Antibacterial (quinolone)
28	Trimeth/sulfameth	Trimeth/sulfameth	Urinary tract infections; acute otitis media in children; prophylaxis of *Pneumocystitis carinii* pneumonitis	Antiinfectant
29	Cardizem CD	Diltiazem	Angina; hypertension	Calcium channel blocker
30	Pravachol	Pravastatin	Hypercholesterolemia	Antihyperlipidemic
31	Biaxin	Clarithromycin	Upper/lower respiratory infections	Antibiotic
32	Propoxyphene N/APAP	Propoxyphene napsylate; acetaminophen	Analgesic	Nonopioid analgesic; opioid analgesic
33	Levoxyl	Levothyroxine	Hypothyroidism	Thyroid hormone
34	Procardia XL	Nifedipine	Angina; hypertension	Calcium channel blocker
35	Prednisone	Prednisone	Severe inflammation; immunosuppression	Glucocorticoid
36	Prevacid	Lansoprazole	Duodenal ulcer; pathological hypersecretory syndromes	Antisecretory; proton pump inhibitor
37	Ultram	Tramadol	Analgesic	Opioid analgesic
38	Alprazolam (Geneva)	Alprazolam	Anxiety; panic disorder	Benzodiazepine

*American Druggist, February 1999.

TABLE 9.9 Top 100 Drugs Prescribed in the United States, 1999 *Continued*

Rank	Brand Name	Generic Name	Common Uses	Pharmacologic Class
39	Ambien	Zolpidem	Insomnia	Nonbarbiturate, nonbenzo-diazepine sedative-hypnotic
40	Amoxil	Amoxicillin	Infections	Antibiotic
41	Accupril	Quinapril	Hypertension	ACE inhibitor
42	K-Dur-20	Potassium chloride	Hypokalemia	Potassium electrolyte
43	Glucotrol XL	Glipizide	Type-II diabetes mellitus (NIDDM)	Oral hypoglycemic
44	Hydrocodone/APAP	Hydrocodone/acetamino-phen	Analgesic	Opioid analgesic; non-opioid analgesic
45	Triamterene/HCTZ	Triamterene/HCTZ	Edema; hypertension	K-sparing diuretic
46	Ortho Tri-Cyclen	Norgestimate/ethinyl estradiol	Oral contraceptive	Oral contraceptive
47	Lotensin	Benazepril	Hypertension	ACE inhibitor
48	Prinivil	Lisinopril	Hypertension	ACE inhibitor
49	Hytrin	Terazosin	Hypertension	Antiadrenergic
50	Veetids	Penicillin VK	Orofacial infection (periapical, periodontal abscess)	Antibiotic
51	Propoxyphene-N/APAP	Propoxyphene acetamino-phen	Analgesic	Opioid analgesic; Non-opioid analgesic
52	Relafen	Nabumetone	Osteoarthritis; rheumatoid arthritis	NSAIA
53	Zyrtec	Cetirizine	Allergic rhinitis	Antihistamine
54	Cardura	Doxazosin	Hypertension	Peripheral alpha-adrenergic blocker
55	Claritin D 12 HR	Loratidine/pseudoephe-drine	Seasonal allergies/decon-gestant	H_1 antihistamine; alpha adrenergic agonist (decongestant)
56	Allegra	Fexofenadine	Seasonal allergies	Antihistamine
57	Pepcid	Famotidine	Ulcers	H_2-antagonist (antiulcer)
58	Triphasil	L-Norgestrel/ethinyl estradiol	Oral contraceptive	Oral contraceptive; estrogen
59	Humulin N	Human insulin-NPH	Type-I diabetes mellitus	Antidiabetic
60	Dilantin	Phenytoin	Seizures	Anticonvulsant
61	Ortho-Novum 7/7/7	Norethindrone/ethinyl estradiol	Oral contraceptive	Oral contraceptive; progestin and estrogen
62	Atenolol (Mylan)	Atentolol	Hypertension; angina prophylaxis	Anti-HTN-selective $Beta_1$-blocker
63	Toprol-XL	Metoprolol	Hypertension; angina	Anti-HTN; selective $beta_1$-blocker
64	Flonase (nasal spray)	Fluticasone	Seasonal allergies	Corticosteroid
65	Lorazepam	Lorazepam	Anxiety; acute alcohol withdrawl	Antianxiety (benzodiazepine)
66	Amitriptyline	Amitriptyline	Major depression	TCA
67	Cefzil	Cefprozil	Tonsillitis; otitis media	Antibiotic (cephalosporin)
68	Depakote	Divalproex	Seizures	Anticonvulsant
69	Imdur	Isosorbide mononitrate S.A.	Angina	Antianginal
70	Viagra	Sildenafil citrate	Erectile dysfunction	Phosphodiesterase enzyme inhibitor
71	Diflucan	Fluconazole	Candidiasis	Antifungal
72	Propulsid	Cisapride	Gastroesophageal reflux disorder	Oral prokinetic
73	Alprazolam	Alprazolam	Anxiety; panic disorder	Benzodiazepine
74	Triamterene HCTZ	Triamterene HCTZ	Edema; hypertension	K-sparing diuretic/thiazide diuretic
75	Atenolol	Atenolol	Hypertension; Angina prophylaxis	AntiHTN; selective $beta_1$-blocker
76	Fosamax	Alendronate	Osteoporosis	Amino biphosphonate
77	Adalat CC	Nifedipine	Angina; hypertension	Calcium channel blocker
78	Cozaar	Losartan	Hypertension	Angiotensin II receptor antagonist

Table continued on following page

TABLE 9.9 Top 100 Drugs Prescribed in the United States, 1999 *Continued*

Rank	Brand Name	Generic Name	Common Uses	Pharmacologic Class
79	Atenolol	Atenolol	Hypertension; Angina prophylaxis	Anti-HTN; selective beta₁ blocker
80	Lescol	Fluvastatin	Hypercholesterolemia	Antihyperlipidemic
81	Hydrocodone w/APAP	Hydrocodone w/APAP	Analgesic	Opiod analgesic; acetaminophen
82	Albuterol Neb Soln	Albuterol	Asthma; bronchospasm	Beta₂-andrenergic agonist
83	Glyburide	Glyburide	Type-II diabetes mellitus (NIDDM)	Oral antidiabetic
84	Wellbutrin SR	Buproprien HCL	Depression; smoking cessation	Antidepressant
85	Vancenase AQ DS	Beclomethasone	Chronic asthma; rhinitis	Glucocorticoid (inhalant)
86	Zithromax Susp	Azithromycin	Respiratory pathogens; alternative antibiotic for prevention of bacterial endocarditis	Antibiotic (macrolide)
87	Clonazepam	Clonazepam	Seizures	Benzodiazepine (anticonvulsant)
88	Naproxen	Naproxen	Analgesic; arthritis	NSAIA
89	Carisoprodol	Carisoprodol	Muscle spasms	Centrally-acting muscle relaxant
90	Daypro	Oxaprozin	Rheumatoid arthritis; osteoarthritis	NSAIA
91	Monopril	Fosinopril	Hypertension, CHF	Ace inhibitor
92	Ceftin	Cefuroxime	Gram-negative bacilli	Antibiotic (cephalosporin)
93	Claritin D 24HR	Loratidine/pseudoephedrine	Seasonal allergies	H1 antihistamine; alpha-adrenergic agonist (decongestant)
94	Hydrochlorothiazide	Hydrochlorothiazide	Edema; hypertension; CHF	Diuretic
95	Acetaminophen/Codeine	Acetaminophen/codeine	Analgesic	Nonopioid analgesic; opioid analgesic
96	Nitrostat	Nitroglycerin	Angina	Vasodilator
97	Atrovent	Ipratropium	Bronchospasm in COPD; emphysema; asthma	Anticholinergic (bronchodilator)
98	Humulin 70/30	Human insulin 70/30	Type-I diabetes mellitus (IDDM)	Antidiabetic
99	Rezulin	Troglitazone	Type II diabetic; hyperglycemic	Antidiabetic agent
100	Lotrisone	Clotrimoxazole/betamethasone	Fungal infections/oral ulcerative inflammatory lesions	Antifungal; corticosteroid

～ CONTENT REVIEW QUESTIONS ～

1. The strength of a drug with regard to its ability to achieve a desired effect is termed:
   A. efficacy
   B. potency
   C. therapeutic effect
   D. tolerance

2. All of the following are sites of drug elimination, EXCEPT:
   A. liver
   B. kidney
   C. colon
   D. lungs
   E. pancreas

3. An adverse reaction to a drug that is predictable and dose related and that acts on target organs is termed a(n):

A. side effect
B. toxic reaction
C. allergic reaction—type I
D. allergic reaction—type III
E. allergic reaction—type IV

4. A patient reveals a history of asthma and uses the following drugs: propranolol, acetaminophen, cephalexin, and isoproterenol. Which of these drugs is used to treat asthma?
   A. propranolol (Inderal)
   B. acetaminophen (Tylenol)
   C. cephalexin (Keflex)
   D. isoproterenol (Isuprel)

5. At his recall appointment, Mr. Jones complains that his oral tissues and teeth are sensitive. He states that he chews gum more often because his mouth is dryer. Upon examination, a caries problem is detected. Mr. Jones reports a medication change since his last

appointment. Which one of the following drugs could account for the change in Mr. Jones' oral condition?

A. nadolol (Corgard)

B. digoxin (Lanoxin)

C. temazepam (Restoril)

D. sulfinpyrazone (Antazone)

6. A recall patient returns after receiving radiotherapy for cancer of the head and neck. The hygienist identifies that the patient has salivary gland hypofunction in the form of xerostomia. The drug that may be prescribed for this condition is:

A. atropine (Atropair)

B. diflunisal (Dolobid)

C. pilocarpine (Salagen)

D. prilocaine (Citanest)

7. An analgesic, antipyretic, and antiinflammatory effect occurs with all of the following drugs, EXCEPT:

A. diflunisal (Dolobid)

B. acetaminophen (Tylenol)

C. naproxen (Aleve)

D. ibuprofen (Advil)

8. The nonopioid drug that patients take to prevent post-MI is:

A. aspirin (Empirin)

B. acetaminophen (Tylenol)

C. ibuprofen (Advil)

D. naproxen (Aleve)

9. A recall patient who is in pain because of a dental abscess is prescribed Tylenol #3. The patient requires diazepam (Valium), an antianxiety drug, before her appointments. A possible drug interaction to be aware of is:

A. decreased sedation

B. increased sedation

C. increased antitussive effect

D. decreased analgesia

10. When respiratory depression occurs because of an overdose of an opioid analgesic agent, a drug that will reverse the respiratory depression is:

A. morphine

B. epinephrine

C. naloxone (Narcan)

D. ammonia inhalants

E. lidocaine

11. All of the following are true about tetracyclines, EXCEPT:

A. they are used to treat localized juvenile periodontitis and RAP.

B. photosensitivity is a side effect of their use.

C. chelation occurs when they are combined with calcium, magnesium, or aluminum.

D. tooth discoloration is not an adverse effect of their use.

E. their use decreases the effectiveness of oral contraceptives.

12. A patient being treated for RAP complains of a metallic taste, black hairy tongue, and xerostomia. The drug that is causing these conditions is:

A. amoxicillin (Amoxil)

B. metronidazole (Flagyl)

C. tetracycline (Tetracyn)

D. cephalexin (Keflex)

E. clindamycin (Cleocin)

13. Mr. Jones reports no medical conditions on his health history but indicates that he takes isoniazid (Nydrazid) and rifampin (Rifadin). These medications indicate that Mr. Jones might have:

A. tuberculosis

B. HIV

C. osteomyelitis

D. candidiasis

14. A patient has RAP and takes chlorpropamide (Diabinese) for NIDDM. The drug of choice for treating the RAP and avoiding adverse interaction with Diabinese is:

A. doxycycline (Doxycin)

B. metronidazole (Flagyl)

C. penicillin V

D. cephalosporin

15. Mr. Harris requires prophylactic antibiotic coverage for rheumatic heart disease before dental treatment. He also takes digoxin (Lanoxin) to treat congestive heart failure. The safest antiinfective agent for Mr. Harris that follows AHA recommendations is:

A. tetracycline

B. clindamycin (Cleocin)

C. erythromycin

D. amoxicillin (Amoxil)

16. Propranolol (Inderal) is used to treat all of the following conditions, EXCEPT:

A. angina pectoris

B. CHF

C. hypertension

D. migraine

E. MI prophylaxis

17. A patient reports that he is being treated for high cholesterol. He most likely is taking which one of the following drugs?

A. propranolol (Inderal)

B. metoprolol (Lopressor)

C. simvastatin (Zocor)

D. atenolol (Tenormin)

E. nifedipine (Procardia)

18. Diazepam (Valium) is used in dentistry for all of the following therapeutic uses, EXCEPT:

A. analgesic

B. antianxiety

C. anticonvulsant

D. muscle relaxant

19. Phenobarbital (Luminal) is used for its anticonvulsant effect and belongs to which one of the following drug groups?

A. benzodiazepines

B. barbiturates

C. nonbarbiturates

D. phenothiazines

E. monoamine oxidase inhibitors

20. A patient reports that he is taking prochlorperazine (Compazine). All of the following are adverse reactions of Compazine, EXCEPT:

A. orthostatic hypotension

B. seizures

C. xerostomia

D. tardive dyskinesia

E. CNS stimulation

21. A patient reports having manic depression. Which one of the following drugs is used to treat this illness?

A. phenelzine (Nardil)

B. amitriptyline (Elavil)

C. lithium

D. chlordiazepoxide (Librium)

22. All of the following are second-generation antidepressant agents, EXCEPT:

A. fluoxetine (Prozac)

B. amitriptyline (Elavil)

C. trazodone (Desyrel)

D. bupropion (Wellbutrin)

23. Mrs. Smith reports that she has epilepsy but cannot remember the drug she takes to treat it. She notices that her gingiva is enlarged. The drug she is MOST likely taking is:

A. cimetidine (Tagamet)

B. fluconazole (Diflucan)

C. phenytoin (Dilantin)

D. diazepam (Valium)

24. Carbamazepine (Tegretol) is used as an anticonvulsant agent. Its other pharmacologic effects include all of the following, EXCEPT:

A. antihypertension

B. anticholinergic

C. antidepressant

D. sedative

E. muscle relaxant

25. Prednisone (Deltasone) is prescribed to treat all of the following conditions, EXCEPT:

A. Crohn's disease

B. rheumatoid arthritis

C. Addison's disease

D. Cushing's syndrome

E. systemic lupus erythematosus

26. A patient with type-I diabetes (IDDM) complains of pain after prophylaxis. The hygienist recommends a nonopioid analgesic. Which of the following medications would have the LEAST interaction with the patient's medication?

A. aspirin (Empirin)

B. acetaminophen (Tylenol)

C. ibuprofen (Advil)

D. diflunisal (Dolobid)

27. A recall patient reveals a recent history of taking Premarin. She states that she has gained weight and the hygienist discovers that the patient's blood pres-

sure is much higher than during previous visits. These symptoms may be the result of:

A. drug interactions

B. allergic reactions

C. adverse reactions

D. toxic reactions

28. A patient who reports taking levothyroxine (Synthroid) has which of the following conditions?

A. hypothyroidism

B. hyperthyroidism

C. Cushing's syndrome

D. Addison's disease

E. Cancer

29. When Mr. Smith arrives for his dental appointment, he complains of itching and a rash on his arm. Mr. Smith reports that he took his prophylactic antibiotic an hour before his appointment. Which of the following drugs will treat this mild type-IV allergic reaction?

A. terfenadine (Seldane)

B. clemastine fumarate (Tavist)

C. prednisone (Deltasone)

D. ibuprofen (Advil)

E. diphenhydramine (Benadryl)

30. A patient with cardiovascular problems has seasonal allergies. Which antihistamine agent has little or no effect on the CVS and can be safely used for this patient?

A. terfenadine (Seldane)

B. nizatidine (Axid)

C. loratidine (Claritin)

D. hydroxyzine (Atarax)

E. famotidine (Pepcid)

31. When oral surgery is performed, a long-acting local anesthetic typically is needed. Which of the following would be the drug of choice?

A. novacaine

B. bupivacaine

C. lidocaine

D. prilocaine

E. mepivacaine

32. Adding a vasoconstrictor to a local anesthetic does all of the following, EXCEPT:

A. creates hemostasis

B. constricts blood vessels

C. increases duration of anesthetic

D. increases absorption into CVS

33. When nitrous oxide is used during dental treatment, which of the following is the desired effect?

A. loss of consciousness

B. conscious sedation

C. general anesthesia

D. respiratory depression

E. local anesthesia

34. After terminating the use of nitrous oxide, a patient complains of a headache. Which of the following has occurred?

A. diffusion hypoxia
B. neuropathy
C. allergic reaction
D. toxic reaction

35. All of the following are inhalation volatile liquids that are used as general anesthetics, EXCEPT:
    A. halothane (Fluothane)
    B. enflurane (Ethrane)
    C. methohexital (Brevital)
    D. isoflurane (Forane)

36. The main adverse reaction that occurs with the use of an opioid agent as a general anesthetic is:
    A. significant cardiovascular change
    B. excessive salivation
    C. hypertension
    D. respiratory depression
    E. bronchospasm

37. Abuse occurs with all of the following CNS depressant drugs, EXCEPT:
    A. alcohol
    B. morphine
    C. Valium
    D. nicotine
    E. Percodan

38. Antineoplastic agents typically produce all of the following oral conditions, EXCEPT:
    A. mucosal pain
    B. gingival recession
    C. gingival hemorrhage
    D. xerostomia
    E. mucosal ulceration

39. An asthmatic patient returns for a recall appointment. The patient forgets to bring her inhaler but remembers that it is a corticosteroid inhaler. The active agent in the inhaler is:
    A. triamcinolone (Azmacort)
    B. albuterol (Proventil)
    C. metaproterenol (Alupent)
    D. isoproterenol (Isuprel)

40. Asthmatic patients may have allergic reactions when they are given local anesthetics that contain vasoconstrictors. Such reactions are caused by which of the following agents in these dental cartridges?
    A. epinephrine
    B. lidocaine
    C. sodium bisulfite
    D. sodium sulfate

REVIEW QUESTION RATIONALES

1. **B** The potency of a drug refers to its strength, which enables it to achieve a desired effect. Efficacy is its ability, not its strength, to produce a desired effect. Therapeutic effect is the clinically desirable action of a drug. Tolerance occurs when no effect takes place because of a decreased susceptibility to the drug after continuous use.

2. **E** The pancreas aids in the digestion of foods and the regulation of carbohydrate metabolism; however, unlike the liver, kidney, colon, and lungs, it does not function to eliminate drugs from the body.

3. **B** Toxic reactions and side effects, unlike allergic reactions, are predictable and dose related. However, toxic reactions, unlike side effects, act on target organs because they are an extension of a drug's pharmacologic effect.

4. **D** Isoproterenol (Isuprel), an adrenergic (sympathomimetic) agent, effects the $beta_2$ receptors in the lungs to enhance bronchodilation. Propranolol (Inderal) is a nonselective beta-adrenergic blocker that is used to treat cardiovascular diseases. Acetaminophen (Tylenol) is a nonopioid analgesic and cephalexin (Keflex) is a cephalosporin antiinfective agent.

5. **A** Nadolol (Corgard) is a nonspecific beta-adrenergic blocking agent. A common adverse reaction is xerostomia, which can cause an increase in caries and sensitivity. Digoxin (Lanoxin), a cardiac glycoside, temazepam (Restoril), a benzodiazepine, and sulfinpyrazone (Antazone), a uricosuric agent, are not associated with xerostomia as an adverse reaction.

6. **C** Pilocarpine is a cholinergic (parasympathomimetic) agent that mimics the action of ACH (a neurotransmitter) on parasympathetic receptors, thereby increasing salivary excretion. Atropine (Atropair) is an anticholinergic agent that decreases salivary excretion. Diflunisal (Dolobid) is a nonsteroidal antiinflammatory agent (NSAIA) that is used for analgesia. Prilocaine (Citanest) is an amide local anesthetic.

7. **B** Acetaminophen (Tylenol) is a nonopioid analgesic with antipyretic but no antiinflammatory effects. The other drug choices are NSAIA nonopioid analgesics that possess all three stated effects.

8. **A** Aspirin is the nonopioid agent that irreversibly reduces platelet adhesiveness. Aspirin is used to prevent unwanted clotting, which aids in reducing the occurrence of MI. The other drug choices also are nonopioid agents but they do not have irreversible platelet effects.

9. **B** Tylenol #3 contains codeine, which is an opioid analgesic that depresses the CNS. Diazepam (Valium) is a benzodiazepine that depresses the CNS. When combined, they produce an additive effect of CNS depression.

10. **C** Naloxone (Narcan) is an opioid antagonist that competes with opioids at their receptor sites; it reverses opioid respiratory depression. Morphine is an opioid analgesic and not an antagonist. Epinephrine, lidocaine, and ammonia inhalants also are not opioid antagonists.

11. **D** Permanent tetracycline staining does occur if the drug is given during enamel calcification.

12. **B** Metronidazole (Flagyl) is an antiinfective agent. It is one of the drugs of choice for RAP that may produce

all three oral effects. Amoxicillin (Amoxil) and tetracycline (Tetracyn) are antiinfective agents that may be used to treat RAP but that do not have all three oral effects. Cephalexin (Keflex) and clindamycin (Cleocin) are antiinfective agents but are not used to treat RAP.

13. **A** Tuberculosis treatments often combine isoniazid (Nydrazid) and rifampin (Rifadin) for their antituberculosis synergistic effects. This drug combination also is used prophylactically in patients who test positive in response to a tuberculosis skin test (Mantoux test).

14. **B** The drugs of choice for RAP are metronidazole (Flagyl) and tetracyclines (doxycycline/Doxycin). Tetracyclines combined with oral sulfonylureas (chlorpropamide/Diabinese) result in hypoglycemia. The only remaining drug of choice for this patient is metronidazole because penicillin and cephalosporin are not appropriate for treating RAP.

15. **D** Amoxicillin (Amoxil), not clindamycin (Cleocin), is the first drug of choice in the AHA regimen. There are no adverse drug interactions between amoxicillin and digoxin (Lanoxin). Combining digoxin with erythromycin may cause increased blood levels of digoxin, which leads to toxicity. Tetracyclines are not a drug choice in the AHA regimen.

16. **B** Propranolol (Inderal) is an antiadrenergic beta blocker (nonselective) agent that can be used to treat angina pectoris, hypertension, and migraines, and can be used for MI prophylaxis. It is not a digitalis glycoside and it cannot be used to treat congestive heart failure.

17. **C** Simvastatin (Zocor) is an antihyperlipidemic agent that is used to treat hyperlipidemia (high cholesterol). Propranolol (Inderal), an antiadrenergic beta blocking (nonselective) agent, metoprolol (Lopressor) and atenolol (Tenormin), antiadrenergic $beta_1$ blocking agents, and nifedipine (Procardia), a calcium channel blocking agent, are all used to treat cardiovascular diseases, not hyperlipidemia.

18. **A** Diazepam (Valium) is a benzodiazepine (sedative/hypnotic) agent that is used for anxiety control, the treatment of seizures, and as a muscle relaxant. It has no analgesic effects.

19. **B** Phenobarbital (Luminal) is a long-acting barbiturate that is used to treat epilepsy.

20. **E** Prochlorperazine (Compazine), a phenothiazine, is an antipsychotic agent that depresses, rather than suppresses, the CNS.

21. **C** Lithium is an antipsychotic agent that is used to treat manic depression. Phenelzine (Nardil), an antidepressant MAO inhibitor, and amitriptyline (Elavil), a TCA, are used to treat depression other than manic depression. Chlordiazepoxide (Librium) is a benzodiazepine that is used to treat anxiety.

22. **B** Amitriptyline (Elavil) is a TCA and not a second-generation antidepressant agent.

23. **C** Phenytoin (Dilantin) is an anticonvulsant agent. Gingival hyperplasia is one of its common adverse

reactions. Cimetidine (Tagamet) is an H_2 antagonist that is used to treat ulcers. Fluconazole (Diflucan) is an antifungal that is used to treat candidiasis. Diazepam (Valium), a benzodiazepine, is used as an adjunct in seizure control and is not associated with gingival hyperplasia as an adverse reaction.

24. **A** Carbamazepine (Tegretol) can create hypertension. It is not classified as a cardiovascular agent.

25. **D** Prednisone (Deltasone), a glucocorticoid with antiinflammatory and immune-suppressing effects, is used to treat the diseases listed, except for Cushing's syndrome. Cushing's syndrome results from a hypersecretion of glucocorticoids by the adrenal cortex; therefore, prednisone is contraindicated for patients with this disease.

26. **B** No adverse drug interaction occurs when acetaminophen (Tylenol) is combined with insulin. Insulin combined with salicylates (aspirin and diflunisal) or NSAIA (ibuprofen) may increase hypoglycemia.

27. **C** Premarin, an estrogen, is associated with several adverse reactions, including nausea, vomiting, uterine bleeding, weight gain, thrombophlebitis, and hypertension.

28. **A** Levothyroxine (Synthroid) is a thyroid gland agent. It is administered to patients who have hypothyroidism and require thyroid replacement therapy. Cushing's syndrome and Addison's disease are associated with adrenal cortex abnormalities. Cancers are treated with antineoplastic agents.

29. **E** Diphenhydramine (Benadryl) is an H_1-receptor antagonist (antihistamine). When a type-IV allergic reaction creates a rash by means of the release of histamine, administration of an antihistamine blocks the histamine and decreases the allergic reaction. Terfenadine (Seldane) and clemastine fumarates (Tavist) are antihistamines that are used to treat seasonal allergies. Prednisone (Deltasone) is a steroid and ibuprofen (Advil) is a nonopioid analgesic.

30. **C** Loratidine (Claritin), terfenadine (Seldane), and astemizole (Hismanal) are second generation H_1-receptor antagonists (antihistamines). Claritin is the only one of the three that has no effect on the CVS and therefore can be administered to patients with cardiovascular problems. Nizatidine (Axid) and famotidine (Pepcid) are H_2 antihistamines that are used to treat ulcers. Hydroxyzine (Atarax) is an antianxiety antihistamine.

31. **B** Bupivacaine and etidocaine are longer-acting amide local anesthetic agents that currently are available. All of the other local anesthetics are considered shorter-acting agents.

32. **D** A vasoconstrictor constricts the blood vessels, thereby decreasing the absorption of a local anesthetic agent into the CVS. This decreased absorption increases the duration of the local anesthetic agent. The vasoconstrictor also creates hemostasis because of blood vessel constriction.

33. **B** Nitrous oxide (an inhalation gas) alone is unsatisfactory as a general anesthetic. When it is used properly, conscious sedation should occur with no significant effect on the respiratory system.

34. **A** Diffusion hypoxia results in a headache if the patient does not receive 5 minutes of 100% oxygen at the termination of the nitrous oxide.

35. **C** Methohexital (Brevital) is an ultra-short-acting barbiturate. It is used as an IV agent and is not an inhalation volatile liquid.

36. **D** The primary adverse reaction associated with opioids is respiratory depression, which can be reversed with an opioid antagonist such as naloxone (Narcan).

37. **D** Nicotine is abused, but it is a CNS stimulant not a depressant.

38. **B** Gingival recession does not occur because of antineoplastic agent use but because of other factors that occur in the patient's oral cavity.

39. **A** Triamcinolone (Azmacort) is a corticosteroid inhaler that achieves significant improvement in pulmonary function. The other agents listed are all adrenergic agonists that create bronchodilation by means of beta$_2$-receptor stimulation in the lungs.

40. **C** Sodium bisulfite is an antioxidant (a preservative) for the vasoconstrictor (epinephrine) in dental local anesthetic (lidocaine) cartridges. This preservative is the catalyst for allergic reactions in asthmatic patients who receive local anesthetics with vasoconstrictors. Sodium sulfate is a natural sulfate found in the body.

References

1. Dajani AS, Taubert KA, Wilson W, et al: Prevention of bacterial endocarditis: Recommendations by the American Heart Association. JAMA 277(22):1794–1801, 1997.
2. Wynn RL, Meiller TF, Crossley HL: Drug Information Handbook for Dentistry, 4th ed. Hudson, New York, Lexi-Comp, 1998–99.

Additional Reading

Gage TW, Pickett FA: Dental Drug Reference. St. Louis, Mosby, 1997.
Haveles EB: Pharmacology for Dental Hygiene Practice, 1st ed. Albany, NY, Delmar Publishers, 1997.
Little JW, Falace DA: Dental Management of the Medically Compromised Patient, 5th ed. St. Louis, Mosby, 1997.
Malamed SF: Handbook of Local Anesthesia, 4th ed. St. Louis, Mosby, 1997.
Requa-Clark BS: Applied Pharmacology for the Dental Hygienist, 3rd ed. St. Louis, Mosby, 1995.
Threlkeld DS, Hagemann RC, editors: Drug Facts and Comparison. St. Louis, Facts and Comparison, 1997.
Wynn RL, Meiller TF, Crossley HL: Drug Information Handbook for Dentistry, 4th ed. Hudson, New York, Lexi-Comp, 1998–99.

Chapter TEN

Dental Biomaterials

Cynthia C. Gadbury-Amyot, R.D.H., M.S.

 ## Clinical Case STUDY

Fifty-nine-year-old Martha Sales is in the office because of a fractured tooth. Upon questioning, Ms. Sales explains that she was at the movies and bit down on a popcorn kernel when she felt her tooth break. Visual examination of tooth #18 reveals a fracture of the mesio-lingual cusp. The remainder of the tooth holds a large mesio-occlusal-distal amalgam restoration. After the dentist removes all of the old amalgam some decay is discovered that must be removed; its removal requires a near pulpal exposure. Ms. Sales has amalgam restorations in teeth #2, 14, 19, and 31, and full gold crowns on teeth #3 and 30.

Clinical Case QUESTIONS

1. What mechanical properties were involved in the fracture of tooth #18?
2. The dentist decides to place a cavity liner before restoring this tooth. Explain what material would be appropriate and why.
3. How should this tooth be restored? Select an appropriate restorative material and include indications and contraindications for different restorative materials.

Clinical Case RATIONALES

1. The first property involved in the fracture was stress; the biting force on the popcorn kernel created both compressive and tensile forces on the tooth. Moreover, the smaller the area over which a force is applied, the larger the value of the stress. In this instance the occlusal surface of #18, which came in contact with the kernel, was relatively small and therefore magnified the stress. The second property involved was strain, or the reaction of tooth #18 to the biting stress, which resulted in the fracture of the mesio-lingual cusp.
2. An appropriate material for lining the cavity would be calcium hydroxide. The advantages of using this material include: (1) it encourages recovery of the pulp by the stimulation of reparative dentin; (2) it protects the pulp; and (3) it is sufficiently strong.
3. This tooth will probably require a full coverage restoration because of the extensive loss of tooth structure. Because the tooth that opposes #18 has never been restored, a full gold crown is indicated; gold would cause minimal abrasion of #15. Porcelain would be contraindicated in this circumstance because it has a high hardness number (480) compared with enamel (343) and would therefore result in the eventual abrasion of tooth #15.

Content Review

General Terminology

Absorption refers to the uptake of a liquid by a solid.

Adhesion is the force of attraction between unlike atoms/molecules on two different surfaces as they are brought into contact.

Adsorption refers to a concentration of molecules at the surface of a solid or liquid.

Alloy is a combination of two different metallic elements.

Amorphous describes a structure that has no regularity or form but possesses many characteristics of a solid (noncrystalline).

Cohesion is the force of attraction between like atoms/molecules within a material that results in a tenacious bond.

Corrosion is a chemical or electrochemical process in which oxidation and reduction reactions occur on a metal surface in the presence of an electrolyte (e.g., saliva), resulting in deterioration of the metal.

Creep is time-dependent deformation of an object that is subjected to a constant stress (related to marginal fractures of dental amalgams).

Hydrocolloid is a suspension of fine particles (e.g., potassium alginate) dispersed in water to produce a viscous solution; reversible hydrocolloid is known as agar, irreversible hydrocolloid is alginate.

Marginal leakage describes the movement of saliva and bacteria between the margin of a dental restoration and the cavity wall.

Polymerization is a chemical reaction that converts small, individual monomer molecules into long, giant polymer molecules.

Polymerization shrinkage is a contraction that accompanies the polymerization reaction, often resulting in microleakage at the margin of the restoration.

Tarnish is a chemical reaction between a metal and its environment that results in discoloration of the metal surface.

Thermal conductivity is the ability of a material to transmit heat; also the rate at which heat is transferred through a material.

Characteristics of Dental Materials

An understanding of the mechanical, physical, electrical, surface, and biological properties of dental materials is important because it enables the dental professional to determine the proper use of dental materials.

Mechanical Properties

Mechanical properties include the reactions of materials to the application of external forces. The magnitude of biting forces is a major reason to study mechanical properties.

I. Forces
A. A tensile force tends to pull an object apart or elongate an object.
B. A compressive force is the downward application of force on an object, which tends to compress the structure.
C. Shear force is characterized by the rotation, twisting, or sliding of one portion of a material by another portion.

II. Stress (Fig. 10–1)
A. Is the reaction with which an object resists an external force. An example would be the stretching or pulling of an orthodontic band. Stress is created because of the wire's being pulled in tension and the wire's ability to resist this external force up to the point of fracture.
B.

$$\text{Stress} = \frac{\text{Force kg/mm}^2}{\text{Area inches/meters}}$$

The smaller the area over which a force is applied, the larger the value of the stress.

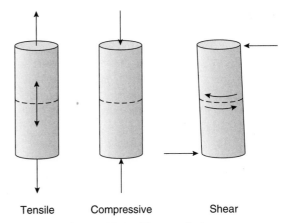

Tensile   Compressive   Shear

Figure 10.1 Types of stress.

C. Stress-related properties
1. Ultimate strength is the highest stress reached prior to fracture.
2. Fracture strength is the point at which a material breaks.
3. Tensile strength is the breaking strength when tested in tension.
4. Compression strength is the breaking strength when tested in compression.

III. Strain
A. Is the deformation or change in the length or dimension of a dental material as a result of applied stress. The stiffer an object is, the greater its ability to resist dimensional change. For example, dental waxes exhibit strain much more quickly than amalgam as a result of character differences in stiffness.
B.

$$\text{Strain} = \frac{\text{Deformation/Change in length (inches/meters)}}{\text{Original length (inches/meters)}}$$

C. Strain-related properties
1. Elastic deformation occurs when material recovers after a load is released or after a material breaks.
2. Plastic deformation is a permanent strain or change in the shape of an object that results when it is stressed beyond its elastic limit.
3. Elongation is the percentage of change in length up to the point of fracture.
4. Ductility is the ability of a material (e.g., gold) to withstand significant plastic or permanent deformation under stress before fracturing.
5. Brittleness characterizes materials (e.g., glass fiber) that fracture before undergoing a significant amount of plastic or permanent deformation when placed under stress; is the opposite of ductility.
6. Malleability is the ability of material to be compressed without fracturing; is similar to

ductility but specifically refers to compressive force applications.

IV. Elasticity

A. Is the property that permits a material to be deformed by an applied load and assume its original shape when the load is removed. The example of orthodontic wires once again illustrates the importance of a material's ability to resist fracture upon manipulation by the dental professional. Other examples include the adjustment of the clasps on partial dentures and the ability of dental bridges to withstand the forces of mastication.

B. The modulus of elasticity is the measure of the stiffness of a material and its ability to resist bending or change in shape.

C. The stress/strain curve diagram is used in the research of dental materials to monitor the change in dimension for a given application and identify important points such as elastic limit/proportional limit and permanent deformation (Fig. 10–2).

D. The elastic limit (proportional limit) is the maximum stress that a material can withstand without being permanently deformed.

E. Inelasticity is permanent deformation as a result of applied force.

V. Hardness (Fig. 10–3)

A. Is the resistance of a solid to penetration. An example would be denture base material and its low abrasion resistance. The dental professional must instruct the patient not to use abrasive cleansing materials in order to prevent excessive abrasion of the denture.

B. Types of hardness tests
   1. Brinell—steel ball (oldest test)
   2. Vickers—square-based diamond point
   3. Knoops test—diamond indenter (widely used in dentistry, can be used with any type of material)

C. The higher the hardness number, the harder the material. Porcelain has a high resistance to abra-

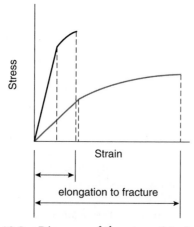

Figure 10.2 Diagram of the stress/strain curve.

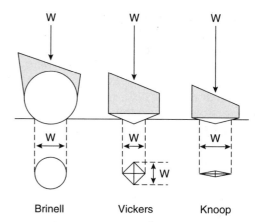

Figure 10.3 Hardness tests.

sion and conversely has the ability to abrade opposing materials with lower hardness numbers (Box 10–1).

Physical Properties

Physical properties depend primarily on the type of atoms and bonding that are present in a material. A good reason for studying physical properties is to determine how a given material will withstand the oral environment (i.e., moistness, temperature fluctuations, biting forces).

I. Thermal Properties

A. Are a material's reaction to temperature changes within the oral cavity and its subsequent expansion or contraction. For example, a rapid change in oral temperature would occur in the individual who eats an ice cream cone immediately before drinking a cup of hot coffee.

B. The coefficient of thermal expansion is the value or measurement of the change in length per unit length for each degree of temperature change.
   1. The higher the coefficient of expansion the greater the degree of contraction/expansion involved when a material is exposed to temperature changes.
   2. Because of the differences in expansion/contraction rates of restorative materials and tooth structures, microleakage of oral fluids between the restoration and tooth can occur (Table 10–1).

C. Thermal conductivity is the ability of a dental material to transmit heat.

BOX 10.1	Hardness of Restorative Materials	
Acrylic		21
Dentin		68
Enamel		343
Porcelain		480

TABLE 10.1	Expansion of Tooth and Dental Materials

Linear Thermal Coefficients of Expansion

Material	Coefficient ($\times 10^{-6}/°C$)
Tooth	11.4
Amalgam	25.0
Acrylic resin	81.0
Composite resin	35.0
Silicone impression material	210.0

1. Enamel and dentin are poor thermal conductors compared with gold alloys and amalgam.
2. Cements are used to insulate the pulp in areas of deep cavity preparations.

II. Electrical Properties
   A. Involve the generation of electrical currents through a variety of means.
   B. Galvanism results from the approximation of dissimilar metals in the mouth and results in small electrical currents. These currents have the potential to create sensitivity by irritating the pulp. (Fig. 10–4)
   C. Corrosion is the deterioration of a metal by a chemical or electrochemical reaction; it can be the result of adjacent restorations that are composed of dissimilar metals.
      1. Roughness and pitting occur as a result of galvanic action.
      2. Also may result from a chemical attack of metals by components in food or saliva.
      3. Tarnish is a surface corrosion that is caused by the reaction of metals in the mouth to components in saliva or food.

III. Color Properties
   A. Are important because they give restorations and prosthetic appliances the appearance of natural teeth and soft tissues (esthetics).
   B. Can be described in terms of three components.
      1. Hue refers to the dominant color of the object (i.e., red, yellow, or blue).
      2. Value refers to the lightness of a color.
      3. Chroma refers to the intensity of a color.
   C. Translucency refers to how light enters the tooth and is affected in several ways:
      1. Part of the light may be transmitted completely through the tooth (the more light that is transmitted through, the more translucent the material).
      2. Part of the light may be reflected from the surface of the tooth and may not penetrate at all.
      3. Part of the light may enter the tooth and subsequently scatter and be absorbed.

4. Composites and ceramics (glass) can be made with varying degrees of translucency by adding opaquing agents to block light penetration.

Surface Properties

Surface properties are associated with the surface of dental materials and include such characteristics as surface tension and absorbability.

I. Matter
   A. Solids
      1. Most materials in dentistry are solids.
      2. Are characterized by a regular arrangement of atoms/molecules (are crystalline or rigid at all temperatures below their melting point).
      3. The atoms are held in position by interatomic forces.
      4. Amorphous structures have no regularity or form but possess many characteristics of solids (noncrystalline). Amorphous substances such as glass do not possess a definite melting or freezing point. For example, dental waxes are amorphous and gradually soften without a definite melting point.
   B. Liquids
      1. Many dental materials are liquids at some point and are changed to solids by cooling or chemical reactions.
      2. Are characterized by an irregular arrangement of atoms/molecules; include reversible hydrocolloid materials that are heated to liquefaction.
      3. The atoms are not held in position, which allows the material to flow easily around oral structures.

II. Attaching Solid Structures
   A. Mechanical bonding
      1. Does not require intimate attraction between the atoms/molecules of the substances involved. Examples include the attachment of two

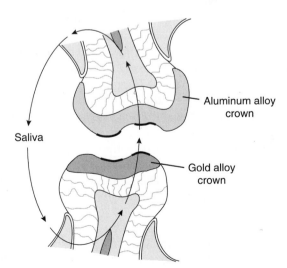

Figure 10.4 Galvanism.

solids by the use of a screw, nail, or bolt. A dental example is the use of dental cements.

2. The retention of a crown is enhanced by the mechanical attachment of the cementing agent. Liquid cement penetrates into irregularities on the internal surface of the crown and into porosities in the tooth structure, thus creating a locking mechanism.

3. Occurs with the use of the acid etch technique for sealants and resin materials. Minute pores are produced in the enamel/dentin when the acid is applied, thus allowing spaces for the interlocking of these materials.

B. Adhesion
   1. Adhesion is the force of attraction between *unlike* atoms/molecules on two different surfaces as they are brought into contact; results in a much more tenacious bond than mechanical bonding (see examples of primary and secondary bonds, below). Cohesion is the force of attraction between *like* kinds of atoms/molecules within a material, which results in a tenacious bond (e.g., the cohesive forces that hold a cement together and prevent fracture within the cement).
      a. A primary bond is adhesion that involves a chemical bond between atoms/molecules (e.g., dyeing cloth).
      b. Secondary bonds (most common bonds) are referred to as van der Waals forces. This type of adhesion involves a physical attraction between atoms/molecules that does not provide as strong a bond as chemical bonding (e.g., in materials with polyacrylic acid, such as glass ionomer cements and polycarboxylate cements).
      c. Adhesion helps control the problem of microleakage around dental restorations.
      d. Effectiveness is determined by:
         1) Wetting—the degree to which an adhesive will spread out on a surface (Fig. 10–5).
         2) Contact angle—the angle between the adhesive and surface that is measured to give a value for wetting. Good wetting is characterized by contact angles of less than 90 degrees; the best are zero degrees (the larger the contact area, the better the chance of adhesion) (see Fig. 10–5).
         3) Surface energy—the higher the surface energy, the greater the attraction of atoms to the surface, resulting in better adhesion. (e.g., metals have high surface energy).
      e. Inhibition is affected by:
         1) Dirty/contaminated surfaces, which result in the reduced surface energy of an adher-

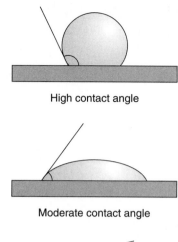

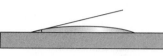

High contact angle

Moderate contact angle

Low contact angle

Figure 10.5 Wetting ability: the lower the contact angle, the greater the adhesion.

ent, thus reducing its ability to attract other atoms/molecules.
         2) Viscosity; adhesives with high viscosity have a high resistance to flow and are less likely to spread out on a surface. If viscosity is too low, it may be hard to control the placement of the adhesive.
         3) Shrinkage of adhesives during hardening, which causes the adhesive to pull away from the tooth or restoration, thus compromising adhesion.

Biological Properties

Biologic properties refer to the biological response of the human body to various materials and the continued examination of the host-foreign body response. The response of both patient and providers is of interest because of allergy, microleakage, and toxicity factors.

I. Allergic Response
   A. Occurs infrequently.
   B. Is elicited in patients who are sensitized to nickel-containing materials.
   C. To latex is receiving a great deal of attention because an allergic reaction can be provoked in both patients and providers.

II. Microleakage
   A. Refers to the inability of materials to adequately seal margins, which allows the leakage of bacteria and their by-products into the area and can lead to:
      1. Secondary caries.
      2. Pain.
      3. Necrosis.

B. Potential can be decreased with the use of poly-acrylic acid (currently the only material able to adhere sufficiently to avoid microleakage).

III. Toxic Effects of Materials

A. Include microleakage, thermal shock, galvanism, and chemical irritation, which can occur during and after the restoration of a carious tooth and may subject the pulp to injury.

B. Can be minimized or eliminated by taking proper steps, (e.g., using insulating bases).

Impression and Replication Materials

The function of impression and replication materials is to accurately record hard and soft tissues in the oral cavity. These impressions subsequently can be used by the dental professional for the construction of restorations to replace missing tooth structure and for the fabrication of preventive devices.

Impression Materials

Impression materials produce a negative reproduction of the area of interest in the oral cavity.

I. Classification of Impression Materials

A. Inelastic materials

1. Are rigid impression materials that are restricted to applications in which no undercuts exist. They include:

a. Compound (modeling plastic), such as tray compound and impression compound.

b. Zinc oxide-eugenol (ZOE) impression paste, which is seldom used and has been replaced by rubber impression materials.

c. Impression plaster, which is rarely used because of its rigidity and ease of fracture; is primarily used to mount casts on an articulator.

B. Aqueous elastomeric materials (hydrocolloid) include:

1. Irreversible hydrocolloid, such as alginate.

2. Reversible hydrocolloid, such as agar.

a. Has been largely replaced by alginate and rubber base impression materials.

C. Non-aqueous elastomeric materials (rubber) include:

1. Polysulfide (mercaptan rubber).

2. Silicone rubber; both condensation and addition (polyvinylsiloxane) types.

3. Polyether.

II. Composition and Chemistry

A. Compound (modeling plastic)

1. Is 40% resin, 7% wax, 3% organic acid, 50% filler, and small amounts of coloring agent.

2. Is thermoplastic (material will reversibly soften on heating and harden on cooling).

3. Tray compound is sold in the shape of a tray; impression compound is provided in small quantities in the form of sticks and cones.

B. ZOE impression paste

1. Is supplied as a 2-paste system.

a. One tube contains zinc oxide, oils, and additives.

b. The other tube contains eugenol, oils, resin, and additives.

C. Irreversible hydrocolloid (alginate) (Table 10–2)

D. Reversible hydrocolloid (agar) (Table 10–3)

E. Polysulfide

1. Is supplied as a 2-paste system.

a. The base contains 80% organic polymer-containing reactive mercaptan groups and 20% reinforcing agents.

b. The catalyst most often is lead dioxide.

F. Silicone rubber

1. The condensation type is supplied as a base and an accelerator; is available in light, regular, and heavy-bodied consistency and as a putty.

a. The base is a silicone liquid called dimethylsiloxane.

b. The accelerator is a tin organic ester suspension and alkyl silicate.

2. The addition type (polyvinylsiloxane) is supplied as a 2-paste or 2-putty system; includes:

a. Silicone

b. Silane hydrogens

G. Polyether

1. Is supplied as a base and a catalyst.

a. The base is polyether.

b. The catalyst is sulfonic acid ester.

TABLE 10.2 Composition of Irreversible Hydrocolloid Alginate Impression Material

Ingredient	Percentage (%)	Function
Diatomaceous earth	60	Filler
Calcium sulfate	16	Reacts with potassium alginate to create gelation
Potassium alginate	15	Reacts with calcium sulfate to create gelation
Zinc oxide	4	Filler
Potassium titanium fluoride	3	Accelerates setting of gypsum
Trisodium phosphate	2	Retarder

TABLE 10.3	Composition of Reversible Hydrocolloid	
Ingredient	**Percentage (%)**	**Function**
Agar-agar	8–15	Substance is extracted from a type of seaweed whose fibrils form a colloid that results in a partially rigid but elastic gel
Water	80–85	Main component that occupies the spaces between the agar-agar fibrils
Borax	Trace amounts	Increases the strength of the gel (also can retard the setting of gypsum; requires the addition of an accelerator)
Potassium sulfate	2	Accelerates the setting of gypsum

III. Characteristics and Properties
   A. Compound
      1. Flow is 85% at 113°F and 6% at mouth temperature (98.6°F); sets up in mouth.
      2. Tray compound is stiffer and has less flow than impression compound.
      3. Is thermoplastic; does not involve chemical change.
      4. Has low thermal conductivity.
   B. ZOE
      1. Soft-set ZOE is tougher and not as brittle as hard-set ZOE.
      2. Both types are classified as rigid; cannot be used to record undercut areas.
      3. Has a setting time that is shortened by the presence of water, high humidity, and high temperatures.
      4. Is accurate; has a dimensional change during setting of approximately −0.1%.
      5. Adheres to tray compound or acrylic tray material, eliminating the need for tray adhesive.
   C. Irreversible hydrocolloid (alginate)
      1. Is a suspension of molecules (colloid) in some type of dispersion medium (water); a liquid colloid is a sol.
      2. Liquid sol is changed into a gel by chemical means, which is an irreversible process.
      3. Normal-set alginate should set in no less than 2 minutes and no more than 4 1/2 minutes (mixing time = 1 minute).
      4. Fast-set alginate sets in 1 to 2 minutes (mixing time = 30 to 45 seconds).
      5. The powder/water ratio effects the setting time; thinner mixes increase the time required for a material to set.
      6. Has 1.5% permanent deformation.
      7. Has increased strength if thick rather than thin mixes are used.
      8. Results in increased tear and compressive strength if impression is left in mouth until fully set.
      9. Is a less accurate impression material than agar or rubber impression materials.
      10. Loses accuracy (dimensional change) if it is stored for more than 1 hour in air because of a process called syneresis (loss of water by evaporation and by exuding fluid).
      11. If stored in contact with water, will absorb water (imbibition), leading to dimensional change.
      12. Is manipulated by:
         a. Proper mixing
            1) Fluffing the alginate powder container or package.
            2) Measuring the appropriate amount of cool water for the required number of scoops of alginate and placing the water in a plastic bowl.
            3) Adding the alginate powder to the water in the bowl, thus helping to eliminate entrapped air in the final mix.
            4) Stirring the powder and water vigorously to wet the powder completely.
            5) Stropping (wiping) the mix against the side of the bowl for 60 seconds to homogenize and remove bubbles.
            6) Visually inspecting the mixture for a creamy, thick consistency.
         b. Filling and seating the tray
            1) Filling the impression tray with mixture by spatula from the posterior regions forward.
            2) Smoothing the alginate surface with a moistened finger and precoating the occlusal and other anatomic areas (i.e., vaulted palate, frenums) for a better impression.
            3) Seating the tray in a posterior to anterior direction.
            4) Bordering the mold by pulling the patient's lips and cheeks over the tray.
            5) Holding the tray in place until the alginate sets.
         c. Removing and pouring the impression
            1) Lifting the lips and cheeks away with fingers to break the seal.
            2) Grasping the handle and pulling the tray away from the teeth with a quick motion (to minimize distortion).

3) Washing the impression under cool water to eliminate saliva and blood.

4) Spraying the impression with disinfectant and sealing in a plastic bag for 10 minutes.

5) Pouring the impression as soon as possible.

D. Reversible hydrocolloid (agar)

1. Sol is changed into a gel by a physical (cooling) reaction and is therefore reversible.

2. Gives a highly accurate impression; must be poured promptly to avoid dimensional changes.

E. Polysulfide

1. Provides excellent reproduction of surface detail.

2. Demonstrates shrinkage of impression material during the first 24 hours, therefore models/dies should be prepared promptly.

3. Materials are highly compatible with model plaster and stone.

4. Has excellent shelf life, which is improved by refrigeration.

F. Silicone Rubber

1. Condensation

a. Has shorter working and setting times than polysulfides.

b. Has less viscosity than polysulfides, making them easier to mix.

c. Has a greater dimension change than polysulfides.

d. Reproduces fine details.

e. Is compatible with model plaster and stone.

f. Has been known to cause allergic reactions.

2. Addition (polyvinylsiloxane)

a. Has a very small dimension change—0.1%; does not require immediate pouring—can be delayed for days.

b. Has lowest level of permanent deformation upon removal from mouth of all impression materials.

c. Is a stiffer material than polysulfides and condensation silicones, which makes removal from undercuts more difficult.

d. Causes less tissue reaction than condensation silicones.

e. Is very hydrophobic material that can cause problems with trapped air bubbles on the surface of the impression when pouring gypsum casts or dies; surfactants are added to make it more hydrophilic.

G. Polyether

1. Has the shortest working time of any of the rubber impression materials.

2. Has a permanent deformation that is greater than that of polysulfides but not as low as that of silicones.

3. Has high stiffness and low flexibility, which can cause problems during removal from mouth.

4. Has a lower dimension change than any other rubber material, except for polyvinylsiloxane.

5. Can cause tissue irritation because of the aromatic sulfonic acid ester catalyst.

IV. Uses

A. Dental compound

1. Tray compound is used for making a primary impression for dentures; another impression material, such as rubber base, is put into the tray to make the secondary or corrective impression.

2. Impression compounds are used for border molding for denture impressions.

B. ZOE impression paste is used as a cementing media; also is used for surgical dressings (after periodontal surgery), temporary restorations, root canal filling material, bite registration paste, and impression material for dentures.

C. Irreversible hydrocolloid

1. Is used in development of study casts, for:

a. Educational purposes.

b. Fabrication of fluoride trays and mouth protectors.

c. Orthodontic appliance construction.

2. Is used to prepare a cast for the development of complete and partial dentures.

D. Reversible hydrocolloid has the same uses as irreversible hydrocolloid but it produces more accurate detail.

E. Polysulfide

1. Is used for inlay and crown impressions.

2. Is used in the development of fixed partial dentures.

3. Is used for secondary impressions for dentures.

F. Silicone

1. Polyvinylsiloxane (addition silicone) has the same uses as polysulfide.

2. Condensation silicone is used for inlay and crown impressions.

G. Polyether has the same uses as condensation silicone.

Replication Materials

Impression plaster and stone are examples of replication materials that are used to produce a positive reproduction.

I. Classification of Gypsum Products (Table 10–4)

II. Composition

A. Gypsum is a dihydrate of calcium sulfate ($CaSO_4 \cdot 2H_2O$); occurs widely in a massive form known as rock-gypsum.

B. Plaster and dental stones are identical chemically (calcium sulfate hemihydrate).

1. Three types of calcium sulfate hemihydrate are manufactured:

a. Plaster, which is made by heating gypsum at

TABLE 10.4	ADA Classification of Gypsum Products
Type I	Impression plaster
Type II	Model plaster
Type III	Dental stone
Type IV	Die stone or high-strength dental stone
Type V	High-strength, high-expansion die stone

atmospheric pressure (results in a porous, irregularly shaped material).

   b. Dental stone, which is made by heating gypsum under steam pressure (results in hemihydrate particles that are less porous and more uniform in shape).

   c. Die stone, which is made by dehydrating gypsum in a 30% solution of calcium chloride (results in the least porous hemihydrate particles).

III. Characteristics and Properties

   A. Hemihydrate

   1. Physical differences in hemihydrate particles determine the manipulative properties for mixing the particles and the use of each.

      a. Mixing (Table 10–5)

         1) The amount of water needed depends on the size, shape, and porosity of the particles.

            a) Porous, irregularly shaped hemihydrate crystals require more water to facilitate wetting and mixing.

            b) High-strength stone requires the least amount of water

            c) Too much water prolongs the setting time and creates a weaker cast/die.

            d) Too little water results in increased expansion.

      b. Setting

         1) When mixed with water, forms a hard substance.

         2) Produces heat through the chemical reaction of hemihydrate with water (exothermic heat).

         3) Common practice is to allow 45 to 60 minutes for gypsum to set before removing the impression from the cast/die.

   B. Accelerators and retarders

   1. Are a more practical method of controlling setting time than varying the water to powder ratio (added by the manufacturer during the manufacturing process).

   2. The accelerator is potassium sulfate; the addition of this salt solution reduces setting time from approximately 10 minutes to 4 minutes.

   3. The retarder, which typically is borax (2%), increases setting time.

      a. Blood, saliva, agar, and alginate also retard setting.

      b. Impressions should be thoroughly rinsed and disinfected (to remove traces of blood, saliva).

   C. Temperature and humidity

   1. Higher water temperatures (during mixing) decrease setting times.

   2. High humidity results in increased setting time.

IV. Uses of Gypsum

   A. Impression plasters (type I)

   1. Are used to make impressions of edentulous patients.

   B. Model plasters (type II)

   1. Are not used intraorally.

   2. Are used to make study casts.

      a. To document conditions in the mouth at the beginning of treatment.

      b. To document the progress of involved/long-term treatment.

      c. For use in forensic cases.

      d. To permit clinicians to examine conditions in the mouth from all views.

      e. To study relationships between adjacent and opposing teeth and to examine, measure, and analyze without discomfort to the patient.

      f. For drawing or performing proposed treatment on models.

      g. To examine occlusal relationships.

      h. To identify factors such as wear facets, open contacts, rotated teeth, and tissue recession when charting existing conditions.

      i. To illustrate existing conditions to the patient during case presentation.

      j. To demonstrate individualized home care procedures and to allow the patient to practice techniques on models.

   3. Are used to mount stone casts in the articulator.

   4. Are stronger than type-I plasters because of a lower water-to-plaster (W/P) ratio (results in less porosity when the material dries).

TABLE 10.5	Water/Powder Ratios of Gypsum Materials*

Gypsum	Water (mL/100 g powder)
Model plaster	37–50
Dental stone	28–32
High-strength dental stone	19–24

*Recommended W/P ratios vary among products and manufacturers.

C. Dental stone (type III)
   1. Is used to make casts of impressions for the production of dentures.
   2. Is used to produce study casts.
   3. Is harder, stronger, and more durable than type-II plaster.
   4. Has greater strength as a result of a lower W/P ratio.
D. Die stone (type IV)
   1. Is used as a die material on which wax patterns of inlays, crowns, and other castings are produced.
E. High-strength, high-expansion die stone (type V)
   1. Is the most recent addition to ADA gypsum.
   2. Resulted from the need for dies with increased expansion to compensate for the greater shrinkage that occurs in newer, higher-melting alloys.
V. Mixing and handling
   A. Dispensing
      1. Powder should be weighed on a scale and water should be measured in a graduated cylinder to get consistent results.
   B. Mixing
      1. Should be performed in a rubber bowl, using a stiff metal spatula.
      2. Is best performed with room-temperature water.
      3. Should involve placing water in the bowl first and subsequently adding powder (which is sifted into water slowly).
      4. Material is spatulated to break up any clumps and to enhance the wetting of the powder.
      5. Is vigorous for 30 to 60 seconds; gypsum should be wiped against the side of the bowl.
      6. Once completed, is followed by vibration to remove remaining air bubbles; the presence of air bubbles results in porosities in the cast, which reduces its strength.
      7. When complete, the mix looks very glossy on the surface and has a smooth, creamy texture (if sandy, grainy, or watery, an incorrect W/P ration has been used or mixing is incomplete).
      8. Can be accomplished using the vacuum mixer technique.
VI. Fabrication of Study Casts
   A. The surface of the impression should be dried (excess water should be removed).
   B. Plaster/stone is dripped into one corner of the impression and gently vibrated to slowly move the mix around the arch and express any air (essentially coat the impression with a layer of plaster/stone).
   C. A second increment of plaster/stone is added and vibrated (excessive vibration should be avoided because it creates air bubbles in the material).
   D. The process is repeated until the entire surface of the impression is coated with plaster/stone and teeth imprints are completely filled.
E. Larger increments of plaster/stone can be added to fill the impression completely.
F. A one-pour technique involves an initial mix of plaster/stone that is large enough to fill the impression and form a base.
G. A two-pour technique involves a second mix of plaster/stone, which is used to form a base.

Direct Restorative Materials

Direct restorative materials can be placed directly in or on a prepared tooth. They are advantageous because of their immediate results and time-saving benefits.

Temporary Restoratives

Many procedures cannot be completed in one appointment because of the need for laboratory work or because of complications of infections. In these instances, a temporary or provisional restoration that is placed over the preparation is indicated. Temporary materials, such as acrylics, stainless steel, composites, or cements occupy the preparation until a permanent restoration can be placed.

I. Acrylics with compositions similar to those used for denture bases are employed.
II. Stainless Steel or Aluminum
   A. Is stiff enough to bear occlusal forces when cemented to a prepared tooth with temporary cement.
   B. Is easy to cut and adjust.
   C. Has poor esthetic qualities.
III. Composite-Type Material
   A. Of intermediate rigidity is somewhat flexible after light curing.
   B. Flexibility allows for easy cutting and removal when permanent restoration is ready for insertion.
IV. ZOE (type III)
   A. Is designed for use as a temporary filling when mixed to a base- or putty-like consistency.
   B. Protects the pulp.
   C. Reduces pulpal inflammation.
   D. Maintains tooth position until a permanent restoration can be placed.

 Clinical Case **STUDY**

Carol, a 47-year-old administrative assistant, presents for oral prophylaxis. A new patient examination reveals the following conditions: porcelain veneers on the maxillary anterior teeth, several posterior amalgams that are fractured, and mandibular anterior composites that show signs of leakage. Upon questioning, the patient states that she has had sporadic dental care during the past 7 years because of her husband's employment changes, which have resulted in numerous family relocations. Carol further states that she is ready for comprehensive treatment that will protect her oral investment.

Clinical Case QUESTIONS

1. What would be the value of fabricating study casts for this patient?
2. Would finishing and polishing her amalgams be appropriate care? Explain.
3. What properties of composite dental materials lend themselves to microleakage?
4. Which topical fluoride would be appropriate for this patient? Explain.

Clinical Case RATIONALES

1. Study casts would allow the dental hygienist to demonstrate the patient's oral conditions (i.e., fractured amalgams, open margins on composites). In addition, the casts could be used to demonstrate home care techniques and allow the patient to practice those techniques on the models.
2. Fractured amalgams are a contraindication to finishing and polishing procedures. Appropriate care would involve the replacement of the worn amalgams.
3. Polymerization shrinkage and thermal expansion. Even with acid etching and the use of bonding agents, stresses from polymerization shrinkage can exceed the strength of the bond between composite materials and tooth structure and fail to prevent marginal leakage. The thermal expansion of composite materials does not match that of tooth structure, therefore a differential expansion occurs that results in the microleakage of fluids between the restoration and the tooth.
4. Neutral sodium. Research has shown that acidulated phosphate fluoride can cause pitting and roughening of porcelain and composite materials. Because the patient has porcelain veneers on her maxillary anterior teeth, acidulated phosphate fluoride is contraindicated. Stannous fluoride can result in staining and also is contraindicated.

Permanent Restorations

Permanent restorations are composed of dental materials whose properties allow them to function in the oral cavity for a greater length of service than that of temporary restorations. They include both tooth-colored and amalgam restorations.

I. Tooth-Colored Restorations
  A. Ceramics
    1. Are compounds formed by the union of metallic oxides and minerals.
    2. Include glass, concrete, fine crystal, and gypsum.
      a. Glass ceramics are used extensively as reinforcing agents or fillers for dental composites and routinely as coatings or veneers to improve the esthetics of metallic dental restorations; also are used in several dental cements and temporary restorations.
    3. Generally are very brittle materials (cannot be bent or deformed without cracking or breaking).
    4. Are characterized by high melting points and low thermal and electrical conductivity.
    5. Are inert, or not chemically reactive, which makes them biocompatible with the patient's body.
  B. Porcelain
    1. Is a specific type of ceramic that is used extensively in dentistry.
    2. Contains three main components: quartz, feldspar (75% to 80%), and kaolin clay (aluminum silicate).
    3. Is fabricated by the dental technician.
    4. Is chosen as a restorative material primarily because of its esthetic qualities; matches adjacent tooth structure in translucence, color, and intensity.
    5. Has a unique ability to emit light when illuminated, which gives it a very natural and vital appearance.
    6. Has a hardness number (Mohs) of 6 to 7; may cause rapid abrasion of opposing enamel, which has a hardness number of 5 to 6.
    7. Is used in restorative dentistry to produce denture teeth, jacket crowns, porcelain-fused-to-metal crowns and bridgework, veneers, and inlays.
  C. Composites
    1. Are used in class-III, -IV, and -V esthetic restorations.
    2. Often are used as veneers to cover teeth stained by drugs or chemicals such as fluoride, to fill spaces between teeth (diastemas), and to enhance the contour of misshapened teeth.
    3. Are composed of three major constituents:
      a. Organic resin matrix composed of monomers called dimethylacrylates and commonly abbreviated as Bis-GMA.
      b. Inorganic filler (quartz, glasses, and colloidal silica particles).
      c. Coupling agent, which chemically bonds the filler to the resin matrix (vinyl silane).
    4. Polymerization
      a. Chemically activated composites involve two containers of composite paste:
        1) One contains a benzoyl peroxide initiator.
        2) One contains a tertiary amine activator.
        3) When mixed, the amine reacts with the benzoyl peroxide and initiates polymerization.
      b. Visible light-activated resins are supplied as a single paste that contains both the photo initiator and the amine activator.
      c. Dual-activated resins contain activation chemicals for both chemical and light-activated resins. When the two pastes are

mixed, a slow chemical activation begins. Exposure to a curing light results in a rapid photoactivation.

5. Composite materials are classified by particle size (Table 10–6).
6. Polymerization shrinkage is the most problematic property of composite materials. Even with the acid etching of enamel and the use of bonding agents, stresses from shrinkage can exceed the strength of the bond between composites and tooth structure, resulting in marginal leakage.
   a. Two techniques for minimizing shrinkage:
      1) Insertion and polymerization of the composite in layers.
      2) Fabrication of composite inlays.
         a) A composite can be cured more fully in a laboratory, which produces a restoration with superior physical and mechanical properties compared with those cured intraorally.
         b) Extraoral processing eliminates concerns about shrinkage away from the tooth structure; the space between the tooth and inlay is filled by a composite cement (after lab fabrication the inlay is cemented at a second appointment, with a dual-cure composite cement).
7. Amount of filler resin
   a. The greater the amount of filler content, the stronger the restoration.
   b. The greater the amount of filler content, the less wearing away of the restoration.
8. Size of filler particles
   a. The smaller the size of the filler particles, the more polishable the restoration.
   b. The larger the size of the filler particles, the more difficult it is to achieve a smoothly polished finish; however, larger filler particles result in a stronger restoration that is able to tolerate more abrasion.
9. Thermal conductivity
   a. Values closely match those of enamel and dentin; composites provide good thermal insulation for dental pulp.
10. Thermal expansion
    a. The more organic matrix, the higher the linear coefficient of thermal expansion.
    b. Microfilled composites have the highest values, which result in the greatest dimension changes in response to oral temperature changes.
    c. Hybrid composites have the lowest values because of their high filler content.
11. Water absorption
    a. Is determined by the organic matrix and results in discoloration by water-soluble stains.
    b. Is greatest for microfilled composites because of their high organic matrix content.
12. Radiopacity
    a. Is caused by heavy metal glasses such as those found in some fine-particle composites and hybrid composites.
    b. Is eliminated in microfilled composites that are filled with silica, and in some fine-particle composites that are filled with quartz.
13. Compression and tensile strength
    a. Are higher in value when the volume of filler is increased.
    b. Are lower in value in microfilled composites because of the percentage of fillers.
14. Bond strengths between composites and acid-etched enamel are approximately twice as great as the bond strengths between composites and acid-etched dentin.

D. Enamel and dentin adhesives
   1. Enamel adhesives

TABLE 10.6	Classification of Composite Materials by Particle Size			
Category	Average Particle Size (μm)	Characteristics	Clinical Recommendations	Commercial Examples
Microfilled	0.02–0.07	High thermal expansion and water sorption; easily polished	Small class III and IV restorations and veneers	Durafill, Kulzer, Heliomolar (RO, Ivoclar/Vivadent)
Small (fine) particle	1–5	Do not polish to as smooth a surface as microfills	Medium class III and IV restorations	P-10 (3M Company)
Hybrid	0.04–5.0	Increase in smaller particles improves polishability; higher filler load results in low thermal expansion and high strength and durability	Large class III and IV restorations	Herculite XR, Kerr, Tetric (Ivoclar)

a. Are unfilled resins that are used to enhance the adaptation and bond of composites to etched enamel surfaces.

b. Have excellent flow properties that allow them to coat and fill acid-etched enamel (enamel tubules) in a more efficient manner than the viscous composite materials.

c. Rely on the mechanical interlocking of the unfilled resin into the enamel rods for adhesion.

2. Dentin adhesives

a. Are necessary for preparations that extend into the dentin.

b. Are developed with regard for the following composition differences between dentin and enamel:

1) In etched dentin only 4% of the dentin surface near the DEJ may contain tubules; near the pulp 30% of the surface area of dentin may contain tubules.

2) Enamel is composed almost entirely of inorganic mineral; 30% of the weight of dentin is organic.

3) A large amount of water exists in dentin tubules.

4) The presence of water and organic components lowers the surface energy of dentin, making bonding more difficult.

c. Attachment to the dentin requires removal of the smear layer—a layer of loosely adhered debris that remains on the dentinal tubules as a result of the cutting action of a dental drill.

1) The object of adhesion is to remove the smear layer while leaving the tubules blocked with debris from the cavity preparation.

2) This removal technique is accomplished with a milder acid (10% vs. 30%) than that used for enamel etching.

3. Basic principles of bonding

a. Isolate the surface to be bonded.

b. Maintain a clean surface.

c. Follow the manufacturer's directions carefully and use a fresh bonding agent.

d. Use a protective liner for deep cavities.

e. Provide mechanical retention in cavity preparations where no enamel is available for etching and retention.

II. Amalgam

A. Is an alloy (a combination of two or more metals).

B. Is composed of mercury (the only pure metal that is liquid at room temperature) mixed with a powder of silver and tin and other trace elements.

C. Has physical properties suitable for dental restoratives.

a. Silver increases setting expansion and strength.

b. Tin has a high solubility in mercury, which facilitates amalgamation and decreases setting expansion.

c. Copper acts much the same as silver; increases the strength of the amalgam, the hardness, and the setting expansion. Amalgam alloys that contain 6% or less copper are low-copper alloys. Amalgam alloys that contain more than 6% copper are called high-copper alloys, generally are superior, and perform better clinically.

d. Zinc often is included to minimize the oxidation of other metals in the alloy.

D. Types of amalgam

1. Low-copper amalgams are seldom used because of their inferior performance.

2. High-copper amalgams produce alloys with greater strength, higher corrosion resistance, less marginal breakdown, and lower creep; universally are the most accepted and used amalgam alloys. High-copper amalgams can be made from lathe-cut or spherical particles, or may be an admixture.

a. Lathe-cut amalgams are powders composed of small shavings or filings produced by a cutting lathe; the final powder is a blend of various-sized particles.

b. Spherical alloys contain alloy particles in the form of small spheres, which result in easier amalgamation (combining of mercury and other alloys); amalgamation is accomplished with a smaller amount of mercury than with lathe-cut amalgams; do not resist condensation forces and therefore require less condensation force and the use of larger diameter condensers.

c. Admixed alloys (a mixture of lathe-cut and spherical alloys)

1) Have a total copper content that ranges from 9% to 20%

2) Adapt better to cavity walls and produce better contacts with adjacent teeth.

d. Single composition (only high-copper alloys) contains powder particles of only one composition (high-copper).

E. Setting reactions

1. Gamma phases

a. The two main types of amalgam alloy composition are silver-tin alloys with or without significant amounts of copper. The difference between the two alloys is the setting reactions with mercury. The reaction that occurs between mercury and amalgam alloy is called amalgamation.

1) The silver-tin phase is called the gamma

(γ) phase and is composed of the unreacted alloy particles. This is the strongest phase in the setting reaction of amalgam.

2) The silver-mercury phase is called the gamma-1 (γ_1) phase.

3) The tin-mercury phase is called the gamma-2 (γ_2) phase. This is the weakest component of the three gamma setting reaction phases; gamma-2 also is more susceptible to corrosion than either gamma or gamma-1.

    a) Low-copper amalgams form a weak tin-mercury phase, resulting in a weaker amalgam with inferior properties.

    b) High-copper amalgams eliminate the tin-mercury phase by forming a copper-tin phase, resulting in a stronger, more superior restoration.

2. Copper content of alloys
  a. Low-copper alloys
    1) The silver and tin (Ag_3Sn) combination in the alloy particle reacts with mercury during trituration (mixing) in the gamma phase (strongest component and strongest phase).
    2) As mercury becomes saturated with silver and tin, the following compounds precipitate:
      a) Silver-mercury (Ag_2Hg_3) compound (gamma 1)
      b) Tin-mercury (Sn_8Hg) compound (gamma 2)
  b. High-copper alloys
    1) Tin has a greater affinity for copper than for mercury, thus a copper-tin compound is formed (eta phase) instead of the tin-mercury compound (gamma 2).
    2) A high-copper alloy contains enough copper to suppress the formation of the gamma 2 phase; results in superior properties.

F. Characteristics and properties
  1. Dimensional changes include:
    a. Shrinkage
      1) Initially is caused by mercury and alloy particles mixing together.
      2) Results in a slight gap between the amalgam and tooth, which allows some leakage of fluids between the amalgam and the wall of the cavity preparation.
      3) Eventually leads to the formation of corrosion products, which seal the tooth from the oral environment.
      4) Results in postoperative sensitivity, often because of fluid movement in unsealed dentin tubules (because the gap allows fluids in).

    b. Creep (flow or dimensional change produced in a material under a constant stress)
      1) Can affect marginal integrity because of chewing forces, which can cause amalgam to creep or flow into open areas, such as margins, and subsequently fracture.
      2) Is influenced by the presence of gamma 2 because it is weak and therefore easily deformed. High-copper amalgams are stronger because gamma-2 does not form.

G. Strength and stiffness
  1. Amalgam is strong, especially during compression.
  2. Amalgam is stiff because it has a relatively high modulus of elasticity.
  3. Amalgam has lower tensile strength and therefore should not be placed in thin layers where it will be exposed to tensile stress.

H. Mixing and handling
  1. Mixing
    a. The goal is to ensure that mercury and alloy are sufficiently mixed to allow the chemical reaction to proceed, thus producing an amalgam that condenses and adapts to cavity preparation with minimal porosity.
    b. Requires mechanical amalgamators to triturate amalgam alloy and mercury.
      1) Amalgam quality is controlled by:
        a) Time, which ranges from 6 to 20 seconds; manufacturer's instructions should be followed.
        b) Speed and force, which can be controlled on variable-speed units (the medium setting is most often used); the efficiency of the unit must be periodically checked to ensure quality.
    c. Characteristics of under-mixed (undertriturated) amalgam include:
      1) Dull appearance
      2) Grainy texture (difficult to manipulate)
      3) Quick hardening
      4) Excess mercury left in restoration, which leads to reduced strength
    d. Characteristics of over-mixed (overtriturated) amalgam include:
      1) Soupy appearance
      2) Inability to hold form
      3) Difficult removal from capsule
    e. Characteristics of correctly mixed amalgam include:
      1) Shiny appearance
      2) Cohesive form
      3) Easy manipulation for condensation
  2. Handling

a. Condensation is the adaptation of amalgam to prepared cavity walls, matrix, and margins; forms a uniform, compact mass with minimum voids and reduction of excess mercury content.
  1) The removal of excess mercury during condensation results in less creep from chewing forces, stronger amalgam, and less dimensional change during setting.
  2) The longer the time lapse between trituration and condensation, the weaker the amalgam will be because of the fracturing of crystal formation.
  3) Begins with the smaller-tipped condenser because greater compacting stress can be generated with the small tip, which also is most effective in the depth and corners of the preparation.
  4) Builds up amalgam in increments to avoid porosities and express excess mercury at each step.
  5) Requires the use of condensers with larger heads as the preparation becomes filled.
  6) Requires over-packing of the restoration; a slight excess of amalgam ensures complete filling.
  7) When performed correctly, has a top layer slightly rich in mercury that is removed during carving.
  8) Moisture contamination must be avoided because it results in excessive expansion.
b. Carving of the amalgam surface to produce the correct anatomy is performed after the amalgam is placed.
c. Burnishing or smoothing the surface and margins, using *light* pressure, follows carving.
  1) Heat generation is avoided during finishing and polishing to prevent the release of mercury and a subsequent reduction in strength.
  2) Polishing is performed at least 24 hours after placement; for spherical high-copper alloys it may be performed during the same appointment.
    a) Should be performed in the presence of water to avoid overheating.
3. Bonding amalgam to tooth
  a. Is performed by specially developed adhesives that bond the amalgam to the tooth structure.
  b. Has advantages, which include fracture resistance, increased strength, and more conservative preparations.
  c. Has disadvantages, which include technique sensitivity, increased time for placement, and increased cost as a result of increased chair time and practitioner training for new technique.
4. Amalgam safety
  a. Involves controlling mercury exposure.
    1) In 1991, the National Institutes of Health (NIH) concluded that for most individuals, the use of mercury in dentistry remains a safe and effective treatment.
    2) Mercury vapor is colorless, odorless, and tasteless, which makes it a hazard for dental personnel.
    3) The maximum safe level of exposure to mercury vapor for dental personnel is 50 μg per cubic meter of air.
    4) Safety precautions include well-ventilated operatories and collection and storage of amalgam scraps in a well sealed container; if mercury contacts skin, it should be washed immediately with soap and water.
    5) Preproportioned capsules of amalgam reduce the risk of mercury exposure; when cutting amalgam, a water spray and high-speed evacuation should be used.
    6) Annual monitoring of actual exposure to mercury vapors is recommended.
    7) Amalgam/mercury waste should be disposed of responsibly in accordance with EPA regulations for the area in which the practice is located.

Classification of Caries and Cavity Preparations

Caries and cavity preparations are designated as class I through class VI, depending on their location.
I. Caries Classification (Fig. 10–6)
  A. Class I
    1. Occur in pits and fissures.
    2. Involve:
      a. Occlusal surfaces of premolars and molars.
      b. Facial and lingual surfaces of molars.
      c. Lingual surfaces of maxillary incisors.
  B. Class II
    1. Occur in proximal surfaces of premolars and molars.
  C. Class III
    1. Occur in proximal surfaces of incisors and canines that do not involve incisal angles.
  D. Class IV
    1. Occur in proximal surfaces of incisors and canines that involve incisal angles.
  E. Class V
    1. Occur in the cervical third of facial or lingual surfaces.
  F. Class VI
    1. Occur on incisal edges of anterior teeth and cusp tips of posterior teeth.
II. Cavity Preparations (see Fig. 10–6)
  A. Nomenclature

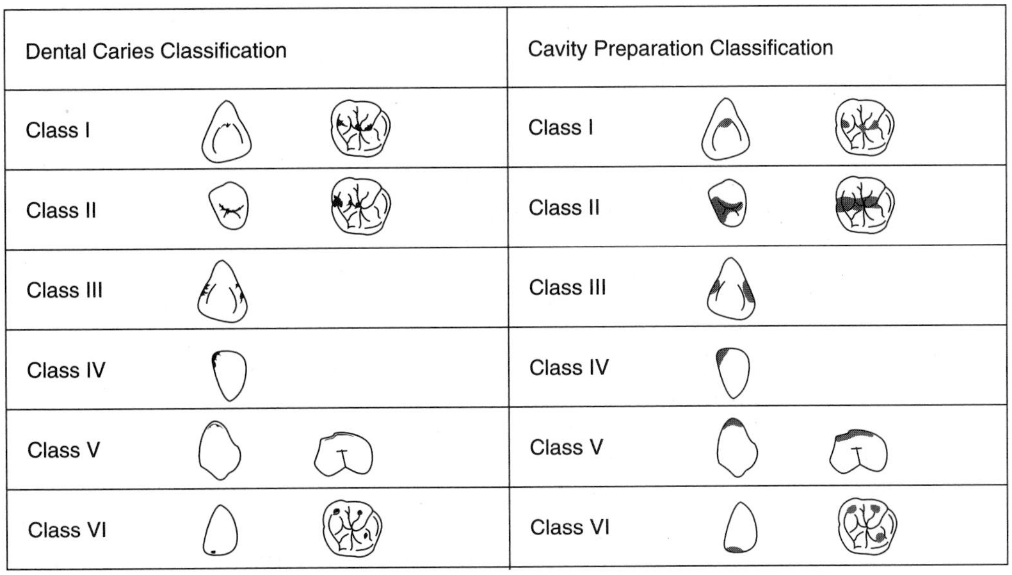

Dental Caries Classification			Cavity Preparation Classification		
Class I			Class I		
Class II			Class II		
Class III			Class III		
Class IV			Class IV		
Class V			Class V		
Class VI			Class VI		

Figure 10.6   Classification of dental caries and cavity preparation.

1. Wall is a vertical or horizontal surface within the cavity preparation that is named according to the closest external tooth surface (e.g., facial, mesial), for the structure it approximates (e.g., pulpal wall), or for its relationship to the long axis of the tooth (e.g., axial wall).
2. Cavosurface is the uncut tooth tissue adjacent to the cavity preparation.
3. Line angle is the line that forms along the junction of two walls or of one wall and the cavosurface; is named according to the walls and surfaces involved.
4. Point angle is the point formed by the junction of three walls within a cavity preparation and is named according to the walls involved.
B. Class-I cavity preparation
C. Class-II cavity preparation
D. Class-III cavity preparation
E. Class-IV cavity preparation
F. Class-V cavity preparation
G. Class-VI cavity preparation

Cements, Bases, Liners, and Varnishes

Dental cements are used for a variety of applications in dentistry. Depending on how they are mixed, cements can serve as luting agents, base materials, or temporary restorations. Liners are applied in a thin layer to seal dentin and varnishes serve as liners under amalgam restorations to seal dentinal tubules and prevent the migration of metallic ions from amalgam to tooth.
I. General Uses (Table 10–7)
  A. Cements
    1. Are primarily used as luting agents (adhere one surface to another) for inlays, onlays, crowns, bridges, and other structures.
    2. Are used to adhere orthodontic bands.
    3. Are used to cement pins and posts to teeth for the purpose of retaining restorations.

TABLE 10.7   Uses of Cement, Bases, Liners, and Varnishes

Material	Product Examples (Manufacturer)	Cement	Base	Liner	Varnish	Temporary Restoration	Permanent Resoration
Zinc phosphate	Flecks (Mizzy)	X	X				
ZOE (type II)	SuperEBA (Bosworth)	X					
ZOE reinforced (type III)	Fynal (Caulk/Dentsply)					X	
Glass ionomer	Ketac-Cem (ESPE-Premier)	X	X				X
Polycarboxylate	Durelon (ESPE-Premier)	X	X				
Calcium hydroxide	Life (Kerr/Sybron)		X	X			
Copal resin varnish	Copalite (Cooley and Cooley)				X		

4. Are used in temporary or permanent restorations.
5. Are mixed creamy and thin for cement.

B. Bases
   1. Are placed in thick layers to provide thermal insulation under deep metallic restorations.
   2. Have therapeutic benefit for the pulp (are soothing).
   3. Are mixed thick and quick (requires incorporation of more powder).

C. Liners
   1. Seal tooth structures against the leakage of irritants present in saliva or restorative materials.
   2. Provide a protective covering to the pulp in deep cavity preparations (pulp capping) or when there has been a pulp exposure.

D. Varnishes
   1. Seal dentin tubules and prevent the migration of agents into the tooth as a result of marginal leakage from a newly placed amalgam.
   2. Prevent the outward migration of metallic ions from the amalgam to the tooth (leads to darkening of tooth structure adjacent to the amalgam); older amalgams are more likely to corrode and cause staining than the more modern amalgams.

II. Types and Characteristics of Cements, Bases, Liners, and Varnishes
   A. Zinc phosphate cement
      1. Composition and chemistry
         a. Contains primarily zinc oxide and 10% magnesium oxide in powder form.
         b. Contains phosphoric acid buffered by alumina in liquid form.
         c. Contains water (33%), which controls the rate at which the powder and liquid react.
         d. Is acidic because of the phosphoric acid.
         e. Is a type-I cement with a film thickness of 25 μm, which permits a thin film for the seating of precision castings.
      2. Uses
         a. Primarily is a luting (cementing) agent for crowns, bridges, and orthodontic bands (mixed thin and creamy).
         b. Secondarily is a base (mixed thick and quickly).
            1) Bases are mixed with a higher powder-to-liquid ratio to obtain maximum strength to enable the material to withstand the forces of condensation.
            2) The higher powder-to-liquid ratio also results in a more rapid setting time.
      3. Manipulation techniques
         a. Include mixing on a cool slab over a wide area to allow the escape of heat (exothermic reaction) because the setting process causes a liberation of heat.
         b. Include adding the powder in small amounts, with thorough mixing of each increment; extends the setting time.
         c. Include mixing with as much powder as possible to reduce acid irritation to the pulp.
         d. Involve controlling the setting time by using a cool slab, which slows down the chemical reaction.
         e. Include reducing any moisture on the mixing slab; moisture accelerates the setting time and has negative effects on the properties of the cement.
      4. Advantages
         a. Has the longest clinical history.
         b. Is useful for multiple restorative procedures.
         c. Has low film thickness, which facilitates easy insertion of restorative work.
         d. Is inexpensive.
         e. Is easy to use.
      5. Disadvantages
         a. Has a low pH of 3.5, which can irritate pulpal tissues.
         b. Is unable to adhere to tooth structure; requires mechanical retention.
         c. Lacks anticariogenic properties.
   B. Zinc oxide-eugenol (ZOE)
      1. Composition and chemistry
         a. Contains zinc oxide powder.
         b. Contains eugenol liquid (oil of cloves), which can irritate connective tissue.
         c. Type II (reinforced cements) may contain EBA (orthoethoxybenzoic acid and alumina).
         d. Has a pH between 7 and 8.
      2. Uses
         a. Type I cements are designed for temporary cementation (e.g., Temp-Bond, Kerr/Sybron); tensile strength is weaker than that of type II, which allows temporary restorative work to be easily removed at a second appointment so that permanent restoration can be placed.
         b. Type II cements (alumina EBA) are designed for permanent cementation (e.g., SuperEBA or Fynal).
         c. Type III are designed for temporary fillings and thermal insulating bases (e.g., IRM).
         d. Type IV are used as cavity liners.
      3. Advantages
         a. Have multiple uses; are used as cavity liners, thermal insulating bases, and temporary or permanent cements; also are used for temporary restoration.
         b. Are the least irritating of dental materials; have a pH of 7.0, which makes them very sedative and palliative to the pulp.
      4. Disadvantages
         a. Lack strength.

b. Are inadequate for use under composite restorations because they interfere with the polymerization process.

c. Are difficult to remove from tissues and mixing surfaces once they are set.

d. Cause sensitivity in some individuals because of eugenol (non-eugenol products, such as Nogenol and GC American, are available).

C. Polycarboxylate cement

1. Composition and chemistry

a. Contains zinc oxide in powder form.

b. Contains polyacrylic acid in water or viscous liquid solution (polyacrylic acid is less irritating to dentin than phosphoric acid in zinc phosphate cement).

2. Uses

a. As a luting agent, often is used in pedodontics for the cementation of stainless steel crowns because of its kindness to pulp.

b. Secondarily, is a non-irritating base, liner, or temporary cement.

3. Advantages

a. Bonds to the tooth.

b. Is kind to the pulp.

c. Is useful in pedodontics because of its kindness to pulp and its ability to bond to stainless steel crowns.

d. Is useful under composites because it does not interfere with their polymerization.

4. Disadvantages

a. Has a short working time.

b. Has limited use because it does not adhere to porcelain, resins, or gold alloys.

D. Glass ionomer cement

1. Composition and chemistry

a. Contains aluminosilicate glass in finely ground powder.

b. Contains polycarboxylate copolymer in water.

c. Has a chemical adhesion to tooth structure (similar to that of polycarboxylate cements).

d. Releases fluoride.

2. Uses

a. Include final cementation of crowns and bridges (type I).

b. Is a high strength base.

c. Is a restorative material for class-V restoration because it releases fluoride (type II).

3. Manipulation

a. Has a mixing time of 30 to 60 seconds.

b. Has a working time of approximately 2 minutes after mixing.

c. Must not contact water or saliva; moisture causes the cement to set too fast.

d. Once hardened, glass ionomer is sensitive to becoming dried out, which results in surface and interior cracks. Two methods to alleviate this problem include:

1) Coating with varnish immediately after the initial hardening has taken place.

2) Placing a layer of unfilled bonding resin over the surface and curing it (more permanent alternative).

4. Advantages

a. Is strong; strength is comparable to that of zinc phosphate cements.

b. Causes less irritation than zinc phosphate.

c. Contains fluoride, which results in anticariogenic property.

d. Is easy to mix.

e. Adheres to tooth structure.

5. Disadvantages

a. High solubility.

b. Complete setting takes approximately one day, thus margins (exposed cement) must be protected for the first 24 hours.

c. Water causes retardation of the set (requires dry field).

d. Requires the use of a base in deep lesions.

E. Calcium hydroxide

1. Composition and chemistry

a. Contains calcium tungstate, calcium phosphate, and zinc oxide in glycol salicylate as a base paste.

b. Contains calcium hydroxide, zinc oxide, and zinc stearate in ethylene toluene sulfonamide as a catalyst paste.

c. Forms an amorphous calcium disalicylate when set.

d. Has a pH that varies from 11 to 12.

2. Uses

a. Include direct and indirect pulp capping.

b. Is a protective barrier under composite restorations (does not interfere with the polymerization of these materials).

3. Manipulation

a. Typically is a two-paste system.

b. Requires dispensing of equal lengths of catalyst and base onto a mixing pad; is mixed to a uniform color.

c. Light-cured cements should be cured by visible light for 20 seconds for each 1-mm layer.

4. Advantages

a. Encourages pulp recovery by stimulation of reparative dentin.

b. Protects the pulp.

c. Has sufficient strength (is stronger than type-IV ZOE cement).

5. Disadvantages

a. Cannot be placed if tooth surface is wet.

b. Proportion is difficult to control with an instrument.

F. Varnish (e.g., Copalite)

1. Composition and chemistry
   a. Contains natural gum, a copal resin dissolved in an organic solvent.
2. Uses
   a. Assists in sealing the cavity preparation, thereby reducing microleakage around the restoration.
   b. Seals dentinal tubules.
   c. Serves as a protective barrier; reduces the possibility of postoperative sensitivity.
3. Manipulation
   a. Involves application to cavity walls in a thin layer with a brush, wire loop, or cotton applicator.
4. Advantages
   a. Seals cavity, reducing microleakage.
   b. Acts as a barrier to cementing material, reducing postoperative sensitivity.
5. Disadvantages
   a. Is not required when nonirritating cements such as ZOE or polycarboxylates are used.
   b. Cannot be used under composite resins because the resin will soften.
   c. Cannot be used with glass ionomer cement because it interferes with bonding to the tooth and the uptake of fluoride from the glass ionomer cement.
   d. Requires a base in deep cavities; varnish does not provide ample protection because of low film thickness.

Finishing and Polishing Materials

The intent of finishing and polishing procedures is to create restorations that fit and maintain occlusal harmony, and to produce a smooth surface that results in less irritation to intraoral tissues, less plaque and calculus adherence, and a decreased potential for the corrosion of metal restorations.

I. Abrasive Procedures
   A. Abrasion is the wearing away or removal of material by rubbing, cutting, or scraping. The object that does the abrading is called the abrasive.
   B. Finishing and polishing are two abrasive procedures commonly used in dentistry; both are wear processes but they differ in intent and degree.
      1. Finishing refers to the process by which a restoration or appliance is contoured to remove excess material and produce a reasonably smooth surface.
      2. Polishing follows finishing and refers to the removal of materials from a restoration or appliance with the intent of producing a smooth, reflective surface that does not contain scratches. The polished surface should resemble the natural surface.

II. Factors That Affect Finishing
   A. Hardness refers to the abrasive's ability to cut.
   B. Size influences the speed of the cut.

1. Larger particles abrade a surface more rapidly.
2. Particles are classified by size in micrometers (μm).
   a. Coarse = 100 μm
   b. Medium = 10 to 100 μm
   c. Fine = 0 to 10 μm
3. Finishing and polishing involves a sequential reduction in the size of abrasive particles.
   C. Pressure
      1. Of the force, when greater, results in more rapid removal of the material.
      2. When greater, creates increased temperature and heat.
      3. Under higher temperatures can lead to distortion or physical changes within the appliance/restoration.
      4. With high temperatures may cause discomfort for the patient because of the transmission of heat to the pulpal tissues.
   D. Speed
      1. When faster, results in faster cutting rates.
      2. When faster, creates greater temperatures.
      3. When faster, creates greater danger of overcutting the appliance/restoration.
   E. Lubrication
      1. Is used to minimize heat build-up.
      2. Facilitates movement of the cutting edge into the surface of the appliance/restoration.
      3. Carries away debris so that the cutting edge does not become clogged.

III. Types and Composition of Abrasives
   A. Diamond
      1. Is composed of carbon.
      2. Is the hardest substance; is an efficient abrasive because it does not wear down or lose sharpness as easily as other abrasives.
      3. Diamond chips of various sizes are bonded to metal shanks (i.e., to create diamond burs).
   B. Carbides
      1. Include silicon carbide, boron carbide, and tungsten carbide.
      2. Silicon and boron for finishing instruments typically are supplied as particles pressed with a binder into disks or wheels for use on a handpiece. They also are attached to steel shanks as burs or stones (i.e., green stones).
   C. Aluminum oxide
      1. Typically is produced as particles bonded to paper disks and strips or impregnated into rubber wheels and points.
      2. Is the abrasive used for white stones.
      3. Has fine particles of aluminum oxide and diamond that can be mixed into a paste to produce smooth, polished surfaces on many types of restorations, including acrylics and composites.
   D. Zirconium silicate
      1. Is a natural mineral.
      2. Is used as a polishing agent in strips and disks.

3. Often is used in prophylactic pastes.
E. Cuttle
1. Is a fine particle form of quartz or sand.
2. Particles are attached to paper disks for use.
3. In the form of beige-colored disks, is used in handpieces to finish gold alloys, acrylics, and composites.
F. Tin oxide
1. Is used as a polishing agent for metallic restorations, especially amalgams.
2. Produces excellent polish of enamel.
G. Pumice
1. Is a natural glass that is rich in silica.
2. Polishes acrylics and enamel.
H. Rouge
1. Is iron oxide.
2. Is a powder that can be formed into a block or cake and used on a rag wheel in a dental lathe/handpiece to polish gold alloys.
IV. Finishing and Polishing Composites
A. Finishing composites
1. Indications include:
a. Surface roughness.
b. Surface discoloration.
c. Flash or overhang.
d. Over-filled restorations.
2. Contraindications include:
a. Open margins.
b. Fractured restorations.
c. Under-contoured proximal contacts.
d. Large overhangs.
e. Recurrent caries.
3. The use of a plastic matrix strip before polymerization minimizes the amount of finishing required to produce a smooth, regularly contoured surface.
4. During initial contouring, water is used to avoid heat build-up and damage to the surface of the restoration; final finishing can be performed dry to facilitate the operator's view of margins.
5. Initial contouring is performed with either a carbide bur (12 flutes) or diamond bur (medium-fine) in a high-speed handpiece, using light pressure to avoid over-contouring.
6. May need further finishing with sandpaper disks, using either a slow or high-speed handpiece.
B. Polishing
1. Involves the use of abrasive sandpaper disks in descending order (coarse to fine); an alternative technique uses rubber points (containing abrasives) on a slow-speed handpiece.
2. Is accomplished with aluminum oxide or diamond pastes that contain particles as small as 1 μm in diameter to create smooth, reflective surfaces.
V. Finishing and Polishing Amalgam
A. Indications include:

1. Newly placed restorations.
2. Irregular margins; flash, creep, and minor ditching.
3. Over-contoured restorations.
4. Poorly defined anatomy.
5. Surface irregularities; pits, scratches, tarnish, and corrosion.
B. Contraindications include:
1. Fractured amalgams.
2. Open margins (deep ditching).
3. Flat proximal contour.
4. Open contacts.
5. Recurrent caries.
6. Large, broad overhangs.
C. Finishing should be performed 24 to 48 hours after placement because of the slow setting of amalgam.
1. A large round finishing bur is used to define gross anatomical features.
2. Green finishing stone removes gross surface irregularities from old restorations.
3. White finishing stone is used to further refine the anatomy of older amalgams.
4. A small round bur is used to define occlusal anatomy; must be followed with a large round bur to smooth out scratches from the small bur.
5. A flame-shaped bur is used on interproximal and gingival margins; burs and stones always move from the restoration to the tooth. Sandpaper disks are helpful for smoothing (coarse to fine).
D. Polish is performed with rubber points impregnated with abrasive particles; interproximal strips are available for polishing interproximal areas.
1. An alternative method of polishing involves the use of pumice slurry, followed by a slurry of tin oxide.

Indirect Restoratives

Many dental procedures require that the restoration be fabricated outside of the mouth and that a cementing media be used for attachment of the restoration to the appropriate oral structures. Inlays, onlays, veneers, crowns, and bridges are indirect restoratives that must be cemented to the teeth.
I. Restorations
A. Inlay restoration is used when the portion of the tooth that must be replaced is within the cusps.
B. Onlay restoration is used when one or more cusps are included but the entire crown of the tooth is not being replaced.
C. Veneer restoration is a cosmetic facing that is bonded to the facial surface of an anterior tooth to improve appearance; porcelain veneers have superior resistance to wear and staining.
D. Crown restorations include two types:
1. Jacket crown—is constructed of all nonmetal components.

	Gold (% Au)	Copper (% Cu)	Silver (% Ag)	Palladium (% Pd)	Uses
TABLE 10.8 ADA Gold Alloy Composition and Use					
Type I (soft)	83	6	10	0.5	Small inlays
Type II (medium)	77	7	14	1.0	Inlays/onlays
Type III (hard)	75	9	11	3.5	Crowns and bridges
Type IV (extra hard)	70	10	11	3.5	Partial dentures

a. Primary limitation is low strength; is brittle and cannot withstand posterior occlusal stresses without breaking.
2. Porcelain-fused-to-metal crown—consists of an outer layer of porcelain bonded to inner alloy casting.
a. An advantage of this type of crown is greater strength.

II. Materials
   A. Gold and alloys (Table 10–8)
      1. Are metals used for inlays and onlays because of their strength and durability.
      2. Type-I and type-II gold alloys are used predominately for inlays and onlays.
      3. Gold comprises the highest percentage of the alloy because of its resistance to corrosion and tarnish.
      4. Disadvantages of these metals include high material and production costs and a lack of esthetics.
   B. Ceramics
      1. Are strong and have been used successfully as inlay and onlay materials.
      2. Are hard but not as abrasive as porcelains; are kinder to the opposing dentition.
      3. Demonstrate superb esthetic results.
      4. The CAD/CAM (computer-assisted design, computer-assisted machining) technique is used to design and cut restorations such as inlays, onlays, and veneers at chairside.
         a. Is used because ceramics do not crack like other glasses and porcelains.
         b. Produces a final restoration that is designed, polished, and cemented in one appointment.
      5. Equipment is expensive; long-term studies are needed to evaluate the longevity of these restorations.
   C. Composites
      1. Two techniques are used for developing composite inlays.
         a. Indirect technique—requires two appointments: one to take an impression and make a die, and a second to cement the inlay onto the prepared tooth.
         b. Direct technique—the composite is placed and cured; the cured inlay is removed and given a secondary cure, using heat to maximize properties; subsequently is cemented onto the prepared tooth.
      2. Curing causes polymerization shrinkage.
         a. Both inlay techniques complete the curing process outside of the mouth, thus providing a better fit than typical composite restoration, in which curing accomplished in the oral cavity results in shrinkage while the composite is bonding to the cavity wall.
         b. Clinical studies suggest that marginal integrity is greater for inlays than for direct composites.
         c. Curing in a laboratory setting allows the use of high temperatures, which:
            1) Enhance the degree of cure.
            2) Enhance mechanical properties, resulting in a stronger restoration.
   D. Porcelain
      1. Has greater resistance to wear and staining (its primary advantage).
      2. Has the advantage of a natural appearance.
      3. Is strong during compression but weak when tensile stresses are applied.
      4. Can cause abrasion to opposing enamel, which must be considered when determining appropriate materials for restorations.

Clinical Case STUDY

Eighty-six-year-old Naomi Aimes is in the office for an examination. She has not seen a dentist for more than 3 years. She complains that her dentures do not fit well. She was sick this winter and lost 20 pounds but is slowly regaining her weight. Visual inspection reveals that her hard palate is very red. Her dentures have a heavy build-up of plaque and food debris. Ms. Aimes explains that she sleeps with her dentures in place and only takes them out after meals to clean them.

Clinical Case QUESTIONS

1. Considering this brief history, what is one possible etiology for Ms. Aimes' red hard palate? What recommendations would you have for this condition?
2. What recommendations should be made regarding the fit of Ms. Amies' dentures? Should her weight loss and gain be a significant factor in immediate recommendations?
3. What home care recommendations should the dental hygienist suggest for Ms. Aimes' dentures?

Clinical Case RATIONALES

1. Ms. Aimes could be suffering from denture stomatitis or denture sore mouth as a result of *Candida albicans*. Use of an antifungal agent is indicated to alleviate the fungal overgrowth. In addition, soaking the dentures nightly in a 10:1 water-to-bleach solution can eliminate fungus on the dentures and maintain a surface compatible with the health of the oral tissues. The patient should be instructed to rinse the dentures thoroughly before placing them in her mouth.
2. When denture fit has been compromised because of weight fluctuation, it is appropriate to recommend a denture adhesive to increase retention. Denture adhesives work by forming a viscous paste with the saliva; the viscosity of the paste between the denture and tissue result in better retention. Her weight loss and gain is a significant factor in immediate recommendations; a more permanent solution would be to add a professional denture liner, but because the patient is regaining her lost weight this should not be recommended.
3. Because Ms. Aimes has explained that she sleeps wearing her dentures, she should be instructed to remove her dentures nightly and soak them in a diluted bleach solution (as described in answer #1); other soaking solutions are commercially available but because she is suffering from fungal overgrowth, the use of diluted bleach is indicated. In addition, a denture brush and instructions on how to brush after each meal can be provided to avoid a heavy build-up of plaque and food debris. The patient should be instructed not to use abrasive dentifrices because they can easily scratch the acrylic plastic of the dentures. To avoid potential breakage, the patient should be instructed to brush her dentures over a sink filled with water or lined with a towel.

Dentures

For patients in whom some or all of the teeth have been removed, dentures are fabricated to provide an appliance that will facilitate the speaking and chewing processes.

Denture Types

   I. A full denture is the prosthetic device used when all of the natural teeth in an arch are lost.

   II. A removable partial denture is used when a number of teeth are missing; clasps are used to attach the partial denture to remaining teeth.

Denture Materials

Dentures must be made of materials that are kind to the soft tissues of the oral cavity, strong enough to withstand the forces of mastication, and yet are aesthetic in appearance.

   I. The denture base is the part of the denture that rests directly on the soft tissues; typically consists of acrylic resins and, most commonly, PMMA (polymethylmethacrylate).

   II. Teeth are made of acrylic resin or porcelain; porcelain teeth are more resistant to wear but are more brittle than those made of acrylic resin.

   III. Clasps (on removable dentures) are silver-colored metals; are primarily composed of nickel, cobalt, and chromium; are strong and highly resistant to corrosion.

Retention of a Denture

Properly fitting dentures do not require the use of adhesives for retention.

   I. Retention is determined by:
      A. The size of the area between the tissue and the denture.
      B. The surface tension of saliva between tissue and denture; patients who have thin, ropy saliva with low surface tension experience problems with retention.
      C. The ability of the saliva to wet the denture.

   II. Denture Adhesives
      A. Have helped to increase the confidence of denture wearers; may not be needed with well-fitting dentures.
      B. Result in viscous pastes when mixed with saliva. Viscous paste between the denture and tissue results in better retention of a poorly fitted denture.

Care of a Denture

Proper denture care is essential to maintaining the denture and the health of the oral cavity.

   I. Patient Care
      A. Dentures should be placed in liquid when they are taken out of the mouth for extended periods to prevent dehydration of the resin.
      B. The use of hot water is avoided because of the risk of distortion to the denture base.
      C. The denture should be brushed after each meal, or at least once daily.

D. A variety of cleansing and soaking agents can be used, including nonabrasive dentifrices, commercial denture cleansers, soap and water, and bleaches (Table 10–9).

E. Patients should be instructed not to use abrasive dentifrices because the acrylic plastic is soft and can be easily scratched and worn away.

F. A solution of 1 teaspoon of bleach and 2 teaspoons of powdered water softener (such as Calgon) in a glass of water is appropriate for occasional overnight cleansing. (This solution should not be used for dentures that contain metal because it corrodes metal components).

G. Metal clasps on a partial denture can be brushed with a denture brush that has a special tufted end for cleansing around the clasp.

H. To avoid potential breakage, the patient should brush the denture over a sink lined with a towel or filled with water.

I. Disclosing solution can be used to check the effectiveness of plaque removal and to provide further instruction as needed.

J. Denture stomatitis can result from the growth of *Candida albicans*. If this condition is present, use of an antifungal is indicated.

K. Alkaline hypochlorites (household bleach) are bactericidal and fungicidal, which makes them useful in treating denture stomatitis and disinfecting dentures.

L. The proper care of containers used for soaking appliances is essential to control the growth of microorganisms such as *Candida*; bleach serves as a good disinfectant for this purpose.

II. Professional Care

A. In-office cleansing involves placing the denture in a 10% bleach solution and vibrating it in an ultrasonic unit; a brush is used after sonication. Any remaining calculus on non-tissue-bearing surfaces is carefully scaled (stain removal solutions are available for ultrasonic use).

B. Plaque control should be stressed, especially for the patient who wears partial dentures, because of the potential for caries and gingival problems around abutment teeth.

TABLE 10.9	Major Ingredients of Commercial Denture Cleansers
Product	**Major Active Ingredients**
Efferdent tablets	Potassium monopersulfate
	Sodium borate perhydrate
Polident tablets	Potassium monopersulfate
	Sodium perborate monohydrate
	Proteolytic enzyme

Denture Liners and Conditioners

Denture liners and conditioners are available to improve the comfort and retention of dentures.

I. Liners and conditioners are used to cover tissue-bearing aspects of the denture to improve fit and comfort for patients who cannot tolerate hard dental acrylic on their mucosa.

II. Liners and conditioners are used for patients with thin alveolar ridges who lack supporting structures for dentures.

III. Materials for lining and conditioning include resilient substances such as acrylics, silicones, and polymers.

IV. The cleaning of liners can be accomplished with the same method that is used for acrylic dentures; however, liners must be cleaned carefully because of their softness and poor abrasion resistance.

V. Homemade liner use should be discouraged; such liners can degrade denture base material, leading to possible improper occlusion and subsequent damage to the oral structures that support the denture.

Preventive Dental Materials

These materials are designed to preserve the integrity of the natural dentition and protect the teeth and supporting tissues from disease or injury. They include dentifrices and other fluoride-releasing agents, pit and fissure sealants, mouth protectors, and fluoride trays.

Dentifrices

Dentifrices are substances used in conjunction with a toothbrush or other applicator to remove bacterial plaque, materia alba, and debris from the teeth and gingiva (Table 10–10).

I. Types

A. Fluoride dentifrices (for cavity protection)

1. Examples include Crest toothpaste, Colgate fluoride toothpaste, and Aqua-fresh fluoride toothpaste.

2. Are a source of fluoride for the tooth surface; control demineralization and promote remineralization.

3. Active ingredients include sodium fluoride (NaF, 0.24% or 1100 ppm) and sodium monofluorophosphate (Na_2PO_3F, 0.76% or 1000 ppm).

4. Should be used at least once daily; individuals at high risk for caries may use several times per day.

B. Tartar control dentifrices

1. Examples include Crest Tartar Protection and Colgate Tartar Control toothpastes.

2. Active ingredients include pyrophosphate (5% in Crest and 1.3% in Colgate) and zinc chloride (which has been used in other formulations to inhibit calculus formation).

TABLE 10.10 Basic Ingredients of Dentifrices

Component	Percentage (%)	Function	Examples
Detergent	1–2	Lowers surface tension, resulting in release of debris from tooth surface	Sodium lauryl sulfate USP, sodium n-lauryl sarcosinate
Cleaning and polishing agent	20–40	Contains an abrasive to clean and a polishing agent to produce a smooth, shiny tooth surface; resists discoloration and bacterial accumulation and retention	Calcium carbonate, calcium pyrophosphate, dicalcium phosphate, dicalcium dihydrate
Binder (thickener)	1–2	Prevents separation of solid and liquid ingredients during storage	Alginates; synthetic derivatives of cellulose
Humectant	20–40	Retains moisture and prevents hardening on exposure to air; stabilizes the preparation	Glycerin; sorbitol; propylene glycol
Flavoring	1–1.5	Makes the dentifrice desirable; masks other ingredients that may have a less pleasant flavor	Essential oils (e.g., peppermint, cinnamon, wintergreen, clove, menthol)
Therapeutic agents	1–2	Contain fluoride for caries protection; decrease root exposure sensitivity; control calculus; control gingivitis	Sodium fluoride, sodium monofluorophosphate; Potassium nitrate, sodium fluoride, strontium chloride; Pyrophosphate, zinc chloride; Stannous fluoride, triclosan, Gantrez copolymer, sodium fluoride
Preservatives, sweeteners, coloring agents	2–3	Preservatives prevent microbial growth in the binder; sweeteners increase patient acceptance; coloring agents increase attractiveness	Artificial noncariogenic sweeteners; vegetable dyes for coloring
Water	20–40	Creates gel/paste consistency	

3. Binds to crystals and prevents them from adhering to the tooth surface, thereby reducing the rate of crystal growth.

C. Gum care dentifrices
1. Examples include Crest Gum Care and Colgate Total.
2. Active ingredients are stannous fluoride (0.454%) in Crest, and triclosan (0.30%), Gantrez copolymer (2.0%), and NaF (0.243%) in Colgate.
3. Reduce gingivitis and bleeding associated with bacterial plaque.

D. Desensitizing dentifrices
1. Examples include Crest Sensitivity Protection, Denquel, and Sensodyne.
2. Active ingredients include potassium nitrate (0.5% KNO$_3$) and sodium fluoride (0.243% NaF) in Crest; potassium nitrate (0.5% KNO$_3$) in Denquel; and strontium chloride (10% SrCl$_2$) in Sensodyne-SC.
3. Reduce the sensitivity of exposed dentin and cementum by plugging/blocking the dentinal tubules, thereby preventing the transmission of sensation through the tubules.

Fluoride-Releasing Agents

Fluoride-releasing gels, varnishes, and dentifrices are agents used by dental professionals to protect the teeth from disease. (Tables 10–11 and 10–12).

I. Professional Topical Fluoride Gels
A. Types
1. Sodium (2% aqueous; pH 9.2)
a. Is the active ingredient in most fluoride oral rinses sold over the counter (OTC).
b. Requires a series of four appointments, 2 to 7 days apart, to provide maximum topical benefits.
c. Is a stable solution; easy to store.
2. Stannous (8% aqueous; pH 2.1 to 2.3)
a. Requires only one application.
b. Has unpleasant taste and can cause staining.
c. Is unstable; must be mixed for each application.

TABLE 10.11 Professional Fluoride Products

Product	Fluoride Concentration	Manufacturer
NUPRO neutral sodium fluoride solution	2.0% NaF gel	Dentsply
Thixo-Set topical gel	1.23% APF gel	Colgate
Oral-B minute-foam	1.23% foam	Oral-B

APF, Acidulated phosphate fluoride.

TABLE 10.12	FDA/ADA Accepted Fluoride Products			
Fluoride	**Office/Daily Use**	**Concentration (%)**	**Product Name**	**Manufacturer**
Acidulated phosphate fluoride	Office use (gel)	1.23	Gel II	Oral-B
	Office use (gel)	1.2	Luride	Colgate-Hoyt, Gel Kam, Division of Colgate-Palmolive
Sodium fluoride	Daily use (gel)	1.1	Thera-Flur Gel-Drops	Colgate-Hoyt
	Daily use (rinse)	0.05	Phos-Flur Supplement	Colgate-Hoyt
Stannous fluoride	Daily use (gel)	0.4	Gel-Kam	Colgate-Hoyt
	Daily use (gel)	0.4	Stop	Oral-B

From The Council on Dental Materials, Instruments, and Equipment and the Council on Dental Therapeutics: Clinical Products in Dentistry: A Desktop Reference. Chicago, American Dental Association, 1993.

3. Acidulated phosphate (1.23% sodium fluoride in 0.1 M orthophosphoric acid; pH 3.0)
   a. Gels for use at home contain 1.1% concentration.
   b. Requires only one application at each recall visit.
   c. Is contraindicated on composite and porcelain materials; causes pitting and roughening.
   B. Application time
   1. Four-minute application is required for maximum fluoride uptake into enamel.
   2. Patients are instructed not to eat, drink, rinse, or brush for 30 minutes after application.
II. Professional Topical Fluoride Foams
   A. Were introduced in 1993.
   B. Are available in 2% NaF and 1.23% APT formulations.
   C. Application time
   1. Four-minute application is required for maximum fluoride uptake into enamel.
   2. Patients are instructed not to eat, drink, rinse, or brush for 30 minutes after application.
III. Home Fluoride Rinses
   A. Daily application of a fluoride rinse is indicated for patients with:
   1. High risk for caries.
   2. Several areas of demineralization.
   3. Root exposures.
   4. Plaque-retentive appliances (e.g., orthodontic braces).
   B. Are available over the counter or by prescription.
   1. OTC rinses are 0.05% NaF (low-potency/high-frequency rinses).
   2. Prescription rinses
      a. Are 0.04% NaF and 0.04% APF (low-potency/high-frequency rinses).
      b. 0.2% NaF rinses (high-potency/low-frequency) are used weekly, most commonly for school fluoridation programs.

   c. Procedure for use of low-potency/high-frequency rinses
      1) Rinse daily with 1 teaspoon after brushing and before retiring.
      2) Swish between teeth for 60 seconds and expectorate.
C. Mechanisms of action
   1. Bacterial inhibition
      a. Rinses lower the metabolism of plaque bacteria.
      b. Also inhibit acid production in plaque.
   2. Decreased adherence
      a. Decrease adherence of materials (e.g., plaque) to fluoride-covered surfaces.
   3. Enamel/fluoride uptake
      a. In pre-eruption states, fluoride replaces some of the hydroxyl ions and forms fluorapatite; fluorapatite is less soluble and therefore more resistant to acids.
   4. Inhibition of demineralization and enhancement of remineralization
      a. Topical fluoride on teeth results in calcium fluoride, which precipitates to provide free fluoride ions. Fluoride acts as a catalyst for the precipitation of hydroxyapatite or fluorapatite and enhances the gain in mineral. This mineral is less soluble and stronger because of higher crystallization.
      b. Ions prevent demineralization by entering partially demineralized crystal to begin remineralization.
D. Toxicity
   1. The Certainly Lethal Dose (CLD) is an estimated dosage range that may cause death.
      a. For an adult, the CLD of NaF is 5 to 10 g taken at one time, or 32 to 64 mg/kg.
      b. For a child, the CLD is 0.5 to 1 g (varies with size and weight of child).
   2. Calculation of amount of fluoride ingested
      a. NaF—(4.5) × (no. mL swallowed) × (NaF concentration [e.g., 0.05%, 1.1%]) = mgF

b. SnF_2—(2.4) × (no. mL swallowed) × (SnF_2 concentration [e.g., 0.4%, 8%, 10%]) = mgF

c. APF—(10) × (no. mL swallowed) × (APF concentration [e.g., 1.23%]) = mgF

3. Signs and symptoms of acute toxicity

a. GI distress includes nausea, vomiting, diarrhea, abdominal pain, increased salivation, and thirst.

b. Systemic distress includes hypocalcemia, convulsions, and cardiovascular and respiratory depression.

c. Emergency treatment:

1) If less than 5 mg/kg is consumed, give calcium orally (milk) to relieve symptoms; observe for a few hours.

2) If more than 5 mg/kg is consumed, induce vomiting, give oral calcium, and admit to hospital for observation.

3) If more than 15 mg/kg is consumed, activate the emergency medical system.

IV. Fluoride Varnishes

A. Currently are available in Europe and Canada.

B. Some varnishes contain sodium fluoride (e.g., Duraphat).

C. Deliver fluoride to teeth in a controlled-release system; are superior to other delivery systems, in which fluoride is washed away by saliva and eating.

V. Fluoride Dentifrices

A. Are a source of fluoride for the tooth surface; control demineralization and promote remineralization.

B. Are part of a total fluoride regimen that includes in-office as well as daily fluoride application.

C. Should be used at least once daily; individuals at high risk for caries may use several times per day.

D. Include abrasives such as calcium pyrophosphate, dibasic calcium phosphate dihydrate, tricalcium phosphate, hydrated alumina, hydrated silica, and sodium metaphosphate.

E. Other ingredients in dentifrices include water, humectants such as glycerin (to keep the paste from drying out), a detergent such as sodium laurel sulfate (to help clean the teeth by improving the wetting on enamel), a binder such as carboxymethylcellulose (to keep the solid and liquid components of the paste from separating), coloring agents such as food dyes, and flavoring agents such as specific oils and extracts.

Pit and Fissure Sealants

Pit and fissure sealants are composed of organic polymers that bind to the enamel surface primarily by mechanical retention.

I. Purpose

A. Act as physical barriers to prevent oral bacteria and their nutrients from collecting within a pit and fissure (and subsequently creating the acid environment essential for the initiation of dental caries).

B. Are relatively ineffective in interproximal spaces and on smooth tooth surfaces.

II. Indications include:

A. Teeth with deep occlusal pits and fissures.

B. High rate of decay; teeth should be sealed as soon after eruption as possible.

C. Sound proximal surfaces.

D. Xerostomic conditions that may lead to decay.

III. Contraindications include:

A. Open occlusal lesions.

B. Caries on proximal surfaces.

C. Adult patient with a low caries/restoration rate.

D. Well-coalesced pits and fissures.

E. Patient behavior that does not allow for a dry field.

IV. Composition

A. Sealants contain the organic monomer Bis-GMA (a reaction product of bis-phenol A and glycidyl methacrylate).

B. For strength, may include a filler of inorganic material such as glass.

V. Polymerization

A. Is the adding together of many molecules to produce a larger molecule (polymer). Polymerization of pit and fissure sealants forms a highly cross-linked polymer network.

1. Autopolymer (chemical reaction)

a. Product is contained in two bottles:

1) Activator—Bis-GMA

2) Initiator—benzyl peroxide

b. Requires that equal drops of each liquid be mixed together; resin liquid hardens in 1.5 to 2 minutes.

2. Photopolymer (visible light-light cured)

a. Has one component system; does not require mixing.

b. The chemical initiator is not activated until it is illuminated by a light source.

c. Has unlimited working time, which reduces the chance of incorporating air into materials and causing air bubbles.

VI. Types

A. Unfilled types consist of the resin component of dental composites.

B. Filled types have inorganic glass filler particles added to reduce occlusal wear from chewing and to increase opacity for easier visualization.

C. Fluoride-releasing types help protect the tooth structure from caries.

VII. Application

A. Clean enamel surfaces with oil-free pumice/air abrasive polisher.

B. Isolate treatment area with:

1. Rubber dam.

2. Cotton roll holders.

C. Etch with phosphoric acid (approximatley 37%) for 30 to 60 seconds.
   1. The acid etch technique (with phosphoric acid) creates micropores in the enamel in which the sealant flows and mechanically locks in.
D. Rinse and dry.
   1. The most common cause of sealant failure is moisture contamination. It is critical that moisture control be employed with the use of rubber dam, cotton roll holders, moisture absorbent dry angles, and similar items.
E. If chemically reactive, mix parts.
F. Apply sealant.
G. If light-curing, illuminate according to directions.
H. Check sealant for complete coverage.
I. Check occlusion.

 ## Clinical Case STUDY

Thirteen-year-old Mike Nelson is in the office for an emergency. Last week, while playing football on his seventh grade team, he was tackled and suffered a head concussion. Visual examination reveals small incisive fractures on teeth #6 and #7. He has a permanent dentition and his twelve-year molars are partially erupted.

Clinical Case QUESTIONS

1. What preventive dental measures might have been recommended to Mike and his parents before Mike's football season? Give the rationale for these recommendations.
2. Because of a busy schedule, the dental hygienist left Mike's alginate impression unwrapped on the laboratory counter until the following day. What result will this have on the final study model?
3. Describe the basic steps for fabricating a custom-made mouth protector.

Clinical Case RATIONALES

1. The use of a mouthguard. Mandatory mouthguard and face mask regulations for high school and junior college football players were first enacted in 1962 by the National Alliance Football Rules Committee (NAFRC) because of the high facial and oral injury rate (50%). The National Collegiate Athletic Association (NCAA) followed suit by adopting a mouth protector rule in 1973. Although the use of mouthguards is mandated, compliance must be achieved for effectiveness. A mouthguard can protect the dentition from direct or indirect trauma. The dental hygienist should discuss not only the fabrication of a mouth protector, but also the consequences of noncompliance in wearing the guard during sporting activities (e.g., chipped and broken teeth, avulsed teeth). The dental hygienist should explain that a custom-made mouth protector is

designed by dental professionals to specifically fit an individual's teeth. As a result, the custom-made appliance feels more comfortable to the patient, reduces gagging, reduces irritation to the oral tissues, and decreases speech impairment. These advantages of the custom-made mouthguard (over the stock, store bought, or mouth-formed item) may contribute to compliance with use.

2. If alginate impressions are stored for more than 1 hour in air, they lose accuracy because of a process called syneresis, or loss of water by evaporation and exuding of fluid. The final study model in this case will be inaccurate.

3. First, an alginate impression of the maxillary arch is needed. Once a good impression is made, a study model is fabricated. The maxillary model subsequently must be trimmed and a thermoplastic sheet of material must be vacuum-formed over the model, trimmed, and finished by buffing the edges.

Content Review

Mouth Protectors/Fluoride Trays

Fluoride trays are designed to hold fluoride gels in close proximity to the teeth. Mouth protectors are designed to prevent head and mouth injuries during sporting events.

I. Fluoride Trays
   A. Are used for the application of fluoride for the patient who has received head and neck radiation with subsequent damage to the saliva glands; also are used for other xerostomic conditions or for patients at high risk for dental caries.
   B. Are formed to cover the entire clinical crown of the tooth.
   C. Are filled with neutral sodium fluoride and are worn for the duration of the high risk period; patients with permanent salivary dysfunction must wear them for life.

II. Mouth Protectors
   A. Are used by participants in sporting activities to protect the dentition from direct or indirect trauma.
      1. Fifty percent of sports injuries involve the oral cavity.
      2. The NCAA adopted a mouth protector rule in 1973.
   B. Types include:
      1. Stock
         a. Are made of rubber, polyvinyl chloride, or polyvinyl acetate-polyethylene copolymer.
         b. Are available at retail shops.
         c. Are manufactured in limited sizes (small, medium, large).
      2. Mouth-formed
         a. Have an outer, harder shell typically made of polyvinyl chloride, and an inner liner made

of acrylic gel, silicone rubber, or polyvinyl acetate.
   b. Are available at retail shops.
   c. Typically are heated and subsequently formed around the teeth.
3. Custom-made
   a. Are fabricated from a thermoplastic resin sheet, which is heated and vacuum processed onto a plaster model of the individual's teeth.
   b. Require four basic steps to fabricate: (1) taking an impression of the arch; (2) pouring the model; (3) forming the thermoplastic material over the model; and (4) trimming and finishing.
   c. Are fit by a dental professional.
   d. Are preferred because they reduce gagging, irritation of the oral tissues, and speech impairment.

Other Supportive Procedures and Techniques

The placement of periodontal dressings is important to the provision of periodontal therapy, particularly during surgical procedures. Today, many patients request teeth bleaching procedures, thus a knowledge of the proper methods and materials for such procedures is vital to the practicing dental professional. Placement of rubber dams and matrices are important supportive techniques that are useful in isolating a tooth or the dentition during restorative procedures. Another supportive technique, margination, is the removal of excessive amalgam in a restoration.

Periodontal Dressings

Periodontal dressings are placed to protect surgical areas and promote healing, thereby increasing postsurgical patient comfort.
I. Materials
   A. The two most widely used types of dressing materials are:
      1. Zinc oxide-eugenol
      2. Zinc oxide-noneugenol
II. Mixing and Application
   A. Lubricate the patient's lips to prevent the moist and sticky dressing material from adhering to the lips during placement.
   B. Mix together equal lengths of each component paste until they are well-blended and the color is homogenous; create two rolls that approximate the length of the surgical area.
   C. Using sterile gauze, gently dry the area to be covered.
   D. Control bleeding before placing the dressing by applying pressure to the area with a sterile gauze sponge until it subsides; if this does not work, hemostatic agents may be necessary.
   E. Place the roll of dressing material so that it wraps around the most distal tooth in the surgical area.
   F. Adapt the dressing to the area by pressing it gently against the wound site and flattening it against the teeth and soft tissues.
   G. The dressing should extend over the entire surgical site, to the most anterior tooth involved.
   H. Apply a roll of surgical material to the opposite side of the surgical area; adapt the material to the teeth and gingiva using a finger wrapped with damp gauze.
   I. Gently compress and flatten the dressing against the teeth and gingiva, adapting the dressing into the interproximal areas using the back of a curette or a cotton plier.
   J. The dressing should be adapted far enough into the interproximal areas that the facial and lingual surfaces of the dressing are joined together to form a mechanical lock between the dressing and the teeth.
   K. Curettes can be used to trim excess dressing carefully from the soft tissues so that interferences are eliminated (i.e., muscle attachments).
   L. The finished dressing should extend no further occlusally than the middle third of the teeth and should not interfere with normal occlusion.
III. Patient Instructions
   A. The patient should be asked to avoid eating, drinking, or rinsing for the first hour after placement to allow the dressing to harden.
   B. Tart or spicy foods should be avoided immediately after surgery.
   C. The dressing should be brushed only with a soft-bristled brush.
IV. Removing the Periodontal Dressing
   A. Gently loosen the dressing from the soft tissues with a pair of cotton pliers and a curette. Lift away from the wound site.
   B. Rinse the area gently with sterile saline to cleanse it of surface debris.
   C. If the dressing was placed over sutures, the suture material may be incorporated into the hardened dressing material. Special care in removal is required:
      1. Remove the lingual portion of the dressing first because sutures typically are knotted on the facial surface of the wound site.
      2. Sutures are cut from the exposed lingual surface; subsequently the suture materials and knots can be removed along with the facial aspect of the dressing.
      3. Cleanse the area and evaluate the tissue.

Bleaching

Tooth bleaching often is the primary treatment for lightening vital teeth stained by fluorosis, tetracycline, and acquired superficial discolorations.
I. In-Office Vital Bleaching
   A. Requires 30% to 35% hydrogen peroxide.

B. Different techniques involve the use of heat, light, gels, and microabrasion.
   1. Heat and light systems use a powerful bleaching light or wand that is calibrated to control bleaching temperatures.
   2. The gel technique is a more conservative chairside approach in which gel is placed on enamel in a 2-mm thick layer for 20 to 30 minutes; can be performed faster if combined with the use of a composite curing light or bleaching unit for 10 minutes.
   3. Microabrasive compounds remove discolored enamel when they are applied using a slow-speed handpiece with a special mandrel.
II. In-Home Vital Bleaching
   A. Generally is performed with a 10% carbamide peroxide solution, which is equivalent to a 3% hydrogen peroxide solution.
   B. Preoperative photographs and tooth shades are recorded.
   C. An alginate impression is made and vacuum-formed mouth tray(s) is (are) fabricated to hold the bleaching gel against the teeth.
   D. The patient is instructed to place bleaching gel on the teeth for 6 to 8 hours per day.
   E. The patient is instructed to report any tissue or tooth sensitivity (critical).
   F. The patient must be seen postoperatively to document changes in tooth shade.
   G. Retreatment may be necessary, depending on the patient's habits (e.g., tobacco, coffee, or tea use). The patient should be informed of this before the initial treatment.

Rubber Dams

Rubber dams are sheets of rubber material that attach to clamps, which are clamped onto teeth for retention in the working area.
I. Indications
   A. Are used to isolate clinical crowns of teeth for restorative procedures.
   B. Retract and control the soft tissues, including lips, cheeks, tongue, and provide limited gingival retraction.
   C. Prevent moisture contamination of the teeth.
   D. Provide optimum visibility of the operative site.
   E. Protect the patient against swallowing or aspirating dental instruments and restorative materials.
   F. Prevent the patient from choking on excess water spray.
   G. Decrease operator contact with saliva and blood, which could be infectious.
   H. Decrease aerosol in the treatment area.
II. Contraindications
   A. Patients with severe breathing or psychological problems.

B. Partially erupted teeth (clamp will not fit).
C. Patients with behavioral problems (i.e., small children).

Matrices

Matrices are materials used in the restoration of teeth to replace missing components of teeth. Matrices allow dental materials to be formed into the shape of the original component or portion of the tooth.
I. Anterior Composite Restorations
   A. Plastic strips (i.e., Mylar strips) are used to place anterior composites; must be clear to allow the transmission of light when polymerizing composite material.
   B. Place the composite first; subsequently place matrix and polymerize. Serves two purposes:
      1. Oxygen inhibits polymerization; covering with plastic, nonporous matrix keeps oxygen out and allows for maximum hardness.
      2. Provides smooth, regularly contoured surface, thus decreasing time required for finishing restoration.
II. Amalgam Restorations
   A. Metal matrix bands are used for amalgam restorations that involve the walls of a tooth.
   B. Matrix bands aid in restoring the natural contours so that the tooth may continue to function properly and maintain adjacent gingival health.

Margination

Margination is the process of removing excess restorative material to establish a smooth margin, to smooth the surfaces of the restorative material, and to recontour functional tooth anatomy.
I. Consequence of Overhanging Margins
   A. Retention of plaque
      1. Can result in recurrent caries.
      2. Can cause periodontal problems such as gingival bleeding and bone loss.
II. Manual Techniques
   A. Amalgam knives are used with short, overlapping, shaving strokes to remove amalgam in small increments and to prevent fracture of the margin.
   B. Files include coarse files for removing the bulk of the amalgam and fine files for smoothing the margins.
   C. Finishing strips are used after gross amalgam has been removed by an amalgam knife/file.
III. Power-Driven Techniques
   A. Finishing burs and stones must be kept in constant motion with light, sweeping movement to decrease the possibility of leaving marks and grooves.
   B. Discs have different abrasivities, which are used according to objectives. Short, overlapping strokes are used diagonally across cavosurface margins;

the disk is rotated from tooth to amalgam to avoid ditching restoration.

C. Ultrasonics effectively remove overhangs; some models have special tips for removal (e.g., reciprocating Profin).

CONTENT REVIEW QUESTIONS

1. The proportional limit of a material is the stress:
   A. beyond which elasticity first begins to occur
   B. at which strain hardening ceases to occur
   C. beyond which plastic deformation begins to occur
   D. at which fracture occurs
2. The amount of deformation or change in the length of a dental material is called:
   A. stress
   B. yield point
   C. strain
   D. galvanism
3. The modulus of elasticity is the measure of a material's _____:
   A. hardness
   B. stiffness
   C. percentage of elongation
   D. ductility
4. The hardness of a material is defined as the resistance of its surface to:
   A. elastic deformation
   B. strain
   C. scratching
   D. indentation
5. Adhesion is defined as the:
   A. type of bonding that does not require intimate attraction between the atoms/molecules of two substances
   B. reaction with which an object resists an external force
   C. attraction between like atoms/molecules on two different surfaces as they are brought into contact
   D. attraction between unlike atoms/molecules within a given material
6. Van der Waals forces refer to which type of bond?
   A. cohesion
   B. primary
   C. secondary
   D. chemical
7. Before adhesion can occur between a liquid and a solid, it is essential that the solid surface:
   A. provide some mechanical interlocking with the liquid
   B. be wetted by the liquid
   C. exhibit a large contact angle with the liquid
   D. enter into some form of chemical reaction with the liquid
8. Which of the following materials is considered an elastic impression material?
   A. ZOE impression paste

   B. reversible hydrocolloid
   C. impression plaster
   D. tray compound
9. The clinician can reduce the potential for permanent deformation when removing an alginate impression from the mouth by:
   A. removing the impression slowly and carefully
   B. removing the impression before it is fully set
   C. having the patient assist in the removal
   D. removing the impression with a quick snap
10. Manufacturers include calcium sulfate as a component of alginate impression material because:
    A. it reacts with potassium alginate to create gelation
    B. it serves as a filler
    C. it acts as a retarder
    D. it accelerates the setting of gypsum
11. Which of the following statements is TRUE?
    A. Agar impression material is composed primarily of diatomaceous earth.
    B. Agar impression material is changed into a gel by a physical reaction.
    C. Agar impression material is changed into a gel by a chemical reaction.
    D. Agar impression material is also known as irreversible hydrocolloid.
12. A disadvantage of polysulfide rubber impression material is:
    A. lacks accuracy in recording detail
    B. has a poor shelf life
    C. lacks compatibility with model plaster and stone
    D. has a strong odor and stains clothing
13. Which of the following is NOT true for polyether rubber impression material?
    A. has the longest working time of any of the rubber impression materials
    B. is the stiffest of any of the rubber impression materials
    C. can cause tissue irritation because of the aromatic sulfonic acid ester catalyst
    D. has great flexibility, which may result in problems when it is removed from the mouth
14. The chemical composition of both plaster and dental stone is:
    A. calcium sulfate dihydrate ($2CaSO_4 \cdot 2H_2O$)
    B. potassium sulfate
    C. calcium sulfate hemihydrate [$(CaSO_4)_2 \cdot \frac{1}{2}H_2O$]
    D. potassium alginate
15. Increasing the water/powder ratio of any of the gypsum materials results in:
    A. decreased setting time
    B. a stronger cast/die
    C. increased setting expansion
    D. increased setting time
16. Plaster requires more water for mixing than stone because:
    A. the hemihydrate crystals are more porous and irregularly shaped

B. its particles are formed by heating gypsum under steam pressure

C. it has the least porous hemihydrate particles of all of the gypsum materials

D. the hemihydrate crystals are more regular in shape and have a smoother surface

17. A high strength dental stone that is used as die material for the fabrication of inlays, crowns, and other castings is:
   A. type-I gypsum
   B. type-II gypsum
   C. type-III gypsum
   D. type-IV gypsum

18. Which of the following could lead to the corrosion of restorative materials?
   A. adjacent restorations constructed of similar metals
   B. an amalgam in close contact with a ceramic restoration
   C. adjacent restorations constructed of dissimilar metals
   D. close contact of a gold onlay and a gold crown

19. Which of the following restorative materials has a thermal expansion closest to that of tooth structure?
   A. acrylic resin
   B. amalgam
   C. gold
   D. composite resin

20. The organic resin matrix used in composite restoration is composed of:
   A. polymethyl methacrylate (PMM)
   B. vinyl silane
   C. polystyrene
   D. bisphenol A-glycidyl methacrylate (BIS-GMA)

21. Current clinical recommendations for composite materials are:
   A. class-III and class-IV restorations
   B. large class-I restorations
   C. class-II restorations
   D. class-V restorations

22. Polymerization shrinkage, the most serious problem associated with dental composites, leads to:
   A. pitting of the composite surface
   B. marginal leakage
   C. wear of the composite
   D. water sorption

23. For dentin adhesives, acid etching is accomplished with:
   A. 30% phosphoric acid
   B. 40% maleic acid
   C. 10% phosphoric acid
   D. 37% EDTA

24. The higher content of which metal increases amalgam strength and superiority?
   A. zinc
   B. silver

C. tin
D. copper

25. For a cavity preparation in which there has been a near pulp exposure, which of the following materials would be used?
   A. polycarboxylate
   B. zinc phosphate
   C. glass ionomer
   D. calcium hydroxide

26. Which of the following is TRUE about the use of zinc phosphate cements?
   A. the powder is added to the liquid all at once
   B. moisture on the slab will accelerate the setting time
   C. the cement is mixed over a small area of the slab
   D. cooling the mixing slab decreases the setting time

27. In a clinical situation in which a patient requires a deep cavity preparation and an amalgam restoration must be placed, which of the following would be the BEST choice for a base?
   A. zinc oxide-eugenol
   B. glass ionomer
   C. polycarboxylate
   D. cavity varnish

28. When a dental cement is mixed for use as a base, which of following is TRUE?
   A. the final mix should be thin and creamy
   B. a low powder-to-liquid ratio should be employed
   C. it will have a slow setting time
   D. a high powder-to-liquid ratio should be employed

29. Which of the following cements actually bonds to tooth structure?
   A. zinc phosphate cement (Flecks)
   B. glass ionomer cement (Ketac-Cem)
   C. calcium hydroxide (Dycal)
   D. polycarboxylate cements (Durelon)

30. The finishing and polishing of amalgams is indicated for which circumstances?
   A. open contacts
   B. fractured amalgams
   C. open margins between tooth and amalgam
   D. surface irregularities

31. The polishing of a newly placed amalgam generally should be performed:
   A. immediately after placement
   B. 24 to 48 hours after placement
   C. 12 hours after placement
   D. 1 month after placement

32. Which of the following is a polishing abrasive?
   A. tin oxide
   B. sand
   C. diamond
   D. alumina

33. A restoration that is used when one or more cusps of a tooth are in need of replacement but a full crown is not indicated is a(n):

A. veneer
B. inlay
C. jacket
D. onlay

34. Which of the following is a disadvantage of using gold for restorative procedures?
    A. lack of esthetic qualities
    B. susceptibility to corrosion and tarnish
    C. poor biocompatibility with oral tissues
    D. high strength and durability

35. Which of the following statements is TRUE regarding the use of porcelain in indirect restorations?
    A. porcelain does not create a natural appearance for the restoration
    B. porcelain can cause abrasion to opposing teeth
    C. porcelain is weak in compression
    D. porcelain stains easily

36. Patients who wear dentures should be instructed to:
    A. use an abrasive dentifrice to remove debris
    B. soak their dentures in full-strength household bleach
    C. use hot water to cleanse their dentures
    D. keep their dentures in water when not in the mouth

37. What is the major etiologic factor of denture stomatitis?
    A. *S. mutans*
    B. papillomavirus
    C. *S. salivarius*
    D. *Candida albicans*

38. The acid etching technique used for the placement of pit and fissure sealants involves:
    A. 10% to 20% boric acid
    B. 30% to 50% phosphoric acid
    C. 40% to 50% maleic acid
    D. 10% to 20% phosphoric acid

39. Retention of pit and fissure sealants is the result of:
    A. chemical bonding to enamel
    B. mechanical retention
    C. adhesion
    D. secondary bonding

40. Pit and fissure sealants are MOST effective in preventing caries:
    A. on occlusal surfaces
    B. on interproximal surfaces
    C. in lingual cingulum
    D. in buccal pits of molars

41. Pit and fissure sealants are indicated for which of the following conditions?
    A. a tooth in which a faulty restoration is present
    B. a tooth in which interproximal caries are present
    C. a tooth that has shallow occlusal pits and fissures
    D. a tooth that has deep occlusal pits and fissures

42. Which fluoride is the active ingredient in MOST over-the-counter fluoride rinses?
    A. stannous fluoride
    B. acidulated phosphate fluoride
    C. hydrogen fluoride
    D. sodium fluoride

43. Which fluoride is contraindicated for use on composite and porcelain restorations?
    A. sodium fluoride
    B. hydrogen fluoride
    C. acidulated phosphate fluoride
    D. stannous fluoride

44. Which of the following is FALSE regarding fluoride varnishes?
    A. they are not washed away by saliva or food
    B. application of varnish requires less cooperation from the patient
    C. sodium fluoride is one of the frequently used fluorides
    D. application of varnish requires more cooperation from the patient

45. Which of the following is NOT true regarding fluoride?
    A. promotes demineralization of the enamel
    B. inhibits acid production in plaque
    C. prevents demineralization of the enamel
    D. decreases adherence of plaque

46. What symptoms might a child exhibit if he or she ingested a toxic dose of fluoride?
    A. caustic burns on mouth and throat
    B. nausea, vomiting, diarrhea, increased salivation, and thirst
    C. sloughing of oral mucosa
    D. syncope

47. Which of the following statements is TRUE?
    A. 50% of sports injuries involve the oral cavity
    B. 10% of sports injuries involve the oral cavity
    C. 90% of sports injuries involve the oral cavity
    D. 5% of sports injuries involve the oral cavity

48. Which of the following is NOT true regarding overhanging margins of restorations?
    A. can result in gingival bleeding, increased pocket depth, and bone loss
    B. may be a cause of periodontal disease
    C. may have a minimal effect on loss of attached gingiva
    D. may result in recurrent caries

49. The material from which custom-made mouthguards are made is thermoplastic, which means that it:
    A. fractures under stress
    B. involves a physical change when converting from a soft to a hard material
    C. involves a chemical change when converting from a soft to a hard material
    D. rebounds to original shape after being deformed

50. Which of the following is a contraindication for the use of a rubber dam?
    A. a patient with severe breathing or psychological problems
    B. prevention of moisture contamination
    C. decreased operator contact with saliva and blood
    D. decreased aerosol in the treatment area

REVIEW QUESTION RATIONALES

1. **C** The proportional limit is the point on the stress/strain diagram at which stress and strain are directly proportionate to one another. If the stress is removed at this point, strain recovers and there is no deformation. Permanent deformation occurs above the proportional limit, when stress and strain are no longer in proportion to one another and the stress is greater than the material can withstand.

2. **B** Strain is defined as the deformation or change in the length/dimension of a dental material that results from applied stress. The stiffness of an object determines its ability to resist dimensional change or strain.

3. **B** The modulus of elasticity is a measure of a material's stiffness. Stiffness is an important issue when selecting restorative materials because large deflections are undesirable under conditions such as biting forces. When materials must withstand the forces of mastication it is preferable that they have a high modulus of elasticity.

4. **D** Hardness is a material's resistance to indentation. The hardness of dental materials is most commonly reported in Knoop hardness numbers. The Knoop hardness test uses a diamond indenter and calculations to create a hardness number. The larger the indentation, the smaller the hardness number. Enamel and porcelain are two of the hardest materials and therefore have two of the highest numbers.

5. **C** Adhesion is the force of attraction between the molecules or atoms on two different surfaces as they are brought into contact with one another. For instance, when an orthodontic bracket is cemented to a tooth it is adhesion between the cement and the tooth surface that holds the bracket in place.

6. **C** Van der Waals forces refer to secondary bonds, which involve a physical attraction between the atoms and molecules of the adhesive and the adherend. A physical attraction does not provide as strong a bond as primary bonds in which a chemical union occurs. The most common type of adhesion involves secondary bonding, which occurs with the use of zinc phosphate cement. Use of this cement does not involve a chemical union between the cement and the tooth.

7. **B** For chemical or physical adhesion to occur, it is essential that the adhesive and adherend be in intimate contact. Therefore, the adhesive typically is a liquid that can easily flow over the entire surface and come in contact with all of the small roughnesses on that surface. The adhesive is said to "wet" the adherend.

8. **B** Impression materials can be classified as either elastic or inelastic. Reversible hydrocolloid (agar) is an elastic material with sufficient flexibility to allow removal from undercuts without permanent deformation.

9. **D** Removing elastomeric impression materials with a quick snap decreases the stress placed on the impression. Reduction of stress results in the decreased likelihood of permanent deformation.

10. **A** Calcium sulfate reacts with potassium alginate to initiate the gelation of alginate impression material. Alginate is placed in the mouth in a liquid state and through a chemical reaction is changed into a gel. This property allows the material to flow around the oral structures when initially placed in the mouth and to harden into a gel for easy removal without deformation.

11. **B** Agar impression material is changed into a gel by a physical reaction that involves water-cooled impression trays. The agar gel is converted to a sol when heated in water (212°F), and becomes a gel when cooled to 110°F. For this reason, agar impression material is also known as reversible hydrocolloid.

12. **D** Polysulfide was the first rubber impression material developed. Although polysulfide has many useful properties, such as accuracy of detail, lead dioxide in the catalyst gives off a strong odor and causes permanent staining of clothing.

13. **D** Polyether impression materials are stiffer than polysulfides or silicones. This stiffness can present problems in removing an impression from undercuts. One way to compensate for this property is to increase the thickness of the material between the impression area and the tray.

14. **C** The chemical composition of both plaster and dental stone is calcium sulfate hemihydrate. Gypsum, the rock from which plaster and stone are formed, occurs widely as calcium sulfate dihydrate. In the manufacturing process, water is driven off to form calcium sulfate hemihydrate. Plaster is made by heating the gypsum at atmospheric pressure; the use of steam pressure results in dental stone.

15. **D** Increasing the water/powder ratio of gypsum materials produces a thinner mix that takes longer to set. Subsequently, a thinner mix results in a weaker cast/die.

16. **A** The more porous and irregularly shaped the hemihydrate crystals, the more water they require for mixing. Plaster is the most porous and irregularly shaped of all of the gypsums. Dental stone is less porous than plaster and has more regularly shaped particles. High-strength dental stone particles are nonporous, dense, and smooth.

17. **D** Gypsum products are classified into five types—two are plaster and three are stone. Type-IV die stone is high-strength, high-hardness, and low-expansion stone that is used as a die material on which wax patterns of inlays, crowns, and other castings are produced. The higher strength is a result of the lower water/powder ratio.

18. **C** Corrosion is the result of a chemical or electrochemical reaction. An electrical current is created by the close proximity of dissimilar metals, which results

in a dissolution of the metals. Dissolution of the metals causes roughness and pitting of the restoration.

19. **C** The thermal expansion of tooth structure is 11.4 and the thermal expansion of gold is 15 ($\times 10^{-6}$/°C). The thermal expansion of restorative materials often does not match that of the tooth. For example, the thermal expansion of composite resin is approximately 35. This differential expansion becomes problematic in dentistry because it results in a leakage of oral fluids between the tooth and restoration, which can lead to decay and discomfort.

20. **D** BIS-GMA is a liquid resin to which the inorganic component, such as silicate or glass particles, is added, subsequently forming a paste or composite material.

21. **A** Clinical trials have shown a high success rate for composite use in anterior teeth. The restoration of class-V lesions has been more problematic because of the need to bond to dentin. Current dentin adhesives have demonstrated greater success than earlier adhesives, but glass ionomer continues to be the more successful restoration for class-V preparations. Additional benefits of glass ionomers are their fluoride-releasing properties.

22. **B** Stresses from polymerization shrinkage can exceed the bond strength and cause a pulling away of the material from the tooth structure, resulting in marginal leakage. Two clinical problems that result from leakage are secondary caries and staining or discoloration of the restoration.

23. **C** Generally speaking, a weaker solution of acid etch is used on dentin than that used for enamel because of the concern for pulpal damage.

24. **D** The tin-mercury compound that is formed when amalgam is mixed results in gamma-2, the weakest of the phases in the setting reaction process. Tin has a greater affinity for copper than mercury, thus the higher copper alloys form a copper-tin compound instead of the tin-mercury compound. This copper-tin compound is sufficient to suppress gamma-2 formation, resulting in a stronger restoration.

25. **D** Calcium hydroxide cement is used for both direct and indirect pulp capping and as a protective barrier beneath composite restorations. One of the unique properties of this cement is that it stimulates the formation of reparative dentin. The pH of the cement is basic.

26. **B** Any moisture on the slab or moisture from condensation results in accelerated setting times and adverse effects on the properties of the cement.

27. **A** Zinc oxide-eugenol cements, because of their neutral pH, have a sedative effect on the pulp. For this reason they are especially useful when deep cavity preparations might lead to post-treatment sensitivity.

28. **D** A high powder-to-liquid ratio is employed to produce a mix that has a thick, putty-like consistency that can be applied to the floor of the cavity preparation with an amalgam condenser. In addition, the high powder-to-liquid ratio results in a quicker settling time and a stronger product.

29. **D** One advantage of the polycarboxylate cements is their ability to chemically bond to tooth structure. The cement adheres through an ionic interaction between negatively charged molecules in the cement and positively charged atoms, such as calcium, in the tooth structure.

30. **D** Finishing and polishing is indicated when there are surface irregularities that might serve as plaque traps or cause irritation to the tissue because of the roughness of the surface. In instances of fractured amalgams, open margins, or open contacts a new amalgam restoration should be placed.

31. **B** Most amalgams are ready for polishing one day after placement. This time lag between placement and polishing allows the amalgam to finish hardening fully.

32. **A** Tin oxide (SnO_2) is a pure white powder that is used extensively as a final finishing/polishing agent for teeth and metallic restorations. The intent of polishing is to create a smooth surface on the restoration or appliance that does not contain scratches. Tin oxide is mixed with water, alcohol, or glycerin and used as a paste. Finishing abrasives are coarse, hard particles and polishing abrasives are fine particles.

33. **D** An onlay often is desirable when full coverage of the tooth by a crown is not necessary. Traditionally only metals were used as restorative materials in the production of onlays because of their high strength and durability. As the demand for esthetics has increased, dentistry has begun to use materials such as ceramics in the production of these restorations.

34. **A** Gold traditionally has been used in dentistry because of superior properties, including the ease with which it can be worked, its resistance to tarnish and corrosion, its ability to withstand the oral environment, and its strength. Demand for more esthetic dentistry has resulted in restorations in which porcelain is fused to metal to give the patient a more natural looking replacement restoration.

35. **B** Porcelains have a greater hardness than enamel, which presents a potential problem when they are placed in opposition to one another. Because porcelain can abrade enamel, it often is used only on buccal or facial surfaces.

36. **D** The acrylic material used in the fabrication of dentures can shrink if it is left in a dry environment. The resulting dimensional change is corrected when water is again absorbed by the denture; however, the dentures will feel tight when first replaced in the oral cavity.

37. **D** A major etiologic factor of denture stomatitis is poor oral hygiene, which results in the formation of mature plaque. Mature plaque contains microorganisms that cause tissue inflammation along with patho-

genic yeast microorganisms, primarily *Candida albicans.* This condition can be provoked or worsened by constant wearing of the denture. Candidiasis can be treated as a localized infection with an antifungal preparation such as clotrimazole and improved hygiene. It may be necessary to soak the denture in an antifungal solution.

38. **B** The etching process involves the use of a 30% to 50% phosphoric acid, which is applied to the pits and fissures to be sealed. The acid removes inorganic materials and creates tiny crevices or micropores into which the sealant material can flow, thus producing a mechanical bonding. Mechanical bonding is the force that holds the sealant to the enamel.

39. **B** Acid etching with phosphoric acid results in the formation of enamel tags, which allows the sealant to penetrate and mechanically bond to the tooth structure.

40. **A** The success of pit and fissure sealants is dependent upon a moisture-free environment when the sealant is applied and proper acid etching to allow for adequate retention. The occlusal surfaces of the teeth are most accessible to acid etching and therefore the effectiveness of sealants is greatest on these surfaces.

41. **D** Fluorides have been least effective at reducing decay on the occlusal surfaces of teeth. The susceptibility of occlusal pits and fissures to caries is directly related to the physical size and morphology of the individual teeth, which provide a shelter for microorganisms. Occlusal surfaces that contain shallow pits and grooves are not as susceptible as those that have very defined anatomy. A full preventive program should include the use of pit and fissure sealants for occlusal protection and fluoride for interproximal protection.

42. **D** Sodium fluoride is the fluoride most commonly used in OTC rinses. Sodium fluoride is a stable solution, which makes it ideal for this type of distribution.

43. **C** Acidulated phosphate fluoride has been shown to cause pitting and roughening of composite and porcelain materials. Therefore the use of sodium fluoride is indicated for patients with extensive restorative work that involves these materials. Stannous fluoride can cause staining and therefore is not recommended. In patients with only minimal restorative work, protective coatings such as petroleum jelly can be applied to the restorations and acidulated phosphate may be used.

44. **D** Fluoride varnishes currently are available in Canada and Europe. One of the major advantages of these varnishes is the fact that they do not require patient compliance with oral health care instructions. Semiannual applications have been used as an alternative for adopting the regimen of regular rinsing with fluoride.

45. **A** Fluoride is effective at preventing caries because of its ability to inhibit the acid production in plaque and decrease the adherence of materials to fluoride-covered surfaces. Fluoride replaces some of the hydroxyl ions in enamel with fluorapatite, which is less soluble and more resistant to acids. Fluoride ions act as a reservoir of fluoride during demineralization to promote the remineralization of enamel.

46. **B** The Certainly Lethal Dose of fluoride is the amount that is likely to cause death if ingested (when no counteragent therapy is applied). The adult dose is 5 to 10 g of NaF taken at one time, and the children's dose is 0.5 to 1 g (depending on the size and weight of the child). Signs and symptoms of acute toxicity include gastrointestinal distress (nausea, vomiting, diarrhea, abdominal pain, increased salivation, and thirst). Systemic distress includes hypocalcemia, CNS convulsions, and cardiovascular and respiratory distress. Emergency treatment includes induction of vomiting and ingestion of large volumes of fluoride-binding liquids such as lime water, milk, and antacids that contain aluminum or magnesium hydroxide. Activation of the emergency medical system is indicated for acute toxicity.

47. **A** Because of this high rate of oral injuries, the NCAA adopted a rule in 1973 instituting mandatory mouth protector use for athletes. The injuries most frequently observed are chipped, broken, or dislodged teeth and concussions resulting from blows to the chin. The NCAA rule was amended in 1990 to require colored mouth protectors. Color makes a mouthguard more visible to coaches and officials who assess compliance; color also makes the item easier to find if lost. Research has shown that athletes who wear mouthguards in college continue to wear them in professional sports.

48. **C** Overhanging margins on restorations result in the retention of plaque and bacteria, which can result in recurrent caries and periodontal problems.

49. **B** Materials that soften when heated and solidify when cooled, without a chemical change, are classified as thermoplastic substances. Examples of thermoplastic materials used in dentistry include impression compounds.

50. **A** The use of a rubber dam is contraindicated for patients with severe breathing or psychological problems, for patients who have behavior problems, and when teeth are only partially erupted and a clamp will not fit securely onto them.

Suggested Readings

Craig RC, O'Brien WJ, Powers JM: Dental Materials: Properties and Manipulation. 6th ed. St. Louis, Mosby, 1996.

Ferrancane JL: Materials in Dentistry: Principles and Applications. Philadelphia, Lippincott, 1995.

Phillips RW, Moore BK: Elements of Dental Materials for Dental Hygienists and Dental Assistants. 5th ed. Philadelphia, WB Sanders, 1994.

Chapter ELEVEN

Clinical Treatment: Planning, Prevention, and Care

Donna Stach, R.D.H., M.Ed. • Janis Keating, R.D.H., M.A. • Robin Applebee Beilby, R.D.H., M.A.

 Clinical Case **STUDY**

Stanley Luck, a 75-year-old man, has lived alone since his wife died 6 months ago. His general health is good. He had heart by-pass surgery 20 years ago and takes Captopril and Hydrochlorothiazide for high blood pressure. Stanley's blood pressure today was 130/86. Clinical and radiographic examinations noted the following: (1) tooth #30 has a swelling on the buccal mucosa, about 6 to 8 mm in diameter; the tooth has a large existing MOD amalgam; the radiograph demonstrates distal root caries, as well as a radiolucency located at the apex of the distal root, and (2) teeth #30 and #31 are in cross-bite with #2 and #3.

Clinical Case QUESTIONS

1. Does Mr. Luck need antibiotic premedication before oral prophylaxis?
2. How should the lesion around tooth #30 be palpated?
3. What are common oral side effects of Mr. Luck's medication? What recommendations can be made to help relieve these symptoms?
4. In describing Mr. Luck's cross-bite, how are the mandibular teeth positioned relative to the maxillary teeth?

Clinical Case RATIONALE

1. A patient with a history of heart by-pass surgery does not require any antibiotic premedication to protect him/her from subacute bacterial endocarditis (SBE). By-pass surgery does not involve the heart valve tissues, which when damaged are at risk for SBE.

2. Before palpating tooth #30 and the adjacent tissues, observe and note any pus or a white pimpled area that indicates a draining fistula. Use digital palpation with light pressure to examine the lesion for tenderness, draining fluid (pus), or any irregular tissue (i.e., hard, firm immovable mass). Bidigital compression and circular movements can also be used to palpate the submandibular area for indications of lymph node drainage and swelling.

3. Xerostomia is a likely problem for Stanley due to the two blood pressure medications he takes. Changes in saliva consistency, amount, and buffering capacity are often associated with aging adults and are most likely associated with medication use rather than physiological changes. Other problems created by xerostomia include increased risk of caries (especially root caries) and irritation or dryness of the mucous membrane that cause difficulties with speaking, taste, and nutrition. Recommending an increase in water consumption, use of artificial saliva, air humidification, water-based lubrication, and sucking on sugarless candies or chewing sugarless gum all help to increase saliva production or relieve mouth dryness. A brush-on or tray prescription-strength fluoride should be recommended at night just before bed with directions to expectorate the excess and not rinse the mouth. Many OTC fluoride rinses contain alcohol and may be contraindicated if the mucous membranes are sensitive as a result of the xerostomia.

4. The mandibular teeth #30 and #31 are buccal to the buccal cusps of the maxillary teeth #2 and #3. Normal occlusion would have #2 and #3 buccal to the mandibular buccal cusps of #30 and #31.

Content Review

The Dental Record

The dental record is a medicolegal document that should be complete, accurate, and legible. From the record it should be possible to recreate the patient's medical and dental history and oral status at their initial presentation along with periodic updates, their treatment needs, the treatment rendered and any recommendations made to the patient. At a minimum the dental record should include the following:

I. Demographic and Insurance Information
II. Assessment Data
   A. Medical history
   B. Dental history
      1. Significant past experiences
      2. Chief complaint
      3. Attitudes about dentistry and possible anxiety
      4. Plaque control and self-care practices
   C. Test results
   D. Abnormal findings from the extra- and intra-oral examination
   E. Dental and periodontal chart
   F. Radiographs and photographs
III. Diagnosis (treatment needs)
IV. Treatment Plan and Record of Informed Consent
V. Treatment
   A. Specific treatment provided by date
   B. Treatment outcomes
   C. Referrals
   D. Recommendations
   E. Future plans
VI. Correspondence
VII. Financial Record

Patient Assessment

Patient assessment is necessary to establish baseline information on the patient's general health, extraoral and intraoral examination, and dental and periodontal evaluations. Obtaining baseline information allows the patient treatment needs to be determined and a subsequent treatment plan developed.

Terminology

Descriptive terminology is used to document abnormal findings recorded in a patient's record

Bulla is a vesicle-like lesion greater than 1 cm in diameter.

Cyst is a fluid-filled, elevated, circumscribed encapsulated palpable lesion.

Corrugated is a rippled surface.

Discrete means separate, does not blend with other lesions.

Ecchymosis is a red-purple discoloration of variable size.

Erosion is a depressed, moist, glistening lesion following rupture of vesicle or bulla.

Fissure is a linear crack or break (angular cheilosis).

Fluctuant is a wave-like motion (mucocele, fluctuant blue swelling).

Herpetic lesion is a fluid-filled lesion that eventually ruptures and coalesces (can occur after dental treatment due to tissue manipulation, latent virus).

Hyperkeratotic is white to grayish in color, thick scaly surface, wrinkled (history of aspirin applied to area, cheek biting, or smokeless tobacco use).

Hyperplastic is an increase in number of cells, tissue overgrowth; possible side effect with Dilantin use.

Hypertrophic is an increase in cell size, causing tissue overgrowth.

Indurated is a hardened tissue area.

Koplik spots are white or blue spots surrounded by inflamed red area on buccal mucosa (commonly seen in German Measles).

Leukoplakia is a whitened, thickened area of the buccal mucosa that doesn't wipe off.

Macule is a flat, nonpalpable, circumscribed lesion, less than 1 cm (e.g. freckle, mole, rubella).

Nodule is a raised, elevated, circumscribed, 1–2 cm.

Papillomatous is a nipple-like growth.

Papule is a raised palpable, firm, circumscribed, less than 1 cm.

Pedunculated means attached to underlying tissue by a stem-like base.

Petechiae are red-purple spots, dot-like, less than .5 cm.

Purpura is a red-purple discoloration or area, greater than .5 cm.

Sessile means the base of lesion is flat; broad base.

Tumor is a solid mass.

Ulceration is the loss of epithelial surface, red border with yellow/gray center, painful (e.g. apthous ulcer, ANUG, traumatic injury).

Vesicle is a raised or elevated, circumscribed, superficial fluid filled lesion of less than 1 cm diameter.

Health History

The health history is useful in gathering information regarding the patient's medical and dental history, behavior, demographics, and vital signs.

I. Medical History
   A. A review of the patient's physical health status includes a statement of the patient's chief compliant, history of present and past illness, and pharmacologic history. The need for physician consultation and premedication must be assessed.
   B. Information obtained by:
      1. Questionnaire versus interview
         a. A questionnaire saves time, is consistent, and potentially more thorough. It has the disadvantage of being inflexible and lacks the opportunity for development of rapport with the patient (impersonal).
         b. The interview is flexible and personable, requires good communication skills, and enhances the relationship-building process be-

tween patient and clinician. It has the disadvantages of being time consuming and may cause the patient embarrassment.

   c. Combining the interview and questionnaire achieves practical results and thoroughness by allowing the clinician to get additional clarification and information on positive responses.

2. Subjective versus objective information

   a. Subjective information includes patient's and dental hygienist's impressions, feelings and attitudes.

     1) Subjective sign: information that the clinician can determine from observing the patient, e.g., flushed skin.

     2) Subjective symptom: information the patient reports about themselves, e.g., nausea.

   b. Objective information is concrete, notes hard facts, data, and test results.

C. Health status

1. Is a notation of patient's existing and previous conditions, including the chief complaint.

   a. Chief complaint is a statement in the patient's own words of why they are seeking dental care.

   b. History of present illness may influence treatment options and setting.

     1) Includes a description of current problem, signs, and symptoms.

     2) Onset, duration, intensity, and location, as well as medication therapies may influence or contraindicate certain dental procedures.

   c. History of past illness includes:

     1) Diseases that could complicate dental and dental hygiene treatment or might require special precautions or premedication before treatment.

     2) Allergic or untoward reactions to drugs.

     3) Diseases and drugs with oral manifestations.

     4) Communicable diseases.

     5) Physiologic state of the patient.

2. Includes common medical condition

   a. Hypertension

     1) Patients who present with elevated blood pressure and may also report symptoms of headache, dizziness or nose bleeds.

     2) Patients report taking antihypertensive and/or diuretic drugs.

     3) Can progress to arteriosclerosis, impaired kidney function, cardiac enlargement, and stroke.

   b. Heart disorders

     1) Valvular heart disease is a deformity of the heart valves due to infection or medication use; increases risk of bacterial endocarditis; requires antibiotic premedication before all invasive procedures.

      a) Rheumatic heart disease is often associated with a prior history of rheumatic fever or scarlet fever.

      b) Phen-fen–related valve disease; associated with the combination use of the diet drugs phentermine (Fastin) and fenfluramine (Pondimin) or the use of dexfenfluramine (Redux); approximately one third of users have valvular damage that puts them at risk of bacterial endocarditis; echocardiogram is recommended to determine damage.[1]

     2) Congenital heart defects

      a) Are structural defects of the heart resulting in a heart murmur.

      b) Patient may report valve replacement or a history of corrective heart surgery; patient is susceptible for bacterial endocarditis.

     3) Coronary artery disease

      a) Involves inadequate blood circulation to heart muscle; results from arteriosclerosis, blocking or narrowing of the blood vessels.

      b) Patient reports angina pectoris, which is caused by muscle pain that radiates to left arm and jaw.

      c) Patient experiences pain with exertion and anxiety; discomfort is relieved by rest and nitroglycerin (vasodilator).

      d) Request patient bring nitroglycerin to dental appointment; have readily available during treatment.

     4) Coronary thrombosis (myocardial infarction)

      a) Results from insufficient blood supply to the heart muscle as a result of atherosclerosis of the blood vessel walls.

      b) Patient may report heart attack and/or use of antianginals and/or antihypertensives.

     5) Congestive heart failure

      a) Occurs when the heart muscle is weak and is unable to pump blood at an adequate rate; blood circulation is poor, resulting in congestion and pooling of blood in the organs and lower extremities.

      b) Patients present with swollen ankles and shortness of breath.

      c) Patients may be taking digitalis and diuretics.

6) Cardiac dysrhythmias
   a) Are irregular heart beats (too slow or too fast).
   b) Patient may have a pacemaker and/or report taking digitalis or calcium channel blockers.
   c) Avoid use of ultrasonic or other dental equipment that may effect the pacemaker's electromagnetic operation.

c. Allergy
   1) Is a reaction to a substance that may be as mild as a skin rash or as severe as a fall in blood pressure and anaphylatic shock (airway obstruction from tissue swelling and/or cardiac arrest).
   2) Patient reports a reaction to known substance e.g. penicillin or sulfa drugs;
   3) Must determine the cause and severity of allergic response.
   4) Latex allergy, see Table 8–2 for details

d. Diabetes mellitus
   1) A disorder of glucose metabolism resulting from a relative or absolute lack of insulin; has a vascular component.
   2) Two types:
      a) Type I—insulin-dependent diabetes mellitus (IDDM); onset in youth; severe and unstable; stems from a lack of insulin produced from the pancreas.
      b) Type II—adult onset, noninsulin-dependent diabetes mellitus (NIDDM), often is not as severe as IDDM and is usually stable; develops slowly with age and is frequently associated with obesity; the pancreas produces adequate insulin but the diabetes is a result of insulin insensitivity of the tissue.
   3) Dental appointment should be scheduled after meal and insulin therapy; have a source of sugar accessible in case of insulin reaction, (juice, glucose or frosting).
   4) Is a risk factor for periodontal disease; more frequent maintenance appointments are required as well as excellent oral hygiene self-care

e. Kidney disease
   1) Renal function is impaired
   2) Patient is maintained by hemodialysis or a kidney transplant
   3) Patient experiences more frequent infections, poor healing and difficulties with bleeding
   4) Patients with surgical systemic shunts may require prophylactic antibiotics.
   5) Some medications remain in circulation longer due to poor kidney function.

f. Blood diseases
   1) Anemia is a deficiency of red blood cells that occurs as a result of vitamin or iron deficiency, bone marrow malfunction, excessive loss of blood or red cell destruction.
   2) Leukemia is a disease of white blood cells that do not function normally (cells are immature and excessive in number); thrombocytopenia may develop from chemotherapeutic treatment
      a) Patients are prone to infection, weakness, and easy bruising.
      b) Patients present with unexplained oral lesions, periodontal disease and xerostomia as a result of chemotherapy
   3) Hemophilia, an inherited disorder, causes excessive bleeding due to lack of one of the coagulation factors (factor VIII, IX, or XI). Von Willebrand's disease, the most common inherited bleeding disorder, results from an inability to utilize factor VIII.[2]
   4) Vitamin K deficiency also interferes with clotting.

g. Sexually transmitted diseases (STD)
   1) STDs, such as syphilis, gonorrhea, and chlamydia, are acquired through sexual intercourse and should be reported on the health history
   2) Note any oral or pharyngeal lesions.
   3) Postpone dental treatment until antibiotic therapy diminishes infection that may be transmitted to others.

h. Hepatitis A, B, or C
   1) Are inflammations of the liver due to viral infection; cause fatigue, nausea, tender joints, and jaundice.
   2) Have a high risk of disease transmission to the dental professional
   3) Dental office staff must follow universal precaution and strict aseptic and sterilization procedures at all times when treating all patients, as carrier status is frequently unknown.
   4) Dental office personnel should follow OSHA recommendations for hepatitis B vaccination prior to treating patients in any clinical setting (for additional information see Chapter 4).

i. Epilepsy
   1) Is a disturbance of electrical brain activity resulting in seizure (convulsions).
   2) Patient usually reports taking phenobarbital, phenytoin or other anticonvulsant medication.

3) Appointments should be made when the patient is rested; confirm medication compliance and keep appointments short; should a seizure occur, do not restrict movement; afterward, turn patient on his/her side and activate Emergency Medical System (EMS)

 Clinical Case **STUDY**

Bob Decker, a 27-year-old man with hemophilia, contracted the AIDS virus 15 years ago during a blood transfusion. Bob has minimal calculus and plaque with slight gingival inflammation.

Clinical Case QUESTIONS

1. What is hemophilia and what are its risks and treatment?
2. What additional information should be known before Bob is treated?
3. Is Bob's sister Rose likely to have hemophilia?
4. Are there any special treatment considerations because of Bob's hemophilia or HIV status?
5. Why were hemophiliacs at risk for AIDS prior to 1985?
6. What HIV symptoms may be discovered during the oral examination?

Clinical Case RATIONALE

1. Hemophilias are a group of disorders involving blood-clotting mechanisms. The diseases are genetic. Persons with these disorders do not produce either factor VIII (hemophilia A), factor IX (hemophilia B or Christmas disease), factor XI, or von Willebrand's factor (vWF). Treatment includes coagulation therapy.
2. Additional information prior to treatment would include the type and severity of the hemophilia, treatment regimen for control of hemophilia, medications, HIV status including CD4 cell counts (a lymphocyte subset cell count), presence of any AIDS-associated conditions (oral manifestations), and any medications to manage his HIV condition
3. Hemophilia A and B are rare in females; von Willebrand's disease does occur in both male and female individuals
4. Universal precautions are followed as they are for every patient. Light debridement and deplaquing is the only instrumentation needed in Bob's case because of minimal deposits and inflammation. Bob should be seen for preventive maintenance every 3 months because of his high-risk status. Excellent OH self-care and preventive therapy reduce his chances for oral infection and bleeding.

5. Prior to 1985, blood utilized for transfusions was not required to be tested for the HIV virus and many hemophiliacs contracted the virus.
6. A thorough intra and extra oral exam is critical for noting the progression of Bob's HIV status, since many early indicators of disease progression are exhibited in the mouth. Palpate for any lymphadenopathy and visually observe for any skin lesions, Kaposi's Sarcoma, purpura or herpes. Check for common oral manifestations of progressing AIDS virus such as candidiasis, Kaposi's Sarcoma, hairy leukoplakia, gingival inflammation (linear gingival erythema or necrotizing ulcerative gingivitis) or periodontal disease.

II. Pharmacologic History
   A. Provides information on medications that may impact oral health, dental treatment and oral hygiene self-care.
   B. Often requires utilization of a reference text, such as the Physicians Desk Reference (PDR), or consultation with a pharmacist for further information
      1. PDR lists all drugs by manufacturer's name, brand name, and generic name
      2. Information regarding drug action, usage, contraindications, adverse reactions, warnings, and precautions are reviewed.
   C. Includes a record of medication taken, noting dosage and the condition being treated; note if the drug has an impact on oral health and any contraindications for dental treatment.
      1. Common medication induced oral side effects
         a. Xerostomia
            1) Is the most common reaction to medication; over 300 medications cause xerostomia
            2) Results in thick and ropy saliva, alters taste, causes loss of buffering action and may cause burning tongue
            3) Increases incidence of root caries; causes difficulty with chewing, swallowing, and speaking
            4) Treatment involves relieving symptoms through increased water consumption, saliva substitutes, tissue lubricants, chewing sugar free gum, air humidification, and home fluoride applications to prevent root caries
         b. Candidiasis
            1) Is an overgrowth of a yeast organism, *Candida albicans*
            2) Is found in individuals with a history of prolonged antibiotic, immunosuppressant, or corticosteroid therapy in immu-

nocompromised health or with denture wear

3) Is characterized by a thick, white coating on the tongue, oral mucosa and palatal tissues that can be wiped off to reveal reddened tissues.

4) Frequently results in painful irritations creating difficulty in chewing, speaking and inability to wear dental appliances

5) Is treated with antifungal medications (Ketoconazole, Nystatin, Clotrimazole)

c. Drug-induced hyperplasia

1) Often results from use of phenytoin, nifedipine (calcium channel blocker) or anti-organ rejection medications (cyclosporin)

2) Is associated with enlarged, bulbous and fibrotic gingival tissues

3) Can be controlled or prevented through adequate oral hygiene self-care, especially if begun before the medication regimen

d. Additional oral manifestations of medications include: glossitis, erythema multiforme, hairy tongue, lichenoid eruptions, and trigeminal neuralgia.

2. Common drugs that impact the dental and dental hygiene appointment

a. Antihypertensives

1) Are used to reduce blood pressure in patients with cardiovascular heart disease

2) Can cause postural hypotension and xerostomia; sit the patient up slowly and keep them seated for several minutes to reduce the dizziness of hypotension. Recommend products for xerostomia relief and home fluoride therapy to prevent root caries. Calcium channel blockers can cause gingival overgrowth.

3) Monitor blood pressure at each visit. Refer patient to physician when blood pressures is higher than 160/95 mm Hg. Do not provide dental treatment when blood pressure is 200/115 mm Hg or higher.

4) Common drugs taken:
   a) ACE inhibitors: Capoten, Vasotec, Captopril, Enalapril
   b) Calcium channel blockers: Cardizem, Procardia, Calan
   c) Beta blockers: Tenormin, Inderal, Lopressor, Propranolol
   d) Diuretics: Dyazide, Maxide, Lasix, Furosemide

b. Diuretics

1) Are used to promote renal excretion in the treatment of congestive heart failure and hypertension

2) Result in frequent urination and xerostomia; impacts planning appointment time and length of appointment

3) Common drugs taken (see antihypertension diuretics).

c. Anticoagulants

1) Are used for the treatment of coronary heart disease to increase blood flow by suppressing or delaying coagulation of blood.

2) Side effects can be prolonged; spontaneous or internal bleeding can occur; hematoma more likely with some local anesthesia injections.

3) Requires obtaining the patient's prothrombin time (PT) from physician before periodontal therapy or other invasive procedures; PT should be 1 to 1½ times normal.

4) Discontinuation of drug may be hazardous to patient due to embolus or thrombus formation; physician consultation is recommended to adjust dosage for dental hygiene treatment.

5) Common drugs taken are Coumadin, Heparin, and Warfarin.

d. Antiseizure medications

1) Are used to reduce the incidence of seizures in epileptic or Down syndrome patients

2) Stimulates gingival growth resulting in gingival hyperplasia or gingival enlargement. The extent of the gingival enlargement is related to the level of inadequacy of oral hygiene self-care

3) Common drugs taken: phenytoin (Dilantin and Diphenylan Sodium)

e. Antianginal medications

1) Are used for the treatment of angina pectoris, to increase the oxygen supply to the heart muscle through vasodilation.

2) Usage pattern by patient should be established prior to each appointment; keep nitroglycerin tablets handy during the dental appointment; make dental appointment short and in the morning.

3) When combined with alcohol can cause severe hypotension

4) Common drugs taken: nitroglycerin (Nitro-Bid, Minitran, Isordil)

f. Thyroid medications

1) Are used to treat hypothyroid disease by increasing the metabolic rate.

2) Have no oral side effects.

3) Common drug name: synthroid (Levothyroxin, Synthroid, Eltroxin)

g. Heart medications

TABLE 11.1	Recommended Regimens for Antibiotic Premedication[3]	
Regimen	**Antibiotic**	**Dosage**
Standard, general prophylaxis	Amoxicillin	Adults: 2.0 g Children: 50 mg/kg orally 1 hr before procedure
Unable to take oral medications	Ampicillin	Adults: 2.0 g IM or IV Children: 50 mg/kg IM or IV 30 min before procedure
Allergic to penicillin	Clindamycin OR Cephalexin	Adults: 600 mg Children: 20 mg/kg orally 1 hr before procedure OR Adults: 2.0 g Children: 50 mg/kg orally 1 hr before procedure
Allergic to penicillin and unable to take oral medications	Clindamycin	Adults: 600 mg Children: 20 mg/kg IV 30 min before procedure

1) Are used with patients experiencing congestive heart failure; they strengthen myocardial contractility.
2) Patient presents with swollen extremities and reports shortness of breath; seat patient in upright inclined position to increase ease of breathing.
3) Common drug names: digitalis (Lanoxin), enalapril (Vasotec), captopril (Capoten)

h. Antinflammatory medications
1) Are used to depress the inflammatory response or process and treat adrenocortical insufficiency, rheumatoid arthritis and respiratory disease (emphysema)
2) Patient is at risk for candida infections and oral ulcerations
3) Common drug names: corticosteriods (Prednisone, Prednisolone, Detrazone)

i. Vasoconstrictor medications
1) Are used to alleviate symptoms of asthma and emphysema; taken as inhalants.
2) Can cause xerostomia; are frequently associated with red gingiva due to mouth breathing (associated with asthma)
3) Common drugs names: epinephrine (Albuteral, Proventil, Ventolin)

j. Tranquilizer medications
1) Long-term use can cause tardive dyskinesia: involuntary facial movements of facial muscles and tongue
2) Can cause occlusal grinding and wear
3) Common drug names: diazepam (Vallium), alprazolam (Xanax)

3. Prevention of bacterial endocarditis
a. Bacterial endocarditis is an invasion of bacteria in the blood stream that can lodge in the heart blood vessels, causing infection and destruction of cardiac tissue.
1) The offending bacteria are vegetative *Streptococcus viridans, Staphylococcus aureus,* *Staphylococcus epidermidis;* alpha hemolytic streptocci are the most prevalent
2) Patients susceptible to bacterial endocarditis have irregular heart valve tissue; patient must be premedicated with antibiotics prior to any invasive tissue manipulation

b. The American Medical Association recommends the following premedication regimen for the prevention of bacterial endocarditis in some medical conditions (Tables 11–1 and 11–2).

c. Conditions that do not warrant premedication but are often questioned: hepatitis, anticoagulant therapy, high blood pressure, coronary artery disease, high cholesterol, epilepsy, bypass surgery after 6 months, angina pectoris, controlled diabetic patients, and mitral valve prolapse without regurgitation.

d. Precautions to utilize for the prevention of endocarditis
1) Identify high and moderate risk patients and premedicate as indicated
2) Confirm that patients comply with antibiotic prophylaxis 1 hour before appointment

 Clinical Case **STUDY**

John Jakes, a 46-year-old man, develops computer software. He has a history of seizure disorder for which he takes 30 mg of phenobarbital and 100 mg dilantin daily. He is allergic to penicillin and Valium. On completion of his dental exam, it is apparent that he clenches his teeth; has moderate gingivitis with fibrotic, enlarged, and bulbous papilla; and plaque covering more than 50% of his teeth. He reports difficulty with flossing, stating "I can't get it between my teeth."

Clinical Case QUESTIONS

1. What are common oral side effects of John's medications and disease? Into what category do these drugs fall?
2. Given John's history of clenching, what clinical signs would one expect to find in his mouth?
3. What recommendations can be made for improving John's oral hygiene self-care?
4. What should the treatment plan include for John?

Clinical Case RATIONALE

1. Phenytoin (Dilantin) can cause gingival overgrowth (hyperplasia). Due to injury from seizure trauma, scars on the lips and tongue and possibly fractured teeth may be found. The two drugs, phenytoin and phenobarbital, are anti-convulsants.
2. Clenching will frequently result in scalloping of the lateral borders of the tongue. The occlusal surface of molars will demonstrate wear, appear shiny, and the dentin may become exposed as the enamel is worn away. Wear is also common on the incisal edges of the anterior teeth.
3. John could improve his oral self-care by using a shred-resistant floss made of polytetrafluoroethylene (PTFE) or thin waxed floss. An automatic toothbrush may help improve his oral hygiene self-care because of built-in timers, ease of technique, and increased access to hard to reach tooth surfaces
4. The treatment plan should include the following: A thorough assessment of the patient's medical history, specifically including most recent seizure, medication regimen and compliance. The dental exam should include, extra and intra oral examination, with special evaluation of the existing periodontal condition. A complete dental and periodontal chart would be obtained, as well as exposing appropriate radiographs. Oral hygiene self-care instructions should involve the patient by having him give a return demonstration of brushing and flossing in order to observe his technique. John will need a thorough prophylaxis including debridement therapy and polishing and reappointment for evaluation in four to six weeks to consider the need for gingivectomy, to assess John's oral hygiene self-care, and to determine the continued care interval.

III. Vital Signs (blood pressure, pulse, respiration, body temperature, and pupil size)
   A. Blood pressure
      1. Is the force the blood exerts on blood vessel walls.
      2. Is measured as millimeters of mercury—mm Hg
      3. Blood pressure is typically recorded systolic/diastolic, e.g., 120/80 mm Hg. (see also Chapter 14).
         a. Systolic pressure is the amount of pressure exerted against the blood vessel walls during ventricular contraction; 120 mm Hg is considered normal, pressures over 140 mm Hg are considered high.
         b. Diastolic pressure is the amount of pressure exerted against blood vessel walls during ventricular relaxation; 80 mm Hg is considered normal, pressures above 90 mm Hg are considered high.
      4. Essential or primary hypertension is of unknown etiology or origin;

TABLE 11.2 Categories of Risk for Bacterial Endocarditis[3]

High Risk (Antibiotic Premedication Required)	Moderate Risk (Antibiotic Premedication Recommended)	Low Risk (Antibiotic Premedication Not Required)
Cardiac valves, including prosthetic and homograft valves	Most other congenital cardiac malformation (other than those listed in other categories)	Isolated secundum atrial septal defect
Previous bacterial endocarditis	Acquired valvular dysfunction (e.g., rheumatic heart disease, Phen-Fen–related damage)	Surgical repair of atrial septal defect, ventribular septal defect, or patent ductus arteriosus (without residua beyond 6 months)
Complex cyanotic congenital heart disease (e.g., single ventricle states, transposition of the great arteries, Tetralogy of Fallot)	Hypertrophic cardiomyopathy	Previous coronary artery bypass graft surgery
Surgically constructed systemic pulmonary shunts or conduits	Mitral valve prolapse with valvular regurgitation and/or thickened leaflets	Mitral valve prolapse without valvular regurgitation Physiologic, functional, or innocent heart murmurs Previous Kawasaki disease without valvular dysfunction

5. Secondary hypertension occurs as a result of a disease such as renal or kidney disease/damage, or diabetes
6. Target organs effected by hypertension are the brain, kidney, heart, and eyes.
7. Risk factors for hypertension are heredity, obesity, race, age, sex, diet (high in fat), smoking and stress
8. Treatment approaches for hypertension usually involve a step program of dietary adjustments and antihypertensive medications given in increments.
9. Measuring techniques (See Chapter 14 Medical and Dental Emergencies)

B. Pulse
1. Measures the rate at which the heart beats.
2. Normal for adults is 60–80 beats per minute
3. Normal for child is 90–120 beats per minute.
4. Is called tachycardia when the pulse is over 150 beats/minute; bradycardia when under 50 beats/minute.
5. Locations for measuring pulse are the radial, brachial, facial, temporal or carotid.
   a. Radial pulse is the ideal point to measure pulse on conscious patient because it is easily accessible.
   b. The carotid pulse is best used for CPR on an adult; brachial artery on an infant.
6. Rate, rhythm and beat characteristics of pulse should be noted
7. Pulse is effected by age, exercise, drugs, diet and emotional state.

C. Respiration
1. Is considered normal when 14–20 respirations and exhalations occur per minute.
2. Rate, rhythm, and quality (strong, labored, shallow or deep) should be noted especially for patients who present with a positive medical history of respiratory symptoms, e.g., asthma, emphysema, congestive heart failure, or allergic reactions.

D. Body temperature
1. Is normally in the range of 97.0°F to 99.6°F, (36.1°C to 37.6°C)
2. When abnormal
   a. Fever is temperature elevated by at least a full degree; occurs with infection or acute inflammation.
   b. Hyperthermia is a temperature above 105.8°F; occurs with infection or overexposure to heat
   c. Hypothermia is a temperature below 96.0°F; occurs with shock or overexposure to cold

E. Pupil examination
1. Evaluate the pupils for signs of constriction, dilation and evenness
2. Dilated pupils are an indication of shock, heart failure, hallucinogens or amphetamine use
3. Constricted or pinpoint pupils occur with use of morphine, heroin or barbiturates

Extraoral and Intraoral Examination

Intraoral and extraoral examination of the soft and hard tissues is part of the total evaluation of the patient. Recognition of abnormal findings may be critical in preserving the overall health of the patient.

I. Examination Technique
   A. Visual observation, palpation, auscultation, and olfaction are all means of assessing tissues of the head and neck
      1. Visual observation uses direct vision and the mouth mirror to examine the intraoral and extraoral structures
      2. To perform:
         a. Inform the patient of the examination
         b. Adopt an organized, sequential pattern to avoid omitting areas
         c. Look for abnormal color (change to red, black, blue, white, dark brown or the spread of color), size (change is sudden or ongoing), or change in appearance (irregular margins, elevation, texture becomes scaly, crusty, or ulcerated)
      3. Palpation is used to examine the tissues and underlying structures of the head and neck; the following are acceptable types of palpation.
         a. Digital palpation—one finger is used to examine tissue (hard palate)
         b. Bidigital palpation—tissue is grasped between finger(s) and thumb (cheeks, alveolar ridges, lips, vestibule, tongue, ducts, floor of mouth, larynx)
         c. Manual palpation—all fingers of one hand are used to grasp tissue (anterior deep and the superficial cervical nodes)
         d. Bimanual palpation—finger(s) and thumb from each hand are applied simultaneously to examine the tissues (floor of the mouth)
         e. Bilateral palpation—bilateral structures are examined simultaneously to detect differences between sides (TMJ, inferior border of mandible); place fingers on the anterior border of the jaw—palpate distally simultaneously on right and left sides
         f. Circular compression—fingers move in circular motion while applying pressure (occipital lymph nodes)
      4. Auscultation is listening to body sounds to determine a change from the normal; Listen for:
         a. TMJ sounds, such as clicking, grinding, or popping; make note if pain is associated with the sounds
         b. Hoarseness/cough, make note of how long it has persisted
         c. Speech disorders, such as slurred speech, stuttering, or extra loud speech

5. Olfaction is the use of the olfactory sense to detect unusual smells; notice:
   a. Halitosis, associated with poor oral hygiene, acute necrotizing ulcerative gingivitis, or gastrointestial difficulties; More than 90% of halitosis comes from the tongue—encourage brushing the tongue
   b. Alcohol breath, associated with recent alcohol consumption or alcoholism
   c. Acetone breath, indicative of diabetes

II. Documentation
   A. Purpose is:
      1. To record findings that may be significant in the overall diagnosis and recommended treatment for the patient
      2. As a legal record in case of a legal claim or patient identification (accident or disaster)
      3. As baseline data for subsequent examination and treatment planning
   B. Standard of recording
      1. Requires adequate space to record in a brief, accurate manner
      2. Includes diagnosis and treatment alternatives and/or recommendations
      3. Summarizes patient's response, listing wants, needs and expectations
      4. Indicates treatment to be rendered
         a. No treatment; patient refuses to follow through with treatment and/or recommendations
         b. Treatment; patient agrees to continue treatment
         c. Consent; documentation of consent including risks, benefits, and alternative treatment options
         d. Referral; patient is referred to a specialist

III. Procedures
   A. Extraoral Examination
      1. Physical appearance is assessed by visual examination for:
         a. Unsteadiness of gait; patient cannot walk at a normal pace and maintain balance
         b. Restricted mobility; patient may limp while walking which may indicate an injury to the hip, leg, knee, or foot or systemic disease; investigate possible surgery that may have required pins or joint repair or prosthesis
         c. Imbalance; patient cannot walk without losing balance; may be due to equilibrium problem, inner ear infection, loss of muscular strength or damage from stroke
         d. Stature; patient may appear stiff while standing, sitting, or walking; may indicate a back problem or arthritis; if patient assumes a slumped position it may be due to lack of muscle tone as a result of a stroke
         e. Difficulty breathing; patient appears out of breath while walking or right after walking; may indicate congestive heart failure, lung disease or other systemic disorder

2. Hair
   a. Unusual amount; loss or thinning of hair may be the result of chemotherapy; excessive hair growth (hypertrichosis) due to hormone disorder
   b. Unusual distribution, as in alopecia, is associated with loss of hair in patches
   c. Lack of luster may be associated with poor nutrition
   d. Scalp lesions; may be associated with psoriasis, previous injury or basal cell carcinoma
   e. Lice are small insects living in the hair and skin; nits appear as tiny, white globules at the hair root; spreads easily from one person to the next

3. Face
   a. Asymmetry is associated with facial paralysis due to stroke or Bell's palsy, lack of eye blinking is also characteristic of Bell's palsy
   b. Drooling, lack of expression and diminished eye blinking are associated with Parkinson's disease
   c. Protruding eyes are associated with hyperthyroidism
   d. Eyes slanting upward and outward and a broad, flat nose and low-set ears are associated with Down syndrome
   e. Puffy and swollen eyes, with a broad nose and edematous eyelids are common with hypothyroidism
   f. Unusual muscle twitchings and loud vocal sounds are associated with Tourette's syndrome
   g. Bruising may be associated with physical abuse, anticoagulation therapy or blood disorder
   h. General expression can indicate the general mood of a patient (happy, sad, angry, indifferent, etc)

4. Skin
   a. Color can indicate general health status; e.g. illness, disease, or trauma; note paleness, redness, acne, rosacea, sunburn, pigmentation
   b. Textures that are unusual should be noted; scarring, clamminess, firmness, swelling, and acne
   c. Lesions should be documented noting color, size, shape, surface texture (note any changes in pigmented nevus)

5. Eyes
   a. Note pupil size; normal, dilated or pin point
   b. Sclera color (yellow may indicate jaundice: red and crusty may indicate conjunctivitis)
   c. Bulging may indicate a possible thyroid disorder

6. Nose
   a. Obstructed airway is associate with congestion and/or a structural defect
   b. Secretions may be clear due to sinus drainage; a yellow/green secretion is indicative of an infection
   c. A "butterfly" shaped lesion over the nose is associated with systemic lupus erythematosus (SLE)
   d. Rhinophyma is an overgrowth of sweat and sebaceous glands; nose appears red and bulbous and is associated with increased alcohol consumption
7. Ear
   a. Hearing loss and use of hearing aids will require the operator to look at the patient while speaking; if using ultrasonic equipment, the patient may need to turn off the hearing aid
   b. Infections may affect patient's ability to hear; may also affect balance
   c. Tinnitis (ringing) may cause humming or buzzing in the patient's ear; is associated with long-term use of aspirin or with infection or environmental noise trauma.
8. Bones, muscles, lymph nodes, and glands
   a. Anterior border of mandible is assessed for tissue asymmetry by bimanual palpation from midline to posterior angle
   b. Temporomandibular joint is assessed for pain, clicking, popping, grinding and restriction in opening or closing; it is evaluated by patient interview (subjective symptoms) and bilateral palpation with index fingers anterior to the outer meatus; have patient open and close several times, slowly; note any deviations or pain
   c. Larynx is assessed for unrestricted movement by bimanual palpation
   d. Mentalis muscle is assessed for smoothness or restriction in swallowing movement; evaluate by digital palpation, rolling the tissue over the mandible
   e. Masseter muscle, and temporalis muscle are assessed for pain, swelling, enlargements, and unusual hardness using bilateral circular compression
   f. Occipital lymph nodes are assessed for pain, swelling, enlargement and unusual hardness using bilateral palpation (with patient's head tilted forward)
   g. Auricular and parotid lymph nodes are assessed for pain, swelling, enlargement and unusual hardness using bilateral palpation
   h. Superficial cervical lymph nodes are assessed for pain, enlargement, and fixed position or mobility by placing the patient's head to the side and palpating with the fingers anteriorly to posteriorly to the sternocleidomastoid muscle
   i. Deep cervical lymph nodes are assessed for pain, enlargement, and fixed position or mobility by placing the patient's head upright and palpating deep tissues along the sternocleidomastoid muscles with the thumb and fingers
   j. Thyroid gland is assessed for asymmetry and enlargement by a combination of bidigital and circular palpation below the "Adam's apple"; can be best felt while patient sits upright and is asked to swallow
   k. Parotid glands are assessed for pain, swelling, enlargement and hardness using bilateral circular compression; salivary flow can be observed at the opening of Stenson's duct when the gland is milked
   l. Submental and submandibular glands are assessed for asymmetry, noncontinuous borders, pain, swelling, enlargement, unusual hardness or difficulty in swallowing by bilateral digital palpation
B. Intraoral exam
   1. Lips are examined for:
      a. Unusual color given the patient's overall pigmentation
      b. Changes in size, may be due to swelling or allergic reaction (latex)
      c. Abnormal texture, lack of firmness or moistness; associated with dehydration and sunburned lips
      d. Chapping, due to mouth breathing, nutritional deficiency or environmental conditions
      e. Cracking, associated with angular cheilosis, candida, or vitamin B deficiency
      f. Blistering, associated with ulcers or herpetic lesions
      g. Irritations, from lip biting or trauma
      h. Limited motion, associated with scarring, trauma, or stroke
   2. Labial and alveolar mucosa are assessed by visual examination and palpated for:
      a. Signs of tissue trauma, due to biting, abrasion, burns; horizontal bruises at commissures may indicate binding or gagging associated with physical abuse
      b. Ulcerated lesions, such as herpetic lesions or apthous ulcers
      c. Tight frenum attachments, can cause gingival defects such as loss of attached gingiva
      d. Torn or lacerated frenum, often associated with forced feedings, binding, gagging (abuse); lingual frenum is typically involved
      e. Amalgam tattoo, blue/black macules, of varying size, found on any area of the soft tissues

f. Smokeless tobacco lesion, hyperkeratinized tissue; white, sometimes corrugated, in appearance

g. Leukoplakia, associated with use of lozenges, medications, and tobacco products held in the lower half of the buccal mucosa on the mandible; careful evaluation of changes is essential

3. Buccal mucosa is assessed by palpation and visual examination for:

a. Linea alba, a white line paralleling the occlusal plane, associated with trauma

b. Trauma from toothbrushing, cheek biting

c. Fordyce granules, slightly raised, yellowish spots frequently found in the oral mucosa and associated with ectopic sebaceous glands; found in 80% of the population

d. Stensen's duct, evaluate bilaterally for enlargements, tumors or calcified areas; milk ducts to confirm function

4. Gingiva is assessed by visual examination and palpation for:

a. Tissue trauma, due to abrasion, burns, or cuts

b. Infection, (redness and swelling) associated with inadequate bacterial plaque removal

c. Fibrosis, associated with chronic gingivitis, medication use, or traumatic toothbrushing

d. Recession, associated with loss of periodontal attachment or vigorous toothbrushing

e. Mucogingival defects, such as:

1) Lack of attached gingiva associated with tooth positioning, hereditary factors, oral habits, and poor oral hygiene

2) Clefts, associated with poor oral hygiene

3) High frenum attachments, associated with muscle pull on attached gingiva

5. Hard and soft palate are assessed by visual inspection and palpated for:

a. Tori, a hard protruding bony structure (benign exostosis), found on the palate; not of significance unless a partial or full denture is being constructed when it may need to be reduced or removed.

b. Petechiae, small red dots on mucous membranes, associated with trauma or systemic disease.

c. Trauma, mechanical or chemical irritation; should heal within 10 days, if not, further investigation is needed to rule out pathology.

d. Stomatitis, ranges from small, red petechiae-like lesions (nicotine and denture stomatitis) to generalized and granular (denture stomatitis) to ulcerative (apthous stomatitis) to intense redness with focal bone loss (necrotizing stomatitis).

e. Ulcerations, fluid-filled lesions surrounded with red halo associated with apthous ulcers or burns.

f. Fistulas, pimple-like lesions associated with a periodontal or periapical abscess.

6. Floor of mouth is assessed by visual inspection and palpation for:

a. Wharton's duct, which can become blocked with mucous plugs or sialoliths and be seen on occlusal radiograph.

b. Varicosities, which are often found sublingual on the aging patient.

c. Limited tongue movement, due to ankylosis of the tongue; may lead to swallowing and speech disorders.

d. Mucous retention cyst or ranula, associated with the ducts of the submandibular and sublingual gland; soft, sessile slowly enlarging mass on one side of the floor of the mouth; painless; once removed, may recur.

7. Tongue is assessed by visual examination and palpation for:

a. Fissuring, associated with the presence of numerous grooves and crevices on the dorsal surface and lateral borders of the tongue; entraps food and bacteria; tongue brushing is necessary to deplaque.

b. Coating indicates varying degree of keratinization of the filiform papilla; food, medications, bacteria, and tobacco causes staining of the area.

c. Common lesions of the tongue

1) Fibroma, associated with trauma

2) Hemangiomas and lymphangiomas, associated with trauma

3) White plaques, indicative of lichen planus, candidiasis, or other systemic disease; definitive diagnosis is needed

4) Ulcers; apthous ulcer is common, also may be associated with systemic disease

5) Malignant lesions, can develop on the lateral border or ventral surface of the tongue; first appear ulcerated and then can develop into a mass infiltrating into the deep layers of the tongue.

d. Macroglossia, symmetric enlargement of the tongue; can be a developmental abnormality or can be associated with cretinism, mongolism, acromegaly or Down syndrome; tongue may appear scalloped from pushing against the teeth.

e. Geographic or migratory glossitis; a common benign condition found on the dorsum and borders of the tongue; the lesions are circinate red areas with white borders; outline of lesions change, heal, and reappear on a different area of the tongue.

f. Hairy leukoplakia, hyperkeratosis of the filiform papillae; results in corrugated appearance; found on the lateral boarders of the tongue; often associated with HIV+.

g. Black hairy tongue, elongation of filiform papillae accompanied by dark staining; often associated with long-term use of certain medications or tobacco use.

h. Median rhomboid glossitis, a flat benign lesion on the dorsum of the tongue, no filiform papillae.

i. Tongue thrust (during swallowing), the anterior portion of the tongue pushes between the teeth; ideally the tongue is positioned on the palate behind the maxillary central incisors while swallowing; retraining of the tongue may be necessary if it is associated with speech disorders or tooth positioning problems.

IV. Tumors of the Oral Cavity and Surrounding Areas
   A. Types
      1. Benign
         a. Papilloma
            1) Clinical features
               a) Cauliflower-like surface
               b) Numerous, small finger-like projections
               c) Well-circumscribed pedunculated tumor
               d) Found on the tongue, lips, buccal mucosa, gingiva, and palate
            2) Histologic features
               a) Extends above the mucosal surface
               b) Continuous layer of stratified squamous epithelium with thin, central connective tissue core
            3) Excision is treatment of choice; if properly removed, recurrence is rare.
         b. Pigmented nevus (mole)
            1) Clinical features of intradermal nevus
               a) Commonly scattered over body; appear smooth/flat or elevated
               b) May have brown pigmentation; frequently have hair growing from surface
            2) Junctional nevus appears clinically similar to the intradermal nevus (differs histologically)
            3) Compound nevus is a interdermal nevus with an overlying junctional nevus
            4) Juvenile melanoma (Spitz nevus)
               a) Occurs mostly in children on the skin of extremities and face
               b) Not found on mucosa
            5) Blue nevus
               a) Present at birth or develops in early childhood and persists throughout life
               b) Color varies from brown to blue and can be found intraorally
            c. Histologic features
               1) Large cells with a vesicular nucleus; grouped in sheets or cords
               2) May contain melanin pigment
            d. Treatment
               1) Removal recommended if nevus is:
                  a) Irritated by clothing or suddenly increases in size
                  b) Becomes ulcerated or undergoes color change
               2) Excision of intraoral nevus recommended as a prophylactic measure due to constant irritation by eating, toothbrushing, etc.
            e. Leukoplakia
               1) Clinical features
                  a) White plaque on the mucosa
                  b) Varies from nonpalpable and translucent to thick fissured indurated lesion
               2) Etiology: tobacco, alcohol, chronic irritation, syphilis, vitamin deficiency and Candidiasis
               3) Histologic feature: dysplasia of surface epithelium
               4) Prognosis: low percentage become malignant
            f. Leukoedema
               1) Clinical features
                  a) An abnormality of the mucosa that resembles early leukoplakia
                  b) Filmy opalescence of the mucosa
                  c) Later stages appear coarsely wrinkled
                  d) Found on buccal mucosa and extends to the oral surface of the lips
               2) Histologic features
                  a) Increased thickness of epithelium
                  b) Intracellular edema
                  c) Superficial parakeratotic layer of cells; broad rite pegs
      2. Malignant tumors
         a. Basal cell carcinoma
            1) Clinical features
               a) Begins as a small, elevated papule
               b) Ulcerates and heals over, then breaks down again
               c) Crusty lesion with smooth, rolled border
               d) Spread laterally beneath skin and can erode deep tissues
               e) Often found in the middle one third of the face
            2) Etiology: ultraviolet radiation
            3) Histologic findings
               a) Group of cells with indistinct cell membranes

b) Cells have little tendency to differentiate
4) Treatment and prognosis
    a) Remove by incising or laser; can recur
    b) If left untreated, can become invasive
b. Squamous cell carcinoma: 90% of these carcinomas found in the oral cavity
  1) Oral sites[4]
    a) Tongue: 52%
    b) Floor of mouth: 16%
    c) Alveolar mucosa: 12%
    d) Palate: 11%
    e) Buccal mucosa: 9%
  2) Clinical features
    a) Intraoral: initially an ulcerated mass (red or white) with mild-to-moderate discomfort
    b) Jaw: swelling, pain, numbness
    c) Hematologic: gingival redness, swelling and bleeding; nonhealing ulcers; secondary infections may be present
    d) Salivary glands: persistent lump; little to moderate pain
    e) Difficulty swallowing or continued hoarseness
  3) Etiology
    a) Smoking
    b) Alcohol
    c) Syphilis
  4) Histologic features
    a) Less differentiated cells: a more aggressive cancer
    b) Red or red with white mucosal lesions develop rapidly and aggressively
c. Malignant melanoma: One of the most deadly of all cancerous lesions
  1) Clinical features
    a) Common sites are skin, oral mucosa, parotid gland, eye, vaginal mucosa, and upper respiratory tract.
    b) Enlarged pigmented area
    c) Color is light brown to deep blue/black
    d) May present as a crusting, bleeding and ulcerated surface
    e) 80% of the oral lesions appear on the maxillary alveolar ridge and palate; also appear on the lower jaw, cheeks, tongue and floor of mouth
    f) Metastases is widespread
    g) Greater risk if there is a family history of malignant melanoma combined with blond or auburn hair; light blue/green eyes; sensitive/fair skin; moles 6 to 10 mm or greater in size.[5–6] Previously diagnosed with malignant melanoma
  2) Etiology

a) 10% to 60% of lesions have a history of injury or irritation; injuries include, but not limited to:
    (1) Blunt injury
    (2) Perforated wounds
    (3) Frostbite
    (4) Chronic irritation along the collar, belt line, and hair line
b) Excessive exposure to sunlight
3) Histologic features
    a) A many-celled lesion extending into the connective tissue
    b) Cells may or may not be uniform in size
4) Treatment and prognosis
    a) Any suspicious nevi should be removed and biopsied due to the serious nature of melanoma cancer.
    b) Common treatment is radical surgery/resection.
    c) The disease is often fatal.
d. Kaposi's sarcoma
  1) Clinical features
    a) Common oral manifestation for patients with AIDS
    b) Red, blue or purple nodular lesion
    c) Common sites are hard and soft palate and gingiva
    d) Lesions may be ulcerated
  2) Histologic features[7]
    a) Represents AIDS diagnosis
    b) Associated with CD4+ cell counts below 200 cells/mm^3
  3) Treatment involves radiation therapy and surgical excision
B. Management of oral cancer
  1. Diagnosis methods
  a. Biopsy
    1) Definitive diagnostic technique: a tissue sample is microscopically examined and evaluated for structure and cell type.
    2) Types
      a) Excisional; the entire suspicious lesion is removed and examined.
      b) Incisional; a representative section of the lesion is removed and examined. Most often used for large lesions.
    3) Indications
      a) Any unusual or suspicious oral lesion that cannot be clinically identified with certainty or has persisted for more than 2 weeks.
      b) Any persistent, thick, white hyperkeratotic lesion.
      c) Any surgically excised tissue should be routinely evaluated.
  b. Exfoliative cytology
    1) Diagnostic aid or screening test: a smear

of surface cells are microscopically examined and evaluated for cell structure.

2) Indications:
 a) No longer a recommended technique in dentistry.
 b) Traditional uses
  (1) When a biopsy is not planned or patient refuses biopsy
  (2) For follow-up examination for patients treated by radiation
  (3) As part of a mass screening project
 c) Technique used is similar to collect material for microscopic examination for a definitive diagnosis of suspected candidiasis; this is not true exfoliative cytology.

3) Limitations
 a) Gives high number of false negatives that seriously limit the diagnostic reliability.
 b) Lacks a definitive diagnosis, so a positive smear must be followed by a biopsy. In highly suspicious lesions, time should not be taken for the exfoliative cytology.
 c) Effectively limited to surface lesions that are not keratinized.

4) Technique
 a) Use a small metal or plastic spatula or moistened tongue blade to gently scrap the entire surface of the lesion to collect surface epithelial cells. Work in only one direction.
 b) Smear the cells evenly over a glass slide.
 c) Fix the cells immediately to preserve them using a commercial fixative, hair spray, or 70% alcohol and air drying in a protected location.
 d) Prepare a second slide in the same manner.
 e) Label the slide with patient's name and date and pack in a laboratory mailing container. In addition to basic demographic information, describe the lesion, its location, and history.

2. Treatment
 a. Pretreatment
  1) Establishment of treatment team
  2) Consultation for recommendation for treatment and expected complications
  3) Assessment of dental/oral needs, to minimize complications during and after therapy
 b. Management during cancer therapy[8]
  1) Radiation side effects
   a) Alteration of taste and decreased salivary flow
   b) Mucositis, oral infections, and increased caries
   c) Altered tooth and jaw development on young growing bodies
   d) Trismus and soft tissue necrosis
  2) Chemotherapy side effects
   a) Nausea/vomiting
   b) Neurotoxicity
   c) Mucosal ulcerations, infection, increased gingival bleeding, decreased salivary flow, and increased dental caries
   d) Odontogenic-like pain
   e) Altered tooth development
  3) Bone marrow transplant side effects
   a) Mucositis
   b) Tissue ulcerations
   c) Increased gingival bleeding and infections
   d) Decreased salivary flow
  4) Managing side effects
   a) Empathy
   b) Nutritional counseling
   c) Cessation of tobacco and alcohol products
   d) Plaque control using an extra-soft toothbrush and nonirritating toothpaste
   e) Oral rinses (avoid rinses with alcohol, phenol, or peroxide)
   f) Salivary substitutes and oral lubricants
   g) Professional deplaquing as needed or tolerated
   h) Home fluoride therapy as tolerated
 c. Management after cancer therapy
  1) Observe postoperative healing
  2) Monitor oral hygiene habits
  3) Continue oral rinses if needed, fluoride therapy, and salivary substitutes
  4) Continue fluoride therapy
  5) Adjust nutritional needs
  6) Monitor oral hygiene needs through restorative rehabilitation
  7) Schedule regular continued care appointments

 Clinical Case **STUDY**

Susan, a 19-year-old college student, returned home for the summer after her first year at State University. At her previous dental examination and oral prophylaxis, 15 months ago, she had one occlusal restoration placed. At this appointment, the clinical and radiographic examinations reveal the following: moderately inflamed gingival

tissues, light calculus on the mandibular anterior teeth and posterior molars interproximally, no plaque, pain in her temporomandibular joint (TMJ) on opening, and new carious lesions on 13 of her posterior teeth (#2-M, #3-D, #4-M, #5-D and O, #12-O, #13-D, #14-M and D, #15-M, #18-M, #19-D, #20-M and D, #30-M, and #31-M and O). Susan has good brushing technique, brushes once a day, and flosses infrequently. When asked about dietary changes, she states she ate well at school until the fall when she began drinking coffee with sugar and 3 to 4 sweetened, carbonated beverages a day.

Clinical Case QUESTIONS

1. What is the most probable reason for Susan's dramatic increase in caries?
2. What techniques should be used to examine the TMJ area? If positive findings, what recommendation should be made?
3. How does Susan's gingival health vary from normal, healthy gingiva with respect to color, consistency, texture, and marginal contour?
4. Why is there tissue inflammation in the absence of any plaque?
5. What oral hygiene self-care regimen(s) is(are) recommended for Susan?
6. Explain any nutritional recommendations that should be made.
7. What type of instrumentation is needed to complete Susan's prophylaxis?

Clinical Case RATIONALE

1. The increase in sugar consumption with coffee and pop is the most likely reason for the increase in interproximal and occlusal caries. Sugar frequency impacts acid production, thereby increasing the risk for proximal and occlusal caries.
2. Utilize bilateral palpation to assess the TMJ. Bilateral palpation involves placing the index fingers of each hand just anterior to the outer meatus of the ear and feeling the joint area as the patient opens and closes. Observation is also required to assess the TMJ for deviations in the functional movements of opening, closing and lateral movements. Use auscultation (listening for sound) to detect clicking/crepitus, popping or grating. Question the patient regarding painful symptoms associated with jaw movements. For positive findings, refer to dentist for further evaluation.
3. Healthy gingiva should appear pale pink, firm, and stippled. The marginal contour should hug the neck of the tooth and be 1 mm above the CEJ, and the papilla would appear pointed or "knife-edge" in the interproximal areas. Susan's gingiva is likely to be red, edematous and spongy with some loss of stippling. The marginal contour will be swollen and possibly bulbous, indicating a diagnosis of gingivitis.
4. Susan is plaque-free at this appointment, most likely because she brushed her teeth more thoroughly just prior to this dental checkup than she typically does. Previous plaque buildup caused the inflammation.
5. At this dental appointment the primary need of the patient, dental caries, should be addressed. Because of the large number of carious lesions, the caries process should be discussed with the patient. The patient should be encouraged to brush 2–3 times per day for 2 minutes each time, using a fluoride toothpaste. A regimen of prescription topical home fluoride applications prior to bedtime (brush-on or tray fluoride) is recommended. Specific directions to not rinse after fluoride application will allow the fluoride to continue to work in higher concentrations. Due to the excessive interproximal decay, it is appropriate to request the patient swish with the home fluoride mouthrinse daily. The patient should schedule another appointment in 3 months for examination, bitewing radiographs, and evaluation of caries management.
6. Discuss the form and frequency of sugar exposures from coffee and pop, explaining that drinking pop for one hour continually bathes the teeth with substrate bacteria use to produce an acid environment. Recommend reducing her sugar exposures by limiting the amount and duration (length of time) of pop and coffee with sugar consumption and by rinsing the mouth with water after eating or drinking in order to reduce the acid environment.
7. Hand instrumentation with anterior and posterior sickles and universal or gracey curets is sufficient to debride and deplaque. Ultrasonic instrumentation using the thin periodontal deplaquing inserts could also be utilized.

Dentition Assessment

The dentition is assessed for caries, attrition, abrasion, erosion, fracture, inflammation, necrosis, restoration, and other problems. These assessments can involve visual, radiographic, and clinical evaluation and a variety of diagnostic tests

I. Dental evaluation includes a written record of the assessment of all teeth using commonly acceptable dental notation, such as identified within this text
   A. The teeth are identified by numbers or symbols
      1. Universal tooth numbering system is the most widely accepted
      2. Permanent teeth are numbered #1–#32 and primary (or deciduous) teeth utilize the letters

A–T. Both permanent and primary identification systems begin in the maxillary right quadrant moving anteriorly to the maxillary left quadrant before progressing to the mandibular left quadrant and ending with the mandibular right quadrant

B. Missing teeth are determined by their clinical absence, radiographic findings, and the patient's reported dental history; are charted with a single vertical line or with an X through the tooth

C. Dental caries are determined by visual, explorer, and radiographic examination; carious lesion is charted in outline and/or colored-in using a red pencil

  1. G.V. Black's Carious Lesion Classification (by location)
     a. Class I—pits and fissures on occlusal, buccal, and lingual surfaces of posterior teeth and lingual of anterior teeth
     b. Class II—proximal surface of molars and premolars
     c. Class III—proximal surface of central and lateral incisors and cuspids
     d. Class IV—proximal surface including incisal edge of anterior teeth
     e. Class V—gingival one-third of facial or lingual surfaces of anterior or posterior teeth
     f. Class VI—cusp tips on molars, premolars and cuspids

  2. Bacterial Influence
     a. Dental caries is caused by *Streptococcus Mutans*, lactobacilli, and *Actinomyces viscosus* bacteria
     b. Enamel caries can begin in the presence of an acidic environment of a pH of 5.0 or less
     c. Root surface caries have an increased incidence in patients over age 65 due to areas of recession, lack of salivary flow, and lack of fluoride; evidence exists that *Actinomyces viscosus* plays an important role in root caries formation

D. Restorations (Fig. 11–1)
  1. Tooth colored restorations may be acrylic, composite resin, glass ionomer cements or porcelain
     a. Composite resins can be placed on anterior or posterior teeth; the material is placed in the preparation, and the material is cured by visible (blue) light; are charted by outlining, shading and noting as "C", CR", "GIC" or "R"
     b. Acrylic jackets are crowns and are charted by outlining, shading and noting as "AJC"
     c. Porcelain is used to fabricate a crown, inlay, or veneer; charted by outlining, shading and noting as "PJC", "PI", or "Ven", respectively; if metal is used as a substructure on the crown, it is noted "PFM" for porcelain-fused-to-metal

  2. A temporary restoration is placed on or in the tooth for a short period of time; is made of cement, preformed aluminum crowns, or chairside-made acrylic crown; is charted by outlining, shading and noted as "T"

  3. A sealant is a resin (clear or tinted) that is chemically or physically bonded to the occlusal pits and fissures of posterior teeth; it is charted by outlining, shading and noting as "S" or "SL"

  4. An amalgam is an alloy commonly used to restore Class I, II, and V dental caries; it is charted by outlining, shading and noting as "A"

  5. A metal casting is a restoration made from a wax pattern of the tooth preparation; depending on the metal content, it is classified as high noble metal, noble metal, or predominately base metal (non-precious); the later is used only for full crowns.
     a. Full high noble, noble and base metal crowns are charted by outlining, shading and noting as "FGC" or GC"
     b. Three-quarter crowns are charted by outlining, shading and noting as ¾GC
     c. An onlay (covers at least one cusp tip) is charted by outlining, shading and noting as "GO"
     d. An inlay (lies between the cusps of the teeth) is charted by outlining, shading and noting as "GI"
     e. A pontic is the part of a bridge that replaces a missing tooth; it is charted by outlining and shading the crown portion of the tooth; a vertical line or an "X" is drawn on the root; double horizontal lines are drawn to abutments (crowns adjacent to the pontic that support the bridge), and abutment crowns are outlined/shaded

  6. A gold foil is a restoration that is condensed or packed into a preparation; it is charted by outlining, shading and noting as "GF"
     a. Cannot withstand heavy occlusal wear because it is a soft material
     b. Seldom used, due to technically demanding and time intensive placement; it may be used as Class I, II, III, IV, V or VI restoration.

  7. An implant is surgically placed into the bone of the jaw. After healing, a prosthesis (crown, bridge, or denture) is constructed over the implant; to chart, an "X" is marked on the root(s) of the tooth/teeth involved, the prosthesis is drawn in and the implant is noted as "I"

E. Other items to be charted
  1. A carious lesion is new decay on a virgin tooth surface; charted by outlining and shading in red
  2. Recurrent caries is new decay around a previously placed restoration; charted by outlining restoration in red

Dental and Periodontal Charting

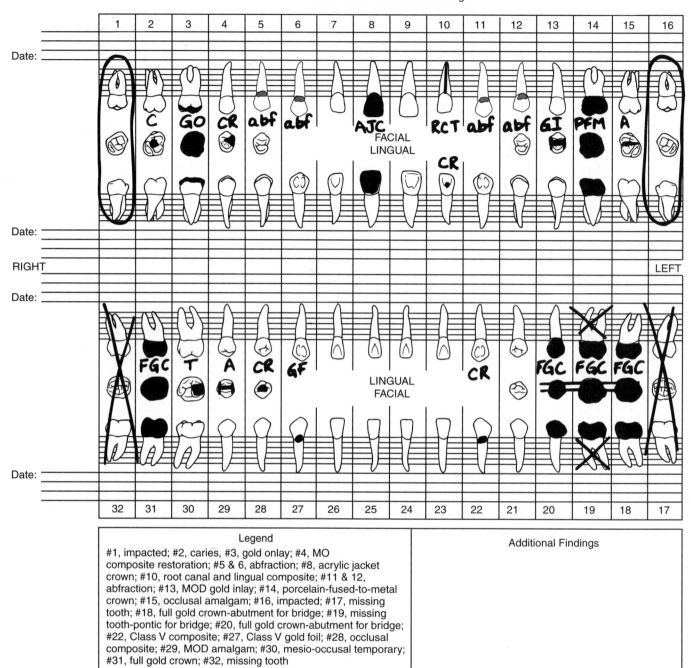

Figure 11.1 Dental charting. Anatomic charting of the permanent dentition, including missing teeth, restored teeth, carious lesions, and additional notations.

3. An overhang is an extension of restorative material beyond the confines of the cavity preparation; its extra bulk makes oral hygiene difficult in the area and may lead to periodontal irritation; is noted with an "O" or "OH" drawn in anatomically (is an example of an iatrogenic restoration)

4. A missing tooth may be one that has never formed (congenitally missing) or has been extracted; is charted with an "X" or a single vertical line

5. Decalcification is an area on the tooth that has started to demineralize; is chalky and soft; note as "decal"; may be shaded in

6. Hypocalcification, or enamel hypoplasia, is an area on the tooth that has not completely calci-

fied; is white or yellow (exposed dentin) in color (pitting may be present); caused by trauma or high fever during tooth formation; especially common in maxillary anterior teeth that developed below a traumatized primary tooth; called Turner's tooth or spot; is noted as "hycal"

7. A supernumerary tooth is an extra tooth; it can be drawn in its general location and is noted as "Su"

8. Abrasion is mechanical wearing of the tooth by a foreign object or substance, other than by mastication; typically caused by aggressive brushing or oral habits like opening pins with one's teeth or biting on a pen; is charted by outlining, shading and noted as "abr"

9. Abfraction is an area at the cervical one third of the tooth that appears as a V-shaped notch; current research associates this defect with occlusal forces; is charted by outlining, shading and noted as "abf"

10. Attrition is the loss of tooth structure caused by tooth-to-tooth contact on occlusal and incisal surfaces; due to excessive horizontal forces such as bruxing and grinding; is charted by outlining, shading and noting with a horizontal line across the affected portion of teeth

11. Erosion is chemical wear of the teeth; it is caused by acid substance (sucking on lemons, frequent vomiting associated with bulimia or acid reflux); it involves several teeth and damage is over a broad surface; the area is bracketed and marked "Ero"

12. Malposed teeth are located out of normal position in the dental arch; it is caused by lack of space or unusual eruption of a tooth; rotated teeth are marked with an arrow pointing towards the surface rotated (usually marked across the facial); teeth in lingual version are noted with arrow pointing from incisal edge away from the facial aspect; teeth in labial version are noted by an arrow pointing toward the coronal aspect of the tooth

13. A fractured tooth is usually the result of some type of trauma; it can be confirmed by using radiograph, illumination, and/or patient's reported history; is noted with a red line that resembles the fracture configuration

14. Ankylosed teeth have roots that are fused to the underlying bone; common on first and second primary molars; generally appear lower than the occlusal plane; sounds hollow when tapped; is noted as "ankl"

15. An open contact is lack of proximal contact between two teeth; due to periodontal disease, unrestored carious lesion, iatrogenic dentistry, or discrepancies in the alignment of the permanent dentition; causes food impaction resulting in increased caries and periodontal irritation; an open contact at the midline is called a diastema; mark with two parallel lines between teeth involved

16. An unerupted permanent tooth, if completely unerupted, is circled entirely; if partially erupted, only that portion that is not exposed to the oral cavity is circled (common with 3rd molars)

17. A full or partial denture is a removable prosthetic appliance; missing teeth are charted with vertical lines and the area the appliance replaces is bracketed; is labeled "PUD" (partial upper denture), "PLD" (partial lower denture), "CUD" (complete upper denture), or "CLD" (complete lower denture) (Fig. 11–2)

18. A root canal is when the pulp tissue has been removed from the tooth (endodontically treated); to chart, place a vertical line through root of tooth and label as "RC"

19. Fusion is the union of two tooth buds involving the dentin along the entire tooth, root or crown; each having separate pulp canals (most common with anterior teeth); is charted by making special note on chart

20. Dilaceration is a distortion of a tooth's root and crown linear relationship usually caused by trauma; is charted by making special note on chart

21. Gemination is the splitting of a single tooth germ; generally having a single root and pulp canal (most common on anterior teeth); is charted by making special note on chart

22. Dens in Dente occurs when an enamel organ is invaginated internally during tooth development (most common on maxillary lateral incisors); can be observed as a tooth-within-a-tooth on radiograph; is charted by making special note on chart

F. Stains are discolorations of teeth.

1. Extrinsic stains occur on the external surface of the tooth and can be removed by scaling and polishing; occur in a variety of colors:
   a. Yellow is due to heavy plaque buildup
   b. Green (at cervical area) is due to poor oral hygiene; can becomes intrinsic to underlying decalcification; difficult to remove; avoid heavy scaling or polishing due to decalcification
   c. Black or black-line is due to iron compounds from oral fluids that get embedded in plaque; found in clean mouths
   d. Tobacco stain is brownish to black in color; consistent with patient history of tobacco use; can become intrinsic
   e. Orange stain is rare; associated with chromogenic bacteria

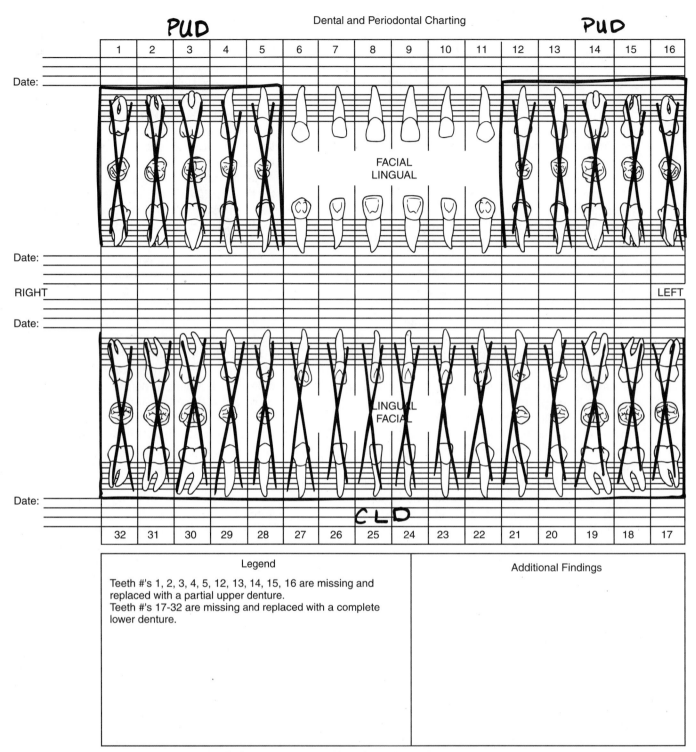

Dental and Periodontal Charting

PUD   PUD

FACIAL
LINGUAL

Date:

Date:

RIGHT   LEFT

Date:

LINGUAL
FACIAL

Date:

CLD

Legend	Additional Findings
Teeth #'s 1, 2, 3, 4, 5, 12, 13, 14, 15, 16 are missing and replaced with a partial upper denture. Teeth #'s 17-32 are missing and replaced with a complete lower denture.	

Figure 11.2 Dental charting of partially edentulous dentition. Anatomic charting that demonstrates bracketing of teeth that are included in the partial, as well as restored teeth, missing teeth, carious lesions, and additional notations.

f. Food stain is tan to dark brown and caused by tea, coffee, colas, vegetables, fruits, nuts, and candies.

g. Drug stain is brown or gray and caused by chlorhexidine use, stannous fluoride, and some antibiotics (e.g., tetracycline).

h. Gray-green stain is associated with marijuana use and appears on cervical third of labial surface.

i. Metallic stain varies in color and is due to ingestion of industrial dust and various foods and water.

2. Endogenous intrinsic stain occurs within the tooth structure.
   a. Fluorosis is white or brown spots, milky opalescence, and in extreme cases, pitting/mottling are possible and is due to excess fluoride intake during tooth development.
   b. Tetracycline stain is yellow/brown or gray/black and is due to ingestion of tetracycline during tooth development.
   c. Traumatized/infected pulp is gray/black and is due to blood leaching into dentin.
   d. Genetic/systemic anomalies
      1) Hypocalcification (white opacities)
      2) Amelogenesis imperfecta (white opacities, pitting)
      3) Dentinogenesis imperfecta (bluish, translucent appearance)
      4) Dentin dysplasia (primary teeth, bluish, translucent appearance)
      5) Porphyria (dark yellow/brown, all hard tooth structures effected)
3. Exogenous intrinsic stain is caused by environmental influences that result in intrinsic (internal) stain.
   a. Caries is white/brown/black and caused by acid-producing plaque.
   b. Pulp necrosis is yellow/black or gray and is due to pulp trauma.
   c. Restorative materials are gray/black and are the result of restorative material (amalgam, pins, posts) showing through enamel.
   d. Fluoride is brown or gray and is due to excessive use of topical stannous fluoride.
   e. Pulpitis is pink and is due to inflammation and internal bleeding within the pulp chamber.
   f. A tooth with internal resorption can also appear pink.

II. Occlusal Evaluation
   A. Defines the contact relationship of the maxillary and mandibular teeth when the teeth are fully closed.
   B. Angle's classification is the most widely used system to describe the relationship of the permanent or primary teeth when they are in centric relation (the most posterior position of the mandibular jaw) (Fig. 11–3)
      1. Class I is the mesognathic position of the permanent teeth; the facial profile is flat, and the chin is in same plane as forehead.
         a. Maxillary arch is larger and facial cusp tips of maxillary teeth lie on facial side of mandibular teeth.
         b. Mesial buccal cusp of maxillary first molar lies in line with the buccal groove of the mandibular first molar.
         c. Maxillary cuspid lies in the facial embrasure of the mandibular first premolar and cuspid.

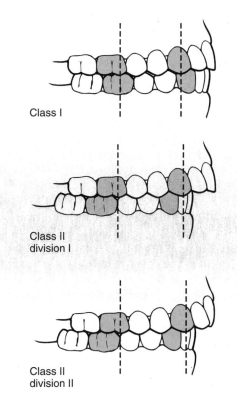

Figure 11.3 Angle's classification of normal occlusion and malocclusion. Class I occlusion: mesognathic positioning of the permanent teeth. Class II division I: retrognathic positioning of the permanent teeth, the mandibular incisors retruded, and the maxillary incisors protruded. Class II division II occlusion: retrognathic positioning of the permanent teeth, the mandibular incisors retruded with laterals more forward than the centrals, and maxillary incisors retruded. Class II occlusion: pronathic positioning of the mandibular jaw.

   d. Interproximal spaces coincide only at the midline.
      2. Class II is the retrognathic position of the permanent teeth; the facial profile is convex, and the chin is retruded.
         a. The mesial buccal cusp of the maxillary first molar lies at least one cusp width mesial of the buccal groove of the mandibular first molar.
         b. Maxillary cuspid lies mesial of the facial embrasure of the mandibular first premolar and cuspid
         c. Division I—mandibular incisors are retruded; maxillary incisors are protruded

d. Division II—mandibular incisors are retruded with the laterals more forward than the centrals; maxillary incisors retruded

3. Class III is the prognathic positioning of the mandibular jaw; facial profile is concave, chin is protruded or forward

   a. The mesial buccal cusp of the maxillary first molars lies at least one cusp width distal of the mandibular first molar buccal groove

   b. Maxillary cuspid lies distal of the facial embrasure of the mandibular first premolar and cuspid

C. Malrelationships

1. Anterior crossbite occurs when the maxillary incisors are lingual to the mandibular incisors

2. Posterior crossbite occurs when the maxillary posterior teeth are lingual or facial to their ideal position (buccal or lingual to the maxillary arch)

3. Edge-to-edge bite occurs when no vertical overlap is present (incisal edge of maxillary teeth meet the incisal edge of mandibular teeth); overbite is 0 mm

4. Open bite is lack of incisal or occlusal contact or overlap between maxillary and mandibular teeth; usually canines, laterals, and centrals

5. Overbite is the vertical overlap between maxillary and mandibular anterior teeth.

   a. Normal overbite is 2–3 mm.

   b. Measure the vertical overlap with a periodontal probe and record in mm; another less detailed way to describe is to determine overlap as slight (overlap in the incisal one third), moderate (overlap in the middle one third), or severe (overlap in the gingival one third)

   c. Over closed, deep bite, or severe overbite are terms used when maxillary incisors overlap into the gingival one third of the mandibular incisors.

6. Overjet is the horizontal distance between maxillary and mandibular incisors.

   a. Normal overjet is 2–3 mm.

   b. Measured as the horizontal distance between the linguals of maxillary anterior teeth and facials of mandibular anterior teeth with a periodontal probe.

7. Labioversion is when a tooth lies labial to its normal position.

8. Linguoversion is when a tooth lies lingual to its normal position.

D. Occlusal evaluation of the primary dentition

1. A terminal plane or mesial step are preferred positioning, since the first permanent molars are guided into position by the distal surface of the primary second molars (Fig. 11–4)

a. A "terminal plane" position is when the maxillary second molars lie end-to-end with the mandibular second primary molars.

b. A "mesial step" is when the maxillary second primary molars are at least a cusp width forward of the mandibular second primary molars.

c. A "distal step" is when the maxillary second primary molars are at least a cusp width behind the mandibular second primary molars.

2. Tooth eruption usually begins between 4–6 months of age and is completed at 2½ to 3 years of age; variability often occurs.

3. Primate spaces are the developmental spaces between primary teeth and are usually located between maxillary lateral incisors and canines and between mandibular canines and first molars.

4. A deep overbite and overjet are often present.

E. Occlusal evaluation of the mixed dentition

1. Both primary and permanent teeth are present in the oral cavity (around 6 to 12 years of age).

2. Successional or succedaneous teeth replace primary teeth.

3. Accessional teeth erupt distal in the arch and do not replace any primary teeth.

4. Leeway space

   a. Sum width of the mesiodistal widths of the primary cuspids through the primary second molars

   b. Usually greater on the maxillary arch

   c. Enhances the development of a normal occlusion in the permanent dentition

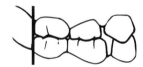

Terminal plane

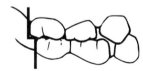

Mesial step

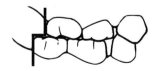

Distal step

Figure 11.4 Terminal plane of deciduous teeth. Lateral view of second primary molar terminal plane in the deciduous dentition.

d. Usually greater than the space needed for successional teeth

F. Occlusal evaluation of the permanent teeth
1. The eruption of all permanent teeth (except third molars) is usually completed by the age of 12.
2. Centric occlusion is the maximum intercuspation of the teeth; it is where the teeth fit "best" when jaws are fully closed.
3. Centric relation is the most retruded (unstrained) relationship of the mandible to the maxilla and is the most reproducible relationship between the maxillary and mandibular jaws and the position from which lateral excursions are made.
4. Protrusive excursion is the forward movement of the lower jaw until the mandibular anterior incisors meet the maxillary incisors edge-to-edge.
5. Lateral excursion is the movement of the mandible from centric occlusion to the right or left until the cuspids on the same side meet cusp tip-to-cusp tip.
6. Occlusal trauma
    a. Occurs when horizontal/oblique force to the long axis of the tooth causes a pathologic change to the periodontium
        1) Primary occlusal trauma occurs from excessive occlusal forces applied to teeth with normal supporting structures.
        2) Secondary occlusal trauma is caused when normal occlusal forces are exerted on a tooth with bone loss and inadequate alveolar bone support; tooth is unable to withstand normal occlusal forces; the following maybe observed:
            a) Widened PDL space
            b) Loss of lamina dura continuity
            c) Bone or root resorption
    b. May become a secondary factor to the progression of periodontal disease when periodontal disease is preexisting; trauma from occlusion does not cause gingivitis or periodontal disease
    c. Is reversible when etiologic factors are removed
        1) Malposed teeth
        2) Tooth-to-tooth habits (clenching, bruxing)
        3) Foreign object-to-tooth habits (holding pin or pipe between teeth, nail biting, finger/thumb sucking)
        4) Oral musculature (tongue thrusting, cheek or lip biting, mouth breathing, abnormal tongue position)
        5) Iatrogenic factors (poorly contoured restorations, improper fit of removable appliance)

III. Pulpal Evaluation for Inflammation or Necrosis
A. Diagnostic categories

1. Normal pulp will typically respond to pain stimulus in a manner consistent with similar teeth.
2. Reversible pulpitis exhibits a quick, sharp hypersensitive response to thermal stimulus that subsides with removal of the thermal stimuli.
3. Irreversible pulpitis is usually indicated by a lingering response to cold temperatures; may give spontaneous pain without stimulation or may be asymptomatic; pulpal damage is not repairable.
4. Necrotic pulp is indicated by an asymptomatic, nonvital tooth.

B. General testing technique
1. Decisions are based on a combination of all available data.
2. Recognize that an individual pulp test can give either a false-positive or false-negative response.
3. The goal is making a distinction between vital and nonvital pulps or determining the existence of an abnormal pulp.
4. Recognize that pulpal pathology can be of dental or periodontal origin.
5. Test both suspected teeth and control teeth (usually the adjacent teeth and the contralateral tooth) for comparison data.
6. Compare readings of all teeth tested to determine results, since the same types of teeth (e.g., molars) give similar readings in the same individual but may vary widely between individuals.
7. Record the results of all tests and other pulpal assessments in the patient's record.

C. Sources of data for pulpal diagnosis
1. Patient's subjective report of symptoms must always be confirmed with objective, clinical information and testing.
2. Intraoral and extraoral examination for evidence of tooth fracture, large carious lesion, large restoration, lymphadenopathy, swelling, pustule (or draining fistula), and tenderness.
3. Dental history related to tooth/teeth in question, as well as trauma, pain, mobility.
4. Radiographic examination by periapical film for pathologic radiolucency, PDL widening, fracture, caries, or deep restorations.
5. Palpation is used for testing for inflammation in the periapical tissues extending into the bone and mucosa.
    a. Technique
        1) Use bidigital palpation of bone in the area of the tooth apex
        2) Use palpation of control teeth for comparison
6. Percussion is used to test for changes in the periodontal ligament
    a. Technique

1) Use the end of a mirror handle or similar instrument to gently tap the teeth in both a vertical and horizontal direction; use only finger pressure rather than tapping with an instrument if the patient reports that the teeth are very sensitive.

2) Ask the patient if any of the percussed teeth feel different or more tender than the other teeth

b. Interpretation
    1) A positive test indicates inflammation in the PDL.
    2) Confirmation of diagnosis by other clinical tests is needed because inflammatory changes in the PDL are not always of pulpal origin.

7. Thermal tests for pulp vitality
  a. May involve use of either cold or hot thermal stimulus to test for pulpal response
    1) Cold test is most frequently used.
    2) Heat test is helpful when the only symptom is heat sensitivity and the offending tooth is not clearly identified.
  b. Cold test technique
    1) Use ice, carbon dioxide (dry ice), or a cotton-tipped applicator coated with refrigerant such as ethyl chloride.
    2) Place the cold agent on the tooth and observe any response.
    3) Remove the stimulus immediately on patient response; leave on the tooth a maximum of 10 seconds (20 seconds for teeth with full crown coverage).
  c. Hot test technique
    1) Lubricate selected teeth to prevent material from sticking.
    2) Heat a small amount of gutta percha or stopping material and place on the tooth.
    3) Remove stimulus immediately on patient response; leave on the tooth a maximum of 10 seconds (20 seconds for teeth with full crown coverage).
  d. Interpretation of test results
    1) An abnormal pulp status is indicated when there is a different response between the suspected and the control teeth.
    2) A diseased pulp is suspected when:
      a) There is no response.
      b) The response is excessively rapid (comparative).
      c) The response is lingering or prolonged (comparative).
      d) The response is of increasing intensity (comparative).
      e) Preexisting pain is alleviated when cold is applied.

8. Electric Pulp Test (EPT) for pulp vitality

a. Technique
    1) Contraindicated for use on patient who wears a cardiac pacemaker
    2) Place a small amount of conducting material on the EPT tip (usually toothpaste).
    3) Start with the control dial at the lowest number (lowest electric impulse), place the electrode on the tooth, have the patient touch the metal handle of the EPT with their fingers to complete the circuit.
    4) Depending on the equipment, the current will automatically increase; instruct the patient to release the handle of the EPT when they feel sensation or manually increase the current dial until the patient gives a prearranged signal, then lift the EPT tip from the tooth.

b. Interpretation of test results is generally all or none
    1) If the patient responds at low electric stimulus level the tooth is vital.
    2) If the patient fails to respond, the tooth is nonvital.
    3) Differing response levels do not indicate different stages of pulp degeneration.

Periodontal Evaluation

Periodontal evaluation is the examining of the soft and hard tissues surrounding the tooth structure. A primary function of the dental hygienist is to help the patient maintain a healthy periodontium by educating the patient about gum disease and treating disease involving these supporting structures of the teeth. Periodontal charts used to document the patient's existing periodontal status include 6-pocket depth readings for each tooth, plus notation of free gingival margin (recession), attachment levels, furcations, and mobility.

I. Healthy Periodontium
  A. Parts of the periodontium (Fig. 11–5)
    1. Free gingival margin is the most coronal aspect of the gingival margin that surrounds the tooth.

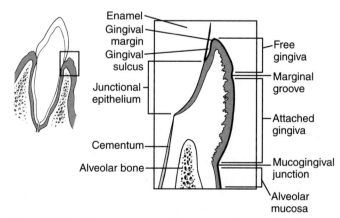

Figure 11.5 Components of the normal periodontium.

2. Free gingiva is composed of stratified, keratinized epithelial tissue and lies between the gingival margin and free gingival groove; its width is 0.5 to 1.5 mm (approximates the level of the base of the gingival sulcus).
3. Free gingival groove is the shallow linear groove that demarcates the free gingiva from the attached gingiva.
4. Attached gingiva is composed of stratified, keratinized epithelial tissue firmly bound to the underlying cementum and alveolar bone; the masticatory mucosa is measured from the free gingival margin to the mucogingival junction; stippling is present in health.
5. Mucogingival junction is the scalloped line that marks the connection between the alveolar mucosa and attached gingiva.
6. Alveolar mucosa is the moveable tissue loosely attached to the underlying bone; it is attached by frena, a band of tissue that attaches a more fixed tissue to a more moveable tissue that may pull or displace tissue when the attached gingival margin is narrow or missing.
7. Gingival sulcus is the space or crevice between the tooth and the free gingiva; its base is composed of epithelium and is not keratinized; the desired depth is 0.5 mm to 3 mm (average depth is 1.8 mm).
   a. Boundaries
      1) inner: tooth surface (enamel and/or cementum)
      2) outer: sulcular epithelium
      3) base: coronal margin of attached tissue, which is the depth of the sulcus or bottom of the pocket
8. Col is the depression between the lingual and facial papilla; consists of non-keratinized tissue that is more susceptible to inflammation (the site of initial periodontal infection); its shape conforms to the shape of the interproximal space
9. Interdental papilla is the tissue that occupies the interdental space between two adjacent teeth; its tip and lateral borders are marginal tissue, continuous with the free gingiva; the center of the papilla consists of attached gingiva; its shape is determined by the amount of interproximal space created by the contact point of adjacent teeth; pointed in the anterior and flatter and wider in the posterior
10. Junctional epithelium or epithelial attachment is the cuff-like band of tissue composed of nonkeratinized, stratified squamous epithelium which is continuous with the sulcular epithelium of the gingival sulcus; it is only a few cells thick at the apical end and widens at its junction with the sulcular epithelium; it is 0.25 mm to 1.35 mm in length

B. Clinical description of healthy periodontium
1. Color is uniform pale to coral pink from the mucogingival attachment to the gingival margin; may be pigmented with melanin which is related to complexion and race
2. Contour and size includes free gingival margins that fit snugly and follow curved lines around the necks of the teeth, papilla are knife-edged, pointed and fill the embrasure space
3. Consistency is firm and resilient
4. Surface texture of attached gingiva is usually stippled due to rete pegs which connect it to the underlying tissue; free gingiva is smooth tissue not bound to underlining tissue
5. Bleeding and exudate are not present
6. The position of the gingival margin is located 1 to 2 mm above the CEJ.

II. Diseased Periodontium
A. Signs of inflammation
1. Acute inflammation
   a. Appears bright red due to dilation of blood vessels and proliferation of blood cells.
   b. Begins in the area of the interdental papilla (initial site is often the col).
   c. Tissue is swollen and edematous in early stages.
   d. Consistency is spongy and soft; tissue indents easily when pressed and hangs away from tooth; there is loss of stippling causing a smooth and shiny look.
   e. Increased infiltration of fluid and inflammatory elements into tissue cells.
   f. Bleeds easily; bleeding on probing is the most objective method of assessing acute inflammation and can identify patients at risk for disease progression.
   g. Suppuration is a sign of acute inflammation and infection; exudate may appear clear, white, or yellow depending on its composition of white blood cells and inflammatory debris.
2. Chronic inflammation
   a. Appears dark red to bluish-red magenta
   b. When extremely chronic will appear fibrotic and near normal in color.
   c. Interdental papilla appears flattened, blunted, or cratered; gingival margins may be rolled; clefts, and festoons may be present.
   d. Consistency is tough and fibrotic with a leathery or hard, nodular-like surface texture.
   e. Bleeding may not be present and is not as obvious as with acute inflammation.
B. Bacterial plaque (causative agent)
1. Composition

a. Acquired pellicle, an amorphous, acellular organic membrane that forms on the tooth within minutes of its complete removal; it provides a highly insoluble coating or barrier against acids and is easily stained by food, chemicals, and chromogenic bacteria.

b. An organized matrix of microorganisms that changes composition with maturity and organic and inorganic solids.

2. Formation
   a. Pellicle formation begins immediately after tooth is completely clean.
   b. Bacterial colonies form layers and continue to multiply.
   c. A matrix forms from saliva and gingival exudate; polysaccharides, glucans, fructan, and levans contribute to the adhesion of plaque to the tooth surface.

3. Maturation
   a. Plaque in a recently cleaned mouth contains leukocytes, epithelial cells, and a few gram positive cocci—*Streptococcus sanguis* and *S. mutans*
   b. Plaque that is 2–7 days old is predominantly cocci with increasing numbers of filamentous bacteria; rods begin to form; leukocytes are present.
   c. Plaque that is 7–14 days old has vibrios and spirochetes; white blood cells increase in numbers and gram-negative anaerobic bacteria increase; signs of gingival inflammation are observable.

4. Association with disease
   a. Attached subgingival plaque is associated with root caries, calculus formation, and adult periodontitis; composed mostly of gram-positive rods and cocci, some gram-negative rods and cocci, gram-negative bacteria and some filaments.
   b. Loosely or unattached subgingival plaque is associated with rapidly progressive periodontal disease; composed of predominately gram-negative rods and cocci, motile organisms and spirochetes.

c. Combination of bacterial plaque and host response to periodontal pathogens influences initiation and progression of periodontal disease (Table 11–3).

d. Microbes, diet, host factors, and time interact to cause dental caries; *S. mutans* and lactobacillus found in plaque form lactic acid; lactic acid causes demineralization of the enamel

5. Mineralization
   a. Results in development of calculus deposits on tooth enamel and cementum, restorations, and prosthetic appliances and is classified by location, either supragingival or subgingival.
   b. Acts as an attachment mechanism for new bacterial plaque
   c. Characteristics
      1) Supragingival calculus derives its minerals from saliva, is white to yellow in color; can be flat or bulky in shape, and is more easily viewed with transillumination and compressed air.
      2) Subgingival calculus derives its minerals from gingival (crevicular fluid) and inflammatory exudate, is generally darker-colored from blood pigments (green-brown-black), can be of any size and shape, and is assessed by form, amount and tenacity

C. Clinical evaluation
   1. Gingival color, contour, size, consistency, and surface texture observed for abnormalities
   2. Radiographs assessed for bone loss, widening of the periodontal ligament space, thinning or loss of definition in the lamina dura, and furcation involvement
      a. In healthy periodontium, the interproximal bone is 1 mm apical to CEJ, the lamina dura is dense, radiopaque, and continuous; there is no furcation involvement.
      b. In diseased periodontium, there is horizontal and/or vertical bone loss, a widened PDL space, and furcation involvement (radiolu-

---

TABLE 11.3 Major Bacterial Species Associated with Periodontal Disease

Gingivitis	Adult Periodontitis	Localized Juvenile Periodontitis
Streptococcus sp	*Streptococcus* sp	*Actinobacillus actinomycetemcomitans*
Actinomyces sp	*Actinomyces* sp	*Prevotella intermedia*
Fusobacterium sp	*Fusobacteium* sp	
Treponema denticola	*Treponema denticola*	
Prevotella intermedia	*Wolinella recta*	
	Porphyromonas gingivalis	

cent); the tooth may have pulpal complications, as well as periodontal pathology.
  c. Limitations
    1) A three-dimensional object is projected on to a two-dimensional film, resulting in less detail.
    2) Buccal and lingual bone is difficult to see through the more dense tooth structure.
    3) Artifacts may be mistaken for pathology.
    4) Angulation of exposure may distort actual bone level.
    5) Exposure and processing errors may decrease the quality of the radiograph.
    6) When bone loss becomes apparent on radiographs, as much as 20% of bone may have already been destroyed.
3. Probe depths of epithelial sulcus from the free gingival margin to the base of the pocket
  a. Depths are recorded on a periodontal chart and include six readings per tooth (three on facial and three on lingual); note bleeding for each reading; note other periodontal concerns such as recession, furcation, reduced attached gingiva, mobility.
  b. Gingival pocket or pseudopocket is formed by enlargement of the gingiva that causes the margin of the gingiva to proliferate in a coronal direction; there is no apical migration; the pocket is suprabony and reversible with good home care and professional intervention.
  c. Periodontal pockets form as a result of disease that causes the junctional epithelium to migrate apically allowing destruction of the attachment mechanism; involves deeper periodontal structures: cementum, periodontal ligament, and bone; in suprabony pockets, the junctional epithelium is below the CEJ but above the crest of the alveolar bone; in infrabony pockets, the junctional epithelium is below the crest of the alveolar bone.
4. Recession, note the level of the marginal gingiva if it is apical to the CEJ, in millimeters, using a periodontal probe.
5. Furcation involvement, classified by extent of bone destruction
  a. Class I: detect concavity but cannot enter it, radiographs show no radiolucency.
  b. Class II: probe can enter furcation but cannot extend through it, radiographs show slight radiolucency or furcation arrow for maxillary proximal furcas.
  c. Class III: probe can pass between facial and lingual, radiographs show obvious radiolucency or furcation arrow for maxillary proximal furcas.

  d. An alternative classification system subdivides class III into 2 categories, furca covered by tissue and furca not covered by tissue
6. Note the width of attached gingiva when it is less than 1 mm or is nonexistent.
7. Mobility: classified by extent of horizontal and vertical movement
  a. Class I: tooth moves up to 1 mm in any direction
  b. Class II: tooth moves more than 1 mm in any direction but cannot be depressed.
  c. Class III: tooth moves more than 1 mm and can be depressed in the socket
D. Additional diagnostic tests that can be used to assess periodontal health or disease are culture analysis and antibiotic sensitivity, DNA probes, enzyme immunoassays (enzymes tested may be derived from the host or the periodontal pathogens), and immunologic tests.

III. Interpretation of the Periodontal Evidence: See Chapter 12
IV. Documentation and Referral
  A. Documentation protocol
    1. Record probing depths, bleeding points, recession, furcations, mobility, reduced attachment level, and bone level.
    2. Determine periodontal status (healthy or AAP periodontal type).
    3. Explain the periodontal status and recommend treatment options to the patient.
    4. Record the patient's response and willingness to proceed with treatment.
    5. Failure to diagnose and properly treat periodontal disease is a leading cause of malpractice lawsuits.
  B. Referral protocol
    1. Establish referral guidelines for the dental office.
    2. Explain the need for special care to the patient.
    3. Assist the patient in scheduling an appointment with a specialist.
    4. Communicate with the specialist and patient to insure continuity of care.
    5. If patient does not follow through with treatment:
      a. Discuss and document reasons for noncompliance.
      b. Answer any additional questions patient may have.
      c. Continue to see patient for regular tissue management appointments.
      d. Monitor periodontal status and continue to encourage patient to seek additional care.
      e. Confirm patient understanding of consequences of noncompliance.

Management of Dental Hygiene Care

Promoting health and disease prevention is a primary objective of the dental hygienist and is most successful when the patient is involved.

Motivation

Motivation is defined as the readiness to act, or the driving force behind our actions. Motivation is influenced by a patient's perception of their responsibility for their own health. Internally motivated people believe they can influence their own lives (they are responsible for success or failure), have control over their own health, and will be motivated to change long-term health behaviors. Externally motivated people feel they have little control over life events, tend to believe in fate (feel they are not responsible for their health), require more supervision and direction, and need an outside source to reinforce positive health beliefs.

Self-Perception of Need or Needs Theories

Patient needs are identified through interview and observation; focusing on a patient's expressed chief concern or complaint helps identify patient's motivational force. Needs theories are useful in determining the motivational process. Maslow's Needs Hierarchy demonstrates that as one need is met, a person is motivated to satisfy the next need in the hierarchy; safety, love, and ego are the needs most often associated with motivating a patient. Basic physical safety needs must be met first (first two levels). Love and belonging, feeling a part of a group, and being a part of a significant relationship are typically met at the third level. Self esteem and ego or a belief in one's self is the fourth level. Self-actualization development, fulfillment of one's ambitions and life's goals, and realizing one's potential is the fifth level.

The dental hygiene human needs conceptual model incorporates concerns about the patient and their environment, specific health and oral health needs, and dental hygiene actions (Table 11–4).

Factors That Influence Motivation

I.   Personal and social needs are major factors in motivating change.

II. Unmet needs serve as motivation for change.

III. Social acceptance and peer group approval are the most common motivating forces and are stronger motivating factors than health promotion.
   A. Stain and plaque accumulated on the teeth affect appearance and serve as motivation for removal.
   B. Malador is socially unacceptable and serves as strong motivation for self-care.

IV. Pain is only an immediate motivation and does not serve as long-term motivation.

V.   Sincerity, concern, and rapport with the health care provider are directly related to the level of motivation for self-care by the patient.

VI. Dental health is frequently neglected due to the nature of the disease being nonthreatening; once the disease becomes more threatening, the patient will perceive a need for action.

VII. Age and level of health belief affects action.
   A. Children: gear motivational efforts toward parent who assists child with oral hygiene tasks

TABLE 11.4 Dental Hygiene Human Needs	
Human Need	**Definition**
Safety	Need to experience freedom from harm or danger related to body structure and environment.
Freedom	Need to be free from physical and emotional discomforts.
Wholesome body image	Need for a positive mental representation of one's own body boundary and how it looks to others.
Skin and mucous membrane—integrity of the head and neck	Need to have an intact and functioning covering of the person's head and neck area.
Nutrition	Need to ingest proper foods required for growth, repair, and maintenance of body.
Biologically sound dentition	Need for intact teeth and restorations to provide for adequate function and esthetics.
Conceptualization and problem solving	Need to grasp ideas to make sound judgments about one's life.
Appreciation and respect	Need to be acknowledged for achievement, worth, service, or merit and receive approval by others.
Self-determination and responsibility	Need of purpose about one's self and accountability for one's behavior.
Territoriality	Need to maintain control of and defend one's own space.
Value system	Need for freedom to develop one's own sense of importance.

Adapted from Darby and Walsh, 1994.[9]

B. Adolescents: gear motivational efforts towards social acceptance

C. Adults: gear motivational efforts toward social acceptance, health maintenance, tooth retention, and cost factors

Communication

Communication is an essential component of managing oral hygiene care. It is continuous, inevitable, and irreversible; is conducted on several levels; and is influenced by the physical setting.

I. Nonverbal communication or behavior skills involve body orientation, posture, facial expressions, gestures, touch, distance/space, tone of voice, and hesitation.

A. The expressed message is 90% to 93% nonverbal.

B. The perceived message of nonverbal communication influences the relationship-building process between patient and health care provider.

C. Effective nonverbal communication connotes interest and involvement, aids in expression of thoughts and feelings, expresses the level of comfort and relaxation, and can give insight into the patient.

D. Body gestures

1. Hand gestures by the patient that give insight are white knuckle grasp, finger pointing, and extending the hand as a sign of welcome.

2. Crossed arms may indicate the patient feels defensive; arms open and relaxed at side may convey patient's willingness to accept information.

3. Voice signals include loudness, intonation or inflection, and can express anger, fear, excitement and cooperation level.

II. Verbal communication involves language and listening skills of both the health care provider and the patient.

A. The health care provider's language should be kept simple, direct, and nonthreatening; use verbiage with meaning so patient understands the disease process and consequences.

B. Listening skills are necessary to achieve good comprehension of the patient's concerns, attitudes, and feelings, as well as their specific health beliefs.

C. Eye contact conveys that you are interested, listening, and fully attentive; it helps the patient relax and feel comfortable; clinician communication is enhanced when eye level is the same.

D. Head nodding and verbal "yes" aid in expressing involvement.

E. Feedback involves paraphrasing what the patient has said; it enhances open communication and allows for expression of thoughts and feelings and also gives the patient an opportunity to validate and/or correct the perception of their verbal and nonverbal behavior.

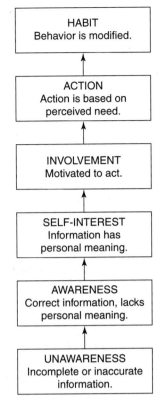

Figure 11.6 The learning ladder. (Modified from Harris and Christensen, 1997.[10])

F. Facilitative or cooperative communication is the give and take between patient and health care provider; it creates a harmonious relationship, builds rapport and gives a sense of empathy, respect, warmth, genuineness, and self-disclosure; it also enables the patient to be involved in the process of care and increases patient compliance.

III. Questioning techniques encourage the communication process.

A. Open-ended questions require an explanation or description—who, what, where, when, why, and how are excellent word choices to begin these questions.

B. Closed questions are also useful to move the conversation along and to get closure, confirmation, or agreement to an action—they require yes, no, or a simple nod of the head.

C. Answers to questions should not be judged; a patient must feel that his answers have value; a provider's acceptance of answers will encourage patient openness.

IV. Learning Principles

A. Learning ladder continuum (Figure 11–6)

B. Principles of instruction

1. Present small amounts of information

2. Organize teaching sessions logically and systematically

3. Use visual aids to enhance learning

4. Let the patient set the pace for learning

5. Present information at an appropriate age level

6. Supervise the patient's skill and habit development by involving the patient through return demonstrations

7. Provide immediate and specific feedback

C. Active participation requires the patient to set goals, fit behaviors into their daily schedule, and decide which dental cleaning aids they are willing to use.

　1. The fewer dental cleaning aids introduced, the greater the chance for compliance

　2. Use of dental cleaning aids should be reevaluated for need, compliance, and skill at maintenance visits

　3. Introducing additional dental cleaning aids should be considered only as skill and compliance are achieved with present aids

V. Planning Individualized Instruction

A. Assess patient needs.

　1. Ask the patient if they have any specific concerns, are experiencing any pain, and what they consider are their current dental needs.

　2. Evaluate the soft and hard tissues for pathology and document findings.

　3. Assess radiographs for pathology and document findings.

　4. Identify risk factors, such as smoking, diabetes, handicaps or disabilities, immunocompromising conditions, and stress.

　5. Identify the patient's health beliefs and dental IQ and apply to treatment planning.

　6. Determine patient's current oral hygiene techniques and effectiveness.

B. Establish a treatment plan by prioritizing needs and treatment.

　1. Plan strategies that account for the patient's dental IQ, health beliefs, and behavior.

　2. Build in reevaluation steps throughout treatment.

C. Implement individualized instruction by explaining the rationale and dental techniques to be utilized; give treatment options; explain needs, and answer questions, initiate oral hygiene techniques by the patient; and initiate treatment.

D. Evaluate treatment by observing and recording plaque levels, changes in tissue health, and skill performance of oral hygiene at each appointment; reinforce oral hygiene technique at subsequent appointments, modifying as needed, assessing the success of the treatment, and retreat as necessary; and document self-care progress/nonprogress in record.

VI. Oral Hygiene Devices and Self-Care Practice

A. Toothbrushes

　1. Manual brush selection and brushing technique

　　a. Choose a toothbrush head size that corresponds with the size of the patient's mouth and tooth accessibility.

　　b. Handles should be easy to grip with minimal slippage and rotation during use (larger handles increase grasp ability for patients with arthritis and other physical disabilities).

　　c. Selection of bristle

　　　1) Bristles ends should be rounded nylon filaments (least damaging to gingival tissues).

　　　2) Filament diameter determines the hardness or softness (thinner filaments are softer and more resilient).

　　　3) Nylon filaments are preferred over natural bristles because they are more resistant to bacterial accumulation, rinse and dry more easily, are durable and maintain their form; their ends are rounded and closed, which repels water and debris.

　　　4) Multitufted bristles support adjacent bristles, allowing for more cleaning action while being less traumatic to the gingival tissues.

　　d. Technique

　　　1) Use light-to-medium pressure to ensure removal of bacterial plaque.

　　　2) Develop a sequence to ensure brushing of all teeth and tooth surfaces.

　　　3) Brush two to three times per day for two to three minutes.

　　e. Tooth brushing methods

　　　1) Sulcular or Bass method

　　　　a) Most widely accepted for removing plaque at gingival margin

　　　　b) Filaments are directed apically at a 45-degree angle, and the brush is vibrated back and forth with a very short small motion; keep the brush tip engaged in the sulci.

　　　　c) Is an excellent method for all patients.

　　　2) Roll method

　　　　a) Is used for removing plaque at the gingival margin and clinical crown.

　　　　b) Filaments are directed apically and then rolled towards the occlusal surface, forcing the filaments interproximally.

　　　　c) Is a good technique for children, although it is easy to miss areas if the brush is improperly placed.

　　　3) Modified Stillman's Method

　　　　a) Uses a vibratory motion to stimulate the tissue while removing bacterial plaque at the gingival margin; the addition of the roll stroke removes the plaque from the buccal and lingual surfaces.

   b) Bristles are directed apically at the gingival margin and a roll stroke and vibratory motion are used.

   c) Is a good technique for all patients.

4) Charter's method

   a) Is most useful for removing plaque that accumulates around orthodontic bands and brackets, fixed prostheses, and recent surgical wounds.

   b) Uses a vibratory motion as the bristles are directed occlusally with the sides of the bristles contacting the gingival margin and tooth surface.

5) Circular method

   a) Is used for plaque removal on the clinical crown.

   b) Uses a rotational motion on the buccal and lingual surfaces.

   c) Good first method for young children, not recommended for adults.

6) Horizontal/scrub method

   a) Is used for plaque removal on the buccal, lingual, and occlusal surfaces.

   b) Uses a horizontal scrubbing motion.

   c) Is generally recognized as detrimental to gingival tissues causing abrasion and recession.

2. Powered brushes are as effective as manual when utilized properly.

  a. Brush motion can be rotational, counter-rotational or oscillating counter-rotational, or sonic.

  b. Technique is product dependent and similar to manual techniques.

   1) Bristle placement is at a 45-degree angle to the gingival margin.

   2) Automatic timer and audible cues help the patient to brush for a specified amount of time (usually 2 minutes) and are useful in encouraging a thorough cleaning.

   3) Smaller brush heads are site specific and require more time to completely clean all teeth.

  c. Recommended for patients with orthodontic appliances, malposed teeth, periodontal disease, arthritis and other grasping disabilities, and care givers (parents, hospital and nursing home personnel).

B. Tongue cleaning is important in reducing bacterial plaque accumulation and malodors caused by sulfa-producing bacteria.

1. Plastic tongue scrapers are commercially-available; use the scraper by placing it on the posterior portion of the tongue and pulling forward to "scrape" the bacterial coating off the tongue.

2. Toothbrushes are effective tools for removing this coating as well; the brush is placed on the posterior portion of the tongue and swept forward (4 to 5 times) to remove bacterial accumulation; brushing without a dentifrice may reduce the gag flex.

C. Interdental care

1. Floss is available in a variety of textures, thicknesses, and materials and should be used daily for effective plaque control.

  a. Types

   1) Unwaxed floss is commonly used by persons with few restorations and with normal contact tightness.

   2) Waxed or polytetrafluorethylene (PTE) coated floss is useful for persons with tight contacts, amalgam overhangs, or rough restorations.

   3) Tufted floss or yarn is excellent for large embrasures spaces and under orthodontic wires.

  b. Technique involves gently inserting the floss between the teeth, wrapping the floss snugly around each proximal tooth surfaces, and using an up and down motion from sulcus to contact to remove plaque.

   1) A floss handle is helpful for those with larger hands or one functional hand.

   2) Floss threaders can be used to get under bridges or orthodontic wires.

2. Interdental brushes are used to cleanse wide embrasures or furcations.

  a. Types

   1) Conical and tapered shaped brushes fixed to a wire and then inserted on a plastic handle.

   2) A single tuft brush with tapered or flat groups of filaments inserted on a plastic handle (also known as an end tuft brush).

  a. For most effective cleaning, use a brush slightly larger than the embrasure.

  b. Can further enhance effect of antimicrobial agent by delivering chemical into embrasure area with interdental brush.

3. Interdental tip can remove excess debris from embrasure area and is used to remove plaque in embrasure area and slightly below the gingival margin.

  a. A soft flexible rubber tip is ideal to adapt into the embrasure space and is less likely to cause trauma than a plastic tip.

  b. Technique involves using the tip to trace along gingival margin and move in and out of the embrasure space.

4. Toothpick in a holder (e.g., Perio-aid) is especially good for removing plaque in periodontal pockets or adjacent to orthodontic appliances.
   a. A round or square-round toothpick is placed in a plastic handle.
   b. Technique involves using the tip to trace along gingival margin and move back-and-forth in the embrasure space; for periodontal patients, the tip is placed on the tooth and traced into the col or furcation area; care is taken not to place excessive force on the gingival tissue; for orthodontic patients, the tip is placed on the tooth and traced around the orthodontic brackets and bands.
5. Wooden interdental cleaner (e.g., Stimudent) is used in areas where papillae are missing.
   a. Triangular shaped; the flat part of triangle is placed toward the tissue.
   b. A burnishing action is used against one side of the embrasure, then the other side.
6. Oral irrigators are used to reduce gingivitis, reduce plaque toxicity by altering microflora, and deliver antimicrobial agents.
   a. Supragingivally, a standard tip provides a steady, low-pressure, pulsating stream of water or other fluid agent to dislodge loosely adherent plaque at or slightly below the gingival margin; tip is directed at a 90-degree angle to the tooth at the gingival margin.
   b. Subgingivally, a sulcus tip (e.g., Pic Pocket) provides a pulsating, low-pressure stream of water or chemotherapeutic agent to the sulcus or periodontal pocket; can dislodge unattached or loosely adherent plaque in the pocket or sulcus; tip is directed at a 45-degree angle with the tip directed into the sulcus; gives deeper subgingival penetration of the water or antimicrobial agent.
D. Chemotherapeutic agents
   1. Dentifrices
      a. Components make the dentifrice effective, long-lasting, palatable, and safe (Table 11-5).
      b. Therapeutic agents added to dentifrices have specific purposes.
         1) Fluoride is added to increase remineralization of enamel, thereby reducing incidence of carious lesions.
         2) Soluble pyrophosphates are used as anticalculus or tartar control agents; they reduce supragingival calculus by changing and weakening the structure of the calculus crystal.
         3) Potassium nitrate, strontium chloride, and sodium citrate are minerals used to reduce dental hypersensitivity; they

TABLE 11.5	Basic Components of Dentifrices[11]
Components	**Amount (%)**
Detergent	1–2
Cleaning and polishing agents	20–40
Binder	1–2
Humectant	20–40
Flavoring	1–1.5
Water	20–40
Therapeutic agent	1–2
Preservative, sweetener, coloring agent	3

Adapted from Wilkins, 1994.[11]

work by causing precipitation or mineralization of the dentinal tubules.
         4) Triclosan is an antimicrobial agent used for the control of gingivitis.
         5) Poloxame 407 (nonionic foaming agent) is added to reduce soft tissue irritation but not resolve inflammation.
   2. Mouth rinses
      a. Components are added to make the rinses palatable, effective, and safe.
         1) Water
         2) Alcohol
         3) Flavoring agents
         4) Sweetener
         5) Active ingredient
            a) Oxygenating (cleansing and antimicrobial)
            b) Astringent (shrinks tissue)
            c) Anodynes (relieves pain)
         6) Buffering agent (relieves pain, reduces oral acidity, dissolves mucinous film)
         7) Deodorizing agent (reduces malador)
         8) Antimicrobial (reduces oral microbial count and bacterial activity)
      b. Types of rinses
         1) Antimicrobial
            a) Chlorhexidine is approved for use in the United States at a 0.12% concentration and is active against gram-positive and gram-negative organisms and fungi.
               (1) Has a prolonged bacteriocidal effect (substantivity).
               (2) Is recommended for short-term use.
               (3) Side effects include staining of teeth and tissues, bitter taste, burning sensation of mucosa, dry and sore mucosa, loss of taste, and tissue ulcerations.
            b) Stannous fluoride is used to reduce bacterial growth and adherence

properties; effective in reducing caries.

   c) Phenolic compounds are antimicrobial agents used to alter the bacterial cell wall (e.g., Listerine). Side effects include burning of mucosa and unpleasant strong taste.

2) Prebrushing rinse

   a) Most commonly used is Plax.

   b) Independent research shows no reduction in bacterial plaque.

   c) Active ingredient is sodium benzoate; not recommend for patients with sodium-restricted diets.

3) Oxygenating rinses

   a) Most commonly used are Amosan, Orthoflur, Oxyfresh, hydrogen peroxide.

   b) Research shows no effect on bacterial plaque.

   c) Short-term use intended for oral wound cleansing and soothing effects.

   d) Long-term use has shown serious side effects including carcinogenesis, tissue damage, ulcerations of the mucosa, hyperkeratosis, and black hairy tongue syndrome.

4) Sanguinarine

   a) Antiplaque agent is composed of benzophenathridine alkaloid

   b) Available as a mouth rinse and dentifrice (most effective when used in combination with one another)

   c) Interferes with bacterial glycolysis and binds to plaque to reduce adherence of microorganisms

   d) Not as effective as chlorhexidine or phenolic compounds

Clinical Case STUDY

Evelyn Haas, a 68-year-old woman, presents to the dental office with a history of Alzheimer's disease in middle stage, congestive heart failure, and pain on chewing in the mandibular left molar area. She wears upper and lower partial dentures. Evelyn's medications include Procardia and Lasix.

Clinical Case QUESTIONS

1. What are the common oral side effects of Ms. Haas' medications?
2. What are the common mental and physical impairments with middle-stage Alzheimer's disease?
3. Describe the procedures for professional cleaning of partial dentures.

4. Describe common oral manifestations seen in Alzheimer's patients.

Clinical Case RATIONALE

1. Nifedipine (Procardia) can cause gingival hyperplasia. Furosemide (Lasix) may contribute to xerostomia and its subsequent sequela.

2. Alzheimer's disease, a nonreversible dementia, impacts thinking, memory, and personality. Patient's in middle stage Alzheimer's experience disorientation, loss of coordination, restlessness and anxiety, language difficulties, sleep pattern disturbances, progressive memory loss, catastrophic reactions, and pacing.

3. To professionally clean partial dentures, place them in a zip-lock plastic bag with tartar- and stain-remover solution. Sonicate the bag with dentures in the ultrasonic bath for 15 minutes. Wash the partial dentures thoroughly with soap and rinse before returning them to the patient. Never use bleach to clean partial dentures as it can corrode the metal framework and clasps.

4. There are no specific oral manifestations seen with Alzheimer's patients; however, oral diseases do develop as Alzheimer's disease progresses. In the late stages of the disease, oral hygiene neglect, resultant decay, periodontal disease, and tissue trauma are common. Because the use of antidepressants is common in this population group, xerostomia can also contribute to oral diseases.

VII. Patients With Special Concerns

  A. Patients may present with a number of special oral conditions that need to be managed as part of comprehensive dental hygiene care.

  B. The following conditions need to be recognized, evaluated and treated appropriately by the dental hygienist, and patients need to be educated about their role in self care and disease prevention.

    1. Rampant caries

      a. Home fluoride use with OTC or prescription mouth rinses or brush-on or tray application of pastes or gels.

      b. Plaque removal with brush, floss, or other aids.

      c. Nutritional counseling to reduce the frequency of ingesting simple-sugar foods; e.g., decrease from three cans of sweetened, carbonated beverages daily to one can, and drink the beverage in 30 minutes, instead of over 3 hours.

      d. Close monitoring

        1) Evaluate patient's ability to remove plaque at 1-week, 1-month, and 3-month intervals.

2) Confirm home fluoride use at each appointment.

3) Have patient keep a diet diary for review at their next appointment.

4) Expose bitewing x-rays at more frequent intervals.

2. Tobacco cessation

a. Dental hygienist is responsible for providing information to encourage patients to quit smoking or using smokeless tobacco.

b. Tobacco cessation program should be available either on-site or by referral.

c. Educational and product information can be made available; e.g., brochures, videos, mint-leaf chew products

3. Dental prostheses and appliances

a. Prosthesis is an artificial replacement for a missing body part. A dental prostheses typically replaces one or more teeth.

1) Removable prostheses include full denture, overdenture with either retained natural teeth or implants, and removable partial denture and obturator.

2) Fixed prostheses include fixed partial denture (also called bridge), dental implant, and implant-supported complete denture (if it cannot be removed by the patient). Individual crowns are considered in this category.

b. Appliances are special devices designed for a specific function or to create a specific therapeutic outcome.

1) Removable appliances include removable orthodontic appliances, such as head gear, retainers, or occlusal splints.

2) Fixed appliances include fixed orthodontic appliances, such as bands, brackets, or palatal expander, periodontal splints, and space maintainers.

c. Prostheses and appliances are subject to accumulation of plaque, calculus, and stain. They need both daily cleaning by the patient and routine, professional maintenance care.

d. Teeth adjacent to or supporting either a removable or fixed prosthesis or appliance typically are more plaque retentive and hard to clean. These teeth are at higher risk for caries and gingival inflammation.

e. Soft tissues under removable prostheses and appliances are more prone to irritation and lesions. To prevent soft tissue damage, removable prostheses and appliances should be kept clean and left out of the mouth for some portion of each day, e.g., leave a denture out overnight.

f. Professional care of full and partial removable denture and orthodontic retainers.

1) The goal is the removal of plaque, calculus, and stain without changing the acrylic or metal surface.

2) One or more of the following cleaning methods is used: ultrasonic bath, careful scaling, polishing, use of a denture or other brush.

3) Special care is needed to prevent abrasions or wear on acrylic surfaces and to avoid bending or breaking partial clasps and retainer wires.

g. Professional care for fixed orthodontic appliances

1) The principals of debridement are the same but the brackets, wires, and ligatures require special adaptation and care.

2) Patients need personalized and often extensive instruction in plaque control methods in order to adapt to all areas of the teeth and appliances. Regular or special toothbrushes, oral irrigators, floss threaders, and toothpicks, with or without adapters, are often used.

3) A daily self-administered fluoride application is highly recommended to prevent decalcification and caries around bands and brackets.

4. The edentulous patient

a. Oral characteristics of the edentulous alveolar ridge

1) The majority of alveolar ridge resorption occurs in the first year.

2) Bone resorption is greater in the mandible.

3) The alveolar ridges continue to change (remodel) throughout life.

b. Reasons for an annual dental visit

1) Soft tissue examination for early identification of cancer or other oral condition(s).

2) Cleaning and maintenance of the denture.

3) Evaluation and reinforcement of good oral self care for both the denture and oral mucosa.

c. Oral lesions associated with denture wear

1) Localized denture sore

a) Red, inflamed or ulcerated appearance underneath or at the margins of the denture

b) Typical causes: trauma from an ill-fitting denture or rough denture surface

2) Generalized inflammation, denture stomatitis, or denture sore mouth

a) Generalized redness of tissue underlying the denture either with or without associated discomfort

b) Typical causes: poor denture hygiene; continuous denture wear; *Candida albicans* infection (once established the acrylic denture is an excellent reservoir for the microorganism); trauma from an ill-fitting denture, occlusion or parafunctional habits; reaction to denture material, inadequately removed cleansing agents, or a combination of these.

3) Papillary hyperplasia

a) A red, bumpy, or pebbly surface, usually located in the palatal vault.

b) Exact cause unknown but is often associated with poor hygiene, ill-fitting denture, and possibly *Candida albicans*.

4) Epulis fissuratum or denture irritation hyperplasia

a) Elongated, single, or multiple folds of fibrotic tissue at the denture border

b) Caused by long-term irritation from ill-fitting denture

5) Angular cheilitis

a) Fissures, ulcerations, or erythema at the corners of the mouth

b) Typically caused from lack of vertical dimension (overclosure), chronic moisture from drooling, *Candida albicans*, frequently associated with riboflavin deficiency

d. A denture needs to be replaced or relined periodically (7–10 years) as the supporting alveolar ridge changes.

e. Dentures should be left out of the mouth for some portion of every day so that the supporting mucosa can have a recovery period. The standard recommendation is to leave them out overnight.

f. Dentures should be permanently marked with the wearer's identification.

5. Infants

a. Infants should not be put to bed with bottle of milk or juice (plain water is good choice) or allowed to sip caries-potentiating fluids indiscriminately, especially once teeth begin erupting.

b. Educate parent about baby-bottle–tooth-decay (BBTD).

c. Instruct parent on the use of soft toothbrushes to brush gums and teeth of infant.

d. No toothpaste should be used.

e. First dental appointment is recommended within 6 months of eruption of first tooth or at one year of age.

6. Children

a. Use no larger than a pea-sized amount of toothpaste at each brushing to minimize fluoride consumption if swallowed.

b. Parent should be involved with brushing and flossing until small motor skills develop and child can become proficient with plaque removal.

c. Short attention span of child demands shorter dental appointments.

d. Explain procedure and equipment at a level a child can understand.

e. Special attention should be given to avoid swallowing fluorides during application as it may cause nausea or cause toxicity (in large doses).

7. Adolescents

a. To promote good hygiene practice, appeal to tooth appearance and acceptance from peers

b. Puberty gingivitis is prevalent during these years; educate teens on their role in self-care.

c. Orthodontic appliance common among this age group; special tools may include electric toothbrush, oral irrigator, tufted toothbrush, floss threaders, Superfloss, and additional fluoride (daily fluoride rinse, brush-on gel fluoride)

8. Pregnancy

a. There are no contraindications for dental hygiene treatment although several precautions are encouraged.

1) Schedule oral prophylaxis appointments during middle trimester for greatest comfort; first trimester is often associated with morning sickness, so patient may gag easily; during the third trimester, the size and position of the fetus may make supine position of the patient uncomfortable.

2) Radiographs can be safely taken at any time if the patient is thoroughly covered, front and back, with a lead apron; many clinicians avoid exposing the pregnant patient to radiation due to patient concerns and possible risk of lawsuit if the infant is born with deformity; reasonable approach is to avoid radiographs unless obvious discomfort or disease demands attention.

3) Pregnancy gingivitis is a local (one or few papilla) or generalized exaggerated response to plaque due to changing hormone levels; results in obvious pap-

illary overgrowth with redness, edema, and bleeding; is reversible when pregnancy ends; frequent oral prophylaxis (3 month) is recommended.

4) Education regarding dental myths: "losing a tooth for every child"; explain how adequate calcium intake during pregnancy will prevent loss of calcium from the bones, calcium is removed from bones before teeth

5) Education regarding early childhood dental care: discuss appropriate brushing and cleansing methods for infants and children, limited amounts of fluoridated toothpaste, need for systemic or supplemental fluoride in fluoride-deficient locations, and timing of first dental visit.

9. Senior patients

a. May have a soft diet, if they wear dentures or their natural teeth are in poor health, which promotes caries.

b. Dry mouth (xerostomia) is more prevalent due to medication use, cancer radiation therapy to the head and neck, and chemotherapy.

c. Root caries is more common due to effects of xerostomia; may not be painful, so patient may be unaware of condition.

d. Recession is common, causing root sensitivity and/or an increased risk for root caries.

e. Physical well-being may be diminishing; patient may have physical impairments such as difficulty with walking, balance, sitting, lying down, hearing, or grasping.

f. Loss of mental alertness is possible due to medication use, depression, dementia, stroke, Alzheimer's disease, or poor health.

10. Implants

a. Cleaning aids should be chosen that are effective, safe (must not scratch the titanium implant), and easy to use.

b. The patient's understanding of proper methods, frequency of use, and techniques of using cleaning aids/adjuncts should be evaluated.

c. Common cleaning aids/adjuncts

1) Tufted or woven fiber floss

2) Plastic elastomeric flange-floss (e.g., Proxi-floss)

3) Interdental brush (must not have exposed wire)

4) Electric or manual toothbrush with tufted end and end-rounded bristles.

5) Gauze strips

6) Cotton swabs saturated with 0.12% chlorhexidine gluconate; short-term use after abutment connection surgery or when inflammation is present.

d. When professionally cleaning an implant, use plastic scalers to remove plaque and calculus, probing should only be done using plastic-tipped probes with a light pressure.

e. For additional detail, see Chapter 12.

11. Dentinal hypersensitivity (see Chapter 12)

Utilizing Preventive Agents

Systemic and topical fluorides and pit and fissure sealants are the major preventive agents used in dentistry today. They are responsible for the sharp reduction in the caries rate in the US population.

Fluorides

Several chemical formulations and delivery agents provide a wide variety of ways to deliver adequate fluoride to the teeth and body.

I. Types of Fluorides

A. Systemic fluoride is the ingestion of fluoride that makes its way into the circulatory system to alter the developing tooth.

B. Fluoride may be naturally occurring, added to drinking water, or taken as a supplement.

1. Ideal concentration is 1 ppm.

2. Ingested fluoride reduces decay 50%–60%.

3. Fluoride added to drinking water is convenient, economical, and very effective in reducing decay.

4. When defluoridation occurs, there is a rapid increase of decay.

5. Fluoridated water over 1 ppm can cause white to brown coloration (mottling), as well as alter the formation of the enamel in the developing tooth.

6. Supplements can be used when fluoridated water is not available (Table 11–6).

a. Most common are liquid drops, tablets, lozenges, and oral rinses.

b. Are prescribed from 6 months to 14 years of age.

c. Supplement needed when water level is <0.7 ppm.

d. Prenatal supplements get fluoride to developing tooth buds.

e. Nursing babies do not require supplements as long as the mother lives in a community with an optimally fluoridated water supply.

C. Fluoridated toothpastes should not be used on small children; eating toothpaste can affect the developing permanent tooth buds causing white spots on the tooth; once the parent is sure the child is not swallowing the toothpaste, fluoridated toothpaste can be used.

TABLE 11.6 Supplemental Fluoride Dosage Schedule By Parts Per Million (PPM) in the Community Water Supply

Years in Age	Less than 0.3 ppm	0.3–0.6 ppm	Greater than 0.6 ppm
6 months–3 years	0.25 mg	0	0
3–6 years	0.50 mg	0.25 mg	0
6–16 years	1.0 mg	0.50 mg	0

D. Topical fluoride is found in toothpastes, gels, and foams (acidulated phophate, stannous, and sodium fluoride) and rinses; the application of fluoride to the erupted tooth, aids in:
  1. Posteruption maturation of the enamel surface
  2. Prevention of demineralization
  3. Remineralization of early decay
  4. Decreasing enamel solubility and maximizing enamel resistance to decay
  5. Alteration of plaque bacteria

II. Administration of Fluoride
  A. Professional application of fluoride
    1. Applied once or twice a year on children 4–18 years of age depending on susceptibility.
    2. Adults may need fluoride treatment depending on decay incidence or xerostomia.
    3. Tray application
      a. Fit Styrofoam trays to the mouth.
      b. Place fluoride gel or foam in the trays.
      c. Dry teeth with air syringe and place trays in mouth for 4 minutes.
      d. Control salivary flow with saliva ejector.
      e. Expectorate fluoride into saliva ejector.
      f. Floss teeth after tray removal and instruct patient not to eat or drink for 30 minutes.
    4. Paint on application.
      a. Isolate teeth with cotton rolls.
      b. Dry teeth with an air syringe.
      c. Paint foam or gel on with cotton-tipped applicator for 4 minutes.
      d. Control salivary flow with saliva ejector.
      e. Expectorate saliva into saliva ejector.
      f. Floss teeth and instruct patient not to eat or drink for 30 minutes.
  B. Self-administered fluoride
    1. May be in the form of a rinse, gel, tablet or toothpaste.
      a. Patient compliance will affect success of decay reduction.
      b. Tablets are generally taken once a day, gels are brushed on once a day, rinses are used after brushing and before bedtime if possible; toothpastes are used as often as the patient brushes his or her teeth.
      c. Patients should refrain from eating or drinking after home fluoride administration for at least 30 minutes.
      d. Parent supervision of fluoride use is necessary until the child has demonstrated ability not to swallow the fluoride; except for tablets, fluoride used in these techniques should not be swallowed.

III. Mechanism Of Action
  A. Metabolism
    1. 86%–97% of ingested fluoride is absorbed in the stomach.
    2. Replaces hydroxyapatite crystals with fluorapatite crystals; makes teeth more resistant to decay
    3. Excess is excreted through kidneys, sweat glands, and feces
  B. Effect of fluoride on tooth formation
    1. Bloodstream carries fluoride to the developing tooth bud.
    2. Fluoride is first deposited at the DEJ.
    3. Excessive intake during formation leads to fluorosis.
  C. Effect of fluoride on erupted tooth
    1. Fluoride uptake on enamel surface remains high for several years.
    2. Mode of delivery is topical.

IV. Toxicology
  A. Concentration of fluoride is regulated by FDA.
  B. Chronic fluoride toxicity
    1. Can cause dental fluorosis, skeletal fluorosis, and kidney damage.
    2. Severity can be influenced by increased intake of naturally fluoridated water, increased intake of food with fluoride, nutritional diseases, and diets low in calcium.
  C. Acute fluoride toxicity
    1. Can cause nausea, vomiting, heavy salivary flow, stomach pain, and diarrhea.
    2. In severe cases, symptoms may also include cramping of the extremities, breathing difficulty, heart failure, dilated pupils, hyperkalemia, and hypocalcemia.

V. Emergency Treatment
  A. If fluoride injection is <5mg/kg body weight
    1. Give milk orally.
    2. Observe for several hours.
  B. If fluoride injection is >5mg/kg body weight
    1. Induce vomiting.
    2. Give milk orally or 5% calcium gluconate.

3. Admit to hospital and observe several hours.

C. If fluoride injection is >15mg/kg body weight
   1. Admit to hospital immediately.
   2. Induce vomiting.
   3. Start calcium gluconate intravenously.
   4. Monitor for heart dysrhythmias.

Pit and Fissure Sealants

Pit and fissure sealants are used to seal deep crevices on the occlusal surfaces of posterior teeth to help reduce the incidence of occlusal caries.

I. Types of Sealants
   A. Self-curing (polymerization occurs chemically)
      1. Has two components that are mixed together.
      2. Material sets in approximately 1 minute.
   B. Light-cured, polymerization occurs when material is exposed to light.
      1. Has a single component; no mixing is required; takes more working time to flow into grooves and pits.
      2. Polymerizes when light is held close to material placed on the tooth for the specified time.

II. Client Selection (Fig. 11–7, A)
   A. Patient demonstrates ability to adequately remove plaque on a daily basis.
   B. Patient does not have a high caries history.

III. Application
   A. Clean tooth of soft and hard deposits.
   B. Isolate tooth with cotton rolls, cheek pads (Dri-Angles), or rubber dam.

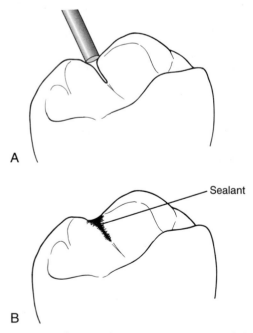

Figure 11.7 Sealants. *A,* Demonstrates inability of a single toothbrush bristle to clean a narrowly fissured groove. *B,* Etched enamel enables sealant material to flow as fingerlike projections into the enamel, allowing the material to become retentive.

C. Apply etchant material to the pits and fissures following manufacturer recommendations (Fig. 11–7, B); if it flows onto soft tissue, rinse immediately, then reapply to tooth.

D. Rinse tooth with copious amounts of water.

E. A dry tooth is essential for successful retention of sealant material; is the primary reason for sealant failure.

F. Apply sealant material into pits and fissures with brush, cannula, or plastic instrument—do not apply an excessive amount (to avoid occlusal discrepancies); taste can be offensive if material touches the tongue

G. Whether the sealant material is self-curing or light curing, follow the manufacturers' time recommendations for curing; if light cured, appropriate shielding of light is required to protect the operator's and assistant's eyes.

H. Evaluate sealant placement checking for voids, bubbles, and adequate seal; check interproximal surfaces with floss for any excess material.

I. Evaluate occlusion with articulating paper; make any necessary adjustment.

J. Instruct patient that chewing ice, hard candies, or other hard objects can fracture the sealant, which can result in leakage; leakage can lead to decay in the tooth.

K. Reevaluate sealants periodically to ensure they are still intact; replace or add to sealant when necessary; if material fails, it is most likely to occur within first 6 months after placement.

IV. Mechanism of Action
   A. Sealants are mechanically bonded to pit and fissures of posterior teeth.
   B. Act as a barrier against bacteria that cause tooth decay.
   C. Can reduce occlusal fillings up to 50% on molars, 10% on premolars.

Clinical Instrumentation

The purpose of clinical instrumentation is to create an oral environment where periodontal health is maintained or where the tissues can return to health. This is accomplished by debridement of the teeth to remove potential periodontal pathogenic microorganisms, their byproducts and calculus deposits or other surface irregularities that harbor microorganisms, and encourage their reaccumulation. Either manual instruments, power-driven instruments, or a combination of the two, can be used to effectively debride the teeth and accomplish this goal.

Positioning

Good positioning of both the patient and the operator are critical to the long-term comfort and effectiveness of the operator.

I. Advantages Of Good Patient And Operator Positioning
   A. Increase patient comfort during appointment.

B. Reduce operator discomfort and fatigue.

C. Reduce possibility of occupational injury such as cumulative trauma injury (also called repetitive strain injury) to neck, shoulders, wrist, and hand.

D. Improve visibility and access to treatment area.

E. Increase treatment efficiency.

II. Principles Of Patient Positioning

  A. Supine position

    1. The chair back is almost parallel to the floor; if the back is adjusted separately for each arch, the chair back is parallel to the floor for the maxillary arch and raised 20 degrees for the mandibular arch.

    2. The patient is almost parallel to the floor.

    3. The patient's head, heart, and feet are at approximately the same height.

    4. This position reduces the possibility that the patient could go into syncope (faint).

    5. Contraindications to this position include congestive heart failure, some severe breathing difficulties, advanced pregnancy, and back injuries.

    6. For additional modifications for specific conditions, see Chapter 15.

  B. Patient's head position

    1. The top of the patient's head should be at the top of the chair to provide the operator good access to the mouth.

    2. The patient's head and neck should be aligned with the spine and supported by the chair and headrest.

  C. Adjustments to improve visibility and access

    1. The patient may be asked to turn their head to the right or left or straight-ahead, depending on the area of treatment.

    2. Treatment of the maxilla

      a. The maxilla should be positioned so that the maxillary occlusal plane is perpendicular to the floor. This is accomplished by adjusting the chair back and/or asking the patient to tilt their head into a chin-up position.

      b. The dental light is positioned over the patient's chest and shines into the mouth at an angle.

    3. Treatment of the mandible

      a. The mandible should be approximately parallel to the floor. This is accomplished by raising the chair back slightly and/or asking the patient to tilt their head into a chin-down position.

      b. The dental light is positioned directly over the patient's mouth and shines straight down.

III. Principles of Operator Positioning

  A. Positioning on the operator's stool

    1. Place feet flat on the floor.

    2. Adjust height so that the thighs are parallel to the floor.

    3. Sit back on the stool so that body weight is fully supported by the stool and the back is against the backrest.

    4. Keep the knees and legs apart to create a tripod effect between the two feet on the floor and the stool base. This gives a good, stable seated position.

  B. Good body mechanics

    1. The head should be centered over the spine for good support. The operator's chin is tilted gently downward for good visibility, but the head is not tilted to the right or to the left.

    2. Eyestrain is reduced by having the patient's mouth at a comfortable focal distance generally about 15 inches from the operator's eyes to the patient's mouth.

    3. The back is straight without being rigid.

    4. Tilt forward from the hips, rather than curling the back or hyperextending the neck when it is necessary to get closer.

    5. Keep body weight evenly centered on the stool.

    6. Shoulders should be relaxed and even; neither raised toward the ears nor rotated forward.

    7. The upper arm should be kept close to the sides, the elbows are bent, and the forearms are generally parallel to the floor.

    8. The patient's chair height is adjusted to place the mouth at the level of the operator's elbows.

    9. The wrist is held straight as much as possible. Pronounced flexion, extension, or deviation to the side should be avoided to prevent excessive stress on the nerves in the wrist area.

    10. The hands should be positioned so that the palms are facing inward toward the operator's midline as much as possible.

  C. Cumulative trauma injuries (also called repetitive strain injuries)

    1. Neuromuscular injuries resulting from the accumulation of many small traumas to the same area are a potential occupational hazard for dental hygienists.

    2. Injuries to the neck, shoulders, hand, wrist, and back have all been reported.

    3. Preventive behavior

      a. Good body mechanics by the operator

      b. Optimum positioning of the patient for the operator's comfort and access

      c. Effective instrumentation to minimize repetitious motions; include using sharp instruments.

      d. Varied activities and positions during an appointment to alternate the muscles used

IV. Basic Operator Positions Or Zones

  A. The area around the patient's head is often portrayed as the face of a clock with 12 o'clock being directly behind the patient (Fig. 11–8).

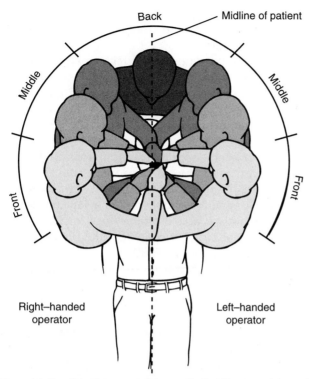

Figure 11.8 Operator positions. *1,* Sealing positions for the operator as related to a clock face. *2,* Right-handed operator sits mainly between 8 and 12 o'clock with the option to sit between 12 and 4 o'clock. *3,* Left-handed operator sits mainly between 12 and 4 o'clock with the option to sit between 8 and 12 o'clock.

B. The majority of patient care is provided with a right-handed operator sitting between 8 and 12 o'clock, a wider range between 8 and 4 o'clock may be used.
C. The majority of patient care is provided with a left-handed operator sitting between 12 and 4 o'clock, wider range between 8 and 4 o'clock may be used.
D. The operator's position should be selected to optimize good body mechanics, plus good access and visibility for treatment.

Manual Instruments

Manual or hand-powered instruments have both basic and specific designs, types, and functions. Commonly used manual instruments include mirrors, explorers, periodontal probes, sickles, and curets.

Basic Instrument Design

Basic instrument design determines the instrument's intended purpose and the location of its use. Specific instrument selections are also based on personal preference and/or ergonomic concerns. Instrumentation with manually activated instruments, both for assessment and treatment, requires a high degree of precision and control, and in some cases, power or force. This can best be accomplished with consistent application of the basic principles of instrumentation.

I. Basic Instrument Design (Fig. 11–9)
  A. Parts of an instrument
    1. Handle
      a. Can be either single- or double-ended.
      b. Varies in diameter; can be either narrow or large.
        1) Compared to narrow handles, larger diameter handles:
          a) Offer better instrument control.
          b) Decrease muscle fatigue and possibly cumulative trauma injury.
          c) Have better transmission of fine vibrations because of their hollowness.
      c. Varies in surface texture
        1) Ranging from smooth to a variety of rough surface textures
        2) When rough-textured, are called knurled or serrated and can:
          a) Reduce the slipperiness of instruments in a wet environment.
          b) Decrease muscle fatigue and possibly cumulative trauma injury by making grasp easier.
      d. Varies in composition; can be metal or high density plastic.
    2. Shank
      a. Connects the working end to the handle.
      b. Functional shank is the portion between the working end and the handle.
      c. Terminal or lower shank is the portion between the working end and the first bend in the shank.
      d. Angles and length largely determine the instrument's use in the mouth.
        1) Angulation may be simple or complex.
          a) Simple, straighter shanks are used primarily on anterior teeth.

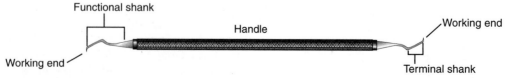

Figure 11.9 Basic instrument design. The parts of an instrument and their relationship.

b) Complex, angled, or bent shanks tend to be used on posterior teeth.

2) Length determines area of access.

a) Shorter shanks are best for use in areas of normal sulcus depth and in anterior regions of the mouth.

b) Longer shanks give better access to deeper pockets and to more posterior teeth; additional length is added to the terminal shank of some instruments designed for access in deep pockets.

e. Thickness determines shank flexibility.

1) Thick shanks are more rigid for removal of heavy deposits.

2) Thinner, more flexible shanks provide for greater tactile sensitivity and are used for finer scaling and for root planing.

3. Working end

a. Is the part of the instrument that does the work.

b. Varies by intended use

1) Curets and sickles, the most common sharp instruments, have a cutting edge formed by the junction of the face and lateral sides.

2) Probes and explorers, the most common assessment instruments, do not have cutting edges; the probe tip is dull or blunt, the explorer tip is sharp.

3) Mirrors and cotton pliers have special functions and designs.

B. A well balanced instrument

1. Is designed with the middle of the working end centered on the long axis of the instrument handle.

2. Makes an instrument easier to use, more comfortable to hold, and provides for better leverage.

II. Manual Instrument Types

A. Functions and area of use are based on the design of the working end.

1. Mirror

a. Design features

1) Front surface mirrors are the most common type; the reflective coating on the face of the glass is easily scratched but does not produce ghost images.

2) Plane or flat mirrors cause double or ghost images.

3) Concave mirrors magnify images and may cause some distortion.

4) Functions are multiple and may be combined.

a) Retraction of the cheek, lips. or tongue improves access and/or visibility.

b) Indirect vision allows observation of a

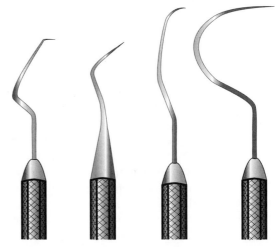

Figure 11.10 Explorers come in a variety of designs. the three on the left are used primarily for calculus detection. The Shepherd's hook on the right is used primarily for caries detection or evaluations or restorations.

reflected image when direct vision is impaired or impractical.

c) Reflected light (indirect illumination) provides illumination of a dark area of the mouth by using light bounced off of the mirror face.

d) Transillumination is light reflected from the mirror through (trans) the tooth to observe shadowing on the teeth as an indication of caries or calculus.

2. Explorers

a. Design features

1) Thin, wirelike working ends taper to a point and are circular in cross-section.

2) Shanks are simple (caries detection) or complex (for calculus and root surface exploration).

3) Have single or paired (mirror-imaged) ends.

4) Several explorer styles are shown in Fig. 11–10.

b. Function as providers of tactile information

1) Assessment of deposits (especially calculus) and irregular tooth surface during all phases of dental hygiene treatment

2) Identification of tooth and pocket characteristics, e.g., concavities, contours of epithelial attachment, and so on

3) Detection of carious lesions (usually with a Shepherd's hook)

4) Assessment of restorations for irregularities or lack of marginal integrity

c. Basic types

1) Shepherd's hook has a single end used for caries detection

2) #17 style has a single end used for calculus/root surface exploration

3) ODU 11/12 has paired ends with complex shanks used for calculus/root surface exploration

4) Pigtail and Cowhorn have paired ends used for calculus/root surface exploration

3: Periodontal probes
  a. Design features
    1) A thin, straight, rodlike, blunt working end that is a miniature measuring device; usually single-ended, although may be combined with explorers or other probes.
    2) Measurements in millimeters; variations occur in the way increments are displayed. Examples 3–6–9 (Marquis) or 1–2–3–5–7–8–9–10 (Williams).
    3) Color coding with dark or light bands improve the ease of reading (some bands are yellow).
    4) Several probe styles are shown in Fig. 11–11.
  b. Functions
    1) Periodontal assessment
      a) Measures sulcular/pocket depth, the distance from the gingival margin to epithelial attachment.
      b) Measures clinical attachment levels, the distance from the CEJ to the epithelial attachment if the gingival margin is at or apical to the CEJ; distance from the gingival margin to the epithelial attachment if the gingival margin is coronal to the CEJ.
      c) Measures recession, the distance from the CEJ to the gingival margin (when margin is apical to the CEJ).

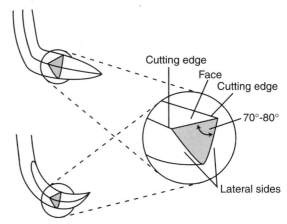

Figure 11.12 Sickle scaler working ends may be either straight or curved. All are triangular in cross-section.

      d) Measure the width of the attached gingiva, the distance from the gingival margin to the mucogingival junction minus the sulcus/pocket depth.
      e) Assesses gingival characteristics, including bleeding on probing (BOP), presence of suppuration and tissue consistency.
      f) Detects calculus or root surface roughness, root anatomy, and pocket topography.
    2) Other uses
      a) Overjet assessment, measures the distance from the maxillary incisal edge to the facial of the mandibular central.
      b) Measures oral lesions.
      c) Overbite assessment.
  c. Special probes
    1) WHO probe is designed with a 0.5 mm ball tip and markings at 3.5, 5.5, 8.5 and 11.5 mm; specifically for periodontal screening and recording (PSR).
    2) Nabor's or furcation probe has a paired curved design with or without millimeter markings; used specifically to identify furcations and examine their topography.
4. Sickles
  a. Design features
    1) Working ends may be straight or curved but are always triangular in cross-section with two cutting edges (Fig. 11–12).
    2) Cutting edges converge to form a sharp point at the tip.
    3) Lateral sides converge to form a pointed back.
    4) Have straight shanks for anterior teeth (single-ended) and contra-angled shanks for posterior teeth (paired).

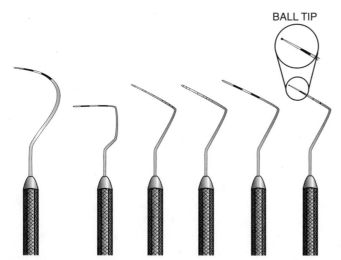

Figure 11.11 Periodontal probes are available in a variety of designs and demarcations. The Nabor's probe on the far left is used to measure furcations.

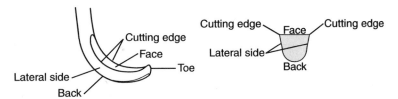

Figure 11.13 The basic design of all curets is rounded toe, rounded back, and a half-moon shaped cross-section.

b. Functions
1) Primarily used for scaling of supragingival deposits.
2) Initial debridement of heavy deposits because of its strength.
3) Removal of calculus in contacts and tight proximal surfaces, due to its thin, pointed tip; the pointed tip also increases the risk of laceration subgingivally or of gouging curved tooth surfaces.

5. Curets
   a. Design features
      1) Rounded toe
      2) Lateral sides that taper to form a rounded back on the working end
      3) A half-moon shape in cross-section (Fig. 11–13)
      4) Simple shanks for anterior teeth and complex shanks for posterior teeth
      5) Paired, mirror-imaged working ends
      6) Two design types; universal and area-specific (Fig. 11–14)
   b. Functions
      1) Versatility; can be used for debridement of both supragingival and subgingival calculus
      2) Usefulness for a wide range of deposit types and areas of the mouth, depending on the thickness, length, and angulation of the shank and working end
      3) Tissue safety: the rounded toe and back make curets the preferred manual instrument for safe and effective subgingival adaptation.

4) Excellent cutting and smoothing abilities for traditional root planing (removal of altered cementum as well as deposits)
   a) Produces the smoothest root surface
   b) Removes the most root structure
c. Design types
   1) Universal curets
      a) Have the curet blade face at 90 degrees to the terminal (lower) shank.
      b) Have two parallel cutting edges per working end.
   2) Treat all surfaces of a tooth with just one instrument by use of all four cutting edges (2 cutting edges per working end and 2 working ends per curet).
   3) Area-specific curets
      a) Are designed specifically to adapt to specific surfaces and teeth.
      b) These include Gracey curets and variations of that design series, e.g., extended shank, mini, and subzero (Table 11–7).
      c) Have a blade face "offset" to a 60- to 70-degree angle to the terminal (lower) shank.
      d) Have one cutting edge per working end (on the longer, lower side of the blade).
      e) Have long shanks and offset angles that allow greater effectiveness in deeper pockets.
      f) To treat all surfaces of posterior teeth requires more than one instrument.

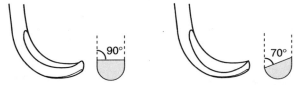

Figure 11.14 Comparison of universal and area-specific curets. Universal curets have a 90-degree angle between the face and the terminal shank, which gives them two functional cutting edges. Area-specific curets have an offset angle with a 70-degree angle between the face and the terminal shank. This makes the lower cutting edge the only one that is used for debridement.

TABLE 11.7	Area-Specific Use of Gracey Curets
Gracey Curet	**Designed Area of Use**
Gracey 1–2 and 3–4	Anterior teeth
Gracey 5–6	Anterior or premolar teeth
Gracey 7–8 and 9–10	Posterior teeth buccal and lingual surfaces
Gracey 11–12 and 15–16	Posterior teeth mesial surfaces
Gracey 13–14 and 17–18	Posterior teeth distal surfaces

6. Hoes (Fig. 11–15)
   a. Design features
      1) Adapts poorly.
      2) A "set" of hoes includes 4 working ends:
         a) One double-ended instrument with contralateral shanks and mirror-imaged working ends
         b) One double-ended instrument with two straight shanks and opposite facing working ends
      3) A bulky working end that gives great strength but makes subgingival access and adaptation difficult
      4) A straight cutting edge that has two sharp corners that can gouge a root surface if poorly adapted; the straight cutting edge makes adaptation to curved areas difficult
   b. Function
      1) Removes heavy supragingival calculus; primarily on the lingual of mandibular anteriors and distal of the most posterior tooth.
      2) Interproximal calculus removal if the adjacent tooth is missing.
      3) Careful adaptation and instrument control are critical to prevent damage from the instrument.
         a) Recommended technique includes vertical, pull strokes and two-point instrument contact with both cutting edge and shank adapted to tooth for increased control.
         b) Currently, hoes are rarely used, since they have been replaced by other instruments such as ultrasonics.
7. Files or periodontal files (Fig. 11–16)
   a. Design features
      1) Working ends have a series of parallel, straight cutting edges; often described as multibladed hoes.
      2) Working ends are thin and rounded.
      3) A thick shank gives it strength.
      4) Requires a special sharpening instrument, either a tanged or a triangular file sharpener.

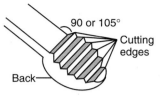

Figure 11.16 Periodontal file has multiple cutting edges. It is a thin instrument that may be used subgingivally when it fits.

      5) Available in sets of two double-ended instruments with configurations the same as described under hoes; also available in a single-ended, straight-shanked design.
      6) Recommended technique includes a vertical, pull stroke with as many blades as possible adapted to tooth/root surface.
   b. Functions
      1) Especially useful on the surfaces of burnished or smooth, dense calculus deposits because the multiple blades crush or fragment the deposit.
      2) Removal of calculus in areas of limited access, e.g., deep, narrow pockets because of small size and flat shape.
      3) Removal of small overhangs at amalgam margins
      4) Careful adaptation of the flat blade is needed when working subgingivally to avoid gouging and root damage.
8. Chisels
   a. Design features
      1) A straight cutting edge that is continuous with the shank
      2) Single or paired ends
      3) Use of a push stroke
   b. Function
      1) Supragingival use on heavy, interproximal calculus; mainly on anterior teeth.
      2) Recommended technique includes pushing from the facial surface through the interproximal surface toward the lingual.
      3) Currently, chisels are rarely used having been replaced by other instruments such as ultrasonics.
9. Implant maintenance instruments
   a. Design features
      1) Made of material that will not scratch the smooth, titanium surface of an implant; working ends made of various forms of plastic or resin (gold plated and titanium instruments exist but have been shown to scratch the implant surface).
      2) Shapes vary; some resemble familiar curets and others are uniquely shaped to adapt to round implant shapes.
   b. Functions

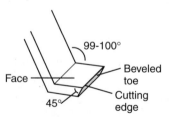

Figure 11.15 The hoe has a straight cutting edge. Since it is a bulky instrument, it is used primarily supragingivally.

1) Removal of plaque and calculus from implant surfaces without scratching; very light, lateral force is all that is normally needed.

2) Recommended technique is similar to a curet.

3) For more information regarding implants and implant maintenance, see Chapter 12.

III. Principles of Manual Instrument Use

A. Grasp

1. Modified pen grasp

a. Technique

1) Is the preferred grasp with manual instruments for both assessment and treatment.

2) Thumb and index finger are placed opposite each other and have the primary grasp or control of the instrument.

3) The instrument handle rests on the hand between the second joint of the index finger and the webbed area formed between the thumb and the rest of the hand.

4) The pad of the middle finger, usually toward the side, but not on the fingernail, is rested lightly at the junction of the instrument shank and handle below the thumb and index finger.

5) The ring finger rests against the middle finger and is used as the fulcrum finger.

6) The thumb and index finger are usually placed on the instrument handle near the shank when using a traditional intraoral fulcrum (tooth surface).

7) For an extraoral fulcrum, all fingers may be moved further up the handle away from the working end.

8) In a variation of the grasp, the index finger is bent more and moved higher on the instrument handle giving a tripod finger placement.

b. Advantages

1) Stable grasp with good control

2) Allows instrument to be rolled in the fingers easily

c. Use during assessment

1) Minimum finger pressure should be exerted against the instrument.

2) The light grasp allows information, especially vibrations, to be sensed by the finger tips, e.g., feeling the explorer bumping over calculus or into furcations or the probe reaching the epithelial attachment.

3) The pad of the middle finger is especially important in sensing vibrations transmitted up the shank of the instrument.

d. Use during treatment

1) Grasp will be light during exploratory strokes made with curets and during the placement phase of the working stroke.

2) Grasp will be moderate to firm during the activation phase of the working stroke.

3) Generally there is a close correlation between the pressure of the grasp and the amount of lateral pressure against the tooth surface.

2. Palm thumb grasp

a. Technique

1) Instrument handle is wrapped in the palm with all four fingers around it.

2) Working end is toward the thumb.

3) Thumb is left free to act as a fulcrum or a special function.

b. Disadvantages

1) Rarely used with debridement instruments.

2) Limits mobility and tactile sensitivity.

c. Uses

1) Air-water syringe

2) Rubber dam clamp holder

3) Instrument sharpening with Nievert Whittler or handpiece mounted stone

4) Porte-polisher for selected areas

B. Fulcrum or finger rest

1. Purpose

a. Provides a point of stabilization.

1) Allows greater control over the instrument and the working stroke, especially the stroke length.

2) Allows greater safety and comfort to the patient.

3) Reduces strain and fatigue for the operator.

b. Is a mechanical leverage point that allows greater force to be exerted at the working end without increased effort; more force and more lateral pressure can be exerted.

1) Reduces muscle strain on the operator.

2. Traditional intraoral fulcrum

a. Fulcrum finger (ring-finger) is placed on a tooth surface (occlusal and facial are most common) near the working area (same arch, same quadrant).

b. Fulcrum finger remains in contact with middle finger.

c. Highly effective and also comfortable for the patient in most circumstances.

d. A rocking or pivoting motion is used.

3. Alternative intraoral fulcrums

a. Used to increase adaptation, improve angulation, or create more effective fulcrum (leverage) location or to create a more physiologically sound wrist position for the clinician.

b. Most common
1) Opposite-arch
2) Cross-arch
3) Finger-on-finger (clinician stabilizes a finger on a finger of the free hand in the patient's vestibule, occlusal surface, or other convenient location, then uses it as a place to rest the fulcrum finger)
4. Extraoral fulcrums
a. Use of an extraoral fulcrum may increase access and effectiveness by improving adaptation and angulation, especially for posterior teeth, in small mouths, and in the deep pockets of periodontally involved teeth.
b. The palm or the back of the fingers or hand are rested against the face; stability is improved by resting on underlying bony structures like the chin or other wide surface area.
5. Reinforced finger rest
a. Used to increase power and control during a working stroke.
b. A finger or thumb of the noninstrumenting hand is pressed against the shank of the instrument.
C. Adaptation
1. Adaptation is the relationship of the working end of the instrument to the tooth surface.
2. Evaluating adaptation:
a. The cutting end should be positioned so that the third of the working end closest to the tip is against the tooth (toe third).
b. The instrument point should be adapted to the tooth as a portion of the toe third. If the point is adapted off of the tooth, it can cause soft tissue laceration and discomfort to the patient.
c. The heel of the working end should be kept close to the tooth to prevent excessive distention of the pocket tissue.
d. The same guidelines for adaptation are used with assessment and treatment instruments.
3. Analyze adaptation difficulties
a. Good adaptation is hardest to achieve on areas of the tooth that are very curved (e.g., line angles) or convex (e.g., mesial maxillary first premolars) or have narrow roots (e.g., lingual mandibular anteriors) or deep pockets, or where teeth and surfaces are hard to access (e.g., third molars).
b. Common solutions to adaptation difficulties
1) Rolling instrument in fingers
2) Moving fulcrum
3) Adjusting hand orientation on fulcrum
4) Changing instruments
5) Altering stroke direction and orientation of the instrument on tooth (e.g., for a line angle, use an oblique stroke with the toe toward apex)

D. Angulation
1. Assessment instruments (explorers and probes)
a. Is the angle formed between the working end of the instrument and the tooth surface.
b. For caries detection, the point of the explorer is pressed into the tooth surface with the terminal portion of the explorer meeting the tooth at a 90-degree angle.
c. For calculus and root surface exploration, the working end of the explorer is angled about 15 degrees from the tooth surface with only the toe (terminal) third lightly touching.
d. The periodontal probe is positioned close (almost parallel) to the tooth surface with the end in contact with the root surface (this might also be considered adaptation).
e. When probing the proximal surface where there is an adjacent tooth, the probe must be angled about 20 to 30 degrees into the col area.
2. For scaling instruments (sickles and curets)
a. The angle formed between the face of the blade and the tooth surface.
b. Angulation for scaling
1) The recommended angulation for debridement is between 45 and 90 degrees.
2) For scaling, the optimum angulation is about 70 to 80 degrees.
3) Scaling at less than 45 degrees results in burnished deposits.
4) For curets only
a) For root planing, the angle becomes more closed, the final strokes are angled between 60 to 45 degrees.
b) For insertion of the instrument into the sulcus/pocket, the angle should be as close to 0 degrees as possible.
3. Angulation for soft tissue curettage is greater than 90 degrees so that the cutting edge is directed toward the epithelial lining of the diseased pocket wall.
E. Stroke
1. Types of instrument strokes differ by the amount of pressure applied to the tooth (lateral pressure) and by the length and direction of the instrument movement.
a. Exploratory stroke
1) The grasp and lateral pressure should remain light throughout the stroke.
2) Strokes should be overlapping and multidirectional.
3) Used with a variety of instruments including explorers, probes, curets, and ultrasonic tips.
b. Probing strokes
1) The grasp and lateral pressure should remain light throughout the stroke.

2) Walking strokes use an up and down motion while moving forward around the tooth in small steps to feel the depth and contour of the epithelial attachment.
c. Scaling stroke—activation phase
   1) Tight or controlled grasp with moderate to heavy lateral pressure, as dictated by the tenacity of the deposit; the lightest grasp and pressure that will remove the deposit is preferred.
   2) Strokes should be overlapping.
   3) Stroke directions vary.
d. Root planing stroke
   1) Grasp is moderate to light.
   2) Stroke length becomes progressively longer and lateral pressure becomes lighter.
   3) Angulation becomes progressively more closed (toward 45 degrees).
   4) Stroke direction is multidirectional and cross-hatched.
2. An instrument stroke has several parts.
   a. Insertion
      1) Position the working end of the instrument at the base of the sulcus or apical to the deposit.
      2) For a bladed instrument, the angle for insertion of curets should be as close to 0 degrees as possible.
      3) Grasp and lateral pressure are light.
   b. Preparation for activation
      1) This will vary depending on the type of stroke that is intended.
      2) Working/scaling stroke:
         a) The grasp is tightened.
         b) The desired angulation is established.
         c) Lateral pressure is increased.
   c. Activation
      1) The movement to accomplish the purpose of the stroke (wrist-rock), e.g., exploration, probing, scaling, and root planing.
      2) Stroke length and direction will vary.
   d. Stroke direction
      1) Selection of stroke direction is based on the anatomy of the individual tooth, access to the tooth/surface, instrument selection, and type of deposit.
      2) Options in stroke direction:
         a) Vertical
         b) Horizontal or circumferential
         c) Oblique
         d) Cross-hatching (combination of vertical, horizontal, and oblique)
   e. Stroke length
      1) Shorter strokes give more control and are typically used for deposit removal.
      2) Longer strokes are typically used for assessment (exploring and probing) and root planing.
      3) There should be an overlap in strokes to ensure that all areas of the tooth surface are instrumented.

Power-Driven Instruments

In recent years, the role of power-driven scalers has changed from gross scaling only, to comprehensive, definitive treatment in periodontal debridement. This is based on a variety of new research findings and on the availability of longer, thinner instrument tips that allow access to deep pockets. This is still a rapidly evolving area for both additional research and technologic advances. Use of power-driven instruments, combined with manual instruments, may give better results in most cases than either one alone.
I. Indications for Use
   A. Prophylaxis
   B. Periodontal debridement (scaling and root planing)
   C. Supportive periodontal therapy (periodontal maintenance)
   D. Overhang removal
II. Power Unit
   A. Sonic scalers
      1. Frequency
         a. Defined as less than 20,000 cycles/sec
         b. Usual range is about 5,000 to 7,000 cycles/sec
      2. Power sources
         a. Compressed air
         b. Attaches to high speed handpiece position on dental unit
      3. Advantages
         a. Does not generate heat, therefore does not require fluid lavage as a coolant (although lavage is still desirable for other reasons).
         b. Highly portable; small, light, and needs only a high speed hook-up.
   B. Ultrasonic instruments
      1. Frequency
         a. Range of 24,000 to 50,000 cycles/sec or Hertz (Hz)
         b. Most machines fall into one of 2 power ranges:
            1) 25,000—30,000 cycles/sec
            2) around 40,000—50,000 cycles/sec
      2. Power source
         a. Electrical energy
         b. Connect to standard electrical outlet
         c. Divided based on the manner of converting electrical power to mechanical movement at the working end of instrument; there are two types
            1) Magnetostrictive, which uses magnetic oscillations
            2) Piezoelectric, which uses crystal oscillations

C. Unit controls
1. Power
   a. Controls the amplitude or size of the instrument tip movement.
      1) A high power setting gives a high amplitude or large movement of the instrument tip.
   b. Power setting selection is based on the patient treatment needs and the instrument tip used.
      1) Medium to high power typically is used for:
         a) Removal of heavy and dense calculus deposits
         b) Heavy or thicker instrument tips
      2) Low to medium power is typically used for:
         a) Light or finishing debridement, root planing, or deplaquing
         b) Sensitive root surfaces
         c) Light or thin instrument tips
2. Tuning
   a. Controls the frequency of the tip movement
   b. Unit types
      1) Autotune—the majority of commercially available units have a built-in control of the tuning or frequency component
      2) Manual tune—these units allow the operator to adjust the tuning of the machine, allowing greater control of the procedure and potentially increasing patient comfort
3. Fluid
   a. The fluid functions as a coolant for those machines that generate heat during operation and provides therapeutic benefits.
   b. Fluid volume
      1) May vary by manufacturers' recommendations
      2) Typically, set to give a fast drip of water from the tip and a halo of fine droplets
   c. Fluid source and type
      1) Water from the dental unit
         a) Hook-up directly to the dental unit provides water as the fluid
         b) Water should be purged through the dental unit and power-scaler for 2–5 minutes at the start of the day and from 30 seconds to 2 minutes between patients (similar to the time used for the air/water syringe.
      2) External fluid supplies
         a) Some units can draw their lavage or coolant fluid from containers that can be filled with any of a variety of fluids.
         b) Sterile water, antimicrobial solutions, or temperature controlled water can have advantages for patient treatment.

III. Instrument Tips
A. Standard tips
   1. Thick, strong tips
   2. Usually shaped like an anterior curet or probe
   3. Used to remove heavier calculus and for initial debridement
   4. May be used for supragingival or subgingival debridement but will not fit to the base of deeper pockets
   5. Often used at a higher power setting
      a. The heavier metal tip does not move as much as a thin tip at the same power setting.
      b. It is used for initial debridement.
B. Thin style or slim style tips
   1. Tips are longer and thinner than standard tips.
   2. Usually shaped like a probe in the terminal portion.
   3. Often used in sets with right and left contra-angled tips and a straight tip.
   4. Used for removing light deposits, plaque, and endotoxin. May follow initial debridement with standard tip.
   5. May be used to the base of deep pockets.
   6. Use at low power to prevent patient discomfort or damage to the tip.
C. Furcation tips
   1. A small ball-like projection at the very end of the instrument tip
   2. May prevent damage to the root when working in tight furcation areas
   3. Available in right, left, and straight thin/slim style tips

IV. Therapeutic Effect
A. Deposit removal
   1. Calculus
      a. Removal is as effective as with manual instruments.
      b. Removal is faster than with manual instruments.
   2. Plaque
      a. Subgingival removal is at least as effective as with manual instruments.
      b. Cell walls are lysed by ultrasonic vibrations and also by fluid cavitation.
   3. Pattern for treatment
      a. With power-driven instruments, treatment begins at the most coronal areas of deposit and moves to the most apical or subgingival deposits.
      b. With manual instruments, deposit removal is from the most subgingival to the most coronal.
B. Detoxification of the root surface

1. Endotoxin or lipopolysaccharide (LPS) is associated with the roots of periodontally diseased teeth.
2. Endotoxin is effectively removed with power-driven instruments using an overlapping stroke.
3. Less root structure is removed with power-driven instruments than with curets.

C. Effect of fluid lavage
   1. The fluid associated with power-driven scalers reaches the base of the pocket.
   2. It serves as an oral irrigator, flushing away:
      a. Some of the microorganisms; loosely attached plaque
      b. Fractured calculus
      c. Hemorrhage products
   3. Cavitation
      a. The fine mist around the tip of a power-driven scaler consists of small bubbles.
      b. When the bubbles burst, it is called cavitation.
      c. When it occurs near microorganisms, cavitation causes a small shock wave that can disrupt or lyse bacterial cell walls.
   4. Acoustic microstreaming
      a. In the confined space of a subgingival pocket, the fluid flow exerts considerable force and turbulence called acoustic microstreaming or acoustic streaming.
      b. It can disrupt the cell walls and kill microorganisms and seems especially effective on highly motile organisms.

D. Healing is comparable between power-driven and manual instrumentation.

E. Furcations at the class II or III level of involvement can be more effectively treated with power-driven instruments than with manual instruments.

V. Comparison of Power-driven to Manual Instrumentation
   A. Advantages of power-driven instruments
      1. Faster than manual debridement
      2. Less operator fatigue and possibly reduced cumulative trauma injury
      3. New thin/slim design instruments, thinner and longer than curets to provide better access to deep pockets
      4. No cutting edges
         a. Less soft tissue trauma
         b. Less soft tissue discomfort for patient
         c. No need for instrument sharpening
         d. No need to achieve an effective scaling angulation
      5. Requires a light touch
         a. Easier to establish a finger rest (fulcrum)
         b. Less tiring for operator and patient
      6. Effective on all sides (less true for piezoelectric and sonic instruments) and in any stroke direction

   7. Effective in a stationary position
   8. Oral irrigation
      a. Reduce microorganisms
      b. Wash field for good visibility
   9. Improved patient comfort in many cases

B. Disadvantages of power-driven instruments
   1. Aerosol carries bacteria, viruses, and hemorrhage products.
   2. Constant water management and evacuation required.
   3. May be a health risk to a few patients.

VI. Principles of the Use of Power-Driven Scalers
   A. Overriding principles that govern use of power-driven scaling instruments, both sonic and ultrasonic, are very similar to those for manual instruments.
      1. Goal for both is to use a technique that is optimally effective and will not create any harm to the patient's dentition or to the clinician.
      2. The main differences stem from the fact that power-driven scalers do not have cutting edges, are active in a stationary position, and are most effective when only light pressure is applied to the tooth.

   B. Grasp
      1. Light pressure should always be used to grasp the instrument.
      2. Grasp may be standard pen grasp or modified pen grasp.

   C. Fulcrum or finger rest
      1. Purpose
         a. Provide a point of stabilization to make instrument movement easier.
         b. Provide a resting and pivoting point for the operator in order to reduce muscle stress and fatigue.
         c. Is *not* used for leverage or increased power of the working stroke.
      2. Fulcrum placement
         a. Select fulcrum location that gives optimum access/adaptation to the treatment area and good body mechanics for the operator.
         b. Traditional intraoral fulcrums
            1) Pressure must be kept light.
            2) Especially useful for mandibular teeth.
         c. Extraoral and alternative fulcrums
            1) May be preferred because soft tissue fulcrums encourage light fulcrum pressure.
            2) Especially useful for maxillary posterior teeth.

   D. Adaptation
      1. Adaptation, the relationship of the working end of the instrument to the tooth surface, is a critical aspect of power-driven instrument use.
      2. Evaluating adaptation

a. The last few millimeters of the instrument tip are most effective and should be positioned against the tooth.

b. The point of the working end should never be directed toward the tooth, especially the root surface. Contact of the point against the root can result in gouging or other damage.

3. Adaptation of effective surfaces
   a. All surfaces of magnetostrictive instruments tips may be adapted and used.
   b. The lateral surfaces of piezoelectric instrument tips are most effective.
   c. The four corner areas of sonic scalers are the most effective.

4. Instrument orientation
   a. Tip parallel to the long axis of the tooth with point pointing toward the apical direction.
      1) The preferred position for most tips and treatment situations
      2) Provides best access to deeper pockets
      3) For debridement of most tooth surfaces
   b. Tip perpendicular to the long axis of the tooth
      1) The side of the tip, and never the point, is used.
      2) For debridement under the contact and at the CEJ, especially a wide or bulbous crown shape which makes the standard adaptation ineffective.
   c. Other
      1) Any orientation may be used as long as the point is not against the tooth.
      2) A greater range of effective adaptations are possible than with manual instruments
         a) An effective working angle need not be achieved
         b) The instrument tips are effective in a stationary position, and for most tips, on all sides.

E. Stroke
   1. Pressure
      a. Light pressure
         1) Only light pressure should be applied against the tooth with the instrument tip during all phases of treatment.
         2) A "feather touch" should be used.
         3) A light grasp encourages the use of light pressure.
      b. Heavy pressure
         1) Reduces effectiveness of the tip
         2) Can cause increased discomfort to the patient
         3) May increase the possibility of root damage
         4) Increases unnecessary wear of the instrument tips
   2. Stroke types

a. A working stoke is performed whenever the instrument tip is applied to the tooth and the power is activated. There is no separate insertion phase to the stroke.

b. An exploratory stroke is used when the tip is moved over the tooth surface but the power is not activated.

3. Stroke direction
   a. Stroke direction is based on tooth anatomy and instrument access.
   b. Options for stroke direction
      1) Vertical
      2) Horizontal or circumferential
      3) Oblique
      4) Cross-hatching
   c. Multidirectional strokes are the most effective in achieving the goal of thorough debridement including root detoxification.

F. Time required for treatment
   1. Reduced working time
      a. Working strokes can be accomplished more quickly because pressure is light and constant, the instrument strokes are effective in both directions, and deposits may be removed more quickly.
      b. Instrumentation is typically reduced by about 25% over manual instrumentation.
   2. Comparable number of working strokes
      a. The effective width of a working stroke is comparable to manual instrumentation.
      b. All surfaces of the tooth/root to be treated need to be thoroughly instrumented.
      c. Approximately the same number of working strokes need to be taken with power-driven instruments as with manual instruments.
   3. Ease of treatment
      a. Physically easier for operators because less pressure and leverage is needed against the tooth.
      b. More comfortable for patients because of reduced pressure against the tooth, reduced trauma to soft tissue, and reduced treatment time.

G. Patient selection and preparation
   1. Patient treatment types
      a. Power-driven instruments may be used for patients with a wide variety of treatment needs.
         1) Gross to fine debridement for initial therapy
         2) Supportive periodontal therapy (SPT) (maintenance treatment)
         3) Prophylaxis or preventive treatment for a healthy mouth
         4) Removal of smear layer following manual instrumentation
      b. May be combined with manual instrumentation.

2. Contraindications
   a. Cardiac pacemakers
      1) Magnetostrictive ultrasonic scalers should not be used with unshielded, usually older, pacemakers.
      2) Medical consult may be indicated.
   b. Immunocompromised and respiratory risk patients
      1) Oral microorganisms will be incorporated into the aerosol that will be inhaled by the patient.
      2) The potential for the development of a respiratory infection exists in susceptible patients.
   c. Restorations
      1) Power scalers are contraindicated for use on porcelain or composite restorations and titanium implants
      2) May be used on adjacent tooth structure but all margins of restorations should be avoided unless purpose is to remove amalgam overhang.
   d. Demineralized areas
      1) Power scalers may remove or damage weakened tooth structure.
   e. May be uncomfortable for patients with pronounced gag reflex or who are obligatory mouth breathers.
   f. Vibrations may be uncomfortable on sensitive roots.
   g. Children
      1) Newly erupted teeth may be susceptible to damage from vibrations.
      2) Large pulp chambers may be more heat sensitive.
   h. Discontinue use if patient reports discomfort.
3. Patient preparation
   a. Provide information to patient about the procedure and secure informed consent.
   b. Drape patient to protect from aerosol spray.
   c. Have patient rinse vigorously with antimicrobial mouthrinse prior to instrument use.
   d. Adjust power for effective debris removal, tip selected, and patient comfort.

Polishing

Polishing of the clinical crowns of all teeth is a traditional part of dental hygiene treatment. In recent years, the efficacy of this procedure, as a routine part of care, has been questioned and selective polishing has been recommended. Polishing can be accomplished by applying an abrasive with a porte polisher, with a cup or brush attached to a prophy angle on a slow speed hand piece or with an air-driven polishing system.

I. The Purposes of Polishing
    A. Improve esthetics by removal of extrinsic stain (main purpose)
    B. Prepare tooth to receive sealants
    C. Remove plaque (can also be accomplished by other methods)
    D. Meet patient's expectations and increase patient satisfaction (of questionable therapeutic value)

II. Contraindications and Precautions
    A. Removal of tooth structure
       1. Repeated polishings can, over time, remove dental structure, even enamel.
       2. Recently erupted teeth are less mineralized, making tooth structure more easily removed by polishing. Avoid polishing the teeth of children.
       3. Cementum and exposed dentin are readily removed by polishing. Ditching has been demonstrated when the pressure on the cup is applied unevenly or is excessively heavy.
       4. Decalcified areas (white or brown spot lesions) are more rapidly abraded than intact teeth and should be avoided.
       5. The outermost layer of the tooth is the most fluoride-rich layer; part of this layer is removed in polishing.
    B. Increased roughness
       1. Use of a coarse abrasive and/or excessive pressure can cause grooving or roughening of the tooth surface. This is especially true of the root but even enamel can be affected.
       2. Some restorative materials can be scratched, dulled or even suffer loss of material with polishing. Rubber cup polish can damage gold, composite, and aesthetic restorations. Air-powder abrasives have been shown to damage all restorative materials, especially composites and other aesthetic materials.
          a. Polishing implants with a cup and very fine abrasive is generally an accepted technique. Use of an air-powder abrasive system on implants is controversial and some studies have shown increased surface roughness and even loss of titanium.
    C. Polishing can cause frictional heat.
       1. Teeth with large pulp chambers, e.g., primary teeth, are susceptible to heat.
       2. Metal restorations can transmit heat to the pulp.
       3. Frictional heat can be reduced by:
          a. Using light pressure against the tooth
          b. Rotating the cup or brush at a slower speed
          c. Decreasing the duration of time of contact between the tooth and cup or brush
          d. Using an abrasive with sufficient wetness to slide over the tooth surface
    D. Contamination from microorganisms
       1. A bacteremia may result from polishing in the presence of gingival inflammation.
       2. An aerosol containing microorganisms is created by all rotary instruments and especially by an air-powered abrasive system. Use of safety glasses by patient and operator, an antimicro-

bial mouthwash pre-rinse, and excellent post-treatment surface decontamination of the operatory is needed.

III. Effect of the Abrasives

A. Abrasive particles can be forced into the pocket or even into the tissue itself during polishing. When treating patients with deep pockets or patients who need extensive instrumentation, it has been suggested that polishing precede the scaling or take place at the reevaluation appointment to prevent the abrasive from being introduced into the tissue and from causing further inflammation.

B. A few individuals will have a negative reaction, either to the fluoride in commercial pastes or abrasive particles or other components of the polishing paste.

C. Studies of changes in blood chemistry following the use of the air-powder abrasive systems have shown varied results. Due to the possible systemic absorption of the sodium bicarbonate powder, its use is generally considered to be contraindicated for patients with a history of any of the following:[12]

1. Hypertension
2. Need for a low sodium diet
3. Renal insufficiency
4. Addison's disease
5. Cushing's syndrome
6. Metabolic alkalosis
7. Taking medications including mineralocorticoid steroids, antidiuretics, or potassium supplements

D. Inhalation of the abrasive particles and the microbially contaminated aerosol by the patient makes the use of air-powder abrasive systems generally contraindicated for a patient with a history of:

1. Respiratory illness
2. Infectious disease
3. Immunosuppression

IV. Selective Polishing

A. Currently the most accepted approach to polishing
B. Only those surfaces of the teeth that have stain or plaque would benefit are polished
C. Iatrogenic damage from polishing is avoided. This is especially important for root surfaces and restorations.

V. Polishing Methods

A. Porte polisher, a manual polishing device
1. Advantages and disadvantages
a. Advantages
1) Use for homebound or bedridden patients where a dental handpiece is not available for conventional polishing.
2) Does not generate an aerosol; indicated for patients with infectious diseases.
3) Does not produce frictional heat so may benefit very sensitive teeth.
b. Disadvantages
1) Technique is time-consuming and stress-ful for the musculature of the clinician's hand and wrist.
2) Equipment
a) Stainless steel handle with contra-angled working end that holds wood polishing point
b) Wood polishing point
(1) Works abrasive polishing agent against the tooth
(2) Commercially available in wedge-shaped and pointed end
(3) Usually made of orange wood or maple
2. Technique
a. Moistened abrasive is worked against the tooth surface to remove stain or plaque.
b. Motion is small circles, especially near the gingival margin, or vertical or horizontal strokes as best adapts to the tooth.
c. Grasp may be either modified pen grasp or palm thumb grasp.

B. Rubber cup or brush attached to prophylaxis (prophy) angle on a slow-speed handpiece
1. Advantage
a. An easy and efficient method of working polishing abrasive over the tooth surface
2. Disadvantages
a. The greater speed of this polishing method can result in excessive abrasion to the tooth surface resulting in loss of tooth structure and ditching if the force on the cup is applied unevenly.
b. Frictional heat can be generated that can cause discomfort to the patient.
c. Care must be taken not to cause trauma to the gingival tissues or pulp.
3. Equipment
a. A slow-speed handpiece provides the rotational energy to power the movement of the prophylaxis angle.
b. Prophylaxis angle
1) A right-angled or contra-angled attachment that attaches to the handpiece and holds the polishing device, usually a rubber cup, bristle brush, or rubber polishing point.
2) May either be a disposable product, or one that can be sterilized between uses.
c. Polishing device moves the abrasive agent over the tooth surface.
1) Rubber cup has a hollow center to hold the abrasive polish and thin edges that flare to adapt to the various smooth tooth surfaces.
2) Bristle brush and abrasive are used for the occlusal surfaces and concave areas of the tooth. Must not be used near the gingiva.

3) Rubber polishing points can apply polishing abrasive to interproximal surfaces if there is adequate space.
4) Dental floss or tape can work the abrasive over the proximal surfaces.
d. Abrasive polishing agent
  1) The abrasive quality of a polishing agent is controlled by:
    a) The size of the abrasive particle, with the smallest particles being the least abrasive
    b) The chemical and physical properties of the abrasive being used (e.g., hardness, particle shape, fracture, and wear characteristics)
  2) Pumice and silicone dioxide are common polishing agents.
  3) Polishing abrasive must always be used in a moist paste form, not dry.
e. Technique
  1) Use the least abrasive polishing agent that will remove the stain. Do not use anything coarser than medium grit.
  2) Use a slowly rotating cup to apply the polishing agent.
  3) Use light pressure
  4) Do not allow the cup to remain on the same area of the tooth.
  5) Keep the cup parallel to the tooth surface to prevent grooving the surface, especially at the cervical area.
  6) Keep the duration of contact between tooth and cup to a minimum.
  7) Flex the cup to adapt the cup edges into the interproximals.
  8) Rinse the patient frequently.
  9) Adapt the bristles of the brush to work the polishing agent into the grooves of the occlusal surfaces.
  10) Use dental floss and polishing agent to clean the interproximals.
C. Air polish, air-powder polish, air-abrasive polish, or airbrasive polish
  1. Are tooth polishing systems that use special air-powered machines to deliver an abrasive slurry that contains sodium bicarbonate powder, water, and air.
  2. Advantages
    a. Removes extrinsic stain and plaque quickly and effectively.
    b. Places less stress on the hand and wrist of the clinician (less pressure and manipulation) than rubber cup or porte polishing.
    c. Some studies show less damage to the tooth surface than is caused by the use of curets or rubber-cup polish.
    d. Superior to rubber-cup polish to prepare occlusal surfaces for pit and fissure sealants.

3. Disadvantages
  a. Causes transient irritation to the gingiva not lasting more than a few days.
  b. Produces an aerosol that contains both sodium bicarbonate and oral microorganisms that have the potential to be inhaled by the patient and clinician and spreads to operatory surfaces (up to 6 feet).
  c. See section III (Effect of the Abrasives), C on contraindications and precautions for a list of specific medical conditions that may contraindicate its use.
  d. Has been shown to alter some restorative materials, especially composites and porcelain.
4. Equipment
  a. The air polish machine uses air pressure from the dental unit to propel a slurry of water, sodium bicarbonate, and air through a small nozzle-like opening.
  b. Common brand names are Prophy-jet or Cavijet (when combined with the Cavitron ultrasonic unit).
  c. A disposable aerosol-reduction device is attached to the evacuation system at one end and fits over the nozzle of the air-polishing device at the other end. It is adapted to the tooth surface and captures the aerosol so that it can be suctioned away. (If available, high-speed evacuation is recommended.)
5. Technique
  a. Both patient and clinician wear protective eyewear and drapes or garments.
  b. Patients should remove contact lenses, use an antimicrobial rinse, and protect lips with an application of lubricant.
  c. For anterior teeth, the tip of the nozzle is directed at a 60-degree angle toward the tooth. For posterior teeth, the angle is 80 degrees; correct tip angulation decreases aerosol production.
  d. Rapid, sweeping strokes are used with the tip held about 4–5 mm from the tooth surface.
  e. Polishing for 5 seconds or less per tooth is usually adequate for stain removal.

Instrument Sharpening

Instruments become dull with use. Instrument sharpening is the technique of grinding or honing one or both of the surfaces that join to form the cutting edge of an instrument blade until a fine, sharp edge is produced. Sharpening is a technically demanding skill that requires precision and reproducibility.

I. Objectives of Sharpening
  A. Maintain a sharp cutting edge
    1. Increases the ease of debridement

2. Increases the quality of debridement
3. Decreases hand fatigue and the potential for occupational injury
4. Decreases time needed for debridement
5. Increases patient comfort because of decreased scaling pressure and reduced number of working strokes needed

  B. Preserve the original instrument shape
1. Maintains effectiveness of instrument design
2. Extends useful life of instrument
3. Reduces instrument replacement costs

II. Need and Frequency of Sharpening

  A. All instruments with a cutting edge need periodic sharpening.
1. The cutting edge is formed by the junction of the instrument face and the lateral side. It has length, but it should not have width.
2. With use, the sharp cutting edge is worn away, becomes rounded and dull, and needs to be sharpened.

  B. The rate at which an instrument becomes dull is determined by:
1. The number of working strokes taken since the last sharpening.
2. The amount of lateral pressure used.
3. The nature of the deposit.
4. The composition of the metal instrument; carbon steel holds an edge longer than stainless steel.

  C. Sharpen at the first sign of dullness. Clinically this is based on:
1. The amount of work or scaling since the last sharpening; the more working strokes and the heavier the calculus, the sooner sharpening is needed.
2. The "feel" of the instrument on the teeth or deposit, e.g., dull instruments have less grab (slip easily), tend to burnish calculus, and have reduced tactile sensitivity during exploring or light scaling.
3. A sharpness test shows the instrument to be dull (see assessment section).

  D. Instruments may need sharpening periodically during a debridement procedure.

  E. Recontouring is an extensive sharpening process that is used when an instrument has become excessively dull or misshapen; the basic process is the same as regular sharpening but more metal is removed, usually from both the lateral sides and the face. There may be selective reshaping to return the instrument to its original design.

III. Equipment/Armamentarium

  A. Sharpening Stones
1. Types
  a. Arkansas stone
    1) Is a natural stone with a fine grit (abrasive particle size).
    2) Is lubricated with a fine oil or petroleum jelly before each use.
    3) May be sterilized by any of the usual methods but may become dry and more brittle with repeated exposure to high heat.
  b. Ceramic stones
    1) Are hard, synthetic stones with a fine to medium grit.
    2) Are lubricated with water or used dry.
    3) Tolerate all sterilization methods well.
  c. India stones
    1) Are synthetic stones with a medium grit.
    2) Recommended lubricants include oil, which is most often recommended, and water; opinions vary on the ideal lubricant.
    3) Tolerate all sterilization methods well.
    4) Tend to groove and show wear with extended use.
2. Shapes/presentation of stones
  a. Flat or wedge-shaped stones
    1) Are the most widely used shapes.
    2) Generally are rectangular; sizes vary.
    3) Wedge-shaped stones have at least one edge that is rounded for use on the face of the instrument.
  b. Cylindric or conical stones
    1) Are unmounted stones.
    2) Sharpen the face of the instrument to supplement sharpening the lateral side as part of recontouring, or to remove a wire edge.
  c. Mandrel-mounted stones
    1) Are usually cylindric or conical-shaped synthetic stone.
    2) Are used with a slow-speed handpiece.
    3) Sharpen the lateral sides or face of the instrument.
3. Sharpening tools
  a. Hand-held (Nievert Whittler)
    1) Is a hand-held sharpening tool.
    2) Uses a hard tungsten carbide steel nib that can be adapted to sharpen all surfaces of an instrument.
  b. Reciprocating honing device (Peri-Perfect, RX Honing)
    1) Has contoured hones to fit different instruments.
    2) Usually has angle guides to assure accuracy.
    3) Can remove excessive amount of metal in inexperienced hands.

  B. Stone maintenance
1. Protect the stone
  a. Use a lubricant matched to the stone type.

b. Use the entire surface of the stone to prevent grooving.

2. Clean the stone before sterilization.
   a. Remove lubricant and metal particles from the stone.
   b. Use soap and a brush or an ultrasonic bath.

3. Sterilize the stone between patients using autoclave, dry heat, or chemical sterilization. All methods are effective on all stones. Natural stones may become dry and brittle with repeated autoclaving or dry heat.

IV. Technique
   A. General principles
      1. The shape of each new instrument should be studied so that it can be preserved during sharpening.
      2. Appropriate angles should be maintained.
         a. The internal angle of 70 degrees (a range from 70–80 degrees may be used) must be preserved in both curets and sickles for maximum effect of the cutting edge.
         b. The angle from the face of the curet or sickle to the sharpening stone should be 110 degrees (a range from 100–110 degrees may be used) (Fig. 11–17)
      3. Selected surfaces are sharpened.
         a. The lateral side is the primary surface to sharpen.
         b. The face may also be sharpened, usually to remove a wire edge or to maintain/recover original shape.
      4. The wire edge is prevented or removed.
         a. Wire edge is an irregular projection that may form from burnished metal particles that extend beyond the surface being sharpened (e.g., when sharpening the lateral surface, the wire edge will project above the face of the instrument).
         b. It is prevented or removed by:
            1) Ending on a stroke away from the cutting edge (this is usually a down stroke)
            2) Taking one or two light sharpening strokes on the adjacent surface (on the face when the lateral surface is sharpened)

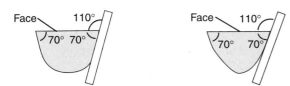

Figure 11.17 Instrument sharpening angles. Angulation for sharpening both curets and sickle scalers are the same. The angle between the instrument face and the stone should be 110 degrees with an internal angle of 70 degrees.

B. All sharpening techniques use the same general principles as stated; several techniques of instrument sharpening are used depending on personal preference.
   1. Instrument stable—lateral surface sharpened
      a. Is the most widely used technique and is described under specific instrument.
      b. Instrument is held steady, either suspended in front of the operator or supported against a counter edge while the sharpening stone is moved up and down.
   2. Instrument stable—face sharpened
      a. Is usually used in combination with sharpening the lateral surface
      b. The instrument is held steady while the stone is moved over the face, usually from the heel toward the toe
      c. Rounded stones or curved edges of flat stones are usually used for curved working ends (curets and some sickles)
   3. Stone stable—lateral surface
      a. Involves a flat stone that is laid on the instrument tray and the instrument is moved across the surface.
      b. Is also used with honing machines and some sharpening devices.

C. Sharpening the lateral sides of sickles and universal curets
   1. Instrument design characteristics
      a. Each working end has two parallel cutting edges that need to be sharpened (if the instrumentation technique used dictates that only one of the cutting edges be used for deposit removal, then only that cutting edge needs to be sharpened).
      b. The face of the blade is positioned at a 90-degree angle to the terminal portion of the shank.
   2. Instrument positioning
      a. The face of the blade is held parallel to the floor or countertop.
      b. The terminal shank is held straight up and down or vertically.
      c. The instrument should be held firmly to prevent movement.
   3. Stone position
      a. The lubricated side of the stone is held against the lateral surface to be sharpened.
      b. An angle of 110 degrees is established between the face of the blade and working surface of the stone (if using clock positions this is equivalent to 4 minutes before or after 12 o'clock).
   4. Stone movement
      a. The stone is moved up and down using the whole arm to create a fluid movement.
      b. The movement in each direction is about one-fourth to one-half inch.

c. In addition to the up and down movement, the stone is rotated very slightly on its long axis. This allows first the heel, then middle, then toe portion of the cutting edge to be sharpened, preserving the instrument's original shape (Fig. 11–18)

5. The opposite cutting edge is sharpened using all of the same techniques.

D. Sharpening the lateral sides of Gracey curets
1. Instrument design characteristics
   a. Each working end has only one cutting edge that needs to be sharpened.
   b. The face of the blade is angled downward to create a 70-degree angle.
2. Instrument position
   a. The toe one-third of the face of the blade is held parallel to the floor or countertop.
   b. The terminal shank is NOT vertical.
3. Stone position is the same as for sickles and universal curets.
4. Stone movement is the same as for sickles and universal curets.
5. The rotation of the stone on its long axis may be very pronounced to accommodate the very curved blade of some Gracey curets.

E. Sharpening the toe of universal and Gracey curets
1. Rounding the toe of a curet is an important step in maintaining the correct shape of the blade.
2. The face of the instrument is held parallel to the floor or countertop.
3. The angle of the stone is opened 25 degrees more than it is for sharpening the lateral surface. This creates a 135-degree angle between the face of the blade and the stone or an internal angle of 45 degrees at the toe of the instrument.
4. The motion of the stone is in small up and down movements while rotating on the long axis of the stone in the shape of a smooth, round curve matching the instrument's round toe.
5. The change in angle from the usual sharpening angle prevents excessive shortening of the instrument blade.

F. Finishing the blade
1. Rounding the back of the curet
   a. After repeated sharpening, a long bevel may form on the lateral sides.
   b. To maintain the original curved shape of the curet back, a few rounding strokes on each side of the back will remove the bevel.
   c. A wire edge should be removed, if present, by smoothing the face with a few sharpening strokes.

V. Assessment or Evaluation for Sharpness
A. Accumulation of the sludge or metal filings
1. During the actual sharpening process, metal

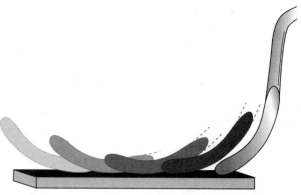

Figure 11.18 Instrument sharpening: stone movement from heel to toe. The entire lateral side of the instrument should be sharpened. This may require a dramatic change in position as the instrument is sharpened from the heel to the toe as shown with this posterior Gracey curet. Or it may be a very slight shift from heel to toe in a universal curet. This adjustment of the stone to instrument relationship is critical for maintaining the original shape of the instrument.

removed from the instrument collects on the face of the blade and is used as a general indication that that portion of the blade is sharp.
2. When using oil as the lubricant, the collection of oil and metal is called sludge; when using water as the lubricant, metal particles collect.

B. Use of a test stick
1. A plastic test stick may be used to evaluate an instrument for sharpness or dullness. It can be part of the standard instrument set-up and sterilized between patients.
2. To use the test stick, apply the instrument at the same angle that would be used against the tooth to be scaled. Press the cutting edge into the test stick and release. Shaving the test stick will dull the blade.
3. A sharp instrument should bite or grab the plastic test stick surface when lightly pressed into the surface and released.
4. Test the entire cutting edge

C. Light reflection or glare test
1. Using good lighting, hold the cutting edge to be evaluated so that it is directed toward the evaluator's eye.
2. A sharp cutting edge is a fine line and will not reflect light.
3. A dull cutting edge has width and will reflect light.

D. Magnification
1. Use of magnification may assist in assessment of the instrument blade for sharpness and contour.
2. Is especially helpful with the light reflection or glare test and when instrument recontouring.

VI. Instrument Recontouring and Replacement
  A. Recontouring
    1. Is used for an instrument that no longer has its original shape but still has sufficient metal bulk in the blade.
    2. Goal is to recreate the original shape of the blade. Use the same principles and techniques as for regular sharpening. Metal is usually removed from both the lateral sides and the face.
  A. Replacement
    1. Rule of thumb is to replace an instrument when the blade thickness has been reduced by 50%. because the blade is at increased risk of fracture during use.
    2. Also recommended when instrument blade effectiveness has been reduced by loss of the original or intended shape.
VII. Instrument Sterilization and Care (see Chapter 8)

CONTENT REVIEW QUESTIONS

1. Subjective information is diagnostic and is obtained through tests and taking measures.
    A. both statements are TRUE
    B. both statements are FALSE
    C. first statement is TRUE, the second is FALSE
    D. first statement is FALSE, the second is TRUE
2. A patient with coronary artery disease will present with all of the following, EXCEPT one. Which one is the EXCEPTION?
    A. usage of nitroglycerin
    B. chest pain with exertion and anxiety
    C. valvular defect
    D. inadequate circulation of blood to the heart
3. Patients with pacemakers may:
    A. report taking digitalis or calcium channel blockers
    B. present with swollen ankles
    C. report taking warfarin
    D. present with dilated pupils.
4. Patients with kidney disease experience all of the following, EXCEPT one. Which one is the EXCEPTION?
    A. need for premedication to prevent bacterial endocarditis when a surgical shunt has been placed
    B. decreased white blood cell formation and function
    C. longer half-life of medications
    D. frequent infections and poor healing.
5. Which one of the following is NOT used in treating hypertension?
    A. ACE inhibitors
    B. nitroglycerin
    C. beta blockers
    D. diuretics
    E. calcium channel blockers

6. All of the following are examination techniques for evaluating the soft tissues of the head and neck, EXCEPT one. Which one is the EXCEPTION?
    A. visual observation
    B. percussion
    C. palpation
    D. auscultation
    E. olfaction
7. All of the following are true of entries made into the dental record, EXCEPT one. Which one is the EXCEPTION?
    A. entries should be lengthy, with detailed recordings of recommended treatments and patient responses
    B. entries should use adequate space to record brief and accurate statements of diagnosis and treatment rendered
    C. entries should summarize a patient's response, noting wants, needs, and expectations
    D. entries serve as a legal document
8. Rhinophyma is best described as:
    A. a butterfly-shaped lesion over the bridge of the nose
    B. an overgrowth of glands causing a red, bulbous nose
    C. numerous infected hair follicles surrounding the nasal septum
    D. a clear drainage from the nose due to an extended sinus infection
    E. an obstructed airway due to a deviated septum
9. A maxillary tori
    A. is of little significance and need not be recorded as a clinical finding
    B. may need to be removed or reduced prior to the fabrication of a full denture
    C. is often removed to improve the patient's ability to clean the lingual surfaces of the maxillary molars
    D. becomes malignant in 15% of the female population
10. All of the following are lesions that can be found on the tongue, EXCEPT one. Which one is the EXCEPTION?
    A. fibroma
    B. hemangioma
    C. mucocele
    D. carcinoma
11. Which one of the following is NOT associated with mucogingival defects?
    A. lack of attached gingiva
    B. clefting
    C. high frenum attachment
    D. tissue trauma
12. A pigmented nevus:
    A. rarely has hair growing from surface
    B. is generally isolated to the posterior dorsum of the tongue

C. is rarely elevated above the surface of the skin

D. may have brown pigmentation

13. A white plaque on the mucosa that can vary from being translucent to forming a thick fissured lesion BEST describes which one of the following?

A. leukoplakia

B. papilloma

C. nevus

D. hemangioma

14. Which of the following is a malignant tumor with etiology directly related to sunlight exposure?

A. squamous cell carcinoma

B. juvenile melanoma

C. basal cell carcinoma

D. intradermal nevus

15. What is the MOST common oral site for the appearance of squamous cell carcinoma?

A. floor of the mouth

B. tongue

C. alveolar mucosa

D. palate

16. Which of the following lesions has the highest mortality rate of all cancerous lesions?

A. basal cell carcinoma

B. squamous cell carcinoma

C. malignant melanoma

D. juvenile melanoma

17. Kaposi's sarcoma is MOST commonly found in patients with which one of the following diseases?

A. uncontrolled NIDDM

B. AIDS

C. syphilis

D. genital herpes

18. A biopsy allows an examination of both surface and deep or internal cells of the lesion. Exfoliative cytology allows an examination of only the surface cells of the lesion.

A. both statements are TRUE

B. both statements are FALSE

C. first statement is TRUE, the second is FALSE

D. first statement is FALSE, the second is TRUE

19. Which one of the following is an advantage of exfoliative cytology?

A. is effective on keratinized lesions

B. indicates need for biopsy

C. gives false-negative results

D. does not involve cutting into the tissue

20. A sealant is placed on permanent molars to help prevent

A. CL I caries

B. CL II caries

C. CL III caries

D. CL IV caries

E. CL V caries

21. A metal casting is a restoration made from which of the following?

A. plastic mold

B. plaster mold

C. metal mold

D. plastic pattern

E. waxed pattern

22. Hypocalcification is an area on the tooth that:

A. needs to be restored

B. has started to demineralize

C. has started to remineralize

D. has not completely calcified

23. Attrition is loss of tooth structure due to which of the following?

A. bacterial influences

B. excessive horizontal forces

C. chemical influences on the cusp tips and incisal edges

D. mechanical wearing

24. Which of the following is NOT associated with anklyosed teeth?

A. first and second primary molars

B. hollow sound on tapping

C. need for extraction

D. subocclusal location

E. roots fused to underlying bone

25. When an enamel organ is invaginated internally during tooth development, it is referred to as which of the following?

A. gemination

B. dens in dente

C. dilaceration

D. fusion

26. Occlusal evaluation defines the contact relationship between the maxillary and mandibular teeth when:

A. anterior teeth are contacting end-to-end

B. teeth are fully closed

C. mandibular teeth are in the most protruded position

D. maxillary and mandibular first molar interproximal spaces coincide

E. contact occurs only on posterior teeth

27. Overbite is which of the following?

A. vertical overlap between maxillary and mandibular anterior teeth

B. horizontal overlap between maxillary and mandibular anterior teeth

C. vertical overlap of the first molars when the anterior teeth are missing

D. horizontal overlap of the first molars when the anterior teeth are missing

28. In the primary dentition, when the maxillary second molars occlude end-to-end with the mandibular second molars, it is referred to as which of the following?

A. mesial step

B. distal step

C. terminal plane

D. end-to-end occlusion

E. CL I occlusion

29. What is the BEST method for identifying a pulpal problem?
    A. comparing the results from the electronic pulp tester to the standardized scores for that tooth type
    B. looking for radiolucent areas at the apex of teeth on periapical films
    C. testing both the suspected and several control teeth by several methods and comparing the results between teeth
    D. using the cold test (usually ice sticks, dry ice, or ethyl chloride)

30. All of the following are true of a percussion test, EXCEPT one. Which one is the EXCEPTION?
    A. it can identify a problem of either periodontal or pulpal origin
    B. if the patient reports a very sensitive tooth, gentle finger pressure is used at first
    C. teeth are tapped or moved in both a horizontal and vertical direction
    D. positive results indicate inflammation in the pulp chamber

31. Which of the following tests is most widely used in conjunction with electronic pulp testing to provide a definitive test for pulp vitality?
    A. heat test
    B. cold test
    C. palpation
    D. percussion

32. An electronic pulp tester should NOT be used on a patient with which of the following?
    A. congestive heart failure
    B. angina pectoris
    C. rheumatic heart disease
    D. cardiac pacemaker

33. The attached gingiva is firmly bound to the underlying:
    A. enamel
    B. dentin and alveolar bone
    C. cementum and alveolar bone
    D. free gingival margin
    E. free gingival groove

34. The base of the sulcus is composed of which of the following?
    A. nonkeratinized epithelial tissue
    B. keratinized epithelial tissue
    C. keratinized connective tissue
    D. keratinized granular tissue

35. Which one of the following is NOT true about junctional epithelium?
    A. composed of stratified squamous epithelium
    B. only a few cells thick at the apical end
    C. composed of keratinized tissue
    D. approximate length is 0.25 mm to 1.35 mm

36. Which of the following is TRUE regarding chronic inflammation?
    A. bleeds spontaneously when probed
    B. appears soft and spongy
    C. appears edematous and bright red
    D. appears leathery and tough

37. Bacterial plaque in a recently cleaned mouth contains
    A. leukocytes, epithelial cells, and a few gram positive cocci
    B. leukocytes, cocci with filaments increasing, and newly formed rods
    C. Gram negative anaerobic bacteria, white blood cells, and spirochetes
    D. Gram negative aerobic bacteria, Gram positive cocci, and spirochetes

38. Which of the following bacteria is associated with localized juvenile periodontitis?
    A. *Streptococcus mutans*
    B. *Actinobacillus actinomycetemcomitas*
    C. *Actinomyces* species
    D. *Treponema denticola*

39. Which statement is TRUE regarding calculus?
    A. by itself, can cause disease
    B. is an attachment mechanism for bacterial plaque
    C. is easily removed with a sharp curette
    D. supragingivally appears darker due to blood pigments

40. Which one of the following is a limitation of the use of radiographs for the assessment of periodontal disease?
    A. artifacts that may be mistaken for pathology
    B. 3-dimensional object projected on a 1-dimensional surface
    C. interproximal areas that are difficult to see on radiographs
    D. age of the patient
    E. amount of gingival enlargement

41. Externally motivated people:
    A. believe in fate
    B. feel they are responsible for success
    C. will be motivated to long term health behavior
    D. require little supervision and direction

42. According to Maslow's Needs Hierarchy, which of the following needs are associated with motivating a patient?
    A. self-actualization and fulfilling one's ambition
    B. need for freedom
    C. safety, love and self-esteem
    D. need to own space and maintain control

43. Which one of the following influences motivation on a short-term basis?
    A. esthetics
    B. malodor
    C. cost
    D. pain

44. When communicating, what percentage of the expressed messaged is nonverbal?
    A. 10%–15%
    B. 28%–30%
    C. 62%–65%
    D. 90%–93%

45. Which one of the following body gestures may indicate the patient has become defensive?
    A. hands gripping the arms of the chair
    B. arms crossed over the chest
    C. hands linked behind the neck
    D. shoulders slumped forward

46. Which one of the following is an example of a "closed question"?
    A. How many times a day do you brush your teeth?
    B. Do you floss your teeth daily?
    C. What kind of toothbrush do you use?
    D. When do you floss your teeth?

47. According to the Learning Ladder Continuum, at what level is behavior modified?
    A. awareness
    B. self-interest
    C. involvement
    D. habit

48. When planning individual instruction, what is the MOST important question to ask?
    A. What can we do for you today?
    B. How long has it been since you have seen a dentist?
    C. How often do you brush your teeth?
    D. When do you want to schedule your dental treatment?

49. Which one of the following characteristics would be LEAST desirable in a toothbrush?
    A. head size that corresponds patient's mouth size
    B. handle that is easy to grip
    C. bristles that are natural
    D. bristles that are multi-tufted

50. What is the MOST widely accepted method of tooth brushing?
    A. roll technique
    B. modified Stillman
    C. Charters
    D. Bass

51. To reduce calculus formation, which one of the following components is added to toothpaste?
    A. potassium nitrate
    B. soluble pyrophosphate
    C. strontium chloride
    D. sodium citrate

52. Chlorhexidine mouthrinse is NOT:
    A. active against Gram-positive organisms
    B. approved in the US in a concentration of 0.12%
    C. an antimicrobial agent
    D. to be used on a long term basis

53. Phenolic compounds do which of the following?
    A. alter the bacterial cell wall
    B. reduce caries

C. promote oral wound cleansing
D. interfere with bacterial glycolysis

54. All of the following are true with regard to the aging patient, EXCEPT one. Which one is the EXCEPTION?
    A. generally has a softer diet
    B. is more sensitive due to recession
    C. is more likely to experience dry mouth
    D. has more interproximal caries than other age groups

55. Which one of the following statements is NOT TRUE for pregnant women?
    A. oral prophylaxis is an accepted treatment during pregnancy
    B. may have gingivitis and require multiple cleanings
    C. dental treatment is best performed during the first and third trimesters
    D. should be educated on early childhood dental health

56. Which one of the following is NOT a dental prosthesis?
    A. single-tooth dental implant
    B. maxillary denture
    C. 4-unit bridge
    D. space maintainer

57. All of the following are examples of dental appliances, EXCEPT one. Which one is the EXCEPTION?
    A. single tooth crown
    B. periodontal splint
    C. orthodontic retainer
    D. occlusal night guard

58. All of the following are reasons for an edentulous patient to have an annual dental visit, EXCEPT one. Which one is the EXCEPTION?
    A. soft tissue exam could identify early cancer or other harmful lesions
    B. dentures need to be relined or replaced annually
    C. dentures need periodic cleaning
    D. self-care of denture needs reinforcement
    E. underlying mucosa of denture need evaluation

59. What is the ideal concentration level of fluoride in drinking water?
    A. 0.5 ppm
    B. 1 ppm
    C. 2 ppm
    D. 4 ppm

60. After application of topical fluoride, the patient should be instructed not to eat or drink for what period of time?
    A. 10 minutes
    B. 15 minutes
    C. 20 minutes
    D. 30 minutes
    E. 60 minutes

61. Emergency treatment for acute fluoride toxicity if ingestion is >5 mg/kg body weight would include all

of the following, EXCEPT one. Which one is the EXCEPTION?
A. giving milk orally
B. inducing vomiting
C. observing patient for several hours
D. monitoring patient for heart dysrhythmias

62. Which of the following is NOT true of self-curing pit and fissure sealants?
A. requires two components that are mixed together
B. has more working time than light-cured sealants
C. tooth needs to be etched prior to application
D. tooth needs to be dried prior to application
E. can reduce need for occlusal restorations of molars by up to 50%

63. Pit and fissure sealants are used to do which of the following?
A. chemically bond to pits and fissures of posterior teeth
B. reduce occlusal caries by 75% on molars
C. act as a barrier against bacteria
D. reduce interproximal caries by 50% on molars

64. Good operator and patient positioning should have all of the following advantages for the operator, EXCEPT one. Which one is the EXCEPTION?
A. reduces the chance of upper body pain and/or injury for the operator
B. reduces the number of instruments needed to complete a full mouth debridement
C. improves visibility of the treatment area
D. reduces the possibility that the patient might faint during treatment

65. A well-positioned patient should have which of the following?
A. top of the head at the top of the dental chair
B. feet higher than head and heart
C. head turned to the right for a right-handed operator
D. chair back at about a 45-degree angle, if the patient has a strong gag reflex

66. When treating the maxillary arch, the patient is typically asked to tilt their chin downward (or chair back is slightly raised) to improve access and visibility. When treating the mandibular arch, the patient is positioned with the maxilla perpendicular to the floor for maximum access and visibility.
A. both statements are TRUE
B. both statements are FALSE
C. first statement is TRUE, the second is FALSE
D. first statement is FALSE, the second is TRUE

67. All of the following are true of the principles of good operator positioning, EXCEPT one. Which one is the EXCEPTION?
A. both feet are kept on the floor except when seated at 7 or 8 o'clock, and the inside leg is crossed over the outside leg to allow seating closer to the patient for improved access

B. the feet and legs are kept apart to create a more stable seated position on the stool
C. the stool height is adjusted so that the operator's thighs are parallel to the floor
D. the body is seated to the back of the stool so that the spine is supported by the back rest

68. The incidence of occupational injury can be reduced by the use of good body mechanics. Which one of the following is NOT good use of body mechanics?
A. keeping the shoulders relaxed and even
B. keeping the upper arms near the body and the forearms parallel to the floor
C. tilting forward and hyper-extending the neck to improve visibility
D. keeping the patient's mouth at a comfortable focal distance of about 15 inches from the operator's eye

69. Curet Q has a shank with complex angles and is designed for use in periodontal pockets. Curet Q is excellent for root planing and removal of light calculus deposits. Which design characteristic would need to be changed in order for instrument Q to be effective in removing moderate calculus deposits?
A. thickness of the shank
B. length of the lower (terminal) shank
C. toe of the blade
D. length of the blade
E. back of the blade

70. A balanced instrument is designed with which of the following?
A. 2 cutting edges
B. 2 mirror-imaged working ends, one on each end of the handle
C. straight or simple shank
D. middle of the working end centered on the long axis of the instrument handle

71. Mirrors are used for many purposes including soft tissue retraction, indirect vision, indirect illumination, and transillumination. Transillumination is the illumination of a dark area of the mouth by bouncing light off the mirror face.
A. both statements are TRUE
B. both statements are FALSE
C. first statement is TRUE, the second is FALSE
D. first statement is FALSE, the second is TRUE

72. The cross-sectional shape of the working end of various instruments helps define the category and function of the instrument. Which one of the following is NOT a correct match between instrument type and cross-sectional shape?
A. explorer—circle
B. universal curet—half moon
C. sickle—triangle
D. area-specific curet—ellipse

73. The primary instruments for assessment of the periodontal status and dental hygiene treatment needs of a patient are various explorers and probes.

A Nabor's probe is designed specifically for identifying and determining the characteristics of furcations.

A. both statements are TRUE
B. both statements are FALSE
C. first statement is TRUE, the second is FALSE
D. first statement is FALSE, the second is TRUE

74. Which of the following would be the BEST choice for removal of calculus around the contacts and adjacent interproximal areas of the mandibular anterior teeth?
A. sickle scaler
B. universal curet
C. area-specific curet
D. chisel

75. Universal curets and area-specific curets share a number of design features. Which of the following is NOT common to both?
A. rounded toe and rounded back
B. 2 cutting edges per working end
C. simple shanks for anterior teeth and complex shanks for posterior teeth
D. paired, mirror-imaged working ends

76. When comparing area-specific curets to all other manual scaling instruments, the area-specific curets have been shown to produce the smoothest root surfaces. Universal curets on the other hand have been shown to remove the most root structure.
A. both statements are TRUE
B. both statements are FALSE
C. first statement is TRUE, the second is FALSE
D. first statement is FALSE, the second is TRUE

77. Which of the following area-specific curets was designed to treat the mesial surfaces of posterior teeth?
A. Gracey 5–6
B. Gracey 11–12
C. Gracey 13–14
D. Gracey 17–18

78. Instruments designed for the debridement of titanium implants:
A. should be made of plastic
B. are standard metal instruments
C. have unique shapes
D. cause light scratches on the surface

79. All of the following are true of the modified pen grasp EXCEPT one. Which one is the EXCEPTION?
A. thumb and middle finger are placed opposite each other on the handle
B. handle rests between the thumb and the second joint of the index finger
C. ring finger rests against the middle finger and is used as the fulcrum finger
D. pad of the middle finger rests on the instrument

80. All of the following are true of fulcrums, EXCEPT one. Which one is the EXCEPTION?
A. effective use of a fulcrum can increase control over the working stroke

B. ring finger is also called the fulcrum finger
C. extraoral fulcrum should be used whenever possible
D. fulcrum is a mechanical leverage

81. The optimum angle of the instrument face to the tooth surface for scaling is between 45 and 60 degrees. The optimum angle for root planing is 70 to 80 degrees.
A. both statements are TRUE
B. both statements are FALSE
C. first statement is TRUE, the second is FALSE
D. first statement is FALSE, the second is TRUE

82. What is the range of movement at the tip of the working end for most sonic scalers?
A. 5,000 to 7,000 cycles/second
B. 25,000 to 30,000 cycles/second
C. 40,000 to 50,000 cycles/second
D. 20,000 to 50,000 cycles/second

83. The two types of machines for ultrasonic scaling are magnetostrictive and piezoelectric. Magnetostrictive ultrasonics convert electrical power to tip movement through magnetic oscillations and have a generally elliptical pattern of tip movement, while piezoelectric units use a crystal to convert electricity to movement and generally have a linear pattern of tip movement.
A. both statements are TRUE
B. both statements are FALSE
C. first statement is TRUE, the second is FALSE
D. first statement is FALSE, the second is TRUE

84. Slim/thin style ultrasonic tips are the BEST choice for which kinds of deposits?
A. heavy calculus and light calculus
B. heavy calculus and plaque
C. light calculus and plaque
D. all deposits

85. When beginning ultrasonic instrumentation on a tooth with both supra and subgingival calculus, one would typically begin on the more apical calculus and end with the more coronal. Subgingival plaque removal is at least as effective with ultrasonic instruments as with manual instruments if you are thorough with both.
A. both statements are TRUE
B. both statements are FALSE
C. first statement is TRUE, the second is FALSE
D. first statement is FALSE, the second is TRUE

86. In deep pockets and hard to reach subgingival areas, curets are the instrument of choice. Because ultrasonic tips do not have a specific cutting edge, there is no need to achieve a specific face to tooth working angle as with a curet or sickle.
A. both statements are TRUE
B. both statements are FALSE
C. first statement is TRUE, the second is FALSE
D. first statement is FALSE, the second is TRUE

87. While not essential for successful treatment, a standard pen grasp and a soft tissue fulcrum are recom-

mended for use with ultrasonic instrumentation because they:
A. foster a lighter working stroke
B. improve penetration of fluid to the base of the pocket
C. are gentler to the soft tissue
D. prevent operator fatigue

88. Why is it critical that the point of the ultrasonic tip never be adapted to the root surface?
A. it can gouge and permanently damage the root surface
B. it generates too much heat
C. it is not effective in deposit removal
D. it is uncomfortable for the operator

89. What is the main reason instrumentation with an ultrasonic takes less time than manual instrumentation?
A. fewer strokes are needed
B. clinician tires less easily
C. less pressure is needed
D. strokes are performed more quickly

90. All of the following may be considered a contraindication for the use of an ultrasonic scaler, EXCEPT one. Which one is the EXCEPTION?
A. implant surface
B. obligatory mouth breather
C. shielded pacemaker
D. newly erupted teeth

91. When used with reasonable skill and care, which of the following is generally considered acceptable to treat with an ultrasonic scaler?
A. amalgam
B. composite
C. porcelain-fused-to-metal crown
D. aesthetic veneer

92. Which of the following is the BEST rationale for polishing?
A. brightening the patient's teeth and smile
B. removing extrinsic stain
C. removing plaque accumulations
D. giving the patient's mouth a clean, fresh feeling

93. As a regular part of the oral prophylaxis, selective polishing has replaced full-mouth polishing for all of the following reasons, EXCEPT one. Which one is the EXCEPTION?
A. repeated polishing can remove cementum, dentin, and even enamel
B. plaque can be removed by other potentially less damaging means
C. fluoride-rich layer is removed
D. treatment time is reduced

94. Which of the following is a potential problem caused by polishing?
A. creation of a bacteremia as a result of abrasive particles being absorbed systemically
B. allergy to ingredients of commercial polishing pastes is more common than is generally believed

C. creation of a microbial-laden aerosol that is inhaled by the patient as well as spread to surrounding surfaces
D. vaporization of mercury during amalgam polishing procedures, even when good technique is used

95. When a patient has a healthy mouth with the gingiva at the CEJ and papilla filling the embrasure spaces, the best way to polish the interproximal surfaces is with an abrasive polishing agent and
A. Porte polisher
B. rubber-cup on a prophy angle
C. air-powder abrasive system
D. dental floss

96. In a rubber-cup polishing system, the slow speed handpiece causes the shaft to rotate in the prophy angle, which causes the rubber cup to turn and move the polishing abrasive over the tooth surface. Regardless of the polishing system used, it is the abrasive agent that produced the polishing action.
A. both statements are TRUE
B. both statements are FALSE
C. the first statement is TRUE, the second is FALSE
D. the first statement if FALSE, the second is TRUE

97. In an air-powder polishing system, polishing is produced by a mixture containing abrasive particles to clean the tooth, water to prevent heating and to dilute the abrasive, and air to provide force to deliver the abrasive to the tooth surface. This system causes more damage to composites and to tooth surfaces than other methods of stain removal.
A. both statements are TRUE
B. both statements are FALSE
C. first statement is TRUE, the second is FALSE
D. first statement is FALSE, the second is TRUE

98. To make air-powder polishing more effective and comfortable, the angle of the tip to the tooth is important. What are the recommended angles?
A. anterior teeth 40 degrees and posterior teeth 60 degrees
B. anterior teeth 60 degrees and posterior teeth 80 degrees
C. anterior teeth 80 degrees and posterior teeth 40 degrees
D. anterior teeth 45 degrees and posterior teeth 15 degrees

99. All of the following are true of sharpened instruments, EXCEPT one. Which is the EXCEPTION?
A. less pressure is needed to remove the deposit
B. more likely to slip during instrumentation
C. less chance of occupational injury
D. more likely to produce a clean tooth surface

100. The cutting edges of scaling instruments dull with use. Dull cutting edges are less effective in removing deposits than sharp cutting edges.
A. both statements are TRUE
B. both statements are FALSE

C. the first statement is TRUE, the second is FALSE

D. the first statement is FALSE, the second is TRUE

101. Which of the following BEST indicates an instrument is dull?

A. the instrument grabs at the root surface

B. light does not reflect off of the cutting edge

C. 10 working strokes have been taken

D. calculus is being burnished

102. An Arkansas stone is a:

A. natural stone that should be lubricated with oil before use and can only be chemically sterilized

B. synthetic stone that does not need to be lubricated before use and can be sterilized by any means

C. natural stone that should be lubricated with oil before use and can be sterilized by any means

D. synthetic stone that should be lubricated with water before use and can be sterilized by any means

103. Which of the following is the most abrasive sharpening stone?

A. ceramic stone

B. Arkansas stone

C. India stone

D. all have a similar abrasive grit

104. Which one of the following is NOT a general principle of instrument sharpening?

A. the angle between the instrument face and the stone is about 110 degrees

B. the original shape of the instrument should be preserved

C. metal is removed equally from the lateral surface and the face

D. the internal angle of the cutting blade of a curet or a sickle must be maintained at about 70 degrees

105. A wire edge is a projection that forms as metal particles are burnished to form an extension beyond the surface being sharpened. It is important to prevent the formation of a wire edge because it is difficult to remove after it is created.

A. both statements are TRUE

B. both statements are FALSE

C. first statement is TRUE, the second is FALSE

D. first statement is FALSE, the second is TRUE

106. When sharpening the lateral sides of a sickle using an instrument-stable technique

A. the face of the instrument is positioned so that it is parallel with the floor or countertop

B. a face-to-stone angle of about 70 degrees is established

C. the stone is moved in an up and down motion ending on the up stroke

D. the stone should not rotate or move in any way except up and down

107. When comparing sharpening technique between a universal and a Gracey curet for an instrument stable technique, which of the following remains the same?

A. rotation of the stone on its long axis is usually the same

B. stone position or angulation is the same

C. terminal shank position is the same

D. number of cutting edges sharpened is the same

108. The "rule of thumb" for determining the need for replacing a dental instrument is when the blade thickness is reduced by

A. 10%

B. 25%

C. 50%

D. 75%

CONTENT REVIEW RATIONALE

1. **A** Subjective information (feelings, perceptions, and attitudes) is obtained from the patient. Objective information is hard fact, the results of tests and measurements. Both objective and subjective information are useful in making a diagnosis.

2. **C** Valvular defects do not impact coronary artery disease. Coronary artery disease causes the arteries of the heart muscle to narrow reducing blood flow to the heart resulting in chest pain that can be relieved by nitroglycerin.

3. **A** Digitalis and calcium channel blockers help to regulate irregular heart beats and are often prescribed to patients after the pacemaker is inserted. Swollen ankles are a common physical presentation of congestive heart failure. Warfarin or coumadin is an anticoagulant taken for chronic heart disease to aid in blood thinning resulting in less pressure being exerted against the arterial walls. Patients with dilated pupils may be using cocaine.

4. **B** Leukemia is a disease of the white blood cells causing poor function and a decreased formation of white blood cells. Kidney disease causes frequent infections and a longer half-life of medications due to the kidney's inability to breakdown medications efficiently. Antibiotic premedication is recommended for kidney disease patients who have had a surgical shunt placed.

5. **B** Nitroglycerin is used for the treatment of angina. ACE inhibitors, beta-blockers, diuretics and calcium channel blockers could all be used to treat hypertension.

6. **B** Visual observation, palpation, auscultation and olfaction are all examining techniques to evaluate soft tissues. Percussion can be used to evaluate teeth.

7. **A** Dental record entries should be brief and accurate, **not** lengthy, and include detailed statements of diagnosis and treatment rendered. They should summarize patient responses and are considered legal documents.

8. **B** Rhinophyma is an overgrowth of sweat and sebaceous glands of the nose, which makes the nose appear red and bulbous. It is associated with heavy

alcohol consumption. Lupus Erythematosus is associated with a butterfly shaped lesion over the nose.

9. **B** Maxillary tori, a benign over-growth of bone, is not of real significance in most people. Should a denture need to be fabricated, tori may interfere with the patient's ability to successfully wear a denture, (rocking or inability to achieve a seal). As a result, tori may need to be surgically removed or reduce prior to denture fabrication.

10. **C** A mucocele is a mucous- or saliva-filled cyst that results from blockage of a salivary duct. It is usually associated with the minor salivary glands found in the labial and buccal mucosa, but not in the tongue. A mucocele under the tongue is often called a ranula.

11. **D** Tissue trauma is associated with irritation from a foreign object, not mucogingival defects. Lack of attached gingiva, clefting, and a high frenum attachment are associated with mucogingival defects.

12. **D** A pigmented nevus lesion may have a brown pigmentation. It often has a hair growing from the surface, may be scattered anywhere over the body, and may be flat or elevated from the surface of the skin.

13. **A** Leukoplakia is a white plaque that may appear translucent or can appear as a thick fissured lesion. A hemangioma is of congenital origin and appears deep red or bluish-purple in color. A papilloma has a cauliflower-like surface with numerous, small projections. A nevus may be flat or elevated and can be pigmented brown.

14. **C** A malignant lesion that is associated with the skin being exposed to the sun is a basal cell carcinoma. Squamous cell carcinoma is associated with smoking, alcohol, and syphilis. Juvenile melanoma and intradermal nevus are not malignant lesions.

15. **B** The most common oral site for a squamous cell carcinoma is the tongue. Less frequently, it may also appear on the floor of the mouth, alveolar mucosa and palate.

16. **C** Malignant melanoma has the highest mortality rate of all cancerous lesions. The mortality rate for squamous cell carcinoma is not as great. Prognosis for recovery from basal cell carcinoma is good when treated early. Juvenile melanoma is not a malignant lesion.

17. **B** Kaposi's Sarcoma is indicative of an AIDS diagnosis. Uncontrolled diabetes, syphilis, and genital herpes are not specifically associated with Kaposi's sarcoma.

18. **A** A biopsy examination includes both surface and deep or internal cells of a lesion. Exfoliative cytology only allows for examination of the surface cells, thus allowing the potential for a false negative result. The statements highlight one of the chief differences between the two types of tests and show the advantage of a biopsy.

19. **D** Patients respond favorably to exfoliative cytology, as it does not involve cutting the tissue. Unfortunately, it has a number of significant disadvantages as a diagnostic tool, such as the limitations on the kinds of lesions it evaluates, frequent false negatives, and the fact that it is not considered definitive.

20. **A** Sealants are placed to help prevent caries in occlusal pits and fissures (Class I caries) of permanent posterior teeth.

21. **E** A waxed pattern is used in development of a metal casting of a restoration. When heated, it evaporates, leaving room for the heated metal to be forced into the empty space.

22. **D** Areas that are hypocalcified have never completely calcified and may never need to be restored. A decalcified area originally was calcified and at some point, started to break down. A remineralized area is tooth structure that has started to break down but has reversed its demineralization process and has hardened.

23. **B** Excessive horizontal forces, such as those caused by bruxing, clenching or grinding can result in attrition of the occlusal/incisal tooth surfaces. Bacterial influences cause caries and periodontal disease. Chemical influences, such as those associated with bulimia, cause erosion (acid destruction of enamel) affecting the lingual of the maxillary anterior teeth. Mechanical wearing is associated with abrasion.

24. **C** Commonly, ankylosed teeth are primary first and second molars and may be identified by a hollow sound produced upon tapping and by their location below the occlusal plane. Many anklyosed teeth have no permanent teeth present to erupt should the anklyosed tooth be extracted. The primary tooth is usually retained for as long as possible.

25. **B** Dens in dente is the term associated with invagination of the enamel organ during tooth development. Gemination is the division of a single tooth germ by invagination resulting in incomplete formation of two teeth. Dilaceration is a distortion of a tooth's root and crown linear relationship, whereas fusion is the union of two tooth buds.

26. **B** The teeth have to be fully closed to evaluate occlusion.

27. **A** The vertical overlap between maxillary and mandibular anterior teeth is called overbite. Overjet is the horizontal overlap between maxillary and mandibular anterior teeth.

28. **C** A terminal plane occurs in the primary dentition when the maxillary second molars occlude end-to-end with the mandibular second molars. Mesial step occurs when the maxillary second molar is at least a cusp width anterior to the mandibular second molar. Distal step occurs when the maxillary second molar is at least a cusp width posterior to the mandibular second molar. An end-to-end occlusion occurs when

the buccal cusps of maxillary and mandibular molars occlude with one another. A Class I occlusion applies to the permanent dentition.

29. **C** There is no one best test for identifying pulp vitality. Any individual test can give a false positive or false negative result. The best system is to use several types of clinical data and to compare findings between several of the patient's teeth.

30. **D** Positive results to a percussion test indicate inflammation in the periodontal ligament that may originate from the pulp or may result from a periodontal problem. Moving the tooth in both directions, (horizontal and vertical) tests all of the different fibers that comprise the periodontal ligament.

31. **B** Electronic pulp testing and thermal testing are the most specific tests for pulp vitality. Cold is a more versatile and therefore more commonly used thermal test than heat. Percussion and palpation also provide information regarding the status of the pulp but are not as definitive as cold and electronic pulp testing.

32. **D** During the use of an electronic pulp tester (EPT), the patient is exposed to a small electrical current that might interfere with the patient's cardiac pacemaker. Use of the EPT is a non-invasive test so a patient with rheumatic heart disease would not be exposed to a potential bacteremia. EPT is not very painful or stressful, so should not pose a particular risk for patients with heart conditions.

33. **C** The attached gingiva is bound to the underlying cementum and alveolar bone. The free gingiva and free gingival groove lie cornonal to the attached gingiva. Attached gingiva does not attach to dentin or enamel.

34. **A** The base of the sulcus is composed of nonkeratinzed epithelial tissue.

35. **C** Junctional epithelium is non-keratinized stratified squamous epithelium that is approximately 0.25 mm to l.35 mm in length. It is only a few cells thick at the apical end.

36. **D** Chronically inflamed tissue will appear tough and fibrotic, often having a leathery appearance. It does not bleed easily and will often look nearly normal in color. Acute inflammation will appear edematous, soft, spongy, and bright red.

37. **A** Bacterial plaque in a recently cleaned mouth contains leukocytes, epithelial cells and a few gram-positive cocci. Plaque that is 2 to 14 days old will contain leukocytes, filamentous cocci, rods, Gram negative anaerobic bacteria, Gram positive cocci, white blood cells, and spirochetes.

38. **B** *Actinobacillus actinomycetemcomitans* is associated with localized juvenile periodontitis. *Streptococcus* species, *Actinomyces* species, and *Treponema denticola* are associated with gingivitis and periodontitis. *S. mutans* is associated with dental caries.

39. **B** Calculus acts as an attachment mechanism for bacterial plaque. By itself, it does not cause disease.

Calculus may be hard to remove regardless of the sharpness of the instrument. Subgingival calculus may appear darker due to blood pigments.

40. **A** Artifacts can be mistaken for pathology on radiographs. Assessment limitation may result from a three dimensional object being projected on a two dimensional surface. The interproximal areas are the easiest areas to assess bone loss. The buccal and lingual areas are difficult to assess due to the density of the tooth structure. Periodontal disease can occur in people of all ages. Enlarged soft tissue is not a major focus and is difficult to detect when evaluating periodontal disease on radiographs.

41. **A** Externally motivated people believe in fate. They are not easily motivated to long term health behavior and require more supervision and direction. Internally motivated people believe they are responsible for their success and will be motivated to long term health behavior. They require little supervision and direction.

42. **C** Safety, love and self-esteem are generally associated with motivating a patient according to Maslow's Needs Hierarchy. Self-actualization and fulfilling one's ambitions are part of the hierarchy, but not associated with motivating patients. Need for freedom, the need for one's own space and the need to maintain control are part of the Dental Hygiene Human Needs Conceptual Model (Darby and Walsh.)

43. **D** Pain is a short term motivating factor. Once the pain leaves, the motivation diminishes. The way one looks to others (esthetics), the smell of one's breath, and the cost of treatment may be considered long-term motivators.

44. **D** The expressed message is 90% to 93% nonverbal. The actual verbal ("words said") message is only 7%.

45. **B** When a patient crosses his arms across his chest, it indicates that he/she has become defensive. Grasping the arms of the chair may indicate apprehension. Linking ones fingers behind their neck shows they are confident. Shoulders slumped forward may indicate lack of confidence or uncertainty.

46. **B** The question "Do you floss your teeth daily?" requires a yes or no answer making it a closed question. Open-ended questions ask the patient who, what, where, when, why or how and require the patient to give more than a yes or no answer.

47. **D** A habit is formed when behavior is modified. Awareness, self interest, and involvement are all steps in forming a habit.

48. **A** The most critical question to ask a patient is "What can we do for you today?" Additional questions may also need to be asked, but only after the patient's major concern (chief complaint) has been addressed.

49. **C** Natural bristles are less desirable than nylon filaments. Nylon filaments cause less damage to the

tissues, rinse and dry more easily, are more durable, and are more resistant to bacterial accumulation. When choosing a toothbrush for a patient, consider head size relative to the size of the patient's mouth and handles that are easy to grip.

50. **D** The Bass or sulcular method of brushing is the most widely accepted toothbrushing method. The bristles are angled at 45 degrees toward the gingival margin. It is efficient in removing plaque and is an excellent method for all types of patients. The roll technique is useful preparatory instruction for modified Stillman. The modified Stillman method incorporates a vibratory stroke followed by a roll stroke. The Charters method, which requires that the bristles be angled toward the occlusal surface, is frequently recommended for orthodontic patients.

51. **B** Anticalculus forming (tartar control) toothpaste contains soluble pyrophosphates. Potassium nitrate, strontium chloride, and sodium citrate are components found in desensitizing toothpaste.

52. **D** Chlorhexidine mouth rinse is intended for short-term use. Chlorhexidine is an antimicrobial agent active against gram-positive and gram-negative organisms, as well as fungi. It is approved for use in the United States at the concentration level of 0.12%.

53. **A** Phenolic compounds, such as *Listerine*, alter the bacterial cell wall. Fluorides reduce caries. Oxygenating agents are intended to cleanse wounds and *sanguinarine* agents interfere with bacterial glycolysis.

54. **D** The aging patient is more likely to experience root caries than any other age group. They are also more likely to experience dry mouth and sensitivity due to recession. Their diet is often of a softer nature.

55. **C** If dental treatment (other than oral prophylaxis) is needed, the best time to provide treatment is during the second trimester. The first trimester is avoided because of the rapidly changing fetus; however, research does not indicate that treatment would be detrimental during this time. Restorative dental care is generally avoided during the first trimester except for emergency treatment. The third trimester is often avoided because the patient may be uncomfortable lying in the dental chair. Multiple cleanings may be necessary during the pregnancy due to hormonal changes that may cause an inflammatory response of the gingiva. This is also a good time to educate the mother-to-be on early childhood dental care.

56. **D** A space maintainer is an appliance. It is a special device designed for a specific function or therapeutic outcome, usually to hold the space of a prematurely lost deciduous molar, preventing the drift of more distal teeth into the open space. When the permanent tooth begins to erupt, the appliance will be removed. A dental prosthesis is defined as an artificial replacement for a missing body part. Good examples are a dental implant, a denture or a dental bridge.

57. **A** A single tooth crown is a fixed prosthesis. It is an artificial replacement for the crown of the tooth. Dental prostheses replace single or several teeth. Periodontal splints, orthodontic retainers, and occlusal night guards are all good examples of dental appliances. They are designed for specific functions or therapeutic outcomes such as stabilizing teeth.

58. **B** Dentures can last many years without replacement or reline especially once the bone support has stabilized after the extraction of teeth. Immediate dentures however, may need to be relined after the first year. Annual examinations are important for denture wearers because of the benefits of a soft tissue examination, denture cleaning, and evaluation and reinforcement of good oral self-care.

59. **B** The ideal concentration level of fluoride is 1 ppm, 0.5 ppm would not be adequate concentration of fluoride in the water. Amounts of 2 ppm and 4 ppm would exceed the recommended concentrations and could result in discoloration and mottling of the enamel.

60. **D** A patient should not eat or drink for 30 minutes following a fluoride application to avoid disturbing the action of the fluoride. Ten or 15 minutes is not long enough and 1 hour is excessive.

61. **D** Monitoring heart arrhythmia is not necessary until fluoride ingestion reaches >15 mg/kg body weight. Drinking milk, inducing vomiting and observing the patient for several hours are all appropriate actions to take for fluoride ingestion >5 mg/kg of body weight.

62. **B** One advantage of light cured sealant over self-cured sealant is the increased working time to place sealant. Self-cured sealants do require the mixing of two components. Both chemical and light cured sealant requires etching and drying.

63. **C** Pit and fissure sealants act as a barrier against bacteria. Etching the tooth with phosphoric acid (35%–50% solution), before the placement of the sealant creates a physical bond. Sealants have been shown to reduce occlusal caries by 54% on molars, they are only effective on occlusal surfaces.

64. **B** Good patient and operator positioning may improve efficiency by providing better visibility and reducing the chance for upper body pain and injury to the operator. It does not change the number of instruments needed to treat all surfaces of the teeth. Good patient positioning reduces the possibility that the patient might faint during treatment.

65. **A** A well-positioned patient should have their head at the top of the chair to give the operator optimum access to the mouth from all clock zone positions. The patient should be in a supine position most of the time with the head, heart, and feet at about the same level. The patient should turn their head as needed for the operator to have the

best access. Patients with a strong gag reflex will do best in a full supine or fully upright position.

66. **B** The first statement describes good patient positioning for the mandibular arch and the second statement describes good patient positioning for the maxillary arch.

67. **A** Sitting with the legs crossed causes stress along the spine and reduces circulation to the legs. It is a less stable seated position than having the body's weight evenly distributed, with legs apart and the back supported.

68. **C** Optimum body position allows for support by the skeletal and muscular system. This includes keeping the head centered over the spine though the chin may be tilted down slightly to look into the patient's mouth from a comfortable distance away. The operator should keep the shoulders and arms down in a relaxed positioned. The operator should consider moving the patient before stressing their own bodies by awkward positioning.

69. **A** The thickness or rigidity of the instrument shank most directly influence the quality of the deposits (tenacity, volume), that the instrument will remove. A thicker shank makes the instrument more rigid and better able to remove bulky or dense deposits.

70. **D** An instrument is considered balanced if the relationship of the working end to the handle makes the instrument comfortable to hold and easy to use. This occurs when the middle of the working end is centered on an imaginary line that also runs through the handle.

71. **C** The four functions of a mirror are soft tissue retraction, indirect vision, indirect illumination (also called reflected lighting), and transillumination. The illumination of a dark area of the mouth with light bounced off the mirror face is indirect illumination. For transillumination, light is reflected off the mirror and directed through the teeth to observe shadows caused by caries or calculus.

72. **D** All curets, whether universal or area-specific, are half-moon shaped in cross-section. The difference between the two is the relationship of the face to the terminal shank. The cross sectional shape of an explorer is a circle and a sickle is a triangle.

73. **A** Explorers and probes are used as the primary instruments of assessment for the dental hygiene treatment plan. Probes, with a variety of numerical demarcations, are used to measure pocket depth, clinical attachment levels, recession, width of the attached gingiva, and to determine a variety of tissue and root characteristics such as BOP and root anatomy. Nabor's probes have a curved design that better fits into furcation areas. Explorers are used to identify calculus and other deposits, root texture and anatomy, and pocket contours. Explorers are also used to identify caries and marginal status of restorations.

74. **A** The sickle scaler tapers to a thin point at the working end. This fits especially well in the tight areas around the contacts and the interproximal. Both types of curets have difficulty fitting into tight contact areas. Chisels are designed for gross debridement of the anterior teeth. They are not suitable for fine scaling either around the contact or the gingiva.

75. **B** Universal curets do have two cutting edges per working end, however, area-specific curets have only one cutting edge per working end.

76. **D** Studies looking at root smoothness and removal of the root structure do not identify a difference between area-specific and universal curets. Both of these statements are true of both types of curet designs. Individual clinicians may have a preference and be more effective with one design type or another but both can be used to effectively instrument the root.

77. **B** Individual area-specific curets are designed to instrument a particular type of tooth, or in the posterior teeth, even a particular tooth surface. Gracey 11–12 and 15–16 were designed for the mesial surfaces of the posterior teeth. Gracey 13–14 and 17–18 were designed to treat the distals of the same teeth. Gracey 5–6 can be used on any of the surfaces of the anterior and premolar teeth.

78. **A** Implant maintenance is a rapidly expanding field. It is critical that titanium implants not be scratched or damaged. Plastic debridement instruments have been shown not to scratch while standard metal instruments do scratch. Plastic instruments may be shaped like curets, sickles or have unique shapes that specifically fit around the implant surfaces.

79. **A** The thumb and index finger are usually placed opposite each other on the instrument handle with the middle finger placed below them on or near the instrument shank.

80. **C** The preferred fulcrum is an intraoral fulcrum placed on a tooth surface near the working area. A fulcrum is a mechanical leverage when used for instrumentation it increases the control over the working stroke. The ring finger is known as the fulcrum finger.

81. **B** The angles have been reversed between these statements. A more open angle is needed for scaling of larger deposits. The optimum is in the range of 70 degrees to 80 degrees. Root planing is a finishing procedure and the blade angle becomes progressively more closed. Optimum is between 45 and 60 degrees.

82. **A** Most commercially available sonic scalers operate in the 5,000 to 7,000 cycles/second range. Most magnetostrictive ultrasonics operate at 25,000 to 30,000 cycles/second, and piezoelectric and some magnetorestrictive ultrasonics generally operate at 40,000 to 50,000 cycles/second. The full range of

ultrasonics is from as low as 20,000 cycles/second to a current high limit of 50,000 cycles/second.

83. **A**   All of this information is accurate and it highlights the chief difference between the two types of ultrasonics.

84. **C**   Slim/thin style tips are very effective in removing light calculus deposits, plaque, and endotoxins. They are generally not as effective for heavy calculus removal as thicker tips.

85. **D**   Ultrasonic debridement is begun at the most coronal deposits and progresses toward the more apical deposits. Both manual and ultrasonic instrumentation are effective in deplaquing the subgingival areas. The ultrasonic may have the advantage.

86. **D**   In deep pockets and hard to reach areas like furcations, ultrasonics are generally considered the superior instrument. The newer long, thin probe-like tips will reach into deep, narrow pockets easily. More advanced furcations have been shown to have a lower bacterial count after ultrasonics than manual instruments. Studies show healing to be at least as good with ultrasonics. Without a cutting edge, angulation of the face of the blade to the tooth is not possible and this makes it easier to use the ultrasonic instruments. Good tip-to-tooth adaptation is still important.

87. **A**   The lighter, more relaxed pen grasp and use of a soft tissue fulcrum result in less pressure of the instrument tip on the tooth and that results in therapy that is more effective and more comfortable. Each of the other answers may occur as a coincidental benefit but improved therapy is the driving rationale. Increased options in fulcrums may lead to better adaptation and therefore, deeper instrumentation which will result in deeper fluid penetration because the fluid follows the tip. A softer, lighter working stroke will be more comfortable to the patient's soft tissue and the operator will be more relaxed and less fatigued.

88. **A**   Adapting the tip of an ultrasonic against the root can result in damage to the root surface. Use of the point is not as effective as adapting the side of the tip. Heat generation is not affected and discomfort is caused to the patient but not the operator.

89. **D**   A comparable number of working strokes are needed to completely treat the root surface but they can be taken more quickly and easily because there is no need to establish a working angle or lateral pressure, and also the strokes are effective in both directions. The action of an ultrasonic stroke is easy and uniform like an eraser motion. The statements that the clinician is less tired and pressure is lighter are true but not the main reasons for the difference.

90. **C**   A shielded pacemaker is protected or shielded from the ultrasonic action and is considered safe for treatment. Titanium implants have shown damage when treated by ultrasonics. An individual who always breathes through their mouth will have a difficult time breathing with the water spray in the mouth. And newly erupted teeth have large pulps that may be heat sensitive and the enamel is not fully mineralized.

91. **A**   Amalgams can be debrided with an ultrasonic scaler if care is used. It is true that amalgam can be removed, in fact, power-driven scalers are an excellent instrument to use for overhang removal but the same could be said of a sickle scaler. Composites have shown surface damage to ultrasonic instrumentation. Porcelain-fused-to-metal crowns and aesthetic veneers can be fractured or loosened with ultrasonic use.

92. **B**   Polishing is an effective and efficient method of removing extrinsic stain. It will brighten the teeth only if stain is present. Polishing will both remove plaque and give the mouth a clean feeling, however, it is potentially damaging to the teeth if repeated too often and there are other less potentially harmful methods of accomplishing these tasks.

93. **D**   Time is not reduced because plaque must be removed by alternative means. Selective polishing is preferred over full-mouth polish because it is more protective of the tooth surface. Repeated polishing can remove tooth structure especially the fluoride rich surface layer. Plaque removal, the traditional reason for full-mouth polish, can be accomplished by other methods that have less potential to damage the tooth.

94. **C**   Polishing always creates a microbial-containing aerosol. A bacteremia may be caused when inflamed gingiva is polished and oral bacteria not abrasive particles are introduced into the body. Allergy to commercial pastes is possible but rare. With good polishing technique, including no frictional heat, mercury should not be released from amalgam restorations.

95. **D**   Dental floss when used with an abrasive agent will effectively polish interproximal surfaces. Floss easily fits into an embrasure space filled with healthy papilla.

96. **A**   The polishing action is accomplished by the abrasive particles. The rubber cup, brush, wood stick, and force of the air in air-powder polish are only a means of applying the abrasive for polishing not the cause of the polishing.

97. **C**   The first statement regarding the components and roles of the ingredients of the polishing slurry is correct. Air-powder polishing systems do cause more damage to composites possibly because the "blasting action" removes some component of the composite material. Regarding tooth structure, air-powder polishing removes less tooth structure than curets when used to remove stain on root surfaces

and cause less abrasion on enamel than rubber-cup polishing.

98. **B** For anterior teeth, the tip of the nozzle is directed at a 60-degree angle toward the tooth and at an 80-degree angle toward posterior teeth.

99. **B** Dull, not sharpened, instruments are more likely to slip during instrumentation. Sharpening improves the quality of debridement and makes treatment more comfortable and effective for both the patient and the clinician.

100. **A** With use, metal is worn away from the cutting edge making the shape rounded at the junction of the face and lateral side where once they formed a sharp edge. The rounded cutting edge is not as effective in engaging and removing deposits since it is dull.

101. **D** A dull instrument is more likely to slide over a deposit, causing burnishing. As the instrument dulls, it will tend to slide on the tooth surface and have less bite or grab than a sharp instrument. The dull or rounded surface will reflect light. A standard rule cannot be made about the number of strokes to take before sharpening because it varies by the amount of lateral pressure being applied, the nature of the deposit, and the metal composition of the instrument.

102. **C** An Arkansas stone is a natural quarried stone. It should be lubricated with fine oil before use and may be sterilized by any of the conventional methods although it may become more brittle with repeated exposures to high heat.

103. **C** The India stone is consistently the most abrasive. Although Arkansas and ceramic stones may vary somewhat, they are less abrasive.

104. **C** Typically, more metal is removed from the lateral surface, rather than the face or the lateral surface and the face equally, when sharpening. Besides making the instrument thinner so that is fits into the sulcus more easily, it is believed that preserving the face to back dimension of the instrument maintains instrument strength best for the pressures and stresses created by scaling.

105. **C** The first statement is an accurate description of how a wire edge is made. It is important not to have a wire edge when the instrument is applied to a tooth because the wire edge fractures easily and the metal can become embedded in the gingival or root surface. It is easily and equally acceptable to prevent or remove a wire edge during sharpening procedures.

106. **A** The sickle is held stable with the face parallel to the floor (the terminal shank is perpendicular to the floor). The internal angel of the curet is 70 degrees, but the visible angle that is formed between the instrument face and the stone is 110 degrees. To prevent a wire edge, it is important to end sharpening of each area with a down stroke so that no metal is burnished above the face.

107. **B** The position and the movement of the stone are the same. Several other aspects of sharpening are not the same because of differences in instrument design. Gracey curets are typically more curved from heel to toe necessitating more rotation of the stone on its long axis. Also, because the blade of the Gracey is offset at a 70-degree angle, the terminal shank is not perpendicular to the floor during sharpening and only one cutting edge is used (or sharpened) on each working end.

108. **C** A dental instrument should be replaced when blade thickness is reduced by 50% because it is at risk of fracturing during use.

References

1. Khan MA, Herzog CA, St. Peter JV, Hartley GG, Madlon-Kay R, Dick CD, Asinger RW, Vessey JT. The prevalence of cardiac valvular insufficiency assessed by transthoracic echocardiography in obese patients treated with appetite-suppressant drugs. N Engl J Med 339:713–718, 1998.
2. Little JW, Falace DA. Dental Management Of The Medically Compromised Patient, 4th ed. St. Louis, Mosby, 1993, pp. 413 and 425–6.
3. Dajani AS, Taubert KA, Wilson W, Bolger AF, Bayer A, Ferrieri P, Gewitz MH, Shulman ST, Nouri S, Newburger JW, Hutto C, Pallasch TJ, Gage TW, Levison ME, Peter G, Zuccaro G Jr. Prevention of bacterial endocarditis. Recommendations by the American Heart Association. JAMA 277:1794–801, 1997.
4. Shafer WG, Hine MK, Levy BM. A Textbook of Oral Pathology, 3rd ed. Philadelphia, W.B. Saunders, 1974, p. 107.
5. http://www.docshop.com/info/melanoma.html.
6. http://www.scfa.edu.au/melanomal.html.
7. Glick M (ed). Clinician's Guide to Treatment of HIV-infected patients. American Academy of Oral Medicine 1996, p. 18.
8. Tyler MT, Lozada-Nur F (eds). Clinician's Guide to Treatment of Medically Compromised Dental Patients. American Academy of Oral Medicine 1995, p. 64–5.
9. Darby ML, Walsh MM. Dental Hygiene Theory and Practice, 1st ed. Philadelphia, W.B. Saunders, 1995, p. 71.
10. Harris NO, Christen AG. Primary Preventive Dentistry, 4th ed. Norwalk, Appleton & Lange, 1995, pp. 378–9.
11. Wilkins EM. Clinical Practice of the Dental Hygienist. 7th ed. Philadelphia, Williams & Wilkins, 1994, pp. 367–8.
12. Gutman ME. Air polishing: A comprehensive review of the literature. JDH 72:47–56, 1998.

Additional Readings

Alvarez KH. Dental Hygiene Handbook. Baltimore, Williams & Wilkins, 1998.

Bricker SL, Langlais RP, Miller CS. Oral Diagnosis, Oral Medicine and Treatment Planning. 2nd edition. Philadelphia, Lea & Febiger, 1994, p. 46–108.

Burns S. It's About Time to Get the Cutting Edge. Chicago, Hu-Friedy, 1995.

Genco RJ (ed). Annals of Periodontology. 1996 World Workshop in Periodontics. Chicago, American Academy of Periodontology, Vol. 1, #1, Nov. 1996.

Green E, Seyer PC. Sharpening Curets and Sickle Scalers. Berkeley, Praxis Publishing Company, 1972.

Hodges KO: Concepts in Nonsurgical Periodontal Therapy, 1st ed, Albany, Delmar Publishers, 1997.

Hu-Friedy: Product Catalog and Reference Guide. Chicago, HuFriedy Manufacturing Incorporated, 1998.

Hupp JR, Williams TP, Vallerand WP. The 5 Minute Clinical Consult for Dental Professionals. Baltimore, Williams & Wilkins, 1996.

Ibsen OAC, Phelan JA. Oral Pathology for the Dental Hygienist, 2nd ed. Philadelphia, W.B. Saunders, 1996.

Langlais RP, Miller CS. Color Atlas of Common Oral Diseases. Philadelphia, Lea & Febiger, 1992.

Mueller-Joseph L, Petersen M. Dental Hygiene Process: Diagnosis and Care Planning. Albany, Delmar Publishers, 1995.

Nield JS, O'Connor GH. Fundamentals of Dental Hygiene Instrumentation, 3rd ed, Baltimore, Williams & Wilkins, 1996.

Pattison AM, Pattison GL. Periodontal Instrumentation, 2nd ed, Norwalk, Appleton & Lange, 1992.

Sonis, ST, Fazio RC, Fang L. Principles and Practice of Oral Medicine, 2nd ed. Philadelphia, W.B. Saunders, 1995.

Savage MG. Patient history in dental treatment planning. In Clark's Clinical Dentistry. St. Louis, Mosby, 1998, pp. 1–12.

Wilson Jr TG, Korman KS, Newman MG. Advances in Periodontics. Chicago, Quintessence Publishing Co, 1992.

Wilson Jr TG. Dental Maintenance for Patients with Periodontal Disease. Chicago, Quintessence Publishing Co, 1989.

Wilson TI, Korman KS. Fundamentals of Periodontics. Chicago: Quintessence Publishing Co, 1996.

Woodall IR. Comprehensive Dental Hygiene Care, 4th ed. St. Louis, Mosby, 1993.

Chapter **TWELVE**

Periodontology

Salme E. Lavigne, R.D.H., M.S.

 Clinical Case **STUDY**

Mary Brown, a 25-year-old patient whom you have been seeing regularly every 6 months for oral prophylaxis, presents with pocket depths that have increased from 3 to 4 mm and a bleeding score of 60%, according to the Ainamo and Bay bleeding index. Additionally, signs of gingival inflammation are present in the form of marginal erythema, generalized bulbous papillae, and rolled margins. This finding is unusual for Mary because she has always exhibited meticulous oral hygiene. Moreover, plaque and calculus are not present in noticeable quantities during this visit. When she is asked about her medical history, Mary reveals that she has quit smoking and that she is expecting her first child in 5 months.

Clinical Case QUESTIONS

1. What is the most likely diagnosis of Mary's condition?
2. What factors are contributing to Mary's condition?
3. How should this condition be treated?
4. What information can be given to Mary to help prepare her for other possible complications?

Clinical Case RATIONALES

1. Chronic marginal gingivitis. Her pocket depths are no greater than 4 mm and most likely are pseudopockets because the signs of inflammation include gingival edema.
2. The predominant factor contributing to Mary's condition is her pregnancy. During pregnancy, increased levels of progesterone have been associated with an increased susceptibility to gingivitis.
3. Thorough professional debridement, elevated plaque control measures, and education regarding the correlation between the condition and the contributing factors will keep the disease under control.
4. Gingivitis associated with pregnancy begins in the second to third months and is most severe in the second and third trimesters. Moreover, localized enlargements in the interdental papillae form tumorlike growths in some individuals and are referred to as pregnancy tumors. If these tumors occur, they will disappear at the end of the pregnancy.

Content Review

Periodontal Tissues

The tissues of the periodontium are made up of gingiva, periodontal ligament, cementum, and alveolar bone.

Functions of the Periodontium

The periodontium functions as an attachment mechanism, a shock absorber, and a line of defense against external agents.

  I. Attaches the tooth to its bony housing (alveolus).
  II. Provides resistance to the forces of mastication, speech, and deglutition.
  III. Maintains body surface integrity by separating the external and internal environment.
  IV. Adjusts for structural changes associated with wear and aging through continuous remodeling and regeneration.
  V. Defends against external noxious stimuli.

Components of the Periodontium

The gingiva, periodontal ligament, cementum, and alveolar bone comprise the periodontium.

  I. Gingiva
    A. Is a component of oral mucous membranes and is classified as masticatory mucosa, which includes the gingiva and hard palate.
    B. Consists of keratinized or parakeratinized stratified squamous epithelium, which is avascular.

C. Underlying the epithelium is the lamina propria, which is the connective tissue layer in the oral cavity.

D. Components
   1. Epithelium
      a. Stratified squamous epithelium provides protective covering and comprises four cell layers.
         1) Stratum basale—The basal layer adjacent to the connective tissue and separated by a basement membrane.
         2) Stratum spinosum—A prickly layer of cells adjacent to the stratum basale.
         3) Stratum granulosum—A granular layer rich in keratohyaline granules, which synthesize keratin for the surface layer.
         4) Stratum corneum—The most superficial layer, which is "cornified" (contains the protein keratin).
      b. Three layers
         1) The oral layer is keratinized/parakeratinized; includes outer free and attached gingivae and papillae. The basal layer is "wavy" and forms deep, fingerlike projections that reach into the connective tissue layer below. These projections are referred to as rete pegs.
         2) The sulcular layer is nonkeratinized; lines the sulcus and is 1 to 3 mm deep in healthy individuals.
         3) The junctional layer is nonkeratinized; attaches to tooth and lies between the base of the sulcus and underlying connective tissue; normally is 0.25 to 1.35 mm long; joins cementum via hemidesmosomes and glycosaminoglycans; attachment consists of a basal lamina comparable to that which exists in epithelial tissue/connective tissue interfaces elsewhere in the body.
   2. Connective tissue (lamina propria)
      a. Contains collagen fibers and cells (e.g., fibroblasts, undifferentiated cells, macrophages).
      b. Gingival fibers primarily consist of collagen (60%) but also comprise reticular, elastic, and oxytalan fibers.
         1) The gingivodental group extends from cementum to free and attached gingiva.
         2) The dentoperiosteal group also embeds in the cementum but extends apically over the alveolar crest and terminates in the alveolar bone.
         3) The circular group encircles teeth that are coronal to alveolar bone.
         4) The transseptal group connects the cementums of two adjacent teeth.
         5) The alveogingival group inserts in the alveolar crest and splays out into free gingiva.
      c. Cells
         1) Fibroblasts synthesize both collagen fibers and glycosaminoglycans or "glue."
         2) Macrophages serve a protective "phagocytic" role.
         3) Mast cells provide necessary histamine during inflammation.
         4) Neutrophils, lymphocytes, and plasma cells are inflammatory cells found in small quantities in healthy gingiva; increase in number during inflammation.
         5) Undifferentiated cells are available to differentiate into any cell type as the need arises.

E. The gingival unit
   1. Marginal gingiva (free gingiva)
      a. Surrounds the tooth like a cuff.
      b. Is knife-edged in anteriors and more rolled in posteriors.
      c. Is separated from attached gingiva by the free gingival groove at the level of the CEJ.
   2. Attached gingiva
      a. Extends from the free gingival groove to the mucogingival junction; is 1 to 9 mm long; also is firm, pink or pigmented, and stippled in healthy individuals.
   3. Interdental gingiva
      a. Is found between two adjacent teeth; typically is pointed.
      b. Its shape is dependent on the contact relationship between adjacent teeth.
      c. The gingival "col" area is found under the contact; is the valley or depression between the facial or lingual peaks of the gingiva.
   4. Alveolar mucosa
      a. Is another component of oral mucous membranes; is separate from the gingiva.
      b. Is found beyond the mucogingival junction.
      c. Is nonkeratinized, flexible, and reddish in color.

II. Periodontal Ligament (PDL)
   A. Together with the alveolar bone, forms the "attachment apparatus."
   B. Is the connective tissue that surrounds the root of the tooth.
   C. Functions
      1. Anchors tooth to alveolar bone.
         a. Has an hourglass shape and ranges in thickness from 0.15 to 0.38 mm.
         b. Protects small vessels and nerves.
         c. Acts as a shock absorber for occlusal forces.
            1) Principal fibers include 4 to 5 groups of collagen fiber bundles:
               a) The alveolar crest group runs from the alveolar crest to the cementum; opposes lateral forces; holds the tooth

in the socket and protects deep layers of PDL.

  b) The horizontal fiber group is found at the coronal 10%–15% of the tooth root and controls lateral (side-to-side) tooth movement.

  c) The oblique fiber group prevents tilting or dislocation of the tooth; is the largest fiber group.

  d) The apical fiber group surrounds the apex of the roots; resists tipping and dislocation; protects the pulp.

  e) The interradicular fiber group presents only in multirooted teeth; resists tipping, torquing, and luxation.

  2) Brush ends of principal fibers (Sharpey's fibers) are embedded in the cementum and alveolar bone.

 2. Is regenerative and formative; serves as periosteum for the alveolar bone and cementum; is responsible for the continued formation, resorption, repair, and/or regeneration of tissues and cells.

 3. Is nutritive; provides blood and lymphatics for nutrition and waste removal.

 4. Is sensory; transmits pressure, pain, and proprioceptive sensations.

D. Blood supply to the periodontium comprises branches from the inferior and superior alveolar arteries.

 1. Apical vessels give off branches that supply the apical region of the periodontium before entering the pulp.

 2. Transalveolar vessels are branches of intraseptal vessels that enter the PDL through the lamina dura.

 3. Vascular supply to the bone enters interdental septa via nutrient canals.

III. Cementum

A. Is a specialized, calcified connective tissue that covers the roots of teeth.

B. Is similar to bone but is 45% to 50% inorganic.

C. Contains Sharpey's fibers, which attach the cementum to the PDL; other Sharpey's fibers are found on the bone side attaching the PDL to the bone. The two sets of Sharpey's fibers comprise the attachment mechanism of tooth to bone.

D. Lacks blood and nerve supply.

E. Types of cementum

 1. Type I is acellular (has no cells) and afibrillar (has no fibers); is located near the CEJ.

 2. Type II is acellular and fibrillar and is located at the coronal third.

 3. Type III is cellular and has intrinsic fibers; is considered secondary or repair cementum.

 4. Type IV is cellular and has extrinsic fibers; is located at the apex and furcations.

F. CEJ

 1. In 60% to 65% of the population, cementum overlaps enamel.

 2. In 30% of the population, an end-to-end butt joint of cementum and enamel occurs.

 3. In 5% to 10% of the population, cementum and enamel fail to meet.

IV. Alveolar Bone

A. Together with the cementum, forms the attachment apparatus.

B. Components

 1. Alveolar bone proper

  a. Houses the root of a tooth (socket).

  b. Is called the cribriform plate anatomically, the bundle bone histologically, and the lamina dura radiographically.

  c. Is composed of compact bone.

  d. Houses Sharpey's fibers.

 2. Supporting alveolar bone

  a. Includes the inner (lingual) and outer (facial) cortical plates, which are compact bone; the thickness of the cortical plates varies, depending on the alignment of the teeth and the angulation of roots and occlusal forces.

  b. Contains cancellous (spongy) bone located between the cortical plates and the alveolar bone proper.

C. Variations in structure/bony defects

 1. Dehiscences are vertical areas of denuded bone on facial surfaces.

 2. Fenestrations are isolated port-hole defects on facial surfaces.

 3. Buttressing bone is an abnormal thickening of bone in areas where trabeculae have been weakened by resorption.

 4. Exostoses are outgrowths of bone that are common on buccal and lingual surfaces of maxillary posterior teeth and facial surfaces of mandibular posterior teeth.

 5. Tori are bony overgrowths in the midline of the palate or on the lingual surfaces of mandibular premolars.

 6. Festooning refers to wavy contouring of the bone between teeth.

Epidemiology

Epidemiology refers to the study of the patterns and dynamics of diseases that affect human populations. Patterns are best identified by variables such as age, sex, race, occupation, place of residence, and social characteristics. Dynamics are concerned with trends, cyclic patterns, and the time of exposure versus the time of onset. This type of information helps to establish a better understanding of the disease process and identifies risk factors that may assist in the control or eradication of the disease. Various indices are used in the gathering of epidemiologic data; these are reviewed in greater detail in Chapter 16.

Prevalence

Prevalence refers to the number of persons affected by a disease at a specific point in time (cross-sectional studies).

I. Most recent US national data[1]
   A. The presence of severe periodontitis is greater in underdeveloped countries than in industrialized countries.
   B. Edentulism is significantly decreasing in the United States.
   C. Gingival bleeding is prevalent in approximately 50% of the population.
   D. Attachment loss is greater as age increases.
   E. Attachment loss is greater in men than in women in the United States.
   F. Approximately one third of all adults have calculus.

II. During the 1996 World Workshop on Clinical Periodontics,[2] a review of the most recent epidemiologic evidence for periodontal disease resulted in the following conclusions:
   A. It is not possible to accurately assess whether the prevalence of periodontal diseases shows a worldwide decline.
   B. Edentulism rates have decreased during the past 20 years.
   C. Retention of the natural dentition is common among older individuals.
   D. Early-onset periodontitis is infrequent among all populations.
   E. Adult periodontitis is prevalent among all populations.
   F. Advanced periodontitis affects limited portions of the population (less than 10% to 15%) but varies with race and geographic region.
   G. Smoking, the presence of specific subgingival microorganisms, and diabetes mellitus have been identified as true risk factors that are independent of other factors.
   H. In some cases, periodontal infections appear to have a systemic impact on the host (i.e., place an individual at risk for coronary heart disease and preterm, low birth weight babies).

Incidence

Incidence refers to the rate of occurrence of a new disease in a population during a given period of time.

Risk Factors

Risk factors affect the prevalence, severity, and development of periodontal disease.

I. Age: the prevalence of periodontal disease increases directly with increasing age as a result of repeated inflammatory episodes during a lifetime.
II. Sex: men tend to have a higher incidence of periodontal disease than women.
III. Race: African Americans have consistently demonstrated a higher prevalence of periodontal disease than Caucasians.
IV. Education: periodontal disease is inversely related to increasing levels of education.
V. Income: periodontal disease also is inversely related to increasing levels of income.
VI. Place of residence: Periodontal disease is slightly more prevalent in rural than in urban areas.
VII. Geographic area: no significant differences have been noted in the United States.
VIII. Genetics: a genetic predisposition to periodontal disease has been related to inherited systemic diseases and to familial occurrences of some periodontal diseases.

Detection Methods

Data are collected with specific measuring systems called indices, which have defined scales that are easily applied to populations. These indices are the methods by which diseases are detected.

I. Data typically are collected by several examiners whose instruments are calibrated in the indices being used.
II. Multiple indices typically are used to evaluate the periodontal status of a population; the association of various signs and symptoms assists in obtaining an overall picture.

Etiology of the Host Response (Immunology)

Bacteria always interact with the host. In healthy individuals, an active host response quickly results in mild inflammation, which destroys the antigens (bacteria). When the host response is impaired, more rapid destruction of the periodontium results.

Defense Mechanisms of the Gingiva

The natural defense mechanisms that exist in the oral cavity comprise the saliva, the intact epithelium, and the gingival crevicular fluid. These mechanisms work together to defend against mechanical, bacterial, and chemical aggression.

I. Saliva
   A. Functions to mechanically cleanse the oral cavity.
   B. Buffers acids produced by bacteria.
   C. Controls bacterial activity.
   D. Contains antibacterial components such as lysosomes and lactoperoxidase.
II. Intact epithelium provides a physical barrier between external noxious substances (e.g., bacterial enzymes and other by-products) and the lamina propria.

III. Gingival Crevicular Fluid (GCF)
   A. Is positively correlated with the severity of gingival inflammation.
   B. Provides an antibacterial action by bringing white blood cells (leukocytes) and antibodies into close proximity with the bacteria.
   C. Supplies complement factors that serve to initiate both vascular and cellular inflammatory responses.
   D. Provides sticky plasma proteins to the sulcus that serve as an adhesive for the junctional epithelium, keeping it intact.
   E. Contains both cellular and organic elements.
   F. Cellular elements include bacteria, desquamated epithelial cells, polymorphonuclear leukocytes (PMNLs), lymphocytes, and monocytes.
   G. Organic components
      1. C3 and C5a, which play a role in the release of histamine; also facilitate chemotaxis and phagocytosis.
      2. IgG and IgM, which function in the activation of the complement system.
      3. IgG, which facilitates phagocytosis.
      4. IgG, IgA, and IgM, which prevent tissue destruction by neutralizing bacterial endotoxin.
      5. IgA, which prevents the penetration of antigens across epithelial barriers.

The Inflammatory Response

Inflammation is the body's natural response to insult and is divided into three phases: acute, chronic, and repair.
I. Acute Phase of Inflammation
   A. Is considered to be the first line of defense and is subdivided into a vascular response and a cellular response.
      1. Vascular response
         a. Develops rapidly following an initial insult.
         b. Provides the plasma proteins and fluid necessary for rapid isolation of the irritant.
         c. The fluid produced during this stage is responsible for associated tissue edema.
         d. Vascular dilation results in an increased blood volume and a decreased velocity, which results in hyperemia.
         e. The initial vasoactive response is produced by the release of histamine and serotonin by mast cells located in the lamina propria.
         f. Vascular permeability is sustained by additional chemical mediators, including:
            1) Kinins.
            2) Prostaglandins.
            3) C3 and C5a from the complement system.
            4) Lysosomal enzymes released from leukocytes.
      2. Cellular response
         a. The primary defense cell released in the acute phase of inflammation is the PMNL.
         b. PMNLs leave the axial stream of the blood vessel and adhere to the endothelial walls (margination or pavementing).
         c. PMNLs escape through the endothelial walls by a process called emigration or diapedesis.
         d. PMNLs migrate to the injured area (migration) by a process called chemotaxis.
         e. The main function of the PMNL is phagocytosis.
         f. Mature PMNLs are capable of living for only a few hours in the highly acidic environment.
         g. After PMNLs die, they release the enzymatic contents of their lysosomes.
         h. Considerable debris accumulates during this stage, requiring the addition of defense cells that are capable of living in an acid environment.
         i. The appearance of monocytes, also called connective tissue macrophages or histiocytes, signals the beginning of the chronic stage of inflammation.
II. Chronic Phase of Inflammation
   A. Often is referred to as the second line of defense.
   B. Predominantly involves chronic inflammatory cells, which are attracted to the area of inflammation by lymphokines. Lymphokines are active proteins released by lymphocytes.
   C. Involves monocyte/macrophage functions to phagocytose or debride the area.
   D. Lymphocytes become the predominant cells, in the form of either T lymphocytes or B lymphocytes.
      1. B lymphocytes are concerned with humoral immunity; they differentiate into plasma cells, which produce specific antibodies targeted at immobilizing specific antigens.
      2. B lymphocytes also produce memory cells that are capable of producing more antibodies on demand.
      3. T lymphocytes are concerned with cellular immunity and consist of:
         a. T4 activator cells.
         b. T8 suppressor/cytolytic cells.
         c. Killer cells.
         d. NK (natural killer) cells.
III. Repair Phase of Inflammation
   A. Begins when macrophages debride the site.
   B. Involves fibroblasts from the surrounding connective tissue that migrate to the injured area and begin to secrete tropocollagen (a precursor to collagen).
   C. Involves endothelial cells that proliferate and provide more oxygen tension.
   D. Involves the development of "granulation tissue," which is composed of fibroblasts, new immature collagen, and new capillaries.

Clinical Signs of Inflammation
Inflammation is identified by several clinical signs, including gingival bleeding and changes in gingival color, contour, and position.
I.   Gingival Bleeding
     A. Is characteristic of the tissue destruction that occurs during inflammation.
     B. Results from vascular engorgement, increased blood flow, loss of vascular wall integrity, and microulceration of the sulcular epithelium, which exposes the lamina propria.
     C. May be spontaneous or may follow provocation.
     D. Is the most reliable sign of inflammation, although it is a late sign.
II. Gingival Color Changes
     A. Occur during both destructive and proliferative stages of inflammation.
     B. Result from a thinning of the epithelial layers, a decrease in keratinization, engorgement of the subepithelial blood vessels, and capillary proliferation.
     C. A bright red color occurs during the acute stage of inflammation and is associated with vascular hyperemia.
     D. A bluish color is associated with chronic inflammation and venous stasis.
III. Changes in Gingival Consistency
     A. Occur during either the destructive or proliferative stages of inflammation.
     B. Include edema, softness, and friability during acute inflammation.
     C. Are primarily caused by the accumulation of tissue fluid during the acute stage of inflammation, the thinning of the epithelial layers, and the loss of keratin.
     D. Result in increases in density during the chronic and repair stages of inflammation, because of a proliferation of fibroblasts, which produce collagen, giving a firm, fibrotic consistency.
IV. Changes in Surface Texture
     A. May include the loss of stippling, when stippling was present during gingival health.
         1. The loss of stippling appears as a shiny surface; is caused by a loss of keratin, thinning of the epithelium, and the accumulation of connective tissue fluid.
         2. The loss of stippling has been recognized as the least reliable sign of inflammation.
V.   Changes in gingival contour occur as a result of either increased tissue fluid (edema) or increased cellular elements (fibrosis) and result in rolled margins and blunted papillae.
VI. Changes in Gingival Position
     A. Are all relative to the CEJ.
     B. Result in an increased height of the gingival margin because of edema or tissue proliferation.
     C. That result in recessed margins have numerous etiologies ranging from edema, to toothbrush abrasion, to malposed teeth.

The Immune Response
The immune response is a complex entity that consists of both nonspecific and specific components. Because of the large numbers of bacteria that inhabit the oral cavity, an effective host response is required to minimize disease and tissue destruction. It is important to recognize that the majority of tissue damage produced during periodontal inflammation is caused by the host's response to bacteria.
I.   Nonspecific host responses often are referred to as innate host defense mechanisms.
     A. The inflammatory response
         1. Is part of the arachidonic acid cascade that produces several biologically active products, including prostaglandins, leukotrienes, thromboxane, and other substances.
         2. The most notable effects of these products are vascular permeability and the attraction of phagocytic cells.
         3. These products also attract antibodies and complement that aid in the destruction of bacteria and their byproducts.
         4. Products of the arachidonic acid cascade are potentially harmful to periodontal tissues and are part of the pathogenesis of periodontal disease.
     B. The complement system
         1. Consists of more than 20 serum proteins that become activated during inflammation and exhibit potent biologic activity.
         2. Is activated through the classical pathway or the alternate pathway.
         3. The effects of activation (by either pathway)
             a. The production of opsonins enhance phagocytosis.
             b. Mast cell release of histamine causes vasodilation.
             c. The release of chemotactic factors causes the migration of PMNLs and macrophages to specific sites.
             d. The production of factors capable of destroying bacterial cell walls.
     C. The phagocytic system
         1. Consists primarily of PMNLs and macrophages.
         2. Phagocytes kill bacteria in two different ways:
             a. In the nonoxygen-dependent system, enzymes and other cationic proteins (e.g., neutral proteases, acid hydrolases), in the lysosomes of PMNLs and macrophages, degrade bacteria after they have been ingested.
             b. In the oxygen-dependent system, bacteria are destroyed in a phagolysosome in the cell itself, by a lysosomal enzyme called myeloperoxidase.

II. Specific Host Responses
   A. Are mediated by lymphocytes.
      1. T lymphocytes provide the cellular immune response.
         a. In this response, T cells release potent products called cytokines, such as interleukin-1, which are capable of inducing bone resorption.
         b. B lymphocytes provide humoral immune responses; produce plasma cells that in turn produce specific antibodies or immunoglobulins, which:
            1) Prevent bacterial cell walls from attaching to oral surfaces.
            2) Trigger activation of the complement system.
            3) Neutralize toxins and enzymes released by bacteria.

Conversion of Gingivitis to Periodontitis

A generally accepted principle supported by animal studies suggests that repeated exposure to gingivitis can lead to periodontal bone destruction or periodontitis.

I. Gingivitis may not result in periodontitis, depending on individual immune responses and plaque composition.
II. Periodontitis is always preceded by gingivitis.
III. Histopathology of Periodontal Disease (Page and Schroeder, 1977).
   A. Consists of four distinct stages; the first three result in gingivitis and the fourth manifests as periodontitis.
   B. Four histologic stages of periodontal lesion development
      1. Initial lesion
         a. Is the initial response of the tissues to bacterial plaque; occurs in the first 2 to 4 days after plaque invasion and is considered subclinical.
         b. Involves initial vasoconstriction followed by subsequent vasodilation and margination; the emigration and migration of PMNLs into the lamina propria results in a slight alteration of the junctional epithelium and an increase in GCF.
      2. Early lesion
         a. Is the acute gingivitis stage, which occurs within 4 to 7 days after an insult.
         b. Results in further invasion of the junctional epithelium, resulting in ulceration of the sulcular epithelium and destruction of the connective tissue fibers.
         c. Involves the appearance of chronic inflammatory cells, such as macrophages and lymphocytes.
      3. Established lesion
         a. Is the chronic stage of inflammation, which occurs after 14 days of initial insult.

      b. Is characterized predominately by plasma cells, bacterial and cell by-products such as collagenase, and other enzymes that are destructive to the periodontal tissues.
      c. May persist from weeks to years.
      4. Advanced lesion
         a. Indicates a stage that occurs only when inflammation invades the supporting periodontal tissues (ligament and alveolar bone); marks the conversion of gingivitis to periodontitis.
         b. Occurs depending on the host response and the presence of specific bacterial species.
         c. Involves bone and attachment loss that becomes evident as destruction and repair results in the formation of fibrotic repair tissue or granulation tissue.

Systemic Modifiers/Risk Factors

Periodontal pathogens alone may not lead to the development of disease. The degree of destruction varies greatly from one individual to another, which suggests that other factors may alter a host's resistance. These factors have been labeled risk factors. Some of these factors, such as genetics and age, are beyond an individual's control but others, such as smoking or psychogenic factors, can be modified. Recent evidence suggests that an increased incidence of periodontal disease may in turn represent a risk factor for cardiovascular disease and cerebral infarction.

Psychosomatic Factors and Stress

Hans Selye's general adaptation syndrome (GAS) identified the relationship between stress and disease more than 50 years ago.
   I. An increased susceptibility to and severity of periodontal disease has been reported during stressful life events such as death, divorce, and war.
   II. Plasma corticosteroids become elevated during exposure to stressful stimuli and act to suppress the immune response.
   III. The strongest example of a correlation between stress and periodontal disease is acute necrotizing ulcerative gingivitis (ANUG).

Tobacco Use

Tobacco is a causative agent for periodontal disease. It is believed that nicotine and other chemicals embed on the root surface and act as toxic irritants, in addition to causing the constriction of blood vessels in the area. The result is that tobacco users are at greater risk for developing periodontal disease and are least likely to heal well after treatment. Thus smoking has been labeled a critical risk factor for the development of refractory periodontitis.
I. Tobacco Smokers
   A. Exhibit deeper pockets, have greater periodontal index scores, show greater bone loss, have higher

rates of attachment loss, and tend to have more calculus (serves as a contributing factor in plaque accumulation and prevents pocket healing) than nonsmokers.

B. Have a higher prevalence of moderate to severe periodontal disease, which is directly related to number of cigarettes smoked per day, to the number of years that the patient has smoked, and to the patient's smoking status.

C. May have an altered host response to various forms of periodontal therapy.

D. Are at greater risk for developing refractory periodontitis, which is characterized by rapid bone loss that continues despite conventional therapy; an unusually high percentage of individuals with this disease are smokers (85% to 90%).

II. Smokeless Tobacco Users

A. Have a well-documented, higher risk of oral carcinoma.

B. May be at greater risk for developing various forms of periodontal disease.

C. Experience local exposure to high concentrations of tobacco products, which may play a role in localized attachment loss.

Nutritional Deficiencies

Poor nutrition lowers resistance to periodontal disease, which makes deficient individuals more susceptible to infection and severe forms of periodontitis.

I. In the United States, nutritional deficiencies are found most commonly among the elderly, low socioeconomic groups, and those addicted to drugs and alcohol.

II. Food consistency also has been recognized as a contributing factor to the accumulation of plaque and the development of periodontal disease.

III. Specific Effects of Nutritional Deficiencies

A. Vitamin A

1. Is involved in the synthesis of epithelial cells, proteoglycans, fibronectin, and procollagen.

2. Deficiency in animals alters tissue integrity and induces keratinization of normally nonkeratinized mucosa; however, this effect has not yet been proven in humans.

3. Retinol (vitamin A_1) is currently under investigation as an antioxidant agent that might assist in the prevention of malignancy, cardiovascular disease, and periodontitis.

B. Vitamin B_2 (riboflavin)

1. Deficiency may affect the oral cavity, causing angular cheilitis, glossitis, and oral ulcerations.

C. Vitamin B_6 (pyridoxine)

1. Is involved in carbohydrate metabolism; a deficiency may induce generalized stomatitis, glossitis, gingivitis, and other oral symptoms.

D. Vitamin B_{12} (cobalamin)

1. Deficiency may result from dietary deficiency or

may result secondary to altered absorption (pernicious anemia).

2. Deficiency may make gingivae more susceptible to epithelial dysplasia or malignant transformation.

3. Deficiency is generally accompanied by a folic acid deficiency; folic acid is of interest to periodontists because it may reduce gingivitis or phenytoin-induced gingival enlargement.

E. Vitamin C (ascorbic acid)

1. Deficiency adversely affects periodontal connective tissue, capillary integrity, and wound healing because vitamin C is essential to collagen biosynthesis.

2. Deficiency (when prolonged) may cause scurvy, which induces severe periodontal changes.

F. Vitamin D

1. Deficiency results in altered levels of plasma calcium and phosphorous, which interferes with the mineralization of organic bone matrix; leads to rickets in children and osteomalacia in adults.

2. Deficiency results in a loss of lamina dura and a thinning of cortical plates (radiographically).

3. Deficiency may cause common dental anomalies, such as delayed development of the permanent dentition, enamel hypoplasia, cemental resorption, open apical foramina, enlarged pulp chambers, and frequent pulp stones.

4. Deficiency in adults may lead to osteomalacia, which destroys the PDL and resorbs alveolar bone; causes replacement fibrous dysplasia.

IV. Antioxidants such as beta-carotene, vitamins A, C, and E, and selenium have been aggressively studied to determine their role in the prevention of diseases.

A. Twenty years of evidence indicates that free oxygen radicals may be involved in cancer, heart disease, and some forms of lung congestion.

B. Antioxidants reduce or prevent diseases caused by free oxygen radicals.

C. May play a role in treating human oral leukoplakia and some forms of oral cancer, although results are inconclusive.

D. Recently have been used to combat the effects of free radicals.

1. Have been shown to be involved in tissue destruction associated with periodontitis and chronic inflammatory osteoarthritis.

2. Are contained in proteases released by inflammatory cells such as PMNLs.

3. Are capable of damaging adjacent tissues during active periodontal disease.

Nutritional Disorders

Good nutrition is linked with overall health. Thus nutritional disorders often manifest themselves not only in other parts of the body, but also in the oral cavity.

I. Osteoporosis
   A. Is a loss of bone mass caused by an imbalance of plasma calcium and phosphorous levels.
   B. Research indicates that the severity of bone loss increases if periodontitis is superimposed on osteoporosis.
II. Protein Deficiency
   A. When severe, significantly reduces host defenses and wound healing.
   B. In its most severe forms, kwashiorkor or marasmus (general starvation) exhibits oral changes such as glossitis, angular cheilitis, xerostomia, increased gingival inflammation, and periodontal bone loss; kwashiorkor also is associated with an increased incidence and severity of necrotizing gingivitis, periodontitis, and cancrum oris (oral ulceration).

Endocrine Disorders

Endocrine glands secrete hormones that regulate the body's cellular metabolism and maintain physiologic homeostasis. Endocrine dysfunctions, such as hyperparathyroidism and diabetes mellitus, have been associated with an increased susceptibility to periodontitis. Fluctuations in sex hormones also have been shown to alter an individual's tissue response to local factors and therefore are risk factors for the development of gingivitis and periodontitis.

I. Hyperparathyroidism
   A. Is the excessive production of parathyroid hormone, which helps control calcium metabolism.
   B. Typically is caused by a benign adenoma or malignancy and results in osteoporosis, multilocular radiolucent jaw lesions, loss of lamina dura, and a ground-glass appearance of the alveolar bone.
   C. Results in a more rapidly demineralized alveolar bone when it occurs in the presence of periodontitis.
II. Alterations in Sex Hormones
   A. Puberty
      1. Involves increased levels of sex hormones, which alter capillary permeability and increase fluid accumulation in the gingiva, resulting in an increased susceptibility to gingivitis in the presence of bacterial plaque.
   B. Menstruation
      1. With its normal, cyclic hormonal fluctuations, has not been shown to increase the risk of gingivitis.
   C. Pregnancy
      1. Has a strong correlation with the development of gingival changes such as gingivitis, gingival enlargements, and pyogenic granulomas.
      2. Results in increased levels of progesterone, which alter capillary permeability and tissue metabolism, making tissues more susceptible to inflammatory changes in the presence of often minimal levels of plaque.
      3. Is associated with elevated levels of anaerobes, such as *Prevotella intermedia*.

   D. Oral Contraceptives
      1. Are drugs that have been shown to elevate hormone levels and thus mimic pregnancy.
      2. Have effects on the gingival tissues that are similar to those of pregnancy; place the individual at risk for gingivitis.
   E. Menopause
      1. Once was believed to be associated with a susceptibility to desquamative gingivitis; currently desquamative gingivitis is believed to be a more likely feature of a mucocutaneous disorder such as erosive lichen planus or mucous membrane pemphigoid.
   F. Diabetes Mellitus
      1. Is a genetically associated, debilitating endocrine disorder characterized by glucose intolerance.
      2. Is associated with increased blood glucose levels that result from decreased insulin levels and create diverse systemic effects, including:
         a. Vascular disease.
         b. Neuropathy.
         c. Retinopathy.
         d. Nephropathy.
         e. Reduced host resistance.
         f. An increased incidence of periodontal disease.
      3. Types
         a. Type-I diabetes (IDDM), which commonly develops before age 30 and must be controlled with insulin therapy.
         b. Type-II diabetes (NIDDM), the most common form commonly occurs after age 40 and may be controlled by diet, oral hypoglycemic agents, or less frequently, insulin therapy.
      4. Oral manifestations include xerostomia, candidiasis, increased caries, burning mouth, altered taste, and progressive periodontitis.
      5. Periodontal disease has been declared the sixth complication of diabetes mellitus.[3]
         a. Defective PMNL chemotaxis, microangiopathy of the periodontal tissues, increased collagen breakdown, and microbial alterations have been cited as rationales for periodontal disease prevalence in diabetes mellitus.
         b. In uncontrolled diabetes mellitus, oral manifestations such as multiple periodontal abscesses, velvety red gingival tissues, and marginal proliferation of periodontal tissues have been noted.

 Clinical Case **STUDY**

Marty Brock, a 38-year-old new patient, indicates that he has severe mouth pain and has been unable to eat for several days. He also admits that he has not been feeling

well lately and has a chronic cough that has persisted for several months. The extraoral examination reveals bilateral lymphadenopathy. Intraorally, several large ulcerations that are red and raw are noted on the hard palate. Additionally, a thick white coating appears on portions of the hard palate and all of the soft palate, extending into the pharynx; when the coating is wiped off with gauze, raw inflamed tissue is exposed. The gingival tissues have a definite red band along the facial gingival margins of the maxillary arch; however, no bleeding is detected.

Clinical Case QUESTIONS

1. What systemic condition is Marty likely to have?
2. What might be causing the severe pain in Marty's mouth?
3. What is the significance of the palatal ulcerations?
4. What treatment for Marty's oral condition should be discussed?
5. What maintenance interval is recommended for Marty, after his acute problems have subsided?

Clinical Case RATIONALES

1. Marty is likely to have HIV/AIDS, based on the lymphadenopathy, generalized malaise, linear gingival erythema (LGE; a classic sign of HIV), probable candidiasis, and oral ulcerations.
2. The severe pain most likely is caused by the open palatal ulcerations. Candidiasis and LGE typically are not painful.
3. The palatal ulcerations most likely are herpetic lesions because they are on tissue overlying bone; aphthous ulcers are found on tissues that do not cover bone. If these are herpetic ulcerations and they persist for longer than 1 month, they are AIDS-defining according to the Centers for Disease Control and Prevention (CDC).[4]
4. Tactful discussion with Marty should include a referral to a physician if he does not reveal his HIV status. His oral condition requires prescriptions for an antiviral drug, such as acyclovir, for the herpetic lesions and an antifungal agent, such as nystatin or ketoconazole, for the candidiasis. Additionally, a povidone iodine rinse would reduce the pain and discomfort the patient is experiencing (chlorhexidine is not recommended when there are open ulcerations because of its alcohol content).
5. All patients with HIV/AIDS should be seen monthly because oral manifestations often are rapid and extremely destructive.

HIV/AIDS

Oral manifestations of HIV infection have been well documented in the literature and often are the first signs of AIDS. The dental hygienist may be the first person to identify such manifestations.

I. The prevalence of periodontal disease and other oral manifestations in patients with HIV/AIDS varies significantly, depending on the decline of the immune system, lifestyle, early recognition, and treatment.

II. Common Oral Manifestations
   A. Oral candidiasis
      1. Is one of the earliest signs of disease in the patient with HIV, although it is not AIDS-defining.
      2. May occur in several forms:
         a. Erythematous
         b. Pseudomembranous
         c. Hyperplastic
         d. Angular cheilitis
      3. Incidence ranges from 43% to 93%.
      4. Increases the risk for HIV-associated gingivitis and periodontitis.
      5. Is caused by long-term use of AZT and other drugs.
      6. Treatment consists of topical application of nystatin or systemic ingestion of either ketoconazole (Nizoral) or fluconazole (Diflucan).
   B. Herpes simplex virus (HSV) lesions
      1. That persist for 1 month or longer are considered AIDS-defining by the CDC.
      2. May be widespread and seldom are confined to the palate.
      3. Treatment consists of oral acyclovir in combination with systemic ganciclovir.
   C. Human papilloma virus infection
      1. Is common in immunosuppressed individuals.
      2. May result in the development of oral warts such as papillomas, condylomas, and focal epithelial hyperplasias.
   D. Atypical ulcerations
      1. Typically are similar to major apthous ulcers (larger than 0.5 cm in diameter), are painful, and are treated with topical corticosteroids.
   E. Oral hairy leukoplakia
      1. Is highly predictive for AIDS.
      2. Is located on the lateral border of the tongue.
   F. Kaposi's sarcoma
      1. Is the most frequently occurring neoplasm in AIDS populations.
      2. Is most commonly found in the head and neck region.
      3. In the mouth, is most commonly found on keratinized tissues such as the palate or gingiva.
      4. Clinically, appears as a multicentric vascular-like neoplasm that presents as red, blue, purple, or black and flat or raised lesions.
      5. Treatment includes excision, radiation, and chemotherapy.
   G. Periodontal conditions
      1. HIV gingivitis or linear gingival erythema (LGE)

is a common occurrence among HIV populations and is manifested as one of the following:
   a. Punctate erythema of the attached gingiva.
   b. Diffuse erythema of the attached gingiva.
   c. A well-defined red band along the free gingival margin, which does not bleed in 50% or more sites in response to probing.
2. HIV-associated periodontitis
   a. Is defined by the presence of LGE, attachment loss, and cratering in the area of the interdental col.
   b. Exhibits severe clefting, which often accompanies recession.
   c. Is treated by conventional nonsurgical periodontal therapy in conjunction with meticulous home care.
3. AIDS-associated necrotizing ulcerative periodontitis (NUP)
   a. Includes criteria for HIV-associated periodontitis in addition to the presence of exposed bone, ulceration/necrosis of the attached gingiva, or complaints of severe, deep bone pain.
   b. Treatment includes 4 to 5 days of metronidazole therapy and povidone iodine irrigation in combination with conventional therapy.

Neutrophil Abnormalities

Current literature has clearly established that the primary etiologic factor in the development of inflammatory gingivitis and periodontitis is bacteria. It is also recognized that the bacteria and the host response must be in balance to avoid disease. One of the prime players in an active host response is the PMNL. When the PMNL response is impaired, bacteria flourish and disease often becomes more severe. Various neutrophil abnormalities that affect periodontal disease are discussed.
I. Neutropenias
   A. Are associated with a decrease in circulating neutrophils.
   B. Are manifested by skin infections, upper respiratory infections, otitis media, stomatitis, early exfoliation of the teeth, and severe gingivitis with ulceration.
   C. May be caused by drugs, radiation, Down syndrome, leukemia, diabetes mellitus, tuberculosis, and autoimmune disorders.
   D. Oral manifestations include gingivitis, early-onset periodontitis, and oral ulcerations.
   E. When systemic, most often are idiopathic.
   F. Cyclic neutropenia is a rare condition characterized by neutropenic episodes that persist for 1 week, occur every 3 weeks, and result in sore gingiva, apthous ulcers, and early-onset periodontitis.
II. Neutrophil Dysfunctions
   A. Adherence defects
      1. Leukocyte adherence defect (LAD)
         a. Is a clinical condition characterized by recurrent bacterial infections, diminished pus formation, prolonged wound healing, and leukocytosis.
         b. Dentally is characterized by generalized prepubertal periodontitis, progressive alveolar bone loss, premature exfoliation of deciduous and permanent teeth, and severe gingival inflammation.
         c. Impairs successful margination of PMNLs, thereby preventing their emigration to sites of infection.
         d. Is a genetic autosomal recessive defect.
   B. Chemotaxis defects
      1. Involve impairment of the directional migration of PMNLs toward attracting molecules such as bacteria.
      2. Include several rare diseases and syndromes that involve defects in neutrophil locomotion and chemotaxis, such as Chédiak-Higashi syndrome, diabetes mellitus, Down syndrome, Job's syndrome, ulcerative colitis, lazy leukocyte syndrome, and Papillon-Lefevre syndrome.
      3. In conjunction with some of the aforementioned diseases, are associated with prepubertal periodontitis.
      4. Have been identified in approximately 75% of cases of localized juvenile periodontitis (LJP).

Adverse Drug Reactions

Drugs may have a variety of adverse effects in the oral cavity, ranging from allergic to toxic reactions and including xerostomia. Although drugs themselves do not cause periodontal disease, they may provide locally irritating conditions that affect plaque control and thus place the individual at risk for periodontal disease.
I. Various drug reactions that place the individual at risk for the development of periodontal disease
   A. Gingival enlargement.
      1. More than 20 medications have been associated with gingival enlargement.
      2. Is caused by commonly used drugs such as anticonvulsants (phenytoin, ethosuximide, mephenytoin, ethotoin, phenobarbital, valproic acid); immunosuppressants used for organ and bone marrow transplants (cyclosporin); calcium channel blockers (felodipine, nitrendipine, isradipine, nifedipine, nicardipine, amilopine, diltiazem, verapamil); and cannabis.
   B. Xerostomia.
      1. Is a side effect of many drugs.
      2. Has been shown to promote the retention of plaque, thus placing the individual at risk for both caries and periodontal disease.

Etiology: Microbiology

The relationship between microbial plaque and periodontal disease has been well documented. However, the constant presence of plaque microorganisms in the oral cavity and its relationship to disease is a complex issue that involves multiple factors, including host response, microbial virulence, and genetics.

Etiology of Periodontal Disease

Periodontal disease is essentially a disease caused by bacteria. However, the mere presence of bacteria does not preclude disease.

I. The host defense mechanism of the individual is the balancing factor in the maintenance of health.
   A. If both bacterial load and host response are in balance, no disease occurs.
   B. If either a critical mass of bacteria is reached or the host response is somehow impaired, disease occurs.
   C. The etiology therefore should be discussed from the perspective of both the bacteria and the host response.

Bacterial Classification and Characteristics

Bacteria can be classified according to their morphotypes, cell wall characteristics, oxygen environment, and metabolism.

I. Several bacterial morphotypes are found in plaque:
   A. Cocci are round in shape and commonly found either singly or in chains (streptococci).
   B. Bacilli or rods are elongated rectangles or are rod-shaped; may have the following characteristics in the oral cavity:
      1. Curved shape.
      2. Uneven diameters.
      3. Club-shaped ends.
      4. Filaments that are thread-like and branching.
      5. Fusiforms that are thread-like with tapering ends.
      6. Spirochetes that are spiral in shape, with one or more axial fibrils embedded in their cell walls.
II. The cell walls of bacteria may be distinguished by their affinity for certain dyes by means of a technique called Gram staining; they may be Gram-positive or Gram-negative.
   A. Gram-positive organisms have an outer capsule composed of a sticky polysaccharide coating called "glucan," which contributes to their adherence to tooth structure.
   B. Gram-negative organisms have an outer wall that contains receptor proteins and complex lipopolysaccharides known as endotoxins; these potent toxins may directly affect host tissue or activate the host response.
III. Bacteria may be classified by their ability to live in particular environments.
   A. Aerobes require oxygen for growth.
   B. Facultative or facultative anaerobic organisms can live in either an oxygen or nonoxygen environment.
   C. Obligate anaerobes cannot survive in an aerobic environment.

IV. Bacteria obtain their energy from different sources.
   A. Saccharolytic bacteria obtain their energy by fermenting sugars into end products such as lactic acids; these bacteria typically are aerobes.
   B. Asaccharolytic bacteria are anaerobic and do not ferment sugars; their energy is derived from amino acids.

Microbial Plaque

Microbial plaque is a living, highly organized, and complex microbial ecosystem composed of more than 300 species of bacteria embedded in a gelatinous matrix. It is classified as either supragingival or subgingival.

I. Types
   A. Supragingival plaque
      1. Is associated with healthy gingiva; is predominantly composed of cocci and rods that are Gram-positive and aerobic.
      2. Is associated with early gingivitis; is characterized by increased numbers of anaerobic, Gram-negative cocci and rods.
      3. Is associated with more intense inflammation; is characterized by increased numbers of anaerobic, Gram-negative, and filamentous organisms, fusobacteria, and spirochetes.
      4. The microbial microcosm increases in complexity by means of progressive, sequential colonization as follows:
         a. Clean tooth
         b. Pellicle
         c. Gram-positive, aerobic, cocci
         d. Gram-negative, anaerobic, rods
         e. Motile organisms (i.e., spirochetes)
   B. Subgingival plaque
      1. In health, is characterized by equal percentages of Gram-positive cocci and actinomyces; less than 15% are anaerobic.
      2. In a diseased area, is more anaerobic because the subgingival area provides less oxygen tension, which is more conducive to anaerobic growth.
      3. During active periodontal disease, the percentage of anaerobes may equal or exceed 90%; the percentage of Gram-negative organisms typically is approximately 75%.
      4. Consists of large numbers of Gram-negative, facultative anaerobic organisms.
      5. May be divided into two categories.
         a. Tooth-associated (attached)
            1) Is located adjacent to the tooth.
            2) Is associated with calculus formation, root caries, and root resorption.
            3) Appears to be composed of coccal or filamentous microorganisms.
         b. Epithelium-associated (unattached)
            1) Is located adjacent to the epithelium.
            2) Predominantly consists of motile, Gram-negative, anaerobic microorganisms.

TABLE 12.1 Microorganisms Associated with Gingivitis

Initial Population	Additional Population
Streptococcus sanguis (Gram-positive)	*Fusobacterium nucleatum*
S. mitis (Gram-positive)	*Treponema* spp.
Actinomyces naeslundii (Gram-positive)	*Prevotella intermedia*
Peptostreptococcus micros (Gram-positive)	*Haemophilus* spp.
	Campylobacter spp.
Veillonella parvula (Gram-negative)	*Actinomyces israelli*

3) In relative proportions are related to the nature of disease activity.
4) Are primarily associated with gingivitis and periodontal disease.

II. Microflora Associated with Gingivitis
   A. Large quantities of microorganisms associated with gingival health (often described as a "critical mass") result in early gingivitis. Microorganisms associated with gingivitis include those in Table 12-1, column 1.
   B. As the microorganisms continue to multiply, other gram-negative species are added to the normally healthy ones (Table 12-1, column 2).
   C. *P. intermedia* in larger quantities is associated with both pregnancy gingivitis and ANUG.
   D. *Treponema* species in larger quantities have been associated with ANUG.

III. Microflora Associated with Periodontitis (Table 12-2)
   A. Chronic adult periodontitis (Table 12-2, column 1)
   B. Rapidly progressive periodontitis (Table 12-2, column 2)
   C. Juvenile periodontitis: a series of studies have shown that the predominant microorganism (as much as 90% of the total cultivable microflora) is *Actinobacillus actinomycetemcomitans*.
   D. Prepubertal periodontitis is associated with profound immunologic abnormalities; for microorganisms associated with localized forms, see Table 12-2, column 3.
   E. Prepubertal periodontitis (see Table 12-2, column 4)

Specific versus Nonspecific Plaque Hypothesis

The specific plaque hypothesis currently is the accepted theory of periodontal disease development. Previously, the nonspecific plaque hypothesis prevailed.

Nonspecific Plaque Hypothesis

The nonspecific plaque hypothesis was accepted theory during the mid-1900s.
   I. Periodontal disease was believed to result from the combination of by-products of all of the plaque in the mouth, rather than from any specific microorganisms.
   II. Resulted in the treatment of all periodontal diseases by controlling plaque accumulation alone.

Specific Plaque Hypothesis

The specific plaque hypothesis was developed in the mid-1970s and currently is the accepted theory of periodontal disease development.
   I. Recognizes the microorganism *A. actinomycetemcomitans* as one of the etiologic agents responsible for LJP, which created a paradigm shift in favor of a more specific plaque hypothesis.
   II. Recognizes only certain pathogens as disease-producing; states that disease occurs only when increased numbers of these specific pathogens accumulate.
   III. This shift in paradigms led to different treatment modalities, including the use of both systemic and locally delivered antibiotics and antimicrobials targeted at destroying very specific microorganisms identified through new microbiologic tests.

Bacteria-Mediated Tissue Destruction

Tissue destruction mediated by bacteria is caused by the release of toxins and enzymes from these microorganisms.
   I. Bacterial enzymes (hyaluronidase, collagenase, ribonuclease) affect host cells and ground substance;

TABLE 12.2 Microflora Associated with Periodontitis

Chronic Adult Periodontitis	Rapidly Progressive Periodontitis	Localized Juvenile Periodontitis	Prepubertal Periodontitis
Porphyromonas gingivalis	*Porphyromonas gingivalis*		*Porphyromonas gingivalis*
Prevotella intermedia	*Prevotella intermedia*		*Prevotella intermedia*
Eikenella corrodens	*Eikenella corrodens*		
Actinobacillus actinomycetemcomitans	*A. actinomycetemcomitans*	*A. actinomycetemcomitans*	*A. actinomycetemcomitans*
Bacteroides forsythus			
Fusobacterium nucleatum			*F. nucleatum*
Campylobacter rectus	*Campylobacter rectus*		
Treponema spp.			
Eubacterium spp.			

proteolytic and hydrolytic enzymes destroy cells and increase the permeability of epithelial and connective tissues.

II. Bacterial cell walls of Gram-negative microorganisms are composed of endotoxins that are released at the time of their destruction.
   A. These endotoxins activate the alternate pathway of the immune complex fixation process.
   B. Side reaction proteins of this process are both chemotactic and cytolytic (C3, C5, and C5a).

III. Lymphotoxins are released when bacteria interact with host defense cells. These bacterial toxins:
   A. Inhibit the chemotactic response of the host cells.
   B. Inhibit host cell phagocytosis.
   C. Create a resistance to killing and digestion within the phagolysosomes of host cells.
   D. Release toxins that are cytolytic and/or cytotoxic.

Occlusion and Temporomandibular Disorders

It is important for the dental hygienist to recognize normal and abnormal occlusal form and function in the treatment of periodontal disease. Occlusal disharmonies can have a profound influence on periodontal disease susceptibility and are considered local contributing factors. Recognizing and recording the signs and symptoms of occlusal dysfunction and subsequently providing referrals for diagnosis and treatment are important components of dental hygiene care.

Trauma from Occlusion

Trauma from occlusion can be defined in two ways: as damage to the periodontium caused directly by stress or as damage caused indirectly by the teeth of the opposing jaw. Occlusal trauma involves pathologic alterations or adaptive changes that develop in the periodontium as a result of undue forces generated by the muscles of mastication.

I. The effect of occlusal forces on the periodontium is dependent on their magnitude, direction, duration, and frequency.

II. Slightly increased forces that result in a nonpathologic form of adaptation are referred to as hyperfunction.
   A. Histologic changes associated with hyperfunction are characterized by an increase in the number of fiber bundles in the PDL; result in an increased width of the PDL.
   B. Hyperfunction also causes an increased thickness of the alveolar bone.
   C. Tooth mobility is not associated with hyperfunction.

III. Injury results when occlusal forces exceed the adaptive capacity of the periodontium.

IV. Histopathologic features of occlusal traumatism result from areas of pressure and tension between the tooth root and the alveolar bone.

V. Clinical signs and symptoms of trauma from occlusion
   A. Radiographic evidence of a widened PDL space.
   B. Tooth mobility.
   C. Evidence of wear facets and/or a history of bruxism.
   D. Occlusal interferences in the excursive movements of the mandible.
   E. Tilted or missing teeth.

Types of Occlusal Trauma

Occlusal trauma may be either primary or secondary in nature, or may result from hypofunction or disuse atrophy.

I. Primary Occlusal Traumatism
   A. Is defined as damage that occurs when the amount of alveolar bone is normal but there is an increase in occlusal forces.

II. Secondary Occlusal Trauma
   A. Occurs when there is a deficiency in alveolar bone support and either normal or excessive forces cause damage.
   B. Occurs most commonly in cases of chronic periodontitis in which the alveolar bone support may be inadequate to withstand the forces of occlusion (whether normal or excessive).

III. Occlusal Hypofunction and Disuse Atrophy
   A. Occurs when occlusal forces are either decreased or removed entirely; a decrease in the production of collagen fibers in the PDL occurs together with a decrease in alveolar bone formation.
   B. Occlusal hypofunction is a nonpathologic form of adaptation characterized by a slight decrease in occlusal forces; a slight reduction in both collagen fibers and bone deposition occurs, resulting in a narrower PDL, which is not sufficient for radiographic diagnosis.
   C. Disuse atrophy is a pathologic process that occurs when all occlusal forces are removed; involves an extreme weakening of the supporting structures.
      1. Is characterized by an obvious reduction in both fibers and bone and results in a radiographically detectable narrowed PDL space.
      2. Radiographic evidence of decreased bone trabeculation in the cancellous bone also is recognizable.
      3. Is always accompanied by increased tooth mobility.
      4. Requires the absence of an occlusal antagonist.

IV. Temporomandibular Disorders (TMDs)
   A. Are conditions that affect the musculoskelature of the joint area; result in pain or dysfunction of the masticatory system.
   B. May affect the muscles only (extracapsular) or the joint itself (intracapsular).
   C. The prevalence of TMDs ranges from 5% to 60%.
   D. The etiology of TMDs is multifactorial. Stress is a frequent factor; other factors include arthritis, psychological problems, and macrotrauma or microtrauma to the joint.
   E. Have four primary diagnostic categories:
      1. Muscle and facial disorders of the masticatory

system, which include trismus, myalgia, spasms, dyskinesia (abnormal movement), and bruxism.

2. Disorders of the TMJ; include conditions that cause internal derangements that impede function of the TMJ (e.g., arthritis).

3. Disorders of mandibular mobility, which include joint adhesions, ankylosis, and muscular fibrosis.

4. Disorders of maxillomandibular growth, which are less common and include both neoplastic and nonneoplastic conditions.

F. Oral habits can be significant factors in the production of TMDs.

1. The amount of damage produced by the habit is relative to its intensity and duration.

2. Bruxism is the most common oral habit; involves grinding or clenching of the teeth and can be recognized by the presence of nonfunctional wear facets.

3. Signs and symptoms of TMDs
   a. Pain and tenderness in the muscles of mastication.
   b. Clicking of the TMJ during function.
   c. Pain and tenderness of the TMJ itself.
   d. Functional limitation of the joint.

Oral Contributing Factors

Although bacterial plaque has been recognized as the prime etiologic factor in the initiation and progression of gingivitis and periodontitis, other oral contributing factors play a role in the retention of plaque. These factors may be divided into local functional factors and local predisposing factors.

Local Functional Factors

Local functional factors include missing teeth, malocclusions, tongue thrusting and mouth breathing habits, parafunctional habits such as chewing on pencils or other foreign objects, and traumatogenic occlusion, which weakens the PDL, widening the PDL space and thus promoting plaque accumulation.

Local Predisposing Factors

Local predisposing factors are those that harbor plaque microorganisms, which are responsible for promoting oral disease. They include calculus, materia alba, dental stains, faulty restorations, and food impaction.

I. Supragingival and subgingival calculus are the most significant among this group of factors because they harbor bacterial plaque and are comprised primarily of mineralized plaque.

II. Supragingival Calculus
   A. Is found above the margins on the clinical crowns of teeth and typically is yellowish-white; may darken with age.
   B. Is found most commonly on the lingual surfaces of the mandibular anterior teeth and on the buccal surfaces of the first and second molars adjacent to the Stensen's duct.
   C. Is composed of inorganic (70% to 90%) and organic (10% to 30%) content.
   D. The inorganic mineral component comprises calcium phosphate (75.9%), calcium carbonate (3.1%), and traces of magnesium, sodium, potassium, fluoride, zinc, and strontium.
   E. The organic component is a mixture of protein-polysaccharide complexes, desquamated epithelial cells, leukocytes, carbohydrates, lipids, glycosaminoglycans, and various types of microorganisms.
   F. The primary crystalline structure is hydroxyapatite; includes smaller amounts of octocalcium phosphate, whitlockite, and brushite.

III. Subgingival Calculus
   A. Is located in pockets below the crest of the marginal gingiva and typically is dense, hard, dark brown or black, and firmly attached to the root surface.
   B. Has a composition that differs slightly from that of supragingival calculus, primarily in the higher ratio of calcium to phosphate and in the increased sodium.
   C. The normal mode of attachment to the tooth is by means of the organic pellicle; mineralization occurs within 24 to 72 hours and maturation occurs in an average of 12 days.
   D. May form a more tenacious attachment by penetrating the cementum and/or mechanically locking into surface irregularities, making removal difficult.
   E. The rate of formation varies among individuals; also may vary among teeth and may be light, moderate, or heavy.

IV. Materia Alba
   A. Is a yellow or grayish-white acquired bacterial coating; is soft, sticky, less adherent than plaque, and can be flushed away with water.
   B. Is composed of microorganisms, desquamated epithelial cells, leukocytes, salivary proteins, and lipids.

V. Food Debris
   A. Although rapidly cleared away, remains on the teeth and mucosa.
   B. Is cleared from the mouth by the effects of salivary flow and the mechanical action of the tongue, cheeks, and teeth.
   C. Adherence varies with food composition.

VI. Faulty Dentistry
   A. Plays a role in plaque retention.
   B. Comprises poorly fitted margins of dental prostheses, overcontoured crowns, rough crown margins, faulty or overhanging restorations, and clasps of partial dentures.

VII. Food Impaction is defined as the forceful wedging of

food into the periodontium by occlusal forces, which leads to plaque retention.

VIII. Dental Stains include a variety of extrinsic stains produced by foods, tobacco products, and poor oral hygiene; may attach to external tooth surfaces, creating a rough surface for the retention of bacterial plaque.

Differential Diagnosis of Gingival Diseases

Gingivitis is the most common periodontal disease and is defined as inflammation of the gingiva. Gingivitis is primarily associated with plaque. Several forms of gingivitis have been identified and are classified as either chronic or acute. The hygienist must be able to identify gingival health before he or she can identify gingival disease.

Gingival Health

Gingival health is characterized by the absence of bleeding in response to probing, the absence of color changes (coral pink in Caucasians), the absence of swelling (knife-edged gingival margins, pointed papillae, and firm, stippled tissues), and the absence of pain.

Chronic Forms of Gingivitis

Chronic forms of gingivitis are characterized by slow onset and slow tissue destruction and are not associated with pain. These forms of gingivitis are associated with chronic plaque accumulation, vitamin deficiencies, leukemia, hormonal changes, allergies, dermatitis, and gingival enlargements.

I. Chronic Plaque-Associated Gingivitis (simple gingivitis)
   A. Is the most common form of gingivitis and is found to some extent in the majority of the population.
   B. Exhibits bleeding in response to probing (its most significant feature).
   C. Is a painless condition; also is typically manifested by redness and swelling of the gingival margins and papillae (i.e., rolled margins, rounded papillae, flabby tissues, and loss of stippling).

II. Gingivitis Associated with Vitamin C Deficiency
   A. Severe vitamin C deficiency results in scurvy; however, a vitamin deficiency alone cannot cause inflammation.
   B. Is exaggerated because a deficiency of this vitamin creates an increased tendency for gingival hemorrhage, degeneration of the collagen fibers, and edema of the gingival tissues.
   C. Clinical characteristics
      1. Bluish-red gingiva.
      2. Enlargement of the marginal gingiva.
      3. Soft, friable, smooth, and shiny gingival surfaces.
      4. Possible pseudomembrane, if necrosis has occurred.

5. A tendency to bleed spontaneously.
6. Gingival pockets or pseudopockets.

III. Gingivitis Associated with Leukemia
   A. Leukemia is a disease of the blood-forming tissues characterized by the production of excessive numbers of immature white blood cells.
   B. Regardless of the form of leukemia, plaque is the primary etiologic agent; the histologic changes associated with leukemia modify and aggravate the inflammatory response to local irritants.
   C. Clinical characteristics
      1. A purplish-blue color caused by blood stagnation.
      2. Enlargement of the marginal or interdental gingivae in the form of tumor-like masses.
      3. Moderately firm to friable tissues.
      4. Shiny surfaces that may have ulcerations, necrosis, and pseudomembrane.
      5. Spontaneous bleeding (in most cases).
      6. Pseudopockets.

IV. Gingivitis Associated with Puberty, Pregnancy, and Menopause
   A. Is caused by bacterial plaque; hormonal alterations tend to exaggerate the inflammatory response.
   B. During puberty, poor diet also may exaggerate the response.
   C. During pregnancy, increased levels of progesterone have been attributed to an increased susceptibility to gingivitis and the presence of *P. intermedia*.
   D. Clinical characteristics
      1. Red to bluish-red gingiva caused by increased vascularity.
      2. Enlarged, edematous gingiva (especially in pregnancy gingivitis).
      3. An increased tendency to bleed.
      4. Puberty gingivitis affects both males and females.
      5. Pregnancy gingivitis begins in the second to the third month and is most severe in the second and third trimesters.
      6. Localized enlargements in the interdental papillae form tumor-like growths, which may be referred to as pregnancy tumors; these tumors are red or magenta, smooth, and shiny and disappear at the end of the pregnancy.

V. Allergic Gingivitis
   A. Is an allergic hypersensitivity that involves an abnormal response of the tissues to specific agents.
   B. May be an oral manifestation of a systemic allergic response, if the sensitivity is to a food or drug.
   C. Also may manifest as a localized contact allergy to dentifrices, mouthwashes, or other dental therapeutic agents.
   D. The antigen (and NOT plaque) is the prime etiologic agent.

E. Clinical characteristics include redness, soreness, gingival necrosis, edema, ulceration, and possible vesicle formation.

VI. Desquamative Gingivitis/Gingivitis Associated With Dermatoses
   A. Is a rare chronic condition that involves the interdental, marginal, and attached gingiva.
   B. Recently has been linked to several dermatologic diseases and drugs, although the exact nature of this condition is unknown.
   C. Dermatoses to which this condition has been linked include pemphigus, pemphigoid, benign mucous membrane pemphigoid, and lichen planus.
   D. Drugs to which this condition is linked include sulfonamides, gold salts, arsphenamine, aminopyrine, antibiotics, barbiturates, salicylates, and numerous others; when the lesions are drug-related, they are referred to as stomatitis medicamentosa.
   E. Clinical characteristics may be mild, moderate, or severe; condition is characterized by redness of the marginal and attached gingiva and periods of exacerbation and remission.
   F. As the severity increases, localized areas of epithelium begin to peel away, exposing painful connective tissues.
   G. In the most severe form, irregular areas of the gingiva are fiery red, smooth, and shiny and exposed connective tissues contain blisters that bleed and are extremely painful.
   H. Mostly affects women and often is associated with menopause.
   I. Is a degenerative condition (not associated with plaque) with only a secondary inflammatory reaction.

VII. Gingival Enlargement
   A. Inflammatory gingival enlargement
      1. Is an increase in the size of the gingival tissues that results from an accumulation of tissue fluid and inflammatory exudate; eventually becomes fibrotic through an increase in the number of collagen fibers.
      2. Overgrowth may be exaggerated by other conditions, such as puberty, pregnancy, mouth breathing, some blood dyscrasias, and medications such as phenytoin, cyclosporins, nifedipine, and diltiazem.
   B. Noninflammatory gingival enlargement
      1. Is not associated with plaque, although inflammation exists.
      2. May be produced by certain drugs, with or without the presence of an inflammatory condition.
         a. Phenytoin, an anticonvulsant drug, produces gingival enlargement in 50% of patients.

            1) Clinical characteristics of phenytoin enlargement include generalized enlargement of the marginal and interdental gingiva, which causes increased sulcular depths; interdental areas become more enlarged and often obscure occlusion.
            2) Enlarged tissues appear firm, fibrotic, pale pink, and resilient; have little tendency to bleed.
            3) Tissues appear lobed and although enlargement is generalized, it frequently is more pronounced in the anteriors.
            4) This condition is more common in younger patients and rarely affects edentulous spaces.
         b. Cyclosporine
            1) Is an immunosuppressive drug used to prevent organ transplant rejection and to treat type-I diabetes and other autoimmune disorders.
            2) Causes enlargements in approximately one third of adults who take the drug and in a greater percentage of children who take it.
         c. Calcium channel blocking drugs
            1) Include such drugs as nifedipine (Procardia) and diltiazem (Cardizem), which are used in the treatment of angina pectoris and produce gingival enlargements similar to those caused by phenytoin in some individuals.
   C. Familial (hereditary) gingival enlargement
      1. Is a rare hyperplastic disease with an unknown etiology; also is referred to as ideopathic gingival hyperplasia.
      2. Exhibits enlarged marginal, interdental, and attached gingiva; affects facial and lingual surfaces of both arches.
      3. Features affected tissues that are pink, firm, resilient, bulbous, and fibrotic without bleeding; tissues may obscure occlusion.
      4. May exhibit inflammatory changes in response to local irritants.

Acute Forms of Gingival Disease

Rapid onset, rapid tissue destruction, and the presence of pain characterize acute forms of gingival disease, unlike chronic forms.

I. Severe and prolonged acute inflammation accounts for the pathologic and clinical findings in this group of diseases, which are always characterized by more rapid tissue destruction than that of the chronic diseases.
II. Acute inflammatory reactions are characterized by the presence of large numbers of neutrophils (PMNLs), which are responsible for the intense tissue destruc-

tion created by the release of large quantities of lysosomal enzymes into the tissues.

III. The two most commonly described acute gingival diseases are ANUG and acute herpetic gingivostomatitis.

   A. ANUG

     1. Occurs in individuals during severe emotional stress or in individuals who exhibit an inability to cope with stress.

     2. Also is associated with patients who exhibit neutrophil chemotaxis and phagocytosis defects.

     3. Exhibits specific combinations of microbes that appear to become pathogenic only when the host defenses are diminished.

     4. Has been associated with the presence of spirochetes and fusiform bacillus.

     5. Has been associated with the following predisposing factors:

       a. Preexisting gingival inflammation

       b. Severe nutritional deficiency

       c. Smoking

       d. Preexisting systemic disease (e.g., leukemia, AIDS, leukopenia, anemia, and ulcerative colitis)

       e. Psychosomatic factors (e.g., stress)

     6. Clinical signs and symptoms associated with ANUG

       a. Pain

       b. Sudden onset

       c. Cratering of interdental papillae (punched-in appearance)

       d. Pseudomembrane formation (created by necrotic epithelial cells)

       e. Spontaneous gingival hemorrhage

       f. Fetid metallic odor (fetor oris)

       g. Lymphadenopathy

       h. Elevated temperature

   B. Acute herpetic gingivostomatitis

     1. Is caused by type-1 herpes simplex virus (HSV1).

     2. Occurs most commonly in children who are less than 5 years old; is the initial episode of type-1 herpes and is more severe than subsequent recurrences.

     3. Is a viral disease and therefore is contagious.

     4. Predisposing conditions

       a. Febrile disease, such as influenza and/or infectious mononucleosis.

       b. AIDS.

     5. Clinical signs and symptoms

       a. Pain.

       b. Small vesicles or clusters of ulcerations on either keratinized or nonkeratinized oral tissues.

       c. Shiny and red marginal and interdental gingivae.

       d. Edematous gingival enlargement.

       e. A tendency toward spontaneous gingival bleeding.

       f. A grayish-white membrane covering the ulcerations.

       g. Moderate to high fever.

       h. Cervical lymphadenopathy.

       i. Generalized malaise.

       j. Difficulty eating or drinking liquids.

Differential Diagnosis of Periodontal Diseases

The inflammatory process associated with periodontitis affects the gingiva, PDL, alveolar bone, and cementum. It is characterized by gingival inflammation, periodontal pocket formation, destruction of the PDL and alveolar bone, and gradual loosening of the teeth.

The Etiology and Pathogenesis of Periodontal Disease

Although gingivitis does not necessarily progress to periodontitis, periodontitis is always preceded by gingivitis. Clinical studies have not demonstrated when or how this transition occurs. The diagnosis of periodontitis is made when inflammation extends into the attachment apparatus, resulting in the loss of clinical attachment and subsequent periodontal pocket formation.

I.   Gingivitis is caused by the invasion of junctional and sulcular epithelia by bacterial plaque.

II.   Vasostagnation, retained tissue fluids, and eventual fibrosis produce gingival enlargement, which results in pocket formation.

   A. If pocket formation is not accompanied by apical migration, the result is a gingival pocket or pseudopocket.

   B. If apical migration occurs, the result is a periodontal pocket.

III. As the inflammatory process destroys the gingival and PDL fibers, apical proliferation and migration of the sulcular and junctional epithelium occurs.

IV. The pocket continues its progression apically; the stimulation of alveolar bone resorption is part of the inflammatory process.

V.   The periodontal inflammatory disease becomes self-perpetuating with the formation of deeper pockets because bacterial plaque, which is the prime etiologic agent, can grow and mature in the more anaerobic environment.

VI. The growth of periodontal pathogens is encouraged as removal by the patient becomes increasingly difficult; if allowed to persist, the chronic infection causes severe destruction and eventual tooth loss.

VII. Research has shown that periodontal disease is site-specific, episodic, and characterized by periods of exacerbation and remission.

VIII. There are two classifications of periodontal pockets.

   A. Suprabony pockets, in which the base of the pocket is coronal to the level of alveolar bone and horizontal bone loss is noted.

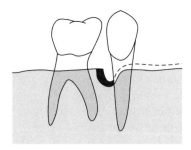

One-walled

Figure 12.1 Infrabony pocket with a one-walled defect.

B. Infrabony pockets, in which the base of the pocket is apical to the level of alveolar bone, exhibiting a vertical pattern of bone loss; are one of three distinct types:
　1. One-walled (Fig. 12–1)
　2. Two-walled (Fig. 12–2)
　3. Three-walled (Fig. 12–3)

Classification of Periodontal Diseases

Although numerous classification systems exist for periodontal diseases, the most commonly used system was developed by the American Academy of Periodontology at the 1989 World Workshop in Clinical Periodontics.[5]
I. 1989 World Workshop in Clinical Periodontics
　A. Classification system
　　1. Adult periodontitis
　　2. Early-onset periodontitis
　　　a. Prepubertal periodontitis (generalized or localized)
　　　b. Juvenile periodontitis (generalized or localized)
　　　c. Rapidly progressive periodontitis
　　3. Periodontitis associated with systemic diseases, including:
　　　a. Down syndrome
　　　b. Type-I diabetes
　　　c. Papillon-Lefèvre syndrome
　　　d. AIDS
　　　e. Chédiak-Higashi syndrome
　　　f. NUP
　　　g. Refractory periodontitis

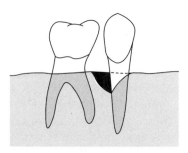

Two-walled

Figure 12.2 Infrabony pocket with a two-walled defect.

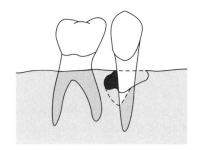

Three-walled

Figure 12.3 Infrabony pocket with a three-walled defect.

Acute Periodontal Diseases

Periodontal diseases generally are considered chronic diseases, with the exception of the acute periodontal abscess.

A periodontal abscess is an acute, inflammatory, localized condition that occurs within a periodontal pocket and is characterized by aggressive tissue destruction.
II. The criteria necessary for the formation of an acute periodontal abscess are:
　A. A periodontal pocket.
　B. Occlusion of the periodontal pocket by foreign matter or by fibrosis of the coronal gingiva.
　C. The presence of virulent microorganisms.
III. The entrapment of virulent organisms leads to large numbers of neutrophils, which result in pus formation, extensive and rapid tissue damage, and abscess formation.
IV. Clinical signs and symptoms of an acute periodontal abscess may include some or all of the following:
　A. Throbbing or pulsating pain
　B. Localized swelling
　C. Exudate (typically pus)
　D. Deep pockets occluded by calculus, food debris, or a fibrotic marginal gingiva
　E. A fistula or drainage tract on soft tissue wall
　F. Tooth mobility
　G. Considerable bone loss that is visible radiographically
　H. Sensitivity of the tooth to percussion
　I. Lymphadenopathy and low-grade fever
　J. A vital pulp that rules out a pulpal origin

 Clinical Case **STUDY**

Forty-four-year-old Ann Larseth recently obtained dental insurance through her employer and is seeking dental care for the first time in more than 15 years. A full-mouth series of radiographs are taken in addition to a complete periodontal assessment. Ann mentions her fear of the dental office and her embarrassment over the condition of her teeth. Examination reveals moderate levels of plaque at the gingival margins, heavy subgingi-

val and supragingival calculus, tobacco staining, and moderate gingivitis. Molars #3, #19, #30, and #31 are badly decayed but are no longer painful. Radiographs indicate a loss of crestal bone throughout the posterior areas of the mouth. Probe readings are 3 to 4 mm in anterior sextants and 4 to 6 mm in posterior areas. Very little recession is evident.

Clinical Case QUESTIONS

1. Identify a likely diagnosis for Ms. Lerseth's condition. What does loss of crestal bone indicate? What AAP classification fits this case?
2. Identify factors contributing to Ms. Lerseth's periodontal condition.
3. Discuss treatment options.
4. What is the prognosis for this disease?

Clinical Case RATIONALES

1. The most likely diagnosis for Ms Lerseth's condition is chronic adult periodontitis, based on the generalized loss of crestal bone, her age, the amount of plaque and calculus, and her lack of routine dental care. The AAP classification for this case most likely is moderate adult periodontitis because the probe readings are generally 4 to 6 mm deep and bone loss is evident on radiographs.
2. Factors contributing to Ms. Lerseth's periodontal condition include inadequate oral hygiene, a lack of professional dental care, and smoking.
3. Appropriate treatment should include thorough periodontal debridement with local anesthetic coverage (preferably by quadrant or arch), toothbrushing and flossing instruction, smoking cessation, and extraction or restoration of the decayed teeth. The patient should return in 4 to 6 weeks for reevaluation of her periodontal health. Any areas with continued bleeding should be debrided and root planed to promote healing. Home care should be assessed and additional instruction should be given as needed.
4. The prognosis for chronic adult periodontitis is good, if the patient refrains from smoking, practices good plaque removal, and complies with appropriate supportive periodontal therapy (typically involving an oral prophylaxis every 3 months).

Chronic Adult Periodontitis

Adult periodontitis is the most common form of periodontitis. Although it may begin subclinically in adolescence, it typically does not become evident until the mid-thirties. Because of its chronic nature, it progresses slowly and is classified by some as "slowly progressive periodontitis."

I. The severity is directly related to the amount of hard and soft deposits on tooth surfaces.

II. Is not associated with an abnormal host or systemic diseases.

III. Is characterized by periodontal pockets, bone loss, and eventual tooth mobility.

IV. Most commonly exhibits horizontal interdental bone loss, which eventually progresses to interradicular areas.

V. Has been subdivided by the AAP into three categories.[5]
   A. Mild adult periodontitis
      1. Is characterized by slight bone loss, involving the alveolar crest, and slight loss of connective tissue (i.e., 2 to 3 mm of attachment loss and 3- to 4-mm pockets).
   B. Moderate adult periodontitis
      1. Is characterized by more advanced bone loss, resulting in 4 to 6 mm of attachment loss and pocket depths of 5 to 7 mm.
      2. May be accompanied by tooth mobility and furcation involvement.
   C. Advanced adult periodontitis
      1. Is a further progression of the disease; results in advanced bone loss, pocket depths of more than 8 mm, and an average of 6 mm or more of attachment loss; is accompanied by increased tooth mobility and furcation involvement.

VI. The degree of periodontal disease activity is directly related to the amount of PDL and bone destruction and is determined more accurately by measures of attachment loss than by measures of probing depth.

VII. Is considered a mixed infection because it involves several bacterial species; *Porphyromonas gingivalis* typically is the most prevalent of these.

VIII. Clinical signs of chronic adult periodontitis
   A. Chronically inflamed gingiva, with color that varies from red to bluish to normal.
   B. Gingiva that varies in consistency from edematous to fibrotic, which gives it an enlarged appearance.
   C. A contour that is rounded at the margins and typically blunted interdentally, exhibiting a loss of stippling.
   D. Evidence of attachment loss and periodontal pockets, with a tendency to bleed in response to probing.
   E. Radiographic signs of bone loss that may include a lack of definition of the lamina dura, fuzzy crestal lamina, horizontal or angular bone loss, or radiolucencies of the bifurcations/trifurcations.
   F. Rough root surfaces, calculus, and exudate that may be purulent (pus).
   G. Tooth mobility, which varies from none to extensive.

Clinical Case **STUDY**

Twenty-one-year-old Sara Berts is a new patient who is scheduled for an oral prophylaxis. Her gingiva appears healthy. She brushes her teeth twice daily and flosses four to five times a week. Probing depths are 2 to 3 mm throughout her mouth, with the exceptions of teeth #3, #14, and #8, which have readings of 6, 6, and 9, respectively. Bleeding is noted in the pockets only. During discussion of the deeper probe readings, Sara indicates that she has no knowledge of previous periodontal disease.

Clinical Case QUESTIONS

1. Identify a likely diagnosis for Ms. Berts' condition. How might radiographs assist in the diagnosis?
2. Identify factors that might have contributed to her periodontal condition.
3. Discuss treatment options.
4. What is the prognosis for this disease?

Clinical Case RATIONALES

1. The most likely diagnosis for Ms. Berts' condition is LJP, which is indicated by the vertical bone loss evident on radiographs of teeth #3, #14, and #8.
2. Contributing factors to her periodontal condition include an inherited neutrophil defect (depressed neutrophil chemotaxis) and a large amount of the pathogen *Actinobacillus actinomycetemcomitans*.
3. This condition typically is treated with a 2-week regimen of antibiotics (tetracycline or a derivative) in conjunction with conventional nonsurgical periodontal therapy. Periodontal surgery may be required to restore periodontal health.
4. The prognosis for this disease is good, except for teeth #3, #14, and #8, because no bleeding is noted and sulcus depths are normal in the rest of the mouth. Prognosis for the areas with pocketing is fair because significant amounts of bone loss already have occurred. Compliance with home and professional dental care should contain the bone loss indefinitely.

Early Onset Periodontitis

Early onset periodontitis refers to a group of aggressive periodontal diseases that are characterized by rapid progression, early onset, and neutrophil abnormalities. These diseases include prepubertal periodontitis, juvenile periodontitis, and rapidly progressive periodontitis.

I. Prepubertal periodontitis is a rare condition that affects both primary and mixed dentitions; may be a localized or a generalized form.
   A. Both forms typically are manifested by white blood cell defects and generally are associated with systemic diseases such as Papillon-Lefevre syndrome, Chédiak-Higashi syndrome, hypophosphatasia, leukemia, Down syndrome, and leukocyte adhesion deficiency.
   B. The onset occurs before 11 years of age.
   C. Is characterized by severe gingival inflammation, rapid bone loss, mobility, and early tooth loss.
II. Juvenile Periodontitis
   A. Occurs in adolescents, is not associated with systemic disease, and typically occurs during puberty, thus affecting the permanent dentition.
   B. Affects more females than males and is suspected to have a genetic basis because it tends to occur in families.
   C. Is associated with depressed neutrophil chemotaxis in most cases.
   D. Affects the anteriors and first molars and is characterized by severe, rapid bone loss, with little evidence of gingival inflammation or plaque and calculus deposits.
   E. The rate of destruction is three to five times faster than that of adult periodontitis.
   F. Occurs in both a localized and a generalized form; the localized form remains confined to the anteriors and first molars and the generalized form affects the entire dentition.
   G. Clinical signs include radiographic evidence of vertical bone loss in the anterior and molar teeth, deep periodontal pockets in these areas, tooth mobility, and drifting of the affected teeth.
   H. Is associated with large numbers of the periodontal pathogen *A. actinomycetemcomitans*.
   I. Is treated initially with antibiotic therapy and conventional nonsurgical periodontal therapy; may be followed by periodontal surgery.
III. Rapidly Progressive Periodontal Disease
   A. Occurs in young adults between 20 and 30 years of age and is believed by some to be related to juvenile periodontitis.
   B. Typically is generalized; exhibits more plaque, calculus, and inflammation than are found in juvenile periodontitis.
   C. Is more difficult to diagnose because the progression of lesions must be documented over a period of at least two time intervals. These intervals can be as short as a few weeks.
   D. May result in very rapid destruction; as much as 60% destruction during a 9-week period has been documented.
   E. May have a genetic component because many affected individuals exhibit defects in neutrophil chemotaxis.
   F. May be associated with autoimmunity.
   G. Associated microorganisms include *A. actinomycetemcomitans*, *P. gingivalis*, *P. intermedia*, *Bacteroides forsythus*, *Eikenella corrodens*, and *Campylobacter recta*.

H. Treatment must be aggressive and is similar to that for juvenile periodontitis.

Periodontitis Associated with Systemic Disease

The majority of cases of generalized prepubertal periodontitis fall into this classification, together with cases involving adults who have chronic diseases associated with immunosuppression (e.g., diabetes, AIDS).

I. Prepubertal periodontitis is associated with the following systemic diseases:
   A. Papillon-Lefèvre syndrome is an inherited autosomal recessive disease characterized by hyperkeratotic skin lesions of the palms, soles, knees, and elbows; may cause severe destruction of the periodontium; onset occurs before age 4.
   B. Down syndrome or trisomy 21 is a chromosomal abnormality characterized by mental retardation, growth retardation, and a high prevalence of aggressive periodontal disease (occurs in almost 100% of affected individuals younger than 30 years of age).
   C. Chédiak-Higashi syndrome is a rare disease that affects the production of cellular organelles; produces partial albinism, mild bleeding disorders, and recurrent bacterial infections, including rapidly destructive periodontitis.
   D. Hypophosphatasia is a rare familial skeletal condition characterized by rickets, poor cranial bone formation, and premature loss of the primary and permanent dentitions.
   E. Other diseases associated with aggressive forms of periodontal disease include neutropenias, acute and subacute leukemias, and leukocyte adhesion deficiency.

II. Diabetic periodontitis occurs most frequently in individuals with uncontrolled diabetes, however, controlled diabetics also have an increased susceptibility to both gingivitis and periodontitis.
   A. Elevated blood sugar levels in the patient with diabetes mellitus may suppress the immune response, thereby increasing the individual's susceptibility to infection and periodontal disease.
   B. The diabetic state is associated with decreased collagen synthesis and increased collagenase activity.
   C. Altered neutrophil function, which has been detected in some individuals with diabetes, increases the risk for periodontal breakdown.
   D. In the presence of periodontal infection, diabetes-induced secondary hyperparathyroidism may stimulate excessive alveolar bone loss.

III. AIDS-associated periodontitis is characterized by a variety of oral manifestations because of a profound impairment of the immune system. Frequently occurring oral manifestations include:
   A. HIV gingivitis or LGE—a distinct erythematous band at the marginal gingiva associated with petechiae that typically do not bleed.
   B. HIV-associated periodontitis, which is defined by the presence of LGE and attachment loss, reverse papillary architecture, cratering in the interdental col area, and frequent severe clefting accompanying the recession.
   C. NUP, which includes the criteria for HIV-periodontitis in addition to the presence of exposed bone, ulceration or necrosis of attached gingivae, or complaints of severe, deep bone pain.
   D. Oral candidiasis, which is one of the early signs of disease in the patient with HIV, may manifest as erythematous, pseudomembranous, hyperplastic, or angular cheilitis; must be treated with antifungal drugs.
   E. HSV lesions that persist for longer than 1 month are AIDS-defining, according to the CDC; often are widespread and severe and may coexist with the cytomegalovirus (CMV).
   F. Oral hairy leukoplakia is a white lesion of the tongue that does not rub off. The Epstein-Barr virus (EBV) has been detected in this lesion in the majority of cases.
   G. Kaposi sarcoma is the most frequently occurring neoplasm in the AIDS population and is most commonly found in the head and neck region.

Necrotizing Ulcerative Periodontitis

Two types of NUP have been described, including a type that is associated with AIDS and a non-AIDS type, which often is seen in cases of extreme malnutrition.

I. Both types have similar features, except that AIDS-associated NUP often results in complications that are rarely seen in the non-AIDS type. These complications may include:
   A. Large areas of necrosis that expose bone.
   B. The sequestration of bone fragments.
   C. Necrotizing stomatitis that involves the vestibule and the palate.

II. Characteristics of both varieties of NUP
   A. Long-standing ANUG, which extends into the bone.
   B. Deep, crater-like osseous lesions.
   C. Osseous lesions that may extend to gangrenous stomatitis or noma.
   D. A lack of conventional periodontal pockets, owing to the removal of tissue by ulcerative necrosis.
   E. Superficial features of ANUG (in some cases).

 Clinical Case **STUDY**

John Gers is a 44-year-old businessman who has returned for his 3-month periodontal maintenance appointment. Two years ago, he was classified as having moderate adult periodontitis and received full-mouth non-surgical periodontal therapy. He always keeps his supportive periodontal therapy appointments. His gingival

tissues appear firm and fibrotic. During his periodontal assessment, generalized bleeding is noted and many pockets exhibit an increased depth. Oral debris assessment reveals little plaque and moderate levels of interproximal calculus. During questioning, Mr. Gers reveals that he has been unsuccessful in his attempts to quit smoking.

Clinical Case QUESTIONS

1. Identify factors that contribute to Mr. Gers' periodontal condition.
2. Identify a likely diagnosis for Mr. Gers' condition.
3. Discuss future treatment options.
4. What is the prognosis for this disease?

Clinical Case RATIONALES

1. Valuable contributing factors include compliance with recommended supportive (maintenance) therapy, low levels of plaque, and a desire to quit smoking. Factors that have contributed to his periodontal disease include smoking and the presence of interproximal calculus.
2. Mr. Gers most likely has refractory periodontitis. This condition typically is associated with smoking and a poor response to conventional periodontal therapy.
3. Because Mr. Gers' periodontal condition is not stable after several thorough periodontal debridement procedures, he should be referred to a periodontist. The periodontist may request a microbial analysis of his periodontal pathogens, prescribe a regimen of antibiotics, and strongly encourage the patient to quit smoking.
4. The prognosis for refractory periodontitis is poor. If Mr. Gers quits smoking, the prognosis will improve.

Refractory Periodontitis

Refractory periodontitis is a classification of periodontal disease that includes cases that have not responded to conventional and appropriate therapy.

I. Must be differentiated from recurrent disease, in which the individual is successfully treated but, after a period of remission, experiences a new exacerbation triggered by the return of irritational factors.
II. Also must be differentiated from maltreated or incompletely treated cases.
III. Deterioration may occur at new sites or at previously treated sites.
IV. May be site-specific or may involve the entire dentition; early-onset periodontal diseases tend to involve the entire dentition but adult periodontitis tends to involve only specific sites.
V. Is associated with high levels of *A. actinomycetem-comitans* at refractory sites, together with other periodontopathic microbes.
VI. Is consistently associated with cigarette smoking.

Clinical Assessment

The clinical assessment is a crucial component of periodontal therapy because it forms the foundation on which an appropriate plan of care can be developed. During clinical assessment, information about the patient's past and present health, personal habits, and clinical findings are compiled to identify all risk factors that affect both patient care and disease etiology.

Medical/Health History

Thorough medical and dental histories must be obtained before the commencement of any intraoral procedures, including the clinical assessment, because they are critical to the provision of appropriate and safe dental hygiene care.

I. Medical and dental histories assist in the following:
   A. Detection of systemic conditions that may require special precautions.
   B. Detection of conditions that may affect periodontal tissue response.
   C. Evaluation of oral manifestations of systemic disease.
II. Histories are used initially to establish whether it is safe to treat the patient. Some conditions that preclude immediate dental treatment include:
   A. Those that require the use of prophylactic antibiotics to prevent endocarditis during the delivery of invasive dental procedures (e.g., organic heart murmurs, most congenital heart malformations, prosthetic cardiac valves, mitral valve prolapse with valvular regurgitation, hypertrophic cardiomyopathy, and rheumatic heart disease).
   B. Heart attack within 6 months of the appointment or hypertension greater than 160/95 (seek medical consult before treatment) or 200/115 (no treatment in any situation).
   C. Immunosuppressive conditions such as HIV/AIDS; diabetes mellitus, depending on the severity, may require prophylactic antibiotics to prevent bacteremia.
III. A history should include a careful evaluation of all medications that the patient is taking before the administration of local anesthesia.
   A. Some tricyclic antidepressants, monoamine oxidase inhibitors (MAOs), antipsychotic drugs, and nonselective beta blockers are contraindicated with epinephrine.
   B. Individuals with significant liver, kidney, or cardiovascular dysfunction may be at severe risk for anesthetic overdose caused by inadequate biotransformation of the drug.
   C. Individuals who are undergoing cancer radiation therapy are at risk for the development of osteo-

radionecrosis; significant periodontal disease should be eliminated and tooth extraction should be completed before radiation therapy. Periodontal therapy after radiation therapy is completed is risky and should be performed with caution.

D. Questioning patients about medication is important because of a rise in the number of medications being taken; according to one study, an alarming 47% of US dental patients take at least one prescription medication.[7] The most commonly used medications are analgesics and cardiovascular agents.

IV. The history is increasingly important because the average dental patient currently is older than in the past; four out of five individuals older than 65 years of age have one or more chronic diseases.[6]

V. A history should be taken during the first visit and should be updated at each subsequent visit. If any major changes occur, a new history form should be completed.

VI. A self-administered written questionnaire should be followed up with verbal questioning by the clinician to clarify any ambiguities and verify responses.

Dental/Personal History

The dental/personal history provides important information about a patient's past dental experiences and indicates why the patient is presenting for care. This history also indicates whether the patient is experiencing symptoms such as pain, how long these symptoms have been present, and whether they are recurrent. The patient's oral hygiene habits should be included and should provide insight into the patient's attitudes toward dental care. The dental/personal history assists in identifying nondental risk factors such as stress, smoking, diet, and alcohol consumption, which may play a role in the patient's periodontal condition.

Extraoral Examination

The extraoral examination should be performed to evaluate jaw movement, identify TMJ dysfunction that may have an impact on therapy, examine the skin for unusual lesions, and identify lymphadenopathy associated with oral pathology.

Intraoral Examination

The intraoral examination is a continuation of the inspection for any suspicious soft tissue lesions that may indicate pathology within the oral cavity.

I. Includes systematic inspection of the lips, vestibular mucosa, floor of the mouth, retromolar pad, surfaces of the tongue (ventral, lateral, and dorsal), hard palate, soft palate, tonsillar pillars, pterygomandibular raphe, and maxillary tuberosity.

II. Is important in identifying oral lesions that have systemic associations (e.g., HIV-associated periodontal disease, acute herpetic gingivostomatitis, desquamative gingivitis).

Periodontal Assessment

The periodontal assessment includes an evaluation of the topography of the gingiva and related structures.

I. Involves identifying the presence of inflammation, which is indicated by:

A. Color changes from "coral pink," which indicates health (varies significantly with differences in pigmentation), to overt signs of redness, which indicate the gingival ulceration and engorgement of blood vessels that occur during the inflammatory process.

B. The contour of the gingiva. In healthy individuals, the gingivae follow the contour of the teeth, the margins are knife-edged (in normal tooth arrangement), and the papillae appear pointed; rolled or rounded marginal and papillary gingivae are suggestive of inflammation.

C. Other changes in contour; often are related to hyperplastic tissues and may include McCall's festoons, which are lifesaver-like enlargements around the free gingival margins, and vertical Stillman's clefts, which are produced by atrophy of the labial gingiva and extensions of adjacent hyperplastic tissue.

D. The texture of the gingiva; is the least reliable sign of inflammation; may appear as a loss of stippling during inflammation.

E. The consistency of the gingiva. In health the gingiva typically is firm and resilient; when inflamed, marginal and papillary gingival tissues become bulbous and flabby, if edematous, or bulky and firm from scar tissue accumulation, if fibrotic.

F. Bleeding; although a late sign, is the most reliable and widely accepted sign of inflammation. A record of bleeding indices establishes a baseline measure from which goals can be established and serves as a powerful motivational tool.

G. Exudate; GCF increases during inflammation; in more severe cases of inflammation becomes milky, contains numerous neutrophils and their by-products, and is referred to as pus.

II. Periodontal probing must be performed to measure the depth of periodontal pockets and the amount of clinical attachment loss; is considered the "gold standard" for determining the extent of periodontal tissue destruction.[5]

A. Both probing depth and attachment loss may be measured with either manual or automated probes; typically involve measurements at six sites per tooth.

B. To encourage all dental practitioners to include routine probing in their patient care, the AAP and the ADA, with the corporate sponsorship of

Proctor and Gamble, developed the periodontal screening and recording (PSR) system.

    1. The PSR system is a modification of the Community Periodontal Index of Treatment Needs (CPITN) developed by the World Health Organization. This system involves probing each of the six routine sites per tooth but recording only the highest reading per sextant and interpreting the findings with a code that determines whether full-mouth recording of all probing depths is required. The presence and distribution of bacterial plaque, calculus, and stain are identified and recorded to assist in setting goals with the patient.

III. Plaque is unquestionably the prime etiologic agent in the development of periodontal disease; its extent and distribution must be determined to facilitate removal.

    A. Several epidemiologic indices assist in recording plaque (see Chapter 16).

    B. Calculus and stain are contributing factors for periodontal disease because they are plaque-retentive, and therefore they should be removed.

    C. The extent and tenacity of calculus deposits and stains determine the length of therapy and thus are important components of treatment planning.

IV. The proximal contact relationships of teeth should be evaluated; open contacts encourage food impaction and tight contacts prevent effective interproximal cleansing.

V. Determining the extent of mobility of teeth and dental implants is an important part of the periodontal assessment; indicates the extent of damage to the supporting structures of the periodontium; is considered a predictor of attachment loss, and as such, a risk factor for the continued progression of periodontal disease.

    A. Mobility is tested with the handles of two instruments or with an automated mobility tester, such as the Periotest by Siemens.

    B. Several mobility scales exist; measurements range from 0 to 3 but with slightly different interpretations.

VI. Determining the presence and degree of furcation involvement is a necessary part of the periodontal assessment; prognosis is poor for teeth with extensive furcation involvement because home care is almost impossible and accessibility during therapy becomes a major obstacle.

    A. Teeth with moderate to advanced furcation involvement are more likely to be lost than teeth without furcations.

    B. Furcation involvement has been labeled a risk factor in the prediction of periodontal breakdown.

    C. A curved, calibrated Nabor's probe is the best instrument for the detection of furcations.

    D. Several scales classify furcation involvement by means of a 1-to-3 or 1-to-4 scale.

VII. The presence of malocclusion or occlusal pathology should be assessed routinely; both are considered risk factors for periodontal breakdown.

VIII. The status of dental restorations and prosthetic appliances should be evaluated to determine whether overhanging margins or poorly contoured crowns exist; both place the individual at risk for periodontal breakdown.

Radiographic Assessment

The radiographic assessment includes an evaluation of the interdental septa, the amount and pattern of bone loss, and furcation involvement.

I. A satisfactory number of diagnostic quality radiographs must be interpreted to determine the extent of bone loss.

II. Includes the use of full-mouth periapical radiographs, panoramic radiographs, or vertical bitewings to accurately assess the periodontal status.

III. Fuzziness of the alveolar crests and breaks in the continuity of the lamina dura are initial signs of periodontal breakdown.

IV. More extensive bone loss is seen as horizontal or vertical/angular and is dependent on the pathway of inflammation.

V. Has limitations in the diagnosis of periodontal disease.

    A. Destruction of the alveolar bone typically is worse than what appears in radiographs.

    B. Destruction of facial and lingual cortical plates is often not detectable in radiographs.

Supplemental Diagnostic Tests

Several adjunctive or supplemental diagnostic tests have been developed to identify the presence of periodontal disease, but none are truly diagnostic. However, these tests play an important role in the identification of risk factors and coupled with clinical parameters, such as bleeding in response to probing and clinical attachment loss, can be strong predictors of future disease progression.

I. Are used primarily as research tools; only a small number are available for use in clinical practice.

II. May be classified as belonging to one of four categories: physical, microbiologic, biochemical, or immunologic.

    A. Physical assessment tests include measures of subgingival temperature and GCF flow rates as they relate to inflammation.

       1. An automated, computerized, temperature-sensitive probe called the Periotemp System (Abiodent) is available for clinical use and functions on the premise that an elevated subgingival temperature is correlated to the presence of inflammation.

       2. The flow rate of GCF has been shown to be

positively correlated to gingival inflammation and thus can be a useful adjunct for monitoring the response to periodontal therapy. The GCF flow rate is measured by an electronic instrument called the Periotron 6000, which is available for clinical use.

B. Microbiologic tests have become popular adjuncts for the identification of bacterial species that may place the individual at risk for aggressive forms of periodontal disease. However, it is important to recognize that these tests are not diagnostic; they should be used solely for identification and monitoring purposes.

1. The culturing of putative periodontal pathogens has been considered the gold standard for the identification and quantification of bacterial species; however, it is impractical and expensive for use in clinical practice and typically is confined to research.

2. Enzymatic methods for identifying the presence of periodontopathic microorganisms have increased in popularity with the release of the BANA test (Knowell Pharmaceuticals) for clinical use. This test has been used extensively in research and identifies the presence of three periodontal microorganisms: *T. denticola, P. gingivalis,* and *B. forsythus.*

3. Immunologic assays such as the ELISA test (enzyme-linked immunosorbent assay) have been used extensively in medicine and in periodontal research for the identification of specific microbes. A promising chairside test (Evalusite) was developed by Kodak for clinical use to identify *A. actinomycetemcomitans, P. gingivalis,* and *P. intermedia;* however, its marketing was short-lived, despite the fact that it had excellent sensitivity and specificity.

4. DNA probes are capable of accurate identification and quantification of microbial pathogens and have the advantage of not requiring a living specimen. Although chairside tests are not yet available (Affirm, MicroprobeCorp), Omnigene (Cambridge, MA) offers a mail-in laboratory service (DMDX) for the identification of as many as six periodontal pathogens, including *A. actinomycetemcomitans, P. gingivalis,* and *P. intermedia.*

C. Biochemical assessments are more sophisticated laboratory tests that have been developed to identify various biochemical markers that are found in GCF and are involved in the host response.

1. Elevated levels of collagenase and other neutral proteases that are positively correlated to clinical attachment loss can be measured through a rapid chairside test (Periocheck) that is commercially available through ProDentec (Batesville, AR). Although the predictive value of this test is yet to be determined, the monitoring system is a useful adjunct to traditional clinical measures.

2. Other biochemical tests (currently used in research only) that have strong diagnostic potential include measurements of prostaglandin E_2 (PGE_2), beta-glucuronidase (BG), and aspartate aminotransferase (AST).

D. Immunologic assessment tests have been developed to identify antibodies to specific periodontal pathogens in either blood serum or GCF. Correlations have been found between elevated antibody levels and active disease; however, the relationship to disease progression has not been established.

1. A chairside serum antibody test is available for office use (PerioAlert; Avitar, Canton, MA).

Interpretation of Evidence, Presumptive Diagnosis, Treatment Planning, and Prognosis

After the health history, personal history, and clinical, radiographic, and adjunctive evidence have been collected, they must be interpreted to determine a differential diagnosis. Only after the differential diagnosis has been established can an appropriate plan of care be devised.

Developing the Differential Diagnosis

All evidence collected during the initial assessment must be considered in developing a differential diagnosis, which subsequently is used to determine the patient's treatment.

I. Developing the diagnosis involves:
  A. Prioritizing immediate extraoral or intraoral problems.
  B. Identifying any systemic component of the disease process.
  C. Reviewing the patient's clinical signs and symptoms.
  D. Looking for radiographic signs of disease.
  E. Evaluating the human needs deficits of the patient.

II. Establishing the differential diagnosis includes:
  A. Determining the health status of the periodontium.
  B. Determining whether the gingivitis, if present, is associated with plaque.
  C. Identifying whether the condition is chronic periodontitis or a more aggressive form.
  D. Making a presumptive diagnosis, which is the "best possibility" after examining all the evidence.

III. Possible diagnostic categories include health, gingivitis, and periodontitis; subsequently a more specific diagnosis can be identified (presumptive diagnosis), which is used to guide the development of the treatment plan.

IV. A final diagnosis can be made only after the completion of initial therapy and reevaluation of the clinical response to therapy. This response guides further treatment planning.

Determining the Appropriate Plan of Action

Determining an appropriate plan of action for each patient involves treatment planning, phases of treatment, AAP classification of case types, the dental hygiene plan of care, obtaining the informed consent of the patient, and prognosis.

I.   Treatment Planning Goals
   A.   Include developing individualized plans based on the specific needs of each patient.
   B.   Include incorporating "evidence" in the development of the plan.
   C.   Include the development of evidence-based, patient-specific treatment protocols.
   D.   Include the determination of methods and the sequence for delivering appropriate treatment.
   E.   Include the elimination and control of etiologic and predisposing factors.
   F.   Emphasize the maintenance of health and prevention of disease recurrence.
II. The phases of treatment have been divided into five groups by Carranza:
   A.   The preliminary phase addresses any dental or periodontal emergencies and involves treatment of all acute and painful oral conditions.
   B.   Phase-I (etiologic phase) therapy, or initial therapy, deals with the control or elimination of etiologic factors and includes:
      1.   Patient education, plaque control instruction, and risk factor counseling.
      2.   Periodontal debridement (including scaling and root planing).
      3.   Recontouring of defective margins of restorations.
   C.   Phase-II therapy is the surgical phase of treatment; involves procedures designed to reduce the effects of disease and also includes regenerative techniques.
   D.   Phase-III therapy includes all restorative procedures, orthodontics, splinting, and occlusal therapy.
   E.   Phase-IV therapy, or supportive periodontal therapy (SPT), is the maintenance phase, which the patient remains in for life. Occasional relapses may require the patient to repeat initial therapy, but the patient always returns to SPT. Appropriate SPT intervals are determined individually, based on tissue response and the home care efforts of the patient.

American Academy of Periodontology (AAP) Classification of Case Types

The AAP classification system is used routinely across the United States to define the severity of disease and is divided into five diagnostic categories:
I.   AAP Case Type I: Gingivitis
II. AAP Case Type II: Early Periodontitis
III. AAP Case Type III: Moderate Periodontitis
IV. AAP Case Type IV: Advanced Periodontitis
V.   AAP Case Type V: Refractory Periodontitis

The Dental Hygiene Plan of Care

The dental hygiene plan of care is developed by the dental hygienist and typically involves phases I and IV of the comprehensive treatment plan.
I.   Must meet individual patient needs and must follow an orderly sequence.
II. Involves determining the number of appointments and the time required for each, depending on the patient's needs.
III. Generally includes planning of 1-hour appointments for each visit; however, variations occur dependent on differing office protocols.
IV. Requires a 1-month reevaluation after initial therapy (for all periodontal patients) to assess the tissue response, determine an appropriate SPT interval, and evaluate the need for referral to a periodontist.
V.   May follow a suggested guideline for determining the number of appointments for the various AAP case types; however, individual needs may alter this model and must always take precedence over any suggested protocols.
   A.   Treatment for AAP case type I typically is completed in one appointment; a recall interval is established at that time.
   B.   Treatment for AAP case type II often requires more than one appointment and may require the use of anesthetics; is followed by a 1-month reevaluation appointment.
   C.   Treatment for AAP case type III typically is divided into quadrants; requires anesthesia and several appointments, including a 1-month reevaluation appointment.
   D.   Treatment for AAP case type IV typically is divided into quadrants or sextants; may require treatment of individual teeth, depending on the extent and tenacity of the deposits; anesthetics are routinely used and a 1-month reevaluation appointment is planned.
   E.   Treatment for case type V may require single or multiple visits, depending on the amount of debridement necessary. More frequent recalls often are required and the adjunctive use of systemic antibiotics may be necessary.

Informed Consent

Informed consent is the verbal or written permission granted by the patient to proceed with a plan of care, and should be obtained before the commencement of treatment in all cases.

Requires that patients be informed of the extent of the disease, all treatment options available, and the consequences of no treatment.

I. Allows patients to choose the treatment option they prefer.

II. To avoid lawsuits, should include the patient's signature to show understanding and acceptance of the treatment plan; if the patient refuses treatment, a signature acknowledges that all consequences of declining treatment have been explained.

Prognosis

Prognosis is the prediction of the duration, course, and termination of a disease and the likelihood of its response to treatment.

I. Is strongly influenced by patient attitude.

II. Is good for gingival diseases, if:
   A. Inflammation is the only pathologic change.
   B. The patient is compliant with oral hygiene.
   C. There are no systemic modifiers.

III. For periodontal disease, is dependent on:
   A. The assessment of past bone response.
   B. The height of remaining bone.
   C. Periodontal attachment loss.
   D. Patient age.
   E. Presence of malocclusion.

IV. For individual teeth, is dependent on:
   A. Loss of attachment, the depth of periodontal pockets, and the width of attached gingiva.
   B. Mobility, furcation involvement, and tooth morphology.

Plaque Control

Because plaque is the prime etiologic factor in the development of periodontal disease, it is critical to the success of periodontal therapy that an effective plaque control program be initiated. Components of plaque control include patient motivation and methods of plaque removal.

Plaque

I. Is the prime etiologic agent for the development of both gingivitis and periodontitis.

II. If limited in amount supragingivally, subgingival plaque formation is reduced.

III. Meticulous control and frequent maintenance appointments, including thorough debridement of all tooth deposits, are necessary components of therapy.

IV. Goals of Plaque Control
   A. Maintenance of gingival and periodontal health
   B. Control of caries
   C. Transfer of responsibility for plaque control to the patient
   D. Management of the complexities of plaque control
   E. Successful motivation of the patient

Patient motivation

Patient motivation is the key to a successful plaque control program yet is a major challenge because most periodontal patients have a history of poor plaque control that preceded disease development.

I. Involves encouraging new oral hygiene procedures that may take more time than the patient is accustomed to spending.

II. Educating the patient regarding the etiology, progression, and long-term effects of disease is mandatory.

III. Includes educating, motivating, encouraging, and reinforcing positive behaviors to effect a change in habits.

Methods of Plaque Removal

Various methods of plaque removal exist and include manual and powered toothbrushing, adjunctive aids, oral irrigation, and the use of chemical agents.

I. Manual Toothbrushing
   A. Scrub technique
      1. Bristles are placed next to the teeth and moved back and forth.
      2. If performed too vigorously, leads to gingival trauma and eventual abrasion of the teeth.
   B. Roll technique
      1. Involves brushing the teeth in the direction that they grow: down on the upper teeth and up on the lower teeth.
   C. Charters technique
      1. Bristles are placed at a 45-degree angle to the tooth, with the bristles pointed away from the gingiva.
      2. Pressure is applied to the gingiva, which forces the bristles interproximally and simultaneously massages the tissues.
   D. Stillman technique
      1. Is used to massage the gingiva; the bristles are placed against the tissues at a 45-degree angle but are pointed apically.
      2. Pressure is applied until the tissues are blanched; subsequently a massaging motion is used, without moving the bristles.
      3. After one area has been massaged, the bristles are removed and placed against the tissues of the next tooth.
   E. Modified Stillman technique
      1. Is the same as the Stillman technique but is followed through with a roll stroke.
   F. Bass technique
      1. Bristle ends are applied to the sulcular area and moved back and forth with short strokes, in a vibratory motion.
      2. The bristles of a soft mutitufted brush are placed at 45 degrees to the long axis of the tooth.
      3. The occlusal surfaces are brushed with back-and-forth strokes.
      4. The lingual areas of the mandibular anteriors are brushed with the heel of the brush.

II. Powered Toothbrushing
  A. Is as effective as manual brushing and has become very popular.
  B. Can be accomplished with a variety of automatic toothbrushes, which are available with different actions (e.g., reciprocating bristle motion, sonic vibrations, rotary motion).
  C. Is an excellent choice for patients who lack dexterity.

III. Interproximal Aids
  A. Dental floss is available in a variety of textures, sizes, thicknesses, and flavors; are equally effective.
  B. Floss threaders are used to thread floss under the pontics of bridges to clean abutment teeth.
  C. Floss holders or floss tools are available for those who are unable to manipulate floss with their fingers.
  D. Interdental brushes are used to cleanse interproximal areas, exposed roots, furcations, and implants; typically have handles and disposable brush ends.
  E. Toothpicks with handles may be useful adjuncts for reaching furcations and areas that are difficult to access with an interproximal or conventional toothbrush; triangular-shaped tooth picks made of balsa wood or plastic are not as useful periodontally but are useful in removing plaque from wider interproximal spaces.
  F. Rubber tip stimulators were originally designed for gingival massage; are useful in interproximal plaque removal.

IV. Irrigating Devices
  A. Are useful adjuncts to plaque removal, particularly for less compliant patients, orthodontic patients, and those who have impaired dexterity.
  B. Have a jet flow that should be directed to the interproximal spaces at a 90-degree angle.
  C. Are contraindicated for patients who require antibiotic coverage for dental procedures or for those who have acute oral conditions.
  D. May have subgingival rubber tips (available with some irrigators) that are placed below the gingiva and directed toward the sulcus.

V. Chemical Antiplaque Agents
  A. Should possess:
    1. Antiplaque action, whether bactericidal or bacteriostatic.
    2. Good substantivity, which is the ability to adhere to tooth structure for long periods of time; enables slow release.
    3. Low toxicity.
    4. Low permeability.
  B. Available agents
    1. Chlorhexidine digluconate 0.12%.
      a. Is available in mouthwash form by prescription only in the United States and Canada.
      b. Significantly reduces plaque and gingivitis (by as much as 60%); exhibits high substantivity and has been researched extensively.
      c. Exhibits side effects that may include dark brown staining of the teeth, increased calculus formation, poor taste, altered taste sensation, and in some patients, reversible desquamation of the oral mucosa.
      d. Recommended use involves rinsing with 15 mL twice daily for 30 seconds.
      e. Contains alcohol (11.6%) and is therefore contraindicated for patients who are sensitive to alcohol.
    2. Phenolic compounds (essential oils).
      a. Contain thymol, eucalyptol, menthol, and methyl-salicylate.
      b. Reduce plaque and gingivitis by 30% and are available without prescription.
      c. Contain high percentages of alcohol (26.4%), have a strong taste, stain the teeth, and may cause a burning sensation in some individuals.
    3. Quaternary ammonium compounds.
      a. Contain cetylpyridinium chloride and also may contain domiphen bromide.
      b. May contain as much as 18% alcohol.
      c. Have slight but not substantive antiplaque activity.
    4. Sanguinarine.
      a. Is a plant alkaloid derived from the bloodroot plant.
      b. Is available in both rinse and paste forms.
      c. Has no significant effects unless both rinse and paste are used together.
      d. Has an alcohol content of 10% to 14%.
    5. Stannous fluoride.
      a. Has exhibited weak antigingivitis effects in some studies.
      b. Is available in paste or rinse form (0.4%) but may stain the teeth.
      c. Contains no alcohol.

VI. Anticalculus Agents (tartar control toothpastes)
  A. Have reduced calculus formation by as much as 40% in some studies.
  B. Active ingredients
    1. Soluble pyrophosphates.
    2. Zinc citrate.
  C. May cause dentinal hypersensitivity[8]

Nonsurgical Periodontal Therapy

Nonsurgical periodontal therapy is a term applied to the initial treatment of gingival and periodontal diseases, which involves eliminating pathogenic microorganisms through definitive instrumentation procedures, plaque control instruction, and other supportive procedures.

Goals of Nonsurgical Periodontal Therapy

The goals of nonsurgical phase-I periodontal therapy (initial therapy) can be divided into short-term and long-term goals.

I. Short-Term Goals
   A. Removal of hard and soft deposits through periodontal debridement procedures
   B. Definitive plaque control instruction (with the patient)
   C. Control of systemic and other risk factors
II. Long-Term Goals
   A. Reduction or elimination of gingival inflammation
   B. Elimination of pockets caused by edema
   C. Restoration of periodontal health

Rationales

The rationales for nonsurgical periodontal therapy include:

I. Removal of the etiologic agent, bacterial plaque, and other local irritants.
II. Initiation of plaque control measures.
III. Modification of risk factors, both local and systemic, wherever possible (e.g., overhang removal).
IV. Reduction or elimination of inflammation.
V. Evaluation of tissue response.
VI. Establishment of supportive periodontal therapy (SPT) or maintenance program.

Procedures and Techniques

Nonsurgical periodontal therapy involves a variety of procedures and techniques.

I. Procedures performed during nonsurgical periodontal therapy may include:
   A. Oral hygiene instruction, which is comprehensive and individualized, to facilitate daily plaque removal.
   B. Scaling for the purpose of supragingival and subgingival calculus removal.
   C. Root planing, which is targeted toward the removal of cementum or surface dentin that is impregnated with calculus, endotoxins, or bacteria; current evidence has led to a more conservative approach to this procedure, thus a glassy, smooth root surface is no longer the goal of root planing.
   D. Periodontal debridement; includes both scaling and root planing, together with subgingival plaque removal and identification of plaque retentive factors; may include the use of adjunctive chemotherapeutic agents.
   E. Closed gingival curettage techniques to remove diseased soft tissues from within the pocket wall; currently is believed to have limited value in nonsurgical periodontal therapy and is used only in selected cases.
   F. Selective coronal polishing to remove retentive supragingival plaque and stains for cosmetic reasons.
   G. Occlusal evaluation for the identification of occlusally-related contributing factors.
II. Clinical techniques employed during nonsurgical periodontal therapy may include:
   A. Hand Instrumentation
      1. A wide range of hand instruments are available for periodontal debridement, including curettes, scalers, and other special instruments such as files, hoes, and chisels.
         a. Curettes may be either universal, with two parallel cutting edges that can be adapted to any tooth surface, or area-specific, with one offset blade designed for use only in a specific area (e.g., Gracey curette).
         b. Curettes currently are available in a wide variety of materials (e.g., stainless steel, carbon steel, and cryogenically treated stainless steel) and creative designs (e.g., longer shanks, shorter blades), which enable better access to challenging root surfaces.
         c. Scalers, such as sickles, which have two blades that converge to a point, are used more often for supragingival calculus removal, as are hoes and chisels; files may be used either supragingivally or subgingivally to crush heavier calculus deposits.
   B. Powered instrumentation
      1. A variety of powered instruments are available for use by dental hygienists, including the EVA device for the removal of overhanging margins of restorations, and sonic and ultrasonic instruments for periodontal debridement.
         a. EVA (EVA Prophylaxis System, Unitek, Monrovia, CA) is a motor-driven system that uses files and points for the removal of overhanging margins of restorations and the interproximal recontouring of restorations.
         b. Sonic scaling devices have been shown to be as effective as ultrasonic and hand instruments and have the advantage of attaching directly to the high-speed handpiece. They generate vibrations of 2000 to 6000 cycles per second.
         c. Ultrasonic scaling devices are separate units that use either magnetostrictive or piezoelectric systems and vibrate between 20,000 to 40,000 cycles per second.
         d. Both ultrasonic and sonic systems have been shown to be as effective as hand scaling in the debridement of tooth and root surfaces and in the achievement of long-term periodontal health.
         e. New slimmer, longer tips that adapt to deeper pockets and furcations have been developed and have proven to be superior

to the older, thicker tips for calculus removal.

f. In individuals who have cardiac pacemakers, the electromagnetic field created by ultrasonic scalers can interfere with the functioning of the pacemaker. Although most pacemakers currently have a shield that protects them from these electromagnetic fields, the use of ultrasonics in patients with pacemakers is not advisable.

Effectiveness

The effectiveness of nonsurgical periodontal therapy, whether performed by hand or with powered instrumentation, has been well documented.

I. Decreased probing depths and reduction in bleeding are expected outcomes of therapy.
II. Gains in attachment in deeper pockets are reasonable expectations.
III. A generally healthier oral environment typically results from successful nonsurgical periodontal therapy.
IV. Close monitoring of all clinical parameters are necessary to prevent or arrest the progression of disease after nonsurgical therapy.

Adjunctive Therapies

Because of the highly infective microbial population present in the diseased periodontal pocket, other therapies, which are used concomitantly with periodontal debridement, may be useful adjuncts to nonsurgical periodontal therapy. These include chemical and antibiotic adjunctive therapies.

I. Chemical Adjuncts
  A. Include antimicrobial rinses that are given before therapy; have not been shown to have significant benefits.
  B. Include subgingival irrigation, which, when combined with scaling and root planing, has been shown in some studies to enhance the success of therapy; controversy regarding its benefits continues to exist.
    1. Irrigation is considered an elective part of therapy.
    2. In order for antimicrobial agents delivered as irrigants to be effective, they must meet the following requirements:
      a. They must reach the base of the pocket.
      b. A bactericidal concentration of agents must be employed.
      c. They must exhibit substantivity.
    3. Methods of delivery
      a. The use of a hand syringe with a cannula tip.
      b. The use of pulsated irrigation devices, with either a rubber tip or a cannula.
    4. Effective irrigants
      a. 0.12% chlorhexidine digluconate
      b. 0.4% stannous fluoride
      c. 0.05% povidone-iodine

C. Include calculus softener agents, which recently have become available to help soften the calculus and enhance the ease of removal; currently there is not enough evidence to support the use of these agents as adjuncts to nonsurgical periodontal therapy.
D. Include desensitizing agents, which are used as adjuncts to nonsurgical therapy; often are recommended because sensitivity after therapy is a commonly reported problem.
  1. Recommended agents
    a. Sodium fluoride compounds
    b. Calcium hydroxide
    c. Cavity varnishes
    d. Potassium oxalate
    e. Ferric oxalate
    f. Iontophoresis and neutral sodium fluoride

II. Antibiotics
  A. Systemic antibiotics
    1. Systemic delivery of antibiotics is sometimes necessary in the treatment of more aggressive forms of periodontal disease because most of these conditions exhibit host impairment.
      a. In all cases the pathogens initially must be identified—by culture and sensitivity, by DNA probing, or by immunofluorescent testing—to determine which antibiotic agent should be prescribed.
      b. Antibiotic agents commonly prescribed as adjuncts to nonsurgical periodontal therapy include amoxicillin, ampicillin, Augmentin, tetracyclines, metronidazole, ciprofloxacin, and clindamycin.
    2. A new form of systemic delivery involves the use of low levels of antibiotics to suppress destructive enzymes produced during the inflammatory process rather than to reduce bacterial numbers. Periostat, which recently was approved for this use by the FDA, is a doxycycline hyclate (20-mg capsule) that is taken orally; is indicated for use as an adjunct to scaling and root planing; is administered as one pill twice daily for up to 9 months; results in decreased pocket depths and attachment loss.
  B. Local delivery of antibiotics (controlled-release)
    1. Is used in cases that do not respond to conventional nonsurgical periodontal therapy.
    2. When used concomitantly with scaling and root planing, has been shown to decrease probing depth and reduce bleeding and microbes.
    3. FDA-approved examples
      a. Actisite fibers; these controlled-release tetracycline-impregnated fibers are placed in pockets greater than 5 mm for 10 days; the fibers are placed in the pocket in successive layers, with a gingival retraction cord packing instrument, and subsequently are sealed with a cyanoacrylate adhesive; the cord is

removed after 10 days; are used as an adjunct to scaling and root planing in adults with periodontitis.
   b. Atridox; a doxycycline hyclate (50 mg), bioabsorbable, two-part formulation is mixed and placed by syringe in a periodontal pocket, where it hardens on contact with saliva and slowly releases the drug for a week; is indicated for use as an adjunct to scaling and root planing in adults with periodontitis; decreases pocket depth, attachment loss, and bleeding; suppresses bacteria by inhibiting protein synthesis.
   c. PerioChip; a chlorhexidine gluconate (2.5 mg), biodegradable, rectangular chip is placed in periodontal pockets greater than 5 mm; releases the drug biphasically (40% initially; the remainder over 7 to 10 days); is indicated for use as an adjunct to scaling and root planing in adults with periodontitis; decreases pocket depth and is bactericidal.
4. Other controlled-release agents that have been researched[2] include:
   a. Chlorhexidine gels; have been tested in 1% and 2% concentrations and have shown limited short-term effects.
   b. Metronidazole gels; have demonstrated promising results in the reduction of bleeding in response to probing; also have reduced pocket depths.
   c. Clindamycin HCL gel, which shows promise in the elimination of periodontal microorganisms.
   d. Other controlled-release films, inserts, chips, membranes, and biosorbable polymers have been tested, such as ofloxacin, doxycycline, tetracycline, chlorhexidine, and methylene blue. All require further studies to substantiate their clinical value.

Surgical Periodontal Therapy

After the completion of nonsurgical periodontal therapy, tissue response is evaluated and the need for surgical intervention is determined. It is important for the dental hygienist to understand the indications and contraindications for basic surgical procedures to reinforce their significance to the patient.

Rationale

The use of periodontal surgical procedures is considered for the reduction of disease progression when nonsurgical interventions have failed. The main goals of periodontal surgery are:
I.   Pocket reduction for better access to home care procedures and professional debridement.
II. The correction of mucogingival defects.
III. The removal of inflamed tissues.
IV. Drainage of periodontal abscesses.
V.   Providing access for restorative dental procedures.
VI. The regeneration of tissue lost to disease.
VII. Improved esthetics.
VIII. The placement of dental implants.

Considerations

Several factors must be taken into consideration before a surgical procedure is recommended by the periodontist. These include probing depths, bone loss, the value of the affected tooth, and a variety of patient factors.
I.   Pocket Probing Depths
   A. Must be greater than 5 mm.
   B. Typically are difficult to debride professionally.
   C. Typically make the performance of home care by the patient difficult.
II. Bone Loss
   A. If more than half of the bone remains, osseous surgery is a viable option.
   B. If less than half of the bone remains, grafting or regenerative techniques may be required.
   C. The choice of procedure depends on the type of bone loss and bony defects (e.g., horizontal, vertical, one-walled, two-walled).
III. Value of the Tooth
   A. Some teeth are less valuable than others and may not be worth saving (e.g., third molar).
IV. Plaque Control by the Patient
   A. The demonstration of adequate plaque control measures by the patient is absolutely necessary before surgical intervention.
V.   Age of the Patient
   A. Is not significant, except in determining the speed of disease progression.
   B. Healing is similar in both young and old patients.
   C. The relationship of surgery to the quality of life should be considered for elderly patients.
VI. Health of the Patient
   A. Poor health contraindicates surgery.
   B. If periodontal disease is contributing to poor health, surgery may be indicated after consultation with the patient's physician.
VII. Patient Preference
   A. Patients must be informed of all risks and benefits of surgery.
   B. Patients must understand the ramifications of not having surgery.
   C. Patients must be willing to increase the frequency of SPT appointments and perform more difficult plaque removal procedures if they opt not to have surgery.

Types of Surgical Procedures

Basic periodontal surgical procedures include gingivectomy, flap procedures, bone modification procedures, and regeneration procedures.
I.   Gingivectomy

A. Is designed to reduce pocket depths by removal of the soft tissue pocket wall.

B. Is indicated in deep gingival pockets that have fibrotic tissue.

C. Is indicated in deep periodontal suprabony pockets.

II. Periodontal Flap Procedures

A. Provide access to and visibility of the root surfaces.

B. Reduce pocket depths surgically.

C. Stimulate regeneration of lost periodontal attachment in periodontal pockets.

D. Are used during procedures that correct mucogingival defects.

E. Are indicated in periodontal pockets that extend to or beyond the mucogingival junction and for infrabony pockets.

F. Two most common flap techniques

1. The modified Widman flap technique involves repositioning of reflected gingival tissues against the tooth at approximately the preoperative position.

2. The apically positioned flap technique involves repositioning the reflected flap more apically, compared with the original position, to reduce the pocket depth.

III. Ostectomy and Osteoplasty

A. Are techniques used to reduce the bony walls of infrabony pockets and to reshape abnormal alveolar contours.

1. Ostectomy refers to the removal of alveolar bone that is directly attached to the tooth via PDL fibers.

2. Osteoplasty refers to the recontouring of the alveolar bone that is not directly supporting the tooth.

B. Are techniques that must be performed in conjunction with the periodontal flap procedure.

C. Treat defects that include:

1. One-walled and two-walled infrabony pockets.

2. Interdental osseous craters.

3. Broad three-walled infrabony pockets.

4. Reversed alveolar bone architecture.

5. Bulbous facial and lingual bony contours.

IV. Periodontal Regenerative Procedures

A. Bone grafting and regeneration procedures

1. Two different techniques for the restoration of periodontal tissues in infrabony pockets and type-II furcations.

a. Guided tissue regeneration

1) Thorough debridement of the area, with flaps reflected.

2) Placement of barrier material (Gortex or collagen) over the defect; flap is closed coronally to the material; the material forms a barrier that prevents epithelial downgrowth and encourages connective tissue reattachment.

b. Bone grafts

1) The placement of various materials in osseous defects before flap closure to encourage the regeneration of lost tissue.

2) Autografts, which consist of bone taken from the patient's body.

3) Allografts, which consist of bone taken from another person (freeze-dried from cadavers).

4) Xenografts, which are created from bone taken from another species (e.g., bovine/cow).

5) Alloplasts, which are created from a variety of synthetic bone minerals (e.g., hydroxyapatite minerals or ceramics).

V. Correction of Mucogingival Defects

A. Types of Defects

1. Type-I defects

a. Pockets extend apically to or beyond the mucogingival junction but a firm keratinized pocket wall exists.

b. The apically positioned flap is the treatment of choice.

B. Type-II defects

a. Alveolar mucosa acts as marginal gingiva, with no zone of attached gingiva.

b. Treatment consists of the transfer of masticatory mucosa from another part of the mouth.

c. A lateral sliding pedicle graft involves moving keratinized tissue from the area immediately adjacent to the defect without completely detaching it from its original spot, sliding it over the defect, and subsequently attaching it with sutures.

d. The double papillae flap involves taking equal amounts of tissue from the two adjacent papillae, sliding them over to cover the defective area, and joining the tissues with sutures.

e. The free autogenous soft tissue graft involves removing a piece of keratinized gingiva from one area of the mouth, such as the palate, and suturing it to the defective region to completely cover the defect.

Postsurgical Procedures

Postsurgical procedures include the placement of sutures and surgical dressings and the provision of postoperative instructions.

I. Sutures

A. Are placed at the end of the surgical procedure to hold the tissues in place.

B. Are made of surgical silk, resorbable gut, or a synthetic material.

C. Are removed between 7 and 14 days after placement.

D. May be interrupted or uninterrupted, but the knot always faces the buccal surface.

II. Surgical Dressing
   A. Includes periodontal packs (surgical dressings) that are placed over the surgical area to protect the wound and increase patient comfort.
   B. Includes several types of dressing materials; the most common type is a zinc oxide/fatty acid compound in the form of a paste, which is mixed and placed on the wound in a thin ribbon.
   C. When placed, must not extend beyond the height of contour of the teeth and should be pressed interproximally for mechanical locking.
   D. Should remain in place for approximately 1 week.
III. Postoperative instructions commonly include:
   A. Directions for the use of mouth rinses, antibiotics, and analgesic medications.
   B. Instructions to eliminate strenuous activity.
   C. Directions regarding continued bleeding.
   D. Recommendation of a soft diet; avoidance of spicy foods.
   E. Directions regarding the periodontal dressing.
   F. Informing the patient that swelling may occur and can be minimized with the use of ice.
   G. Directions for home care; including brushing with a soft- bristled toothbrush and gently debriding the dressing area.
   H. A reminder to return for suture removal.
   I. The telephone number of the office.

Effectiveness

The effectiveness of periodontal surgery is dependent on the patient's long-term thoroughness in plaque control. Thoroughness should be reinforced at each SPT appointment. Many studies have shown that compliance with ongoing supportive therapy is the single most important factor in the success of surgical and nonsurgical therapy.
   I. Healing of the surgical wound commences immediately after surgery with the formation of a blood clot to protect the wound and allow for healing to begin.
   II. Epithelial healing is accomplished within 7 days, at which time the sutures and pack may be removed.
   III. Osseous healing does not begin until 1 month after surgery; complete healing and remodeling does not take place until 4 to 6 months after surgery.
   IV. Gingivectomy wounds take slightly longer to heal than flap procedures because the healing is by secondary intention rather than by primary intention.

The Dental Hygienist's Role in Periodontal Surgery

The dental hygienist serves several roles when periodontal surgery is discussed, explained, and performed for patient.
   I. Includes discussing the advantages and disadvantages of surgical treatment with the patient.
   II. Includes acting as a patient advocate by asking questions and providing answers to concerns that the patient may not be able to verbalize.

III. Involves postoperative suture and dressing removal.
IV. Includes postsurgical plaque removal, follow-up wound care, and providing home care instructions.
V. Includes motivating the patient to engage in long-term maintenance of plaque control.
VI. Involves providing SPT at regular intervals.

Supportive Periodontal Therapy (SPT)

The success of periodontal therapy hinges on the successful maintenance of health and the prevention of recurring disease. To accomplish this healthy state for any length of time, regular maintenance or recall appointments are required at relatively short intervals to reinforce home care and to control the accumulation of plaque-retentive deposits. These routine maintenance visits are referred to as SPT.

Rationale for SPT

Because the primary goal of dentistry is to "attain and maintain" a healthy dentition for a lifetime, the rationale for routine periodontal maintenance visits or SPT is to help the patient achieve this primary goal. Preservation of the stability achieved during active nonsurgical periodontal therapy can be accomplished only through repeated maintenance visits.

Objectives of SPT

To prevent the recurrence of disease and preserve the dentition for a lifetime, several objectives must be met. These include the preservation of clinical attachment levels, the maintenance of bone height, the control of inflammation, and the control of plaque.
   I. The preservation of clinical attachment levels includes:
      A. Monitoring probing depths at SPT appointments, which can predict attachment loss, signaling the return of disease, or can indicate stability.
      B. The recording of clinical attachment levels, which should take place periodically at maintenance appointments for baseline comparison.
   II. Maintenance of Alveolar Bone Height
      A. Periodic radiographic evaluations of bone levels are necessary for comparison with baseline levels.
         1. Radiographs do not indicate active disease; they only illustrate historic bone loss.
      B. Evidence of continued bone loss is indicative of disease progression.
      C. A primary goal of SPT is to prevent further bone loss, which can lead to eventual tooth loss.
   III. Control of Inflammation
      A. To halt disease progression, inflammation must be eliminated.
      B. Repeated evaluation of the gingival tissues for signs of inflammation at SPT appointments enables the dental hygienist and patient to effectively control disease progression.

C. All bleeding sites must be recorded because bleeding has been shown to be the most reliable sign of inflammation.

IV. Evaluation and Reinforcement of the Patient's Oral Hygiene

    A. Compliance with oral hygiene procedures requires frequent reinforcement.

    B. Regular observation and recording of plaque scores assist in motivating the patient.

    C. Direct observation of the patient's home care techniques can assist the dental hygienist in behavior modification.

    D. Plaque control education is as important and as difficult as the technical aspects of therapy.

V. Maintenance of Optimal Oral Health

    A. All aspects of oral health must be evaluated at each SPT appointment; should include the identification of new hard and soft tissue lesions, significant systemic disease that might effect oral health, and any other disharmonies or discrepancies that may affect the health of the patient.

The Effectiveness of Supportive Periodontal Therapy

Both surgical and nonsurgical periodontal therapies have been shown to be effective in eliminating active disease but only if routine maintenance at regular intervals is performed.

    I. Periodontal therapy in the absence of regular maintenance may result in attachment loss and loss of alveolar bone.

    II. Meticulous plaque control and professional debridement results in the eradication of disease in most cases.

Compliance

Compliance with SPT appointments and plaque control measures are the keys to successful therapy.

    I. Compliance is a major challenge for the dental hygienist; studies have revealed low compliance rates with SPT.

    II. The hygienist must spend time explaining the significance of SPT to the maintenance of the patient's oral health.

    III. The reasons for noncompliance are complex and may include:

        A. Fear.

        B. Economics.

        C. The interpretation of chronic disease as not life-threatening.

        D. Perceived indifference on the part of the dental hygienist.

        E. The socioeconomic status of the patient.

        F. The influence of friends and family.

        G. A failure to understand its significance.

    IV. The success of periodontal therapy rests on the performance of adequate plaque control by the patient.

A. The dental hygienist is responsible for educating and motivating the patient to perform these procedures routinely.

B. Compliance with oral hygiene has been shown to diminish within 30 days of its commencement.

C. The more aids that are introduced, the less compliant a patient is likely to be.

D. Interproximal aids are difficult to use and lead to a lack of compliance.

E. New types of electric toothbrushes have been shown to increase patient compliance.

Significance of Noncompliance

Noncompliance with either SPT appointments or the maintenance of oral hygiene results in continued disease progression.

    I. Techniques for Enhancing Compliance

        A. Simplify explanations.

        B. Accommodate program to suit patient needs; satisfied patients are more compliant.

        C. Remind patients of appointments.

        D. Keep compliance records for legal purposes and to guide behavior modification.

        E. Write down oral hygiene regimens to serve as reminders.

        F. Provide positive reinforcement.

        G. Identify noncompliers before the commencement of initial therapy and discuss the consequences of noncompliance.

Components of the SPT Appointment

The primary aims of the SPT appointment are to evaluate the stability of the results of initial therapy; to thoroughly debride all tooth surfaces; to eliminate any factors that may support the persistence of disease-producing microorganisms; and to evaluate and reinforce plaque control.

    I. The length of a typical SPT appointment is 1 hour.

    II. Procedures performed at the SPT appointment

        A. Medical and dental history updates.

        B. Oral and dental examinations.

        C. The evaluation of:

            1. Pocket probing depths.

            2. Clinical attachment loss.

            3. Gingival recession.

            4. Bleeding in response to probing.

            5. Suppuration.

            6. Tooth mobility.

            7. Furcations.

            8. Mucogingival involvement.

        D. Radiographic examination as necessary.

        E. A plaque control evaluation, which involves:

            1. A plaque index score.

            2. Education, motivation, and reinforcement regarding plaque control.

        F. The provision of oral hygiene instructions, including:

1. A review of toothbrushing and interdental cleansing techniques.
   2. Reinforcement of the significance of daily home care.
   G. Periodontal debridement.
   1. Includes the removal of all supragingival and subgingival plaque and calculus.
   H. Selective polishing, if rationale for it exists.
   I. Fluoride therapy, if warranted.
   J. Desensitization as needed.
   K. Referral to an appropriate specialist, if warranted.
   L. The establishment of appropriate SPT intervals that meet the patient's individual needs.

Recurrence of Disease

Recurrence of periodontal disease is common.
I. Causes of recurrence
   A. Insufficient plaque control.
   B. Incomplete removal of deposits during therapy.
   C. Faulty restorations and/or prostheses that foster plaque accumulation.
   D. A lack of compliance with regular SPT intervals.
   E. Systemic conditions that affect the host response.
II. Sometimes, despite appropriate therapy and compliance, the disease remains active or "refractory" (occurs in 10% of all periodontal patients).
III. The return of disease requires that initial therapy be repeated, results be reevaluated, and decisions be made regarding surgical alternatives; also requires referral to a specialist.
IV. Other treatment modalities may include microbiologic monitoring and/or antibiotic therapy.

Root Caries

Because of the attachment loss that occurs during periodontal therapy, exposed root surfaces become more susceptible to the development of root caries.
I. Are soft, progressive lesions of the root surfaces that are caused by microbial plaque.
II. Contain *Actinomyces viscosus*, which is the predominant microorganism.
III. Can lead to a rapid loss of teeth, despite valiant SPT efforts.
IV. Formation is precipitated by conditions that cause root surface exposure, including:
   A. Periodontal disease.
   B. Malocclusion.
   C. Orthodontic tooth movement.
   D. Surgery.
   E. Mechanical trauma.
V. Significant risk factors involve attachment loss, age, the number of teeth, the presence of coronal caries, the level of oral hygiene, water fluoridation, years of education, and xerostomia.
VI. Are a common outcome when xerostomia is present; xerostomia is a significant risk factor because the preventive washing action of saliva is diminished. Risk factors for xerostomia include:
   A. Radiation therapy.
   B. Some systemic medications.
   C. Pathologic conditions.
VII. May be avoided by use of the following:
   A. Fluoride therapy.
   B. Effective plaque control.
   C. A noncariogenic diet.
   D. Reduced intake of cariogenic foods to decrease the accumulation of substrate.
VIII. Can be controlled effectively with fluoride therapy; the multiple approach is most effective and includes the use of:
   A. Water fluoridation.
   B. Fluoride rinses.
   1. 0.2% sodium fluoride (once a week).
   2. 0.05% sodium fluoride (once daily).
   3. 0.2% acidulated phosphate-fluoride (APF) (once daily).
   C. Professionally applied and self-applied topical gels or solutions.
   1. Professionally applied forms
      a. 1.23% APF.
      b. 2% neutral sodium fluoride.
      c. 8% stannous fluoride.
   2. Self-applied forms
      a. 0.5% APF.
      b. 1.1% sodium fluoride.
      c. 0.4% stannous fluoride.
   3. Fluoride dentifrices
      a. 0.24% sodium fluoride.
      b. 0.76% sodium monofluorophosphate.
      c. 0.45% stannous fluoride.

Dentinal Hypersensitivity

Dentinal hypersensitivity is pain caused by cold or hot sensations, sweet or sour foods, dentifrices, toothbrushes, or toothpicks. It is a common occurrence among periodontal patients.
I. Affects an estimated one in seven adult patients.
II. Associated pain may be sharp, intermittent, and of short duration, or a dull chronic pain.
III. Is best explained by the hydrodynamic theory:
   A. Stimulation of open dentinal tubules at the root surface causes movement of the fluid within the tubules.
   B. This movement transmits signals to the nerves in the pulp chamber.
   C. Results in pain.
IV. The tooth root after periodontal surgery is frequently sensitive; is caused by exposure of the root surface and an eventual dissolution of the smear layer approximately 7 days after exposure.
V. The root after scaling and root planing is frequently sensitive; because removal of the cementum exposes the dentinal tubules.

VI. May result in a spontaneous remission of hypersensitivity without therapeutic intervention (in 20% to 45% of cases).

VII. Management may be performed professionally or at home.

    A. The professional application of the following has proven to be effective:

       1. Antiinflammatory agents (corticosteroids).

       2. Protein-precipitating agents (e.g., silver nitrate, zinc chloride, strontium chloride, formaldehyde).

       3. Tubule-occluding agents (e.g., calcium hydroxide, potassium nitrate, fluorides, sodium citrate, iontophoresis with 2% sodium fluoride, potassium oxalate).

       4. Physical sealing of the tubules with composites, resins, glass ionomers, varnishes, and sealants may be used if chemical applications do not provide relief.

       5. A variety of desensitizing toothpastes are available for home use and contain one of the following active ingredients:

          a. Strontium chloride

          b. Potassium nitrate

          c. Sodium citrate

The Role of the Dental Hygienist in SPT

The dental hygienist is the primary provider of supportive periodontal care. This role is critical to the success of periodontal therapy.

I. The dental hygienist must work in collaboration with the dentist and periodontist in the provision of quality oral health care.

II. The dental hygienist also must function as a co-therapist, serving as both a teacher and a coach; must encourage the patient to assume ultimate responsibility for the maintenance of periodontal health.

Emergency Treatment

An important part of delivering quality oral health care is practicing effectively as a team. Identifying conditions that require immediate care and bringing them to the attention of the dentist or periodontist is an example of effective teamwork.

Emergency situations must be addressed before the commencement of other therapies, thus their identification by the dental hygienist is imperative. The treatment of several common periodontal emergencies follows.

Periodontal Abscess

These abscesses are caused by the entrapment of bacteria in a periodontal pocket through occlusion of the pocket by foreign debris, such as a popcorn kernel, or incomplete scaling and root planing. The periodontal abscess may be acute or chronic and is associated with preexisting periodontal disease.

I. Is characterized by an acute inflammatory reaction that results in suppuration (pus or exudate).

II. Is characterized by redness, swelling, pain, rapid onset, and rapid bone loss.

III. An acute abscess sometimes stabilizes by draining through either the sulcus or a fistula in the adjacent tissues; becomes a chronic abscess that often is painless.

IV. Treatment of the periodontal abscess includes:

    A. Drainage of the abscess, typically through the pocket; is accomplished by scaling, root planing, and curettage of the soft tissue wall.

    B. Irrigation with an antimicrobial agent such as povidone iodine or chlorhexidine.

    C. Antibiotics may be required if fever or lymphadenopathy is present.

V. If diagnosed and treated early, the prognosis is excellent and lost bone typically regenerates.

Gingival Abscess

Gingival abscesses typically occur as a result of injury caused by the forceful occlusion of a foreign object in the gingiva. They tend to occur on marginal gingiva and are not associated with deeper periodontal pockets or with disease.

I. Is characterized by a raised, painful area of acute inflammation that is accompanied by suppuration.

II. Treatment consists of:

    A. Incision, drainage, and irrigation with antimicrobials.

    B. Warm salt water rinses after surgery.

    C. Scaling and root planing of the teeth in the adjacent area.

Periapical Abscess

Periapical or endodontic abscesses are caused by trauma, caries, and the spread of infective microorganisms to the pulp. In most cases they result in pulpal necrosis.

I. Often is difficult to distinguish from the acute periodontal abscess.

II. Is characterized by pain, tenderness, and swelling; the presence of suppuration depends on the drainage pathway.

III. Radiographically is seen as a radiolucency at the apex of the tooth, unless drainage has occurred through other channels, such as the PDL.

IV. In most cases, involves a nonvital tooth; the pain differs from that of a periodontal abscess in that it is sharp and intermittent rather than dull and continuous.

V. Treatment typically consists of either endodontic therapy or extraction.

Combination Abscess

These lesions are coined combination abscesses or endo/perio lesions and are difficult to diagnose.

I. May involve a pulpal abscess that spreads through accessory canals to the periodontium or vice versa.

II. Cause severe damage and may cause tooth loss if left untreated.

Pericoronitis

Pericoronitis is an abscess that occurs most commonly in the distal region of partially or fully erupted mandibular third molars that are covered, partially or fully, by a flap of tissue referred to as the operculum.

I. Is the direct result of the entrapment of food and bacteria under the operculum, which ultimately becomes inflamed and painful.

II. Most commonly occurs in young adults between the ages of 17 and 26.

III. Exhibits as pain, fever, and purulent exudate; trismus also may be present.

IV. Treatment

    A. On the first day gently debride and irrigate the area under the operculum with an antimicrobial such as diluted hydrogen peroxide.

    B. If fever is present, include a prescription for antibiotics.

    C. Recommend plenty of rest, fluid intake to avoid dehydration, and warm salt water rinses.

    D. On the second day, area should show signs of improvement; can be flushed again and more thoroughly debrided.

    E. Educate the patient regarding plaque control.

Acute Herpetic Gingivostomatitis

Acute herpetic gingivostomatitis typically is an oral manifestation of a primary infection with HSV1.

I. Occasionally is a manifestation of HSV2 (genital herpes) infection.

II. Is seen primarily in infants and children; however, is becoming more common among young adults infected with HSV2.

III. Is symptomatic in only 10% to 20% of persons infected with HSV1.

    A. Is characterized by:

        1. Fever, malaise, headache, irritability, and lymphadenopathy.

        2. Oral lesions that begin as small, yellow vesicles and coalesce to form larger, round ulcers with gray centers and bright red borders.

        3. Lesions that may appear on any oral mucous membranes, including the lips, tongue, gingivae, and buccal mucosa.

        4. Serious to extreme pain that restricts eating and drinking and may threaten the patient's health.

IV. Treatment

    A. Primarily involves supportive care because the disease is viral and typically runs its course in 7 to 10 days.

    B. Because this is an extremely infectious disease, instrumentation should not be performed.

    C. Poses a major risk to dentists and dental hygienists because transmission of the virus through an inadvertent puncture results in herpetic whitlow.

    D. Involves patient and parent education in gentle plaque removal, diet, and in particular, the importance of fluid intake to prevent dehydration.

 Clinical Case **STUDY**

Nineteen-year-old Pete Begley has arrived for an emergency appointment. He complains of a very sore mouth. After further questioning, Pete indicates that he has had a fever and has been feeling run down since he completed his final exams 2 days ago. During visual examination, his gingiva appear fiery red and swollen. The interdental papilla are grayish-white and ulcerated. A strong malodor is noted.

Clinical Case **QUESTIONS**

1. Identify factors that have contributed to Mr. Begley's periodontal condition.
2. Identify a likely diagnosis for Mr. Begley's condition.
3. Discuss treatment options.
4. What is the prognosis for this disease?

Clinical Case **RATIONALES**

1. Factors that have contributed to his oral disease include stress and inadequate oral hygiene (spirochetes and Gram negative organisms). Other contributing factors may include smoking, fatigue, and inadequate nutrition.

2. Mr. Begley most likely has ANUG. This is an opportunistic bacterial infection that often occurs in young individuals who are under stress and have not been taking good physical care of themselves. Inadequate care may include smoking, drinking, inadequate nutrition and plaque removal, and a lack of sleep.

3. Mr. Begley needs a series of treatments. The immediate concern should be to gently debride the areas infected with bacteria. This is accomplished with ultrasonic or sonic instruments because they gently flush the area with oxygenated water. Topical or local anesthetics may be needed if the debridement causes discomfort. If fever or lymphadenopathy is present, systemic antibiotics may be prescribed. A 0.12% chlorhexidine rinse should be prescribed (for use twice daily). Plaque control methods and the need for adequate sleep and nutrition should be discussed with the patient. Mr. Begley subsequently should be seen within a few days to assess the gingival healing, remove more plaque and calculus, and reinforce home care. At a third appointment, scheduled 3 to 5 days later, an assessment of healing, the removal of remaining

plaque and calculus, and the reinforcement of oral hygiene instructions should take place. Referral to a periodontist is recommended if the gingival architecture requires correction.

4. The prognosis for ANUG is good. After Mr. Begley completes therapy and begins to take better care of his health, the condition will improve. In a few cases, surgery is required to repair gingival contour.

Acute Necrotizing Ulcerative Gingivitis (ANUG)

ANUG is an opportunistic infection that is associated with stress, poor nutrition, poor oral hygiene, fatigue, and other lifestyle factors, such as smoking.

I. Also has been associated with immunosuppressive diseases such as HIV, blood dyscrasias, and Down syndrome; in these cases, the necrosis typically exceeds gingival boundaries and is more accurately described as acute necrotizing ulcerative periodontitis (ANUP).

II. Predominant microorganisms are spirochetes and Gram negative organisms.

III. Characteristics
  A. Necrotic papilla with cratered, punched-out appearance.
  B. Gray pseudomembrane covering the necrotic area.
  C. Gingivae that are red and painful and bleed spontaneously.
  D. Foul odor (fetor oris).
  E. Possibly fever and/or lymphadenopathy.
  F. The infection is not communicable.

IV. Treatment
  A. Involves several appointments because pain prevents immediate comprehensive debridement.
    1. The first appointment consists of:
      a. Superficial, gentle debridement with ultrasonics.
      b. The use of either local or topical anesthetics.
      c. Administration of systemic antibiotics, if fever or lymphadenopathy is present.
      d. Extensive plaque control instruction and counseling on the significance and control of lifestyle risk factors.
      e. Prescription of oral rinses to be used twice daily, with either 0.12% chlorhexidine or diluted 3% hydrogen peroxide.
    2. The second visit should occur within 1 or 2 days; significant improvement should enable:
      a. More thorough plaque and calculus removal.
      b. Reinforcement of oral hygiene and other recommendations.
    3. The third visit should occur 3 to 5 days after the second; all instructions should be reinforced and remaining debridement should be completed (if possible). Hydrogen peroxide rinses,

if prescribed, should be discontinued at this time to avoid the development of black hairy tongue.

4. Subsequent follow-up appointments may involve the correction of local plaque-retentive factors (e.g., defective amalgam margins) and possible referral to a periodontist for the surgical correction of gingival architecture.

5. After the completion of emergency treatment, the patient should be reevaluated to determine appropriate SPT intervals to prevent recurrence.

Dental Implants

Since the advent of the osseointegrated implant, the placement of such devices has increased tremendously and has become an accepted treatment alternative. Because implants are vulnerable to bacterial invasion and subsequent failure, the dental hygienist can play an important role in both patient education and professional maintenance.

Types of Implants

Several types of implants exist. They include endosseous, subperiosteal, and transosteal implants.

I. Implants are designed for several uses:
  A. To support dentures in edentulous mouths.
  B. As abutments in partially edentulous mouths to support fixed bridgework.
  C. To replace single teeth.

II. Several types of implant systems are available, of which the endosseous is the most popular.

III. Endosseous implants are placed directly in the bone; may be either root form or blade form.
  A. The root form is more common than the blade form and may be conical, cylindrical, threaded-screw, perforated, or hollow baskets.
  B. Typically are made of titanium; however, polymers, ceramics, and other metals also are used.
  C. May be made of smooth titanium or may be sprayed or coated with other materials, such as plasma of titanium, aluminum oxide, hydroxyapatite, or single-crystal sapphire.

IV. Subperiosteal implants are positioned over the bone and consist of a cast framework, with projections protruding through the mucosa that are designed to support a complete removable denture.

V. Transosteal implants or staple implants are surgically placed through the mandible and provide anchorage for a removable lower denture; often are made of gold or Vitallium instead of titanium.

Implant Surgery

Implant surgery involves the placement of an implant and typically is completed in two steps.

I. Involves placing the implant in the jaw by drilling a

hole through the bone. This procedure is referred to as an osteotomy.

II. Involves covering the implant with gingiva and allowing 3 to 6 months for healing; osseointegration is expected to occur during this time.

III. During the second surgery, the implant is exposed and placement of the abutment fixture, which protrudes above the gingiva, is made.

IV. Subsequently, final "loading" is performed, which involves the placement of the prosthesis onto the abutment.

V. Success is dependent on:
  A. Careful selection of the candidate. Individuals with the following should be avoided:
    1. A history of blood dyscrasias, diabetes, or other diseases that compromise health.
    2. Poor oral health (e.g., gingivitis, periodontitis).
    3. Poor oral hygiene practices.
    4. Poor quality and quantity of bone.
  B. Careful preparation of the implant site; overheating of the bone should be avoided.
  C. If the bone overheats, necrosis may occur and may result in fibrointegration rather than osseointegration.
  D. Accurate sizing of the placement site.
  E. Preserving ample keratinized tissue around the implant.
  F. Parallel placement of multiple implants, which allows the prostheses to be attached with screws.
  G. Allowing time for healing and osseointegration (3 to 6 months) before loading the implant.

Osseointegration

Osseointegration refers to direct contact or integration of the bone to the dental implant and provides the most stable attachment. If connective tissue grows between the bone and the implant, it is referred to as fibrointegration and is less likely to exhibit long-term success.

Tissue Interface

The tissue interface consists of the gingiva surrounding an implant; it is similar to that which surrounds a normal tooth except there are no dentogingival or PDL fibers between the gingiva and the bone.

I. The sulcular epithelium is nonkeratinized and cells at the base of the sulcus form a junctional epithelium that attaches to the implant by means of a basal lamina and hemidesmosomes.

II. This interface or biologic seal prevents the penetration of bacteria and their toxins to the osseointegrated implant surface.

III. Implant sulcus depths range from 1.3 to 3.8 mm.

IV. The area between the junctional epithelium and the bone is composed of connective tissue, which touches the implant surface directly and contains collagen fibers that run parallel (rather than perpendicular) to the implant surface.

Periimplantitis

Periimplant tissues are as susceptible to invasion by microorganisms as natural periodontal tissues; thus affected implants are said to have periimplantitis rather than periodontitis.

I. Microbiota found in an implant sulcus are similar to those found in natural sulcus, in both health and disease.

II. Because of their susceptibility to periimplantitis, the maintenance of implants is of prime concern.

Professional Implant Maintenance

Professional maintenance procedures include assessing tissues, probing implant sulcus depths, checking for mobility, assessing plaque, removing plaque and calculus, and obtaining annual radiographs.

I. Only plastic instruments should be used for the removal of hard and soft deposits and for probing; conventional metal instruments scratch the titanium surface of implants, making them less biocompatible with the surrounding tissues and more conducive to plaque accumulation.

II. Sonic and ultrasonic instrumentation, air-powder polishing, and the use of any metallic instruments, including gold and titanium, should be avoided.

III. Rubber cup polishing with a fine powder, such as tin oxide, or with a fine-grit commercial polishing paste may be performed selectively, as with natural teeth.

IV. The implant-supported prosthesis should be removed yearly to permit thorough debridement and to check for stability.

V. A 3-month recall interval should be established for at least the first year after implant placement.

Home Care Instructions

Individualized plaque control regimens must be developed for patients with implants because each implant system is unique. Depending on whether the prosthesis can be removed, plaque control may present difficult challenges for the patient.

I. If an overdenture is present, it must be removed daily for cleansing and soaking and plaque must be removed from around the abutments.

II. If the prosthesis is not removable, plaque removal becomes more difficult; requires the use of a variety of oral hygiene aids.

III. Recommended Oral Hygiene Aids
  A. Traditional toothbrushes, end-tuft brushes, interproximal brushes with nylon core tips (rather than metal core tips), and powered interproximal brushes (Rotadent, ProDentec Corp).
  B. Tufted floss, floss threaders, yarn, gauze folded into a ribbon, floss cords (Postcare, John O. Butler Co.) and dental tape/ribbon (G-Floss, 3i Implant Innovations).

C. Wooden interdental cleaners, plastic interdental cleaners, and rubber-tipped stimulators.

D. Rinsing or swabbing the implant interface with 0.12% chlorhexidine often is recommended.

IV. Home care methods and techniques should be reviewed thoroughly at each SPT appointment.

Implant Failure

Because approximately 5% to 15% of implants fail, the dental hygienist should be able to recognize a failing implant.

I. Is characterized by:

A. Pocketing, bleeding in response to probing, exudate, and progression of bone loss.

B. Mobility.

C. A dull sound on percussion.

D. Radiographic evidence of periimplant radiolucency.

II. Treatment requires removal of the implant.

∼ CONTENT REVIEW QUESTIONS ∼

1. The functions of the periodontium include all of the following, EXCEPT:
   A. attaching the tooth to the bony socket
   B. resisting forces generated by mastication and speech
   C. defending against external noxious stimuli
   D. protecting the tooth against cariogenic bacteria

2. Oral epithelium is classified as:
   A. simple squamous epithelium
   B. stratified squamous epithelium
   C. pseudostratified columnar epithelium
   D. simple cuboidal epithelium

3. Sulcular or crevicular epithelium is:
   A. keratinized
   B. parakeratinized
   C. pseudokeratinized
   D. nonkeratinized

4. Attached gingiva is found between:
   A. the mucogingival junction and the free-gingival groove
   B. the alveolar mucosa and the marginal gingiva
   C. the marginal gingiva and the free gingival groove
   D. the teeth

5. The connective tissue of the gingiva is called the:
   A. lamina dura
   B. lamina propria
   C. lamina lucida
   D. lamina densa

6. Which one of the following descriptors does NOT pertain to the alveolar mucosa?
   A. nonkeratinized
   B. found beyond the mucogingival junction
   C. flexible
   D. component of gingiva

7. The thickness of the PDL ranges from:
   A. 0.15 to 0.38 mm
   B. 0.40 to 0.56 mm
   C. 0.62 to 0.81 mm
   D. 1.00 to 1.50 mm

8. Brush ends of the fibers of the PDL, which are embedded in both the cementum and alveolar bone, are referred to as:
   A. oblique Fibers
   B. Sharpey's fibers
   C. principal fibers
   D. transseptal fibers

9. Type-I and type-II cementum is acellular and typically is located on the:
   A. coronal third of the root
   B. middle third of the root
   C. apical third of the root
   D. furcation area of the root

10. CEJs occur in many forms. The most common configuration of the CEJ is:
    A. enamel overlapping cementum
    B. cementum overlapping enamel
    C. an end-to-end joint
    D. a gap without a joint

11. The compact bone that surrounds the roots of the tooth and forms the lining of the tooth socket is known as all of the following, EXCEPT:
    A. alveolar bone proper
    B. cribriform plate
    C. lamina dura
    D. lamina propria

12. The supporting alveolar bone is made of:
    A. compact and cancellous bone
    B. cortical and spongy bone
    C. cancellous and spongy bone
    D. cortical, cancellous, and spongy bone

13. The most recent national epidemiologic data on the prevalence of periodontal disease indicates all of the following, EXCEPT:
    A. severe periodontitis is more prevalent in underdeveloped countries than in industrialized countries
    B. edentulism is significantly decreasing in the United States
    C. attachment loss is greater in women than in men in the United States
    D. gingival bleeding is prevalent in 50% of the US population

14. The rate of occurrence of a new disease in a population during a given period is referred to as its:
    A. incidence   — new
    B. prevalence — # of persons affected at time
    C. patterns
    D. severity

15. All of the following statements are true, EXCEPT:
    A. the prevalence of periodontal disease does not increase with age
    B. Blacks consistently demonstrate a higher incidence of periodontal disease than Whites

C. periodontal disease is inversely related to levels of education

D. the prevalence of periodontal disease is higher in rural than in urban areas

16. Which of the following groups of risk factors for periodontal disease have the capacity to be modified?
   A. age, genetics, and race
   B. smoking, sex, and HIV
   C. diabetes, nutritional deficiencies, and neutrophil abnormalities
   D. stress, smoking, and pregnancy

17. Which of the following is the strongest indication of a correlation between stress and periodontal disease?
   A. acute herpetic gingivostomatitis
   B. ANUG
   C. refractory periodontitis
   D. LJP

18. A significant possible complication of smoking is:
   A. HIV periodontitis
   B. ANUG
   C. refractory periodontitis
   D. acute herpetic gingivostomatitis

19. Nutritional deficiencies are considered risk factors for periodontal disease because they:
   A. contribute to the accumulation of plaque
   B. promote bone loss
   C. lower the host response
   D. are associated with lower socioeconomic groups

20. Oral side effects of a deficiency in Vitamin B_6 (pyridoxine) include all of the following, EXCEPT:
   A. gingivitis
   B. glossitis
   C. stomatitis
   D. candidiasis

21. An antioxidant agent that currently is under investigation for its beneficial effects in the prevention of periodontitis, cardiovascular disease, and malignancy is:
   A. vitamin A
   B. beta-carotene
   C. vitamin C
   D. vitamin E

22. A deficiency in this vitamin, which is responsible for the biosynthesis of collagen, will adversely affect periodontal connective tissues and wound healing:
   A. vitamin A
   B. vitamin B
   C. vitamin C
   D. vitamin D

23. When vitamin D deficiency occurs in adults, the resulting effects on the periodontium include all of the following, EXCEPT:
   A. resorption of the alveolar bone
   B. destruction of the PDL
   C. fibrous dysplasia of the bone
   D. hyperplasia of the gingiva

24. Which of the following nutritional deficiencies has been associated with an increased incidence of necrotizing gingivitis?
   A. osteoporosis
   B. osteomalacia
   C. marasmus
   D. kwashiorkor

25. Oxygen-free radicals may play a role in the tissue destruction associated with all of the following, EXCEPT:
   A. periodontal disease
   B. heart disease
   C. cancer
   D. systemic lupus erythematosus

26. Multilocular radiolucent jaw lesions, the loss of lamina dura, and a ground-glass appearance of the alveolar bone are characteristics of:
   A. a vitamin D deficiency
   B. hyperparathyroidism
   C. osteomalacia
   D. Paget's disease

27. During puberty an adolescent is more susceptible to the development of gingivitis because of:
   A. poor oral hygiene habits
   B. altered capillary permeability
   C. decreased levels of sex hormones
   D. altered chemotactic response

28. Recent evidence indicates that desquamative gingivitis is most likely a feature of all of the following, EXCEPT:
   A. menopause
   B. erosive lichen planus
   C. mucous membrane pemphigoid
   D. pemphigus

29. The rationale for the prevalence of periodontal disease in patients with diabetes mellitus includes all of the following, EXCEPT:
   A. defective PMNL chemotaxis
   B. microangiopathy of the periodontal tissues
   C. increased collagen breakdown
   D. increased fibrosis of the periodontal tissues
   E. microbial alterations

30. Multiple periodontal abscesses, velvety red gingivae, and marginal proliferation of the gingivae are common oral manifestations of:
   A. type-I diabetes
   B. type-II diabetes
   C. uncontrolled diabetes
   D. controlled diabetes

31. If treating a patient with AIDS who had pseudomembranous candidiasis, which of the following drugs would the dentist or physician MOST LIKELY prescribe?
   A. acyclovir
   B. corticosteroid
   C. ketoconazole
   D. chlorhexidine

32. The neoplasm most frequently found in patients with AIDS is Kaposi's sarcoma. The most common oral site for this neoplasm is the:
    A. floor of the mouth
    B. tongue
    C. soft palate
    D. keratinized tissues *ging. & hard palate.*

33. The most common form of gingivitis among patients with AIDS is:
    A. linear gingival erythema
    B. chronic marginal gingivitis
    C. acute necrotizing gingivitis
    D. desquamative gingivitis

34. A decrease in circulating neutrophils results in:
    A. spontaneous gingival hemorrhage
    B. oral herpetic lesions
    C. an impaired host response
    D. leukemia

35. Neutropenia is present in all of the following, EXCEPT:
    A. Down syndrome
    B. diabetes mellitus
    C. autoimmune disorders
    D. CNS dysfunction

36. A leukocyte adherence defect (LAD) that impairs successful margination of PMNLs and prevents their emigration to sites of infection typically results in generalized:
    A. prepubertal periodontitis
    B. juvenile periodontitis
    C. adult periodontitis
    D. chronic marginal gingivitis

37. Cyclosporin, diltiazem, phenobarbital, and nifedipine are drugs that:
    A. belong to the beta-blocker category
    B. cause xerostomia
    C. cause gingival enlargement
    D. suppress the immune system

38. The prime etiologic factor in periodontal disease is:
    A. bacteria
    B. host response
    C. bacteria and host response
    D. poor oral hygiene

39. Filaments, fusiforms, and curved microbes are classified as:
    A. cocci
    B. rods
    C. spirochetes
    D. vibrios

40. Gram-negative organisms are characterized by:
    A. an outer capsule composed of glucan
    B. the absence of an outer cell wall
    C. cell walls containing exotoxins
    D. cell walls containing endotoxins

41. Microorganisms that cannot survive in oxygen environments are classified as:
    A. aerobes
    B. facultative aerobes
    C. facultative anaerobes
    D. obligate anaerobes

42. Plaque associated with gingival health typically is composed of:
    A. Gram-positive aerobic cocci and rods
    B. Gram-negative aerobic cocci and rods
    C. Gram-positive rods and spirochetes
    D. Gram-negative rods and spirochetes

43. Which microorganisms are seen more frequently during ANUG?
    A. *P. intermedia*
    B. *P. gingivalis*
    C. *Treponema* ssp.
    D. *A. actinomycetemcomitans*

44. When a patient has been diagnosed with rapidly progressive periodontitis, one would expect to see which of the following combinations of microorganisms?
    A. *F. nucleatum, P. gingivalis,* and *A. actinomycetemcomitans*
    B. *P. gingivalis, P. intermedia,* and *A. actinomycetemcomitans*
    C. *B. forsythus, P. gingivalis,* and *C. rectus*
    D. *Treponema* ssp., *E. corrodens,* and *P. intermedia*

45. The current paradigm or belief system associated with the development of periodontal disease is the:
    A. multiple burst theory
    B. single burst theory
    C. specific plaque hypothesis
    D. nonspecific plaque hypothesis

46. Bacterial enzymes that can affect host cells and ground substance include all of the following, EXCEPT:
    A. hyaluronidase
    B. collagenase
    C. ribonuclease
    D. lipase

47. Bacterial endotoxins are primarily responsible for:
    A. host cell destruction
    B. activating the complement cascade
    C. releasing enzymes
    D. killing bacteria

48. All of the following are antibacterial components found in saliva, EXCEPT:
    A. lysozyme
    B. lactoperoxidase
    C. macrophages

49. Which of the following (is) are not (a) chemical mediator(s) of vascular permeability?
    A. histamine and serotonin
    B. kinins and prostaglandins
    C. thyroxin
    D. C3 and C5
    E. lysosomal enzymes

50. When PMNLs leave the axial stream and begin to adhere to endothelial walls during the period of vascular dilation, this is referred to as:
    A. margination

B. emigration

C. migration

D. chemotaxis

51. The first cell to appear in chronic inflammation that constitutes the body's second line of defense is the:
    A. PMNL
    B. macrophage
    C. lymphocyte
    D. basophil

52. All of the following types of lymphocytes are responsible for cellular immunity, EXCEPT:
    A. T4 activator cells
    B. T8 suppressor cells
    C. NK (natural killer) cells
    D. B cells

53. The chronic inflammatory cells responsible for humoral immunity are:
    A. macrophages
    B. B lymphocytes
    C. T lymphocytes
    D. monocytes

54. The appearance of fibroblasts and new capillaries are characteristic of which stage of inflammation?
    A. the acute stage
    B. the chronic stage
    C. the remission stage
    D. the repair stage

55. The primary tissue destruction that occurs during the inflammatory phase of periodontal disease is produced by the by-products of:
    A. bacterial cell walls
    B. complement proteins
    C. antibodies
    D. arachidonic acid cascade

56. The release of chemotactic factors that cause the migration of PMNLs and macrophages to specific sites is controlled by the:
    A. phagocytic system
    B. complement system
    C. arachidonic acid cascade
    D. kinin system

57. The cytokine released by T cells that is capable of inducing bone resorption is:
    A. arachidonic acid
    B. prostaglandin
    C. interleukin-1
    D. myeloperoxidase

58. According to Page and Schroeder, within 4 to 7 days after plaque accumulation, the lesion that occurs is the:
    A. initial lesion
    B. early lesion
    C. established lesion
    D. advanced lesion

59. Histologically, when a lesion extends into the PDL and alveolar bone, it is classified as an:
    A. initial lesion
    B. early lesion

C. established lesion

D. advanced lesion

60. The clinical signs and symptoms of occlusal traumatism include:
    A. radiographic evidence of a narrowed PDL space and clinical evidence of tooth mobility
    B. radiographic evidence of a narrowed PDL space and clinical evidence of tooth extrusion
    C. radiographic signs of a widened PDL space and clinical evidence of tooth mobility
    D. radiographic evidence of a widened PDL space and clinical evidence of tooth extrusion

61. Damage that occurs when the amount of alveolar bone is normal but there are excessive occlusal forces present is referred to as:
    A. primary occlusal traumatism
    B. secondary occlusal traumatism
    C. hyperfunction
    D. hypofunction

62. Muscle and facial disorders of the masticatory system that impede mobility include:
    A. dyskinesia, myalgia, and trismus
    B. arthritis, neoplasms, and bruxism
    C. joint adhesions, ankylosis, and muscular fibrosis
    D. spasms, myalgia, and bruxism

63. During inspection of the patient's mouth, several wear facets on the teeth are noted and determined to be nonfunctional. This sign is indicative of:
    A. decay
    B. TMJ disorder
    C. trismus
    D. bruxism

64. Subgingival calculus, in the etiology of periodontal disease, is a:
    A. prime etiologic factor
    B. local predisposing factor
    C. local functional factor
    D. systemic contributing factor

65. Calculus is primarily composed of:
    A. inorganic matter
    B. organic matter
    C. microorganisms
    D. protein polysaccharide complexes

66. A soft, sticky, yellow or grayish-white substance that partially adheres to the teeth is referred to as:
    A. bacterial plaque
    B. materia alba
    C. food debris
    D. acquired pellicle

67. The most commonly occurring form of periodontal disease is:
    A. gingivitis
    B. adult periodontitis
    C. early onset periodontitis
    D. refractory periodontitis

68. The most significant feature of chronic gingivitis is:
    A. marginal redness

B. edema of the gingival margins

C. bleeding in response to probing

D. a loss of stippling

69. A deficiency in vitamin C causes all of the following, EXCEPT:
    A. gingival inflammation
    B. an increased tendency for hemorrhage
    C. the degeneration of collagen fibers
    D. poor healing

70. A 17-year-old male patient presents with purplish-blue gingiva, tumor-like masses around several papillae, shiny gingival surfaces with ulcerations, and spontaneous bleeding. The patient looks pale and says that he has been tired, has not felt well for a while, and is undergoing some medical tests. A possible diagnosis might be:
    A. ANUG
    B. primary herpetic gingivostomatitis
    C. leukemia
    D. pregnancy gingivitis

71. Localized, enlarged interdental gingiva that form tumor-like growths may accompany:
    A. leukemic or pregnancy gingivitis
    B. pregnancy gingivitis or ANUG
    C. ANUG or diabetic gingivitis
    D. diabetic gingivitis or AIDS

72. A patient presents with a complaint that her gums are very sore in the lower right posterior region of her mouth. Her oral hygiene is meticulous and there is no visible plaque. Her tissues appear very healthy, except for the region surrounding her first molar, which appears red and edematous and has several small vesicles on the marginal gingiva surrounding the full nonprecious metal crown. A diagnosis of this condition might be:
    A. desquamative gingivitis
    B. menopausal gingivitis
    C. allergic gingivitis
    D. apthous ulcers

73. Desquamative gingivitis frequently is linked with all of the following EXCEPT:
    A. pemphigus
    B. pemphigoid
    C. lichen planus
    D. drugs
    E. pregnancy

74. Desquamative gingivitis is most commonly seen in:
    A. pregnant women
    B. menopausal women
    C. adults of all ages
    D. equal numbers of males and females

75. Inflammatory gingival overgrowth is associated with all of the following, EXCEPT:
    A. bacterial plaque
    B. phenytoin
    C. cyclosporin
    D. calcium channel blockers
    E. bulimia

76. Occasionally, severe enlargement of the entire gingiva, including both facial and lingual surfaces, occurs with no apparent explanation. This condition is most likely caused by:
    A. the use of cyclosporin
    B. the presence of type-1 diabetes
    C. a rare hereditary or familial condition
    D. epilepsy

77. The rapid tissue destruction commonly associated with acute gingival disease is primarily caused by large numbers of:
    A. P. gingivalis
    B. macrophages
    C. A. actinomycetemcomitans
    D. PMNLs

78. A nineteen-year-old college student presents for emergency care complaining of pain in the gingiva, spontaneous bleeding, and a bad metallic taste in his mouth. During inspection, a fetid odor, punched-out papilla covered with a gray pseudomembrane, and the spontaneous bleeding are noted. This patient most likely has:
    A. acute herpetic gingivostomatitis
    B. leukemia
    C. ANUG ← Treponema
    D. AIDS

79. Which microorganism is most commonly associated with the condition described above?
    A. spirochetes · Treponema
    B. P. intermedia
    C. S. sanguis
    D. P. gingivalis

80. Mrs. Jones arrives in a panic with her 3-year-old daughter, whom she claims has been feverish, very whiny, and unable to eat for the past 24 hours because of multiple painful ulcerations in her mouth. The marginal and interdental gingivae appear red and swollen and appear to have a gray pseudomembrane that covers the numerous ulcerations. The presence of cervical lymphadenopathy is also detected. This child most likely is suffering from:
    A. ANUG
    B. acute myelocytic leukemia
    C. primary herpetic gingivostomatitis
    D. acute gingival abscesses

81. A periodontal pocket whose base is coronal to the level of the alveolar bone is referred to as a:
    A. pseudopocket
    B. relative pocket
    C. suprabony pocket
    D. infrabony pocket

82. Prepubertal periodontitis, according to the 1989 AAP World Workshop in Clinical Periodontics, is categorized as:
    A. adult periodontitis
    B. early-onset periodontitis
    C. periodontitis associated with systemic disease
    D. chronic periodontitis

83. A patient with moderate adult periodontitis received scaling and root planing of the maxillary right arch 2 weeks ago. The patient returns for treatment of the mandibular right quadrant but complains of a dull, throbbing pain around the maxillary right molar area. During inspection, an 11-mm pocket depth and accompanying suppuration on the mesial facial surface of tooth #2 is found. The chart indicates that the pocket depth before scaling was 6 mm. This patient most likely has developed:
    A. a periodontal abscess
    B. a periapical abscess
    C. an endo/perio lesion
    D. pericoronitis

84. The most common form of periodontitis, which is characterized by periodontal pocket formation, bone loss, and eventual tooth mobility, with no abnormalities of the host defense system is:
    A. early onset periodontitis
    B. juvenile periodontitis
    C. prepubertal periodontitis
    D. adult periodontitis

85. The color of chronically inflamed gingiva associated with adult periodontitis may be any of the following, EXCEPT:
    A. red
    B. pink
    C. blue
    D. white

86. Early onset periodontal disease includes any of the following, EXCEPT:
    A. juvenile periodontitis
    B. rapidly progressive periodontitis
    C. refractory periodontitis
    D. prepubertal periodontitis

87. Which of the following forms of periodontal disease are most likely to be associated with systemic diseases?
    A. adult periodontitis
    B. prepubertal periodontitis
    C. LJP
    D. generalized juvenile periodontitis

88. A periodontal condition that appears during puberty and is characterized by severe, rapid vertical bone loss in the anterior and first molars, depressed neutrophil chemotaxis, and little evidence of gingival inflammation is known as:
    A. rapidly progressive periodontitis
    B. refractory periodontitis
    C. prepubertal periodontitis
    D. juvenile periodontitis

89. The microorganism MOST commonly associated with juvenile periodontitis is:
    A. *A. actinomycetemcomitans*
    B. *P. gingivalis*
    C. *P. intermedia*
    D. *T. denticola*

90. Of the more aggressive periodontal diseases, which one of the following seems to be MOST closely linked with juvenile periodontitis?
    A. prepubertal periodontitis
    B. rapidly progressive periodontitis
    C. refractory periodontitis
    D. periodontitis associated with systemic diseases

91. A systemic condition characterized by hyperkeratotic skin lesions of the palms, soles, knees, and elbows, severe destruction of the periodontium, and onset before age 4 is:
    A. Chédiak-Higashi syndrome   · Albinism
    B. hypophosphatasia   - rickets
    C. Papillon-Lefèvre syndrome
    D. Down syndrome

92. LGE is associated with:
    A. diabetic gingivitis
    B. leukemic gingivitis
    C. AIDS-associated gingivitis
    D. chronic gingivitis

93. The risk factor MOST consistently associated with refractory periodontitis is:
    A. poor oral hygiene
    B. genetic predisposition
    C. smoking
    D. alterations in host response

94. Prophylactic antibiotics are required for the prevention of bacterial endocarditis in all of the following conditions, EXCEPT:
    A. mitral valve prolapse with valvular regurgitation
    B. hypertrophic cardiomyopathy
    C. prosthetic cardiac valves
    D. organic heart disease
    E. functional heart murmurs

95. During the medical history, a patient reveals that he currently is taking a tricyclic antidepressant. What alterations to the patient's treatment plan must be made?
    A. only early morning appointments should be made
    B. prophylactic antibiotics should be prescribed
    C. blood pressure should be monitored very closely
    D. no epinephrine should be administered

96. You discover that your patient has been diagnosed with thyroid cancer and must undergo radiation therapy. How should you plan his periodontal therapy?
    A. perform all necessary periodontal therapy immediately, before his radiation therapy
    B. wait until after his radiation therapy has been completed and the cancer has been eliminated before proceeding with his periodontal therapy
    C. ask the patient whether he wishes to have his periodontal therapy before or after radiation therapy
    D. do noninvasive therapy before his radiation treatments and complete the more invasive care after he is feeling better

97. The personal history is important for the identification of all of the following nondentally related risk factors, EXCEPT:
    A. smoking
    B. alcohol consumption
    C. diet
    D. stress
    E. social status

98. Lifesaver-like enlargements surrounding the free gingival margins are referred to as:
    A. rolled margins
    B. Stillman's clefts
    C. McCall's festoons
    D. marginal hyperplasia

99. The "gold standard" for determining the extent of periodontal tissue destruction is the measurement of:
    A. clinical attachment loss
    B. periodontal pockets
    C. bleeding in response to probing
    D. bone loss through radiographic analysis

100. The periodontal screening and recording (PSR) system is a modification of the:
    A. Ramfjord index
    B. Russell index
    C. CPITN (WHO)
    D. Loe and Silness index

101. It is important for a dental hygienist to examine the condition of tooth proximal contact areas because:
    A. drifting may occur if contacts are not tight
    B. contact areas affect a patient's home care abilities
    C. contact areas affect a patient's occlusion
    D. extrusion may change a contact point

102. Tooth mobility, furcation involvement, malocclusions, overhanging margins of restorations, and the status of prosthetic appliances are all important because they are classified as:
    A. etiologic factors for periodontal disease
    B. systemic risk factors for periodontal disease
    C. local risk factors for periodontal disease
    D. primary risk factors for periodontal disease

103. The use of supplemental periodontal diagnostic tests should be reserved exclusively for:
    A. the identification of risk factors
    B. definitive periodontal diagnosis
    C. treatment planning purposes
    D. identifying unusual periodontal diseases

104. The BANA test, ELISA test, and DNA probe are all used for the measurement of:
    A. biochemical markers in gingival crevicular fluid
    B. bacterial enzymes
    C. bacterial species
    D. bacterial antibodies

105. The "presumptive diagnosis" refers to the:
    A. initial list of possibilities
    B. patient's presumptions

106. Treatment planning must be all of the following, EXCEPT:
    A. evidence based
    B. applied randomly
    C. patient specific
    D. defined by methods and sequence of care
    E. geared toward health and the prevention of disease recurrence

C. final diagnosis
D. best possibility after examining the evidence

107. According to Carranza, the phase of periodontal treatment that involves the elimination of etiologic factors is:
    A. phase I therapy
    B. phase II therapy
    C. phase III therapy
    D. phase IV therapy

108. The AAP classifies early adult periodontitis as:
    A. case type I
    B. case type II
    C. case type III
    D. case type IV
    E. case type V

109. All periodontal patients who have received initial therapy require an evaluation after:
    A. 1 to 2 weeks
    B. 4 to 6 weeks
    C. 2 to 3 months
    D. 4 to 6 months

110. An assessment of Mr. Forbes identifies his condition as AAP case type III, with average pocket depths of 5 to 6 mm and moderate to heavy subgingival calculus in most areas. His initial therapy should most closely resemble which of the following treatment sequences?
    A. one 1-hour appointment for completion of all debridement
    B. two 1-hour appointments, without an anesthetic
    C. two 1-hour appointments, with an anesthetic
    D. four 1-hour appointments, with an anesthetic

111. Prognosis refers to:
    A. the planning of care
    B. the identification of disease
    C. the prediction of an outcome
    D. posttreatment assessment

112. The key to a successful plaque control program is:
    A. accurate instruction
    B. an appropriate length of instruction
    C. patient motivation
    D. multiple reinforcement appointments

113. The toothbrushing technique in which the bristles are applied to the sulcular area and moved back and forth with short strokes in a vibratory motion is the:
    A. Stillman's technique
    B. modified Stillman's technique
    C. Charter's technique
    D. Bass technique

114. Furcation areas are best cleansed with:
    A. dental floss and interdental brushes
    B. toothpicks with handles and dental floss
    C. interdental brushes, toothpicks with handles, and end-tuft brushes
    D. dental floss, interdental brushes, and toothpicks with handles

115. Supragingival irrigating devices are contraindicated for patients with:
    A. orthodontic appliances
    B. conditions requiring prophylactic antibiotic coverage
    C. cardiac pacemakers
    D. periodontal disease

116. The mouth rinse that has the highest substantivity and also has been shown through extensive studies to reduce plaque and gingivitis is:
    A. chlorhexidine digluconate
    B. phenolic compounds
    C. cetylpyridinium chloride
    D. sanguinarine
    E. stannous fluoride

117. Toothpastes that contain soluble pyrophosphates or zinc chloride are labeled:
    A. antigingivitis dentifrices
    B. antiplaque dentifrices
    C. antisensitivity dentifrices
    D. antitartar dentifrices

118. Rationales for nonsurgical periodontal therapy include all of the following, EXCEPT:
    A. the need for surgical access
    B. the modification of risk factors
    C. the removal of bacterial plaque (etiologic agent) and other local irritants
    D. the initiation of plaque control measures
    E. the evaluation of tissue response

119. Current research suggests that the purpose of root planing is to:
    A. remove all plaque, plaque-retentive materials, and endotoxins from the root surface with minimal damage
    B. remove only plaque from the root surface
    C. create a glassy, smooth root surface
    D. create a smooth surface for the reattachment of connective tissue

120. Closed gingival curettage is a technique:
    A. that has limited value in nonsurgical periodontal therapy
    B. whose use is limited to periodontists and dentists only
    C. that is a useful adjunct to conventional scaling and root planing
    D. that is used in conjunction with tetracycline fiber placement

121. Sonic scaling devices have been shown to be as effective as ultrasonic devices and hand scaling. These sonic devices operate at:
    A. 600 to 1000 cycles per second
    B. 2000 to 6000 cycles per second
    C. 8000 to 15,000 cycles per second
    D. 20,000 to 40,000 cycles per second

122. Subgingival irrigation combined with scaling and root planing:
    A. should be performed in all cases of nonsurgical periodontal therapy
    B. has been shown in numerous studies to have significant benefits
    C. remains controversial and should be an elective part of therapy
    D. has not been shown to have any significant benefits in most studies

123. Sodium fluoride compounds, calcium hydroxide, potassium oxalate, and ferric oxalate are all agents commonly used in:
    A. calculus softening products
    B. tooth desensitizing products
    C. tartar control dentifrices
    D. anticavity products

124. Antibiotic agents that are commonly prescribed systemically for more aggressive forms of periodontitis include:
    A. penicillin, metronidazole, and cephalexin
    B. amoxicillin, ciprofloxacin, and erythromycin
    C. tetracyclines, metronidazole, and amoxicillin
    D. ampicillin, cephalosporin, and tetracyclines

125. Which one of the following is NOT a goal of periodontal surgery?
    A. reducing pocket depths for better access to home care
    B. correcting mucogingival defects
    C. retaining inflamed tissues
    D. regenerating tissues lost to disease

126. A surgical procedure that reduces pocket depths by removing the soft-tissue pocket wall in supragingival pockets is referred to as a:
    A. gingivectomy
    B. modified Whitman flap
    C. guided tissue regeneration
    D. ostectomy

127. One-walled and two-walled infrabony pockets are treated with which of the following procedures?
    A. ostectomy
    B. osteoplasty
    C. osteotomy
    D. ostectomy and osteoplasty
    E. osteoplasty and osteotomy

128. Bone grafting material that is taken from another person (freeze-dried from cadavers) is referred to as a(n):
    A. allograft
    B. autograft
    C. xenograft
    D. alloplast

129. A type-II mucogingival defect refers to a defect in which:
    A. alveolar mucosa acts as marginal gingiva, without a zone of attached gingiva
    B. pockets extend to or beyond the mucogingival junction
    C. the gingiva is recessed beyond the mucogingival junction
    D. a port-hole defect is present in the alveolar mucosa

130. Periodontal surgical dressings are placed over a surgical wound for protection and should remain in place for:
    A. 3 to 5 days
    B. 7 to 10 days
    C. 12 to 14 days
    D. 18 to 21 days

131. Which one of the following is not a goal of SPT?
    A. preservation of clinical attachment levels
    B. maintenance of alveolar bone height
    C. control of inflammation
    D. evaluation and reinforcement of the patient's oral hygiene
    E. correction of mucogingival defects

132. The most significant challenge for the dental hygienist is:
    A. subgingival deposit removal
    B. compliance with plaque control measures
    C. compliance with SPT appointments
    D. B and C
    E. all of the above

133. Studies have shown that compliance with oral hygiene measures decreases within
    A. 1 month
    B. 2 months
    C. 3 months
    D. 4 months

134. Which of the following procedures is not a part of the SPT appointment?
    A. complete periodontal evaluation
    B. quadrant scaling and root planing with anesthesia
    C. oral hygiene instructions
    D. tooth desensitization as needed

135. During one of Mrs. Smith's routine SPT appointments, increases in pocket depths in several areas, multiple areas of bleeding in response to probing, and moderate to heavy calculus deposits in several molar areas are detected. The best approach would be to:
    A. review oral hygiene more thoroughly, emphasizing the effects of noncompliance
    B. treat the areas that exhibit breakdown
    C. repeat initial therapy by quadrant and reevaluate after 4 weeks
    D. refer Mrs. Smith to a periodontist for surgical intervention

136. Xerostomia caused by radiation, medications, or pathology is of concern to the dental hygienist because this condition places the patient at great risk for the development of:
    A. oral cancer
    B. calculus
    C. periodontal disease
    D. root caries

137. The most effective approach for controlling root caries is:
    A. water fluoridation
    B. fluoride rinses
    C. fluoride gels or solutions
    D. fluoride dentifrices
    E. combination fluoride therapy

138. Dentinal hypersensitivity occurs frequently in periodontal patients. Spontaneous remission without therapeutic intervention can be expected in:
    A. 10% to 20% of patients
    B. 20% to 40% of patients
    C. 50% to 60% of patients
    D. 60% to 70% of patients

139. Agents that have been shown to be effective desensitizers include all of the following, EXCEPT:
    A. strontium chloride
    B. zinc citrate
    C. potassium nitrate
    D. zinc chloride

140. The acute periodontal abscess should be treated with:
    A. drainage of the abscess through scaling and curettage
    B. antibiotics
    C. tooth extraction
    D. tetracycline fiber placement

141. A raised, painful area of acute inflammation on the marginal gingiva, with no accompanying periodontal pockets and no radiographically visible bone loss, most likely is a(n):
    A. acute periodontal abscess
    B. periapical abscess
    C. gingival abscess
    D. combination abscess

142. If a patient presents with pericoronitis, the dental hygienist's role in caring for the patient may include all of the following, EXCEPT:
    A. irrigation of the area under the operculum
    B. gentle debridement under the operculum
    C. providing a prescription for antibiotics
    D. providing oral hygiene instruction

143. The most important instruction that a dental hygienist can provide to the parents of a patient with acute herpetic gingivostomatitis is:
    A. to keep the child isolated because the virus is contagious
    B. to engage in gentle, daily plaque removal
    C. to follow diet instructions
    D. encourage fluid intake

144. A 19-year-old college student presents for emer-

gency care complaining primarily of pain in the gingiva, spontaneous bleeding, and a bad metallic taste in his mouth. During inspection a fetid odor, punched-out papillae with a gray pseudomembrane, and the areas of spontaneous bleeding are noted. This patient MOST likely has:

A. acute herpetic gingivostomatitis
B. leukemia
C. ANUG
D. AIDS

145. If a patient with ANUG or a patient with pericoronitis has been prescribed a hydrogen peroxide rinse, the patient should discontinue the rinse after:

A. 3 days
B. 7 days
C. 14 days
D. 21 days

146. A root-form or blade-form implant placed directly into the bone is classified as a(n):

A. endosseous implant
B. subperiosteal implant
C. transosteal implant
D. staple implant

147. The purpose of two-step implant surgery is to allow for:

A. fibrointegration
B. osseointegration
C. bone regeneration
D. settling to occur

148. The interface or biologic seal found around an implant is created by the formation of a long junctional epithelium that is attached to the implant surface by:

A. glycosaminoglycans
B. connective tissue
C. hemidesmosomes
D. gap junctions

REVIEW QUESTION RATIONALES

1. **D** Protection against cariogenic bacteria has not been shown to be a function of the periodontium. The functions of the periodontium include attaching the tooth to its bony housing; providing resistance to the forces of mastication, speech, and deglutition; maintaining body surface integrity by separating the external and internal environments; and defending against external noxious stimuli.

2. **B** Oral epithelium consists of keratinized or para-keratinized stratified squamous epithelium. Simple epithelia, pseudostratified columnar epithelia, and simple cuboidal epithelia typically are found in other areas of the body but not in the lining of the oral cavity.

3. **D** Sulcular or crevicular epithelium is nonkeratinized. Only the tougher portions of the oral cavity, such as the gingiva and hard palate, are keratinized

or parakeratinized. No areas of the mouth are considered pseudokeratinized.

4. **A** The attached gingiva is the portion of the gums that is firmly bound to the underlying bone and is located between the free gingival groove and the mucogingival junction. The free gingival groove demarcates the part of the sulcus that is not attached to the tooth. Alveolar mucosa is loose and moveable. Connective tissue of the PDL is the only tissue that attaches to the tooth.

5. **B** The lamina propria is the connective tissue of the gingiva that contains collagen fibers, fibroblasts, undifferentiated cells, and macrophages. The lamina dura is the radiographic term for the alveolar bone proper, which surrounds the tooth root. The lamina lucida and lamina densa are components of the PDL.

6. **D** The alveolar mucosa is nonkeratinized, flexible, and located beyond the mucogingival junction. However, it is a separate part of the oral mucous membranes and is not classified as gingiva.

7. **A** The thickness of the PDL ranges from 0.15 to 0.38 mm and is shaped like an hour glass.

8. **B** The brush ends of the principal fibers that are embedded in both the cementum and alveolar bone are referred to as Sharpey's fibers. The oblique, transseptal, and principal fibers span across the entire PDL space; they do not refer to just the embedded portions of the fibers.

9. **A** Both type-I and type-II cementum are acellular and are located in the coronal third of the root. The middle and apical thirds of the root are more likely to house cellular cementum.

10. **B** Studies have shown that cementum overlaps enamel in 60% to 65% of the population, and that a butt end-to-end joint occurs in 30%. In 5% to 10% of the population, the enamel and cementum fail to meet.

11. **D** Lamina propria is the name for oral connective tissue. The alveolar bone proper is the compact bone that forms the housing of the root or tooth socket. Histologically this bone is referred to as the cribriform plate; anatomically it is the bundle bone; and radiographically it is the lamina dura.

12. **A** The supporting alveolar bone contains both compact and cancellous bone. The facial and lingual cortical plates are compact and the spongy bone between these plates is cancellous.

13. **C** According to the most recent national data, attachment loss is greater in men than in women in the United States. The other statements are all consistent with this national data.

14. **A** Incidence refers to the rate of occurrence of a new disease in a population during a given period of time. Prevalence refers to the number of persons affected by a disease at a specific point in time. Patterns are formed when data repeats itself over time. Severity refers to the extent of a disease.

15. **A** Although age does not necessarily preclude

periodontal disease, studies have shown that the prevalence of periodontal disease increases directly with age, most likely because of repeated exposures to bacterial infection over a lifetime.

16. **D** Although age, sex, genetics, and neutrophil abnormalities are not modifiable, it is possible to minimize or control stress and quit smoking. Because pregnancy is a temporary condition, it is considered modifiable.

17. **B** For decades, ANUG has been linked to stress. A virus causes acute herpetic gingivostomatitis, and both refractory periodontitis and LJP are bacterial infections that may be associated with neutrophil defects.

18. **C** Studies have shown that an unusually high number of patients (85% to 90%) with refractory periodontitis are smokers. HIV periodontitis occurs only in individuals infected with the HIV virus. Acute herpetic gingivostomatitis also has a viral etiology, and ANUG has been correlated with stress and immunosuppression.

19. **C** Poor nutrition results in lowered resistance (host response) to infections, including periodontal diseases. Individuals with nutritional deficiencies are therefore more susceptible to severe forms of periodontal disease; however such deficiencies have not been shown to contribute to plaque accumulation, bone loss, or lower socioeconomic status.

20. **D** Vitamin B_6, or pyridoxine, deficiency is not associated with the development of candidiasis. Vitamin B_6 is involved in carbohydrate metabolism and deprivation may result in generalized stomatitis, gingivitis, glossitis, and other oral symptoms.

21. **A** Retinol, or Vitamin A, currently is under investigation as an antioxidant agent that could have beneficial effects in the prevention of malignancy, cardiovascular disease and periodontitis.

22. **C** Vitamin C is essential to collagen biosynthesis; a deficiency adversely affects periodontal connective tissue integrity and wound healing. Vitamin A is associated with the synthesis of epithelial cells. Vitamin B is a group of vitamins with multiple roles. Vitamin D is involved in maintaining calcium and phosphorus levels.

23. **D** Vitamin D deficiency is not associated with the development of gingival hyperplasia. In adults, a deficiency in vitamin D is called osteomalacia, which is characterized by destruction of the PDL, resorption of alveolar bone, and replacement fibrous dysplasia.

24. **D** Severe protein deficiency, or kwashiorkor, has been associated with an increased incidence and severity of necrotizing gingivitis. Marasmus (general starvation), osteoporosis, and osteomalacia have not been linked with necrotizing gingivitis.

25. **D** No connection between systemic lupus erythematosus and free oxygen radicals is known. Evidence suggests that free oxygen radicals are involved in the tissue destruction associated with periodontitis and chronic inflammatory osteoarthritis. Moreover, these free radicals are thought to play a role in cancer and heart disease.

26. **B** Multilocular radiolucent jaw lesions, the loss of lamina dura, and a ground-glass appearance of the alveolar bone are characteristics of an excessive production of parathyroid hormone or hyperparathyroidism. This combination of lesions is not characteristic of the other conditions listed.

27. **B** Increased, rather than decreased, levels of sex hormones alter capillary permeability and increase tissue fluid accumulation in the gingiva, resulting in an increased susceptibility to gingivitis in the presence of bacterial plaque. An altered chemotactic response has not been demonstrated in cases of puberty gingivitis.

28. **A** It was once believed that desquamative gingivitis was associated with menopause. However, recent studies have ruled out that association and indicate that it is more likely a feature of mucocutaneous disorders, such as lichen planus or mucous membrane pemphigoid and pemphigus.

29. **D** Increased fibrosis of the periodontal tissues is not a common occurrence in diabetic patients and is not related to prevalence. Defective PMNL chemotaxis, microangiopathy of the periodontal tissues, increased collagen breakdown, and microbial alterations have been cited as rationales for the prevalence of periodontal disease in individuals with diabetes mellitus. Moreover, periodontal disease has been declared the sixth complication of diabetes mellitus.

30. **C** In uncontrolled diabetes mellitus, oral manifestations such as multiple periodontal abscesses, velvety red gingivae, and marginal proliferation of the periodontal tissues have been noted. Although susceptibility to periodontal breakdown exists in controlled cases of type-I or type-II diabetes, oral manifestations can be controlled with frequent supportive therapy.

31. **C** Recommended treatment for pseudomembranous candidiasis consists of either topical or systemic ingestion of an antifungal agent, such as nystatin, ketoconazole, or fluconazole. Acyclovir is reserved for viral infections, and Lidex, a corticosteroid, often is used to soothe the pain of oral ulcerations. Chlorhexidine frequently is prescribed to patients with HIV/AIDS to assist in controlling the bacterial load intraorally.

32. **D** Kaposi's sarcoma, a neoplasm that occurs most frequently in the AIDS population, is most likely to occur on keratinized tissues such as the gingiva or the hard palate. It also is most commonly located in the head and neck area.

33. **A** The most commonly occurring form of gingivitis in the HIV population is LGE. It was previously coined HIV gingivitis and was renamed because of

its characteristic, well-defined red band along the free gingival margin.

34. **C** Although it is well established that periodontal disease is caused by bacterial plaque, it is also recognized that an impairment in the host response increases susceptibility to periodontal breakdown. Because neutrophils are key players in the host response, a shortage of these PMNLs results in an increased susceptibility to periodontal infections.

35. **D** The cause of neutropenia is multifactorial but is not associated with CNS dysfunction. Because the term neutropenia refers to reductions in the neutrophil count, conditions such as Down syndrome, diabetes mellitus, and a variety of autoimmune disorders are all capable of producing neutropenic states.

36. **A** LAD is clinically characterized by recurrent bacterial infections, diminished pus formation, prolonged wound healing, and leukocytosis. Dentally, it is characterized by generalized prepubertal periodontitis, progressive alveolar bone loss, premature exfoliation of the primary and permanent dentitions, and severe gingival inflammation. The other conditions listed have not been associated with LAD.

37. **C** The only thing that cyclosporin (an immunosuppressant), phenobarbital (an anticonvulsant), and diltiazem and nifedipine (calcium channel blockers) have in common is their ability to produce gingival overgrowth.

38. **A** It is a well established fact that the prime etiologic agent in the development of periodontal disease is bacterial plaque. However, the host response is recognized as the balancing factor because the mere presence of bacteria does not preclude disease.

39. **B** Filaments, fusiforms, and curved microbes are forms of rods. Cocci are rounded microbes; spirochetes and vibrios are more curved or corkscrew-like in appearance.

40. **D** Gram-negative microorganisms have an outer cell wall composed of receptor proteins and complex lipopolysaccharides known as endotoxins. Gram-positive microbes contain an outer capsule made of glucan, which is referred to as exotoxin.

41. **D** Obligate anaerobes cannot survive in oxygen environments. Aerobes require oxygen for survival; facultative aerobes and anaerobes can live in either an oxygen or nonoxygen environment.

42. **A** Plaque associated with gingival health typically is composed of Gram-positive, aerobic cocci and rods. Gram-negative microorganisms increase in numbers as gingivitis and periodontitis progress. Spirochetes are Gram-negative organisms.

43. **C** Although other species may be present, *Treponema* species have been identified in large quantities in individuals with ANUG.

44. **B** Elevated levels of *P. gingivalis, P. intermedia, A. actino-mycetemcomitans, E. corrodens,* and *C. rectus* have been associated with rapidly progressive periodontitis.

45. **C** Current thought focuses on the specific plaque hypothesis, which recognizes specific pathogens as disease-producing and often treatable by antibiotics and antimicrobial agents. Belief in the nonspecific plaque hypothesis prevailed before the 1970s. The multiple burst theory has been proposed by some researchers recently but has not been substantiated. No single burst theory exists.

46. **D** Lipase is an enzyme that aids fat metabolism, not a bacterial enzyme. Proteolytic enzymes such as hyaluronidase, collagenase, and ribonuclease affect the host cells and ground substance by increasing the permeability of epithelial and connective tissues and outwardly destroying cells.

47. **B** Bacterial endotoxins are responsible for activating the alternate pathway of the immune complex fixation process known as the complement cascade. Side reaction proteins of this process are both chemotactic and cytolytic.

48. **C** Macrophages are large defense cells that appear in larger numbers during chronic inflammation and are typically not found in saliva. Saliva contains antibacterial components such as lysosomes and lactoperoxidase.

49. **C** Histamine, serotonin, kinins, prostaglandins, C3 and C5, and lysosomal enzymes are ALL mediators of vascular permeability, unlike thyroxin.

50. **A** The process by which PMNLs leave the axial stream and adhere to the endothelial cell walls of blood vessels is called pavementing or margination. Emigration, migration, and chemotaxis follow as the cells escape through the endothelial walls into the connective tissues and move along chemical gradients to the attracting microorganisms.

51. **B** The monocyte or connective tissue macrophage signals the beginning of the chronic stage of inflammation. Soon afterward, lymphocytes arrive at the scene and eventually become the predominant cell. Basophils typically are present only in allergic conditions. The PMNL is the predominant cell in acute inflammation.

52. **D** B cells are responsible for humoral immunity. The cells that are responsible for cellular immunity are T4 activator cells, T8 suppressor cells, and NK (natural killer) cells.

53. **B** The B lymphocyte is responsible for humoral immunity and the T lymphocyte is responsible for cellular immunity. The macrophage and/or monocyte is the phagocytic cell that appears first during chronic inflammation.

54. **D** The combination of fibroblasts, new immature collagen, and new capillaries comprise granulation tissue that is formed during the repair stage of inflammation.

55. **D** Products of the arachidonic acid cascade are potentially harmful to periodontal tissues and are

part of the pathogenesis of periodontal disease. Antibodies and complement proteins are later attracted and also assist in the destruction.

56. **B** The complement system is responsible for the release of chemotactic factors that cause the migration of PMNLs and macrophages to specific sites. The phagocytic system is composed of PMNLs and macrophages. The arachidonic acid cascade and the kinin system are responsible for other aspects of the immune response.

57. **C** As part of the process of cellular immunity, T cells release potent cytokines, such as interleukin-1, that are capable of causing bone resorption. Arachidonic acid has the potential for tissue destruction and prostaglandin is a mediator of vascular permeability. Myeloperoxidase is found in the saliva and is a protective enzyme.

58. **B** The initial lesion occurs in the first 2 to 4 days, the early lesion occurs in 4 to 7 days, the established lesion occurs after 14 days, and the advanced lesion occurs only after the inflammation invades the supporting periodontal tissues.

59. **D** The advanced lesion, however, is characterized by an invasion of the periodontal tissues, the PDL, and the alveolar bone. The initial, early, and established lesions do not typically involve the PDL and alveolar bone.

60. **C** Clinical signs and symptoms of occlusal traumatism always include radiographic evidence of a widening of the PDL space and clinical evidence of tooth mobility. Tooth extrusion typically is related to the lack of an opposing tooth. A narrowed PDL space is associated with a lack of occlusal contact.

61. **A** Primary occlusal trauma is defined as damage that occurs when the amount of alveolar bone is normal but there is an increase in occlusal forces. Secondary occlusal trauma occurs when there is a deficiency in the amount of alveolar bone support. Neither hyperfunction or hypofunction result in irreversible damage.

62. **C** Disorders of the temporomandibular joint that impede mobility include joint adhesions, ankylosis, and muscular fibrosis. Conditions such as myalgia and bruxism do not necessarily affect mobility.

63. **D** Bruxism is the most common oral habit; it involves grinding or clenching of the teeth and can be recognized by the presence of nonfunctional wear facets. Wear facets are not associated with decay, TMJ disorder, or trismus.

64. **B** Bacterial plaque is considered the prime etiologic factor in the development of periodontal disease; however, several contributing factors have been identified that make the individual more prone to plaque retention and thus disease susceptibility. One such factor is subgingival calculus, which is considered a local predisposing factor. Missing teeth, malocclusions, and traumatogenic occlusion are considered local functional factors. Systemic

contributing factors include those conditions that lower the host response of the individual and raise the susceptibility to disease.

65. **A** Calculus is composed of approximately 70% to 90% inorganic matter and 10% to 30% organic matter. The organic component is a mixture of protein polysaccharide complexes, desquamated epithelial cells, leukocytes, carbohydrates, lipids, glycosaminoglycans, and various types of microorganisms.

66. **B** Materia alba is a yellowish or grayish-white acquired bacterial coating that is soft, sticky, and less adherent than plaque. Both plaque and acquired pellicle are visible only if stained with a dye. Food debris may be any color or texture, depending on the nature of the retained food.

67. **A** The most commonly occurring form of periodontal disease is gingivitis, which is defined as inflammation of the gingivae. Adult periodontitis is the second most common form of periodontal disease; early onset periodontitis and refractory periodontitis are less common.

68. **C** The most significant feature of chronic gingivitis is marginal bleeding; marginal redness, edema, and a loss of stippling may or may not be found.

69. **A** Vitamin C deficiency alone cannot cause inflammation; however, a deficiency in vitamin C causes an increased tendency for gingival hemorrhage, degeneration of the collagen fibers, and poor healing.

70. **C** The clinical characteristics of leukemia include purplish-blue gingivae, interdental tumor-like masses, and shiny gingival surfaces that may have ulcerations and spontaneous bleeding. ANUG should be ruled out because purplish-blue gingivae and tumor-like masses are not common characteristics. Pregnancy gingivitis must be ruled out because the patient is male. Because of his age, primary herpetic gingivostomatitis, which typically occurs during the first 5 years of life and is not associated with tumor-like masses, also should not be a consideration.

71. **A** Localized tumor-like growths on the interdental gingivae are commonly found in both leukemic gingivitis and pregnancy gingivitis. However, these enlargements are not characteristic of ANUG, diabetic gingivitis, or AIDS.

72. **C** Allergic hypersensitivity involves an abnormal response of the tissues to specific agents, which typically manifests as redness, pain, edema, ulceration, and possible vesicle formation. This patient has an allergy to the nonprecious metal crown on #30. No mention was made of desquamating tissues or tissues that were peeling away, which rules out desquamative gingivitis. Menopausal gingivitis has not been established as an acceptable term and apthous ulcers should be ruled out because they occur only in the soft tissues, and not on tissues overlying bone.

73. **E** Pregnancy is associated with pyogenic granu-

loma rather than desquamative gingivitis. Although the exact nature of desquamative gingitivis is unknown, recent links to several dermatologic diseases and drugs have been made, including pemphigus, pemphigoid, and lichen planus.

74. **B** Although desquamative gingivitis may occur in any individual, this condition most often affects women during menopause.

75. **E** The eating disorder, bulimia, is associated with enamel erosion rather than gingival overgrowth. Drugs such as phenytoin, cyclosporin, and calcium channel blockers initially cause gingival overgrowth. When bacterial plaque accumulates on the enlarged gingival tissues, the inflammatory response ensues and results in inflammatory gingival overgrowth.

76. **C** A rare hyperplastic disease with unknown etiology, which is referred to as idiopathic gingival hyperplasia, is believed to be familial or hereditary. No association has been established between this condition and diabetes, epilepsy, or the use of drugs.

77. **D** The large numbers of neutrophils (PMNLs) are responsible for the intense tissue destruction created by the release of large quantities of lysosomal enzymes into the tissues during acute inflammation. *P. gingivalis*, *A. actinomycetemcomitans*, and macrophages have not been associated with this type of rapid destruction.

78. **C** The spontaneous bleeding, metallic taste, fetid odor, punched-out papillae, and gray pseudomembrane are all typical characteristics of ANUG. Acute herpetic gingivostomatitis, leukemia, and AIDS-associated gingivitis do not exhibit the characteristic punched-out papillae.

79. **A** Both spirochetes and fusiform bacilli have been associated with ANUG. *P. intermedia*, *S. sanguis*, and *P. gingivalis* have not been found in large quantities in this condition.

80. **C** The young age of the patient, the multiple ulcerations, and the lymphadenopathy indicate acute herpetic gingivostomatitis rather than the other options. The characteristic punched-out papillae of ANUG; the characteristic bluish-purple gingivae of leukemia, and the absence of the gingival enlargement that is indicative of acute gingival abscess are all absent from the case description.

81. **C** Periodontal pockets are classified as either suprabony or infrabony. If the base of the pocket is coronal to the alveolar bone, it is a suprabony pocket. However, if the base of the pocket is apical to the alveolar bone crest, the pocket is infrabony. Both pseudopockets and relative pockets are gingival and not periodontal pockets.

82. **B** According to the 1989 AAP World Workshop in Clinical Periodontics, prepubertal periodontitis is categorized as an early-onset periodontal disease. Adult periodontitis and periodontitis associated with systemic disease are separate classifications that do not include prepubertal periodontitis.

Chronic periodontitis is a descriptive term and not a classification or category of periodontal disease.

83. **A** The rapid pocket destruction (from 6 mm to 11 mm within a few weeks) and the presence of suppuration are suggestive of periodontal abscess. The entrapment of virulent microorganisms after an incomplete scaling procedure results in pus formation and rapid tissue destruction. A periapical abscess results in intermittent sharp pain with localized swelling. The combination (endo/perio) lesion has characteristics of both periapical & periodontal abscesses; pericornitis is a severe, localized infection associated with terminal molars.

84. **D** Adult periodontitis is the most common form of periodontal disease and is characterized by slow progression, pocket formation, bone loss, and eventual tooth mobility. The host response generally is normal and does not implicate a systemic disease. Early-onset periodontitis, juvenile periodontitis, and prepubertal periodontitis generally are characterized by some type of defect in host response.

85. **D** White-colored gingiva is not associated with periodontal disease. The clinical signs of chronically inflamed adult periodontitis may include gingival coloration that ranges from red to bluish to normal. Gingival color is not a reliable sign of periodontitis.

86. **C** Refractory periodontitis is associated with chronic forms of periodontitis that do not respond well to treatment and is not considered an early-onset disease. Early-onset periodontitis is a group of aggressive periodontal diseases that are characterized by rapid progression, early onset, and neutrophil abnormalities. These diseases include prepubertal periodontitis, juvenile periodontitis, and rapidly progressive periodontitis.

87. **B** Prepubertal periodontitis is a rare condition that affects both primary and permanent dentitions and typically is manifested by white blood cell defects and systemic diseases, such as Chédiak-Higashi and Papillon-Lefèvre syndromes. Adult periodontitis and juvenile periodontitis are not linked with systemic disease.

88. **D** Juvenile periodontitis occurs during puberty and is characterized by rapid vertical bone loss in the anterior and first molar regions, with little evidence of inflammation. Prepubertal periodontitis has a much earlier onset; rapidly progressive and refractory periodontitis occur in early to middle adulthood.

89. **A** The association between high numbers of *A. actinomycetemcomitans* and juvenile periodontitis is well documented in the literature. Elevated numbers of *P. gingivalis*, *P. intermedia*, and *T. denticola* have not been demonstrated in juvenile periodontitis.

90. **B** Rapidly progressive periodontitis occurs in young adults between 20 and 30 years of age and is believed to be related to juvenile periodontitis. Prepubertal and refractory periodontitis and peri-

odontitis associated with systemic disease are unrelated to rapidly progressive periodontitis.

91. **C** Papillon-Lefèvre syndrome is characterized by hyperkeratotic skin lesions of the palms, soles, knees, and elbows, and involves severe destruction of the periodontium before age 4. Chédiak-Higashi syndrome produces partial albinism, mild bleeding disorders, and periodontal diseases. Hypophosphatasia is characterized by poor bone formation, rickets, and the premature loss of the dentition. Down syndrome, or trisomy 21, manifests as mental and growth retardation and is characterized by a high prevalence of aggressive periodontal disease.

92. **C** LGE was previously referred to as AIDS-associated gingivitis and typically is associated with patients who have HIV or AIDS. The characteristic red band of marginal gingiva that rarely bleeds has not been demonstrated in diabetic, leukemic, or chronic gingivitis.

93. **C** Smoking has been consistently associated with refractory periodontitis. Studies have demonstrated that 85% to 90% of patients with this disease are smokers. No such linkage has been established with poor oral hygiene, genetic predisposition, or poor host response.

94. **E** Functional heart murmurs involve no tissue damage and therefore no risk of bacterial endocarditis. The American Medical Association recommends that prophylactic antibiotics be given before any invasive dental procedure for patients with mitral valve prolapse with regurgitation, hypertrophic cardiomyopathy, prosthetic cardiac valves, and organic heart disease.

95. **D** Tricyclic antidepressants, MAO inhibitors, antipsychotics, and some nonselective beta blockers are contraindicated with the use of epinephrine. The other distractors are not relevant to the use of this drug.

96. **A** Individuals undergoing cancer radiation therapy are at risk for the development of osteoradionecrosis and should have any significant periodontal disease eliminated and teeth extracted before radiation therapy. Continuing periodontal therapy after radiation treatment begins is extremely risky.

97. **E** Social status is not an important characteristic to gather from the personal history unlike other non-dentally related risk factors such as stress, smoking, diet, and alcohol consumption, which may play a role in the patient's periodontal condition.

98. **C** Life-saver-like enlargements surrounding the free gingival margins are referred to as McCall's festoons. Stillman's clefts are narrow, slit-like areas where the marginal gingiva has receded. Rolled margins are less enlarged than McCall's festoons and marginal hyperplasia demonstrates greater overall enlargement.

99. **A** Clinical attachment loss is considered the gold standard for determining the extent of periodontal tissue destruction. Pocket depths may vary according to the amount of edema or hyperplasia. Bleeding in response to probing is an indicator of active disease but does not indicate the extent of damage. Bone loss through radiographic analysis is less reliable because of associated distortion and magnification issues.

100. **C** The AAP and the ADA developed the PSR to encourage general practitioners to probe routinely. The system is a modification of the CPITN, which was developed by the World Health Organization (WHO). The other indices are measurements of plaque, debris, calculus, and gingivitis.

101. **B** The condition of tooth proximal contact areas should be evaluated because open contacts encourage food impaction and tight contacts prevent effective interproximal cleaning. This is of major concern to dental hygienists, who develop home care strategies for their patients to facilitate the cleansing of these difficult areas.

102. **C** Tooth mobility, furcation involvement, malocclusions, overhanging margins of restorations, and the statuses of prosthetic appliances are considered local risk factors for the development of periodontal disease. Plaque is considered the primary etiologic factor; systemic diseases, host response factors, and genetic predispositions are considered systemic risk factors.

103. **A** Although supplemental diagnostic tests were developed to diagnose specific periodontal diseases, none have been truly diagnostic. These tests play an important role in the identification of risk factors and, coupled with clinical evidence, can be strong predictors of future disease progression.

104. **C** These tests measure bacterial species. The BANA test measures the presence of *B. forsythus*, *T. denticola*, and *P. gingivalis*. The ELISA and DNA tests measure the quantities of *P. gingivalis*, *P. intermedia*, and *A. actinomycetemcomitans*.

105. **D** The presumptive diagnosis is determined to be the best possibility after the evidence has been examined. The initial list of possibilities is called the differential diagnosis. The patient's presumptions typically are not taken into serious consideration. The final diagnosis is not determined until after the completion of initial therapy and the reevaluation of tissue response.

106. **B** Treatment planning must be based on individual need, must incorporate "evidence" in the development of the plan, must define methods and establish the sequence of delivering appropriate care, and must be geared toward health promotion and disease prevention. These principles should be consistently—not randomly—applied in practice.

107. **A** Phase-I therapy is considered the etiotrophic stage, which deals with the elimination of etiologic factors. Phase II is considered the surgical phase, phase III is the restorative and orthodontic phase,

and phase IV is concerned with maintenance therapy or SPT.

108. **B** The AAP classification defines gingivitis as case type I, early periodontitis as case type II, moderate periodontitis as case type III, advanced periodontitis as case type IV, and refractory periodontitis as case type V.

109. **B** All periodontal patients require a 1-month (4–6 weeks) reevaluation after initial therapy to assess the tissue response and to establish an appropriate SPT interval or determine whether referral to a periodontist for further treatment is necessary.

110. **D** For moderate to heavy calculus deposits and 5- to 6-mm pocket depths, quadrant scaling and root planing with anesthesia would be the best possible treatment option. Thorough debridement of the deeper pockets, which is likely to involve some inadvertent curettage to allow proper access to the junctional epithelium, is a definitive process that requires time and operator skill.

111. **C** Prognosis is the prediction of the duration, course, and termination of a disease and its response to treatment (treatment outcome). The planning of care refers to the treatment plan. The identification of the disease is the diagnosis. Posttreatment assessment generally is referred to as reevaluation.

112. **C** Patient motivation is the key to a successful plaque control program. Although the accuracy of instruction, the amount of time spent, and multiple reinforcement appointments are all important, all efforts will be futile if the dental hygienist is unable to motivate the patient to comply with the regimen.

113. **D** The Bass method of brushing involves placing bristles in the sulcular area and moving them back and forth in a vibratory motion. The Stillman's and modified Stillman's techniques involve placing the bristles on the marginal gingiva and moving them in a vibratory motion. The Charter's technique advocates pointing the bristles away from the gingiva.

114. **C** Furcation areas are difficult to cleanse with conventional toothbrushes and dental floss. Special disposable interdental brushes, toothpicks attached to the ends of handles, and end-tuft brushes have been shown to be most effective in these difficult-to-access areas.

115. **B** Patients who require antibiotic coverage for dental procedures or those with acute oral conditions should not use irrigating devices. However, these devices are recommended for patients with orthodontic appliances and for those with some forms of periodontal disease. No known contraindications for the use of oral irrigating devices exist for patients with cardiac pacemakers.

116. **A** Extensive research has shown that chlorhexidine digluconate significantly reduces plaque and gingivitis by as much as 60% and that it exhibits high substantivity. Phenolic compounds, cetylpyridinium chloride, and sanguinarine have not been shown to exhibit substantivity or significant antiplaque qualities. Stannous fluoride has demonstrated weak antigingivitis effects in some studies.

117. **D** Anticalculus agents or tartar control dentifrices contain either soluble pyrophosphates or zinc citrate as an active ingredient.

118. **A** The need for surgical access is a rationale for surgical therapy. The rationales for nonsurgical periodontal therapy include the modification of risk factors, the removal of etiologic agents, the initiation of plaque control, and the evaluation of tissue response.

119. **A** The removal of plaque and plaque-retentive factors, such as calculus, with minimal damage to the root surface is the current standard of care. Root planing in the past was targeted at the removal of cementum, surface dentin impregnated with calculus, endotoxins, and bacteria. Current evidence suggests a more conservative approach, which no longer aims for glassy-smooth root surfaces.

120. **A** The closed gingival curettage technique, which is used to remove diseased soft tissues from within the pocket wall, currently is believed to be of limited value in nonsurgical periodontal therapy and is therefore not considered a useful adjunct to either scaling and root planing or the placement of tetracycline fibers. However, this technique is a legal dental hygiene procedure in most states.

121. **B** Sonic scaling devices generate vibrations of 2000 to 6000 cycles per second. Ultrasonic scaling devices operate at 20,000 to 40,000 cycles per second.

122. **C** Subgingival irrigation combined with scaling and root planing has been shown to enhance the success of therapy. However, because controversy over its benefits continues to exist, its use should be elective.

123. **B** Sodium fluoride, calcium hydroxide, potassium oxalate, and ferric oxalate are compounds that are commonly used for desensitizing root surfaces.

124. **C** Tetracyclines, metronidazole, amoxicillin, ampicillin, ciprofloxacin, and clindamycin have been shown to be effective adjuncts to nonsurgical periodontal therapy in more aggressive forms of periodontitis. Penicillin, cephalexin, erythromycin, and cephalosporins have no demonstrable effectiveness in the treatment of periodontal diseases.

125. **C** Retaining inflamed tissues is not a goal of periodontal surgery. Periodontal surgery goals are to reduce pocket depths, provide better access for home care, correct mucogingival defects, remove inflamed tissues, and regenerate tissues lost to illness.

126. **A** The gingivectomy procedure is designed to reduce pocket depths by removing the soft tissue pocket wall in suprabony pockets. The modified Widman flap exposes the periodontium to provide access for other procedures. Guided tissue regener-

ation involves the placement of barrier materials to prevent the downgrowth of epithelium and stimulate the reattachment of connective tissues. Ostectomy involves the removal of alveolar bone.

127. **D** Ostectomy and osteoplasty are used to treat one-walled and two-walled infrabony pockets. Osteotomy refers to the sectioning and repositioning of bone and is employed during mandibular advancement surgery.

128. **A** Freeze-dried bone from cadavers that is used as grafting material is referred to as an allograft. Autografts involve donor bone taken from the patient's own body and xenografts are bone specimens obtained from other species (e.g., cows). Alloplast materials are synthetic substances that are used for bone grafting procedures.

129. **A** A type-II mucogingival defect refers to a defect in which the alveolar mucosa acts as marginal gingiva without a zone of attached gingiva. Type-I defects occur when pockets extend to or beyond the mucogingival junction but have a firm keratinized pocket wall.

130. **B** Periodontal surgical dressings are placed over the surgical wound for protection and should remain in place for at least 7 days to allow for adequate healing. Dressing and suture removal typically are performed concomitantly.

131. **E** Correcting mucogingival defects is not a goal of SPT, rather the goal is to maintain optimal oral health through the preservation of clinical attachment levels, the maintenance of alveolar bone height, the control of inflammation, and the evaluation and reinforcement of patient oral hygiene.

132. **D** Compliance with both SPT appointments and plaque control measures are the keys to successful therapy. Subgingival deposit removal, no matter how meticulously performed, does not affect the success of therapy unless the patient is motivated to perform adequate plaque control and attend regular SPT appointments.

133. **A** Compliance studies have shown that oral hygiene decreases within 30 days of instruction, which suggests a major challenge for the dental hygienist regarding patient motivation.

134. **B** Quadrant scaling and root planing with anesthesia are performed during initial therapy, not during SPT appointments. Complete periodontal examination, oral hygiene instructions, and periodontal debridement, including targeted root planing of areas with active disease, are routinely performed at SPT appointments. Tooth desensitization typically is performed based on need during SPT appointments.

135. **C** With the return of active disease, initial therapy should be repeated by quadrant with anesthesia, followed by a reevaluation in 4 weeks. At the reevaluation appointment, the appropriate course of action should be determined and may include referral to a specialist, return to SPT intervals, or other treatment options such as antibiotics or surgery.

136. **D** Xerostomia presents a significant risk for the development of root caries when the preventive washing action of the saliva is diminished. Oral cancer, calculus, and periodontal disease are unaffected by xerostomia.

137. **E** Combination or multiple-approach fluoride therapy has proven to be the most effective treatment in the control of root caries. This approach involves using several or all methods of fluoride treatment, from the ingestion of fluoridated drinking water to the application of prescription fluoride gels.

138. **B** Although dentinal hypersensitivity occurs frequently after periodontal therapy, spontaneous remission without further intervention has been shown to occur in approximately 20% to 45% of patients.

139. **B** Zinc citrate is most effective as an anticalculus agent rather than a desensitizing agent. Strontium chloride, potassium nitrate, and zinc chloride have demonstrated effective desensitizing properties.

140. **A** The treatment of a periodontal abscess includes drainage through scaling, root planing, curettage of the pocket wall, and antimicrobial irrigation. Antibiotics are prescribed only if lymphadenopathy and/or fever are present. Tooth extraction and tetracycline fiber placement are rarely considered.

141. **C** Gingival abscesses are not associated with bone loss or deeper periodontal pockets but periodontal abscesses are always associated with both. Periapical and combination abscesses involve periapical bone loss; combination abscesses also may be characterized by deeper periodontal pockets.

142. **C** If fever and lymphadenopathy are present, the dentist (not dental hygienist) may opt to prescribe an antibiotic. The dental hygienist's role would involve gentle debridement, irrigation of the area under the operculum with an antimicrobial agent, and the provision of oral hygiene instruction.

143. **D** The painful lesions associated with this condition often prevent the child from eating and drinking. Dehydration in a child may be life threatening, therefore it is essential that the significance of fluid intake be stressed to the parent.

144. **C** This patient most likely has ANUG because all of the classic signs, including the presence of punched-out papilla, are present. Acute herpetic gingivostomatitis, leukemia, and AIDS share several of the signs but do not typically include punched-out papilla.

145. **B** The use of hydrogen peroxide intraorally must be discontinued in 7 to 10 days to prevent the development of black hairy tongue.

146. **A** Endosseous implants are shaped in the form of roots or blades and are directly implanted into the

bone. Subperiosteal implants are in the form of a metal framework that is placed over the alveolar bone to provide support for complete and removable dentures. Transosteal or staple implants are surgically placed through the mandible to provide an anchor for a removable lower denture.

147. **B** After the initial placement of the implant, the surgical site is covered for approximately 3 to 6 months to allow for osseointegration (implant to bone integration) to take place; this process leads to the most stable attachment. Fibrointegration should be avoided because implant failure typically follows. Bone regeneration and settling are not related factors.

148. **C** Cells at the base of the implant sulcus form a junctional epithelium that attaches to the implant by means of a basal lamina and hemidesmosomes. Glycosaminoglycans constitute intercellular "glue." Hemidesmosomes are part of the basal lamina or basement membrane that forms between the tooth and the epithelium and therefore are not part of the connective tissue. Gap junctions are cell-to-cell attachment mechanisms that typically are found in epithelial tissues.

References

1. Miller AJ, Brunelle J, Carlos J et al: Oral Health of United States Adults: National Findings 1985–86. Washington, DC, US Department of Health and Human Services, 1997.
2. American Academy of Periodontology: Annals of Periodontology: 1996 World Workshop in Periodontics. Chicago, American Academy of Periodontology, 1996.
3. Loe H: Periodontal disease: The sixth complication of diabetes mellitus. Diabetes Care 16:329–334, 1993.
4. Lavigne SE: Oral Care of the Patient with HIV/AIDS. Periodontal Management July:2(2), 1996. Professional Audience Communications, Yardley, PA.
5. American Academy of Periodontology: 1989 World Workshop in Clinical Periodontics. Chicago, American Academy of Periodontics, 1989.
6. Niesen LC, Mash LK, Gibson G: Practice management considerations for an aging population. JADA 124:55–60, 1993.
7. Miller CS, Kaplan AL, Guest GF et al: Documenting medication use in adult dental patients: 1987–1991. JADA 123(11):41–48, 1992.
8. Lavigne SE, Gutenkunst L, Williams KB: Effects of tartar-control dentifrice on tooth sensitivity: A pilot study. J Dent Hyg 71(3):105–111, 1997.

Additional Readings

American Academy of Periodontology: 1989 World Workshop in Clinical Periodontics. Chicago, American Academy of Periodontics, 1989.

Carranza FA, Newman MG: Clinical Periodontology, 8th ed. Philadelphia, WB Saunders, 1996.

Fedi PF, Vernino AR: The Periodontic Syllabus, 3rd ed. Baltimore, Williams and Wilkins, 1995.

Hodges KO: Concepts in Nonsurgical Periodontal Therapy, 1st ed. Albany, Delmar Publications, 1997.

Lavigne SE: Oral manifestations. In Muma RD, Lyons BA, Boruski NJ, Pollard RB, editors: HIV Manual for the Health Care Professional, 2nd ed. Stamford, Conn, Appleton and Lange, 1997.

Perry DA, Beemsterboer PL, Taggart EJ: Periodontology for the Dental Hygienist. Philadelphia, WB Saunders, 1996.

Wilson TG, Kornman, KS: Fundamentals of Periodontics, 1st ed. Chicago, Quintessence Books, 1996.

Wilkins E: Clinical Practice of the Dental Hygienist, 7th ed. Baltimore, Williams and Wilkins, 1994.

Chapter THIRTEEN

Pain Management

Alisa D. Feugate, R.D.H., M.A.

 ## Clinical Case STUDY

Alice, a 35-year-old woman, has not been to the dentist's office for 10 years. During her last dental experience she had two third molars extracted and the anesthetic did not work. Repeated injections did not improve the situation but did make Alice more anxious and uncomfortable. Lately, her gums have been bleeding and sore. Her husband persuaded her to have a thorough exam and cleaning. Her treatment plan suggests quadrant dental hygiene therapy with local anesthetics. On the day of her appointment with the dental hygienist, Alice calls and cancels.

Clinical Case QUESTIONS

1. What is the major problem confronting Alice?
2. Identify the most effective methods for treating Alice's condition.
3. What is the difference between fear and a phobia?

Clinical Case RATIONALES

1. Anxiety related to past dental experiences is the problem that Alice is most likely confronting.
2. First, the patient must visit the dental office to be fully informed about the necessary dental procedures. Next, the dental hygienist should help the patient identify problems that occurred before and explain choices that will decrease the likelihood of similar occurrences during dental hygiene treatment. The patient needs to feel in control of the situation.
3. A phobia is excessive fear that leads to inaction, which can be detrimental to a person's health and well-being.

Content Review

Anxiety

Anxiety keeps many people from receiving necessary dental treatment because of fear of pain or discomfort. Understanding dental fear can help the dental hygienist select appropriate methods for alleviating patient discomfort.

Causes of Dental Anxiety or Fear

Anxiety and fear are common occurrences in the dental office and can be managed by a variety of techniques.
I. Definitions
    A. Anxiety is a state of apprehension or a reaction to the unknown.
    B. Fear is excessive apprehension or anxiety.
    C. A phobia is excessive fear that promotes inaction (failure to seek necessary dental treatment).
II. Etiology of Dental Anxiety or Fear
    A. Anxiety and fear typically are based on past experiences associated with a dental office.
        1. May be based on fearful experiences related by others (friends or family).
        2. Fearful experiences portrayed by the media (movies, TV, newspaper, cartoons) can increase dental anxiety.
    B. Iatrogenic causes arise from an individual's personal experiences with dental situations and personnel (typically during childhood).
        1. The two greatest dental fears are of needles and of the dental drill.
        2. Feeling a loss of control can increase dental anxiety and fear.
III. Treatment of Dental Anxiety, Fear, and Phobias
    A. The use of relaxation techniques in the dental environment decreases anxiety.

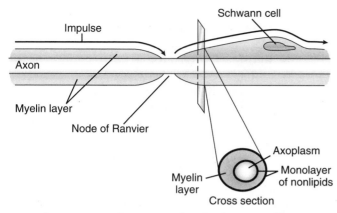

Figure 13.1 Structure of a single nerve fiber.

1. Relaxation techniques include the use of headphones or other distracters, the use of a calming voice, and the use of biofeedback; adhering to a time schedule reduces anxiety.
2. Increasing patient control during treatment sessions decreases the fear of helplessness and increases a sense of trust.
3. Explaining procedures thoroughly decreases the fear of the unknown.

B. Using systemic desensitization (small doses of positive experiences) for highly anxious patients increases their tolerance for dental encounters.

C. Conscious sedation with nitrous oxide and oxygen can increase relaxation (sedation), increase pain threshold (analgesia), decrease the awareness of time (amnesia), and increase a sense of well-being (euphoria).

The Anatomy and Physiology of Peripheral Nerves

The PNS comprises sensory (afferent) nerves that carry sensations of pain to the CNS, and motor (efferent) nerves that transmit messages from the CNS to muscles and glands. An understanding of sensory nerve anatomy and physiology and the action of local anesthetics is essential to the provision of pain management (see Chapter 2).

Sensory Nerves

The sensory nerves are afferent nerves that carry sensations of pain to the CNS.

I. Anatomy of a Nerve
  A. Myelinated nerves (comprise most nerves in the body)
    1. Are divided into three zones.
      a. The dendrite zone (free nerve endings) reacts to stimuli in the tissues.
      b. The axon is the pipeline that delivers impulses to the CNS.
      c. Terminal nerve endings (arborization) synapse with CNS nerves.
  B. Structure of single nerve fiber (Fig. 13–1)
    1. The myelin sheath covers the axon and is composed of approximately 20% proteins and 75% lipids.
      a. The proteins act as channels to allow some ions (Na^+, K^+) to pass through the nerve membrane.
      b. The lipid layers act as barriers to some molecules and as binding sites for lipophilic components of local anesthetics.
    2. The nodes of Ranvier are constrictions that are 0.5 to 3 mm apart; nerve impulses travel from node to node.
  C. Structure of a nerve bundle (Fig. 13–2)
    1. Many peripheral nerves have hundreds to thousands of tightly packed axons in bundles called fasciculi.
    2. Layers of a nerve bundle

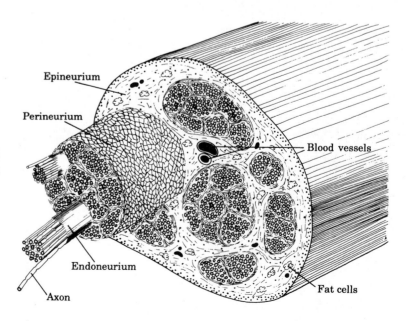

Figure 13.2 Structure of a nerve bundle. (From Jastak, JT, Yagiela, JA, Donaldson D: Local Anesthesia of the Oral Cavity. Philadelphia, WB Saunders, 1995, p. 8.)

a. The epineural sheath is the outer layer; is not a barrier to anesthetics.

b. The epineurium is a connective tissue layer; carries fasciculi, blood vessels, and lymphatic vessels; anesthetic solution diffuses through the epineural sheath and blood vessels begin to eliminate the anesthetic.

c. The perineurium surrounds the fasciculi; is the greatest barrier to a local anesthetic.

d. Fasciculi

1) Mantle bundles, which are on the outside of a nerve bundle, receive anesthetic solution first; innervate proximal areas (molars) and lose anesthetic properties first.

2) Core bundles, which are on the inside of a nerve bundle, receive anesthetic solution last and in a lower concentration due to distance from anesthetic source and more blood vessels; innervate distal areas (anterior teeth) and lose anesthetic properties last.

II. Physiology of a Nerve

A. A nonstimulated nerve has Na^+ ions outside the membrane, K^+ ions and negative ions inside, and a resting potential of -70 mV.

B. Stimulation of a nerve is caused by mechanical (instrument in the soft tissue), chemical, thermal, or electrical means; starts the depolarization process, which permits the movement of ions across the nerve membrane; electrical potential changes from between -50 and -60 mV to $+40$ mV; as electrical potentials change, the impulse moves along the nerve from node to node.

C. Repolarization occurs when Na^+ ions begin to move back across the nerve membrane to increase negative potential inside the nerve; from stimulation to repolarization the process takes approximately 1 msec.

Action of Local Anesthetics

The action of a local anesthetic depends on its chemical structure and the pH of the solution and body tissues.

I. Chemical Formula (Fig. 13–3)

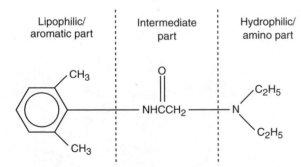

Lipophilic/aromatic part | Intermediate part | Hydrophilic/amino part

Figure 13.3 Chemical formula for a local anesthetic.

A. The aromatic group, also known as the lipophilic (hydro*phobic*) component, has an affinity for the lipid portion of the myelin sheath, which helps the local anesthetic attach to the nerve membrane and block the nerve impulse.

B. The intermediate chain is either an ester (—COO—R) or an amide (NHCO—R) group; determines the mode of biotransformation or metabolism.

1. Esters are hydrolyzed in plasma; leave the system faster and therefore are not as likely to be toxic.

2. Amides are metabolized in the liver; are slower to leave the system and therefore potentially more toxic.

C. The amino end (hydro*philic* component) makes an anesthetic injectable; amides dissolve poorly in water and are unstable on exposure to air, therefore hydrochloride (HCL) is added to produce a salt that is soluble and more stable.

II. pH

A. Definition

1. pH is a mathematical measure of a substance's acidity or alkalinity, expressed as a negative logarithm.

2. Acidic substances have higher concentrations of hydrogen (H+) ions and therefore can give up more H+ ions; alkaline (base) substances have lower concentrations of H+ ions and can accept more H+ ions.

B. The pH of tissues

1. The pH of normal tissue is 7.4.

2. The pH of inflamed tissue is between 5 and 6 (more acidic).

a. Decreased extracellular pH does not decrease nerve action; the internal pH of a nerve is constant.

b. Decreased extracellular pH does decrease the action of an anesthetic.

C. The pH of local anesthetics

1. The pH of an anesthetic without epinephrine (vasoconstrictor) is 5.5.

2. The pH of an anesthetic with epinephrine is approximately 3.3.

a. Manufacturers acidify anesthetics to inhibit the oxidation (breakdown) of epinephrine.

b. Anesthetic solutions may burn on deposition because of the difference between the pH of the solution and the pH of tissues.

c. The more acidic the anesthetic, the slower its onset.

Dissociation of Local Anesthetics

The ability of a local anesthetic to dissociate is indicated by its pK_a number.

I. The pK_a Number

A. Is a constant that characterizes the equilibrium of a particular compound; also measures the molecule's affinity for H$^+$ ions.

B. Equilibrium equation
   1. The pK$_a$ equation: RNH$^+$ $\Leftrightarrow$ RN + H$^+$
   2. The cation: RNH$^+$ is a positively charged molecule that is responsible for binding at the receptor site and decreasing the Na$^+$ that enters the nerve.
   3. The free base: RN is an uncharged molecule that is responsible for the diffusion of anesthetic through surrounding tissues and the nerve sheath.

C. Clinical implications of the pK$_a$ number
   1. Each anesthetic has a pK$_a$ number.
   2. The lower the pK$_a$ number (below 7.5), the more lipophilic free base molecules (creates greater diffusion, quicker onset) but the fewer cations available to bind the anesthetic.
   3. When the pH of an anesthetic is the same as the pK$_a$ number, equal amounts of base and cation exist.

Diffusion, Onset, and Duration of Local Anesthetics

The clinical implications of dissociation are the diffusion, onset, and duration of local anesthetics.

I. Equilibrium Shifts
   A. Shifts left (cation state) when there are more hydrogen ions (low pH).
   B. Shifts right (free base state) when there are fewer hydrogen ions (high pH).

II. The more free base molecules available, the greater the diffusion of anesthetic through tissues and membrane, and therefore the faster the onset of action.

III. The pH of an anesthetic solution is lowered with the addition of epinephrine (pH 3.3).
   A. When more cations exist, more Na$^+$ is bound at the nerve receptor, which creates greater binding power.
   B. Less free base leads to less diffusion and slower onset.
   C. Surrounding tissues buffer more acidic solutions.

IV. The pH of inflamed tissues is low (5 to 6).
   A. More cations exist and therefore more Na$^+$ is bound at the nerve receptor site.
   B. Less diffusion into surrounding tissues causes slower onset or leads to ineffective anesthesia.
   C. Surrounding tissues are not able to buffer more acidic solutions because of the lower pH.

Pharmacology of Local Anesthetics and Vasoconstrictors

Understanding the metabolism, action, dosage calculations, and specific functions of topical and local anesthetics and vasoconstrictors helps the practitioner to use these agents more safely and efficiently (see Chapter 9).

Biotransformation (metabolism)

Ester and amide local anesthetics are metabolized differently, which affects their potential for causing overdose reactions.

I. Types of Local Anesthetics
   A. Esters
      1. Are biotransformed to paraaminobenzoic acid (PABA) in blood plasma by the enzyme pseudocholinesterase.
      2. The half-life (rate at which 50% of the anesthetic is eliminated from the blood) is 2 to 8 minutes.
      3. Have a low potential for overdose (toxicity).
      4. Increased the chance of an allergic reaction to PABA.
   B. Amides
      1. Are biotransformed primarily in the liver.
      2. The half-life is 50 to 120 minutes.
      3. Have a greater potential for overdose because higher blood levels of amides occur (until the anesthetic reaches the liver for biotransformation).
      4. Are less likely to cause an allergic reaction because methylparaben, which causes allergic reaction, has been eliminated as a local anesthetic preservative.

II. Distribution and Elimination of Local Anesthetics
   A. After they enter the blood stream, local anesthetics permeate all body tissues.
   B. Local anesthetics are vasodilators; thus vasoconstrictors are added to decrease vasodilation.
   C. Esters and amides are eliminated mostly through the kidneys.

Systemic Action of Local Anesthetics

Local anesthetics have effects on the CNS, the CVS, and the respiratory system.

I. Effects of Local Anesthetics on the CNS
   A. Low levels have no effect on the CNS but can provide anticonvulsive properties by raising the seizure threshold; are used to treat epileptic seizures.
   B. Preconvulsive levels can elicit slurred speech, shivering, twitching, a flushed feeling, a dream state, lightheadedness, blurred vision, and tinnitus.
      1. Lidocaine may cause mild sedation or drowsiness, which are good indicators of possible toxic reaction.
      2. Therefore, an anesthetized patient should never be left alone, since onset occurs in 5 to 10 minutes.
   C. Convulsive levels elicit convulsions, CNS depression, respiratory depression, and respiratory arrest.

II. Effects of Local Anesthetics on the CVS
  A. Low levels exhibit no effects.
  B. High (non-overdose) levels cause mild hypotension by relaxing smooth muscles.
  C. Overdose levels can produce profound hypotension, which causes decreased myocardial contractions, decreased cardiac output, and decreased peripheral resistance.
  D. Lethal levels exhibit cardiovascular collapse caused by massive peripheral vasodilation, decreased heart contractions, and a decreased heart rate.
III. Effects of Local Anesthetics on the Respiratory System
  A. Non-overdose levels relax the action of bronchial smooth muscles.
  B. Overdose levels can lead to respiratory arrest secondary to CNS depression.

Vasoconstrictor Action

Vasoconstrictors act on alpha and beta receptors in the body tissues, causing the constriction or dilation of blood vessels.
I. Chemical Structure of a Vasoconstrictor (Fig. 13–4)
  A. A benzene ring with two OH groups in the third and fourth positions is a catechol.
  B. A benzene ring with an amine group in another position is a catecholamine.
  C. Most vasoconstrictors are catecholamines.
    1. Epinephrine, norepinephrine, and dopamine occur in nature.
    2. Levonordefrin and isoproterenol are synthetics.
II. Adrenergic Receptors
  A. Are present in most body tissues.
  B. Include two types of receptors:
    1. Alpha (α) activation causes the contraction of smooth muscles in blood vessels.
    2. Beta (β) activation
      a. β_1 activation in the heart and small intestine is responsible for cardiac stimulation and lipolysis.
      b. β_2 activation in the bronchi, vascular beds, and uterus produces bronchodilation and vasodilation.
  C. Most vasoconstrictors that are used in dentistry exert action on adrenergic receptors.
    1. Epinephrine acts on both α and β receptors, but primarily on the latter.
    2. Norepinephrine acts on both α and β receptors, but primarily on the former.

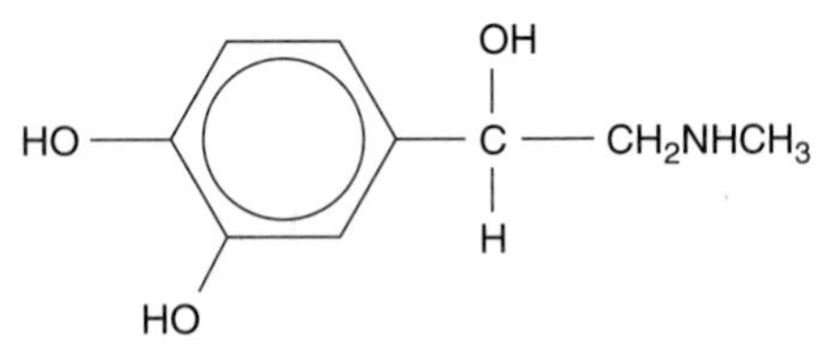

Figure 13.4 Chemical structure of a vasoconstrictor.

    3. Levonordefrin, a synthetic, acts on both α and β receptors, but primarily on the former.
III. Types of Vasoconstrictors
  A. Epinephrine (Adrenalin)
    1. Is the most potent and most widely used in dentistry; is found in both natural and synthetic forms.
    2. In skeletal muscle and blood vessels, epinephrine produces both vasodilation (small amounts act on β_2 sites) and vasoconstriction (large amounts act on α receptors).
  B. Norepinephrine (Levarterenol)
    1. Is one fourth as potent as epinephrine and demonstrates less systemic action.
    2. Is used in other countries with 4% propoxycaine/2% procaine in a 1:30,000 concentration.
      a. The activation of alpha (α) receptors in the smooth muscles of palatal blood vessels can cause ischemia and subsequently tissue necrosis.
      b. Neither norepinephrine or 4% proxycaine/2% procaine are currently used in the United States.
  C. Levonordefrin (Neo-Cobefrin)
    1. Is one fifth as potent as epinephrine and demonstrates less systemic action.
    2. Is used with 2% mepivacaine in a 1:20,000 concentration.
IV. Selection of Vasoconstrictors
  A. Medical considerations that contraindicate the use of vasoconstrictors
    1. Cardiovascular concerns include heart attack within the last 6 months, high blood pressure (> 200/115 mmHg), or daily angina.
    2. Other systemic concerns include patients taking tricyclic antidepressants (neither norepinephrine or levonordefrin should be used) and patients with uncontrolled hyperthyroidism.
  B. Duration of appointment
    1. The addition of a vasoconstrictor increases the length of anesthetic effects.
    2. The concentration and type of vasoconstrictor affect the duration of a local anesthetic.
  C. Hemostasis
    1. A vasoconstrictor should be close to the area of bleeding to be effective.
    2. Epinephrine acts as a vasoconstrictor in large quantities; in smaller quantities it becomes a vasodilator that has the potential to increase bleeding postoperatively.

Dose Calculations (Table 13–1)

Dose calculations for local anesthetics are based on the size and general health of the patient and on the type and concentration of the anesthetic agent and vasoconstrictor.
I. Dose Calculations for Local Anesthetics
  A. Depends on

TABLE 13.1 Local Anesthetic Dose Calculations

Questions

A. How many mg/mL of anesthetic in solution = % grams anesthetic?
B. How many milligrams of local anesthetics are there per cartridge?
C. What is the MRD in cartridges of local anesthetic allowed per patient?
1. To change % grams of local anesthetic to milligrams, first divide by 100, then multiply by 1000.
2. To find milligrams/milliliter of local anesthetics per cartridge multiply by 1.8 mL/cartridge.
3. To find maximum recommended dosage of local anesthetic multiply patient's weight by established MRD in milligram/pound.
4. To find milliliter of anesthetic solution divide by MRD in milligram by milligram/milliliter of local anesthetic solution.
5. To find number of cartridges in MRD milliliter of anesthetic solution by 1.8 mL/cartridge.

Example: Local Anesthetic Dose Calculation: 2% Lidocaine

1. 2% ÷ 100 = .02g × 1000 = 20mg/mL
2. 20 mg/mL × 1.8 mL/cartridge = 36 mg/cartridge
3. 2 mg/lb (MRD/manufacturer) × patient's weight (e.g., 120 lb) = 240 mg MRD/patient
4. 240 mg ÷ 20 mg/mL = 12 mL
5. 12 mL ÷ 1.8 mL/cartridge = 6.7 cartridges
Fast Tip: Eliminate steps 4 and 5 by dividing mg MRD/patient by 36 mg/cartridge.

1. The maximum recommended dosage (MRD) for each anesthetic.
2. The weight of the patient.
3. Anesthetic percentage
B. Calculation (Table 13–1)
II. Concentration of Vasoconstrictors
A. Depends on
1. The ratio of vasoconstrictor to milliliters of solution.
2. The MRD of epinephrine:
a. For the healthy patient is 0.2 mg.
b. For the patient with heart disease is 0.04 mg.
3. The MRD of levonordefrin:
a. For all patients is 1 mg per appointment.
B. Calculation (Table 13–2)

Selection of Local Anesthetics and Vasoconstrictors

Vasoconstrictors and local anesthetics must be chosen carefully, based on the patient's medical concerns and the type of dental procedure to be performed.
I. Selection Considerations
A. Medical concerns (if vasoconstrictor used, see Selection of Vasoconstrictors)

1. True allergy to a local anesthetic is rare.
2. Cardiovascular considerations include heart attack within the last 6 months.
B. Onset and duration
1. The onset is determined by the properties of a local anesthetic, including its dissociation.
2. The duration (short-, medium-, or long-acting) is determined by the site of injection, the type of anesthetic, the addition of a vasoconstrictor, and the patient's idiosyncrasies.
C. Local anesthetics with and without vasoconstrictors
1. Lidocaine is used with a vasoconstrictor and without a vasoconstrictor.
2. Mepivacaine is used with a vasoconstrictor and without a vasoconstrictor.
3. Prilocaine is used with a vasoconstrictor and without a vasoconstrictor.
4. Bupivacaine is used with a vasoconstrictor.
5. Etidocaine is used with a vasoconstrictor.

TABLE 13.2 Calculation of Vasoconstrictor Concentration

Concentration of Vasoconstrictors

1. Ratio = 1 gram of drug to milliliters of solution, therefore, to change grams to milligrams multiply by 1000
2. To find mg of vasoconstrictor drug per mL of solution divide 1000 mg by mL of solution
3. To find mL of solution divide MRD of vasoconstrictor by mg/mL
4. To find number of cartridges divide MRD mL by 1.8 mL/cartridges

Calculation of Concentration of Vasoconstrictors: 1:100,000 Epinephrine/mL of Solution

1. Ratio: 1:100,000 = 1 g of drug per 100,000 mL of solution
2. 1 g = 1000 mg of drug per 100,000 mL of solution
3. 1000 mg ÷ by 100,000 mL = 0.01 mg/mL

Example: Vasoconstrictor Dose Calculation for Healthy Adults and Heart Patients

MRD: Healthy adult: 0.2 mg per 1:100,000 epinephrine
MRD: Heart patient: 0.04 mg per 1:100,000 epinephrine
How many cartridges of anesthetic with epinephrine can a healthy adult have?
   0.2 mg of drug ÷ by 0.01 mg/mL = 20 mL ∴ 20 mL ÷ by 1.8 mL/cartridge = 11.11 cartridges.
How many cartridges of anesthetic with epinephrine can a heart patient have?
   0.04 mg of drug (heart patient) ÷ by 0.01 mg/mL = 4mL
   4 mL ÷ by 1.8 mL/cartridge = 2.2 cartridges
Levonordefrin (Neo-Cobefrin) = 1 mg vasoconstrictor/any patient/visit.

| TABLE 13.3 | Short-Acting Local Anesthetics |

Local Anesthetics	Onset (min)	Duration: Pulp (min)	Duration: Soft Tissue (hr)	Dose/ Cartridge (mg)	MRD/Body Weight (mg/lb)	MRD for Healthy Adult (mg)	Maximum Cartridges
2% Lidocaine HCL	2–3	5–10	1–2	36	2	300	8.3
3% Mepivacaine HCL (Carbocaine)	1.5–2	20–40	2–3	54	2	300	5.5
					3*	400*	7.4*
4% Prilocaine HCL (Citanest, Plain)	2–4	10–20	1.5–2	72	2.7	400	5.5

Data from Malamed, Astra, and Cook-Waite. Revised May 1998.
MRD, Maximum Recommended Dose.
*Manufacturers' recommendation.

Maximum Dosage of Local Anesthetics

Local anesthetics may be short-acting, medium-acting, or long-acting (Tables 13–3, 13–4, and 13–5). An anesthetic is selected based on whether its duration is appropriate to the procedure being performed.

Topical Anesthetics

Topical anesthetics are useful for providing light, localized anesthesia to the first 2 to 3 mm of the mucosa just before the injection of a local anesthetic by means of a needle.

I. Action
   A. Most topical anesthetics are higher concentrations of injectable anesthetics and thereby increase diffusion of the active ingredients through mucous membranes or open wounds to free nerve endings lying 2 to 3 mm below the surface.
      1. Topical anesthetics do not contain vasoconstrictors.
      2. Efficient diffusion leads to faster onset.
      3. Increased water solubility increases diffusion and onset; water insolubility decreases diffusion

| TABLE 13.4 | Medium-Acting Local Anesthetics |

Local Anesthetics	Onset (min)	Duration: Pulp (hrs)	Duration: Soft Tissue (hrs)	Dose/mg Cartridge (mg)	MRD/Body Weight (mg/lb)	MRD for Healthy Adult (mg)	Maximum Cartridges
2% Lidocaine/1:100,000 Epinephrine (Epi)	2–3	55–65	3–5	36	2	300	8.3
					3*	500	13.8*
2% Mepivacaine 1:20,000 Levonordefrin	1.5–2	1–1.5	3–5	36	2	300	8.3
					3*	400*	11*
4% Prilocaine/1:200,000 Epinephrine	2	1–1.5	3–8	72	2.7	400	5.5

Data from Malamed, Astra, and Cook-Waite. Revised May 1998.
*Manufacturers' recommendation.

| TABLE 13.5 | Long-Acting Local Anesthetics |

Local Anesthetics	Onset (min)	Duration: Pulp (hrs)	Duration: Soft Tissue (hrs)	Dose/ Cartridge (mg)	MRD/Body Weight (mg/lb)	MRD for Healthy Adult (mg)	Maximum Cartridges
0.5% Bupivacaine/1:200,000 Epi (Marcaine HCL)	3–10	1–2	5–9	9	0.6	90	10
1.5% Etidocaine/1:100,000 Epi (Duranest HCL)	1.5–3	1.5–2	4–9	27	3.6	400	14.8

Data from Malamed, Astra, and Cook-Waite. Revised May 1998.

and onset but increases duration by retaining the topical anesthetic at the site.

4. Without vasoconstrictors, duration is decreased but the potential for overdose is increased because of the faster uptake of local anesthetic into the bloodstream.

5. Higher concentrations increase the potential for overdose because the uptake of local anesthetic into the vascular system is greater.

II. Types of Topical Anesthetics (Table 13–6)

Armamentarium

Preparing the armamentarium for the delivery of local anesthetics involves knowledge of the syringe, needle, and anesthetic cartridge, proper set-up procedures, care of the equipment, safe handling, and management of associated problems.

Syringe

Dental syringes, which come in a variety of types and sizes, must be maintained with care for proper function.

I. Types of Syringes
   A. Dental syringes that are used most frequently include:
      1. Breech-loading, cartridge-type, aspirating, or nondisposable.
      2. Metal or plastic construction.
      3. Harpoon (Fig. 13–5) or self-aspirating (Fig. 13–6).
         a. Use of the self-aspirating syringe
            1) The metal projection presses on the rubber diaphragm of the cartridge.
            2) Pushing on the thumb disk or pushing forward on the thumb ring increases the pressure of projection on the diaphragm and thereby increases pressure inside the cartridge.
            3) Aspiration occurs when the operator releases the pressure.
   B. Other syringe types
      1. Pressure syringe
         a. Is used for PDL (membrane) injections; permits a measured dose of solution; overcomes tissue resistance.
         b. May cause trauma to tissue and tooth if increased solution (under pressure) is forced into the periodontal membrane space.
      2. Safety syringes (UltraSafe aspirating syringe and Septodont Safety Plus)
         a. Reduce the risk of needlestick injury.
         b. Pose environmental concerns because of disposable plastic.
II. Care and Handling of Syringes
   A. Before use, should be checked for rust, harpoon sharpness, and working piston.

B. All threaded joints should be lubricated periodically.

III. Problems with Syringes
   A. Leakage during injection is caused by offset needle placement into rubber diaphragm or loose needle
   B. Broken cartridge is caused by too much pressure when engaging harpoon or bent harpoon
   C. Disengagement of harpoon during aspiration is caused by dirty, dull, or broken harpoon or harpoon not securely engaged in cartridge rubber stopper

Needles

Needles are stainless steel, disposable, presterilized, and sharp to decrease the potential for cross-contamination.

I. Parts of the Needle (Fig. 13–7)
   A. The bevel is designed to penetrate soft tissue without resistance and is short, long, or multibeveled.
   B. The shank
      1. The length is measured from the tip of the bevel to the hub.
         a. Long shanks range from 1.13 to 1.6 inches or 30 to 40 mm.
         b. Short shanks range from 0.75 to 1.0 inches or 20 to 25 mm.
      2. The gauge is the measure of the inside diameter of the lumen; the larger the number, the smaller the needle.
         a. The standard needle used in dentistry ranges from 25- to 30-gauge.
         b. Smaller needles (30-gauge) deflect more when penetrating tissues, are more likely to show false-negative aspiration, and therefore are used primarily for maxillary palatal injections.
            1) Deflection of the needle in tissues reduces the accuracy of an injection because solution is deposited away from the intended site.
            2) A smaller lumen increases the possibility of clogging the needle with blood cells and showing a false negative aspiration.
         c. Larger needles (25-gauge) are easier to aspirate and are used primarily for mandibular injections.
            1) Produce less defection.
            2) A larger lumen increases true-negative aspiration.
   C. The hub/needle adapter
      1. Because plastic adapters are not prethreaded, the operator must push the needle onto the syringe and then tighten it.
      2. Metal adapters are prethreaded; are tightened by turning gently.

TABLE 13.6 Topical Anesthetics

Topical Anesthetic	Delivery System	Concentration	Onset of Action	Duration	Side Effects/ Contraindications	Benefits
ESTERS						
Benzocaine: Hurricaine Cetacaine	Liquid, gel, ointment, or spray	6% to 20% (20% typically is used before injection)	30 seconds with 20% strength	5 to 15 minutes	No toxic effects; Contraindicated in patients with allergy to esters	Quick onset of action
Tetracaine: Cetacaine	Liquid, ointment, or spray	0.2% to 2%	2 minutes	45 to 60 minutes	Potential for toxicity due to high solubility in water (maximum dose = 20 mg for healthy adult)	Rapidly absorbed; most appropriate for small areas
AMIDES						
Lidocaine base: Alphacaine Xylocaine	Ointment or spray	5% ointment; 10% spray	Dissolves poorly in water; may take as long as 3 minutes	15 minutes	No toxic effects; contraindicated in patients with allergy to amides	Can be used on non-intact tissues (abraded or ulcerated)
Lidocaine hydrochloride: Lidocaine	Liquid or gel	4% or 5% liquid; 2% or 5% gel	Water soluble; approximately 2 minutes	15 minutes	Potentially more toxic due to higher water solubility; contraindicated in patients with allergy to amides	Quicker onset than lidocaine base topical anesthetics
Lidocaine transoral delivery system: DentiPatch	Mucoadhesive patch	10% or 20% 46.1 mg/patch (2 cm²)	5 to 15 minutes	45 minutes	Tissue reactions occur at site; contraindicated in patients with allergy to amides	Lower blood level concentrations
EMLA: Eutectic mixture of local anesthetics	Cream	5% (with 25 mg lidocaine and 25 mg prilocaine)	5 to 30 minutes	30 to 40 minutes	Minimal toxic effects; contraindicated in patients with allergy to amides	Oil-in-water emulsion that provides intact skin anesthesia
KETONE						
Dyclonine hydrochloride: Dyclone	Liquid	0.5% or 1%	2 minutes	30 to 60 minutes	Can be irritating to tissues at application site; children require smaller doses	Can be used by patients with allergies to esters or amides

HARPOON ASPIRATING SYRINGE

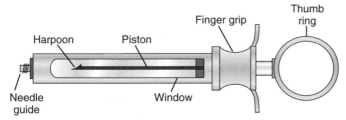

Figure 13.5 Harpoon aspirating syringe.

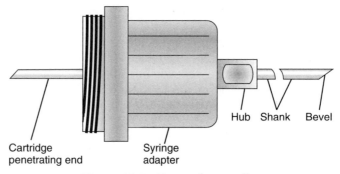

Figure 13.7 Parts of a needle.

3. Some needle adapters have bevel indicator dots (e.g., ACCUJET by Astra).
D. The cartridge-penetrating end is sharp and is produced with or without a bevel to penetrate the rubber diaphragm of the cartridge.
E. A plastic casing with an intact seal indicates an unused needle; the cap is used to recap the needle by means of the scoop technique.

Cartridges

Anesthetic cartridges are glass containers that hold anesthetic solution for placement in the dental syringe.
I. Components (Fig. 13–8)
   A. The cylindrical glass tube holds 1.8 mL of solution.
   B. The rubber stopper
      1. Is coated with silicone to ease movement.
      2. Is engaged by the harpoon.
      3. Is pushed by the piston to dispel solution.
      4. Is color-coded by the manufacturer to distinguish types of anesthetic solutions.
   C. The aluminum cap holds the rubber diaphragm in place.
   D. The rubber diaphragm acts as a seal to prevent anesthetic from leaking around the needle, as long as the needle penetrates the diaphragm squarely and not on an angle.
II. Contents
   A. HCL (hydrochloride) is added to a local anesthetic to create an acidic salt for better water solubility; increases diffusion of the anesthetic to the nerve; makes the anesthetic solution injectable.

B. A vasoconstrictor, when added, increases the duration of the drug and decreases the potential for overdose.
C. Sodium bisulfite is an antioxidant that is added to preserve the vasoconstrictor by reacting with oxygen to produce sodium bisulfate (sodium bisulfate is more acidic and therefore increases burning during injection).
D. Sodium chloride is added to make the solution more isotonic with soft tissues.
E. Distilled water provides the remaining volume.
III. Care and Handling of Cartridges
   A. Read drug package insert and cartridge label.
   B. Local anesthetics that contain vasoconstrictors have a shelf-life of 18 months; without vasoconstrictors the shelf-life is 24 months.
   C. To maintain viable anesthetic solutions, do not autoclave, soak cartridges in disinfectant, or keep cartridges in direct sunlight or in warmers.
IV. Problems with Cartridges
   A. Bubbles in a cartridge that are small (1 to 2 mm) are acceptable; however, larger bubbles may mean that the solution was frozen, which causes chemical changes.
   B. An extruded stopper can be caused by freezing the cartridge or by storing it in a disinfectant.
   C. Burning during injection is a normal response to the pH of the drug; however, cartridges containing

SELF-ASPIRATING SYRINGE

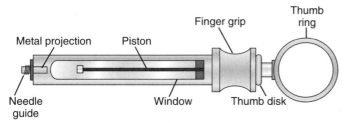

Figure 13.6 Self-aspirating syringe.

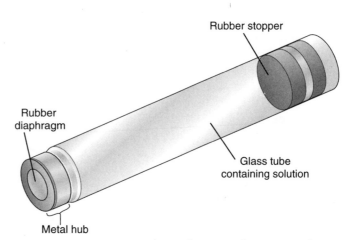

Figure 13.8 Components of an anesthetic cartridge.

disinfectant or vasoconstrictors and overheating can cause burning during injection.

D. A sticky stopper is not common with the use of a silicone lubricant; however, cartridges that are cold may cause difficulty in stopper movement.

E. A corroded or rusty cap can be caused by cartridge breakage in a round tin container (10-cartridge blister packs decrease breakage) or by immersion in disinfectant (metal cap in solution).

Preparation of the Armamentarium

It is important to properly assemble the armamentarium for the local anesthetic injection before the injection. This involves the proper selection of equipment, anesthetic, and vasoconstricting agents, the proper assembly of the syringe and needle, and preparation of the injection site.

I. Preinjection
   A. Review the patient's medical history for contraindications, determine the appropriate anesthetic solutions, and check the patient's blood pressure.
   B. Review the patient treatment plan for injections to be performed to determine appropriate needle lengths and anesthetic solutions.

II. Armamentarium Set-Up
   A. Select the appropriate syringe (harpoon, self-aspirating, or pressure).
   B. Select the appropriate cartridge.
      1. According to patient treatment and medical needs.
      2. According to date and physical appearance; should have no large bubbles, a clear color, a rust/corrosion-free cap, and a rubber stopper without needle punctures.
   C. Select the appropriate needle according to scheduled injections.
   D. Place hemostat or locking cotton pliers on tray for potential retrieval of a broken needle.
   E. Select appropriate topical anesthetic and amount (large doses can produce toxicity).

III. Syringe Set-Up
   A. Place cartridge in the syringe; subsequently place the needle in the syringe so that the cartridge penetrating end passes through the diaphragm and into the anesthetic solution.
   B. Engage the harpoon in the rubber stopper with firm, gentle motions (the self-aspirating syringe has no harpoon).
   C. Rotate the needle bevel so that on penetration it faces the bone, to prevent scraping the periosteum.
   D. Dispel some solution to ensure correct needle placement in the cartridge.
   E. Aspirate to ensure that the harpoon is engaged (for harpoon syringe only).
   F. Remove bubbles from the cartridge.

IV. Site Preparation
   A. Inspect site for lesions (avoid lesions if present).

B. Dry tissues with a patting motion to decrease abrasions.

C. Place the topical anesthetic for at least 1 minute; subsequently wipe gently.

Clinical Case STUDY

During an initial dental hygiene appointment, the dental hygienist observes blood in a cartridge (positive aspiration) while administering an inferior alveolar nerve (IAN) block (2% lidocaine with 1:100,000 epinephrine). A large amount of blood fills the cartridge quickly. Tom, a 35-year-old engineer and a patient with AAP case type-III periodontitis, reports no medical conditions and exhibits no significant need for dental restoration.

Clinical Case QUESTIONS

1. What is the most likely cause of the positive aspiration?
2. How should the dental hygienist handle this situation?
3. Are positive aspirations preventable?

Clinical Case RATIONALES

1. If the tip of the needle is located in a large artery during aspiration, blood will quickly flow into the cartridge. The artery that is most likely to be penetrated is the inferior alveolar artery. Veins are more passive and typically cause blood to enter the cartridge more slowly and in smaller amounts.

2. The dental hygienist should stop the injection and remove the syringe from the patient's mouth. The cartridge should be changed and the injection should be repeated. If the positive aspiration is small enough so that the operator can see if more blood enters the cartridge on a second aspiration, indicating a blood vessel was punctured, the operator may proceed with the injection without changing the cartridge.

3. No, the purpose of choosing a needle with appropriate lumen size is for the very purpose of getting a positive aspiration when the needle inadvertently enters a blood vessel. For patient safety, the dental hygienist must prevent the deposition of solution in a blood vessel while administering an anesthetic in a vascular area. This is accomplished by continually aspirating and checking for blood in the cartridge before and during the injection process, especially in highly vascular areas.

Safety

The safe delivery of local anesthetics depends on a thorough knowledge of proper injection techniques, signs of overdose or allergy, and the proper handling and disposal of equipment.

I. During Treatment
   A. Injection technique
      1. Keep the syringe out of the patient's view.
      2. The window should face the operator to ensure the ability to see positive aspirations.
         a. Blood that enters the cartridge may indicate that the needle has entered a blood vessel.
         b. Blood that enters the cartridge may indicate that the needle is in hematoma-induced, blood-filled tissue.
      3. Change the needle when barbed, or after several injections, because the needle becomes dull.
      4. Ensure the correct point and depth of penetration; to prevent the loss of a broken needle, do not bury the hub in soft tissue.
      5. Aspirate a harpoon syringe by retracting the piston/harpoon; aspirate a self-aspirating syringe by pushing forward and then releasing pressure.
      6. Aspirate in two planes to ensure that the needle has not entered a blood vessel and drawn up the vessel wall during aspiration; it may lead to a false-negative aspiration.
      7. Inject slowly, at the rate of approximately 1 minute per cartridge, to decrease the potential for overdose.
      8. Deposit the appropriate amount of anesthetic, according to the patient's treatment plan.
      9. Evaluate the success of the injection; if necessary, repeat the injection with appropriate adjustments.
      10. Observe aseptic technique; avoid touching nonsterile surfaces or picking up debris (gauze) on the needle.
      11. Use the scoop technique or other needle holders to recap the needle to decrease the potential for needlestick injuries.
   B. Monitor the patient during and after injection for signs of adverse reactions.
      1. Allergic reactions must be handled immediately, according to protocol.
      2. Overdose (toxicity) reactions must be handled according to protocol.
      3. For the treatment or prevention of vasodepressor syncope (the most common adverse reaction), the patient should be placed in a supine position.
   C. Dispose of the needle/cartridge in an appropriate sharps container (cartridges are biohazardous waste because they contain aspirated body fluids, including blood).
II. Posttreatment Chart Entry
   A. Record health history findings including blood pressure and pulse rate including regularity.
   B. Record the type of injection, including the type and amount of anesthetic solution that was administered. Record any complications that need immediate or delayed attention (e.g., hematoma or trismus).

Injection Technique

Appropriate injection techniques are based on the teeth that must be anesthetized and the anatomical landmarks of the area.

Anatomy

The maxillary and mandibular divisions of the trigeminal nerve often are landmarks for local dental anesthesia (see Chapter 3).

I. Maxillary Division of the Trigeminal Nerve (CNV_2) (Fig. 13–9)
   A. The maxillary division exits the cranium via the foramen rotundum; in the pterygopalatine fossa, it divides into three branches.
      1. The pterygopalatine nerve gives rise to the greater palatine and nasopalatine nerves.
      2. The zygomatic nerve supplies the zygomatic arch and skin on the side of the forehead.
      3. The superior alveolar nerve gives off the posterior superior alveolar nerve before entering the infraorbital canal; subsequently it passes through the infraorbital canal, giving off two branches (the middle superior alveolar and anterior superior alveolar nerves) before the terminating branches pass through the infraorbital foramen.
   B. All maxillary division nerves are sensory nerves.
   C. The maxillary cortical plate is thin; allows local anesthetic solution to penetrate through the cortical plate to anesthetize the maxillary nerves.
II. Mandibular Division of the Trigeminal Nerve (CNV_3) (Figs. 13–10 and 13–11)
   A. The mandibular division exits the cranium via the foramen ovale; in the infratemporal fossa, it separates into anterior and posterior divisions.
   B. The mandibular division contains both sensory and motor nerves.
      1. The anterior division is primarily motor; innervates muscles of mastication; the only sensory nerve is the buccal nerve.
      2. The posterior division is primarily sensory; contains only two motor branches.
         a. Sensory branches include the lingual nerve and the IAN with its terminal branches being the incisive and the mental nerves.
         b. Motor branches include the mylohyoid and anterior digastric nerves.
   C. The mandibular cortical plate is thicker than that of the maxillary cortical plate, especially in the posterior region; block injections are more successful than infiltrations in this region.

Maxillary Technique

Maxillary injection techniques include those of the posterior superior, middle superior, and anterior superior

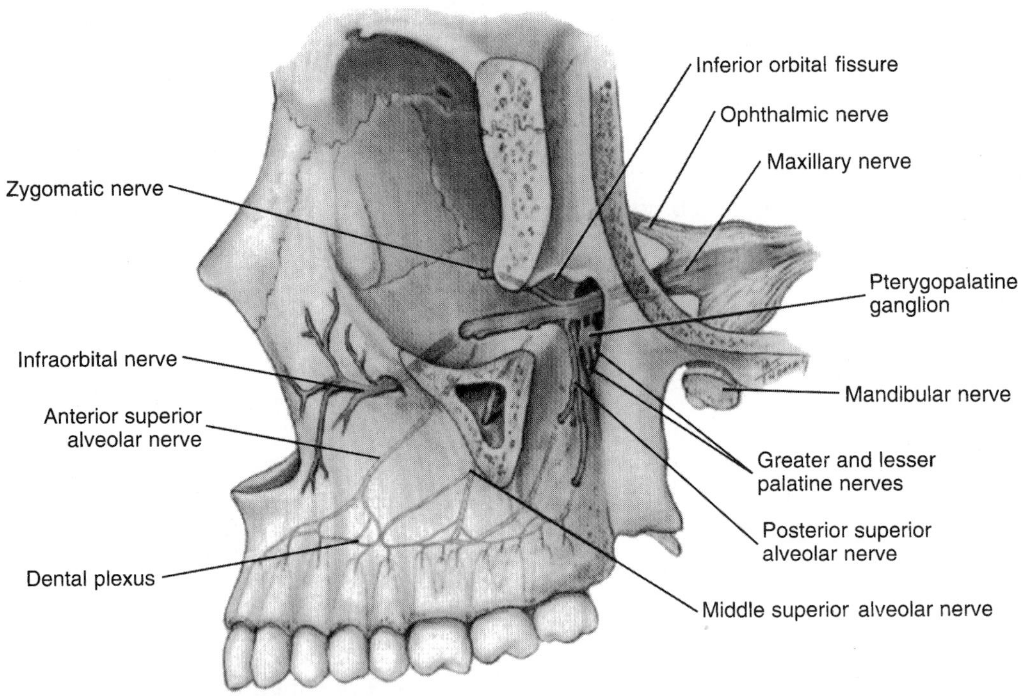

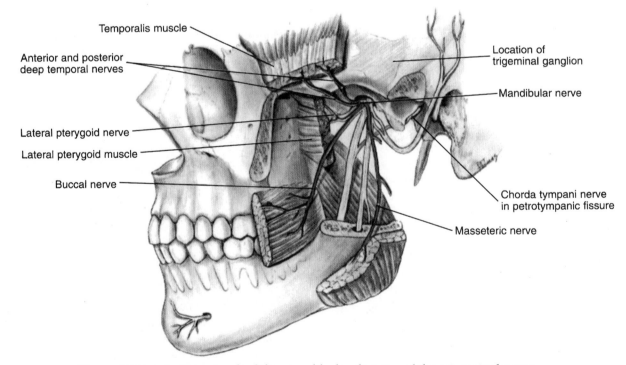

Figure 13.9 Maxillary division of the trigeminal nerve. (From Fehrenbach MJ, Herring SW: Illustrated Anatomy of the Head and Neck. Philadelphia, WB Saunders, 1996, p. 201.)

Figure 13.10 Anterior trunk of the mandibular division of the trigeminal nerve. (From Fehrenbach MJ, Herring SW: Illustrated Anatomy of the Head and Neck. Philadelphia, WB Saunders, 1996, p. 204.)

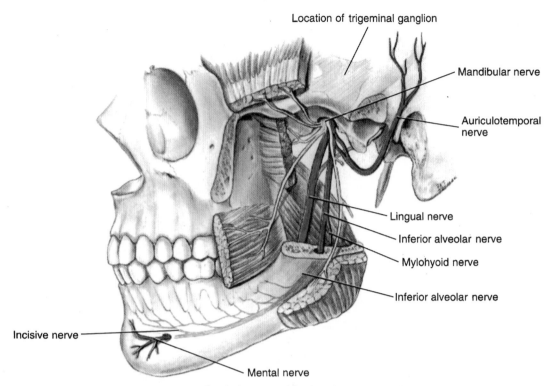

Figure 13.11   Posterior trunk of the mandibular division of the trigeminal nerve. (From Fehrenbach MJ, Herring SW: Illustrated Anatomy of the Head and Neck. Philadelphia, WB Saunders, 1996, p. 205.)

alveolar injections and the greater palatine, nasopalatine, and anterior middle superior alveolar injections.

I. Guide to Maxillary Injections (Table 13–7)

II. Injection Technique Complications

A. Of the posterior superior alveolar (PSA) nerve block

   1. May include inappropriate anesthesia or failure of anesthesia.

     a. Mandibular anesthesia occurs when the vertical angle (45 degrees to the occlusal plane) is too close to zero degrees (flat).

     b. Infiltration occurs when the horizontal angle (45 degrees to the midsagittal plane) is too close to zero degrees (flat).

     c. A deposition site that is too shallow decreases the anesthetic effect.

   2. A deposition site that is too deep increases the potential for hematoma caused by entering the pterygoid plexus of veins.

B. Of the middle superior alveolar (MSA) and anterior superior alveolar (ASA) nerve blocks

   1. MSA and ASA nerve blocks may cause soft tissue anesthesia without pulpal anesthesia when the deposition sites are either too coronal or too far away from the cortical plate.

   2. Pain occurs when the needle hits the zygomatic arch or the nasal spine.

C. Of the greater palatine (GP) and nasopalatine (NP) nerve blocks

   1. A greater palatine nerve block may cause soft palate anesthesia when the deposition site is too posterior and the lesser palatine nerve is inadvertently anesthetized.

   2. A nasopalatine nerve block (only dental nerve block that anesthetizes both right and left sides of mouth) may provide palatal soft tissue anesthesia on only one side of the maxillary anterior teeth, or may fail to provide anesthesia when penetration is too shallow.

   3. Palatal tissue is very tightly adapted to underlying bone, thus the injection of even small amounts of anesthetic solution is difficult or painful; the solution that drips from the site of injection has a bad taste.

III. Anterior Middle Superior Alveolar (AMSA) nerve block (palatal approach)

A. Areas that are anesthetized by the AMSA nerve block include the pulp and palatal soft tissue of the teeth from the bicuspids to the midline.

B. Administration of the anesthetic is best accomplished using The Wand, but traditional syringe systems can be used.

   1. The penetration site for the extra-short 30-gauge needle is just distal to the first premolar

TABLE 13.7 Guide to Maxillary Injections

Injection Techniques	Posterior Superior Alveolar (PSA)	Middle Superior Alveolar (MSA)	Anterior Superior Alveolar (ASA)	Infiltration	Greater Palatine (GP)	Nasopalatine (NP)
Anatomy anesthetized	Molars (all but mb root 1st molar); pulpal and buccal soft tissue	Premolars, pulpal and buccal soft tissue, and mb root 1st molars	Canine, lateral, central; pulpal and buccal soft tissue	Single tooth; pulpal and buccal soft tissue	Premolars and molars; lingual soft tissue only	Cuspids, laterals, centrals bilaterally; lingual soft tissue only
Needle gauge and length	25- or 27-gauge; short	27-gauge; short	27-gauge; short	27-gauge; short	27-gauge; short	27-gauge; short
Depth of penetration	1/2 to 3/4 short needle (12–19 mm)	1/4–1/2 short needle (12 mm)	1/4–1/2 short needle (12 mm)	Depth to above apex	3–5 mm	2–3 mm
Landmarks	Distal buccal root, maxillary 2nd molar, height of mucobuccal fold, zygomatic arch	Height of mucobuccal fold, maxillary bicuspids	Canine eminence, mucobuccal fold, lateral, canine	Mucobuccal fold, long axis of tooth	Mid-saggital suture, gingival margin, palatal fat pad, 1st and 2nd molars	Incisive papilla
Site of penetration	Distal buccal 2nd molar, 45° to occlusal plane and 45° to mid-sagittal plane	Above 2nd premolars at height of mucobuccal fold	Above lateral, angled toward canine fossa	Above tooth to be anesthetized	Between 1st and 2nd molars, half way between gingival margin and mid-sagittal suture	Side of incisive papilla
Site of deposition	Posterior surface of maxilla	Above premolars	In canine fossa	Apex of tooth	Just anterior to greater palatine foramen	Just anterior to nasopalatine foramen
Cartridge amount 1.8 mL cartridge	1.3 mL (3/4 cartridge)	0.45 mL (1/4 cartridge)	0.45 mL (1/4 cartridge)	0.45 mL (1/4 cartridge)	0.45 mL (1/4 cartridge) or until blanching	0.3 mL or until blanching
Complications	Trismus of lateral pterygoid; hematoma; mandibular anesthesia if angle too flat	Pain, if needle hits zygoma	Hematoma of anterior facial vein; hitting nasal spine	Inadequate pulpal anesthesia if below apex of tooth or too far away from cortical plate	Ballooning of tissues; anesthesia of soft palate (lessor palatine nerve)	Pain
Advantages	Atraumatic, high rate of success; fewer injections	No fear of eye damage	Easy technique	Easy technique; anesthetizes only one tooth	Minimizes both volume and needle penetration	Minimizes both volume and needle penetration
Disadvantages	Hematoma; trismus; may require two injections	Nerve not present in 28% of population	Discomfort; may hit nasal spine	Not a good substitute for block anesthesia of quadrant	Soft palate may be anesthetized; swallowing is difficult; discomfort	Discomfort; solution is difficult to place

on the palatal aspect, and is midway between the gingival margin and the mid-palatine suture.
2. With the bevel toward the palatal tissue, the needle is inserted until it touches bone.
3. 0.6 mL of anesthetic solution is administered.
4. Tissue will blanch; the injection must be stopped if tissue in the area looses all pink color.

C. Buccal soft tissue in the area may be anesthetized but not the lip and muscles of facial expression.
D. A very shallow injection at the height of the mucobuccal fold may be necessary to anesthetize buccal soft tissue.

 ## Clinical Case STUDY

Alison, a 30-year-old woman, presents in the dental office for extensive root debridement therapy. She has had very limited dental care. Her periodontal assessments reveal AAP case type-III periodontitis with moderate inflammation and generalized 4- to 6-mm pocket depths. Only three small caries are noted. There are no significant medical considerations. The dental hygienist begins the periodontal treatment appointment by administering the right IAN, lingual nerve, and long buccal nerve blocks. When the dental hygienist proceeds with root debridement in the lower right quadrant, tooth #30 is sensitive to both hand and ultrasonic instrumentation. All other teeth in the quadrant exhibit profound anesthesia.

Clinical Case QUESTIONS

1. What is the most likely cause of the sensitivity in tooth #30?
2. Identify the most effective ways to handle this sensitivity.
3. What should the dental hygienist do to prevent this situation in the future?
4. Identify other major causes of mandibular anesthesia failure.

Clinical Case RATIONALES

1. The most likely cause is accessory sensory nerve innervation (of the mylohyoid nerve). The mylohyoid nerve branches off V_3 superior to the mandibular foramen. This nerve runs down and forward along the mylohyoid groove on the medial surface of the mandible. Terminal branches may penetrate the ramus to innervate the posterior mandibular teeth.
2. An alternative mandibular block, such as the Gow-Gates (G-G) technique, may be used to anesthetize the mylohyoid nerve, which can give accessory innervation to the mandibular molars—especially the mesial root of the mandibular first molar.

3. Prevention includes taking a thorough dental history and recording the sensitivity in the patient treatment record for subsequent appointments. The accessory sensory innervation may be bilateral.
4. Other major causes of mandibular anesthesia failure include anatomical variations, infections, needle deviation, and improper type, placement, or amount of anesthetic.

Mandibular Technique

Mandibular techniques of local dental anesthesia include inferior alveolar, lingual, mental, and buccal nerve blocks.
I. Guide to Mandibular Injections (Table 13–8)
II. Injection Technique Complications
   A. Of the inferior alveolar nerve/lingual nerve (IAN/L) block
      1. May include inappropriate anesthesia or failure of anesthesia.
         a. Deposition sites that are too low (below mandibular foramen) decrease the anesthetic effect.
         b. Deposition sites that are too shallow (outside of pterygomandibular space) decrease the anesthetic effect to the IAN but may anesthetize the lingual nerve.
         c. The IAN/L nerve block may be successful except for the mandibular first molar, which may receive innervation from the mylohyoid or accessory nerves; this problem may be corrected with the use of a PDL injection or the G-G technique.
         d. Crossover innervation from the opposite side can be eliminated by means of a PDL injection or opposite mental injection.
      2. Touching a nerve during penetration causes the patient to react (sudden movement); the operator should reassure the patient while redirecting the needle.
         a. When the lingual nerve is touched during penetration, the operator should stop and subsequently question the patient regarding "tingling" sensations down the tongue.
         b. When the IAN is touched during penetration, the operator should stop and subsequently question the patient regarding "tingling" sensations down the jaw.
            1) If bone is contacted after the penetration of less than half of the long needle, the affected structure most likely is the internal oblique ridge; the operator should back off, bring the syringe over the anterior teeth, continue to penetrate until beyond the ridge, reposition over the opposite bicuspids, and continue to penetrate to the IAN site while injecting.

TABLE 13.8 Guide to Mandibular Injections

Injection Technique	Inferior Alveolar Nerve/Lingual (IAN/L)	Buccal (B)	Incisive/Mental (I/M) Combination	Gow-Gates (G-G)	Akinosi (AK)	Periodontal Ligament (PDL)
Anatomy anesthetized	(IAN): Molars to midline; pulpal, buccal soft tissue; premolars to incisors; (L): lingual soft tissue	Molars: buccal soft tissue only	(I): Premolars to midline, pulpal, (M): buccal soft tissue, lower lip and chin	Molars to midline, pulpal and buccal/ling soft tissue, mylohyoid, auriculotemporal	Molars to midline, pulpal buccal/lingual soft tissue, mylohyoid nerve	Pulpal and soft tissue and nerve endings in area of injection
Needle gauge and length	25- or 27-gauge; long	27-gauge; short or long	27-gauge; short or long	27-gauge; long	27-gauge; long	30-gauge; short, extra short, or ultra short
Depth of penetration	25 mm (3/4 long needle)	a: 2–3 mm; b: 2–6 mm	2–5 mm	25–30 mm (3/4 long needle to before hub)	25 mm (3/4 long needle)	Base of pocket until resistance is met
Landmarks	Contralateral bicuspids, pterygomandibular raphe, occlusal plane	Occlusal plane, external oblique ridge, coronoid notch, buccal cusps	Mental foramen, height of mucobuccal fold	Mesial lingual cusp of 2nd maxillary molar, tragus of ear, head/neck of condyle	Mucogingival junction, external oblique ridge	Pocket area, mesial or distal of root
Site of penetration	Between internal oblique ridge and pterygomandibular raphe, at height of coronoid notch	a: Medial to external oblique ridge at height of coronoid notch; b: In facial vestibule, lateral to ramus at or below level of buccal cusps	Between 1st molar and 2nd bicuspid (slightly distal to mental foramen)	Distal to terminal molar at height of ML cusp of 2nd molar	Distal to terminal molar at height of mucogingival junction	Long axis of root on mesial or distal with bevel toward root
Deposition site	Above mandibular foramen	a: Retromolar triangle; b: Lateral to ramus or in buccal triangle	Distal to mental foramen	Lateral region of condylar neck	Medial of ramus, higher than IAN and lower than G-G	Base of pocket
Cartridge amount (1.8 mL/cartridge)	1.5 to 1.8 mL	0.45 mL (1/4 cartridge)	0.9 mL (1/2 cartridge)	1.8 to 3.6 mL	1.5 to 1.8 mL	0.2 mL
Complications	Transient facial paralysis; high + aspiration; trismus of medial pterygoid muscle; hematoma	Bone discomfort in response to touch, ballooning tissues	Ballooning of tissues; hematoma of mental blood vessels	Failure to connect with condylar neck; deposition of solution in masseter muscle	Hitting ramus or alveolar bone	Pain; injection pain if solution deposited too rapidly
Advantages	Single penetration permits quadrant treatment	Easy technique; many methods of injection; high success rate	High success rate; good for crossover innervation	Single injection for IAN, L, and LB; used for accessory nerve innervation	Single injection for IAN, L, LB; useful when mouth cannot open	Minimal dose required; no unnecessary structures anesthetized
Disadvantages	Hematoma; low success rate (85%); may require two injections	More uncomfortable if bone is touched	May balloon tissue or cause hematoma	Difficult to see landmarks	Difficult to see penetration site	Leakage of anesthetic; difficult to deposit with nonpressure syringe

2) If bone is contacted after penetration of less than half to three quarters of the long needle, the affected structure most likely is the lingula; the operator should back off, redirect the needle, continue to penetrate until past the lingula, reposition the syringe over the opposite bicuspids, continue to penetrate, and inject when the IAN site is reached.

3) If bone is contacted after penetration of three quarters or more of the long needle, the affected structure most likely is the medial surface of the ramus; the operator should back off and inject.

3. When a patient has trismus of the medial pterygoid muscle (mastication) and cannot open his or her mouth, the Akinosi technique is recommended.

Complications

Several complications of local anesthetic use or technique are possible. Some cause systemic difficulties, such as allergy or overdose, and others are local, such as needle breakage or trismus (see Chapter 14).

Systemic Complications

Systemic complications of local anesthetic/vasoconstrictor use include overdose, allergy, and syncope.

I.   Types of Adverse Drug Reactions
   A. Reactions caused directly by the effects of drugs include side effects and overdose.
   B. A reaction may be caused by a sensitivity that is unique to the patient because of:
      1. Disease (e.g., methemoglobinemia).
      2. Emotional disturbance (e.g., psychogenic syncope).
      3. Allergy to the local anesthetic (rare).
II. Factors in Local Anesthetic Overdose (toxicity)
   A. Patient factors include age, weight, sex (e.g., pregnancy), disease, and genetics (e.g., deficient pseudocholinesterase).
   B. Drug factors include vasoactivity, concentration of the anesthetic, dose, route of administration, rate of injection, vascularity of the site, and the presence of a vasoconstrictor.
III. Causes of Local Anesthetic Overdose
   A. A total dose that is too large; the dose is determined by a patient's weight, physical status, and age.
   B. Rapid absorption into the blood; the rate of absorption is decreased by the use of a vasoconstrictor.
   C. Intravascular injection; occurs most often (in both veins and arteries) with IAN and PSAN blocks; operator must be sure to aspirate and inject slowly (60 sec/mL).

D. Slow biotransformation (>30 minutes); is caused by systemic diseases such as atypical pseudocholinesterase and liver disorders.
   E. Slow elimination (>30 minutes); is caused by renal dysfunction.
IV. Mild to Moderate Overdose
   A. Signs and symptoms include talkativeness, excitedness, slurred speech, apprehension, stutter, muscle twitching, increased blood pressure, increased heart rate, increased respiration, lightheadedness, dizziness, inability to focus, tinnitus, drowsiness, and disorientation.
   B. Treatment includes reassuring the patient, administering oxygen (prevents acidosis), and monitoring vital signs; if the operator is appropriately trained, may include performing venipuncture and administering diazepam (anticonvulsant) slowly (5 mg per minute); if the reaction is delayed, the patient's hepatic and renal functions should be checked; the cause should be determined before anesthetics are given again.
V.   Moderate to High Overdose
   A. Signs and symptoms include seizures, decreased blood pressure, decreased heart rate, unconsciousness with or without convulsive seizures, and CNS depression that leads to respiratory depression.
   B. The most likely cause is intravascular injection of the local anesthetic.
   C. Treatment includes placing the patient in a supine position, protecting the patient from convulsive injury, maintaining basic life support (BLS), and administering oxygen; if the operator is appropriately trained, may include injecting anticonvulsants and vasopressors.
VI. Epinephrine Overdose
   A. Signs and symptoms include:
      1. Fear, anxiety, tenseness, restlessness, headache, tremor, perspiration, weakness, dizziness, pallor, and respiratory difficulty.
      2. Increased blood pressure and heart rate and possible cardiac dysrhythmias, including tachycardia and fibrillation.
   B. Likely causes include:
      1. A concentration of epinephrine that is too high (the optimum safe concentration is 1:100,000 or lower).
      2. Administering too much epinephrine at one time (gingival retraction cord).
      3. Injecting an anesthetic with epinephrine into a blood vessel.
   C. Treatment
      1. No treatment is necessary if the overdose is short in duration.
      2. If an epinephrine overdose is prolonged, terminate the procedure, seat the patient upright to decrease CVS effects, reassure the patient,

and give oxygen (unless the patient is hyper-ventilating).

VII. Allergy to Local Anesthetics
   A. Signs and symptoms
      1. Dermatologic
         a. Urticaria, including wheels (smooth patches) and itching
         b. Angioedema (i.e., localized swelling)
      2. Respiratory
         a. Bronchial asthma is a classic sign; includes respiratory distress, dyspnea, wheezing, flushing, cyanosis, perspiration, tachycardia, and anxiety.
         b. Laryngeal edema; associated swelling can block the upper airway.
   B. Causes of local anesthetic allergy
      1. Allergy is a hypersensitive state caused by exposure and subsequent reexposure to an allergen.
      2. Individuals are more likely to experience allergic reactions to esters than to amides because esters breakdown into PABA.
         a. Many people are allergic to PABA.
         b. Sodium bisulfite (an antioxidant) is used to preserve epinephrine.
      3. Topical ester anesthetics have allergy potential because they breakdown into PABA.
   C. Treatment of Allergies
      1. Assume the presence of an allergy until it is disproved.
      2. Postpone routine care until the cause is known.
      3. Refer the patient to an allergist if necessary.
      4. Use amides for patients who are allergic to esters.
      5. Immediate allergic reaction (occurs in less than 60 minutes)
         a. Administer 0.3 mL epinephrine (1:1000) intramuscularly (IM) or IV every 5 minutes as needed.
         b. Administer 50 mg diphenhydramine hydrochloride (antihistamine) IM or IV once allergic reaction subsides. Helps prevent relapse.
         c. Observe the patient for at least 60 minutes.
         d. Obtain a medical consult before discharging the patient.
      6. Delayed reaction (occurs after 60 minutes)
         a. Administer 50 mg diphenhydramine hydrochloride IM, or prescribe tablets (50 mg qid for 3 or 4 days).
         b. Obtain a medical consult.

Local Complications

Needle breakage, hematoma, pain, paresthesia, lip chewing, facial nerve paralysis, and trismus are some of the complications of dental local anesthesia.

I. Needle Breakage (occurs rarely with the use of disposable needles)

   A. Causes
      1. Sudden movement, especially when the hub is in tissue.
      2. Smaller gauge needles (30-gauge) break more easily.
      3. Bent needles break more easily.
   B. Prevention
      1. Use larger gauge (27- or 25-gauge) needles.
      2. Do not bury the hub.
      3. Do not redirect the needle inside tissue.
   C. Management includes the use of a hemostat or locking cotton plier to remove the broken needle from tissue; an embedded needle may require referral to an oral surgeon.

II. Pain or Burning When Penetrating or Injecting Anesthetic Solution
   A. Causes
      1. Careless technique or a callous attitude.
      2. A dull needle or multiple injections.
      3. Rapid deposition of the anesthetic.
      4. Difference between the pH of tissues and that of the anesthetic and vasoconstrictor.
      5. Contamination of cartridges with alcohol or sterilants.
      6. Anesthetic is too cold.
   B. Prevention
      1. Employ proper technique.
      2. Use topical anesthetics before penetration.
      3. Replace barbed needles.
      4. Use sharp needles.
      5. Inject slowly.
      6. Use anesthetics at appropriate temperatures.

III. Persistent Anesthesia (paresthesia)
   A. Causes
      1. Trauma caused by a solution that is contaminated (e.g., with alcohol) or by needles.
      2. Pressure caused by excessive bleeding at the site of injection
   B. Prevention
      1. Includes the use of proper technique and the proper handling of cartridges.
   C. Management
      1. Reassure the patient.
      2. Explain that the affected area is likely to require 2 to 12 months to regenerate nerves.
      3. Examine the patient every 2 months until paresthesia is gone; if paresthesia last longer than 1 year, refer the patient to an oral surgeon or neurologist.
      4. Paresthesia is more likely to affect the lingual nerve than the IAN.

IV. Trismus
   A. Characterized by motor disturbances of the trigeminal nerve, especially spasms of the masseter muscle, which cause difficulty in opening the mouth.
   B. Causes

1. Trauma to muscles or vessels caused by repeated penetrations or hitting a nerve.
   2. Infection from contaminated cartridges.
   3. Increased hemorrhage from a hematoma.
   4. Excessive volumes of anesthetic injected into tissue.
C. Management
   1. Includes the use of heat therapy, analgesics, and muscle relaxants.
   2. Encourage patient to exercise muscles by chewing gum (sugarless).
   3. If improvement does not occur in 48 hours, prescribe antibiotics for 7 days.
   4. If improvement does not occur after the use of antibiotics, refer the patient to an oral surgeon.
V. Hematoma
   A. Effusion of blood into extravascular spaces
   B. Cause
      1. Nicking a blood vessel
         a. Artery—tissue vessel rapidly increasing in size
         b. Vein—perhaps nothing
   C. Prevention
      1. Review knowledge of anatomy, strive for good technique, and minimize penetrations.
      2. Use a short needle for PSA nerve block, never probe with a needle, and penetrate slowly.
   D. Management
      1. Apply direct pressure with ice for at least 2 minutes.
      2. Inform the patient of possible side effects, including cosmetic effects, soreness, and limited movement.
VI. Tongue, Lips, and Cheek Trauma
   A. Cause
      1. Long-acting anesthetics provide opportunities for children or mentally challenged people to inadvertently chew on the lip or side of the tongue.
   B. Management
      1. Place a cotton roll between the lips and teeth.
      2. Warn the patient or caregiver about the need to avoid drinking hot foods and chewing until the anesthesia dissipates.
VII. Facial Nerve Paralysis
   A. Cause
      1. Temporary paralysis may occur in response to an infraorbital injection; when the facial nerve is inadvertently anesthetized, the result is temporary facial nerve paralysis that dissipates when the anesthesia wears off.
      2. Inadvertent injection into a deep lobe of the parotid gland during administration of an IAN block also may cause paralysis.
   B. Prevention
      1. Use MSA and ASA blocks instead of an infraorbital nerve block.

2. Use proper technique for an IAN block by placing the syringe over the contralateral bicuspids before injecting.
   C. Management
      1. Instruct patient to close eyelid manually to keep eye moist.
      2. Reassure the patient that the paralysis will disappear when anesthetic effects subside.

Nitrous Oxide and Oxygen Conscious Sedation

Fearful dental patients can benefit from the relaxing effects of conscious sedation with nitrous oxide and oxygen. This sedative is used alone and in combination with local dental anesthesia.

Pharmacology

Nitrous oxide is a colorless, tasteless, sweet-smelling gas that is not flammable but does support combustion (see Chapter 9).
   I. Is commercially prepared by heating ammonium nitrate crystals in an iron retort at 240°C and storing it as a liquid at 650 to 800 pounds pressure per square inch (psi).
   II. As an inhaled gas, nitrous oxide does not chemically combine with body tissues but does cause depression of the CNS.
   III. Nitrous oxide is not metabolized in the body but is eliminated by diffusion properties from the lungs.
   IV. Nitrous oxide is highly soluble in blood plasma and therefore has analgesic properties in concentrations as low as 20%.
   V. Higher altitudes increase the demand for nitrous oxide concentrations because of an increased need for oxygen in the blood.

Mode of Action

The uptake, distribution, and elimination of nitrous oxide sedation by inhalation involves a series of equilibriums that must be reached to provide effective analgesia.
I. Equilibrium Series
   A. The first equilibrium that must be reached is between the machine and the lungs; occurs rapidly (1 to 2 minutes).
   B. The second equilibrium occurs between the lungs and the blood (3 minutes) and is dependent on respiratory output, concentrations of the gasses, and cardiac output.
   C. The third equilibrium occurs between the blood and the brain (approximately 3 minutes); 3 minutes should elapse between changes in concentrations to decrease the adverse effects of too much nitrous oxide.

Administration

The proper administration of nitrous oxide/oxygen sedation involves proper patient selection and the appropriate management of the sedation unit.
I. Patient Selection

A. Nitrous oxide/oxygen sedation is most beneficial for fearful patients who do not have conditions that contraindicate its use.
B. Contraindications include:
  1. Recent myocardial infarction (within the past 6 months).
  2. Chronic obstructive pulmonary disease (e.g., emphysema, chronic bronchitis).
  3. Pregnancy, especially in the first trimester (research indicates that continuous exposure can lead to spontaneous abortion).
  4. Upper respiratory conditions, including active asthma, upper respiratory infection, or nasal obstruction.
  5. An inability to communicate or follow directions (e.g., young children or mentally challenged individuals).
  6. Individuals with a history of substance abuse.
  7. Individuals with a history of epilepsy.
II. Preparation of the Nitrous Oxide/Oxygen Unit
  A. Turn on the unit and determine the appropriate liter flow for the patient (most adults breathe 4 to 6 liters per minute).
  B. Explain the procedure to the patient; also explain potential sensations associated with the gas.
  C. Adjust the nose piece and scavenger system while the patient breathes pure oxygen.
  D. At 3-minute intervals, decrease the oxygen flow by the same amount that nitrous oxide flow is increased until the patient acknowledges appropriate effects.
  E. Continue to monitor the patient for signs of nitrous oxide intolerance, including nausea, diaphoresis (perspiration), unconsciousness, or changes in behavior.
  F. When nitrous oxide is no longer needed, have the patient breathe pure oxygen for at least 5 minutes, until the effects of sedation disappear.

Safety Procedures for the Administration of Nitrous Oxide/Oxygen

For the safe administration of nitrous oxide/oxygen, the patient must be screened and monitored for contraindications to its use and the sedation unit must be checked for leaks and other faults.
I. Patient
  A. Take a thorough medical history.
  B. Monitor the patient during the administration of gas to determine consciousness and intolerance.
  C. Instruct the patient to refrain from talking to decrease the amount of nitrous oxide exhaled into the room air.
  D. Record the time and amount of nitrous oxide administered and any complications encountered.
II. Nitrous Oxide/Oxygen Unit
  A. Thoroughly check the unit for leaks and unsafe equipment.
  B. Monitor "fail-safe" features.

  1. The minimum flow of oxygen is 2 liters/minute.
  2. A sound occurs when oxygen quits or else nitrous oxide shuts off when oxygen quits.
  3. A universal color scheme is used for oxygen and nitrous oxide tanks (blue = nitrous oxide; green = oxygen).
  4. Tanks for various gasses are not interchangeable.
  5. The scavenger system removes exhaled gases from the nose piece and room air.
  6. The flush system is available to provide 8 or more liters of oxygen to the patient if signs of intolerance are observed.

Complementary Pain Management Techniques

Several other techniques for pain management are available. These include hypnosis and new local and topical anesthesia delivery systems and products.
I. Hypnosis
  A. Professional hypnosis should not be performed by individuals who do not have an appropriate educational background.
  B. Nonprofessional hypnosis for apprehensive patients can be accomplished by:
    1. Using a quiet, calm, monotone voice.
    2. Allowing the patient to have control.
    3. Demonstrating confidence in dental techniques.
    4. Remaining calm and controlled in anxious situations.
    5. Providing the patient with soothing music (via head phones or in office).

Anesthesia Delivery Systems

Electronic and transcutaneous dental anesthesia systems use electrical stimulation to block nerve sensation. Computer-controlled delivery systems block sensations with the use of local anesthetics.
I. Computer-Controlled Local Anesthesia Delivery System (The Wand)
  A. Was developed by Milestone Scientific. The computer-assisted syringe uses traditional cartridges and needles; provides controlled amounts of anesthetic solution for all types of injection techniques.
  B. The handpiece is held with a pen grasp and is lighter than traditional syringes. As the needle penetrates the skin, the operator steps on a pedal to activate the flow of anesthetic solution ahead of the needle path.
  C. Has an auto-aspiration feature that can be used for any type of injection; the amount deposited for most injections is 0.6 to 0.9 mL.
II. Electronic Dental Anesthesia (EDA)
  A. A 120-Hz frequency is used to stimulate increased blood levels of serotonin and beta-endorphins (analgesics that raise the pain threshold); EDA-stimulated analgesics take approximately 10 min-

utes to reach an effective blood level and last approximately 2 hours.

B. Involves the placement of electrodes, either intraorally or extraorally, and patient control of the amount of analgesia administered.

C. Dental hygiene indications include:
 1. The administration of local anesthetics.
 2. Periodontal therapy.
 3. Needle phobic patients.

D. Hygiene contraindications include:
 1. Medically compromised patients (e.g., those affected by stroke, epilepsy, pacemakers, or transient ischemia).
 2. Patients with a decreased ability to communicate.

III. Transcutaneous Electrical Nerve Stimulation (TENS)
 A. Is used for chronic pain reduction (EDA is used for chronic and acute pain reduction).
 B. Operates at a frequency of 2 Hz.

Anesthetic Delivery Products

Transoral delivery of lidocaine is available by means of a patch for site-specific soft-tissue anesthesia.

I. Lidocaine Transoral Delivery System (DentiPatch)
 A. Patch contains 46.1 mg of lidocaine; onset of action occurs in 5 to 10 minutes; duration of action is approximately 45 minutes.
 B. Patch delivers site-specific anesthesia for soft-tissue therapy and preinjection topical anesthesia.
 C. Is applied by:
  1. Removing the plastic backing.
  2. Isolating and drying the targeted area for 30 seconds.
  3. Applying the patch with pressure for 30 seconds.
 D. Hygiene indications include:
  1. Preinjection anesthesia, especially in palatal areas.
  2. Soft-tissue therapy.
  3. Substitution for an injection, when an injection is contraindicated.

CONTENT REVIEW QUESTIONS

1. In a sensory neuron, the dendrite zone functions to:
 A. synapse with CNS nerves
 B. support metabolism
 C. receive a stimulus
 D. direct ion movement

2. Which of the following anesthetic agents is most appropriate if both severe and prolonged postoperative dental pain are expected?
 A. bupivacaine with epinephrine (Marcaine)
 B. lidocaine with epinephrine (Xylocaine)
 C. mepivacaine (Carbocaine)
 D. prilocaine with epinephrine (Citanest Forte)

3. Which of the following is false with regard to local anesthetic metabolism?

A. procaine is metabolized primarily in plasma
B. lidocaine is not metabolized in individuals with atypical pseudocholinesterase
C. some local anesthetic passes unchanged in urine
D. amides are primarily broken down in the liver

4. Levarterenol (norepinephrine):
 A. is contraindicated when injecting the palate
 B. is twice as potent as epinephrine
 C. relaxes bronchial smooth muscle in a manner similar to that of epinephrine
 D. is commonly used as a local anesthetic agent

5. Nitrous oxide:
 A. requires a long time for recovery
 B. is used to induce stage-III anesthesia quickly
 C. is both flammable and explosive
 D. is the safest of all analgesics

6. Trismus is:
 A. extremely rare
 B. a total lack of sensation
 C. a motor disturbance of the trigeminal nerve
 D. a sensory disturbance of the trigeminal nerve

7. *Initial* treatment for injection-induced hematomas includes which of the following?
 A. ice and pressure
 B. surgical removal
 C. heat
 D. aspirin

8. With regard to the dissociation of local anesthetics:
 A. the more base molecules ($RN + H^+$) available, the better the diffusion properties
 B. the more cation molecules (RNH^+) available, the better the diffusion properties
 C. the fewer base molecules ($RN + H^+$) available, the weaker the binding properties
 D. the fewer cation molecules (RNH^+) available, the greater the binding properties

9. Which anesthetic agents are more concentrated?
 A. injectable anesthetics
 B. topical anesthetics

10. When a patient experiences vasodepressor syncope, the best response is to:
 A. activate EMS.
 B. begin cardiopulmonary resuscitation
 C. place the patient in a supine position
 D. administer 1:1000 injectable epinephrine

11. The pH of a local anesthetic (2% lidocaine) is approximately 6.8; when a vasoconstrictor is added, the pH drops to approximately 4.2. Which of the following explains the drop in pH?
 A. the epinephrine is acidic
 B. the epinephrine is basic
 C. the preservative (sodium bisulfite) is acidic
 D. the preservative (sodium bisulfite) is basic
 E. the tissue has a pH of 5.5

12. The half-life of a local anesthetic is which of the following?
 A. the rate at which the local anesthetic is eliminated from the blood

B. the rate at which the local anesthetic effects the blockage of the nerve impulse

C. the length of time an anesthetic can be stored before it is no longer effective

D. the average length of time it takes for anesthesia to wear off

13. Positive aspiration indicates all of the following situations, EXCEPT:
    A. the needle is in a blood vessel
    B. a hematoma developed
    C. poor technique was employed
    D. an appropriate needle gauge was used

14. A patient receives 2% lidocaine with 1:100,000 epinephrine and subsequently experiences symptoms of local anesthetic overdose approximately 30 minutes after the injection. The most likely cause of this overdose reaction is:
    A. an excessive dose of lidocaine
    B. injection of the solution into a blood vessel
    C. liver dysfunction or renal impairment
    D. rapid injection of the solution

15. The part of its chemical structure that makes a local anesthetic agent hydrophilic is the:
    A. amino group
    B. aromatic ring
    C. intermediate chain
    D. benzene ring

16. An anesthetic solution must form a salt to:
    A. enable the anesthetic to penetrate the nerve membrane
    B. enable the anesthetic to diffuse through the tissue to the nerve
    C. decrease the acidic properties of the solution
    D. increase the shelf life of the solution

17. All injectable local anesthetic drugs used in dentistry are:
    A. vasoconstrictors
    B. vasodilators
    C. neither vasoconstrictors or vasodilators
    D. both vasoconstrictors and vasodilators

18. During an IAN injection, the patient gives a sudden jump and complains of a tingling sensation shooting downward in the jaw. This is most likely caused by:
    A. injecting too rapidly
    B. injecting into the inferior alveolar artery
    C. contacting the lingual nerve
    D. contacting the inferior alveolar nerve

19. A leaky cartridge is most likely caused by
    A. piercing the cartridge diaphragm on an angle
    B. failing to screw the needle tightly onto the syringe
    C. bubbles in the cartridge
    D. corrosion on the metal cap

20. Aspiration in two planes is necessary to:
    A. prevent the needle from entering a blood vessel
    B. ensure that the bevel is facing the bone
    C. reduce the internal pressure of the cartridge
    D. ensure that a blood vessel wall is not drawn against the bevel during aspiration

21. An IAN block will NOT provide anesthesia if the solution is deposited too:
    A. medially
    B. laterally
    C. superiorly
    D. inferiorly

22. The depth of penetration for a maxillary infiltration injection is determined by the:
    A. length of the needle
    B. root length of the tooth
    C. gauge of the needle
    D. location of the zygomatic bone

23. During the administration of a right IAN block, the syringe is over the left bicuspid at the height of the coronoid notch. As penetration occurs (less than half of the long needle), resistance is met. The resistance is most likely caused by which anatomical structure?
    A. medial pterygoid muscle
    B. internal oblique ridge
    C. pterygomandibular raphe
    D. medial surface of the ramus

24. In the same case as Question 23, which of the following is the best way to proceed?
    A. continue to penetrate tissue until the needle insertion depth reaches the hub
    B. retract the needle slightly and deposit the solution
    C. withdraw the needle, reinsert the needle superiorly, and penetrate until bone is recontacted
    D. back off slightly, redirect the needle laterally, and penetrate until bone is recontacted

25. Trismus is a complication that may occur during the administration of an IAN block; it involves which of the following muscles?
    A. buccinator
    B. lateral pterygoid
    C. masseter
    D. medial pterygoid

26. All of the following are fail-safe components of the nitrous oxide unit, EXCEPT:
    A. the minimum flow of nitrous oxide is 2 liters/minute
    B. different universal colors are used to label oxygen and nitrous oxide
    C. oxygen and nitrous oxide tanks cannot be interchanged
    D. a scavenger system is used to decrease exhaled gasses

27. The Akinosi technique is indicated in which of the following situations?
    A. as an alternative to the PSA nerve block
    B. when trismus decreases a patient's ability to open the mouth
    C. for young children or mentally handicapped adults
    D. when bilateral anesthesia of the mandible is required

28. The deposition site for the ASA nerve block is:
    A. apical to the lateral incisor
    B. at the apex of the canine
    C. in the canine fossa
    D. over the central incisor
29. For which of the following injections does tissue blanching indicate an adequate deposition of local anesthetics?
    A. posterior superior alveolar nerve block
    B. anterior superior alveolar nerve block
    C. nasopalatine nerve block
    D. mental nerve block
    E. inferior alveolar nerve block
30. To determine the maximum recommended dose (MRD) of a local anesthetic for a particular patient, the clinician must do which of the following?
    A. multiply the age of the patient by the dose/cartridge
    B. multiply the manufacturer's number for mg/lb by the weight of the patient
    C. divide the mg/cartridge of the local anesthetic by the weight of the patient
    D. divide the maximum cartridges allowed by the mg/cartridge of local anesthetic
31. A fearful dental patient presents for extensive dental hygiene treatment. The best way to approach this patient is to:
    A. perform treatment quickly to reduce the time that the patient is stressed
    B. tell the patient that nitrous oxide/oxygen sedation is available
    C. give little information about the procedures to avoid frightening the patient
    D. increase the patient's control of the treatment session

REVIEW QUESTION RATIONALES

1. **C** The dendrite zone is composed of small nerve endings at the terminal ends of nerves. These free nerve endings receive stimuli from tissues. When the clinician places a curette in a pocket and the nerve endings of the dendrite zone receive the stimulus, they send an impulse along the nerve to the CNS, which interprets the sensation as pain.
2. **A** Bupivacaine with epinephrine (Marcaine) is a long-acting local anesthetic that lasts 1 to 2 hours as an infiltration and 5 to 9 hours as a nerve block. The epinephrine concentration is 1:200,000. The other anesthetics listed are shorter-acting varieties.
3. **B** An individual with *atypical* pseudocholinesterase cannot metabolize ester anesthetics. Normally, ester-type local anesthetics are metabolized in the blood plasma by the enzyme pseudocholinesterase. Because lidocaine is an amide local anesthetic and is metabolized (hydrolyzed) in the liver, it is safe to use for individuals with atypical pseudocholinesterase. All other statements are true.

4. **A** Levarterenol (norepinephrine) is a vasoconstrictor not a local anesthetic; it acts primarily on α receptors that constrict smooth muscle in blood vessels. When norepinephrine is used on the palate, the constriction of blood vessels may cause ischemia and eventually necrosis of the palatal tissues. It has 25% of the potency of epinephrine.
5. **D** As an inhaled gas, nitrous oxide/oxygen does not combine chemically with body tissues and thus is the safest of all analgesics. The gas is taken in and eliminated in the same state, and recovery is quick. Nitrous oxide/oxygen supports combustion but is not flammable or explosive. In the dental office setting, it should not be used to induce stage-III anesthesia.
6. **C** Trismus is a motor, not sensory, disturbance of the trigeminal nerve (C-V). It disturbs motor nerves that affect the muscles of mastication and increases difficulty in mastication and in opening and closing the mouth. Trismus is common and seldom involves a complete loss of sensation.
7. **A** Tearing a blood vessel causes a hematoma. Initial treatment includes applying ice to the area with direct pressure for 2 minutes to decrease blood flow. The hematoma does not need surgical removal because it will dissipate with time. Initially, heat and aspirin should not be used because they may increase bleeding in the area. Heat may be applied after 4–6 hours or the next day to increase healing.
8. **A** Base molecules (RN) are uncharged ions and are responsible for the diffusion properties of the local anesthetic; the more free base molecules available, the better the diffusion properties. The number of cation molecules (RNH) determines the anesthetic's binding ability; the more cations, the longer the anesthetic remains in the targeted area.
9. **B** Topical anesthetics require a higher concentration to diffuse the agent through the mucous membranes. A 2% solution of injectable lidocaine has a concentration of 20 mg/mL or 36 mg/cartridge of local anesthetic. A lidocaine topical anesthetic typically has a concentration of 5%, which equals 50 mg/mL. Concentrations of injectable anesthetics are generally lower than those of topical agents.
10. **C** Vasopressor syncope is fainting that is caused by a pooling of blood in the muscles, which decreases the blood flow to the brain. Placing the patient in a supine position, with the head and feet parallel to the floor, increases the blood flow to the brain and prevents syncope. Activating the EMS, beginning CPR, or administering epinephrine are not appropriate choices for this emergency.
11. **C** Vasoconstrictors require preservatives to extend their shelf-life to approximately 18 months. The preservative added by the manufacturer (sodium bisulfite) makes the local anesthetic solution more acidic.
12. **A** Half-life is defined as the rate at which ½ of the local anesthetic is eliminated from the blood stream. For example, lidocaine has a half-life of 96 minutes,

which means that 50% of the agent is eliminated from the body in 96 minutes.

13. **C** A careful technique is important but does not eliminate the chance of positive aspiration. Aspiration is the act of drawing fluids into a syringe. If the needle tip is in a blood vessel, blood will flow into the cartridge. If the needle tip is not in a blood vessel, interstitial fluids will flow into the cartridge. However, if blood flows into the tissues from a hematoma (tearing of the blood vessel) and the clinician aspirates, blood will flow into the cartridge, giving a positive aspiration. Positive aspiration is an indication that the needle lumen size was inadequate for aspiration.

14. **C** A slow rise (30 minutes or more) in blood levels of lidocaine indicates that the amide anesthetic is not undergoing proper elimination from the body, typically because of liver dysfunction or renal impairment. A rapid rise in blood levels of lidocaine can be caused by an excessive dose of local anesthetic, by injecting too quickly, or by injecting anesthetics into a blood vessel.

15. **A** The hydrophilic portion of the local anesthetic is the amino group. The hydrophilic portion determines the diffusion properties of the anesthetic. If an amino group does not exist, the anesthetic cannot be injected into tissues. The aromatic or benzene rings provide the lipophilic portion of the anesthetic, which increases nerve penetration. The intermediate chain determines whether the anesthetic is an ester or an amide.

16. **B** Local anesthetics must be combined with hydrochloride to form a salt. As a salt, the anesthetic is more soluble in water (diffuses through tissue) and thus more injectable. Salt does not increase the anesthetic's shelf life, affect acidic properties, or enable the anesthetic to penetrate the nerve membrane.

17. **B** Local anesthetic agents used in dentistry act as vasodilators of the blood vessels in surrounding areas. Vasoconstrictors are added to these anesthetic agents to increase the duration of the agent and to decrease the potential toxic effects of too much anesthetic in the blood stream.

18. **D** One major complication of the IAN block is caused by the close proximity of the IAN and the potential for touching this nerve during penetration. When the nerve is touched, the patient feels a tingling along the nerve that enters the ramus at the mandibular foramen. Injecting too rapidly will cause discomfort during the injection not tingling. Injecting into the IA artery may cause an overdose reaction. Contact with the lingual nerve may cause the tongue to tingle.

19. **A** The needle must pierce the diaphragm so that the diaphragm is able to make a tight seal around the needle. If the needle pierces the diaphragm on an angle, making the hole ovoid in shape, a faulty seal will result and cause leakage of the anesthetic solution. A loosely tightened needle may cause the needle to fall off but will not cause leakage of the solution. Solution in cartridges exposed to freezing temperatures may exhibit bubbles and should be discarded. Corrosion of the metal cartridge cap indicates that its outer surface has been exposed to a solution (either disinfectant or an anesthetic solution); thus it should be discarded.

20. **D** If the needle is in a blood vessel during aspiration, the blood vessel wall can be drawn in against the bevel, giving a false-negative aspiration. Rotating the needle 45 degrees and aspirating again increases the likelihood of accurately determining the needle location. Injecting a local anesthetic into a blood vessel greatly increases the potential for overdose reactions. Aspiration will alert (not prevent) one to the possibility of entering a blood vessel. Observation of the needle bevel prior to insertion is necessary to prevent scraping of the periosteum. Aspiration increases rather than decreases internal pressure of the cartridge.

21. **D** If the anesthetic is deposited below the mandibular foramen, the IAN will not be anesthetized. Deposition of the anesthetic at a higher deposition site will provide anesthesia. Deposition superiorly, medially, and laterally may slow the speed of onset but will result in anesthesia.

22. **B** To anesthetize a single tooth (infiltration), the anesthetic solution must be deposited at or above the apex of the root. It is important to know the length of the tooth root to provide adequate anesthesia to an individual tooth. Neither the length or gauge of the needle nor the location of the zygomatic bone are necessary to determine depth of penetration for infiltration anesthesia.

23. **B** One of the first bony landmarks for the IAN block is the internal oblique ridge. If positioning is too low, this landmark will be contacted almost immediately during insertion, or as soon as approximately half of the needle progresses through the tissue. Contact with the medial pterygoid muscle may occur but offers little resistance. The pterygomandibular raphe is the landmark used for insertion during the IAN block. Contact with the medial surface of the ramus should occur when bone is contacted after penetration of three fourths or more of the needle.

24. **D** The depth of penetration for the IAN block is approximately three quarters of the long needle. The medial surface of the ramus should be contacted prior to depositing any solution, not just contact with any bone.

25. **D** On the medial surface of the ramus, the medial pterygoid muscle (a muscle of mastication) runs superiorly from the posterior, inferior angle of the ramus and covers the mandibular foramen and IAN. Penetration of this muscle may cause trismus. The buccinator is not a muscle of mastication, whereas the

pterygoid and masseter muscles are not located near the site of IAN injection.

26. **A** The minimum flow for oxygen (not for nitrous oxide) is 2 liters/minute. This fail-safe component ensures that the patient does not inhale nitrous oxide without oxygen. Color-coding, noninterchangeable tanks, and scavenger systems are all fail-safe components.

27. **B** The Akinosi technique (an alternative mandibular block) is indicated when the patient cannot open his or her mouth. This technique is not specifically indicated for young children, mentally-handicapped adults, or for bilateral mandibular injections.

28. **C** The ASA nerve is a branch of the maxillary division of the trigeminal nerve (CNV). The terminal nerve endings are located within the alveolar process in the area of the canine fossa.

29. **C** For the nasopalatine nerve block injection, the amount of anesthetic deposited should be just enough to blanch the tissues. The other injections listed require the deposition of solution in milliliters.

30. **B** For each type of local anesthetic, the manufacturer establishes a MRD (in milligrams per pound). To determine the maximum dose for a patient, the clinician should multiply the MRD/lb by the weight of the patient. The MRD for 2% lidocaine is 2 mg/lb; thus a 140-lb patient could safely receive 280 mg of lidocaine.

31. **D** Increasing a fearful patient's control decreases fear by allowing the patient to determine his or her comfort level. Fearful dental patients require more than quick appointments and limited information about procedures and pain control methods.

References

Astra: Prescribing Information Dental. Wesborough, MA, Astra Pharmaceutical Products, 1990.

Cook-Waite: Cook-Waite Anesthetics: Average Durations. Eastman Kodak Company, 1993.

Additional Reading

Febrenbach MJ, Herring SW: Illustrated Anatomy of the Head and Neck. Philadelphia, WB Saunders, 1996.

Feugate AD: Topical anesthetics: An important pain control technique. Dental Hygienist News 8(1):14,17, 1995.

Evers H, Haegerstam G: Introduction to Dental Local Anesthesia, 2nd ed. Philadelphia, Kin Keong, 1995.

Genco RJ, Newman MG: Annals of Periodontology, Vol. 1, No. 1. American Academy of Periodontology, November, 1996.

Jastak JT, Yagiela JA, Donaldson D: Local Anesthesia of the Oral Cavity, 9th ed. Philadelphia, WB Saunders, 1995.

Krochak M, Rubin JG: An Overview of the Treatment of Anxious and Phobic Dental Patients. Compendium of Continuing Dental Education 14(5): 604–613, 1995.

Malamed SF: Handbook of Local Anesthesia, 4th ed. St. Louis, Mosby, 1997.

Woodall IR: Comprehensive Dental Hygiene Care, 4th ed. St. Louis, Mosby, 1993.

Chapter FOURTEEN

Medical and Dental Emergencies

Beverly J. Kennedy, R.D.H., M.A.

 Clinical Case **STUDY**

Thomas, a 34-year-old man, is in the dental office for his first oral prophylaxis appointment in 7 years. He appears apprehensive and states that he hates coming to the dentist and hopes that no problems are found. He takes no medications and has no allergies or medical conditions. After the treatment procedures for the appointment are explained, Thomas asks the dental hygienist to stop because he feels hot and dizzy. Perspiration is apparent on his forehead.

Clinical Case **QUESTIONS**

1. What emergency situation is the patient probably experiencing?
2. What treatment should be initiated at this time?
3. If the patient loses consciousness, what steps should be followed?
4. What has caused this emergency to occur?

Clinical Case **RATIONALES**

1. The patient most likely is experiencing syncope or fainting. The dizziness indicates that he is still in the presyncope stage.
2. At this time, the patient should be positioned in the Trendelenburg position.
3. If the patient becomes unconscious, it is essential to open the patient's airway using the head-tilt chin-lift technique. This is indicated for any patient who is losing consciousness to prevent the tongue from obstructing the airway. An ammonia inhalant can be used to stimulate the patient's breathing, if necessary. Oxygen also may be administered. No further dental treatment should be performed at this time and the patient should be released.

4. The stress indicated by the patient's apprehension about the appointment is the likely psychogenic cause of syncope in this case.

Content Review

Terminology

ASA physical status classification—Classification devised by the American Society of Anesthesiologists (ASA) to categorize the physical status of patients; considered invaluable for determining risks and necessary modifications before treatment; currently includes six categories of physical status.

Anaphylaxis—Severe, sometimes fatal, allergic reaction that results in shock.

Angina pectoris—Chest pain caused by a lack of oxygen to the heart muscle; is common in individuals with blocked arteries; may or may not result in a heart attack; is treated with nitroglycerin.

Angioedema—Localized, large swellings without the well-defined borders of hives; an allergic reaction to a food or medicine; affects the tissues of the hands, face, and genitals.

Antigen—Foreign substance that causes an immune response.

Arteriosclerosis—Hardening of the arteries caused by an accumulation of plaque.

Atherosclerosis—Arteriosclerosis of the coronary arteries.

Avulsion—Traumatic removal of a tooth from its socket.

Bradycardia—Slower than normal pulse rate; less than 60 beats per minute for an adult.

Cerebrovascular accident (CVA)—A stroke caused by cerebral hemorrhage, embolism, thrombosis, or infarction.

Clonic—Convulsive movements characterized by the contraction and relaxation of muscles.

Cyanosis—Blue coloration of an area, particularly of the lips, caused by a lack of oxygenated blood.

Dyspnea—Difficult or labored breathing.

Embolism—A blood clot, unattached to a blood vessel, that is carried through the blood stream.

EMS—The emergency medical system within a community; consists of trained personnel and communication, transportation, and medical facilities to provide emergency medical care; is activated in most communities by telephoning 911; sometimes is referred to as Phone First.

Gingival hyperplasia—An overgrowth of the connective tissue component of the gingiva; occurs in direct response to medication use (e.g., phenytoin [Dilantin]) and plaque accumulation.

Hemorrhage—Uncontrolled bleeding.

Hyperglycemia—High blood sugar.

Hypertension—Higher than normal blood pressure; for an adult, a systolic reading greater than 140 mm Hg and/or a diastolic reading greater than 90 mm Hg.

Hyperventilation—An increased rate and depth of respirations that results in a decreased level of carbon dioxide.

Hypoglycemia—Low blood sugar.

Hypoxia—Deficiency of oxygen in the air being breathed.

Ictal—Relating to a convulsion.

Insulin shock—Low blood sugar.

Ketones—Excess amounts of acetone and acetoacetic acid in the blood and urine of individuals with diabetes; contributes to an increased frequency of urination.

Kussmaul breathing—Heavy, labored breathing that may be either rapid or slow; occurs during a hyperglycemic incident.

Myocardial infarction (MI)—A heart attack.

Orthostatic hypotension—Low blood pressure that results from remaining in one position for a significant length of time; may be characterized by dizziness, light-headedness, a loss of balance, or syncope.

Pericoronitis—Inflammation of the soft tissue that surrounds an erupting tooth.

Postictal—Relating to the final stage of a seizure (e.g., grand mal seizure); often involves extreme exhaustion and sleep.

Prodromal—Relating to an initial phase of a seizure (e.g., grand mal seizure) during which an aura may be sensed.

Pruritus—Itching; typically is associated with allergy.

Syncope—Fainting; is caused by decreased blood flow to the brain.

Tachycardia—Faster than normal pulse rate; more than 100 beats per minute for an adult.

Thrombosis—A blood clot attached to a blood vessel.

Tonic—Stiff and rigid movements caused by muscle contraction.

Tonic-clonic—Describes the sudden muscle contractions followed by convulsive movements during a seizure.

Transient ischemic attack (TIA)—A temporary stroke; also is termed incipient stroke; does not result in permanent neurological damage, although its occurrence indicates the presence of cerebrovascular disease.

Trismus—Difficulty in opening the mouth.

Urticaria—Hives; appear as raised areas of edema and erythema and are accompanied by pruritus.

Vasodilator—A medication or drug that causes the arteries to dilate (e.g., nitroglycerin).

Emergency Prevention

The combination of pain, stress, and anesthesia that a patient experiences in the dental office may contribute to the occurrence of an medical emergency. Emergencies may be minimized or prevented by the pretreatment evaluation of a patient's health status. Such evaluation includes the completion of a comprehensive health history, an assessment of vitals signs, and thorough office preparation.

Medical-Dental Health History

The medical-dental history is crucial to the diagnosis and treatment of and prognosis for conditions experienced by dental patients. Modifying dental treatment as indicated by the medical-dental health history dramatically decreases the occurrence of emergencies in the dental office.

   I. Identifies changes in medications and/or conditions that may require antibiotic premedication (e.g., valvular damage, synthetic replacement); for antibiotic premedication regimens, see Table 9–3.

   II. Identifies precautions, allergies, or conditions that may contraindicate or alter treatment.

   III. May assist in the identification of oral manifestations associated with some medications.

   IV. Assists in planning treatment according to the patient's physiologic and psychological status.

   V. Includes a record of vital signs.

   VI. Serves as a legal record.

Vital Signs

Blood pressure, pulse, and respiration are obtained as a baseline for the patient and are performed as a health service.

   I. Blood pressure is measured in terms of the air pressure that is required to compress a large artery to the point of shutting off flow to the artery.

     A. Is recorded in fractions of millimeters of mercury (mm Hg).

     B. Systolic pressure

       1. Is the pressure in blood vessels when the heart contracts.

       2. Typically is 100 to 140 mm Hg for adults.

       3. Is the first pulse sound that is heard when pressure is released from the cuff.

     C. Diastolic pressure

       1. Is the pressure in blood vessels when the heart dilates.

       2. Normally is 60 to 90 mm Hg for adults.

3. Is the last pulse sound that is heard when pressure is released from the cuff.

D. Technique
   1. The instruments used to measure blood pressure include a stethoscope and a sphygmomanometer (cuff size is determined by the size of a patient's arm).
   2. The cuff is placed snugly 1 inch above the antecubital fossa, with no clothing between the cuff and the arm.
   3. The cuff is pumped until the radial pulse is no longer felt; the operator notes this point (the estimated systolic number) and releases the pressure.
   4. The cuff subsequently is repumped to 10 to 30 mm Hg above the previously recorded point (maximum inflation level).
   5. The pressure is released slowly; the operator notes the first pulse sound or systole.
   6. The operator continues to release pressure slowly until the last pulse sound or diastole is heard.
   7. The patient is informed of the reading, and the reading is recorded in the patient's record.

E. High blood pressure or hypertension
   1. Is indicated by sustained readings that are greater than 140/90 mm Hg.
   2. Systolic readings of 140 to 160 mm Hg and diastolic readings greater than 90 to 95 mm Hg must be rechecked for accuracy.
   3. Medical consultation is indicated when a patient has a systolic reading higher than 160 mm Hg and/or a diastolic reading higher than 95 mm Hg.
   4. No dental treatment, routine or emergency, should be performed when a patient's blood pressure level is 200/115 or higher.

F. Blood pressure is affected by exercise, eating, stimulants, pain, stress, anxiety, and patient positioning. Moreover, recordings taken from the right and left arms may differ.

II. The Pulse (Fig. 14–1)
   A. Is taken for 30 seconds if within normal range (this number is multiplied by two and recorded); if abnormal, is taken for 1 minute.
   B. Is taken from the radial artery in normal situations and from the carotid artery in emergencies.
   C. A normal pulse for adults is between 60 and 90; for children a normal pulse is between 80 and 110; it is necessary to note both the rate and the rhythm of the pulse.
   D. The pulse is affected by exercise, stress, stimulants, fasting, and long-term illness.
   E. Pulse beats that are alternately weak and strong are known as pulsus alternans.
   F. Premature ventricular contractions are identified when there is a longer than normal pause or skip

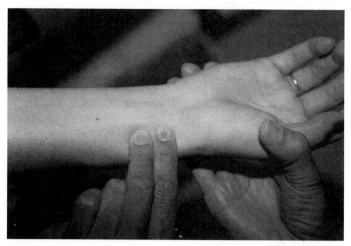

Figure 14.1 The radial artery is used for taking a routine pulse.

between beats; if more than 5 per minute occur, they are a cause for concern.

III. Respirations
   A. Are obtained by counting the number of breaths for 30 seconds (the number is multiplied by two and recorded); one exhalation and one inhalation together count as one breath.
   B. The rate will be altered if the patient knows that breathing is being observed.
   C. In the adult, the range normally is between 14 and 20 breaths per minute; in children the range normally is between 18 and 30 breaths per minute.
   D. The rate may be affected by pain, excitement, and/or the presence of a fever.

 Clinical Case **STUDY**

Jody Weets, a 37-year-old woman who is new to the dental practice, has completed the medical history. She has indicated that she has diabetes, which is well controlled by Orinase, diet, and exercise. No other medications or conditions are reported. She states that because of her anxiety about the dental appointment, she forgot to eat breakfast. At mid-morning, near the end of the hour-long appointment, the patient complains of a headache, reports feeling weak, and becomes more nervous and somewhat confused.

Clinical Case **QUESTIONS**

1. What type of diabetes does Jody have?
2. What is the ASA classification of this patient?
3. What emergency situation has begun to occur during this appointment?
4. Describe the steps that should be followed to manage this situation.

5. How could this emergency situation have been avoided?

Clinical Case RATIONALES

1. Jody has NIDDM, which most often is controlled by diet and exercise, and in some cases, an oral hypoglycemic medication such as Orinase.
2. The physical status of this patient (mild systemic disease such as NIDDM) indicates an ASA II classification.
3. The emergency that has occurred is hypoglycemia or low blood sugar. This condition most often is associated with a lack of food intake; in this case the patient missed breakfast because of anxiety associated with the dental appointment. Headache, weakness, nervousness, and confusion are symptoms of hypoglycemia. This condition typically occurs rapidly for the patient who requires insulin; the onset of symptoms is slower for the patient who is taking an oral hypoglycemic.
4. Dental treatment must be stopped and the patient must be positioned upright. A source of sugar (such as orange juice or a chocolate bar) should be supplied. If the situation is allowed to progress, the patient may become unconscious, in which case the administration of Glucagon will be indicated.
5. Both the lack of breakfast and the stress related to the appointment contributed to the occurrence of hypoglycemia. It is essential to thoroughly explain all dental procedures to this patient to alleviate anxiety for future appointments and encourage eating before the appointment.

Office Preparation

When emergency situations occur, it is essential that all office personnel know the procedures to be followed, the location and use of the emergency kit and oxygen, and basic life support management.

I. Emergency Kits
  A. Can be homemade or manufactured.
    1. A homemade kit is more likely to contain articles that meet the needs of a particular office.
    2. Office personnel are more likely to be familiar with a kit that they have organized.
  B. All staff must be trained to use an emergency kit's contents.
  C. Contents
    1. Equipment must include an oxygen delivery system, disposable syringes, a rubber tourniquet, and a pocket mask.
    2. Noninjectable drugs must include nitroglycerin or a nitrolingual spray, a bronchodilator, aromatic ammonia, and a sugar source (e.g., oral glucose gel (e.g., glucose 15) or decorative cake icing).
    3. Injectable drugs must include epinephrine and diphenhydramine (Benadryl).

II. Oxygen
  A. An oxygen cylinder (size E) should be available to deliver 100% oxygen for 30 minutes.
  B. For the patient who is not breathing, delivery requires a mask and a demand-valve resuscitator. An alternative to the demand valve is the ambu-bag.
  C. Full masks of clear material that provide a tight seal are necessary.

III. The primary management of emergency situations involves basic life support; the use of drugs is secondary.

IV. The ASA physical status classification of a patient is used to determine risks and necessary modifications before treatment.
  A. ASA I indicates a normal, healthy patient.
  B. ASA II indicates a patient with a mild systemic disease, which may include:
    1. A cold, flu, or hayfever.
    2. Pregnancy, noninsulin-dependent diabetes mellitus (NIDDM), or asthma (without attacks); an individual with well-controlled diabetes and without associated diseases, such as hypertension or cardiovascular disease, would be placed in this category.
  C. ASA III indicates a patient with a more severe systemic disease that limits activity yet is not incapacitating, which may include:
    1. Angina or exercise-induced asthma.
    2. Stroke or myocardial infarction that occurred at least 6 months previously.
  D. ASA IV indicates a patient with a severe systemic disease that is a constant threat to life.
    1. A patient in this category is not an acceptable risk for surgery or dental care.
    2. This category includes patients with worsening angina and those who have experienced stroke or myocardial infarction within the past 6 months.
    3. Others in this category include patients on constant oxygen and those with severe congestive heart failure.
  E. ASA V indicates a moribund patient who is not expected to live longer than 24 hours.
  F. ASA VI indicates a patient who has died and whose organs are to be harvested.

V. Drug references (e.g., *Physician's Desk Reference, Mosby's Dental Drug Reference,* and *Lexi-Comp's Drug Information Handbook for Dentistry*) are used in the dental office to assist in the identification of medications taken by patients; indicate contraindications to treatment.

 Clinical Case STUDY

Ms. Foster dreads dental appointments but currently experiences less anxiety because she has been following a 6-month oral prophylaxis schedule and her appointments take less time. Her dental health is good. After her medical history is updated and her vital signs are obtained, bitewing radiographs are taken. While the dental hygienist leaves to process the radiographs, Ms. Foster remains seated in an upright position. Upon returning, the dental hygienist notes that Ms. Foster is breathing rapidly. The patient complains of a tightness in her chest and tingling in her fingers.

Clinical Case QUESTIONS

1. What is Ms. Foster most likely experiencing?
2. How should this emergency situation be handled?
3. Is oxygen indicated? Why or why not?

Clinical Case RATIONALES

1. The patient is probably experiencing hyperventilation, which is indicated by her increased rate of respiration, dizziness, chest tightness, and the tingling in her fingers. Hyperventilation most often occurs in the dental office because of anxiety. Ms. Foster's anxiety about dental appointments always has been apparent, although she believed it had lessened.

2. Treatment includes calming the patient and keeping her positioned upright. A rapid rate of breathing results in a decreased level of carbon dioxide. To restore the carbon dioxide, Ms. Foster should inhale, hold her breath, and subsequently exhale. If this is ineffective, she should breathe into a paper bag 6 to 10 times per minute. It is important to allow her to hold the bag in position.

3. Hyperventilation is one emergency in which the administration of oxygen is not indicated. Although oxygen would not harm the patient, it also would not benefit her.

Office Emergencies

Medical and dental emergencies, ranging from fainting or puncture wounds to cardiovascular difficulties or anaphylaxis, may occur in the dental office. Knowledge of basic life support and other emergency management techniques enables the dental professional to react appropriately in emergency situations.

Medical Emergencies

Medical emergencies that may occur in the dental office include hyperventilation, syncope, allergic reactions, airway obstruction, angina, myocardial infarction, cerebrovascular accident, seizures, hyperglycemia, and hypoglycemia.

I. Syncope or fainting
  A. Is the most common dental office emergency.
  B. As with all emergency situations that involve an unconscious patient, may lead to airway obstruction and death if improperly treated.

C. Is most often associated with a form of stress.
D. Is caused by decreased oxygen flow to the brain, which in turn is caused by:
  1. Psychogenic factors, such as stress, unwelcome news, or the sight of a needle or blood (the most common cause in dental offices).
  2. Nonpsychogenic factors, which include poor health or exhaustion.
  3. Orthostatic hypotension may occur when a patient sits up quickly from being in a supine position; this may result in syncope. The use of hypertensive drugs predisposes a patient to orthostatic or postural hypotension.
E. The presyncope stage is characterized by:
  1. Pallor, dizziness, and nausea.
  2. Lowered blood pressure and an increased pulse rate.
F. Syncope is characterized by:
  1. The loss of consciousness, shallow breathing, and dilated pupils.
  2. Lowered blood pressure and a thready pulse.
G. Treatment includes:
  1. Placing the patient in the Trendelenburg position (supine with feet elevated); typically this ensures recovery (Fig. 14-2).
  2. Placing a pregnant patient on her side before her feet are elevated.
  3. Maintaining an open airway to prevent airway obstruction by the tongue; is imperative for the unconscious patient.
  4. The use of ammonia inhalants, as needed, to provide a stimulus for breathing; caution during use is necessary to prevent the burning of tissue.
  5. The administration of oxygen.
  6. Careful monitoring of the patient until vital signs return to baseline; is essential because syncope is likely to recur soon after recovery;

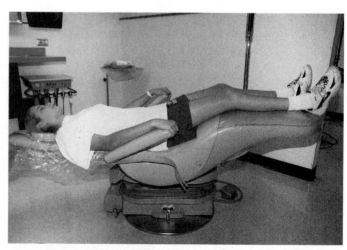

Figure 14.2 The Trendelenburg position. The patient is in a supine position with feet elevated.

vomiting commonly occurs after unconsciousness.

7. No further dental treatment should take place for 24 hours after syncope.

II. Hyperventilation

A. That occurs in the dental office typically is related to anxiety.

B. Is characterized by an increased rate and depth of respirations, which results in a decreased level of carbon dioxide.

C. Other symptoms include tightness of the chest, a sensation of suffocating, dizziness, and tingling in the fingers.

D. Typically does not occur in children because they release anxiety by other means (e.g., crying).

E. Treatment

1. Calm the patient and place the patient in an upright position (respiratory emergencies should be managed with the patient upright, if conscious).

2. Restore carbon dioxide by:

a. Having the patient inhale, hold the breath, and subsequently exhale.

b. Having the patient breathe into a paper bag or headrest cover (not plastic); the patient should hold the bag and breathe 6 to 10 times per minute (Fig. 14–3).

3. This is the only emergency situation in which oxygen does not benefit patient; it further decreases carbon dioxide levels and slows the return to normal.

4. The dentist may administer diazepam (Valium) in severe cases.

F. Prevention involves correct patient management and the ability to recognize signs of anxiety. For this reason, hyperventilation is an emergency that should not occur twice for the same patient.

III. Allergic reactions

A. Are caused by an increased sensitivity to an antigen that has entered the body; the immune system subsequently releases chemicals, such as histamine, which result in varying degrees of reactions.

B. Skin reactions generally are not considered true emergencies yet they must be monitored for potential advancement.

C. The severity and type of reaction is related to the type and amount of allergen exposed to.

1. If the reaction occurs immediately after exposure, it typically is more severe.

2. When the reaction occurs more than 60 minutes after exposure, the reaction is less severe.

3. Reactions may be localized or generalized.

D. Types of reactions

1. Contact dermatitis

a. Occurs when the skin is exposed to an allergen; results in erythema, edema, and vesicle formation.

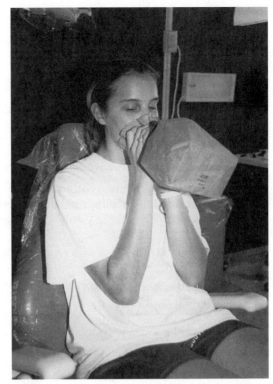

Figure 14.3 During hyperventilation, carbon dioxide level can be restored by breathing into a paper bag.

b. Typically is acute and localized but can spread.

c. Treatment includes removing the cause; a physician may administer an antihistamine such as diphenhydramine (Benadryl) or chlorpheniramine (Chlor-Trimeton) to reduce reaction.

2. Urticaria (hives)

a. Is caused by the ingestion of food or medicine or by direct skin contact with the allergen.

b. Appears as raised areas of edema and erythema and is accompanied by pruritus.

c. Treatment involves removing the cause; a physician may administer an antihistamine, such as diphenhydramine (Benadryl) or chlorpheniramine (Chlor-Trimeton) to reduce reaction.

3. Angioedema

a. Initially may be mistaken for hives.

b. Is characterized by localized, large swellings without the well-defined borders of hives.

c. Is an allergic reaction to a food or medicine.

d. Affects the tissues of the hands, face, and genitals.

e. Rarely results in pain or itching.

f. Treatment includes removing the cause and administering an antihistamine, such as diphenhydramine (Benadryl) or chlorpheniramine (Chlor-Trimeton) to reduce reaction.

4. Localized, mild allergic reactions should be treated with an oral histamine blocker for 3 days.

5. Anaphylactic reaction (anaphylaxis)
   a. Is a severe allergic reaction that is related to the amount of allergen exposed to, acquired sensitivity, and the route of entry.
   b. Occurs almost immediately after exposure to the antigen.
   c. May be fatal despite treatment.
   d. Symptoms affect different body systems and may occur separately or simultaneously.
      1) Begins rapidly as a skin response (pruritus, urticaria, angioedema); angioedema in the mouth may result in airway obstruction.
      2) The gastrointestinal system may respond with spasms, cramps, nausea, and diarrhea.
      3) The respiratory system exhibits varying degrees of laryngeal edema, which is the most common cause of death from anaphylaxis.
      4) Circulatory system involvement includes hypotension, shock, and cardiac arrest.
   e. Treatment includes:
      1) Placing the patient in a supine position and administering oxygen.
      2) Providing basic life support as needed.
      3) Activating the emergency medical system (EMS) by calling 911.
      4) Administration of epinephrine (0.3 mg every 5 minutes) by the dentist, when the diagnosis is definite.
      5) Administration of an antihistamine during recovery.
      6) Hospitalization is essential for this patient.

6. Asthma attack
   a. Is a respiratory emergency that affects individuals of all ages and often is triggered by anxiety.
   b. May occur suddenly or slowly and may be allergic or nonallergic in nature.
   c. Identification requires distinguishing asthma (wheezing upon expiration) from airway obstruction (wheezing upon inspiration). If the patient's medical records indicate a history of asthma, it is more likely that the patient is experiencing an asthmatic attack.
   d. Involves a narrowing of the bronchioles (airway) in response to an overproduction of mucus and smooth muscle contraction, which results in difficulty breathing.
   e. Symptoms
      1) Sweating, coughing, nervousness, and tightness of the chest.
      2) The patient struggles for air (wheezing upon expiration).
   f. Treatment includes:
      1) Positioning the patient upright.
      2) The use of a bronchodilator.
      3) Administering oxygen and allowing the patient to position the mask.
      4) Administration of epinephrine by the dentist if the bronchodilator is not effective.
      5) Providing basic life support, if necessary.

7. Allergy to local anesthesia
   a. Occurs rarely; less than 1% of patient reactions to anesthesia are allergic.
   b. When reported, it must be determined if a true allergic reaction occurred or if some other adverse reaction occurred.
   c. Occurs more often in response to ester local anesthetics (procaine); allergic reactions to amide local anesthetics are rare.
   d. Is characterized by inflammation, edema, pruritus, and papule formation.
   e. Can be severe enough to cause anaphylaxis.
   f. Is treated in the same manner as other allergic reactions, depending on the symptoms.

IV. Airway Obstruction or Foreign Body Airway Obstruction (FBAO)
   A. Occurs more easily in the dental office because of the reclining position of the patient; objects that can be aspirated into the airway and cause obstruction include cotton rolls, whole teeth or fragments of teeth, crowns, amalgams, and veneers.
   B. Types of FBAO include:
      1. Partial obstruction with adequate air exchange.
         a. Occurs when the airway is not completely blocked.
         b. Allows the patient to cough forcibly and talk.
         c. Requires no treatment but must be monitored closely.
      2. Partial obstruction with poor air exchange.
         a. Is indicated when the patient is unable to cough forcibly and wheezing occurs during inhalation.
         b. May lead to complete airway obstruction and should be treated as such.
      3. Complete airway obstruction.
         a. Is indicated when the patient is unable to talk; the patient may exhibit the universal distress signal (hands clasped at the throat; Fig. 14–4).
         b. Symptoms include cyanosis and a loss of consciousness when the object is not removed.

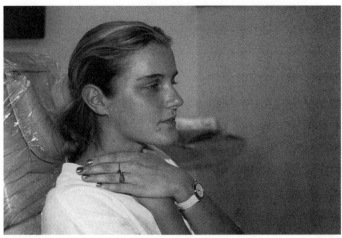

Figure 14.4 The universal distress signal for airway obstruction (choking).

c. Treatment for the conscious adult or child with complete obstruction or partial obstruction with poor air exchange is the same and includes:

 1) Asking the patient "Are you choking?" and "Can you speak?"

 2) Performing the Heimlich maneuver, which involves standing behind the patient, wrapping both arms around the victim, and delivering abdominal thrusts. The flat portion of one fist is positioned between the navel and the bottom of the rib cage. The other hand is wrapped around this fist; the rescuer subsequently pushes inward and upward until the object is removed or the patient becomes unconscious.

  a) For the pregnant or obese patient, chest thrusts are performed by standing behind the patient and positioning the fists in the same manner on the lower portion of the sternum; inward thrusts are given until the object is expelled or the patient becomes unconscious.

d. Activate the EMS if the patient becomes unconscious.

 1) Help the patient to the floor or perform abdominal thrusts in the chair.

 2) Position yourself by straddling the patient's hips or standing close to the hips at one side (if patient remains positioned in dental unit) (Figure 14–5).

 3) Place the heel of one hand between the navel and the bottom of the rib cage; position the other hand above the first, interlacing fingers.

 4) Push inward and upward five times; subsequently move to the head of the patient and open the airway. Look for the object, sweep in an attempt to remove it, and attempt to ventilate.

 5) If no breath goes in, reattempt ventilation, then continue with five abdominal thrusts, look, sweep, and attempt to ventilate. Continue this cycle until help arrives or air goes in.

 6) If air does go in, give two additional breaths to stimulate breathing and check the patient's pulse. Begin cardiac compressions if a pulse is not present (Table 14–1).

 Clinical Case **STUDY**

Arthur Mack, a 54-year-old man, is in the office for his recall oral prophylaxis appointment. He currently takes medication for hypertension and carries nitroglycerin for occasional angina. He had a heart attack 5 years ago, at which time coronary bypass surgery was performed. Arthur reports feeling fine and is anxious to have his teeth cleaned because it has been almost a year since his last appointment. His blood pressure today is 158/94 and his pulse is 92. Shortly after the patient is placed in a reclining position and treatment is begun, Mr. Mack asks to be positioned upright. He appears pale, is short of breath, and says that his chest hurts.

Clinical Case QUESTIONS

1. What term describes the pain in the patient's chest?
2. How should this condition be treated?
3. What is indicated by the continued presence of chest pain after the use of nitroglycerin tablets?
4. What type of drug is nitroglycerin?
5. Describe how this situation is managed if the patient loses consciousness.

Clinical Case RATIONALES

1. The chest pain is angina pectoris and is caused by a decreased oxygen supply to the heart. Hypoxia refers to a deficiency of oxygen in the air being breathed in. Dyspnea is another term for difficult or labored breathing.
2. The treatment of angina includes the administration of nitroglycerin beneath the patient's tongue. It is best to follow the patient's instruction for administering this drug, if possible. Relief often results within 90 seconds. While the patient is experiencing angina, he should be positioned in whatever way he is most comfortable. Oxygen should be administered to any patient who is experiencing chest pain.
3. When angina is not relieved after three nitroglycerin tablets or sprays, a myocardial infarction or heart attack may occur. Other terms for myocardial infarction include coronary thrombosis and coronary occlusion.

TABLE 14.1 Airway Obstruction		
	Adult	**Child**	**Infant**
If conscious	• Ask victim "Are you choking?" • Perform Heimlich maneuver; repeat until effective or victim becomes unconscious.	• Ask victim "Are you choking?" • Perform Heimlich maneuver; repeat until effective or victim becomes unconscious.	• Check for breathing difficulty (e.g., no crying, blue lips) • Give 5 back blows, then 5 chest thrusts until effective or victim becomes unconscious.
If unconscious	• Activate EMS—call 911 • Look into mouth for object; sweep to remove. • Attempt to ventilate. • If breath does not go in, reposition head, try again. • If unable to ventilate, kneel astride victim's thighs and give 5 abdominal thrusts, recheck mouth for object, attempt to ventilate. • If still unable to ventilate, continue with 5 abdominal thrusts, followed by attempts to ventilate. • If ventilation goes in, give 2 additional breaths and check the pulse. • If no pulse, begin compressions.	• Activate EMS—call 911 • Look into mouth for object; sweep only if object is visible. • Attempt to ventilate. • If breath does not go in, reposition head, try again. • If unable to ventilate, kneel astride victim's thighs and give 5 abdominal thrusts, recheck mouth for object, attempt to ventilate. • If still unable to ventilate, continue with 5 abdominal thrusts, followed by attempts to ventilate. • If ventilation goes in, give 2 additional breaths and check the pulse. • If no pulse, begin compressions.	• Activate EMS—call 911. • Look into mouth for object; sweep only if object is visible. • Attempt to ventilate. • If breath does not go in, reposition head and try again. • If still unable to ventilate, give 5 back blows followed by 5 chest thrusts. • If ventilation goes in, give 2 additional breaths and check the pulse. • If no pulse, begin compressions.

Although this patient does exhibit predisposing factors for a stroke (hypertension, cardiovascular disease), the presence of angina is characteristic of myocardial infarction and not of CVA.

4. Nitroglycerin is a vasodilator and the most effective drug in the treatment of angina. Normally it increases blood flow to the coronary arteries by decreasing coronary artery resistance.

5. If the patient loses consciousness, management includes basic life support as follows: activate the EMS system by calling 911 or having another individual call; position the patient supine, open the airway, and assess breathing; give two ventilations if breathing is not present; check for the carotid pulse, and begin chest compressions as needed. A demand-valve system can be used to supply ventilations but breathing must be assessed initially. Chest compressions are given on the lower half of the sternum.

VI. Angina pectoris
   A. Refers to chest pain caused by a decreased oxygen flow to the heart.
   B. Symptoms
      1. Include chest pain, which may spread to the jaws and teeth, and possibly to the edentulous arches.
      2. Lasts 3 to 5 minutes after the cause of the pain is removed.
      3. The patient remains still in an attempt to relieve the pain.
   C. Types of angina
      1. Stable angina
         a. Often is caused by emotional upset or physical exertion.
         b. Is characterized by a constant duration and intensity of pain.
         c. Is relieved by the administration of nitroglycerin.
      2. Unstable angina
         a. Can occur when the victim is at rest.
         b. Is characterized by greater intensity, longer

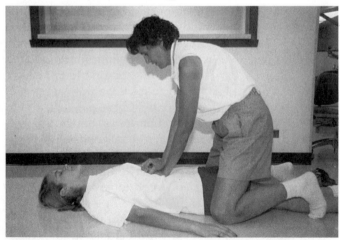

Figure 14.5 Abdominal thrusts are administered when airway obstruction results in a loss of consciousness.

duration, and more frequent occurrence compared with stable angina.

c. Is not relieved by the administration of nitroglycerin.

D. Treatment for either type of angina includes:

1. Calming the patient and positioning the patient as comfortably as possible.
2. The administration of oxygen, as needed.
3. The administration of nitroglycerin beeath the tongue, as needed.

   a. Nitroglycerin works as a vasodilator; the emergency kit should contain a tablet or spray form of the drug.

      1) The tablet form has a short shelf life; may be used for 6 months after the container is opened.
      2) The nitrolingual spray has a much longer shelf life; one spray is equal to one tablet.
      3) Amyl nitrite also is a vasodilator and is used as an inhalant; is crushed and held beneath the patient's nose; provides significant vasodilation in 10 seconds. Side effects are greater with this type.
      4) Ointment or patch forms of nitroglycerin may be prescribed by the patient's physician to prevent or reduce the number of angina episodes; are not recommended for rapid treatment of angina because they work slowly; patients must use sublingual nitroglycerin for quick relief.

   b. Normally 1 to 3 sublingual tablets or the same number of nitrolingual sprays relieve the pain in 1 to 2 minutes; it is best to follow the patient's instructions for nitroglycerin use; the pain should not return.

   c. Side effects include orthostatic hypotension and headache.

   d. If no relief occurs after three nitroglycerin tablets or sprays or if the angina returns after relief, myocardial infarction may be occurring.

VII. Myocardial Infarction (MI)

A. Is more commonly known as heart attack, coronary thrombosis, or coronary occlusion.

B. Involves the death of a portion of the heart muscle; is caused by a decrease in or lack of oxygen flow to that part of the heart muscle.

C. May be caused by atherosclerosis of the coronary arteries or by thrombosis in the artery that supplies the heart muscle.

D. Most often occurs while the victim is at rest.

E. May follow a preexisting anginal condition.

F. Symptoms

1. Diffuse pain in the chest, arms, neck, and/or lower jaw.

2. Pain is of greater intensity and duration than angina.

3. The patient typically moves around in an attempt to alleviate discomfort.

4. Other symptoms include dizziness, shortness of breath, cold and clammy skin, weakness, fatigue, anxiety, and the denial of a possible MI.

G. Treatment includes:

1. Positioning the patient however he or she is most comfortable.
2. Administering nitroglycerin.
3. Activating the EMS by calling 911.
4. Providing oxygen.
5. Providing basic life support management as indicated.

H. Angina that is not relieved by nitroglycerin may lead to cardiac arrest.

I. Considerations after the occurrence of an MI

1. No dental treatment is recommended during the first 6 months after the episode; the patient's cardiologist must be consulted before treatment.
2. The patient may begin to take anticoagulants, digitalis, and/or nitroglycerin.

VIII. Cardiac Arrest or Sudden Death

A. Refers to the abrupt, unexpected cessation of breathing and circulation.

B. Causes

1. Cardiovascular disease
2. Drug overdose
3. Electrocution
4. Drowning
5. Anaphylactic shock
6. Hypoxia

C. Symptoms

1. No pulse or respiration
2. Cyanotic tissues and dilated pupils
3. Unconsciousness

D. Treatment for an adult

1. Provide basic life support

   a. Determine unconsciousness and activate the emergency medical system (EMS) by telephoning 911.

   b. Position the victim on a hard surface or place a CPR board beneath the victim's back on the dental chair.

   c. Open the airway with the head-tilt chin-lift method and determine breathlessness; look, listen, and feel for moving air for 7 to 15 seconds (Fig. 14–6).

   d. Ventilate twice; each breath should last 1 to 1½ seconds.

   e. Check for the presence of a pulse, using the carotid artery, for 5–10 seconds.

   f. If there is no pulse, find the landmark for external compressions, which is two finger widths above the xiphoid process. Place the

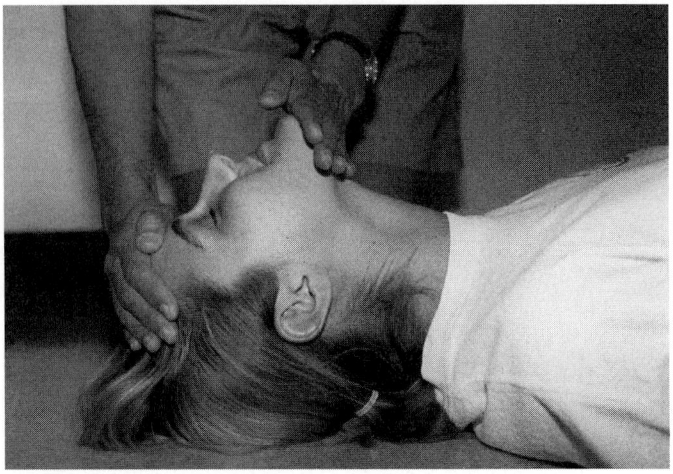

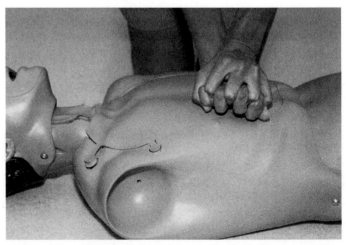

Figure 14.6 The airway is opened using the head-tilt chin-lift technique.

heel of one hand on this point and the other hand above it, interlacing fingers. Be sure that the xiphoid process is not compressed.

   g. Press down 1½ to 2 inches for 15 compressions in 9 to 11 seconds (Figure 14–7).

   h. Give two ventilations and resume compressions.

   i. Continue with 15 compressions and 2 breaths for a total of four cycles; subsequently recheck the pulse. If there is no pulse, continue with the compressions and ventilations until help arrives or the pulse returns.

2. Replace the first rescuer with a second rescuer
   a. A second rescuer should identify self and state "I know CPR, I can help."

   b. Should call 911, if necessary; subsequently checks the patient's pulse.

   c. Begins compressions and rescue breathing; the first rescuer assesses efforts by watching for the chest to rise during rescue breaths and checking for a pulse during compressions.

   d. The rescuers alternate roles (as each tires) until help arrives.

3. CPR with two rescuers
   a. Begins with one rescuer, who determines unresponsiveness, calls for help (second person), opens the airway, checks for breathing, gives two rescue breaths, and checks the carotid artery for a pulse.

   b. If there is no pulse, the second rescuer gives five compressions at the correct landmark, which are followed by one slow rescue breath given by first rescuer. Cycles of five compressions and one breath continue.

   c. Between 80 and 100 compressions should be given in 1 minute.

   d. The pulse should be checked after 1 mi-

nute; if there is no pulse, compressions and rescue breathing should continue.

E. Other considerations
   1. If the victim has a pulse but is not breathing, provide rescue breaths at a rate of 12 per minute, or once every 5 seconds, and continue checking for the presence of a pulse.

   2. The emergency medical system (EMS) must be activated immediately by calling 911; if the heart is in fibrillation, defibrillation is necessary to make the compressions effective.

   3. Gastric distention (excess air in the stomach) may occur, even with correct technique; there is no treatment for this.

   4. Broken ribs, a lacerated liver, or punctured lungs may occur, even with correct technique.

F. CPR for children (1 to 8 years of age)
   1. Cardiac arrest in children most often occurs as a result of respiratory difficulty; therefore, the heart will not be in fibrillation. If no other person is available to call 911 immediately, CPR can be performed for 1 minute, followed by activation of the EMS.

   2. The technique is the same as for an adult victim, with the following exceptions:
     a. Only the heel of one hand is used for compressions, compared with the use of two hands for an adult (Fig. 14–8).

     b. Compressions are only 1 to 1½ inches in depth.

     c. Five compressions are followed by 1 breath; 100 compressions should be given in 1 minute. The ratio of compressions to breaths is 5:1 for the child, compared with 15:2 for the adult.

     d. When rescue breathing is necessary, it is performed once every 3 seconds or 20 times per minute.

Figure 14.7 If no pulse is detected, chest compressions are begun; the rescuer presses 1½ to 2 inches on the lower half of the sternum.

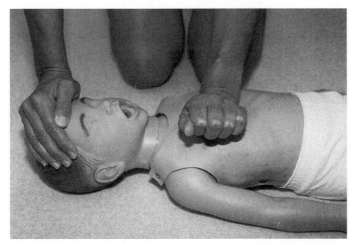

Figure 14.8 For the child, the heel of one hand is used for compressions.

G. CPR technique for the infant (less than 1 year of age)
  1. Tap or gently shake the infant to establish unresponsiveness.
  2. When the infant is turned, the head and neck must be supported. Open the airway using the head-tilt chin-lift method and determine breathlessness (look, listen, and feel).
  3. If the infant is not breathing, give two gentle rescue breaths while maintaining an open airway. The rescuer's mouth should cover the mouth and nose of the infant. Each breath should be given for 1 to 1½ seconds.
  4. Check for the presence of a pulse using two fingers of one hand at the brachial artery (inside the upper arm) while maintaining the head tilt with the other hand. The pulse check should take 5 seconds (Fig. 14–9).
  5. If there is no pulse, begin chest compressions by first finding the correct landmark: draw an imaginary line between the nipples and position the index finger on this line. Place the middle and ring fingers below the index finger and make compressions with the pads of these two fingers at a depth of ½ to 1 inch. Compressions must not be given on the xiphoid process.
  6. Five compressions are given for one breath, at a rate of at least 100 compressions per minute (five compressions are given in 3 seconds). After approximately 1 minute, check for a pulse. If alone, activate the emergency medical system and continue with cycles of compressions and breaths until help arrives or a pulse returns.
  7. The infant's head must be supported at all times (Table 14–2).

TABLE 14.2	Basic Life Support		
	Adult CPR	**Child CPR**	**Infant CPR**
Assessment	• Establish unresponsiveness; activate EMS—call 911.	• Establish unresponsiveness; call for "help."	• Establish unresponsiveness; call for "help."
Airway	• Open airway using head-tilt, chin-lift.	• Open airway using head-tilt, chin-lift.	• Open airway using head-tilt, chin-lift
Breathing	• Determine breathlessness (Look, Listen, Feel).	• Determine breathlessness (Look, Listen, Feel).	• Determine breathlessness (Look, Listen, Feel).
	• No breathing: give 2 ventilations (1–1½ seconds per breath).	• No breathing: give 2 ventilations (1–1½ seconds per breath).	• No breathing: give 2 ventilations (1–1½ seconds per breath).
Circulation	• Check carotid pulse	• Check carotid pulse	• Check brachial pulse
	• If no pulse, begin compressions, pressing 1½ to 2-inches on lower ½ of sternum using both hands.	• If no pulse, begin compressions, pressing 1–1½-inches on lower ½ of sternum using both hands.	• If no pulse, begin compressions, pressing ½ to 1-inches, one finger-width below the nipple line, using pads of middle and ring fingers.
	• Give 80–100 compressions per minute; 15 compressions followed by 2 breaths	• Give 100 compressions per minute, 5 compressions followed by one breath.	• Give 100 compressions per minute, 5 compressions followed by one breath.
	• After 4 cycles, recheck pulse	• After 20 cycles, call 911, recheck pulse.	• After 20 cycles, call 911, recheck pulse.
	• If no pulse, continue with compressions and breathing until help arrives	• If no pulse, continue with compressions and breathing until help arrives	• If no pulse, continue with compressions and breathing until help arrives.
	• If pulse returns but victim is not breathing, provide rescue breathing	• If pulse returns but victim is not breathing, provide rescue breathing	• If pulse returns but victim is not breathing, provide rescue breathing.
Ventilation	• 1 breath every 5 seconds (12 per minute).	• 1 breath every 3 seconds (20 per minute).	• 1 breath every 3 seconds (20 per minute).
	• Continue monitoring pulse.	• Continue monitoring pulse.	• Continue monitoring pulse.

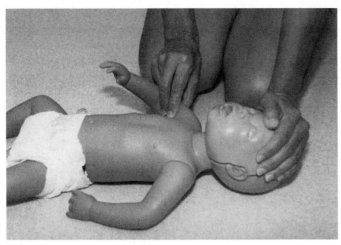

Figure 14.9 For the infant, the pulse is checked by placing two fingers on the brachial artery while maintaining the head tilt.

 Clinical Case **STUDY**

Mr. Jamison, a 65-year-old man, is following a 6-month recall schedule for oral prophylaxis and examination. He currently takes medication for high blood pressure and insulin for his diabetes, which is well controlled. No other conditions are reported. Mr. Jamison's vital signs during this appointment include a pulse rate of 82, a respiration rate of 16 breaths per minute, and a blood pressure reading of 144/86 mm Hg.

Clinical Case QUESTIONS

1. Which of Mr. Jamison's medical conditions are associated with potential emergency situations?
2. Describe potential emergency situations that the dental hygienist should be aware of for this patient.
3. Are the vital signs recorded for this appointment within normal range?

Clinical Case RATIONALES

1. Hypertension, diabetes, and the use of antihypertensive drugs each pose risks and may lead to the development of an emergency situation.
2. Several emergency situations are possible. Antihypertensive drugs increase the chance of syncope caused by orthostatic hypotension (a lowering of the blood pressure from remaining in one position for a significant period). Mr. Jamison may experience dizziness, lightheadedness, a loss of balance, or syncope when he is raised from the supine position. It is important to raise the patient slowly and allow him to sit upright before he is dismissed.

   The potential for hypoglycemia or hyperglycemia is of concern for patients who have diabetes. Individuals with insulin-dependent diabetes are more likely to experience hypoglycemia. Conscious patients who experience hypoglycemia demonstrate quickly occurring symptoms of a cold sweat, headache, trembling, weakness, a personality change, and confusion. A source of sugar, such as orange juice or a chocolate candy bar, should be ingested by the patient to reverse the symptoms. If unconsciousness occurs because of hypoglycemia, the patient will be unable to swallow a sugar source and an injection of Glucagon will be necessary. When hyperglycemia occurs, the patient presents dry, warm skin, Kussmaul breathing, a fruity breath odor, and increased thirst and urination. Factors that increase the need for insulin, such as stress, illness, or infection, will precipitate hyperglycemia. If these symptoms occur, dental treatment should be stopped and a medical consultation should be sought.

   The presence of both hypertension and diabetes also is a concern. A cerebrovascular accident (stroke) does not commonly occur in the dental office, but two predisposing factors (hypertension and diabetes) increase a patient's risk for this occurrence.

3. A pulse rate of 82 is within the normal range of 60 to 90 beats per minute for adults. The respiration rate of 16 is within the normal range of 14 to 20 breaths per minute. The blood pressure reading of 144/86 indicates a higher than normal systolic reading (normal range is between 100 to 140) but the diastolic is within normal range (60 to 90 mm Hg). Because the systolic reading is above 140, a second blood pressure reading should be taken to check accuracy. This patient's reading is below the level that necessitates a medical consultation (160/95 or greater).

VIII. Cerebrovascular Accident (CVA) or Stroke
   A. Is classified according to its cause.
   B. May be caused by cerebral embolism, hemorrhage, infarction, or thrombosis.
   C. Symptoms include the presence of a headache together with confusion, impaired speech, paralysis, and unconsciousness; they vary in relation to the area affected and the type of CVA and do not regress.
   D. Treatment
      1. If the patient is conscious, allow him or her to remain upright; if unconscious, position the patient supine, with the head slightly elevated.
      2. Activate the EMS.
      3. Monitor vital signs (blood pressure will be elevated).
      4. Administer oxygen to the unconscious patient; for conscious patients, administer oxygen only when respiratory difficulty exists.
      5. Provide basic life support as needed.
   E. Other considerations

1. CVAs are characterized by a high incidence of recurrence; thus patients with this history pose a greater risk in the dental office. Management involves recording vital signs at each appointment; elevated blood pressure readings are of concern.
2. No elective dental treatment should be performed within 6 months after a CVA.
3. Physical limitations are a common result of stroke.
4. A cerebrovascular accident is not a common dental office emergency; predisposing factors include hypertension, diabetes mellitus, cardiovascular disease, and a history of transient ischemic attacks.

F. Transient ischemic attack (TIA)
1. Is similar to a stroke yet lasts for only a few minutes; symptoms regress and no permanent neurologic damage results; also is referred to as a temporary or incipient stroke.
2. TIAs indicate the presence of significant cerebrovascular disease.
3. May advance to cerebral infarction and result in a stroke.
4. The patient is conscious during a TIA yet experiences confusion.

IX. Seizures
A. May be caused by epilepsy; other causes include a prolonged high fever, alcohol or drug withdrawal, trauma to the head, congenital abnormalities, and an imbalance of body fluids. In the dental office, seizures caused by epilepsy may be triggered by stress.
B. Seizures are categorized according to the area of the brain affected and associated symptoms.
1. Grand mal seizure
a. Is the most common type of seizure (approximately 90% of patients with epilepsy experience this type).
b. Has three phases.
1) The prodromal phase (an early symptom of disease)
a) Occurs before seizure activity.
b) May result in a personality change.
c) May include the experience of an aura (a scent, a flicker of light, or a noise) that is unique for that person.
d) May last for a few seconds or several hours.
2) The convulsive or ictal phase
a) Is characterized by the loss of consciousness.
b) Is associated with an epileptic cry caused by air rushing from the lungs.
c) Is characterized by tonic movements that occur as the body becomes rigid (10 to 20 seconds).
d) Also is characterized by clonic movements that result from the contraction and relaxation of muscles and cause the patient to jerk violently.
e) Typically lasts for 2 to 5 minutes.
3) The postictal stage
a) Occurs after seizure activity and lasts for 10 to 30 minutes, during which time the patient sleeps soundly.
b) Basic life support is critical at this time. Snoring during the sleep indicates that the airway is partly blocked; a gurgling sound indicates that the airway must be suctioned for vomitus or blood.
c) Is characterized by confusion and disorientation; full recovery takes several hours.
2. Petit mal seizure
a. Also is known as an absence seizure.
b. Occurs more often in children than in adults.
c. Involves a loss of awareness of surroundings for a few seconds; the victim stares blankly and experiences twitching or rapid blinking.
3. Partial seizure
a. Is characterized by a jerking of one side of the body because only one hemisphere of the brain is involved.
b. Is characterized by a trance-like appearance and engagement in a purposeless activity.
4. Hysterical seizure
a. Occurs when there is an audience and is used to manipulate others, which indicates that this seizure can be triggered by emotions and anxiety.
b. Involves movements that are more controlled (e.g., the repeated up-and-down movement of one arm).
5. Status epilepticus
a. Is characterized by the same symptoms that are present during the convulsive stage of a grand mal but the symptoms last longer than 5 minutes; is uninterrupted, with no recovery between episodes; may last for hours or days.
b. Is the major cause of death related directly to seizures.
C. Treatment
1. Main objectives include:
a. Preventing the patient from hurting himself or herself.
b. Providing support after the seizure.
2. Other considerations include:
a. Removing dental objects from the patient's mouth if possible.

b. Clearing the area surrounding the patient.

c. No attempt should be made to restrain patient.

d. Placing the patient on his or her side after the seizure.

e. For the unconscious patient, placing the patient in a supine position and maintaining an open airway.

f. The patient should not be given anything to eat or drink; also should not be permitted to drive after the episode.

g. Medical assistance must be summoned if injury occurs during the seizure or if no breathing is present.

D. Medications may include anticonvulsants, such as phenytoin (Dilantin) or phenobarbital, which may result in gingival overgrowth.

E. Removable appliances are not recommended because they may cause trauma or may be aspirated during seizure activity.

X. Hypoglycemia

A. This office emergency is more likely than others to occur if a patient has a history of diabetes.

1. Types of diabetes

a. Type I or IDDM

1) Accounts for 10% of cases of diabetes.

2) Is the more severe form.

3) Is treated with daily administration of insulin, by means of injection or infusion pump.

b. Type II or NIDDM

1) Is most common among middle-aged, obese individuals (accounts for 80% of cases of Type II diabetes).

2) Most often is controlled with diet and exercise; in some cases may require an oral hypoglycemic medication such as Orinase.

B. Also is known as insulin shock or low blood sugar. Although low blood sugar can be experienced by anyone, a much higher incidence occurs among individuals with IDDM.

C. Can be caused by a skipped meal, excess insulin, increased exercise, or a change in routine; onset is rapid for the patient who requires insulin; symptoms occur more slowly for individuals who take an oral hypoglycemic medication such as Orinase.

D. Is characterized by a cold sweat, headache, trembling, weakness, a possible personality change, nervousness, and confusion; the confusion may be mistaken for inebriation.

E. Treatment

1. Includes supplying sugar; orange juice, a chocolate bar, cake icing, or glucose gel from a tube may be used if the patient is conscious.

2. If the patient becomes unconscious, he or she should be positioned supine, with feet elevated. Normally, breathing and circulation are maintained; the pulse rate is more rapid but blood pressure is not affected. Because a sugar source cannot be administered to an unconscious patient, Glucagon, a hormone that changes stored sugar to a usable form, is given intramuscularly. A response to Glucagon occurs in 10 to 15 minutes; if parenteral administration is not possible, small amounts of honey, decorative cake icing, or glucose gel can be placed in the lining of the mucobuccal fold.

3. When the patient is unconscious for more than 30 seconds, seizure activity is more likely to occur. If a seizure occurs, it must be managed before the hypoglycemia is treated.

XI. Hyperglycemia

A. Occurs in response to little or no insulin or when an individual's glucose level is too high; may occur in patients with diabetes or in those with undiagnosed diabetes. Urine samples indicate a high glucose level and the presence of ketones.

B. Is an emergency situation; if untreated may lead to unconsciousness (diabetic coma or ketoacidosis). Infection, stress, illness, failure to comply with therapy, and other factors that increase the need for insulin may precipitate this condition.

C. Is characterized by increased thirst and urination, a loss of appetite, nausea, vomiting, Kussmaul breathing (heavy, labored breathing), dry, warm skin, and a fruity, sweet odor of the breath. The heart rate is rapid and weak, and blood pressure is lower than normal. When these symptoms are present, no further dental treatment is performed and a medical consultation is indicated.

D. The patient typically is seen immediately by a physician or is hospitalized. This condition may advance to diabetic coma; before the use of insulin, diabetic coma was the major cause of death from diabetes.

E. When it is not known whether the nature of the emergency is hyperglycemia or hypoglycemia, the condition is treated as hypoglycemia by emergency medical personnel. Hypoglycemia, if not treated quickly, may lead to serious damage or death. Alternately, permanent disability or death from hyperglycemia takes much longer to occur (Table 14–3).

Dental Emergencies

Dental emergencies occur as a result of dental treatment or because treatment is needed. These emergencies include acute pericoronitis, necrotic socket, avulsed tooth, displaced tooth, postsurgical hemorrhage, broken instrument tip, foreign body injuries, and common injuries to the patient or operator.

TABLE 14.3	Quick Check Chart of Medical Emergencies	
Emergency	**Important Features**	**Treatment**
Syncope	Pallor, dizziness, nausea	Position in Trendelenburg position Maintain open airway (if unconscious) Administer ammonia inhalant, oxygen
Hyperventilation	Increased rate, depth of breathing	Position upright Have patient breathe into paper bag (6–10 times per minute) Administer diazepam (severe cases)
Asthma	Wheezing on exhalation; difficulty breathing	Position upright Administer bronchodilator, oxygen Provide BLS, as needed Administer epinephrine (if bronchodilator is ineffective)
Anaphylactic reaction	Affects skin, respiratory GI, and circulatory systems	Position supine Provide BLS, as needed Administer epinephrine
Cerebrovascular accident	Severe headache, confusion, slurred speech, paralysis	Conscious • Position upright • Administer oxygen (if dyspnea) Unconscious • Position supine with head slightly elevated • Adminsiter oxygen • Activate EMS, BLS
Angina pectoris	Chest pain; may radiate to jaws, teeth, edentulous arch; may advance MI	Position comfortably Administer nitroglycerin, oxygen
Myocardial infarction (MI)	Diffuse pain in chest, arms, neck, and jaw—of longer duration, greater intensity than angina	Position comfortably Administer nitroglycerin, oxygen Activate EMS, BLS
Partial airway obstruction	Patient able to speak or cough	Monitor situation
Complete airway obstruction	Inability to speak , cough forcibly; wheezing on inhalation	Administer Heimlich maneuver If unconsciousness, administer abdominal thrusts, open airway.
Grand mal seizure	3 stages: prodromal, convulsive, prodromal	Keep patient from hurting self Offer support after seizure activity Maintain airway if patient is conscious
Cardiac arrest/ sudden death	Sudden, unexpected cessation of breathing, circulation; tissue cyanotic, pupils dilated, patient unconscious	Activate EMS Provide BLS
Hypoglycemia	Weakness, dizziness, pale and moist skin, shallow respirations, confusion, personality change (diabetic and nondiabetic patients)	Conscious • Supply sugar source Unconscious • Position supine • Give glucagon injection
Hyperglycemia	Increased thirst, urination, Kussmaul breathing, fruity acetone breath caused by insufficient insulin (insulin-dependent diabetes)	Conscious • Seek medical consult • Terminate dental treatment Unconscious • Position supine • Provide BLS and medical assistance

BLS, basic life support.

I. Acute Pericoronitis
   A. Is an inflammation of the soft tissue that surrounds the crown of an erupting tooth.
   B. Is most often associated with erupting mandibular third molars and typically is accompanied by an infection.
   C. Symptoms
      1. Include localized tenderness and erythema.
      2. May progress to severe soreness and edema, with lymph node involvement and the presence of a fever.
      3. The patient may experience trismus or difficulty in opening his or her mouth when the mandibular third molar is involved.
   D. Treatment includes:
      1. Irrigation with a saline rinse to clean the area.
      2. The use of hot saline soaks by the patient at home.
      3. Antibiotics, as prescribed by the dentist, to treat lymphadenopathy and fever.

II. Dry-Socket or Acute Osteomyelitis
   A. Is a painful condition that occurs after the extraction of a tooth.
   B. Is caused by the loss of a blood clot in the area; results in the exposure of bone.
   C. Symptoms
      1. Severe pain in the extraction area or referred pain 3 to 5 days after extraction.
      2. The lack of a blood clot in the extraction site.
      3. A strong mouth odor.
   D. Treatment
      1. Debriding the area with a saline solution.
      2. Isolating and drying the area and subsequent placement of a dressing that contains germicide and analgesic.
      3. Retreatment, as needed. When a gauze packing is used, it must be removed after treatment.

III. Avulsed Tooth
   A. Refers to a tooth that has been completely removed from its socket because of trauma.
   B. May involve moderate pain or no pain.
   C. Treatment
      1. Immediate examination of the patient in the office.
      2. Asking the patient to bring the tooth to the office in a wet handkerchief, milk, or water, or in the patient's buccal vestibule (preferred mode of transport).
      3. Radiographing the area to identify any remaining fragments.
      4. Reimplantation of the tooth and placement of a splint in the area.
      5. A better prognosis results when there is a short time between avulsion and reimplantation.
      6. Root canal therapy, as indicated.
      7. Observation of other trauma.
   D. A tetanus booster may be indicated.

IV. Displaced Tooth
   A. Refers to a tooth that has loosened in the socket and visibly moves.
   B. Typically is associated with pain.
   C. Treatment
      1. Immediate dental treatment.
      2. Radiographing the area to check for root fracture.
      3. Applying a splint, depending on the severity of the displacement.
      4. Instructing the patient not to chew or bite with this tooth.
      5. Observation of other trauma.
      6. Identifying the need for a tetanus booster.
      7. The application of cold packs to minimize external swelling.

Clinical Case STUDY

Ben Martin visits the dental office on Wednesday morning for an extraction of tooth #15. The extraction is simple and no complications are expected. After the extraction, sterile gauze is placed over the wound and Mr. Martin is instructed to bite the gauze for 30 minutes. Verbal instructions for care of the extraction site are given before Ben is released. On Thursday afternoon, Ben calls the office because the extraction site has begun to bleed. Upon further questioning, he indicates that he continued to smoke after the extraction because it helped him relax.

Clinical Case QUESTIONS

1. What verbal instructions should have been given to Ben after the extraction?
2. Is the bleeding that occurred on Thursday considered primary or secondary bleeding?
3. Describe the appropriate treatment for this situation.
4. What could the patient have done to prevent the recurrence of bleeding?
5. What could dental personnel have done to prevent the situation?

Clinical Case RATIONALES

1. The patient should have been given verbal instructions to avoid all of the following for at least 24 hours: strenuous activity, rinsing the mouth, drinking from a straw, smoking, and drinking alcohol.
2. Bleeding that occurs 24 hours after extraction is considered secondary bleeding. Bleeding that occurs within the first 24 hours is termed primary bleeding.
3. The treatment of postsurgical hemorrhage includes returning to the dental office if occlusion on gauze

does not halt the bleeding. Because bleeding has recurred, the patient should not drink from a straw or rinse the area with warm saline rinses for 24 hours.

4. The patient's smoking after the extraction most likely was the cause of the secondary bleeding.

5. In cases of surgical tooth extraction, written instructions in addition to verbal instructions should be given to the patient. Although the patient may indicate that he understands the procedures to be followed, he may not hear or remember all instructions. In this case, he did not adhere to the instruction regarding smoking.

V. Postsurgical Hemorrhage
   A. Occurs when bleeding returns or continues after an extraction and is not halted by occlusion on gauze; the patient must return to the office.
   B. Can be controlled at home by biting on folded gauze, folded tissue, or on a tea bag.
   C. Is considered primary bleeding when it occurs within 24 hours after the extraction.
   D. Is considered secondary bleeding when it occurs 24 or more hours after the extraction.
   E. Prevention involves:
      1. Awareness of medical conditions that could cause problems (updating medical history).
      2. Instructing the patient to refrain from tobacco or alcohol use after the extraction.
      3. Advising the patient to avoid rinsing the area or drinking from a straw for 24 hours after the extraction.
      4. Advising the patient to avoid strenuous exercise for 24 hours after the extraction.
      5. Providing the patient with both written and verbal instructions.
VI. Broken Instrument Tip
   A. Requires removal from the patient's mouth.
   B. Requires that the operator stop procedures, keep the patient calm, and ask the patient not to swallow.
   C. Recovery
      1. Visually examine the area first, and subsequently drying the area with a cotton roll (not with the air syringe).
      2. Examine the sulcus with gentle strokes of a curette in a spoon-like manner; the tip should not be pushed into the base of the sulcus.
      3. Expose a periapical radiograph of the suspected location of the broken tip (if the tip is not located).
      4. Request medical consultation and radiographs of the patient's chest and gastrointestinal area (if the tip is not located and secured).

D. Office policy is essential for the management of this emergency situation; should include an outline of the steps to be followed. All office personnel should be familiar with this policy.
VII. Foreign Body Injuries
   A. Are injuries caused by objects that are foreign to a particular part of the body; in dentistry, these injuries most often affect the eyes or respiratory tract.
   B. Typically involve polishing agents, calculus, restorative materials, cements, displaced crowns, chemicals, or extracted teeth.
   C. Prevention
      1. Protective eyewear should be worn by the patient during treatment.
      2. The operator must have knowledge of the equipment being used and the rotation direction of the rubber cup when polishing.
      3. The patient should be informed of all procedures and their role in prevention.
      4. The operator must use care when handling instruments and polishing pastes; pastes and other solutions should not be held directly over a patient's face.
      5. Thin instruments should be replaced to prevent breakage.
      6. Children must be attended to at all times.
      7. A rubber dam should be used as needed during treatment.
   D. Treatment
      1. For cases involving aspiration, radiographs of the chest and gastrointestinal area may be necessary to locate the object.
      2. If an object enters a patient's eye (the eye reacts by tearing and blinking):
         a. Ask the patient to look down and position the upper lid over the lower lid for 1 second; subsequently pull lid upward.
         b. If the object or particle can be seen in the lower lid, use a moistened cotton applicator to retrieve the object and flush the eye using an eye cup or an eye washing station.
         c. Medical assistance is necessary if the object cannot be removed; to prevent the patient from rubbing the eye, stabilize gauze over the eye with adhesive tape.
VIII. Common injuries to the operator include skin wounds, burns, and foreign bodies in the eye.
   A. Wounds that break the skin
      1. Are caused by:
         a. The slippage of instruments during treatment or clean-up.
         b. The use of dull instruments.
         c. Sudden patient movement.
         d. A needlestick.
         e. A bite.

2. Prevention includes:
   a. Maintaining a stable fulcrum on a dry surface during instrumentation.
   b. Maintaining sharp instruments.
   c. Using the "scoop technique" or a commercial device to recap needles.
   d. Wearing protective eyewear.
3. Treatment
   a. Cleaning the wound with soap and water; it may be necessary to force a puncture wound to bleed.
   b. Placing an ice pack on the area to reduce swelling.
   c. Applying firm pressure to control the bleeding of a laceration.
   d. When cross-infection or contamination is a concern:
      1) Have the source tested for hepatitis B surface antigen (HBsAg) and for antibodies to the human immunodeficiency virus (anti-HIV) on the same day. If this is not possible, the operator must be tested.
      2) If the operator has completed the hepatitis B vaccine and postvaccine titer levels are adequate, testing for the hepatitis B virus (HBV) is not necessary. If the titer level is not adequate, a single dose of hepatitis B immunoglobulin (HBIG) is indicated.
      3) When the operator is tested for HIV, testing should occur on the same day, at 6 weeks, at 12 weeks, and at 6 months. If no antibodies are detected at 6 months, the exposure did not result in HIV infection.
      4) The operator's tetanus vaccine should be current.
B. Burns that occur in laboratories or in sterilization areas are most often caused by Bunsen burners, autoclaves, or dry heat sterilizers.
   1. Are classified according to their source (e.g., heat or chemicals).
   2. Also are classified according to their depth.
      a. Superficial burns or first degree burns involve only the top layer of skin; such burns are red, dry, and painful.
      b. Deep burns or second- and third-degree burns involve both the epidermis and dermis layers of skin; are red and have blisters that may open and weep, causing a wet appearance. Swelling results and the burn is painful; scarring may occur during healing.
   3. Basic steps of treatment
      a. Small superficial burns should be immersed in cool water to stop the burn (ice can be used for this type of burn only). The area should be cleaned and can be covered with an antibiotic ointment; most often this burn does not require medical attention.
      b. Second- and third-degree burns require immediate cooling of the area with large amounts of cool water. Clothing should be removed from the area carefully; cloth that sticks to the burn should not be removed. If the burn has exposed nerve endings, it will be sensitive to air. A dry, sterile bandage should be used to cover the burn loosely to prevent infection.
      c. Ointments, butter, oil, and other remedies should not be placed on a deep burn that requires medical attention. Blisters should be left intact to help prevent infection. A large deep burn can cause shock from pain and body fluid loss. The patient must not become chilled or overheated. If possible, the burned area should be elevated above the heart. Medical attention is essential.
      d. Chemical burns will continue to burn as long as the agent is in contact with the skin. The affected area should be flushed with water (but not forcefully; vigorous flushing may further damage the area), and soaked clothing should be removed. If an eye is affected, the required OSHA eye washing station should be used to flush the eyes for 15–20 minutes; the head should be tipped so that the affected eye is lower than the other. If chemicals have been inhaled, medical attention is required (Table 14–4).

CONTENT REVIEW QUESTIONS

1. The pressure in the blood vessels when the heart contracts is known as:
   A. diastolic pressure
   B. systolic pressure
   C. pulse pressure
   D. ventricular pressure
2. During an emergency, which artery is used to check the pulse for an adult?
   A. femoral
   B. brachial
   C. carotid
   D. radial
3. Premature ventricular contractions (PVCs) refer to:
   A. a longer than normal pause or skip between beats
   B. a slower than normal pulse rate
   C. alternately strong and weak beats
   D. a faster than normal pulse rate
4. The most important step in treating an anaphylactic reaction consists of administering:
   A. oxygen
   B. epinephrine

TABLE 14.4	Quick Check Chart of Dental Emergencies

Emergency	Features	Treatment
Acute pericoronitis	Localized tenderness, erythema, edema, trismus, enlarged lymph nodes, fever)	Rinse with saline solution Prescribe antibiotic (if fever or lymphadenopathy)
Necrotic or dry socket (acute osteomyelitis)	Pain, strong mouth odor 3–5 days after extraction	Debride with saline solution Place germicide and analgesic dressing Retreat as necessary
Avulsed tooth	Tooth loss due to trauma; other trauma possible	Bring tooth to office immediately in wet handkerchief, milk, or patient's buccal vestibule. Radiograph area to check for tooth fragments Reimplant and splint as needed Determine need for tetanus booster
Displaced tooth	Tooth visibly loose; pain, other trauma possible	Radiograph area to check for tooth fracture Splint as needed Advise patient to avoid chewing or biting with tooth Apply cold pack to minimize swelling Determine need for tetanus booster
Postsurgical hemorrhage	Bleeding not halted by pressure from biting on gauze	Instruct patient to bite on gauze, tea bag, folded tissue Evaluate in office
Broken instrument tip	Occurs during treatment	Cease procedure Inform patient not to swallow Examine area visually, dry with cotton roll Use curet in spoonlike manner to examine sulcus Radiograph area if fragment not recovered Request medical consult if fragment does not appear on radiograph
Foreign body injury (patient)	Injury to eye, respiratory tract	If aspiration occurs, request medical radiograph of chest, GI tract If eye injury occurs, ask patient to look down, position upper lid over lower for 1 second before pulling upper lid upward (causes tearing) • Object visible in lower lid, remove with cotton applicator and flush eye • Object not visible or removed, consult physician
Wound breaking skin (operator)	Due to instruments, needlestick, patient bite	Clean with soap and water Force puncture wound to bleed Apply ice packs to reduce swelling Apply firm pressure to control bleeding If cross-contamination is likely, test source for HBsAg and anti-HIV; if not possible, test operator (unless HBV vaccine titer levels are adequate) Determine need for tetanus booster
Burns to operator	Classified by source, depth: • Superficial (first degree) • Deep (second or third degree) • Chemical burns continue to burn as long as agent contacts skin	Immerse burn in cool water Clean area and cover with antibiotic ointment Cool area immediately with large amounts of cool water Remove clothing from burn unless sticking Loosely cover burn with sterile bandage Observe signs of shock; seek medical attention Flush area with mild stream of water Remove soaked clothing Flush eyes (if affected) at eye-wash station Seek medical attention

C. corticosteroids

D. antihistamines

5. A possible side effect of Dilantin that affects dental health is:

A. gingival hyperplasia

B. dry mouth

C. an increased chance of syncope

D. a decreased prothrombin time

6. Erythema and small vesicle formation on the hands in response to wearing latex gloves is an example of:

A. pruritus

B. urticaria

C. contact dermatitis

D. angioedema

7. Warm saline rinses would benefit which emergency?

A. acute pericoronitis

B. postsurgical hemorrhage

C. foreign body injury

D. chemical burn

8. Those who are least likely to hyperventilate include:

A. males

B. children

C. elderly

D. females

9. The emergency oxygen tank or cylinder in the dental office should be which size?

A. H

B. B

C. C

D. E

10. If the mask becomes fogged when oxygen is delivered to a patient, it indicates which of the following?

A. the flow meter is set too high

B. the mask does not fit the patient correctly

C. the tank is empty and no further oxygen is available

D. the patient has started breathing

11. The primary advantage of using a "homemade" emergency kit in the dental office is that:

A. office personnel are more familiar with the contents

B. it is less expensive than manufactured kits

C. there is no advantage; manufactured kits are always superior and more effective

12. When blood pressure is taken, the cuff is initially inflated to 110 mm Hg, the point at which the pulse is no longer felt. To which level should the cuff be inflated next?

A. 90 to 110 mm Hg

B. 100 to 110 mm Hg

C. 130 to 140 mm Hg

D. 150 to 160 mm Hg

13. Which of the following is indicated for the patient who is experiencing an asthma attack?

A. aspirin

B. bronchodilator

C. glucagon

D. diazepam

14. Which emergency situation is NOT triggered by stress?

A. insulin shock

B. hyperventilation

C. epileptic seizure

D. asthma attack

E. anaphylaxis

15. An aura may be experienced during which type of seizure?

A. petit mal seizure

B. partial seizure

C. grand mal seizure

D. hysterical seizure

16. The initial treatment for syncope involves:

A. positioning the patient upright

B. the administration of oxygen

C. the use of ammonia inhalants

D. placing the patient in the Trendelenburg position

17. Patients with diabetes who require daily insulin are at risk for the following emergency, which is characterized by increased thirst and urination, Kussmaul breathing, and a fruity, acetone breath:

A. hyperglycemia

B. insulin shock

C. hypoglycemia

18. The following applies to the treatment of any emergency in the dental office:

A. the patient always should be moved from the dental chair

B. the use of a manufactured drug kit ensures greater success

C. basic life support is considered primary management; the administration of drugs is considered secondary

D. oxygen must be administered

19. For the victim with partial airway obstruction and poor air exchange:

A. manage the situation as for a complete airway obstruction

B. do not intervene; allow the patient to cough and expel the obstruction

C. administer back blows as needed until the object is expelled

D. do nothing until the victim becomes unconscious

20. When performing basic life support on an adult victim with no pulse or respiration, the chest compressions are accomplished by pressing down _____ on the lower half of the sternum:

A. ½ to 1 inch

B. 1 to 1½ inches

C. 1½ to 2 inches

D. 2 to 2½ inches

21. The ratio of compressions to breaths for an adult victim during one-rescuer basic life support is:

A. 5:1

B. 5:2

C. 15:1

D. 15:2

22. For a child who requires only rescue breathing during basic life support, ____ breaths should be given within 1 minute:
    A. 5
    B. 10
    C. 12
    D. 15
    E. 20

23. After determining that an adult victim is unconscious, the next step in this emergency situation is to:
    A. activate the EMS
    B. perform CPR for 1 minute and then call 911
    C. determine whether the victim is breathing
    D. open the airway

24. For a child who requires chest compressions:
    A. the heel of one hand is used
    B. one hand is placed above the other, with fingers interlaced
    C. the pads of two fingers are used

25. A patient is being transported to the dental office after an accident during volleyball practice that resulted in an avulsed tooth. The BEST method of transporting the tooth is:
    A. in a dry cloth
    B. in a glass of water
    C. in the patient's vestibule
    D. in the patient's hand after it has been wiped dry

26. During scaling, an instrument tip breaks. Initially the operator should:
    A. examine the area closely, after drying it thoroughly with air
    B. ask the patient to help locate the tip with his or her tongue
    C. exam the sulcus, using a curette and gentle strokes
    D. expose a radiograph of the area

27. You have been performing the Heimlich maneuver for a victim for some time without being able to dislodge the obstruction. As the individual becomes unconscious, you help him to the floor and activate the EMS. It is now necessary to:
    A. straddle the victim's hips, administer five abdominal thrusts, and attempt to ventilate
    B. continue administering the Heimlich maneuver, with the victim positioned on his side
    C. kneel beside the victim's hips and administer 6 to 10 chest compressions
    D. do nothing further until emergency assistance arrives

28. For the patient who has experienced a heart attack within the last 6 months:
    A. patient positioning is important; the patient should be more upright
    B. the operator should be ready to perform basic life support as needed
    C. dental treatment should be performed only after consulting with the patient's cardiologist

    D. the operator must determine whether angina is present

29. At which blood pressure level is a medical consultation indicated?
    A. 110/68
    B. 120/76
    C. 150/92
    D. 164/96

30. Conditions that predispose a patient to cerebrovascular accident include all of the following EXCEPT:
    A. diabetes
    B. hypertension
    C. previous TIA
    D. cardiovascular disease
    E. epilepsy

31. An epileptic cry, caused by air rushing from the lungs, may occur during which stage of a grand mal seizure?
    A. prodromal stage
    B. convulsive stage
    C. postictal stage
    D. an epileptic cry is characteristic of the hysterical seizure and not the grand mal seizure

32. A seizure may be caused by all of the following EXCEPT:
    A. prolonged high fever
    B. trauma to the head
    C. congenital abnormalities
    D. drug withdrawal
    E. myocardial infarction

REVIEW QUESTION RATIONALES

1. **B** Systolic pressure is the pressure in the blood vessels when the heart contracts. Diastolic pressure is the pressure in the blood vessels when the heart dilates. Pulse pressure is found by subtracting the diastolic reading from the systolic reading. Ventricular pressure applies to pressure within the ventricular chambers of the heart, not within the blood vessels.

2. **C** The carotid artery is used to check the pulse for an adult in an emergency situation. The brachial artery is used during an emergency situation for an infant. The radial artery is used during routine appointments. The femoral artery is not commonly used to check pulse in an adult.

3. **A** Premature ventricular contractions refer to the presence of longer than normal pauses or skips in the heart beat when the pulse is taken. Bradycardia refers to a slower than normal pulse rate. Alternate strong and weak beats are termed pulsus alternans. Tachycardia is the term given to a faster than normal pulse rate.

4. **B** Epinephrine is the drug of choice when treating severe allergic reactions such as anaphylaxis. Its rapid effect after administration makes it extremely useful when time is crucial. As with most emergency situa-

tions, oxygen can be administered but will not stop the reaction. Epinephrine is a vasopressor and bronchodilator and has antihistamine actions. Corticosteroids and antihistamines can be used in nonlife-threatening allergic reactions.

5. **A** The use of Dilantin can result in slight to severe gingival hyperplasia and may affect the patient's oral hygiene. Other possible side effects of Dilantin include skin rash, drowsiness, gastric distress, and restlessness. Dry mouth may result from the use of antihistamines and other drugs. An increased chance of syncope results from orthostatic hypotension, which commonly occurs with the use of antihypertensive medications. A decreased prothrombin time may occur with an increased use of aspirin.

6. **C** Contact dermatitis, which is characterized by erythema and small vesicle formation on the hands, is a localized allergic reaction. Pruritus, urticaria, and angioedema are other types of allergic reactions.

7. **A** Acute pericoronitis refers to the inflammation of the soft tissue surrounding the crown of an erupting molar. Treatment of the localized tenderness includes the use of warm saline rinses by the patient at home. Warm saline rinses do not benefit postsurgical hemorrhage, foreign body injury, or chemical burns.

8. **B** In the dental office, hyperventilation in response to anxiety is least likely to occur in children because they release their anxiety in other ways (e.g., by crying, refusing to cooperate).

9. **D** Oxygen tanks that are part of the emergency equipment in dental offices should be at least size E, which supplies 100% oxygen for 30 minutes.

10. **D** When the oxygen mask becomes fogged during use, it indicates that the patient has started breathing. A full mask made of clear material should be used, and it should fit the patient to provide a tight seal. Setting the flow meter too high, an empty tank, or the improper fit of a mask does not cause the mask to fog.

11. **A** Office personnel will be more familiar with the contents of an emergency kit that they have assembled to meet the needs of their particular office. Although a homemade kit is likely to be less expensive, the cost is not an issue. The effective use of an emergency kit is the most important factor.

12. **C** When blood pressure is taken, the cuff is initially inflated until the radial pulse is no longer felt. This is the estimated systolic number and is mentally noted as an aid in hearing the first systolic sound; the cuff is then reinflated 10 to 30 mm Hg above this point. If the pulse is no longer felt at 110 mm Hg, the cuff is subsequently inflated to 130 to 140 mm Hg. Inflating to only 90 to 110 mm Hg would result in the loss of the first systolic reading; inflating to 150 to 160 is unnecessary and is uncomfortable for the patient.

13. **B** An asthma attack is a respiratory emergency that often is triggered by anxiety. It is characterized by an overproduction of mucus and the contraction of smooth muscles, which narrows the bronchioles and makes breathing difficult. Treatment includes the use of a bronchodilator, which acts directly on the bronchial smooth muscle. The patient should be allowed to use his or her own bronchodilator if possible. Aspirin may cause an asthma attack in those who are allergic to it. Glucagon is administered to the unconscious patient who is experiencing hypoglycemia. Diazepam (Valium) can be administered by the dentist for the treatment of severe hyperventilation.

14. **E** Anaphylaxis is caused by exposure to an allergen and is not associated with stress. Insulin shock, hyperventilation, epileptic seizure, and asthma attack may be triggered by stress; thus it is necessary to lower anxiety as much as possible by explaining all procedures thoroughly, attending to patients promptly, and closely monitoring patients.

15. **C** An aura, such as a flicker of light, a certain smell, or a noise may occur during the prodromal phase of a grand mal seizure. It is characteristic only of the grand mal seizure; it is not characteristic of the petit mal, partial, or hysterical seizure.

16. **D** Syncope is caused by a decreased oxygen supply to the brain. Placing the patient in the Trendelenburg position (supine with feet elevated) typically ensures recovery by increasing blood flow to the brain and thereby replenishing oxygen. If such positioning does not result in recovery, ammonia inhalants can be used to stimulate breathing, and oxygen can be administered.

17. **A** Hyperglycemia is an emergency situation that affects patients with diabetes who require daily insulin. It results when there is little or no insulin available and may be caused by a failure to adhere to therapy, increased exercise, or an infection. This emergency is characterized by increased thirst and urination, Kussmaul breathing, and the presence of a fruity odor on the breath. Loss of appetite, nausea, and vomiting also may be present. Urine samples indicate high glucose levels and the presence of ketones. Hypoglycemia and insulin shock occur when the level of glucose in the blood is low and have different characteristics.

18. **C** During the treatment of any emergency, basic life support is considered primary management and the administration of drugs is considered secondary. For an unconscious patient, it is imperative to maintain an open airway and to administer breathing and/or chest compressions as indicated to supply the necessary oxygen to the brain. It is not always necessary to move the patient from the chair; the positioning of the patient depends on the type of emergency. Using a manufactured drug kit does not

guarantee successful recovery. Oxygen may be beneficial but not necessary for all emergencies (e.g., hyperventilation).

19. **A** When an individual exhibits partial airway obstruction and poor air exchange, it indicates that he or she is unable to cough forcibly in an attempt to remove the object. This situation must be managed in the same manner as complete airway obstruction: the Heimlich maneuver should be performed until the obstruction is expelled or the victim becomes unconscious. Back blows are not part of the Heimlich maneuver; they are employed as part of the protocol for the obstructed airway of an infant. Only when the victim can cough forcibly is it correct NOT to intervene. Doing nothing until a patient becomes unconscious is not an appropriate choice for any emergency situation.

20. **C** For an adult who requires basic life support, chest compressions are performed by interlacing the hands and pressing with the heel 1½ to 2 inches on the lower half of the sternum. For an infant, compressions are ½ to 1 inch deep; for a child, compressions are 1 to 1½ inches deep; 2–2½ inches is not considered an appropriate compression depth for any person during CPR.

21. **B** During one-rescuer basic life support for an adult victim, 15 chest compressions are followed by 2 breaths. For one-rescuer life support for a child or infant victim or for two-rescuer CPR for the adult, the rate changes to 5:1 (five compressions followed by one breath); 15:1 and 5:2 are not appropriate compression to breath ratios for any person during CPR.

22. **E** For the child who is not breathing yet has a pulse, rescue breathing is performed at a rate of 20 breaths per minute, or one breath every 3 seconds. This rate is identical for an infant in the same situation; an adult would require 12 rescue breaths or one every 5 seconds.

23. **A** As soon as unconsciousness is established in an adult victim, the next step is to activate the EMS by calling 911. Afterward, the airway is opened and the rescuer determines whether the victim is breathing. If the victim is not breathing, two full breaths are given and the carotid artery is used to determine whether a pulse is present. When no pulse is present, chest compressions are begun. It is necessary to activate the EMS as quickly as possible. During cardiac arrest, the heart may undergo fibrillation and require the use of special equipment transported by emergency medical personnel. Such equipment defibrillates the heart and allows effective compressions.

24. **A** For the child who requires chest compressions, the heel of one hand only is sufficient to compress the sternum the required 1 to 1½ inches. For an adult, the hands are interlaced and both are used. For an infant, only the pads of two fingers are necessary to perform chest compressions.

25. **C** The best mode of transportation for an avulsed tooth is in the patient's own buccal vestibule. Other choices include a wet handkerchief, milk, or water. For reimplantation with the best prognosis, it is best not to dry the tooth.

26. **C** When an instrument tip breaks during scaling, the primary objective is to remove the tip from the patient's mouth. It is important for the operator to remain calm and examine the area using gentle strokes with a curette in the sulcus. To dry the area, a cotton roll should be used. The patient should not swallow or attempt to locate the broken tip with their tongue. If the tip is not retrieved, a radiograph should be used to aid in the location of the tip.

27. **A** When airway obstruction results in unconsciousness, the victim should be helped to the floor. The operator subsequently should straddle the victim's hips and administer five abdominal thrusts with an upward and inward motion in an attempt to dislodge the obstruction. The thrusts are followed by an attempt to ventilate. This routine is continued until the object is expelled and the operator is successful in ventilating. Two additional ventilations are subsequently given to stimulate breathing and the pulse is checked.

28. **C** Dental treatment within the first 6 months after a heart attack should be performed only after consulting with the patient's cardiologist. Patient positioning is not the primary consideration. Any patient who experiences angina and carries his or her own nitroglycerin should have easy access to nitroglycerin. The operator should be prepared to provide basic life support for any patient, not just those with a recent history of heart attack.

29. **D** A medical consultation is indicated when the systolic reading is higher than 160 and the diastolic is greater than 95 mm Hg. The blood pressure reading of 150/92 should be rechecked for accuracy. Readings of 110/68 and 120/76 and are considered within normal range.

30. **E** Epilepsy does not predispose one to cerebrovascular accident. Diabetes, hypertension, previous TIAs, and/or cardiovascular disease all increase the risk of experiencing a cerebrovascular accident.

31. **B** The epileptic cry, which is caused by air rushing from the lungs, occurs during the convulsive stage of a grand mal seizure. An aura is characteristic of the prodromal stage; the patient regains consciousness during the postictal stage. Petite mal seizures do not have stages.

32. **E** A myocardial infarction typically does not cause seizures. A seizure may be caused by a prolonged high fever, trauma to the head, congenital abnormalities, and alcohol or drug withdrawal. Other causes include epilepsy and an imbalance of body fluids.

Suggested Reading

American Heart Association: Basic Life Support Heartsaver Guide. Dallas, 1997.

American Red Cross: First Aid Responding to Emergencies, 2nd ed. St. Louis, Mosby Lifeline, 1996.

Chernega JB: Emergency Guide for Dental Auxiliaries, 2nd ed. Albany, NY, Delmar, 1994.

Malamed SF: Handbook of Medical Emergencies in the Dental Office, 4th ed. St. Louis, Mosby, 1993.

Malamed SF: Managing medical emergencies. J Am Dent Assoc 124:40, August, 1993.

Ohman SM: Medical Emergency Management. ADHA self-study course sponsored by Block Drug. Chicago, 1990.

Wilkins EM: Clinical Practice of the Dental Hygienist, 7th ed. Malvern, Penn, Williams and Wilkins, 1994.

Chapter FIFTEEN

Special Needs Patient Care

Debralee McKelvey Nelson, R.D.H., M.A. • Gerry Barker, R.D.H., M.A. • Kimberly Krust Bray, R.D.H., M.S.

 ## Clinical Case STUDY

Kevin Watkins, a 17-year-old developmentally disabled patient, is scheduled for an oral prophylaxis appointment. Kevin is wheelchair bound, has spastic movements of his extremities, and has difficulty keeping his mouth open for prolonged periods of time. He lives with his family on weekends but lives at a school for the developmentally disabled during the week. During oral examination, generalized moderate gingivitis is noted. Kevin has not had dental radiographs taken for 2 years.

Clinical Case QUESTIONS

1. What developmental disability does Kevin have?
2. What barriers or risks does Kevin face in receiving adequate professional dental care?
3. Recommend home care products and procedures for Kevin.
4. What specific procedures should the dental hygienist be prepared to provide while treating Kevin?

Clinical Case RATIONALES

1. Kevin has cerebral palsy, a developmental disability present since birth and typically caused by exposure to a virus prenatally or a lack of adequate oxygen intake immediately after birth.
2. Physical barriers Kevin may face include a lack of wheelchair access to the building and in the building. Communication barriers also are likely with spasticity because speech-making is difficult. Transportation and financial responsibility lie with the parent, school, and government, and should not be a barrier for him. Risks associated with the provision of professional care include accidental injury from involuntary movement of the patient.
3. Recommendations for home care should include as much emphasis on self-care as possible. If Kevin is unable to adequately clean his mouth or if brushing

causes trauma because of his spasticity, his caregivers must perform toothbrushing procedures. Adaptive aids, such as a lengthened toothbrush handle and fixed toothpaste cap, in addition to powered toothbrushes and oral irrigators, may be helpful.

4. Communication difficulties may be present and may affect interaction between the dental hygienist and patient. The parent or caregiver can provide a useful link when communications are ineffective. The dental hygienist should be prepared to safely handle a wheelchair transfer to the dental chair. A relaxed atmosphere and good patient rapport will help reduce spastic movements associated with emotional distress. Spastic movements can be risky for both the patient and the operator, so solid instrumentation fulcrums are required. Mouth props, body wraps, and head restraints may be needed. Extra cushioning and/or frequent repositioning can reduce patient discomfort. Because Kevin is 17 years old, a panoramic radiograph may be indicated to check development of the third molars and other oral structures. Bitewing radiographs can be taken by having a parent or caregiver stabilize Kevin's head with one arm and hold the film and holder in his mouth with the other hand.

Content Review

Basic Principles of Care for Special Needs Patients

Special needs patients have some type of disability or condition that requires individual consideration in planning treatment. These patients may have physical, medical, psychological, and/or mental limitations.

Disabilities

A disability is defined as a permanent or long-term condition that limits an individual's ability to perform usual tasks.

I. Types of Disabilities
   A. Developmental disabilities may be present at birth (as a result of a genetic defect, brain damage, or a nutritional or other deficiency during prenatal development) or they may occur before adulthood; are considered permanent conditions.
   B. Acquired disabilities are obtained from external forces during adulthood, such as those related to illness or injury.
II. Classifications of Disabilities
   A. Developmental disabilities
     1. Are present from birth.
     2. Include mental retardation, autism, epilepsy, cerebral palsy, and muscular dystrophy.
   B. Communication disabilities
     1. Often are related to neurologic damage to parts of the brain responsible for language or speech development.
     2. Include aphasia, apraxia, and dysarthria.
   C. Cognitive disabilities
     1. Are associated with reduced mental capabilities.
     2. Include mental illnesses, Alzheimer's disease, eating disorders, and cerebrovascular disorders.
   D. Medical disabilities
     1. Are associated with conditions that affect major organs of the body.
     2. Include arthritis, heart disease, cancer, diabetes, drug and alcohol abuse, respiratory disease, kidney disease, endocrine disease, and blood disorders.
   E. Orthopedic disabilities
     1. Are conditions associated with use of the legs and arms.
     2. Include paralysis and the loss of limbs.
   F. Sensory disabilities
     1. Are conditions associated with the senses.
     2. Include varying degrees of blindness and hearing loss.
   G. Nervous system disabilities
     1. Commonly involve degeneration of the nervous system.
     2. Include disorders such as myasthenia gravis, Parkinson's disease, Alzheimer's disease, Bell's palsy, and multiple sclerosis.

Prevalence

Approximately 50 million Americans (15% to 19%) have some form of functional disability [1,2]; half of these have a severe disability[2] that limits their daily activities (e.g., climbing, lifting).
   I. These individuals may require modified dental treatment planning; awareness of the limitations of these patients and their impact on the provision of dental care can help dental hygienists provide appropriate care.

II. Many of these individuals rely on Social Security benefits for their livelihood.

Levels of Function

The assessment of a patient's functional level involves an evaluation of the patient's ability to perform activities of daily living (ADL) such as bathing, eating, dressing, speaking, and walking. The higher the functional level, the greater a patient's ability to take care of himself or herself. ADL assessments have different rating scales and levels. Typically the first level refers to the highest level of function and the last refers to the lowest level of function.
I. High Function Category
   A. Is limited to individuals who are able to attend to most of their ADL needs with some supervision or encouragement.
   B. Patients typically require a daily reminder to brush the teeth and encouragement to go slowly and thoroughly; may require assistance with transportation.
   C. Is typically categorized as level I or II.
   D. Patients typically are capable of giving informed consent.
II. Moderate Function Category
   A. Is limited to individuals who need supervision or assistance with some of their care.
   B. May require the use of gestures or demonstration, or the use of adaptive equipment for communication.
   C. Is typically classified as level III.
   D. Patients typically are unable to give informed consent; power of attorney or guardianship documentation must be obtained to determine with whom to discuss patient treatment.
III. Low Function Category
   A. Is limited to individuals with little or no ability to perform ADLs themselves.
   B. Patients require a second or third party to provide daily care.
   C. Patients typically are homebound.
   D. Is typically classified as level IV.
   E. Patients typically are unable to give informed consent; power of attorney or guardianship documentation must be obtained to determine with whom to discuss patient treatment.[3]

Common Barriers to Healthcare

The Americans with Disabilities Act of 1992 helped improve access to care for many disabled Americans. Some of the improvements that resulted from this act include wheelchair access to public buildings and rest rooms, barrier-free public buildings, and improved telecommunications for hearing- and vision-impaired individuals. Special needs patients face many barriers.

I. Communication Barriers
   A. Include attitudes of health care workers about treating and communicating with disabled individuals, and patient and family attitudes toward dental care.[3]
   B. Involve hearing and visual losses and speaking difficulties.
      1. Always talk directly to the patient, even when the caregiver is present, unless the patient is unable to communicate.
      2. Patient consent is required (when the patient is cognizant) before patient care can be discussed with caregivers or others.[3]

II. Physical Barriers
   A. Include
      1. Stairs
      2. Narrow doorways
      3. Heavy doors
      4. Distant parking
      5. Area rugs or other floor coverings that could cause tripping
      6. Lack of elevators
      7. Narrow rest room stalls
      8. Restricted access to drinking fountains, telephones, and rest rooms
   B. Are addressed by the Americans with Disabilities Act, which requires dental offices to have[3]:
      1. Ramped access to the office building
      2. Room for wheelchair transport in the waiting room, operatory, and rest rooms
      3. Parking spaces for disabled individuals

III. Transport Barriers
   A. Are common for disabled individuals.
      1. Many of these individuals prefer the safety of their homes to the problems associated with public or private transportation.
   B. Related to public transit include:
      1. Difficulty accessing public transit, including:
         a. Reading time schedules
         b. Finding the appropriate bus or train
         c. Getting to and from the station
   C. Can be eased through:
      1. Senior citizen buses or similar transportation
      2. Private transportation
         a. Requires reliance on family members or friends to provide rides to appointments or stores
         b. Can influence a disabled person's ability to reach important destinations

IV. Economic Barriers
   A. Are the greatest limitations to receiving necessary dental care
      1. Many disabled people have only Social Security or other governmental programs as a means of economic support.
      2. Those who are employed typically earn low wages.
      3. Any money received is needed for primary needs such as shelter and food.
      4. Medical and dental care often are relegated to the bottom of the list of needs.
      5. Those on Medicaid or Medicare have difficulty finding providers who are willing to accept less than customary fees for their services.
   B. Make paying for dental services difficult because most are paid out of pocket and are not covered by insurance.

V. Motivational Barriers
   A. Are common among the disabled, who rely on others for partial care.
   B. May be complicated by communication difficulties.
      1. Although cognizant, disabled individuals may be unable to communicate their needs to caregivers.
      2. Some disabled individuals also may be forgetful; written instructions in addition to verbal instructions should be given to both patient and caregiver.[3]

Special Needs Conditions

Individuals with special needs include the developmentally disabled, the communication disabled, the sensory disabled, the elderly, the patient with an eating disorder, the medically disabled, the patient with cancer, the patient with an orthopedic disorder, the patient with nervous system degeneration, the patient with cleft palate or Bell's palsy, the abused patient, and the pregnant patient.

 Clinical Case **STUDY**

Sarah is an 8-year-old girl with Down syndrome. She attends special education classes in second grade at her local elementary school. She is able to read. Sarah communicates best by sign language but communicates verbally with people she is comfortable with.

Clinical Case **QUESTIONS**

1. Down syndrome is known by another name. What is it? Identify several physical characteristics of this syndrome.
2. What significance does this syndrome have in dentistry?
3. Down syndrome and other forms of mental retardation are associated with a number of medical manifestations. Identify several of these.
4. Describe how to provide brushing instructions to Sarah.

Clinical Case **RATIONALE**

1. Trisomy 21 is another name for Down syndrome. Individuals with this disorder inherited an extra copy of

chromosome 21 in their cells. Common physical characteristics of this syndrome include small skull, simian crease on the palm, flattened nose, large protruding tongue, and extra skin folds under the eyelids.

2. Patients with Down syndrome often have delayed tooth eruption, have small and irregularly shaped teeth, are mouth breathers and tongue thrusters, have cracked lips, and are at increased risk for developing gingivitis and periodontal diseases.

3. Medical manifestations associated with mental retardation include unusual physical appearance, increased risk of leukemia, congenital heart abnormalities, infectious hepatitis (in institutionalized individuals), neuromuscular disorders, and respiratory infections.

4. Sarah is able to comprehend simple, repetitive brushing instructions. Demonstration of technique is a particularly important means of communication.

The Patient with Developmental Disabilities

Developmental disabilities are those that a person is born with. Common disabilities include mental retardation, cerebral palsy, autism, epilepsy, and cleft lip or palate.

I. Mental Retardation
   A. Is the most common developmental disability.
   B. Is below average intellectual functioning (IQ below 70 to 75) caused by chromosomal disturbances; by infection, trauma, or disturbance during fetal development; by trauma or infection during birth; or by trauma or nutritional deficiencies during childhood.
   C. Affects 3% of the US population.[3, 5]
      1. Down syndrome (trisomy 21) is a form of mental retardation that is particularly significant in dentistry because of associated intraoral anomalies (short, narrow palate; large, fissured tongue) and risk factors for periodontal disease (Fig. 15–1).
      2. Fetal alcohol syndrome (FAS) is a disorder associated with prenatal exposure to alcohol. It is characterized by mental retardation, poor coordination, behavioral disorders, growth disturbances, and abnormal facial features (epicanthal folds, low nasal bridge, small head, and small mouth [micrognathia]).
   D. Medical manifestations tend to be more extensive in more severely retarded individuals.
      1. Affected individuals tend to have characteristic physical traits; body stature, head, face, eyelids, ears, and nose may be malformed, depending on the syndrome and its severity.
      2. Other medical problems are commonly associated with mental retardation, including:
         a. Leukemia.
         b. Congenital heart abnormalities.

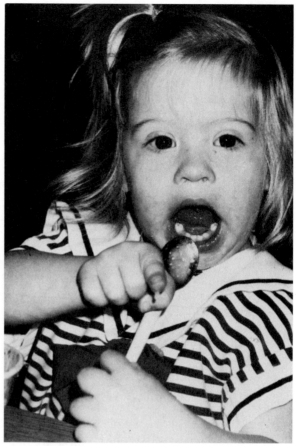

Figure 15.1 Child with Down syndrome.

         c. Infectious hepatitis.
         d. Epilepsy.
         e. Respiratory infections.
         f. Neuromuscular disorders.
   E. Oral manifestations
      1. Delayed or irregular tooth eruption
      2. Small, cone-shaped, fused, or missing teeth
      3. Malocclusion
      4. Repercussions of mouth breathing and tongue thrusting
      5. Cracked lips
      6. Increased risk of gingivitis and periodontal disease
      7. Caries
   F. Risk factors include:
      1. Susceptibility to infection because of a weakened defense system.
      2. Increased risk of hepatitis B infection if the patient has been institutionalized.
      3. Difficulty modifying behavior.
      4. Poor coordination.
   G. Barriers to care include:
      1. Dependence on the caretaker to make and keep dental appointments.
      2. The cost of dental care.
      3. Mental limitations.
         a. Build patient's trust.

b. Communicate at his or her developmental level.

c. Speak simply.

d. Reward good behavior; restraints and sedation to manage behavior are recommended only when absolutely necessary.

H. Professional and home care includes:

1. Frequent oral prophylaxis to reduce the risk of periodontal disease.

2. Lubrication of lips to reduce the risk of cracking.

3. Awareness that the gag reflex may be strong.

I. Patient/Caregiver education emphasizes:

1. Repetition of simple, demonstrable home care procedures with the patient and caregiver.

   a. The caregiver supervises and/or performs oral hygiene procedures depending on the abilities of the patient.

2. Discussion of periodontal risk and the need for excellent daily home care, frequent progressive oral prophylaxis, and examination.

II. Cerebral Palsy

A. Is a developmental, neuromuscular disorder that results in an inability to control muscular movement (spasticity); limitation ranges from mild to severe.

B. Is caused by a variety of injuries to the brain (e.g., infection, trauma, poisoning, anoxia) either before, during, or not long after birth.

C. Affects 0.2% of the US population.[3, 5]

D. Medical manifestations include chronic contraction of muscles, poor coordination and dexterity, mental retardation (in 33% to 50% of affected individuals),[3, 5] and learning disabilities caused by sensory (hearing and vision) and possibly respiratory impairment.

1. Affected individuals who have seizure disorders (20% to 30%)[3] take appropriate medications.

2. Communication often is difficult because of motor difficulties.

E. Oral manifestations of the condition include:

1. Lack of control of facial muscles, which makes speech (dysarthria), chewing, and swallowing (dysphagia) difficult.

2. Difficulty keeping mouth open during dental appointments.

3. Temporomandibular dysfunction.

4. Tongue thrusting.

5. Mouth breathing.

6. Bruxing.

7. Attrition.

8. Caries and periodontal disease related to the inability to practice good oral hygiene measures because of limited coordination.

9. Gingival hyperplasia in those taking phenytoin; the degree of hyperplasia is related to the level of plaque control (i.e., as plaque increases, so does hyperplasia).

F. Risk factors include inadequate fluoride intake, soft diets, poor motor control, and the inability to properly maintain own oral care.

G. Barriers to care include:

1. Communication difficulties between patient and dental professional; low self-esteem may influence desire to communicate also.

2. Unfamiliarity of dental office; causes emotional distress and thereby increases spastic movement.

3. Dependence on the caregiver.

4. Lack of mobility.

5. Inability of the dental professional to provide thorough treatment because of the patient's physical limitations.

H. Professional and home care include:

1. Building trust.

2. Desensitizing the patient to dental routines.

3. Encouraging complete communication.

4. Avoidance of injury to the patient or operator from uncontrolled movements of the patient during instrumentation (fulcrums are a must).

5. Protecting patient from aspiration of water or other materials placed in the oral cavity.

6. Assisting the patient during seizures (during seizure activity, the patient should not be moved; the area should be cleared of items that may hurt the patient during convulsive movement).

7. Wheelchair transfer.

8. Realizing that communication barriers do not indicate incomprehension.

9. Involvement of the caretaker.

10. The use of an assistant during treatment to avoid injury and to expedite treatment.

11. The use of sedation and general anesthesia (only as needed).

12. Consultation with a medical physician regarding a change in medications if hyperplasia is a concern.

I. Patient/caregiver education should emphasize:

1. Adaptations of toothbrushes or floss handles as needed (Fig. 15–2).

2. Evaluation of the need for mechanized cleaning devices (toothbrushes and oral irrigators).

3. Explanation and demonstration of all home care procedures; great patience may be necessary but most patients are willing to learn.

4. Daily disclosing of plaque.

5. Assistance with daily plaque removal if the patient is unable to thoroughly cleanse own mouth.

6. The use of fluoride and chlorhexidine to control disease as needed; chlorhexidine gluconate sprays effectively reduce plaque when they are used twice daily.[8]

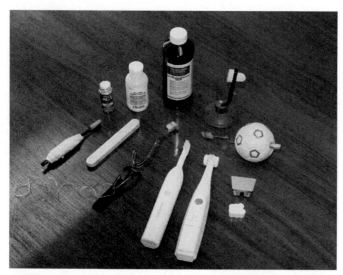

Figure 15.2 Adjunctive and adaptive aids for patients with disabilities: modified toothbrush handles, powered toothbrushes, floss holder, mouth props, antimicrobial rinses, saliva substitute, and fluoride rinse.

    7. Explanation of the need for frequent oral prophylaxis.

III. Autism

  A. Is a lifelong, behavioral developmental disability of unknown cause.

  B. Has a prevalence of 0.1% among the US population[3] and affects many more males than females.

    1. Approximately 80% of affected individuals have some degree of mental retardation.[3]

    2. The disability commonly becomes evident during the first 3 years of life.

    3. Is identified by an inability to communicate appropriately.

      a. The autistic person does not interact or communicate at an age-appropriate level, making behavior management quite difficult.

      b. Autistic individuals prefer routine (e.g., same foods, same way of doing things) and often perform repetitive motions (e.g., hand wringing, head banging).

      c. Autism may be present alone but many autistic individuals also experience mental retardation, seizures, and other problems.

      d. The disability is treated by behavior modification, speech and play therapy, medication, and psychotherapy.

  C. Medical manifestations include:

    1. Injuries caused by repetitive motions such as head banging and biting.

    2. Metabolic disorders.

    3. Nutritional deficiencies (because diet typically is limited to foods that are familiar to the patient).

  D. Oral manifestations:

    1. Typically are no different for these patients than for others, unless patient has received insufficient care.

    2. May include a tendency for oral trauma because some patients may be aggressive or injure themselves when brushing.

    3. May include an increased risk of caries if patient has a high carbohydrate intake.

  E. Risk factors include:

    1. A fear of procedures and not understanding the need to sit still.

    2. Inadequate nutrition because of strong food preferences.

  F. Barriers to care include:

    1. The stress of the dental visit.

    2. Communication difficulties because of poor behavior control (caregivers may be embarrassed about child's behavior).

      a. Managing behavior may include:

        1) Desensitization over multiple appointments.

        2) Reinforcing good behaviors.

        3) Using physical restraint when safety is a concern.

        4) Sedation and/or and general anesthetics (if other methods fail).

        5) Reliance on the caregiver to make and keep appointments.

  G. Professional and home care includes:

    1. Consistency in care and among care providers; the patient's preference for routine dictates that the same dental team member should see the patient at each visit.

    2. Shorter, more frequent appointments in a quiet, calm environment are preferable to longer, infrequent visits; noises, movement, and other changes are disconcerting to the patient and should be avoided or introduced slowly as needed.

    3. Involving the caregiver in preparing the child for the dental visit.

      a. Procedures should be explained to the caregiver so that some can be practiced at home in preparation for the dental visit.

      b. Home care instructions should be performed consistently on a daily schedule.

  H. Patient/Caregiver education should emphasize:

    1. The use of both verbal and nonverbal techniques of communication to demonstrate simple oral care instructions.

    2. Discussion with the caregiver about the patient's need to eat fewer cariogenic foods.

    3. The need for frequent preventive dental visits to create routine and avoid the need for extensive treatment.

IV. Epilepsy
   A. Is a central nervous system disorder; convulsions and/or loss of consciousness are common symptoms.
   B. Affects approximately 0.8% of the US population.[3]
      1. Eighty percent of individuals with this disorder live normal lives because their illness is controlled by medication.[5]
   C. May be caused by head trauma, infection, genetic predisposition, brain tumor, or vascular disease and may be present from birth or may occur at any age.
   D. Seizure (convulsive) activity is managed by prescription medications such as phenytoin, phenobarbital sodium, carbamazepine, primidone, and valproic.
   E. May require emergency procedures (e.g., prevention of injury, basic life support) if seizures occur during dental appointment.
   F. Medical manifestations may include:
      1. An aura or predication of an oncoming seizure.
      2. Seizures
         a. May be simple and characterized by staring and trembling or jerking motions with no loss of consciousness
         b. May be complex and characterized by a trance-like stage, impairment of consciousness, and involuntary motor movements followed by confusion, irritability, extreme fatigue, and no memory of the seizure
   G. Oral manifestations include:
      1. Gingival hyperplasia secondary to phenytoin use; plaque control is vital to the prevention and limitation of gingival overgrowth.
      2. Trauma from seizure activity such as cheek, tongue, or lip-biting, falling, and tooth chipping (from biting instruments or clenching).
   H. Risk factors include:
      1. Trauma from seizure activity during dental procedures.
      2. Development of gingival hyperplasia because of phenytoin use.
      3. Drowsiness from medications, which may inhibit memory.
      4. Drug interactions (e.g., between phenytoin and barbiturates, doxycycline, and other medications).[5]
   I. Barriers to care include:
      1. Economic cost, particularly if the disability affects employability.
      2. Lack of transportation, if the patient is unable to drive.
      3. Lack of communication, if fear of or embarrassment about having a seizure in public is strong.
   J. Professional and home care includes:

      1. Frequent (even monthly) oral prophylaxis, depending on the severity of the gingival condition.
      2. A calm atmosphere.
      3. Careful preparation for dental appointments; a medical kit or medical consult may be necessary.
      4. Demonstration and explanation of thorough home care procedures; should include sulcular brushing and flossing.
      5. Consultation with physician regarding medication change if gingival overgrowth is excessive or uncontrollable; surgical excision of gingival overgrowth may be required.
   K. Patient/Caregiver education should emphasize:
      1. Discussion of oral health and the need for excellent plaque control.
      2. Repetition of instruction if patient's memory is impaired by medication.
      3. Positive reinforcement to bolster self-esteem.
V. Muscular Dystrophy (MD)
   A. Is an inherited, progressive skeletal muscular disorder.
      1. Duchenne (severe) MD presents during early childhood and results in death by age 20; primarily affects males (1 in 3500 male births).[6]
      2. Becker (mild) MD presents during middle to late childhood and does not result in early, premature death; affects both males and females.
   B. Medical manifestations include progressive muscle weakness caused by the replacement of skeletal (and eventually heart and lung) muscle with fibrofatty tissues; patients have difficulty walking, standing, speaking, and eating as the disease progresses.
   C. Oral manifestations are related to a loss of muscle control and may include injury or infection. Irritated gingiva may be caused by an open mouth; poor oral hygiene may occur because of a reduced ability to provide self-care.
   D. Risk factors include trauma from injury (e.g., falling, difficulty swallowing, choking) because of a loss of muscle control; oral infection may be caused by inadequate plaque removal.
   E. Barriers to care include:
      1. Economic issues; caregivers are needed to provide full care as the disorder progresses.
      2. Dependence on the caregiver to make and keep dental appointments.
      3. Lack of communication; speech difficulties occur as muscle weakness affects muscles of the head and neck.
      4. Immobility or difficulty controlling movement.
   F. Professional and home care includes:
      1. Frequent oral prophylaxis to reduce the risk of infection.

2. Short dental appointments.
3. The use of a bite-block to keep the mouth open after muscle loss prevents it.

G. Patient/Caregiver education should emphasize:
   1. Supervision and/or performance of oral hygiene procedures by the caregiver if the patient is unable.
      a. Power-assisted devices enable the patient to continue self-care.
      b. Adaptive aids accommodate muscle weakness.
   2. Discussion with the patient and/or caregiver about the risk of infection and the need for excellent daily home care, frequent professional oral prophylaxis, and examination.
   3. The use of petrolatum on lips and oral tissues irritated by open mouth.

VI. Cleft Lip and Palate
   A. Is a craniofacial deformity that ranges from a mild unilateral clefting of the lip to a wide, bilateral clefting of the lip and palate; typically is not life threatening but requires much care (minor clefting associated with the uvula and soft palate requires little if any medical care); defect is associated with inadequate fusing of the lip, palates, or uvula during the 4th to 12th weeks of gestation.
   B. Is the second most common birth defect in the United States; affects approximately 0.2% of live births.[7, 8, 9]
   C. The cause is unknown, but genetics and exposure to environmental factors such as medications or toxins (cigarettes, retinoic acid analogues, alcohol, anticonvulsants)[8] during early prenatal development are believed to play a large role. Affects more males than females; is more common in Asian and Native American populations than in white or black populations.[9] Results in imperfect fusion of the medial and lateral nasal processes with the maxillary process.
   D. Medical manifestations include one or more of the following:
      1. Facial or palatal deformities that require surgical intervention.[9]
         a. Lip closure (adhesion) is performed before the 3rd month of life.
         b. Palatal closure is performed between the ages of 1 and 5.
         c. Bone grafting, orthodontics, and speech and hearing evaluation and treatment occur between the ages of 6 and 15.
         d. Final plastic surgical procedures and the replacement of teeth occur after the age of 15, when physical growth is complete.
      2. Medical anomalies such as heart, ear, skeletal, and genitourinary tract deformities also may occur.
      3. Oral manifestations include an increased risk of oral infection (including periodontitis and dental caries) from malpositioning of the teeth, wearing of a dental appliance (obturator), mouth breathing, and oral deformity, which also make oral hygiene procedures more difficult.

   E. Risk factors include upper respiratory and middle ear infections and inadequate nourishment (before completion of surgical procedures).
   F. Barriers to care include:
      1. Economic issues; multiple oral and facial surgeries and care by professionals from different disciplines are required to correct the defect and associated conditions.
      2. Difficult communication, because of inadequate speech production, hearing loss related to the defect, or self-consciousness.
   G. Professional and home care includes:
      1. Frequent oral prophylaxis (3 to 4 times annually) to reduce the risk of infection.
      2. When the premaxilla is unfixed or immediately after surgical procedures, fulcruming in the site should be avoided or limited.
      3. Fluoride treatment to reduce the incidence of dental caries.
   H. Patient/Caregiver education should emphasize:
      1. Caregiver supervision and/or performance of oral hygiene procedures, depending on the age and abilities of the patient.
         a. Care of the teeth and gums involves the use of a soft-bristled toothbrush and dental floss to remove plaque.
         b. Care of the dental prosthesis is similar to care of the partial denture; involves removal after meals to cleanse thoroughly and reduce halitosis.
      2. Discussion with patient or caregiver and patient about the risk for infection and the need for excellent daily home care, frequent professional oral prophylaxis, and examination; a daily fluoride rinse or gel is recommended.

The Patient with Communication Disorders

Patients with communication disorders are either unable to make speech sounds, because of structural disease or damage, or unable to understand language or form thoughts into words.

I. Types of Communication Disorders
   A. Aphasia
      1. Is the inability to put thoughts into words or to understand language.
      2. Is caused by neurologic damage or an organic brain disorder such as dementia.
      3. Affects approximately 1 million (0.4%) Americans.[3]
   B. Apraxia
      1. Is an inability to properly form speech sounds because of a CNS lesion or organic brain disorder such as dementia.

C. Dysarthria
  1. Is a motor speech disorder that often is associated with cerebrovascular accident (CVA), cerebral palsy, or Parkinson disease.
  2. Results in the slurring of speech patterns as a result of damage to the CNS or PNS.
II. Oral manifestations depend on the severity of the condition and the loss of muscle control; difficulty in clearing food and an inability to adequately clean the teeth may cause an increased risk of caries and periodontal disease; difficulty swallowing and an inability to perform or understand the need for good oral hygiene also may complicate oral health.
III. Risk factors may include choking when swallowing is difficult.
IV. Barriers to care include economic cost if the disability affects employment, transportation if the patient is unable to drive, and communication when speech-making or comprehension is difficult.
V. Professional and home care should include maintenance of adequate home care, with assistance as needed.
VI. Patient/Caregiver education should emphasize discussion about oral health and the need for excellent plaque control. Caregivers who provide oral care should hear instructions.

The Patient with Sensory Impairment

The patient with sensory impairment has a loss of sight or hearing that makes communication and other daily living issues difficult. Sensory impairments often occur as a result of infection, trauma, or disease but some may be inherited.
I. Types of Sensory Impairment
  A. Hearing impairment
    1. Affects approximately 9% of noninstitutionalized Americans[3]; affects individuals of all ages.
      a. Approximately 30% of older adults have hearing loss.[3]
      b. Severity can range from slight to total deafness.
    2. Can occur as a result of infection, trauma, disease, medication, or heredity.
      a. In adults, is commonly noise-induced.
      b. In children, is associated with heredity, pregnancy or birth complications, or meningitis.[3]
    3. May be indicated by inappropriate responses to questions or lack of interest in verbal communication.
    4. Hearing aids may help restore some hearing acuity.
  B. Visual loss or blindness
    1. Affects 2% to 3% of noninstitutionalized Americans; affected individuals are unable to read with correction.[3]
      a. Few legally blind individuals are totally blind.

b. Blind individuals may exhibit sensitivity to light.
II. Oral manifestations are not directly associated with visual or hearing impairment; poor oral hygiene and accompanying oral disease are common and may occur because of inadequate presentation of oral hygiene instruction.
III. Risk Factors
  A. For the visually impaired, include an inability to see objects in their path or to visualize instructions.
  B. For the hearing impaired, include an inability to understand instructions or fear or shock in response to unexplained procedures.
    1. The patient may feel discomfort when hearing aids are on during noisy procedures.
    2. Patients should be asked to turn off hearing aids during the use of powered devices such as a high-speed handpiece or an ultrasonic/sonic scaler.
IV. Barriers to Care
  A. Physical obstacles such as doorways and stairs; finding one's way in new surroundings is particularly difficult for the blind individual.
  B. Lack of transportation; arranging transportation and/or relying on a caregiver for scheduling and transportation is cumbersome.
  C. Lack of communication, which is more difficult for sensory-impaired individuals; health care workers may be apprehensive about communicating with sensory-impaired individuals.
  D. Economic issues; good employment opportunities may be more limited for the sensory-impaired person.
V. Professional and Home Care
  A. For the visually impaired individual includes:
    1. Positioning of caregivers and others to the visual advantage of the patient (typically directly in front of the patient).
    2. The use of large visual aids and materials.
    3. Avoiding shining of the operatory lamp in the patient's eyes.
  B. For the hearing impaired individual includes:
    1. Elimination of loud or background noises when attempting to communicate.
    2. If some hearing is present, directing speech to that ear.
    3. Positioning of caregivers and others so that the patient can see the facial features (particularly the lips and tongue) of the person speaking.
    4. The use of sign language, a message board, or an interpreter if the patient is unable to read lips (speech).
VI. Patient/Caregiver Education
  A. For the visually impaired
    1. Extremely descriptive explanations are important because they make use of other senses

(particularly hearing), which are better developed.

2. Use appropriate changes in tone of voice when providing information since facial expressions may not be seen.
3. Involves explanation and demonstration (on the hand) of each procedure; the patient should handle visual aids to improve understanding; the caregiver should be involved as needed.

B. For the hearing impaired
   1. The use of demonstration is particularly effective when explaining techniques of oral care.
   2. May involve the use of an interpreter, sign language, or a message board to explain things that are not easily demonstrated.
   3. Includes take-home written instructions for effective reinforcement.

The Geriatric Patient

Aging baby boomers and an increased life expectancy will greatly expand the proportion of elderly individuals between the years 2010 and 2039. Projections indicate that the percentage of Americans who are older than 65 years of age will increase from 13% to more than 21% of the total population by the year 2030.[10]

I. Three generally recognized gerontologic stages are:
   A. "Young old" (ages 65 to 74)
   B. "Old" (ages 75 to 84)
   C. "Old old" (ages 85+)

II. Medical manifestations include several chronic diseases. The occurrence of chronic diseases and multiple disease processes increases with age. Diseases in the elderly can include:
   A. Cardiovascular disease, which accounts for more than half of all deaths among the elderly. Oral complications and treatment plan alterations vary based on the type and severity of the disease.
   B. Dementia/Alzheimer disease, in some form. The incidence of these disorders increases with age; they affect 5% of individuals 65 to 75 years old and more than 20% of individuals older than age 85.[11]
      1. Oral complications and alterations in dental hygiene care are frequently associated with medications that are used to control the disease.
      2. Ensuring suitable personal daily oral care is a primary concern.
      3. Patients with Alzheimer disease who experience seizure disorders may experience phenytoin-associated gingival hyperplasia.
   C. Arthritis, which is experienced by approximately 53% of the older adult population.[12]
      1. Is a common source of discomfort and disability among older adults.
      2. Modified oral hygiene aids, such as powered toothbrushes and floss holders, are the most common oral care alterations.

D. CVAs result in coordination and mobility impairments that may require adaptive aids or assistance with personal oral hygiene care.
E. Diabetes is the seventh leading cause of death among older adults.[13]
   1. Individuals with diabetes are at increased risk for periodontal disease.
   2. Uncontrolled disease may require antibiotic premedication before dental treatment.
   3. Appointments ideally should take place mid-morning, after a meal, when blood sugar is stable.
F. Sensory defects
   1. Include visual impairments, which affect 23% of the aging population, and hearing loss, which is experienced by 40% of the elderly.[13]
   2. Modification of oral hygiene aids and practices often is necessary to accommodate the impairment.
G. Oral adverse drug reactions
   1. Medication use among the elderly is high; 88% to 93% of older adults take at least one medication.[13]
   2. Eighty percent of the elderly take a medication with potential adverse reactions.[13]
      a. Xerostomia is the most common medication-induced oral condition (56%).[13]
      b. Abnormal homeostasis (52%), soft tissue reactions (23%), taste changes (11%), alterations in host responses (9%), and gingival overgrowth (5%) also occur with the use of medications.[13]
      c. Patients should be advised and educated about the need to discuss alternative prescriptions with their medical doctors.
H. Osteoporosis
   1. Is thinning and weakening of the skeletal structure, which leads to loss of bone density and possible fracture.
   2. Women are four times more susceptible to this condition than men, particularly after menopause.[14]
   3. Evidence of loss of bone density may be apparent in the bones of the jaw in severe cases.

III. Oral Manifestations
A. The prevention of dental disease during the past three decades has resulted in an increasing number of older adults retaining their natural teeth. Many oral conditions once believed to be a normal part of aging currently are recognized as sequela to disease.
   1. Age-related oral changes (normal)
      a. Include darkening of the teeth, attrition, and gingival recession.
   2. Disease-related oral changes
      a. Drug-induced oral conditions
         1) Xerostomia (dry mouth); although once believed to be a normal process asso-

ciated with aging, is most commonly caused by medication use.
  2) Gingival hyperplasia
  3) Oral candidiasis
  4) Stomatitis
  5) Glossitis
  6) Hairy tongue
  7) Trigeminal neuralgia
 b. Dental decay, particularly of root surfaces, becomes increasingly more frequent in seniors because of gingival recession from periodontal disease or improper brushing; xerostomia often is a contributing factor.
 c. Periodontal disease increases in severity with age, due to the accumulated lifelong attachment loss associated with this chronic disease process.
  1) Slight gingival recession (1 to 2 mm) is considered a normal part of aging.
  2) Recession in excess of 1 to 2 mm most likely is a result of past or present periodontal disease activity.
 d. Oral cancer
  1) More than one half of oropharyngeal cancers and the majority of related deaths in the United States occur in adults older than 65 years of age.
  2) Oral cancer is more common in older men than in women and is associated with alcohol and tobacco use.
IV. Barriers to Care
 A. Income limitations are an obstacle to dental care for seniors.
  1. Few seniors have dental insurance.
  2. Medicare does not reimburse dental services; typically discretionary income is used to cover the cost of dental care.
 B. Education is positively correlated with seeking adequate dental care.
  1. As a general rule, older populations have less formal education than younger populations.
  2. The young old are better educated and are more likely to demand quality health care than the old old.
 C. Residential status affects an older individual's ability to seek or receive dental care.
  1. The majority (67%) of the elderly live in family settings (are homebound).[15]
  2. Approximately one in four seniors can expect to spend some time in a nursing home.[15]
  3. Some seniors are homebound but continue to live at home with assistance.
 D. The use of dental services varies among the elderly.
  1. An estimated 40% of all seniors visit the dentist annually.[16]

2. Individuals with natural teeth are more than four times as likely to seek dental care.[16]

The Patient with an Eating Disorder

Patients with serious eating disorders typically are classified as anorexic, bulimic, or bulimorexia. Adolescents and young adult females are primarily affected, although men and adults of all ages can be afflicted. Serious cases require psychiatric treatment.
I. Types of Disorders
 A. Anorexia nervosa
  1. Is a syndrome that involves extreme loss of weight (more than 15% below ideal weight) as a result of starvation, excessive exercise, and/or the chronic use of laxatives or suppositories in response to a distorted body image; its cause is unknown but the disorder is associated with psychosocial pressures; affects 1% of adolescent girls and 10% of cases prove fatal.[17] Outpatient treatment, in conjunction with antidepressants and antianxiety medications, is common.
  a. Is most common among women.
  b. Malnutrition and dehydration are common.
  c. Often occurs in individuals with a family history of depression or bipolar disorder.
  d. May cause dry skin and nails.
  e. Excessive growth of facial and appendage hair is common.
  2. Oral manifestations include dental caries, xerostomia, and oral lesions from malnutrition.
  3. Risk factors include medical crises and emotional stress.
  4. Barriers to care include lack of communication because of patient denial, guilt, fear of gaining weight, and lack of compliance; may include economic barriers because of the cost of repairing damage caused by the eating disorder.
  5. Professional and home care include multidisciplinary care (dental, medical, and nutritional consultations) because of the severity of the disorder. Fluoride in a custom tray is recommended if xerostomia or vomiting is a problem.
  6. Patient education should be based on the prevention of further damage to the teeth. Should involve discussion of the influence of diet on caries; daily fluoride use (rinse or gel) should be recommended.
 B. Bulimia nervosa
  1. Is a compulsive disorder that involves periods of starvation and bingeing and a perceived lack of control over eating behavior; affected individuals engage in an average of two episodes a week; its cause is unknown but is likely to be stress-related. Affects 2% to 3% of young women.[17]
  a. Bingeing may be followed by purging activity in those who are fearful of gaining weight. Purging is responsible for most of the oral and medical complications associated with

this disorder, including erosion, anemia, heart problems, gastric disturbances, renal failure, and failure to ovulate.

b. Diuretic use can cause a reduction in salivary flow and the development of angular cheilitis; laxative use can lead to metabolic acidosis and dependence on laxatives for adequate bowel function.

c. Body weight is normal or slightly overweight.

d. Malnutrition, dehydration, and cardiac dysrhythmias are common.

e. A family history of alcoholism and drug abuse is common.

2. Oral manifestations include:

a. Enamel erosion (perimolysis) on maxillary anterior teeth from vomiting (restoration margins appear raised), dishing of lingual surfaces, and the appearance of an anterior open bite.

b. Dental caries from stomach acids.

c. Dry mouth from diuretic use.

d. Salivary gland enlargement.

e. Palatal trauma lesion from forced vomiting.

f. Sensitivity to temperature changes and acids if dentin is exposed.

g. Square appearance of the jaw from enlargement of the salivary glands; a round appearance is caused by parotid gland enlargement.

h. Xerostomia from prescribed antidepressants.

3. Risk factors include denial of the problem, emotional stresses, xerostomia, and vomit acid.

4. Barriers to care

a. A lack of communication because of patient denial, guilt, fear of gaining weight, and lack of compliance; also results from an inability to gain the trust and confidence of the patient or failure to refer the patient to a physician or psychiatrist.

b. Economic barriers may be involved because of the cost of repairing damage caused by the eating disorder (Fig. 15–3).

5. Professional and home care should include the restoration of decayed teeth with a glass ionomer restorative (to leach fluoride ions) where possible, sealing of eroded areas with composite resins, and assessment of the progression of erosion (whether by study models or intraoral photos).

6. Patient education should emphasize:

a. Discussion of oral and medical problems associated with purging, diuretics, and laxative use.

b. The need to neutralize vomit acid by rinsing with tap water, a sodium bicarbonate, or a magnesium hydroxide and water rinse.

c. Discouragement of toothbrushing immediately after vomiting in order to reduce abrasion.

d. The use of saliva substitutes or sugarless gums to increase salivary flow.

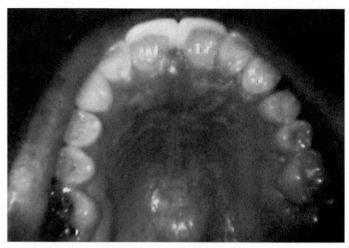

Figure 15.3 Porcelain veneers used to restore tooth structure lost to erosion in a bulimic patient.

e. The daily use of fluoride supplements in rinse or gel form.

f. Daily vitamin and mineral supplementation may be recommended when gingival tissue appears unhealthy or when angular cheilitis is present.

C. Bulimorexia

1. Is a combination of anorexia and bulimia (binge eating followed by starvation); involves signs and symptoms of both anorexia and bulimia.

2. Medical manifestations, oral manifestations, risk factors, barriers to care, professional care, and patient/caregiver education are the same as for anorexia nervosa and bulimia.

 Clinical Case **STUDY**

Nina Jane, a 12-year-old girl, recently has been diagnosed with leukemia. She is scheduled for intensive chemotherapy. During dental examination, gingival bleeding, poor oral hygiene, three carious lesions, and two nearly exfoliated teeth are observed.

Clinical Case QUESTIONS

1. What information must be obtained from Nina's medical oncologist before any dental treatment can be given?

2. What dental procedures should be completed before chemotherapy?

3. When during the several months of chemotherapy should dental treatment be scheduled?

Clinical Case RATIONALES

1. Before dental treatment, the medical oncologist should be consulted regarding CBCs with differential, clotting/bleeding factors, placement of the central

venous catheter, when chemotherapy will begin, and the expected length of immunosuppression.

2. If the blood counts are adequate and time is available before chemotherapy, all loose teeth and teeth close to exfoliation should be removed, carious teeth should be restored, oral hygiene instructions and the need for meticulous oral hygiene should be stressed, and oral prophylaxis should be completed.

3. Dental treatment can be scheduled whenever blood counts have returned to safe levels. Safe levels are most common just before a scheduled round of chemotherapy.

The Patient with a Medical Disability

I. Arthritis, a common disorder of the musculoskeletal system that causes painful swelling of the body joints, affects 14% of Americans.[18] Approximately half of older Americans have some form of arthritis.[7] The disorder may be caused by infection, allergy, trauma, drug reactions, or heredity; it results in fatigue and the loss of mobility and hand strength. Common forms include rheumatoid arthritis, juvenile rheumatoid arthritis, and degenerative joint diseases (osteoarthritis) (Fig. 15–4).

A. Oral manifestations include an increase in bleeding and oral infection from the use of antiinflammatory drugs; temporomandibular joint pain may be present.

B. Barriers to care include transportation difficulties because of a loss of mobility; long appointments and keeping the mouth opened can be uncomfortable; irritability is common in those with chronic pain.

C. Risk factors include the effects of medications and difficulty with motor activities.

D. Professional and home care considerations include assessing the need for antibiotic premedi-

cation in cases of joint replacement, the need for short appointments with frequent opportunities to close the mouth, and the patient's need to shift positions in the chair to relieve discomfort.

E. Patient/Caregiver education involves discussion of the oral side effects of arthritis medications; recommendation of powered toothbrushes and other adaptive aids (enlarged toothbrush handles, floss holders) as needed; and recommendation of frequent recall so that appointments are quicker and easier on the patient.

II. Alcoholism is a chronic but treatable disease that involves the compulsive abuse of ethanol-containing substances. Causes of the disease may include genetic, psychological, and environmental factors. An estimated 43 million Americans are considered binge or heavy drinkers.[19]

A. Medical manifestations include:
1. Nutritional deficiencies.
2. Cirrhosis of the liver.
3. Oral cancer (in individuals also addicted to tobacco products).
4. Reddened nose, forehead, and cheeks.
5. Jaundiced (yellow) skin and puffiness of the eyes.

B. Oral manifestations include:
1. Xerostomia.
2. Reduced ability to taste.
3. Glossitis.
4. An increased risk of both dental caries and periodontal disease from poor oral hygiene.
5. Leukoplakia.
6. Odor of alcohol on breath.
7. Enlargement of the parotid gland and the tongue.
8. An increased risk of oropharyngeal cancer.
9. Facial and dental trauma from falls and injuries.

C. Risk factors include nutritional deficiencies, infections, trauma, and oral cancer (especially if tobacco is also used); caution should be used when administering amide local anesthetics and nitrous oxide sedation.

D. Barriers to care include:
1. Communication difficulties; patient may not appear for appointments when actively drinking.
2. Transportation problems, if the alcoholic does not drive or has lost driving privileges and must rely on others.
3. Economic problems, if the patient is unable to hold a job or is on a fixed income.

E. Professional and home care involves:
1. The use of nonalcoholic mouth rinses.
2. Possible bleeding problems from liver damage.
3. The need for oral cancer evaluation.

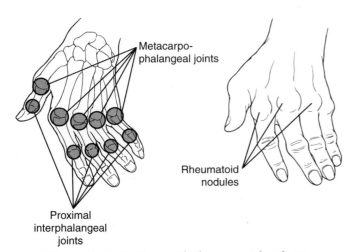

Metacarpo-
phalangeal joints

Rheumatoid
nodules

Proximal
interphalangeal
joints

Figure 15.4 Patient with rheumatoid arthritis.

4. Fluoride treatment and daily supplementation as needed.
5. Dealing with patient's intoxication and difficulties in keeping appointments.

F. Patient/Caregiver education should emphasize the need for frequent recall, fluoride supplementation, saliva substitutes, and the need for practicing good home care because of the risk of infection.

III. Blood disorders include anemia, leukemia, and hemophilia and are caused by inadequate numbers of specific blood parts or components. The disorders range from mild and easily treatable to severe and incurable.

A. Anemias are disorders of red blood cell production, hematocrit, or hemoglobin concentrations. The limited number of cells or blood parts results in inadequate oxygen delivery throughout the body.

1. Causes of anemia include nutritional deficiency, blood loss, the destruction of red blood cells, and the failure of bone marrow to produce enough cells.
2. Medical manifestations include a pale appearance and tiredness; anemia is most common in women of menstruating age who have inadequate dietary iron intake.
3. Oral manifestations include pallor of the oral mucosa, glossitis or burning tongue, and angular cheilitis. In cases of sickle-cell anemia, the gingiva may have a yellow tone and individuals may be prone to bleeding and periodontal disease.
4. Risk factors include excessive bleeding and trauma.
5. Barriers to care may be nonexistent; in severe cases, fatigue may discourage patients from keeping appointments.
6. Professional and home care should focus on observation of the signs and symptoms of anemia and appropriate referral; for sickle cell anemia, consultation with a physician and antibiotic premedication is recommended.
7. Patient/Caregiver education should emphasize the appropriate care of anemia through following physician's orders and the practice of good oral hygiene to decrease the risk of infections.

B. Leukemias are malignant overgrowths of immature white blood cells that are most likely caused by viral infection, ionizing radiation, chemicals, or heredity. Leukemia can be acute or chronic in nature.

1. Oral manifestations are more common in acute than in chronic cases and include:
   a. Susceptibility to bacterial, viral, and fungal infection.
   b. Gingival bleeding, bluish-red gingival color, and gingival hypertrophy (see cancer section for effects of cancer therapy).
   c. Full-body lymphadenopathy.
   d. Toothaches.
   e. Changes in maxillary and mandibular alveolar bone.
2. Risk factors include susceptibility to infection, bleeding, and risks associated with cancer therapy.
3. Barriers to care include the need to schedule appointments during periods of remission.
4. Professional and home care involves:
   a. Scheduling dental appointments during periods of remission.
   b. Consultation with the oncologist.
   c. Frequent prophylaxis and oral examination as per consultation with oncologist.
   d. Treatment of acute problems (e.g., bleeding, candidiasis, inflammation) as they occur.
5. Patient/Caregiver education should include discussion of:
   a. Preventive procedures
   b. The need for meticulous home care to prevent infection
   c. Meticulous cleaning of dental appliances
   d. The use of antimicrobial rinses as needed
   e. Fluoride rinses or gels
   f. Pit and fissure sealants
   g. The need for frequent dental evaluation, especially during active treatment

C. Hemophilias are inherited, congenital disorders of the blood clotting mechanism. There are three distinct versions of hemophilia: A and B (which affect only males) and von Willebrand's disease (which affects both sexes).

1. The primary medical manifestation is difficulty with uncontrolled bleeding (varies in severity with extent of disease).
2. Oral manifestations include gingival bleeding associated with poor oral hygiene (because of fear of causing bleeding during home care procedures) or caused by trauma.
3. Risk factors include susceptibility to bleeding and potential for acquiring infectious disease (AIDS, Hepatitis) from blood transfusions.
4. Barriers to care include:
   a. Communication difficulties, if the dental professional has fear regarding treatment of a patient with hemophilia or if the patient has suffered mental or intellectual impairment from bleeding or from the stresses of dealing with the disease.
   b. Economic difficulties because of the life-long cost of infusions, laboratory tests, and physician consultations.

5. Professional and home care should include:
    a. Consultation with a physician regarding the severity of the disease and medication use.
    b. Preparedness for potential bleeding (including treatment with factor replacement immediately before any dental procedures that may cause bleeding).
    c. Prevention of infectious disease transmission.
        1) When gingival tissues are greatly inflamed, tissues should be supragingivally cleaned in small segments over several appointments and allowed to heal before subgingival therapy is begun.
        2) Avoid trauma to tissues during scaling, radiography, or any other dental procedures.
6. Patient/Caregiver education should include discussion of the need for frequent recall, procedures to prevent infection and associated bleeding, and the need for soft-bristled brushes, gentle flossing, and antimicrobial rinses.

IV. Cardiovascular disease comprises a variety of diseases of the heart and the blood vessels and affects an estimated 17% of the US population.[18] These include congenital heart diseases, heart valve diseases, cardiac dysrhythmias, hypertension, ischemic heart disease, and congestive heart failure.

A. Types
1. Hypertension is a symptom of disease or pathology that is expressed as an abnormally high blood pressure (systolic >140; diastolic >90).
    a. Affects approximately 15% of the US population.[18]
    b. Is treated with a wide variety of antihypertensive medications in conjunction with changes in diet and activity level. Common medication types are diuretics, vasodilators, and sympatholytic agents.
    c. May lead to hypertensive heart disease because of the stress that high blood pressure places on the heart muscle.
    d. Primary hypertension is most common and its cause is unknown.
    e. Secondary hypertension comprises approximately 10% of cases of hypertension and is associated with some underlying disease.
2. Congenital heart disease is a malformation of the heart and blood vessels that occurs during fetal development. Examples are defects of the ventricular septum, atrial septum, and patent ductus arteriosus, and displacement of the great vessels of the heart.

a. Is caused by heredity, mother's infection with rubella, or drugs taken by the mother during pregnancy.
b. Patients may have difficulty with exertion and may have inhibited growth.
c. May require antibiotic premedication.

3. Heart valve disease is caused by damage to the heart valve after rheumatic fever or the use of diet drugs (fenfluramine or dexfenfluramine).
    a. Rheumatic fever is caused by a beta-hemolytic streptococcal infection that affects the heart, joints, skin, central nervous system, and subcutaneous tissues during its course. The heart may sustain permanent damage.
    b. At this time, the exact mechanism of valvular damage as a result of taking fenfluramine or dexfenfluramine remains unknown. An estimated 14 million prescriptions for these drugs were written between 1995 and 1997. Based on preliminary data, as many as one third of individuals who took these drugs may have valvular heart damage.[20]
    c. Patients with valvular damage require antibiotic premedication before all invasive dental procedures that may cause bacteremia.

4. Cardiac dysrhythmia is an irregular heart beat caused by an unreliable sinoatrial node, cardiac arrest, various dysrhythmias, heart blockage, or other disease.
    a. Treatment consists of medications and/or the implantation of a pacemaker.
    b. Antibiotic premedication during the first 6 months after implantation of a pacemaker is required.
    c. Avoid use of or proximity to dental equipment with an electrical current (e.g., ultrasonics, mechanical toothbrushes, pulp testers) when a patient has a pacemaker.

5. Ischemic heart disease (coronary heart disease) occurs when blood supply to the heart is partially or fully blocked and the heart is deprived of oxygen.
    a. Typically is caused by atherosclerosis of the blood vessel walls.
    b. May lead to angina pectoris, myocardial infarction (heart attack), congestive heart failure, or death.
    c. Treatment includes lifestyle changes (diet and exercise), medication (diuretics, beta and channel blockers, vasodilators, and antidysrhythmics), and surgery (bypass, angioplasty).

6. Congestive heart failure is failure of the dis-

eased heart to meet the needs of the body; causes fluids to build up in body tissues.

    a. Failure of the heart muscle typically is related to underlying heart valve damage or ischemic heart disease.

    b. Causes of sudden death include dysrhythmias, pulmonary embolism, acute myocarditis, and acute hypertensive crisis.

B. Oral manifestations of cardiovascular diseases typically are no greater than for other patients, unless the patient is severely debilitated; some medications (calcium channel blockers) are associated with the development of gingival hyperplasia (Fig. 15–5).

C. Risk factors include infection (rheumatic heart disease and congenital heart disease), side effects of medication, and vasoconstrictors (should be used with caution).

D. Barriers to care include transportation difficulties when the condition restricts the patient's mobility; patient may need to rely on others. Economic barriers may be present if income is restricted because of disability or fixed income.

E. Professional and home care should include:

    1. Consultation with a physician regarding the need for antibiotic premedication and carefully documented medication needs.

    2. Caution when administering local anesthetics because of possible interactions with medications.

    3. Adjusting chair appropriately because some patients are unable to recline in a supine position.

F. Patient/Caregiver education should include emphasis on daily meticulous home care, frequent dental recall, and the need to take antibiotic premedication and heart medications as prescribed.

V. Cerebrovascular accident (stroke) is a temporary or permanent loss of brain function caused by a loss of blood flow to the brain via a clot, constriction, or rupture of a blood vessel supplying the brain. An estimated 2% to 3% of Americans have had a stroke.[3]

A. Underlying diseases (e.g., hypertension, diabetes, drug abuse, atherosclerosis) typically are the cause of the constriction or tear. Preventive treatment consists of aspirin or ticlopidine.

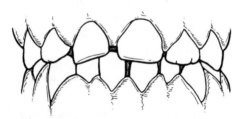

Figure 15.5 Severe gingival overgrowth in a diabetic patient taking nifedipine.

B. Oral manifestations of cardiovascular diseases typically are no greater than for other patients, unless the patient is severely debilitated.

C. Risk factors include continued high blood pressure and receiving dental treatment within 6 months of a stroke.

D. Barriers to care include transportation difficulties, when the condition restricts the patient's mobility, and economic problems, if income is restricted because of disability or fixed income.

E. Professional and home care should include:

    1. Consultation with a physician regarding the need for antibiotic premedication and careful documentation of medication needs.

    2. Caution when administering local anesthetics because of possible interactions with medications.

    3. Adjusting the chair appropriately for patients unable to recline in a supine position.

F. Patient/Caregiver education should include emphasis on daily meticulous home care, frequent dental recall, and the need to take antibiotic premedication and heart medications as prescribed.

VI. Diabetes are associated with inadequate insulin production or utilization, which causes glucose intolerance. These diseases have a hereditary basis and are related to a reduced production of insulin, hyposensitivity to insulin, and/or excessive glucose production. When blood sugars are uncontrolled, oral insulin or injectable insulin may be needed.

A. Types

    1. Type I is termed juvenile diabetes or insulin-dependent diabetes mellitus (IDDM) and requires daily injection of insulin because of a severe reduction in insulin production.

    2. Type II is called noninsulin-dependent diabetes mellitus (NIDDM) and often can be controlled through diet and exercise.

B. Medical manifestations

    1. Hyperglycemia, or high levels of glucose in the blood; occurs when inadequate levels of insulin or insulin resistance prevents proper utilization of available glucose; may result in coma.

    2. Hypoglycemia, or low levels of glucose in the blood, occurs after injection or oral intake of insulin when a meal is not eaten or when excessive amounts of insulin are taken; symptoms include sweating, palpitations, weakness, lightheadedness, and trembling; patient should be given a high-carbohydrate snack.

C. Oral manifestation severity is related to the level of control of the blood glucose; common conditions include:

    1. Dry or cracked lips.

    2. A mild increase in caries because of de-

creased salivary flow or high carbohydrate intake.

3. Periodontal disease because of poor healing.
4. Parotid gland enlargement.
5. Ulcerated and reddened mucosa.
6. Candida.

D. Risk factors
1. Poor healing, which results in an increased risk of bacterial, viral, and fungal infection.
2. Local anesthetics with vasoconstrictors are recommended for all but the most complicated procedures.[18]
3. A disturbance in the balance between glucose and insulin; occurs when the diabetes is uncontrolled or if dental procedures are major and require large amounts of anesthetics.

E. Barriers to care are no greater than for unaffected patients unless complications exist.

F. Professional and home care includes:
1. Scheduling short dental appointments soon after morning meals.
2. Thoroughly assessing oral health.
3. Preparing for diabetic emergency (sugar, glucose gel or tablets, or orange juice must be available).
4. Consultation with the treating physician is necessary and prophylactic antibiotics are advised in cases of uncontrolled diabetes or extensive infection.

G. Patient/Caregiver education should emphasize:
1. Preventive oral health procedures.
2. The need for frequent recall.
3. Daily fluoride supplementation.
4. Control of infection.

VII. Substance abuse is the use of illegal or prescribed drugs for nonmedicinal purposes; abuse can lead to psychological, chemical, or physical addiction to a drug.

A. Alcohol abuse affects approximately 7% of Americans,[21] and drug abuse affects approximately 5% of the population.[19]

B. Examples of abused drugs include heroine, marijuana, nitrous oxide, LSD, cocaine, and amphetamines. (Alcohol abuse is also considered substance abuse and is covered in the section on alcoholism).

C. Oral manifestations may include trauma, mucositis, xerostomia, extrinsic stain, high rates of dental caries, gingival lesions, and periodontal disease, often from poor oral hygiene.

D. Risk factors include drug interaction with local anesthetics (vasoconstrictor use should be avoided in cocaine or marijuana users) and the ineffectiveness of local anesthetics in drug abusers. The risk of bacteremia is higher in IV drug users, thus antibiotic premedication may be indicated. Patients also are at risk for infection with hepatitis and HIV because of risky behaviors.

E. Barriers to care
1. Communication problems related to denial of drug abuse and disordered behavior (careful attention to behavior and physical appearance may help identify the condition).
2. Transportation problems, if patient is unable to drive.
3. Economic problems related to drug habit costs and possible unemployment.

F. Professional and home care includes:
1. Careful assessment of patient behavior and appearance (needle marks, sniffing, agitation, dull expression, careless dress and hygiene, dilated/constricted pupils, bloodshot eyes).
2. Thorough intraoral examination.
3. Awareness that patient may request pain or nitrous oxide sedation because of a drug habit.
4. Caution with the use of local anesthetics to prevent reactions with illegal drugs.

G. Patient/Caregiver education should emphasize:
1. Responsibility for maintaining good oral hygiene and for keeping scheduled recall appointments.
2. That prevention of oral infection is particularly important in IV drug users because of the risk of bacteremia.

VIII. The HIV-Positive/AIDS Patient
A. HIV infection affects more than 600,000 individuals in the United States.[22] HIV refers to the human immunodeficiency virus, which infects human T-helper lymphocytes and CD4 lymphocytes and causes acquired immunodeficiency syndrome (AIDS), a usually fatal disease.
1. The disease is transmitted by sexual contact, blood contact, or perinatally and is characterized by immune suppression and opportunistic infections.
2. The latency period after infection can last as long as 12 years.
3. According to statistics from the Centers for Disease Control through December 1997, more than 600,000 cases of AIDS were reported in the United States. Of the individuals affected, approximately 78% are men, 22% are women, and 1% are children.[22]
4. AIDS cases are rising among Hispanics, Blacks, and women.
5. Neurologic and physical symptoms present as CD4+ lymphocyte counts decrease.
6. Death typically occurs from infections caused by the immunodepressed state.

B. Oral manifestations include:
1. Persistent and generalized lymphadenopathy.
2. Candidiasis.
3. Hairy leukoplakia (which is strongly associated with HIV infection).

4. Angular cheilitis.
5. Recurrent and severe aphthous and herpetic infections.
6. Severe and chronic gingival and periodontal infection.
7. Oral warts.
8. Kaposi sarcoma.
9. Tooth erosion from frequent vomiting (a side effect of AZT use).
10. Xerostomia (medication-induced) and caries.

C. Risk factors include vomiting and xerostomia from infection or medication use and risk of infection when CD4+ lymphocyte counts are low.

D. Barriers to care include:
1. A lack of communication; the patient may be afraid to provide accurate or thorough medical information; the attitudes and fears of dental professionals who work with AIDS patients also may interfere with communication.
2. Transportation problems, if the patient is debilitated.
3. Economic difficulties, because of the high costs of medication, medical visits, and hospitalizations; also may be caused by loss of employment.

E. Professional and home care should include:
1. Consultation with the patient's physician regarding blood counts and the risk of bleeding.
2. Careful oral examination for signs of infection and a focus on maintenance of oral health.
3. Frequent professional oral prophylaxis and dental examination to reduce the opportunity for secondary infections.
4. Avoiding the creation of aerosols during instrumentation.
5. Diet counseling, if xerostomia and vomiting occur, should emphasize adequate nutrition with noncariogenic foods to reduce the risk of dental caries.
6. Tobacco cessation counseling, as needed, to reduce the risk of periodontitis.
7. Treating the patient and caregivers with respect, kindness, and compassion.
8. Providing literature regarding AIDS and the importance of good oral care; such literature is free (call the AIDS hotline at 1–800–342–2437).

F. Patient/Caregiver education should emphasize:
1. Meticulous, frequent daily home care, including flossing and brushing; self care may be impossible during later stages of the disease.
2. Prevention of dental disease to promote oral and systemic health.
3. The use of daily chlorhexidine rinse and systemic antibiotics if severe gingivitis or periodontitis is present.

IX. Renal disease is disease of the kidney, which alters the kidney's filtering ability and is caused by infection, autoimmune disease, or a developmental disorder. It affects approximately 3% of Americans.[18]

A. Patients with renal disease have unusually high levels of toxic urine components in their blood. As the disease worsens, the patient may need dialysis to clean the blood and prevent death.

B. Oral manifestations include:
1. Mucositis.
2. Candidiasis.
3. Hemorrhage and petechiae.
4. Halitosis.
5. Enamel hypocalcification.
6. An increase in dental caries and periodontal disease if oral hygiene is poor.
7. An increase in calculus development.

C. Risk factors include infections, malnutrition, and possible drug-drug interactions (the use of local anesthetics should be limited).

D. Barriers to care are economic; finances may be limited because of high medical costs and the patient's inability to maintain employment.

E. Professional and home care should emphasize:
1. The need to check vital signs and prevent drug interactions.
2. Consultation with a physician to determine the need for antibiotic or steroidal premedication (patient may have arteriovenous shunt or organ transplant).
3. The tendency for bleeding.
4. Possible interactions with local anesthetics.
5. Slow healing.

F. Patient/Caregiver education should emphasize:
1. Meticulous oral hygiene to reduce the incidence of infection.
2. Frequent recall appointments for examination and prophylaxis.
3. Daily fluoride supplementation.
4. Toothpastes with antigingivitis, anticaries, and anticalculus properties, unless mucosal irritation results.

X. Chronic respiratory diseases include chronic obstructive pulmonary disease, active tuberculosis, and lung cancer. These diseases may have a variety of causes, including allergy, cigarette smoking, infection, pollutants, and heredity.

A. Types
1. Chronic obstructive pulmonary disease (COPD) (Table 15–1)
   a. Collectively refers to pulmonary disorders associated with chronic irreversible obstruction of airflow, including asthma, chronic bronchitis, and emphysema; affects an estimated 13.5 million people and is the fifth leading cause of death in the United States.[23]

TABLE 15.1 Distinguishing Features of COPDs			
	Asthma	**Chronic Bronchitis (Blue Bloaters)**	**Emphysema (Pink Puffers)**
Age of onset	< 30 years	> 50 years	> 50 years
Smoking history	+	+	+
Course	Paroxysmal	Progressive	Progressive
Allergy history	Frequent	Infrequent	Infrequent
Chest x-ray	Normal	Increased marking	Hyperinflammation
Dyspnea	Mild to moderate	Mild	Severe
Hypoxia	No	Yes	No

Modified from Kaliner M, Lemanske R: JAMA 268:2807–2829, 1992.

1) Asthma refers to a bronchiolar inflammation with secondary hyperresponsiveness and narrowing,[24, 25] which leads to coughing and wheezing symptoms.
   a) Symptoms are worse at night, after physical exertion, and upon exposure to allergens or airway irritants.
   b) Contemporary therapy emphasizes an antiinflammatory approach that often combines inhalation bronchodilation therapy with an aerosolized corticosteroid or mast cell stabilizer; candidiasis often results, thus rinsing with water after inhaler use is helpful.
2) Chronic bronchitis is a progressive respiratory disorder characterized by excessive sputum production that is not associated with local disease; results in cough upon respiration for at least 4 months of the year for more than 2 consecutive years.
   a) The resulting airway obstruction (on both inspiration and expiration) is caused by the narrowing, mucous plugging, and collapse of peripheral airways; is almost always associated with cigarette smoking.
   b) Treatment involves smoking cessation, the avoidance of air pollutants, and the use of bronchodilators and antibiotics.
3) Emphysema is the anatomic permanent distention of the air space beyond the terminal bronchiole, accompanied by the destruction of alveolar septa[26]; diagnosis often is based on clinical presentation because the anatomic change in the terminal bronchioles can be detected only by autopsy.
   a) Is commonly associated with smoking; the barrel-chested appearance of the patient is caused by the use of accessory muscles for respiration.
   b) Treatment involves smoking cessation, breathing exercises, and low-flow oxygen therapy as needed.
   b. Treatment is difficult because there is no known cure; general treatment principles that help improve quality of life and further disease progression include:
      1) Smoking cessation, a critical element of management and elimination or reduction of respiratory allergens and irritants.
      2) Proper nutrition and exercise.
      3) Annual influenza and pneumococcal vaccinations (palliative measures).
      4) Inhalation therapy, the cornerstone of therapy regardless of the type of COPD; may consist of the use of any combination of beta-adrenergic bronchodilators, corticosteroids, and/ or methylxanthines; an estimated 25% to 75% of patients use their metered dose inhalers incorrectly.[27] If misuse is suspected, refer for proper instruction.
   c. Dental management focuses on the prevention of respiratory depression.
      1) A more upright chair position may be necessary.
      2) Involves the avoidance of nitrous oxide/oxygen sedation from respiratory depressive effects of high oxygen administration (no contraindication to the use of local anesthetics exists).
      3) Rubber dam use may result in the feeling of compromised air exchange.
      4) Patients with concurrent heart disease may require special management.
   d. Oral manifestations of COPD are medication-related and may include candida and xerostomia.
2. Active tuberculosis
   a. Is a chronic, infectious disease that causes

fibrosis and the calcification of granulomas in the lungs; also can involve the liver and kidneys; is caused by *Mycobacterium tuberculosis*; is more common among HIV-positive individuals.

b. Symptoms include fever, night sweats, chills, malaise, cough, and lymphadenopathy of the cervical and submandibular lymph nodes; weight loss is common.

c. Treatment involves diagnosis by chest x-ray after a positive skin test; multi-drug treatment includes isoniazid (INH) and rifampin, streptomycin, and ethambutol use for months to years, which eliminates infectiveness quickly; drug-resistant strains are increasing.

3. Lung cancer

a. Is typically squamous cell carcinoma, adenocarcinoma, small cell carcinoma, or large cell undifferentiated carcinoma; either develops in the lungs or metastasizes to the lungs from lymph nodes or other sites (such as the oral cavity); most often is associated with tobacco use (cigarette or pipe smoking and the use of smokeless tobacco) although other pollutants (e.g., uranium, asbestos) may be implicated; is more common in men than in women.

b. Symptoms include chronic coughing, coughing up blood, frequent pulmonary infections, Cushing's syndrome, clubbing of fingers, dyspnea, and weight loss.

c. Treatment involves cessation of tobacco use, surgical removal of the cancerous site, chemotherapy, and/or radiation therapy.

B. Oral manifestations may include xerostomia and candidiasis from inhalants or the use of other medications, ulcerations, and lymphadenopathy.

C. Risk factors include:

1. Infections, especially among patients who take steroids for long intervals.

2. Exposure to asthma-provokers, such as sulfites or stress.

3. Difficulty breathing in the supine position.

4. Persistent coughing.

5. A risk of lung infection with the aspiration of aerosols from ultrasonics because of immunosuppression; aerosol use should be minimized and the patient's condition should be observed at all times.

6. The use of sedatives, antihistamines, and aspirin should be avoided.[18]

7. Valium, nitrous oxide, and general anesthetics should be used only with caution.[18]

D. Barriers to care

1. Lack of communication because of patient's embarrassment about the condition (e.g., TB, emphysema).

2. Transportation difficulties, if the patient has difficulty walking even short distances.

3. Weather may exacerbate certain respiratory conditions and may require the rescheduling of appointments.

E. Professional and home care involves:

1. Recognition of the communicability of tuberculosis and the need to avoid aerosol production.

2. Awareness of and the ability to deal with respiratory difficulties associated with asthma and COPD.

3. The need for a relaxed dental environment to prevent asthmatic or other complications.

4. The placement of medications and bronchodilators in close proximity to the patient.

5. The avoidance of vasoconstrictors in local anesthetics.

F. Patient/Caregiver education should emphasize the need for meticulous oral hygiene, daily fluoride supplementation as needed, and the use of saliva substitutes for patients with xerostomia.

XI. Thyroid Disorder

A. Hyperthyroidism, an overproduction of thyroid hormones, may be caused by tumors (benign or malignant), autoimmune disease (Grave's disease)[29] or pituitary gland disease; is a common condition (affects 0.4% of US population),[6] particularly among 30- to 40-year-old women; also is called thyrotoxicosis.

1. Causes thyroid gland enlargement (goiter), lymph gland enlargement, and exophthalmos; nervousness, fast pulse rates, hypertension, tremors, weight loss, anxiety, sweating, heat intolerance, frequent bowel movements, heart palpitations or dysrhythmias, rosy complexion, eye discomfort or vision disturbance, and fine hair growth are common symptoms and signs.

2. Oral manifestations include:

a. In children—premature loss of primary dentition and eruption of permanent dentition accompanies premature physical maturity.

b. In adults—rapidly progressing periodontitis, dental caries, osteoporosis, and a burning sensation of the tongue; salivation may be increased.

3. Treatment includes the administration of radioactive iodine (most common) or antithyroid medications, such as methimazole or propylthiouracil; may involve surgical removal of part of the gland.

4. Risk factors include thyroid storm, an emergency situation characterized by fever, heart dysrhythmia and tachycardia, and hypermetabolism, which can result in death; the use of vasoconstrictors should be avoided.

5. No barriers to care are specific to this condition.

6. Professional and home care involves thorough extraoral and intraoral inspection for increases in thyroid gland or lymph node size; the use of home and professional fluoride to reduce the incidence of decay; and frequent examination and oral prophylaxis to manage bone loss, caries, and periodontal infection.

7. Patient/Caregiver education should emphasize instruction in plaque removal methods to prevent periodontitis; adequate diet to reduce the risk of osteoporosis; and the use of home fluoride gels or pastes.

B. Hypothyroidism (inadequate production of thyroid hormone) initially may be associated with hyperthyroidism, which eventually leads to thyroid gland destruction; common causes are autoimmune (Hashimoto's disease), radioactive iodine therapy or thyroid surgery, developmental disturbances, iodine deficiency (uncommon in US, where salt is iodized), pituitary disease, or medication; the disorder is much more common among 30- to 50-year-old women than among men; in children, it is referred to as cretinism, in adults as myxedema.

1. Is manifested in adults as a symmetrically enlarged thyroid gland, which may have nodules; signs and symptoms include myxedema (fatigue and weight gain from slow metabolism), skin dryness, hair coarseness, face puffiness, intolerance to cold temperatures, constipation, muscle cramping, mental slowness, low blood pressure, and slow pulse; delayed development (physical and mental) occurs in infants and children.

2. Treatment includes thyroid hormone supplementation (e.g., with levothyroxine sodium).[29]

3. Oral manifestations include:
   a. In children—enlarged tongue and lips and delayed tooth eruption.
   b. In adults—enlarged tongue; chronic, severe periodontal disease; and slow, hoarse speech.

4. No significant risk factors exist.

5. Professional and home care involves thorough extraoral and intraoral inspection for increases in thyroid gland or lymph node size and frequent oral examination and prophylaxis.

6. Patient/Caregiver education should emphasize instruction in thorough plaque control and the need for frequent oral prophylaxis to reduce the incidence of periodontal destruction.

Clinical Case STUDY

A 55-year-old man with stage III squamous cell carcinoma of the retromolar trigone and left lateral tongue, with metastasis to the left neck, is scheduled to receive a 7000-cGy dose of radiation therapy. The radiation field will include the entire neck, mandible, TMJ, and posterior of the maxilla. The patient has a well-fitting maxillary partial denture. Teeth #6–#11 have type-II periodontal involvement and teeth #19 through #29 have type-III periodontal involvement. The plaque level is moderate, with heavy calculus and stain. The patient drinks occasionally and smokes two packages of cigarettes daily. He brushes his teeth twice daily and rinses with Listerine once each day.

Clinical Case QUESTIONS

1. Identify five acute complications that this patient may experience as a result of radiation therapy.
2. Name common long-term complications associated with radiation therapy to the head and neck.
3. What dental and dental hygiene treatments should be completed before the initiation of radiation therapy?
4. Two years after radiation therapy, the patient complains of pain in the left mandible and an open sore beneath his denture. What may be the problem?

Clinical Case RATIONALES

1. Five acute complications that the patient may experience as a result of radiation therapy include thickened saliva (which causes dry mouth), an alteration in taste sensation, mucositis (inflamed tissue), candida infection, and muscle tightness (trismus).

2. Common long-term complications associated with radiation therapy to the head and neck include xerostomia (dry mouth), osteoradionecrosis (nonhealing tissues and bone), trismus that limits mouth opening, TMJ pain, and rampant caries in remaining teeth.

3. Before the initiation of radiation therapy, all mandibular teeth should be extracted and the bone and tissues should be allowed to heal; all remaining teeth should be thoroughly scaled and root planed as needed. The maxillary denture must be cleaned and the patient should be instructed on the importance of meticulous home care, including toothbrushing and flossing. Custom fluoride trays should be fabricated and tobacco cessation counseling is encouraged.

4. The patient complains of pain in the left mandible; the open sore beneath his denture most likely is from denture irritation and osteoradionecrosis. The patient should be referred to an oral surgeon who is aware that the patient has undergone radiation therapy.

The Patient with Cancer

Approximately 40% of Americans will develop cancer in their lifetimes. Each year, approximately 30,000 individuals develop oral cancer.

I. Types of Cancer
   A. Oral and pharyngeal carcinoma
   1. Ninety percent of these cancers are squamous cell carcinoma.
      a. Are most commonly found on the tongue and floor of mouth.
      b. Signs and symptoms include erythroplakia, leukoplakia, ulcers that do not heal, hoarseness, bleeding, difficulty swallowing, and/or a lump or mass.
   2. Risk factors include tobacco use, heavy alcohol use, age, race, and exposure to sunlight (lip cancer).
   3. Barriers to care include:
      a. A delay in diagnosis and treatment by a doctor.
      b. Psychosocial factors such as alcoholism, patient's denial of disease, and patient's disadvantaged mental and social status.
   4. Disease manifestations include pain, dysphagia (difficulty swallowing), nutritional deficiency, and speech alteration.
   5. Treatment manifestations
      a. Surgery
         1) Acute complications include pain, fistula formation, speech alteration, nutritional deficiency, infection, and psychosocial impact.
         2) Long-term complications include pain, disfigurement, malocclusion, temporomandibular disorder, speech alteration, nutritional deficiency, infection, and psychosocial impact.
      b. Radiation therapy to the oral cavity and salivary glands.
         1) Acute complications include loss of taste, xerostomia, mucositis, infection, and nutritional deficiency.
         2) Long-term complications include xerostomia, caries from radiation, trismus, and osteoradionecrosis; altered growth and arrested tooth development occur in children.
      c. Chemotherapy
         1) Acute complications include mucositis, myelosuppression, and infection.
         2) No long-term complications occur after chemotherapy is completed and acute complications are resolved.
   B. Non-Head and Neck Cancer (requiring chemotherapy and/or bone marrow transplantation)
   1. Chemotherapy for malignancies other than squamous cell carcinoma of the head and neck

   a. Forty percent overall incidence of oral complications.
   b. There is a higher risk for oral complications in patients with leukemia, lymphoma, and solid tumors as opposed to patients on chemotherapy for other malignancies.
   2. Complications associated with intensive chemotherapy and bone marrow transplantation
      a. Cytotoxic drug effects include temporary destruction of healthy tissues, including oral mucosa (mucositis).
      b. Myelosuppression results in a low white blood cell count, which increases the risk for oral and systemic infections; hemorrhage in response to low platelet counts and clotting factors also may occur.
      c. Include temporary xerostomia, loss of appetite, nausea, pain, fatigue, and graft-versus-host disease in bone marrow transplant patients.
   3. Barriers to oral care
      a. Physicians often tell patients to stop brushing teeth when blood counts are low and discourage dental visits to avoid the risk of infection.
      b. Psychosocial manifestations, treatment schedules, and fatigue disrupt dental recall schedules.

II. Dental Hygiene Care
   A. Before cancer treatment:
   1. Assess condition of teeth, periodontal structures, oral hygiene, previous interest in dental care, and psychosocial factors.
   2. Patients scheduled for radiation therapy to the jaw bones
      a. Teeth can never be extracted safely from irradiated bone.
      b. Determine, with the dentist, which teeth can be maintained for the life of the patient.
   3. Oral hygiene education should emphasize bacterial plaque control and the use of oral rinses.
   4. Nutrition and dietary counseling are essential.
   5. Tobacco cessation counseling is recommended.
   6. Fluoride
      a. Patients scheduled for radiation therapy to the salivary glands need daily prescription-strength fluoride gel in brush-on form or in custom fluoride trays.
      b. Patients with temporary xerostomia during chemotherapy may benefit from an over-the-counter fluoride rinse or gel.
   7. Instrumentation should include scaling, root planing, removal of overhangs, and smoothing of rough restorations.
   B. During cancer treatment:
   1. Design alternative plaque control measures for patients with mucositis and for patients forbidden by a physician to use a toothbrush and floss.

2. Encourage continued fluoride application.

3. Suggest measures to relieve xerostomia, and topical anesthetics/coating agents for mucositis.

4. Assist with the selection of nonirritating and noncariogenic foods.

5. Counsel patients with dentures on daily cleansing and removal before sleep.

6. Continue to assist with tobacco cessation.

C. After cancer therapy:

1. For patients who receive radiation therapy to the salivary glands and jaw bones

   a. Encourage frequent recalls, scheduled according to individual patient need, for prophylaxis and home care evaluation.

   b. Reinforce the need to continue daily fluoride applications.

   c. Encourage excellent home care.

   d. Encourage palliative measures for xerostomia and stimulation of saliva.

   e. Recommend daily jaw exercises to prevent trismus.

   f. Provide tobacco cessation counseling.

   g. Caution patient to avoid all future surgical procedures to irradiated bone.

2. For patients who receive chemotherapy or bone marrow transplantation

   a. Monitor blood counts until patient recovers from immunosuppression; subsequently place patient on regular dental hygiene recall.

   b. Encourage excellent oral hygiene.

   c. Consider fluoride rinse or gel until xerostomia is resolved.

   d. Provide tobacco cessation counseling.

Patients with Spinal Cord or Limb Disorders

Patients who have suffered damage to the limbs or spinal column may have difficulty caring for themselves because of their injuries. Teaching self-care techniques is particularly important to their dental health.

I. Types

A. Amputation is the removal of a limb or appendage either through accidental injury or surgical procedure. The amount of functional disability is dependent on the type and extent of amputation.

B. Paralysis is the loss of motor, sensory, and autonomic function of parts of the body located below the area of the spinal cord injury.

   1. The paralysis may be caused by trauma, congenital defect, infection, hemorrhage, or infarction.

   2. Approximately 0.7% of Americans have some form of paralysis.[30]

C. Spinal cord injuries typically result in partial or complete paralysis from trauma to the spinal cord.

   1. Occur in 0.08% of Americans[30]; victims often are children or young adults.

2. Common causes include auto accidents, violent crime, and sporting accidents.

3. The amount of injury is related to the location and extent of the injury. Generally, all motor, sensory, and autonomic function is lost below the point of the injury.

4. Types

   a. Spina bifida is a congenital defect of the spinal column in which some of the spinal cord is displaced through an opening in the spinal column.

      1) Partial or full paralysis is common.

      2) Hydrocephalus, an excessive accumulation of spinal fluid in the brain that causes excessive skull growth and brain compression in infants, often occurs.

         a) Seizure may occur.

         b) Antibiotic premedication is necessary when patient has a shunt for draining excessive fluid from brain.

   b. Traumatic injury results from physical trauma that causes compression, fracture, or severing of the spinal column. An example is a compression neck injury suffered during a diving accident.

II. Oral manifestations are related to the patient's ability to care for his or her own oral health; may include dental caries and periodontal disease if oral hygiene is poor or if diet or motor function is restricted.

III. Risk factors include:

A. Respiratory difficulty from an inability to cough.

B. Pressure (decubitus) sores.

C. Infection.

D. Spasms.

E. Inability to maintain body temperature.

F. Autonomic dysreflexia, a serious increase in blood pressure from bowel or bladder irritation; is an emergency and requires immediate referral for medical treatment.

IV. Barriers to care include:

A. Lack of communication, when learning disabilities (spina bifida), depression, and poor self image (paralysis) are present.

B. Transportation difficulties because of ambulatory disability.

C. Economic loss from reduction in or loss of employment because of severe disability.

V. Professional and home care involves:

A. Providing thorough dental hygiene care in a comfortable, relaxed environment.

B. Antibiotic premedication is required for the patient with a shunt.

C. Awareness of the risk for respiratory difficulty from accidental airway blockage when motor dysfunction such as spasticity and tremor occur.

D. Familiarity with wheelchair transfer procedures is essential.

E. Maintenance of good oral hygiene and the use of fluorides to prevent dental caries.

F. Encouragement and empathy, which are extremely important to developing patient rapport.

VI. Patient/Caregiver education should emphasize:

A. Adaptive equipment and aids, including powered toothbrushes and oral irrigators.

B. Emphasis on self-care, although assistance of caregivers may be sought when efforts to maintain good oral hygiene are not feasible.

C. The need for fluoride supplementation.

The Patient with Nervous System Degeneration

Nervous system degeneration is caused by a variety of diseases and often has devastating consequences. Common diseases of this type include Alzheimer's disease, multiple sclerosis, myasthenia gravis, and Parkinson's disease. Bell's palsy, which typically is a temporary disorder, is also discussed.

I. Types

A. Alzheimer disease affects 1% of the US population and is a common form of dementia[30]; primarily affects individuals older than 65 years of age.

1. The disease tends to strike in the middle to later years and causes an increasing loss of mental function as the years pass.

a. Its cause is unknown but genetics, virus, brain injury, and metal toxicity are suspect.

b. Affected individuals have difficulty with cognition, depression, bladder and bowel control, tiredness, emotional control, weight loss, and other medical conditions.

c. Affected individuals may take antipsychotic (neuroleptic) medications that increase the risk of bleeding, candida, and other infections.

2. Oral manifestations include speech difficulties and poor oral hygiene because of a loss of cognitive abilities; may include trauma from falls or elder abuse.

3. Risk factors include:

a. Emotional stress and generalized depression.

1) Patients are easily confused and function better in a quiet, familiar environment.

2) Behavior may be uncooperative; caregivers should speak in short, simple sentences and move slowly.

b. The use of epinephrine and atropine should be avoided to prevent drug interactions with neuroleptics.[30]

4. Barriers to care include:

a. Difficult communication because of cognitive difficulties.

b. Lack of transportation; patient must rely on others when unable to transport self.

c. Economic obstacles, because of an inability to hold a job or because of a fixed income.

5. Professional and home care involves:

a. Scheduling short, relaxed appointments during the patient's most alert times.

b. Reintroducing staff and procedures to enhance familiarity.

c. Home care instructions that are concrete; must be repeated because of patient's memory and behavior difficulties.

d. Reminders to brush and/or assistance with oral care tasks as the dementia increases.

6. Patient/Caregiver education should emphasize:

a. Gaining assistance of caregivers when the patient is unable to maintain appropriate oral cleanliness.

b. The importance of frequent dental recalls.

c. Empathy with the difficulties the caregiver faces in caring for a loved one.

B. Multiple sclerosis is an incurable, chronic, and progressive disease that is distinguished by demyelination of CNS nerve sheaths.

1. The disease, in which sclerotic plaques replace the nerve sheaths, tends to occur in individuals who are 20 to 40 years of age and who live in northern regions of the United States.[6]

a. The cause is unknown, although autoimmune disease or virus infection is suspected.

b. The average person with MS lives 25 years beyond the date of diagnosis.

c. Symptoms include general fatigue, weakness, and numbness of body parts during periods of activity; facial pain may occur along with heat sensitivity.

d. The disease involves relapses and remissions and is treated with medication.

2. Oral manifestations include facial pain, speech disorders, and facial paralysis in severe cases.

3. Risk factors include:

a. Physical or emotional stresses, such as infections, emotional stress, inadequate rest, and excessive exercising.

b. Side effects of medications.

c. Diet restrictions caused by muscle dysfunction.

4. Barriers to care include:

a. Communication difficulties, from dysfunction of the muscles of speech.

b. Transportation difficulties, because of ambulatory problems and the need to use canes, walkers, or wheelchairs; patients eventually must rely on others.

c. Economic issues, when income is restricted because of reduction in or loss of employment.

5. Professional and home care involves:

a. Scheduling short, relaxed appointments for the patient, preferably during times of remission.

b. Keeping the patient at a comfortable temperature.

c. Attention to proper cleansing when facial paralysis and weakness reduce the patient's ability to cleanse the cheeks and tongue.

d. Home care instructions related to frequent cleansing of the oral cavity; powered toothbrushes, adaptive aids, and oral irrigators may be recommended for those who have difficulty manually cleaning the oral cavity.

6. Patient/Caregiver education should emphasize:

a. Family assistance in maintaining good daily oral hygiene after the patient is no longer able to do so.

b. Daily fluoride supplementation.

c. Maintenance of an adequate diet.

C. Myasthenia gravis affects approximately 0.005% of the population; is an autoimmune disease that affects the neuromusculature of the body.[30]

1. A decrease in the number of acetylcholine receptors results in a decreased transmission of nerve impulses.

a. Causes a generalized feeling of exhaustion from muscle fatigue and weakness.

b. Causes paralysis in its most severe form.

c. Affects younger women and older men.

d. Is treated by anticholinesterase medication, surgical removal of the thymus gland, or steroidal hormones.

2. Oral manifestations include effects on the facial and cervical musculature, which lead to a loss of control of facial muscles and result in smiling, eating, swallowing, speaking, and vision difficulties; when severe, can cause respiratory distress.

3. Risk factors that cause a crisis include infection, emotional stress, and surgery. Two types of crises include:

a. Myasthenic crisis, which causes a loss of swallowing and speaking ability and difficulty breathing and seeing; is caused by under-medication, underlying illness or risk factors, or a worsening of the disease.

b. Cholinergic crisis, which is related to over-medication with anticholinesterase and occurs within an hour of medication use. Symptoms include increased muscle weakness, gastrointestinal upset, and respiratory difficulties. Both crises require immediate medical attention. Airway should be maintained and/or ventilated until help arrives.

4. Barriers to care include:

a. Communication difficulties, if patients experiences facial weakness or paralysis (patient may hold chin with hand to speak).

b. Transportation difficulties; generalized fatigue affects the patient's ability to get to the dental office.

c. Economic issues for those on fixed incomes.

5. Professional and home care involves:

a. Scheduling appointments during the patient's most active periods of the day—generally soon after medication is taken and after a good night's sleep.

b. The availability of emergency equipment for respiratory distress during appointments.

c. Home care instructions related to preventing oral infections, which are risk factors for crisis development. Powered toothbrushes and oral irrigators are recommended for patients who have difficulty manually cleaning the oral cavity.

d. Careful attention to proper nutrition, which becomes more important when food selections are limited by an inability to chew or swallow some foods.

6. Patient/caregiver education should emphasize keeping the oral cavity in excellent condition to reduce the risk of crisis. Family members may be enlisted to assist in frequent, daily oral care procedures and transport of the patient to the dental clinic when the patient is no longer able.

D. Parkinson's disease affects 1% of the US population older than 50 years of age and is a slow, progressive degeneration of basal ganglion neurons; results in a loss of control of voluntary musculature.[30] The inability to produce adequate levels of dopamine, a brain chemical, is related to the degeneration, although the exact cause is unknown. Possible causes are exposure to environmental toxins, such as pesticides and mercury, or head injury. The disease affects more men than women and tends to occur during the middle to later years of life (ages 50 to 65). Symptoms include a pill-rolling motion of the fingers, a masked facial appearance, and muscle rigidity.

1. Oral manifestations include drooling, difficulty swallowing, tremors, and a reduced ability (or inability) to properly care for the mouth because of motor dysfunction, which may result in oral infection; speech may be stammered and monotone; xerostomia is a common side effect of medication.

2. Risk factors include difficulty in swallowing, a restricted diet because of eating difficulties, and difficulty in walking.

3. Barriers to care may include:

a. Communication difficulties, because of the patient's embarrassment about the condition; slurred speech from motor dysfunction occurs later in the course of disease.

b. Transportation difficulties, including ambulation problems and the need to rely on others as the disease progresses.

c. Economic difficulties associated with the loss

of employment or reliance on a fixed income during the later years.

4. Professional and home care involves making the patient comfortable during appointments, the use of stable instrumentation to deal with tremors, and active listening and encouragement, which are important to the patient's sense of well being.

5. Patient/Caregiver education should emphasize frequent and proper care of the oral cavity, with emphasis on the use of adaptive aids as needed; as the disease progresses, family assistance should be requested to maintain oral health; frequent dental recall is recommended.

 Clinical Case **STUDY**

Naomi Bishop is a 26-year-old woman in her 5th month of pregnancy. She has come to the office because her gums are bleeding and swollen. Naomi does not have routine dental examinations; she prefers to wait until she has a dental problem before making an appointment. Her mother lost a tooth for every child she bore, and Naomi is concerned that she will do the same.

Clinical Case QUESTIONS

1. In what trimester of pregnancy is Naomi? What fetal development occurs during this trimester?
2. What special precautions, if any, are recommended when treating a pregnant patient?
3. What is the most likely cause of the bleeding and swollen gums? What recommendations should be made?
4. Does Naomi need to worry about losing a tooth for every child? Why? Why not?

Clinical Case RATIONALES

1. Ms. Bishop is in her second trimester of pregnancy. During this developmental period, the organs of the fetus mature and growth continues. This is considered the best trimester for dental treatment because developmental disturbances of the fetus are less likely and the patient can still sit comfortably in the dental chair.
2. Radiographs generally are postponed during pregnancy, unless an emergency condition indicates a need for them. Medications are not recommended at any time during pregnancy. Special consideration during dental treatment should be made regarding the potential for nausea or hypotension.
3. The patient appears to be experiencing pregnancy gingivitis, a hormonally influenced, exaggerated response to bacterial plaque. Recommendations should include oral prophylaxis and meticulous home care, including toothbrushing and flossing.

4. The loss of a tooth for every child is a myth. If inadequate calcium intake occurs during pregnancy, calcium is removed from the mother's skeletal and alveolar bones, not from the teeth. Naomi should be informed of the need for adequate calcium in the diet and the myth should be dispelled. Most teeth are lost because of unrestored caries or periodontal disease, which is the most likely explanation for Naomi's mother's lost teeth.

Patient during Pregnancy

Full-term pregnancy is defined as the 40-week-long developmental period of the fetus.

I. Pregnancy is divided into first, second, and third trimesters; each has its own focus.
   A. During the first trimester the fetal organ systems develop. The lips, palate, and tooth buds form, and mineralization is initialized toward the end of the trimester; is a critical period of development, during which birth defects may occur from infection, prescription or illegal drug use, alcohol use, or nutritional deficiency.
   B. During the second trimester the fetal organ systems mature and fetal growth continues.
   C. During the third trimester the fetus becomes fully mature and gains weight; the average birth weight is 7 to 8 pounds.
II. Medical Manifestations
   A. The pregnant patient undergoes system-wide changes during pregnancy; may have difficulty with nausea and vomiting (typically first trimester) that predispose the patient to malnutrition because of appetite loss; caries also may result from acid in vomit contacting teeth and oral structures; is the best period for preventive dental examination.
   B. The second trimester typically is the best time to schedule routine dental care appointments for several reasons: the patient typically is over morning sickness, the risk for developmental disturbances of the fetus is lower, and the fetus is small enough that the patient can still sit comfortably in the dental chair.
   C. The third trimester is undesirable for treatment only because the patient may have difficulty sitting or lying in the dental chair for the entire appointment.
III. Oral Manifestations
   A. Erosion of enamel may occur in response to frequent vomiting, which accompanies severe morning sickness; small, frequent meals of healthy, noncariogenic foods should be recommended; the mouth should be rinsed thoroughly with water after vomiting and fluoride should be applied daily; frequent intake of fermentable carbohy-

drates for nausea puts the patient at high risk for caries; gagging and nausea may lead to inadequate performance of home care.

B. Tetracycline and its derivatives are contraindicated during pregnancy and early childhood to avoid staining effects during mineralization of the teeth.

C. Inadequate oral home care can predispose the patient to gingival inflammation; although pregnancy itself does not cause the inflammation, the elevated hormonal influences of estrogens and progesterone during pregnancy can exaggerate the gingival response to microorganisms; the inflammation abates somewhat after the pregnancy terminates. Proper plaque removal can prevent inflamed tissues.

1. Pregnancy gingivitis is generalized gingival enlargement with the overall appearance of sore, reddened, swollen, bleeding gums. *Prevotella intermedia* frequently is associated with pregnancy gingivitis; plaque control instruction and thorough instrumentation are essential.

2. Pregnancy tumor is a localized area of gingival enlargement, typically on the interdental papilla; also is called epulis gravidarum, pregnancy granuloma, or pyogenic granuloma. It is a painless, mushroom-shaped hyperplasia that bleeds easily and typically diminishes after birth; plaque control instruction and thorough instrumentation are essential.

D. Recent research has found a relationship between periodontal disease and low-birth-weight infants. It is believed that some periodontal pathogens stimulate uterine contractions and may cause premature labor.

IV. Risk Factors

A. Radiographs are avoided unless necessary to the provision of dental care; if radiographs are needed, use the paralleling technique, limit the number of radiographs, and use a lead apron with a thyroid collar to cover the patient's front and another lead apron to cover the patient's back (to eliminate both primary and secondary radiation to the fetus). Local anesthetics may be used during the second and third trimesters. General and nitrous oxide analgesia is contraindicated during pregnancy.

B. Extensive or elective restorative, scaling, and root planing procedures should be postponed until after the birth. Routine preventive and restorative dental procedures can be performed safely at any time during the pregnancy.

V. Barriers to care

A. During pregnancy: include morning sickness (gagging, nausea, lack of appetite); inability to sit comfortably for long periods (backache, frequent urination, fatigue, dizziness); and economic difficulty because of increased medical costs

and possible reduction in or loss of employment income.

B. After pregnancy: include lack of time (return to work, family obligations) and economic difficulty because of increased costs associated with child rearing and possible reduction in or loss of employment income.

VI. Professional Care

A. Should be based on the patient's needs, in terms of both frequency of care and level of care; more frequent care (every 3 months) may be necessary for those with less-than-desirable home care, those with periodontal disease, or those whose morning sickness results in frequent vomiting.

B. Should include routine oral prophylaxis and root planing; avoid taking radiographs or giving medications.

C. Should be provided in limited, shorter appointments as required for patient comfort. Allow patient to shift position as needed, preferably to the left side when orthostatic hypotension presents. Supine positioning must be avoided if hypotension persists.

VII. Patient/Caregiver education should emphasize:

A. General health and well-being during pregnancy and a well-balanced diet that meets the needs of both mother and fetus. Adequate consumption of protein, calcium, folic acid, and vitamins A, B-complex, C, and D is particularly important.

B. Plaque-induced and hormone-influenced inflammatory effects on gingiva and the effect of vomiting on enamel erosion; rinsing with water instead of brushing after vomiting should be recommended.

C. The dispelling of myths (e.g., about loosing a tooth for every child); when the diet contains inadequate amounts of minerals, calcium and phosphorus are removed from the mother's bones (including alveolar and all other skeletal bones), not from the teeth. Nursing bottle syndrome and its prevention should be discussed.

D. Meticulous plaque control; includes proper toothbrushing and flossing daily.

E. Fluoride application via dentifrices, gels, or rinses as needed, depending on the patient's risk for the caries.

F. Fluoride supplementation should be provided only for the benefit of the mother; no studies have found a link between prenatal fluoridation and a reduction in the rate of dental caries in children.

 Clinical Case **STUDY**

Six-year-old Daniel Gates visits the dental office for his annual examination, oral prophylaxis, and fluoride treatment. His father walks him to the dental chair, kisses the

top of his head, and returns to the reception room. Daniel's teeth are very clean and show no evidence of caries or gingivitis. During inspection of the oral mucosa, a purplish bruise the size of a quarter is observed along the midline, in the posterior third of the hard palate. When asked about the bruise, Daniel indicates that he is unaware of its cause. Daniel is well behaved while his teeth are being cleaned, although he gags whenever the clinician touches his tongue or gingiva in the molar regions. Because of his strong gag reflex, taking bitewing radiographs is difficult and giving a fluoride treatment is impossible. At the end of the appointment, Mr. Gates is shown the bruised area and asked whether he is aware of its cause. Mr. Gates indicates that he has no idea why the area is bruised.

Clinical Case QUESTIONS

1. What are possible causes of the purplish bruise on Daniel's hard palate? How old is the bruise? What evidence is there to support your theory of the cause?
2. What causes a gag reflex? Identify ways to manage a gag reflex while taking radiographs or giving a fluoride treatment.
3. Is any follow-up of the palate lesion necessary, and if so, why?

Clinical Case RATIONALES

1. A palate bruise is caused when a hard object strikes the palate with enough force to cause superficial blood vessels to rupture and blood to pool in the area. This type of bruise can be caused innocently when a person falls with a candy sucker, pen, or other hard object in the mouth, forcing the object against the palate. However, it may indicate sexual abuse, in which the penis is forced against the hard palate. Because neither child nor father can recall an injury to the palate, the bruising is recent, and a strong gag reflex is exhibited, it is prudent to suspect that the bruising may be a sign of sexual abuse. The parent and child most likely would recall a recent traumatic incident with enough force to cause a large area of bruising.
2. A gag reflex is caused when oral tissues, particularly in the posterior regions, are hypersensitive to films, instruments, or fingers that are moved across oral tissues or are retained in place for long periods. It also may be associated with previous unpleasant experiences, such as poor clinical technique or sexual abuse. Techniques to manage gagging include calming the patient by explaining all procedures; working efficiently and confidently; providing distraction by having the patient breath through the nose, bite on a bite block, or concentrate on another object; or, in severe cases, applying a local anesthetic gel, salt, or ice to desensitize the area just before the procedure. The radiograph films

should be quickly placed in the mouth, after the tubehead is focused, and removed immediately upon exposure. The fluoride treatment should be left in the mouth for 1 minute only (or less if not tolerated well) and the patient should be complimented on the ability to maintain the trays for that long (the major benefit of the fluoride is received and tolerance can be increased as patient confidence rises).

3. The palatal lesion should be examined by the dentist, photographed if possible (no parental permission is required if abuse is suspected), described and documented in the patient record, and examined one week later for signs of resolution. When abuse of any type is suspected, authorities (the Department of Social Services, police department, or other such agency) should be notified while the child is in the operatory, if possible, or immediately afterward, if not. The health professional should not attempt to confront the caregiver regarding concerns of abuse.

The Abused, Dependent Patient

The dental hygienist should be aware of the signs of dependent abuse or neglect. Dependents include children, disabled adults, and the elderly—any person under the care of another. Abuse occurs in cases of physical neglect or abuse, emotional deprivation or abuse, and sexual abuse or exploitation. It is estimated that hundreds of thousands of elderly Americans[31] and between 1 and 2 million children[32] are abused or neglected each year.

I. Types of Abuse
   A. Physical neglect is the failure to provide a healthy environment for a dependent. This includes the provision of adequate food, clothing, supervision, health care, living environment, personal hygiene, and education. Neglect can be either deliberate or the result of ignorance.
      1. Dental neglect is the willful failure of the caregiver to provide appropriate treatment for dental disease when the disease causes pain, discomfort, or delays in growth and development.
      2. Common dental conditions related to neglect include rampant caries, untreated oral or facial trauma, and untreated oral infection.
   B. Physical abuse is nonaccidental biting, striking, burning, lacerating, or other type of conduct that results in injury.
   C. Emotional deprivation is the failure to provide for the emotional needs of a dependent. It can include withholding love, lack of caring, alienation, and chronic criticism (is common in immature parents or caregivers).
   D. Emotional abuse is the purposeful use of demeaning, vengeful, demanding, or aggressive be-

haviors to control a dependent. It can also include role-reversal, whereby the child or dependent controls the caregiver (is common in immature parents or caregivers).

E. Sexual abuse is the purposeful use of a dependent for nonconsensual sexual acts, or sexual acts with a dependent who is unable to give informed consent.

F. Sexual exploitation is the purposeful use of a nonconsensual dependent or a dependent who is unable to give informed consent to provide some form of sexual act for the sexual or monetary gain of the caregiver.

II. Medical Manifestations of Abuse

A. Signs of physical neglect may include:

1. An unkempt appearance, which can include soiled clothing; dirty hair, hands, and skin; poor personal hygiene; inappropriate clothing or clothing in need of repair; and a lack of dental or medical care.

2. Lack of appropriate supervision, which can include allowing the dependent unrestricted freedom to roam the streets, leaving a dependent home alone, and failing to provide needed assistance in proper oral or personal hygiene.

3. Improper or inadequate nutrition, which can include: allowing indiscriminate eating and drinking of junk foods and beverages, restricting dietary choices, or providing too little food to give adequate nutrition.

B. Signs of physical abuse

1. Bruising
   a. On areas of the body where bruising typically does not occur
      1) Accidental bruising (not associated with abuse) typically occurs in areas overlying bone (shins, forehead) or areas that protrude (knees, elbows).
      2) Nonaccidental bruising (associated with abuse) tends to occur in areas unlike those mentioned and may take on the shape of the object used to hit or pinch (fingers, hands, paddle, bat, belt buckle, teeth). Bruising tends to occur on the buttocks, thighs, face, neck, and upper arms. Be suspicious if:
         a) A patient exhibits discomfort when sitting or lying in the dental chair.
         b) Multiple and multi-stage bruises are evident.
         c) Bruises are visible only where clothing shifts during movement (e.g., top of thighs).
         d) The description of an incident does not match the visual evidence.
         e) The patient wears clothing that is unseasonable and may be used to cover bruising (i.e., long-sleeved or legged garments in warm weather).
   b. In various stages of healing
      1) May be a strong indicator of abuse because accidental injury typically does not occur frequently enough to cause bruising in different stages.
      2) Are indicated by:
         a) New bruises that are reddish-purple in color.
         b) Week-old bruises that are greenish in color.
         c) Two-week-old bruises that are yellowish in color.
         d) Two-to-four-week-old bruises that are brownish in color.

2. Lacerations tend to occur on the lips, eyes, or face; a lacerated maxillary labial frenum can indicate forced feeding.

3. Bites
   a. Anywhere on the body (unless obviously made by a toddler) are signs of abuse.
   b. Greater than 3 cm from canine puncture to canine puncture indicate that they were made by an adult.
   c. Are useful for identifying the perpetrator; bite marks are very individual.
   d. Caused by humans create puncture/pressure-type wounds that leave a mark; animal bites typically cause tearing of the flesh.

4. Burns that appear suspicious and have no reasonable explanation; often are made by cigarettes, immersion in hot water, or by rope (in cases of confinement).

5. Hitting
   a. Is the purposeful delivery of blows.
   b. Is associated with bruising, fractures, and internal injuries (brain hemorrhage, retinal hemorrhage, and laceration or rupture of internal organs).
   c. To the face and head can result in fractured jaws, broken or avulsed teeth, and lacerated lips.

6. Hair pulling is indicated by bald patches or thinning hair.

7. Head banging may be evidenced by bruising of the back of the head, loss of consciousness, and retinal hemorrhage (as in shaken baby syndrome).

8. Inappropriate behavior is common in the abused. It may include:
   a. Inappropriate fearfulness and crying.
   b. Abrupt changes in behavior when separated from a caregiver.
   c. Delays in language or growth development in infants and children.
   d. A withdrawn, unhappy character.

C. Signs of emotional deprivation or abuse
  1. Improper behavior of a caregiver, including displays of anger, a condescending attitude, and criticism of a patient in front of others.
  2. Improper behavior of the patient, including extreme displays of fear, dependence, and withdrawal.
D. Signs of sexual abuse and exploitation
  1. Sexually explicit behavior in a child
  2. Severe gag reflex
  3. Oral lesions of sexually transmitted diseases
  4. Refusal to allow clinician to enter mouth
  5. Bruising of the palate not associated with accidental injury
  6. Discomfort of the genital-rectal area upon sitting
  7. Discomfort of the genital-rectal area when walking
III. Oral Manifestations of Abuse
  A. Facial trauma, as evidenced by bruising, lacerations, bite marks, or burns in unlikely locations or associated with an unlikely cause.
  B. A torn maxillary labial frenum, which often is associated with forced feedings.
  C. Severe caries or oral infections that remain untreated after the caregiver is notified of need for treatment.
  D. Oral lesions associated with sexually transmitted diseases.
  E. Palatal bruising, which is associated with forced oral sex.
IV. Risk factors include a fear of dental procedures, inappropriate behavior in the dental office, and an inability to control gagging during procedures.
V. Barriers to care include communication difficulties with both patient and caregiver. The dental professional may feel unprepared or uneasy dealing with abuse situations, the patient may be fearful of reporting abuse to anyone, and the caregiver may be in denial of any wrongdoing. An abusive caregiver who feels threatened with discovery may fail to keep appointments or may switch doctors.
VI. Professional and home care involves:
  A. Building trust with the patient by explaining all procedures and encouraging appropriate behavior.
  B. Immediately reporting suspicion of abuse to supervising dentist or appropriate agency.
    1. National requirement for reporting abuse
      a. Currently, all states have a mandatory reporting law for the abuse of children under the age of 18. Most states also mandate reporting the abuse of dependent adults.
      b. Any person in a paid position of providing care or services to a person suspected of being abused must report suspicions of abuse. Dentists are mandated to report

indications of child abuse in all states and dependent abuse in most states.
    2. Local requirements for reporting abuse
      a. In some states, the law requires dental hygienists to report suspected abuse of a child or other dependent.
      b. In other states, dental hygienists are not required to report but are encouraged to report suspected abuse of a child or other dependent.
  C. Discussing superficial treatment of injured areas; refer patient to a physician as needed.
VII. Patient/Caregiver education should include discussion of the need to reevaluate the injured area at a later date.

Positioning and Stabilization

Effective patient positioning and stabilization serve to provide for the well-being of the patient and the efficiency of the operator by providing a comfortable, safe environment.
I. Includes stabilization and positioning of the patient chair and the patient's head and body.
II. Requires knowing for which conditions a patient is more comfortable sitting upright than lying supine for proper care. Patients prone to decubitus ulcers, such as paraplegics, require careful readjustment of body position and the use of additional cushioning during long appointments.
III. Support and Restraint Devices
  A. Most commonly used for patients with neuromuscular disorders or extreme behavioral problems that put the patient and/or operator at physical risk from movement during instrumentation; should not be used routinely. Sedation is another option but is reserved as a last resort.
  B. Mouth props typically are rubber materials that are used to hold the mouth open for patients who are unable to do so themselves. Some are placed in a closed position and gradually opened as needed; others place the jaws in an open position at all times.
  C. Head stabilization involves the use of the clinician's arm to surround the patient's head, cup the chin, and hold it still during procedures.
  D. Wraps tend to be used for young children when full-body restraint is necessary. Sheets and blankets are similarly used to wrap and secure the patient with straps.
  E. Papoose boards are boards with padded straps that are used to secure patients of any size during operatory procedures.
IV. Wheelchair transfer is important to know because approximately 0.6% of Americans are wheelchair bound.[33] Several methods are available. Before transfer, determine whether special padding should be transferred, whether a urine-collecting device is pre-

sent, and whether there is a need to secure the limbs because of spastic movements.[3] Depending on the severity of the disability, some patients can assist in some or all of the transfer (Fig. 15–6).

A. Secure a transfer belt around the patient's waist.

B. Clear the area.

C. Position the dental chair at the same height as the wheelchair or lower; face the wheelchair in the same direction and at a slight angle to the dental chair.

D. Remove or release the dental chair and wheelchair armrests.

E. Set the brake.

F. Determine whether any special equipment must be transferred or might be in the way.

G. Lift the footrests.

H. While facing the patient, place your feet on either side of the patient's feet.

I. With the clinician's knees holding the patient's legs stable, grasp the patient under the arms and around the back to grasp the transfer belt.

J. Place the patient in a standing position.

K. Rotate the patient into the dental chair in a smooth movement.

L. Position the patient on the dental chair; place padding as needed and straighten clothing.

V. Behavior management involves familiarity with the special characteristics and needs of the patient, inclusion of caretakers in discussions of behavior management, and patience with and empathy for the patient. Dental visits are more successful if the patient is familiarized with the office by frequent, short visits during which procedures are demonstrated.

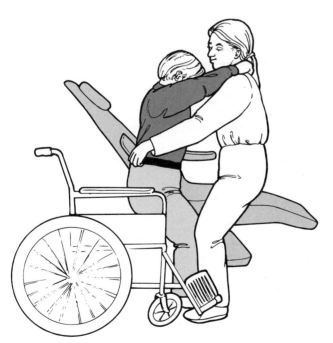

Figure 15.6 Wheelchair transfer of a patient to the dental chair.

CONTENT REVIEW QUESTIONS

1. Developmental disabilities include all of the following, EXCEPT:
   A. mental retardation
   B. cerebral palsy
   C. multiple sclerosis
   D. autism

2. Aphasia, apraxia, and dysarthria are examples of _____ disabilities.
   A. communication
   B. developmental
   C. cognitive
   D. sensory
   E. nervous system

3. All of the following are examples of nervous system disabilities, EXCEPT:
   A. Parkinson's disease
   B. myasthenia gravis
   C. Alzheimer's disease
   D. multiple sclerosis
   E. muscular dystrophy

4. Patients who can bathe, feed, and dress themselves but may need to be reminded to brush their teeth and hair are considered _____ functioning.
   A. high
   B. moderate
   C. low
   D. not

5. The least likely oral manifestation of mental retardation is:
   A. early tooth eruption
   B. fusion of teeth
   C. malocclusion
   D. tongue thrust
   E. missing teeth

6. When discussing home care procedures with the mildly mentally retarded individual:
   A. speak directly to the caregiver
   B. use simple demonstrations
   C. send home printed materials
   D. discuss the risk of periodontitis

7. The patient with cerebral palsy is likely to have difficulty with all of the following, EXCEPT:
   A. controlling movement
   B. communicating
   C. dental caries
   D. oral hygiene
   E. comprehension

8. When treating the patient with autism, one should:
   A. use nonverbal instructions
   B. follow a consistent routine
   C. speak in a louder tone of voice
   D. schedule longer visits

9. A central nervous system disorder in which loss of consciousness is common is:
   A. autism
   B. cerebral palsy

C. epilepsy

D. mental retardation

10. An aura is commonly associated with:

A. epileptic seizure

B. myocardial infarction

C. anorexia nervosa

D. Sjögren's syndrome

11. A secondary effect of phenytoin use is:

A. gingival hyperplasia

B. ulcerative gingivitis

C. desquamative gingivitis

D. gingival atrophy

12. The inability to properly form speech sounds is termed:

A. apraxia

B. aphasia

C. dysarthria

D. ataxia

13. When providing oral health care instructions to a visually-impaired individual, it is MOST important to:

A. talk more loudly

B. speak more slowly

C. face the patient

D. use visual aids

14. Which of the following diseases or disorders is NOT associated with aging?

A. cardiovascular disease

B. hypertension

C. diabetes mellitus

D. senile dementia

E. muscular dystrophy

15. Which one of the following oral manifestations is a result of normal aging?

A. xerostomia

B. attrition

C. stomatitis

D. glossitis

E. periodontitis

16. In older individuals, decay is MOST commonly located on _____ surfaces.

A. occlusal

B. proximal

C. root

D. lingual

17. The majority of elderly individuals:

A. live in family homes

B. live in nursing homes

C. have dental insurance

D. visit the dentist annually

18. The most common barrier to care for the patient with an eating disorder is:

A. communication

B. transportation

C. economic

D. physical

19. The most devastating oral effects of eating disorders are related to:

A. excessive exercising

B. binge eating

C. frequent purging

D. malnutrition

E. laxative use

20. Which of the following should immediately follow a purging incident?

A. rinsing with tap water

B. brushing with baking soda

C. brushing with fluoride gel

D. flossing

21. All of the following are oral manifestations associated with arthritis, EXCEPT:

A. angular cheilitis

B. gingival bleeding

C. oral infections

D. TMJ discomfort

22. Which one of the following adaptive aids would MOST benefit the patient with arthritic joints of the hands?

A. an extended-handle toothbrush

B. a textured-handle toothbrush

C. an enlarged-handle toothbrush

D. a curved-handle toothbrush

23. All of the following are conditions associated with alcoholism, EXCEPT:

A. reddened nose

B. puffy eyes

C. yellow skin

D. dry mouth

E. fruity breath

24. Angular cheilitis, pale oral mucosa, and glossitis are signs of:

A. anemia

B. leukemia

C. hemophilia

D. jaundice

25. When treating the patient with hemophilia, one should do all of the following, EXCEPT:

A. consult with the patient's physician

B. treat with replacement factor

C. prevent infectious disease transmission

D. clean teeth in small segments over several appointments

E. scale the entire mouth in one appointment

26. Which of the following is FALSE regarding rheumatic heart disease?

A. is caused by infection with hemolytic streptococcus

B. involves damage to the heart's valves

C. requires antibiotic premedication before dental procedures

D. is an outcome of rheumatic fever

E. permanently affects the joints of the body

27. Which of the following should be avoided when a patient with cardiac dysrhythmia has a surgically implanted pacemaker?

A. rubber cup polishing
B. subgingival scaling
C. ultrasonic scaling
D. flossing

28. The patient with a cardiac condition:
A. may have difficulty breathing in a supine position
B. should not be administered local anesthetics
C. is at high risk for developing oral candidiasis
D. may have difficulty communicating

29. A cerebrovascular accident:
A. is a sudden loss of blood flow to the heart
B. is caused by a restriction in or rupture of a blood vessel
C. often is preceded by rheumatic heart disease
D. requires no modification of dental procedures after the incident

30. Patients with type-I diabetes mellitus:
A. have noninsulin-dependent diabetes
B. can control the disease with oral insulin
C. are at increased risk for infection
D. typically have low blood glucose levels

31. Which one of the following in NOT a common oral manifestation of diabetes mellitus?
A. parotid enlargement
B. candida infection
C. xerostomia
D. atrophic tongue
E. periodontitis

32. When treating the patient with diabetes, one should do all of the following, EXCEPT:
A. schedule appointments before a meal
B. consult with the treating physician
C. limit the length of the appointment
D. be prepared for an emergency

33. Common oral manifestations of substance abuse include all of the following, EXCEPT:
A. xerostomia
B. trauma
C. lichen planus
D. extrinsic stain
E. mucositis

34. When treating a patient who is a suspected substance abuser, the safest pain control modality is:
A. local anesthetic
B. local anesthetic with vasoconstrictor
C. nitrous oxide analgesia

35. HIV is the acronym for:
A. human acquired immune virus
B. human immunodeficiency virus
C. acquired immunodeficiency virus

36. All of the following are common oral manifestations of AIDS, EXCEPT:
A. hairy leukoplakia
B. candidiasis
C. Kaposi's sarcoma
D. angular cheilitis
E. lichen planus

37. The major barrier to care for the patient with HIV/AIDS is:
A. communication
B. transportation
C. economic
D. physical

38. Which of the following is a common oral manifestation of renal disease?
A. herpes
B. lichen planus
C. halitosis
D. angular cheilitis

39. A physician consult is necessary before treating the patient with renal disease. Which one of the following is NOT a reason for consultation?
A. premedication needs
B. bleeding tendency
C. drug-drug interactions
D. HIV status

40. Common causes of respiratory disease include all of the following, EXCEPT:
A. cigarette smoking
B. allergy
C. cystic fibrosis
D. infection
E. diabetes mellitus

41. The dental patient with respiratory disease is at risk when exposed to all of the following, EXCEPT:
A. aerosols
B. sulfites
C. stress
D. inhalants

42. All of the following are risk factors associated with oral cancer, EXCEPT:
A. denture irritation
B. heavy alcohol use
C. age
D. tobacco

43. Patients who undergo chemotherapy for acute leukemia are not at an increased risk for oral infections. All patients who undergo chemotherapy for cancer will experience oral complications that are directly related to drug activity.
A. the first sentence is true, the second is false
B. the first sentence is false, the second is true.
C. both sentences are true
D. both sentences are false

44. Patients who have suffered spinal cord injuries may have difficulty performing oral care. When teaching oral health care measures, one should emphasize:
A. self care
B. proper nutrition
C. good oral hygiene
D. caregiver assistance

45. The level of paralysis or dysfunction associated with a spinal cord injury is most closely related to:
A. the type of traumatic injury

B. the severity of traumatic injury

C. the location of the traumatic injury

D. the cause of traumatic injury

46. All of the following are nervous system disorders, EXCEPT:

A. Parkinson's disease

B. multiple sclerosis

C. Sjögren's syndrome

D. myasthenia gravis

E. Alzheimer's disease

47. Which of the following statements regarding the patient with Alzheimer's disease is TRUE?

A. Alzheimer's disease is a form of dementia that tends to affect the oldest of the old.

B. Patients with Alzheimer's disease often are confused by change and prefer quiet surroundings.

C. When scheduling dental appointments, a single long appointment is preferable to several short appointments.

D. Most patients can take care of their oral health needs without the assistance of a caregiver.

48. The disease that affects the myelin sheath and results in fatigue and numbness is:

A. muscular dystrophy

B. multiple sclerosis

C. Parkinson's disease

D. Bell's palsy

E. myasthenia gravis

49. All of the following disorders may result in facial paralysis, EXCEPT:

A. multiple sclerosis

B. Alzheimer's disease

C. Bell's palsy

D. myasthenia gravis

50. During which trimester of pregnancy is it most advantageous to schedule a dental appointment?

A. first trimester

B. second trimester

C. third trimester

D. any trimester

51. Morning sickness puts a woman at risk for:

A. caries

B. malnutrition

C. periodontal disease

D. constipation

52. Which of the following is contraindicated during pregnancy?

A. flossing

B. tetracycline

C. mouth rinses containing alcohol

D. frequent meals

53. Which one of the following is NOT associated with morning sickness?

A. vomiting

B. enamel erosion

C. high carbohydrate snacks

D. nausea

E. periodontitis

54. When taking radiographs of a pregnant patient, one must do all of the following, EXCEPT:

A. use the paralleling technique

B. cover patient's back with a lead apron

C. limit the number of radiographs

D. cover patient's front with a lead apron

E. recline the chair in a supine position

55. The "loosing a tooth for every child" myth is based on the premise that:

A. calcium needed for the baby's growth is removed from the mother's teeth as needed

B. constant vomiting in the first trimester causes demineralization of tooth enamel

C. gagging leads to poor oral hygiene and caries

D. pregnancy tumors cause displacement and eventual loss of teeth

56. The failure of a caregiver to provide dental care for a dependent when obvious signs of dental decay are present is considered:

A. physical neglect

B. physical abuse

C. emotional abuse

D. emotional deprivation

E. sexual abuse

57. Which one of the following is commonly associated with physical abuse?

A. bruising along the shins

B. abrasions on the knees

C. tearing of the maxillary frenum

D. fracture of the tibia

58. Bruising associated with physical abuse often is:

A. red and purple

B. green

C. green and yellow

D. red, green, yellow, and brown

59. Which of the following conditions may indicate the need for a patient to be repositioned frequently during a dental appointment?

A. spina bifida

B. multiple sclerosis

C. Down syndrome

D. Parkinson's disease

60. This device is used specifically for the full-body restraint of young children:

A. mouth prop

B. head stabilization

C. wraps

D. papoose boards

61. When performing a wheelchair transfer, one must do all of the following, EXCEPT:

A. clear the area of any obstacles

B. secure a transfer belt to the patient

C. raise the chair above wheelchair height

D. stabilize the patient's legs

E. grasp the patient under the arms and around back

CONTENT REVIEW RATIONALES

1. **C** Mental retardation, cerebral palsy, and autism are all developmental disorders that are present at birth. Multiple sclerosis a nervous system disorder that typically is acquired during adulthood.

2. **A** Communication disabilities are those related to neurologic brain damage that disturbs language and speech development. Aphasia is an inability to put thoughts into words or to understand language; apraxia is the inability to form speech sounds; and dysarthria results in slurred speech patterns.

3. **E** Muscular dystrophy (Duchenne's) is an x-linked recessive disorder of the musculoskeletal system that results in wasting of the skeletal muscles. No neurologic effects occur with the disease. The disease manifests itself in young childhood and death commonly occurs within 15 years. Parkinson's disease, myasthenia gravis, Alzheimer's disease, and multiple sclerosis are all disorders of the nervous system.

4. **A** Assessment of functional levels is from high (requires little assistance with ADL) to low (caretaker provides most or all care). A high-functioning patient can bath, dress, eat, communicate, and ambulate well enough to function with only minimal assistance. The patient may require reminders to perform tasks.

5. **A** Individuals with mental retardation often exhibit delayed (not early) tooth eruption; fused, pegged, or missing teeth; malocclusion; and tongue thrusting and mouth breathing.

6. **B** When discussing home care procedures with the mentally retarded individual, use simple and demonstrable instructions. Include the caregiver so that the caregiver can repeat the instructions as needed. Sending home printed materials and discussing risks for periodontal disease may be beneficial to the caregiver but are not appropriate for educating the patient.

7. **E** Individuals with cerebral palsy typically are able to comprehend instructions; fewer than half are mentally retarded and in need of simpler instructions. Those with cerebral palsy have difficulty with motor control, speaking, and performing home care procedures. Poor home care often results in caries.

8. **B** Patients with autism prefer routine and familiar procedures and surroundings. Instructions should be both nonverbal and verbal and kept simple. The tone and loudness of the voice should be normal. Shorter dental visits are preferred.

9. **C** Loss of consciousness is associated with epilepsy, as are convulsive episodes. Individuals with cerebral palsy, mental retardation, or autism, alone, are not prone to convulsions or loss of consciousness.

10. **A** An aura (or predication) often precedes an epileptic seizure and is not typically associated with myocardial infarction, anorexia nervosa, or Sjögren's syndrome.

11. **A** Gingival hyperplasia is a common effect of phenytoin use. Phenytoin often is prescribed as an anticonvulsant. Excellent plaque control measures can prevent and control gingival overgrowth. Ulcerative gingivitis, desquamative gingivitis, and gingival atrophy are not associated with phenytoin use.

12. **A** Apraxia is the inability to properly form speech sounds. Aphasia is the inability to understand language or put thoughts into words, and dysarthria is the slurring of speech patterns. Apraxia, aphasia, and dysarthria are all considered communication disorders. Ataxia is not a communication disorder but is a motor disorder that affects ambulation.

13. **C** Always face the patient when providing oral health care instructions to a visually impaired individual. Speaking more loudly or more slowly is more appropriate for dealing with hearing impairment. Visual aids may be used but must be enlarged to be of benefit.

14. **E** Aging is associated with many disorders and diseases. Cardiovascular disease, hypertension, diabetes mellitus, and senile dementia are common among aging individuals. Muscular dystrophy is an inherited disorder that causes weakness and deterioration of the muscles and often is evident in childhood.

15. **B** Attrition, darkening of the teeth, and gingival recession are the only oral manifestations that are considered a result of normal aging. Xerostomia, stomatitis, glossitis, and periodontitis often are seen in the aging population but are associated with illness and/or medication use rather than with aging itself.

16. **C** Decayed root surfaces are especially problematic for older individuals and are directly related to increased incidences of gingival recession, periodontal disease (which exposes the roots to the oral environment), and xerostomia (often medication induced; reduces salivary flow and its pH-neutralizing effects). Decay on occlusal, proximal, and lingual surfaces are not specifically related to age unless they are located at or below the gingival margin.

17. **A** The majority (67%) of elderly individuals live in a family home. Twenty-five percent of seniors will live in a nursing home, at least for a while. Few elderly have dental insurance or visit their dentist annually.

18. **A** Communication is the most common barrier to care for the patient with an eating disorder. Denial, shame, guilt, lack of compliance, and fear of weight gain are typical reasons the patient may have for not wishing to discuss the eating disorder. Transportation and physical barriers are insignificant but economic considerations may be problematic when the dentition has been damaged from behaviors associated with eating disorders, particularly vomiting.

19. **C** Frequent purging (vomiting) is responsible for the most devastating oral effects of eating disorders. It is associated with severe erosion of enamel surfaces,

a high incidence of caries, and sensitivity to sweets and temperatures. Excessive exercising, binge eating, malnutrition, and laxative use have fewer direct effects on the oral cavity.

20. **A** Immediately after a purging incident, the individual should rinse with tap water (sodium bicarbonate or magnesium hydroxide may be added) to neutralize the vomit acid. Brushing and flossing are contraindicated immediately after vomiting because the tooth enamel is weakened and brushing and flossing may abrade the surface.

21. **A** Gingival bleeding and oral infections are associated with medications that are used to treat arthritis. TMJ discomfort occurs when the disease has affected the joint. Angular cheilitis is associated with denture wearing, malnutrition, and candidal infection but not with arthritis.

22. **C** A toothbrush with a larger handle would be more beneficial for the patient with arthritic joints of the hands. Many arthritics have difficulty with grip strength. A larger brush handle would allow greater control. An extended-handle toothbrush is unnecessary unless the patient has difficulty raising the arms. A texture-handle toothbrush is helpful to prevent slipping but only if on a larger handle that improves the gripping ability of the arthritic. A curved-handle toothbrush is appropriate for reaching molar areas for patients with limited arm movement.

23. **E** Fruity breath is not one of the conditions associated with alcoholism. Reddened nose, puffy eyes, yellow skin, and dry mouth are associated with alcoholism.

24. **A** Angular cheilitis, pale oral mucosa, and glossitis are signs of anemia. Leukemia is manifested by gingival bleeding, susceptibility to infection, and gingival hypertrophy. Hemophilia is associated with excessive gingival bleeding. Jaundice is associated with yellow skin tones from hemoglobin breakdown or liver disease.

25. **E** When providing dental care for the patient with hemophilia, especially when procedures may cause bleeding or when inflammation is present, the entire dentition should NOT be scaled in one appointment. To minimize bleeding, the dentition should be cleaned in a series of small segments over several appointments. Before treatment, the patient's physician should be consulted, replacement factor should be given (according to physician recommendation), and infectious disease transmission protocols should be in place.

26. **E** Rheumatic heart disease does not permanently affect the joints of the body, although rheumatic fever temporarily does. Rheumatic heart disease is one outcome of rheumatic fever, an infection with hemolytic streptococcus that results in damage to the heart's valves. Patients with heart valve damage require antibiotic premedication whenever bacteremia is anticipated and particularly before oral prophylaxis.

27. **C** Ultrasonic scaling should be avoided when a patient has a cardiac pacemaker because high frequency vibrations may disrupt the pacemaker signal and cause a cardiac emergency. It is not necessary to avoid rubber cup polishing, subgingival scaling, or flossing.

28. **A** The patient with a cardiac condition may have difficulty breathing in a supine position, thus the patient chair should be adjusted upright. Caution should be taken when administering local anesthetics because of possible drug-drug interactions; however, most individuals with cardiac conditions have no difficulty with local anesthetics and vasoconstrictors. Patients with heart disease are not at high risk for developing oral candidiasis or communication difficulties.

29. **B** A restriction in or rupture of a blood vessel causes a cerebrovascular accident. It involves a sudden loss of blood flow to the brain, not to the heart. It is not associated with rheumatic heart disease and often is preceded by underlying diseases such as hypertension, diabetes, drug abuse, and atherosclerosis. Consultation with the patient's primary care physician is important because some modification of dental procedures may be necessary, particularly within the first 6 months after the incident.

30. **C** Patients with type-I diabetes mellitus (IDDM) are at increased risk for infection. They require daily injections of insulin to reduce their high blood glucose levels.

31. **D** An atrophic tongue is not a common oral manifestation of diabetes mellitus. The tongue often is edematous and the parotid gland may be enlarged. Xerostomia and candida infection are common. All diabetics are at increased risk for developing periodontitis.

32. **A** Schedule appointments for a patient with diabetes after the morning meal, when blood glucose is more stable, to reduce the possibility of an emergency. Before treatment, consult with the treating physician regarding the level of blood glucose control and the need for antibiotic premedication. Appointments should be short. Keep glucose, sugar, or orange juice on hand in case of diabetic emergency.

33. **C** Common oral manifestations of substance abuse include xerostomia, oral and facial trauma, extrinsic stain, and mucositis. Lichen planus is an inflammatory disease of unknown origin that is associated with systemic diseases such as hypertension and diabetes.

34. **A** With a suspected substance abuser, one should avoid the use of epinephrine because it may interact with cocaine and other drugs. The safest pain control modality is a local anesthetic without a vasoconstrictor. Nitrous oxide analgesia is safe to use but does have the potential for abuse and for transmission of infectious diseases (hepatitis B) if the tubing is not sterilized.

35. **B** HIV is the acronym for human immunodeficiency virus, the virus that causes AIDS (acquired immunodeficiency syndrome).

36. **E** Hairy leukoplakia, candidiasis, Kaposi's sarcoma, and angular cheilitis are common oral manifestations of AIDS. Lichen planus is a chronic inflammatory disease of unknown cause that often is associated with systemic diseases such as diabetes mellitus and hypertension. It is not commonly associated with AIDS.

37. **A** Communication is the major barrier to care for the patient with HIV or AIDS. Fear of health care providers' attitudes may prevent a patient from fully disclosing his or her health status. Transportation, economic, and physical barriers may present as the patient becomes more debilitated with the disease.

38. **C** Halitosis is a common oral manifestation of renal disease. Herpes is a common viral infection that is not specifically associated with renal disease. Lichen planus is a chronic inflammatory disease associated with systemic diseases such as hypertension and diabetes mellitus. Angular cheilitis is associated with nutritional deficiency, candidal infection, and immunocompromised states but not specifically with renal disease.

39. **D** A physician consult is necessary before treating the patient with renal disease. The physician should indicate the need for antibiotic or steroidal premedication, the patient's tendency to bleed, and any drug-drug interactions. The HIV status of the patient is only of peripheral significance.

40. **E** Common causes of respiratory disease include cigarette smoking, allergy, cystic fibrosis, and infection. Diabetes mellitus is not associated with respiratory disease.

41. **D** Inhalers contain medicaments that help dilate the bronchioles and result in easier breathing for the patient. The dental patient with respiratory disease is at risk for breathing difficulty when exposed to aerosols (from ultrasonic scalers), sulfites (which provoke asthma), and stress (which also can provoke asthma).

42. **A** Denture irritation never has been proven to cause squamous cell carcinoma. Patients with oral cancer can experience denture sores or trauma from intraoral changes associated with cancer. Age, heavy alcohol use, and tobacco have been identified as major risk factors for oral squamous cell cancer.

43. **D** Both sentences are false. Patients with acute leukemia undergo myelosuppressive chemotherapy, which causes suppression of the immune system. Approximately 40% of patients who receive chemotherapy experience oral complications. Certain chemotherapy drugs have little effect on the mucosal tissues and do not cause significant immunosuppression.

44. **A** Patients who have suffered spinal cord injury should be taught oral self-care. Depression and low self-esteem often accompany this disorder. The use of adaptive aids, powered toothbrushes, and oral irrigators gives patients some control over their own care. Discussion of proper nutrition and good oral hygiene also is important. When necessary, the caregiver can offer assistance to the disabled patient.

45. **C** The location of the traumatic injury to the spine is most closely related to the degree of paralysis or dysfunction associated with the spinal cord injury. The type, severity, and cause of injury influence the injury in its location (vertebral level).

46. **C** Sjögren's syndrome is an inflammatory autoimmune disease that results in destruction of the exocrine glands. Parkinson's disease, multiple sclerosis, myasthenia gravis, and Alzheimer's disease are all nervous system disorders.

47. **B** Alzheimer's disease, a form of dementia, often affects individuals in their middle-to-later years. These individuals often are confused by change and prefer quiet surroundings. For this reason, shorter, more frequent appointments are preferable to single, longer appointments. The appointments should be relaxed and involve familiar routines. Oral health care instructions should be repetitious and simple. Although most patients can take care of their oral health needs with just a reminder from a caregiver during the early stages of the disease, during later stages the caregiver will need to take over more of the care.

48. **B** Multiple sclerosis is the disease that affects the myelin sheath and results in fatigue and numbness. Muscular dystrophy is an inherited disease in which muscles atrophy and death may result. Myasthenia gravis and Parkinson's disease are disorders of the nervous system. Bell's palsy is a disease involving facial paralysis and typically is of unknown cause, although any trauma to the facial nerve may result in this paralysis.

49. **B** Alzheimer's disease affects cognition and is not associated with paralysis. Multiple sclerosis, Bell's palsy, and myasthenia gravis are disorders that may result in facial paralysis.

50. **B** The second trimester of pregnancy is the best time to schedule a dental appointment because nausea associated with the first trimester and discomfort-upon-reclining associated with the third trimester are not present.

51. **B** Morning sickness puts a woman at significant risk for malnutrition. Caries can be a result of morning sickness if vomiting is present and frequent. Periodontal disease and constipation are not directly associated with morning sickness.

52. **B** Tetracycline, an antibiotic, is contraindicated during pregnancy. It is associated with brownish-yellow staining of the dentition and should be avoided during pregnancy and early childhood. Flossing and frequent meals (low in simple carbohydrates) are recommended. Alcohol mouth rinses are acceptable for patient use as long as they are not swallowed.

53. **E** Periodontitis is NOT associated with morning sickness, unlike vomiting, enamel erosion, ingestion of high carbohydrate snacks, and nausea.

54. **E** Unnecessary radiographs should be avoided during pregnancy. If radiographs must be taken, a paralleling technique should be used, the patient's front and back should be covered with lead aprons, and the number of radiographs taken should be limited to those that are absolutely necessary. Reclining the chair in a supine position is unnecessary and may be uncomfortable for a pregnant patient.

55. **A** The "loosing a tooth for every child" myth is based on the premise that the calcium needed for the baby's growth is removed from the mother's teeth as needed. Skeletal bones (including the alveolar bones) supply calcium for the baby that is not provided in the diet. Constant vomiting in the first trimester may indeed cause demineralization of tooth enamel and gagging may lead to poor oral hygiene; both may increase the risk of dental caries but the effects can be reduced by daily use of fluoride gels or rinses. Pregnancy tumors are gingival inflammatory lesions associated with raised hormonal levels and inadequate plaque removal. The tumors do not cause displacement or loss of teeth and do regress at pregnancy's end.

56. **A** Failure of a caregiver to provide dental care for a dependent with obvious dental decay is considered dental neglect, a form of physical neglect. Emotional abuse and emotional deprivation are harmful behaviors that affect the emotional needs of a person. Sexual abuse involves nonconsensual sexual acts.

57. **C** Tearing of the maxillary frenum, which is commonly associated with forced feeding, is a type of physical abuse. Bruising along the shins and abrasions of the knees are common injuries in children and are not typically associated with abuse. Fractures of the tibia and other long bones can occur from falls and are not typically a sign of abuse.

58. **D** When physical abuse occurs frequently, bruising in various stages is apparent. Variations in coloration (red, green, yellow, and brown) may indicate numerous abuse incidents, ranging from days to weeks apart. A new bruise is reddish-purple; subsequently it turns green, then yellow, and finally brown, during the course of two weeks.

59. **A** Spina bifida, a defect of neural tube development, often results in paralysis below the point of the defect. Paraplegics, and others with paralysis, often need to be repositioned frequently during a dental appointment. Additional cushioning also helps prevent decubitus (pressure) ulcers. Patients with multiple sclerosis, Down syndrome, or Parkinson's disease typically do not suffer from pressure ulcers unless they are bedridden or confined to a wheelchair for long periods.

60. **C** Wraps are devices used specifically for the full-body restraint of young children. They often are sheets or blankets that are wrapped around the child, from neck to toes. Mouth props and head stabilization secure only the jaws or head. Papoose boards are another method of full-body restraint and can be used to secure patients of any age.

61. **C** When performing a wheelchair transfer, one must clear the area of any obstacles, secure a transfer belt to the patient, and lower the chair at or below the wheelchair height. While facing the patient, stabilize the patient's feet with your feet and legs with your knees, grasp the patient under the arms and around the back, and lift and rotate the patient to the dental chair.

References

1. National Institute on Disability and Rehabilitation Research ISSN: 0732–2623; Vol. XIV, No. 8. Office of Special Education and Rehabilitative Services, Department of Education, Washington, DC, 1993.
2. Vital and Health Statistics, Series 10, No. 193. Current Estimates from the National Health Interview Survey, 1994.
3. Module 1: Rehabilitation of the Dental Patient with a Disability. Seattle, WA, University of Washington School of Dentistry, 1995.
4. Module 5: Anxiety and Pain Control for the Patient with a Disability, Unit A, Behavior Modification. Seattle, WA, University of Washington School of Dentistry, 1986.
5. Module 2: Dental Treatment of the Patient with a Developmental Disability. Seattle, WA, University of Washington School of Dentistry, 1992.
6. Harruff, RC: Pathology Facts. Philadelphia, JB Lippincott, 1994.
7. Shoaf, SC: Coordinating the care of the patient with a cleft lip and palate: Early needs and lifelong challenges. Physician Assistant, June:41–49, 1993.
8. NIDR: Meeting the challenges of craniofacial-oral-dental birth defects. J Am Dent Assoc 127 (May):681–682, 1996.
9. Yetter III, JF: Cleft lip and cleft palate. Am Fam Physician 46(4):1211–1216, 1992.
10. Spencer G: Projections of the Populations of the United States by Age, Sex, and Race 1983–2080. US Bureau of Census. Current Population Report Series P-25, No. 952, May 1984.
11. LaPlante MP: Data on Disability from the National Health Interview Survey 1983–85. Washington, DC, US National Institute on Disability and Rehabilitation Research, 1988.
12. Fowler DG: A Profile of Older Americans. American Association of Retired Persons, Washington, DC, 1988.
13. National Center for Health Statistics: Current Estimates From the National Health Interview Survey: United States, 1981, Series 10, No. 141. Public Health Service Publication No. 82–1569. Hyattsville, MD, 1982.
14. Niessen LC, Gibson G: Aging and oral health: Implications for women. Compendium of Continuing Education in Dentistry 14(12):1542–1554, 1993.
15. National Institute on Aging Publication No. 88–2899. Washington DC, 1988.
16. Center for Dental Information: Monograph 7: Oral Health and Aging, Princeton Dental Resource Center, Princeton NJ, 1992.
17. Hoffman L: Eating Disorders: Decade of the Brain. NIH Publication No. 94–3477, National Institute of Mental Health (NIMH), US Department of Health and Human Services, 1993.
18. Module IV: The Medically Compromised Patient in Dental Practice. Seattle, WA, University of Washington School of Dentistry, 1993.
19. 1996 National Household Survey on Drug Abuse, Substance Abuse, and Mental Health Services Administration. Office of Applied Studies, US Department of Health and Human Services, August, 1997.
20. Cardiac Valvulopathy Associated with Exposure to Fenfluramine or Dexfenfluramine: US Department of Health and Human Services Interim Public Health Recommendations, Report 1061, November 1997. MMWR 46(45).
21. The Physicians' Guide to Helping Patients with Alcohol Problems, NIH Publication No. 95–3769. The National Institute on Alcohol and Alcoholism, US Department of Health and Human Services, Public Health Service, 1995.

22. HIV/AIDS Surveillance Report, Year-End Edition, 9(2). US Department of Health and Human Services, Public Health Services, Centers for Disease Control and Prevention, Atlanta, Ga, June 30, 1997.

23. Centers for Disease Control: Mortality Patterns—United States, 1989. MMWR 41:121–125, 1992.

24. McFadden ER, Gilbert IA: Asthma. N Engl J Med 327:1928–1937, 1992.

25. Barnes PJ: A new approach to the treatment of asthma. N Engl J Med 321:1517–1527, 1989.

26. Jacobs M: The Office Management of Obstructive Lung Disease. Stanford University School of Medicine Primary Care Teaching Module 1–8, 1998.

27. Li JTC, Reed CE: Proper use of aerosol corticosteroids to control asthma. Mayo Clin Proc 64:205–210, 1989.

28. Kaliner M, Lemanske R: Rhinitis and asthma. JAMA 268:2807–2829, 1992.

29. Singer PA, Cooper DS, Levy EG et al: Treatment guidelines for patients with hyperthyroidism and hypothyroidism. JAMA 273:808–812, 1995.

30. Module IX: Dental Management of Patients with CNS and Neurologic Impairment. Seattle, WA, University of Washington School of Dentistry, 1989.

31. Holtzman JM, Bomberg T: A national survey of dentist's: awareness of elder abuse and neglect. Special Care in Dentistry 11(1):7–11, 1991.

32. The Third National Incidence Study of Child Abuse and Neglect (NIS-3). US Department of Health and Human Services, September 1996.

33. Advance Data From Vital and Health Statistics, Assistive Technology Devices and Home Accessibility Features: Prevalence, Payment, Need, and Trends, No. 217. National Center for Health Statistics, US Public Health Service, Hyattsville, Maryland, 1995.

Additional Readings

Darby ML, Walsh MM: Dental Hygiene Theory and Practice, Philadelphia, WB Saunders, 1995.

Wilkins EM: Clinical Practice of the Dental Hygienist, 7th ed. Baltimore, Williams and Wilkins, 1994.

Woodall IR: Comprehensive Dental Hygiene Care, 4th ed. St. Louis, Mosby, 1995.

Hupp JR, Williams TP, Vallerand WP: The 5 Minute Clinical Consult for Dental Professionals. Baltimore, Williams and Wilkins, 1996.

Tamparo CD, Lewis MA: Diseases of the Human Body, Philadelphia, FA Davis, 1995.

Center Against Sexual Abuse: www.syspac.com.

Bites, Bruises and Other Signs of Child Abuse: Guidelines to Determine Symptoms of Abuse; PANDA, Delta Dental Plan of Missouri.

Chapter SIXTEEN

Community Oral Health

Carrie Carter-Hanson, R.D.H, M.A.

 ### Clinical Case STUDY

Mrs. Anderson, a dental hygienist, is conducting a dental needs assessment on 12-year-old children in a small, nonfluoridated community. Most of these children have not had regular dental care for several years. Clinical findings indicate that most of the children have moderate marginal inflammation and plaque. In addition, decay is present on many occlusal surfaces and along the gingival margin in some of the children. Survey results show that a large number of these children frequently consume candy and sugared sodas and that their home care is poor (the average child brushes with a fluoride toothpaste once daily and flosses sporadically).

Clinical Case QUESTIONS

1. Identify two indices that would be most appropriate for assessing the children's oral condition and for use as motivational tools.
2. Should these children receive systemic fluoride? If so, what type and dosage should be recommended?
3. Describe two other dental/oral public health care measures that might be recommended.

Clinical Case RATIONALES

1. The DMFS (decayed, missing, filled surfaces) index would be appropriate for identifying specific caries activity and restorative needs and it has greater sensitivity than the DMFT (decayed, missing, filled teeth) index. In addition, for both the children and their parents, it may be used as a visual tool to identify patterns of caries and areas that need concentration. The O'Leary plaque index would be appropriate for identifying the plaque present and providing the children with an opportunity to see exactly which surfaces have plaque. This index also gives the patient a good visual display of areas that require attention (e.g., plaque

along the margins, which can be removed by brushing, and/or in interproximal areas, which must be removed by flossing).

2. Yes, these 12 year olds should be receiving systemic fluoride. Systemic fluorides are recommended through 16 years of age, since all teeth are not fully developed until then. In a nonfluoridated community, the supplemental dosage for a 12 year old is 1.0 mg per day in tablet form. Tablets are recommended because they provide both topical and systemic effects.
3. Two dental/oral public health measures to recommend for these children are sealants and brush-on fluoride gel. Because most of these children have several areas of occlusal decay, sealants are recommended for the occlusal surfaces that remain caries free. A brush-on fluoride gel is recommended to strengthen the outer layer of enamel and to protect and decrease areas of decalcification along the margins. The use of topical and systemic fluoride in combination with sealant placement will help to decrease smooth surface and pit and fissure caries activity.

Content Review

Terminology

To fully comprehend the components of community dentistry, one must grasp the meanings of specific terms related to and commonly used in the field.[1, 2]

Community dentistry encompasses the dental health of the public and the knowledge and use of dental services by the public; involves identifying and addressing the oral health needs of a particular population or community through assessment, planning, implementation, and evaluation processes.

Health is an ever-changing state that encompasses external and internal physical, spiritual, emotional, and social function. These components overlap and each influences the others in a continuum.

Public health is the concern for the health of a people, group, community, state, or nation. Public health is peoples' health.

Dental public health is the promotion of oral health and prevention of dental disease, including the control of dental disease through organized community efforts; the community is the patient; involves the dental health education of the public, the application of dental research, the administration of group dental care programs, and community efforts to prevent and control dental diseases.

Health education involves providing enough health information to enable individuals to make informed decisions; may or may not initiate behavior changes.

Health promotion facilitates a voluntary adaptation of health seeking behaviors through any combination of learning opportunities; involves behavior changes produced by advice and counseling.

Community oral health is oral health education and promotion aimed at meeting the specific oral health needs of a people, group, community, state, or nation.

Primary prevention includes techniques designed to prevent the onset of disease, reverse the initial stages of disease, or arrest a disease process before treatment is needed.

Secondary prevention includes techniques designed to terminate disease and restore tissues to near normal function.

Tertiary prevention includes techniques designed to replace lost tissues and rehabilitate to near normal function.

Characteristics of the Ideal Public Health Measure

I. Proven to reduce the target disease
II. Medically and dentally safe
III. Easily and efficiently implemented
IV. Easily administered by nondental personnel
V. Attainable by all regardless of socioeconomic status, education, income, race, age, or sex
VI. Available to and accessible by a large number of individuals
VII. Inexpensive; affordable for the majority of individuals
VIII. Easily learned by users
IX. Receives maximum acceptance by the patient
X. Requires minimum compliance by the patient

Characteristics of a Public Health Problem

I. A public health problem is a condition or situation that is widespread or has the potential to cause morbidity or mortality.
II. A public health problem is one that is perceived by the public, government, or public health authority as an existing problem.

Utilization of Dental Services

The demographics of the US population are rapidly changing. The population's growth, age, gender, socioeconomic status, race, and ethnicity each play a vital role in the use of dental services by the public. Ultimately, these changes will impact the practice of dentistry in the future.

Need and Demand

The need for dental services typically exists when a specific oral health disease has been identified in the community. The demand for services is related to the perception of need and the desire to receive treatment.

I. Two Types of Need
    A. A perceived need refers to the public's perception that they have a need for dental care; is a personally perceived need.
    B. A normative need is a professionally perceived need; refers to the quantity of dental treatment required for a community to become orally healthy.
II. Existence of Demand
    A. Occurs when individuals actively seek dental care services in response to a perceived need for care.
    B. Is the expression of a desire to receive dental care because of a perceived need.

Use of Dental Services

The use of dental services is defined as the proportion of the population who receive dental care services within a given period of time.

I. In 1993, 61% of the US population had seen a dentist in the past year.[3]
II. The use of dental services is disproportionate among population groups.

Factors Affecting Use

Dental service use is not evenly distributed across the population and is affected by several factors. Currently, the individual who most regularly uses dental services can be described as a white, college-educated woman with a higher than average income, who lives in a suburban area, has dental insurance, and possesses the characteristics of good general and oral health. Factors that affect the frequency with which an individual seeks dental care are age, gender, economics, ethnicity, geographic location, general health status, and the acquisition of dental insurance. These factors influence and impact each other; their interrelationship makes it difficult to determine the exact influence of each component.

I. Age
    A. Teenagers have the highest utilization rate of dental services, followed by people in early adulthood; in 1993, 74% of teenagers visited the dentist compared with 60% of young adults.[3]
    B. The population is aging, which will lead to a change in the type of restoratives used in dentistry.
    C. The use of dental services tends to decrease with increasing age; however, an increase in use among the elderly population has occurred during the past several years.

1. Among persons 64 years of age or younger, 60% to 67% saw a dentist in the past year, compared with 45% to 56% of those 65 years of age and older.[3]
    2. The decreasing use of dental services that occurs with age is most likely due to the loss of teeth in later years and the elderly individual's perception that dental care is unnecessary.
    3. It has been shown that those who remain dentate as they age continue to seek dental care; their use remains approximately the same as when they were younger.
    D. The use of dental services is lowest during the preschool years; in contrast, the use of medical services is highest during the preschool years.
II. Gender
    A. More females (63%) than males (58%) visited the dentist in the past year.[3]
    B. The more frequent use of dental services among women is consistent across all countries and parallels the trend whereby more women than men seek medical care.
    C. The "like views" of women are believed to affect their health-seeking behaviors.
III. Socioeconomic Status (SES)
    A. Is a measure of an individual's income and education.
        1. Average incomes among the US population and poverty levels by education and race (1996; Table 16–1)
        2. US poverty levels by region (1996)[4]
            a. South: 38% of individuals live at or below poverty level.
            b. West: 25% of individuals live at or below poverty level.
            c. Midwest: 11% of individuals live at or below poverty level.
            d. Northeast: 13% of individuals live at or below poverty level.

TABLE 16.1	Average Income of US Population and Poverty Level by Education and Race		
Race/Ethnicity	Average Income	Education (≤12 years or ≥13 years)	Poverty Level
Asian/Pacific Islander	$43,000	65% ≤12 years 35% ≥13 years	15%
White, nonHispanic	$39,000	67% ≤12 years 33% ≥13 years	9%
Hispanic	$25,000	86% ≤12 years 14% ≥13 years	29%
Black, nonHispanic	$23,000	82% ≤12 years 18% ≥13 years	28%

B. Influences the use of dental services; use increases with an increase in SES.
    1. Among individuals who live above poverty level, 64% visited a dentist in the previous year, compared with 36% of those who live below poverty level.[3]
    2. Among those with 12 years of education, 59% sought dental services in the previous year, compared with 38% of those with less than 12 years of education.[3]
    3. Family income was a better predictor of dental use than race, although Whites were somewhat more likely than Blacks or Hispanics to seek dental services in the previous year at all income levels.[4]
C. Trends are similar to those in other industrialized countries.
D. The relationship between SES and dental service use
    1. Elderly individuals who are well educated and remain dentate continue to seek dental services as they age.
    2. Edentulous individuals tend to be from lower SES backgrounds and therefore use dental services less.
    3. Fewer dentists practice in lower SES areas, which limits access to dental care in such areas; even when care is available, individuals with a low SES typically cannot afford dental care.
    4. Values and attitudes among lower SES populations influence the frequency with which they seek dental care.
    5. Individuals from lower SES backgrounds who use dental services less are models for future generations, who tend to repeat their behavior.
IV. Ethnicity
    A. Percentage of Use of Dental Services
        1. Caucasians (64%) were more likely to seek dental services than Blacks (47%) or Hispanics (46%).[3]
        2. Native-American (Navajo, Lakota), African-American, and Hispanic adults who participated in a WHO study were less likely than Whites to have sought dental services during the previous 12 months.[5]
        3. Race and ethnicity also are related to SES, cultural values, and geographic location, which makes it difficult to differentiate reasons why dental care services are used less among ethnic minorities.[6]
        4. Few dental practitioners are of ethnic minorities (1995-1996 data).[4]
            a. 68% are White (nonHispanic).
            b. 21% are Asian.
            c. 6% are Black (nonHispanic).
            d. 5% are Hispanic.
            e. 1% are American Indian.

B. SES is the most likely reason for decreased use of dental services by Blacks and Hispanics; lack of dental insurance is another common reason.[7]

C. Individuals with higher SES use dental services more frequently than those with lower SES, regardless of race.[4]
   1. 62% of Blacks (nonHispanic) with middle to high income used dental services in the past year, compared with less than 47% of those with lower income.
   2. 59% of Hispanics with middle to high income used dental services in the past year, compared with less than 42% of those with lower income.
   3. 72% of Whites (nonHispanic) with middle to high income used dental services in the past year, compared with less than 48% of those with lower income.

V. Geographic Location[6]
   A. The use of dental services in three geographic areas (1986)
      1. Suburban residents use dental care services most often; slightly more than 61% seek dental care.
      2. Slightly more than 54% of central city (midtown) residents seek dental care.
      3. Only 52% of rural area residents seek dental care.
   B. Variations throughout the United States
      1. The West, Midwest, and Northeast are similar in their use of dental services; slightly more than 60% of these residents seek dental care.
      2. The South uses fewer dental services; slightly more than 50% of residents seek dental care; concomitantly, the southern part of the country is characterized by the lowest SES and the smallest population of dental practitioners compared with other regions.

VI. General Health
   A. Is related to age, education, mobility, and SES.
   B. White and middle-aged adults are more likely to believe in the benefits of preventive practices.[8]
   C. Women, individuals with higher educational levels, and those with better health (self-rated) are more likely to hold positive oral health beliefs.[8]
   D. Conversely, males, individuals with less education, and those who self-report poorer health are least likely to hold positive oral health beliefs.[8]

VII. Insurance
   A. Dental service-seeking behaviors are strongly related to whether or not an individual has dental insurance; individuals with dental insurance are twice as likely to seek preventive dental care.[9]
   B. Most dental services are paid for on an out-of-pocket basis, compared with medical services, which are primarily reimbursed through third-party plans.

C. In 1996, nearly half of the US population (46%) had some form of dental insurance.[10]
   1. Managed dental care (30% of the dental benefits market covers 13% of the US population)
      a. Dental HMOs hold nearly 18% of the dental benefits market.
      b. Dental PPOs hold 12% of the dental benefits market.
   2. Dental referral networks hold nearly 2% of the dental benefits market and cover 1% of the US population.
   3. Dental indemnity holds nearly 69% of the dental benefits market and covers 31.3% of the US population.
D. According to the 1995 Behavioral Risk Factor Surveillance System (BRFSS), a national survey, 69% of individuals in the United States had obtained dental services in the past year; only 44% of individuals had dental insurance at the time.[11]
E. The possession of dental insurance is strongly related to SES. White-collar workers, union employees, and professionals typically are the populations who have dental insurance; BRFSS data indicates that nearly two thirds of those who earn less than $25,000 per year per household are without dental insurance, compared with fewer than one third of those who earn $35,000 per year per household.[11]
F. An individual is less likely to acquire dental care without insurance to help cover the costs.

Financial Considerations

Government expenditures for dental services have been decreasing rapidly during the past several years. This fact combined with the large percentage of out-of-pocket payments by patients and the limited number of individuals with dental insurance paints a grim picture for the financing of dental care services in the United States. However, hope is on the horizon with the advent of more dental insurance coverage and the development of managed care programs.

The Increasing Cost of Care

The costs of both medical and dental care are rising and are related to multiple factors.
I. Rising Cost of Health Care
   A. In 1965, 5.7% of the gross domestic product (GDP) was spent on health care.[4]
   B. In 1996, 13.6% of the GDP was spent on health care.[4]
   C. Reasons for rising costs include:
      1. Substantial rises in the incomes of health care workers during the past several years.
      2. The practice of defensive medicine (procedures used to protect the practitioner from legal suits).
      3. Unbalanced economic scales; to increase the amount of care, manpower must be increased at the same rate, which increases cost.

4. An increase in the elderly population; elderly individuals possess more critical medical problems and use more health care services.

5. New developments in technology; advances in treatment technology require more money for research and implementation strategies.

6. The increased costs of third-party payment plans.

7. The public's increasing expectations regarding the types and amount of services offered (e.g., the demand for transplants, cosmetic services, and esthetic surgery).

II. Rising Cost of Dental Care[12]

A. Health care expenditures in the United States in 1996 were $1,035,080 million, which is more than 13% of the GDP.

B. Of total US health care expenditures in 1996, 4.6% were spent on dental services (nearly $48 million), at an average expense per capita of $173.00.

1. In 1970:

a. Nearly 96% of total expenditures for dental care were paid for by private funds, whether by the patient (93%) or by health insurance (4%); government funding paid for 4% of all dental expenditures (federal and state/local governments each contributed half).

b. In comparison, patients and health insurance paid 63% of total health care expenditures, and federal and state/local governments paid nearly 37% of these total costs.

2. In 1996:

a. Nearly 96% of total expenditures for dental care were paid for by private funds, whether by the patient (49%) or by health insurance (51%); government funding paid 4% of all dental expenditures (federal and state/local governments each contributed half).

b. In comparison, patients and health insurance paid 54% of total health care expenditures, and federal and state/local governments paid 46% of these total costs.

3. In 2005 (projected)

a. Nearly 94% of total expenditures for dental care (an estimated $79 billion) are expected to be paid for by private funds, whether by the patient (53%) or by health insurance (47%); government funding is expected to continue to pay 4% of all dental expenditures (federal and state/local governments each paying approximately half).

b. In comparison, patients and health insurance are expected to continue to pay 54% of total health care expenditures, and federal and state/local governments are expected to pay 46% of these total costs.

C. The government's (federal, state, and local) share of expenses for dental care has continued to be approximately 4%.

D. Out of pocket expenditures by dental care consumers is 49% of total dental care expenditures and is expected to rise during the next decade.

E. The government pays much more for health care than for dental care.

Paying for Dental Care

Dental services are paid for by several means, including fees for service, third party plans, UCR (usual, customary, and reasonable) fees, capitation plans, dental service corporation plans (Delta Dental), indemnity plans, direct reimbursement, managed care plans, and public financing.[1]

I. Fee-for-Service Payment

A. A two-party plan whereby the individual who receives dental services pays the fee directly out of pocket to the provider (dentist).

II. Third-Party Plans

A. Include both not-for-profit and for-profit plans.

B. Involve a contract between the dental office (first party), the patient (second party), and the insurance company (third party).

C. Involve the collection of premiums from the patient by the third party, which in turn pays the dental provider for services rendered.

D. Regard the third party as the insurance company, carrier, insurer, underwriter, or administrative agent.

E. The insurance holder may be the patient's employer, a union group, a government agency, or a welfare fund.

F. In 1991, 50% of Americans (more than 100 million) had dental insurance; most of the coverage was provided through employer groups and not directly by individuals.[1]

G. A 1990 survey found that 92% of 944 US companies surveyed offered some type of dental plan to their employees.[1]

III. UCR Fees

A. Are a method of reimbursement used in a prepayment plan; are usual, customary, and reasonable fees.

B. The usual fee is the fee that is most frequently charged by dentists for a particular dental service.

C. The customary fee is the maximum benefit payable under a particular plan for a specific procedure; is determined by the administrator of the dental insurance benefit plan and is based on submitted fees. This maximum benefit may or may not correlate with the patient's submitted fee.

D. The reasonable fee is the actual fee charged by the dental provider for a particular procedure; is modified according to each patient's specific circumstances; may or may not differ from the dentist's usual fee or the insurance company's customary fee.

IV. Capitation Plans
  A. Are defined by the ADA; a dentist contracts with an insurance program to provide most or all dental services covered by the dental benefit program. The dentist is given payment on a per-capita basis.
  B. Characteristics
    1. Involve fixed, monthly payments to the providing dentist.
    2. Payments are based on the number of patients assigned to the dentist by the benefit program.
    3. Patients are assigned to the dentist to receive care.
    4. Monthly payments are received by the dentist whether or not the patients assigned to him or her require treatment.
    5. The insurance benefit program assumes that some members will require a significant amount of care and that others will not seek care.
  C. By 1990, copayments and yearly maximums were features of these plans.
V. Dental Service Corporations
  A. Originated in 1954 for the International Longshoremen and Warehousemen Union-Pacific Maritime Association, which joined forces with the Seattle District Dental Society to develop and implement a comprehensive dental program for children under 14 years of age.
  B. Include the Delta Dental Plans, which are the most common examples.
    1. Are provided by the Dental Service Corporation
      a. Is a not-for-profit organization that negotiates and provides dental care contracts.
      b. Is incorporated state by state and is sponsored by each state's constituent dental society.
      c. Is governed by the insurance laws of each participating state.
      d. Provides dental treatment for clients in private practice facilities.
      e. Assists dentists in providing group purchase of dental care through traditional practice.
      f. Is available throughout the United States and Puerto Rico.
      g. Quality assurance is provided by a committee of nonparticipating dentists who conduct posttreatment evaluations to ensure acceptable quality.
      h. Payments to dentists are made through the customary fee structure.
VI. Indemnity Plans (commercial)
  A. Are traditional insurance plans that operate by means of a submittal and reimbursement method.

B. Operate for profit.
C. Require no filing of UCR fees by dentists.
D. Are based on an insurance company-generated "fee profile" that reflects the fees most often charged.
VII. Direct Reimbursement
  A. Occurs when an employer agrees to pay for a portion of an employee's dental treatment.
  B. Allows an employee to seek dental care with a dentist of his or her choice.
  C. Involves direct payment of fees to the dentist by the employee/patient.
    1. The employee/patient pays for the dental service and submits the record of treatment to the employer.
    2. The employer reimburses the employee/patient according to the agreed upon reimbursement schedule.
VIII. Managed Care
  A. In 1994, approximately 14 to 17 million Americans participated in some type of managed care plan.[1]
  B. Types of managed care plans:
    1. Health maintenance organization (HMO)
      a. Characteristics
        1) Was developed in 1973 by the HMO Act.
        2) Allowed federal funds to provide an alternative to customary fee-for-service payment.
        3) Was designed primarily to help lower the cost of health care.
        4) Participants prepay a "fixed" premium for health care services.
        5) Currently is operated by both for- and not-for-profit organizations; no longer has federal constraints or dollars.
        6) The number of participants in some managed care programs has risen dramatically.
      b. Advantages
        1) HMOs claim to reduce health care costs for participants by reducing hospitalization and the use of costly services; involve an increased use of ambulatory care.
        2) Provide a range of health care services; offer increased convenience.
      c. Disadvantages
        1) Dental care typically is limited or is only a supplemental service that is subject to a separate fee or premium.
        2) No real difference between an HMO and a prepaid group practice.
        3) Some in the dental community are concerned that HMOs may lead to organized dentistry and may decrease the patient's freedom to choose a particular provider.
    2. Preferred Provider Organizations (PPOs)

a. Characteristics
1) PPOs are defined as contracts between practitioners and their insurers to provide health care services for lower-than-average fees.
2) Practitioners agree to provide services through a PPO primarily because it allows competition for patients.
3) A PPO is a fee-for-service plan.
4) Patients may choose a participating provider to render a covered service; the service subsequently is paid for by the PPO.

IX. Public Financing
A. Federal, state, and tribal government provides health care for groups such as the military, the Coast Guard, American Indians, Native Alaskans, and federal penitentiary inmates.

The Government's Role in Oral Health Care

The philosophy of the United States government gives the responsibility for seeking and receiving oral health care services to each individual. Most health-related programs administered by the federal government are conducted through the Department of Health and Human Services (HHS).

Two Oral Health Care Activities Conducted by HHS

The federal government developed two programs for the express purpose of improving the nation's capacity to provide improved oral health protection and oral health care services.
I. Group I: programs designed to improve the nation's capability to provide improved oral health protection.
A. Biological research.
B. Disease prevention and control.
C. The planning and development of oral health programs.
D. Education and services research.
E. Regulation and compliance functions such as quality assurance and assessment.
II. Group II: programs concerned with the provision of oral health care services. Examples include:
A. Oral health care services rendered to specific groups by the US Public Health Service (PHS).
1. The PHS are commissioned officers of the Dental Corps who provide services to the following:
a. The Indian Health Service (IHS)
b. Prisoners in federal penitentiaries
c. Personnel of the Coast Guard
d. Personnel of the US Merchant Marines
e. Underserved populations
B. The PHS also administers research, prevention, resource planning, and development programs by the National Institute of Health (NIH).
1. The NIH is the largest single source of monetary support for health research and development.

2. The dental component of the NIH is called the National Institute of Dental Research (NIDR).
a. The NIDR is the chief sponsor of oral health research.

Federally Funded Services

Federally funded services include services for maternal and child health, Head Start programs, Medicaid, Medicare, and the National Health Service Corps.
I. Maternal and Child Health Services (MCH)
A. Provides services
1. For women of child-bearing age.
2. For children less than 21 years of age.
3. For individuals with low incomes.
4. Through grants to improve health care for mothers and children.
B. The dental component of MCH provides health care services that include:
1. Maternity and infant care projects.
2. Children and youth projects.
3. Dental health projects for children.
4. Crippled children services.
5. The Women, Infant, and Children (WIC) program.
C. Head Start
1. Developed in 1965 by the Office of Economic Opportunity.
2. Provides educational, health, and social services to low-income preschool children; enables them to enter school on a level equal to that of their peers from higher-income families.
3. Is required to provide dental services to all enrolled children. Such services include:
a. Oral health screening.
b. Oral health education programs.
c. Sealant programs.
II. Medicaid (Title 19 of the Social Security Act)
A. Is a federal program, enacted in 1965, that distributes funds to states for the provision of health care services to the indigent.
B. Dental care is an option, but is not required; dental benefits, if included, typically are limited.
C. The early periodic screening, diagnosis, and treatment program (EPSDT) provides the following:
1. Oral health care services for individuals under the age of 21.
2. Periodic screening for health defects.
3. Any necessary diagnosis and treatment determined by screening.
III. Medicare (Title 18 of the Social Security Act)
A. Covers individuals 65 years of age and older.
B. Covers some disabled individuals.
C. Provides insurance protection against the cost of health care.
D. Consists of two parts
1. Part one
a. Basic plan for hospital and related care.

b. Dental payments for routine dental care are *excluded*.
2. Part two
   a. Is the voluntary supplementary plan for physician services and other health care services.
   b. Dental payments for routine dental care are *excluded*.
E. Dental services are limited to those that are medically necessary, such as oral/maxillofacial needs related to a medical condition.

IV. National Health Service Corps
A. Is a federal health labor deployment program.
B. Deploys commissioned officers and civil service employees of the PHS to render health services in geographic areas that are underserved because of health care shortages.

V. State Health Agencies (agencies or departments headed by a state or territorial office)
A. Provide dental services that typically are limited to the following:
   1. Preventive services for children under 18 years of age.
   2. Restorative and emergency services.
   3. Screening.
B. A very small number of states provide specialty services such as orthodontics, prosthetics, or correction or repair of cleft palate.

 ## *Clinical Case* STUDY

Children of a Native American tribe between the ages of 12 and 14 were assessed for the need for sealants. The children live in a rural, nonfluoridated community. An alphabetized list of names of school-aged children was used to select participants. Of the 980 children on the list, every twentieth child was selected for the study. Among the 49 youth examined, 155 tooth surfaces had restorations, 42 surfaces had decay, and no teeth required extraction.

Clinical Case QUESTIONS

1. What method of sampling was used in this study?
2. Identify the best index to use for assessing the sealant needs of this population.
3. What do the results of the study indicate?
4. Is fluoridation of the school water supply an example of primary, secondary, or tertiary prevention?
5. Identify the best way to promote the sealant project. Should professional fluoride treatments be a part of the project? If so, when should they be given?

Clinical Case RATIONALES

1. A systematic method of sampling was used in this study because every twentieth child was selected from

an alphabetized list. Other methods of sampling include random sampling, in which every element in a population has an equal chance of selection; convenience sampling, which involves a selection made for convenience that may not be representative of the general population; stratified sampling, in which members are randomly selected within subgroups; and single-subject sampling, which involves the study of one or a few subjects who exhibit a special condition.

2. The best index to use for assessing the sealant needs of this population is the DMFS because it assesses the decayed, missing, and filled surfaces of teeth. This index would be helpful in identifying pit and fissure surfaces in need of sealants. DEFT and DEFS are indices that identify decayed, extracted, and filled teeth or surfaces of deciduous teeth; they would not be appropriate for studying decayed pits and fissures in the teeth of elementary school-aged children because sealants are not routinely placed on deciduous teeth.

3. The study results indicate that there is a need for both sealant placement and school water fluoridation because the DMFS is 4.1 (D = 0.9, M = 0, and F = 3.2). Water fluoridation would decrease the number of smooth surface caries, and sealants placed on remaining caries-free surfaces would reduce the number of pit and fissure caries.

4. Fluoridation of the school water supply is an example of primary preventive dentistry. It can prevent the onset of disease (caries), reverse the initial stages of disease (demineralization), and arrest the process before treatment is indicated. Secondary and tertiary prevention, respectively, are associated with restoring tissues to near normal function and with replacing lost tissue and providing rehabilitation.

5. The best way to promote the sealant project is to involve community leaders. Involving community leaders allows the project to take on value and priority. Other methods of promoting the project include informational meetings for parents, teacher-student discussions, radio advertising, and informational flyers. Professional fluoride treatment should be given immediately after sealant placement.

Biostatistics

Biostatistics is the tool by which research data are analyzed and results are defined.

Sampling

Sampling provides a representation of the general population and is used in research to manage the time and cost involved in conducting the research.
I. Random Sampling
   A. Every member in the population has an individual and equal chance of being selected.

B. A table of random numbers may be used to select a sample or participants may be chosen by lottery.

C. Prevents researcher bias.

II. Stratified Sampling

A. Is a modification of random selection.

B. Divides the population into subgroups before selection to ensure that all subgroups are sampled.

C. Typically involves random selection within each subgroup (stratified random sampling).

D. Prevents bias because it eliminates the possibility that members of a subgroup will not be selected.

III. Convenience Sampling

A. Is the simplest method.

B. Involves selecting a convenient group (e.g., classroom, church, club members).

C. May encourage bias because of the sampling of a select group; results may not be applicable to the general population.

IV. Systematic Sampling

A. Is similar to, but is not truly, random sampling because all members of a population do not have the same chance of being selected.

B. Typically begins by determining that every nth member on a list will be selected; a starting number is drawn and every nth member that follows the starting number is selected; another method involves systematically choosing every even-numbered individual and excluding all odd-numbered individuals.

Descriptive Statistics

Statistics are used to make inferences about a population. Descriptive statistics involve frequency distribution, graphs, central tendency, and variability.[1]

I. Frequency Distribution

A. Is a group of scores arranged from lowest to highest that contains the frequency with which each score occurs; scores can be grouped, ungrouped, or cumulative.

1. Relative frequency is expressed as the frequency with which a specific score is earned (e.g., 15 students scored an 80 on an exam); can be expressed as a percentage.

2. Relative percent can be expressed as the percentage of students who receive a particular score (e.g., three students scored 77, or 9.1% of the 33 students who took the exam).

3. Cumulative frequency is expressed as the frequency of occurrence of scores, up to and including any value in the data set; is most useful for data grouped by class intervals (e.g., 88 students scored in the range of 75% to 79% or below).

4. Cumulative percent is expressed as the percent frequency of occurrence of scores, up to and including any value in a data set. (e.g., 96% of students scored 90 or below on the exam).

B. Is most commonly expressed as a normal (bell) curve.

1. Exhibits a symmetric grouping of scores around the mean or center of the curve.

2. Assumptions are made regarding the focal center of the curve.

3. Has a total area of 1 (100%); its mean, median, and mode are equal and are located in the center of the distribution.

a. The total area is divided into segments called standard deviations.

b. The area between the mean and one standard deviation to the right is 34.13%, and to the left is 34.13% (the total is approximately 68.26% of the total distribution).

c. The area between the first and second standard deviations on the right is 13.59%, and on the left is 13.59% (the total is approximately 27.18% of the total distribution).

d. The area between the second and third standard deviations on the right is 2.15%, and on the left is 2.15% (the total is approximately 4.30% of the total distribution).

II. Graphs are used to visually represent the distribution of scores along the y and x axes.

A. The Y axis typically represents the frequency of scores and typically is vertical.

B. The X axis typically represents the scale that measures a specific variable.

C. Types

1. The bar graph, which is a two-dimensional representation of discrete data.

2. The histograph, which is a representation formed directly from a frequency distribution.

III. Central Tendency[1]

A. Is a measure of the average score; is a summary or typical score of a distribution.

B. The mean is the arithmetic value that is computed by dividing the total by its members (e.g., 450 students/3 schools = 150; the mean is 150 students per school); can be influenced by extreme scores.

C. The median is the point that divides a score distribution into two equal parts, with 50% of the scores falling below and 50% of the scores falling above that point (e.g., 22, 56, 57, 78, 79, 80, 83, 84, 85, 90, 100; the median is 80 because 5 scores fall below it and 5 fall above it); is least influenced by extreme scores.

D. The mode is the value that occurs with the most frequency in a distribution (e.g., 1, 1, 3, 3, 3, 3, 3, 4, 5, 6, 7, 7, 7, 7, 8, 9; the mode is 3); more than one mode can occur; is useful for quick computation.

IV. Variability is useful for describing the spread, range, or distribution of scores.[1]

A. The range is the difference or distance between the highest and the lowest scores (e.g., the range is 4 when scores range from 8 to 12); is not stable with extreme scores because it only uses the highest and lowest scores.

B. The variance is a measure of the average spread of scores around the mean; the greater the dispersion around the mean, the greater the variance; is more useful than the range because it considers all scores.

C. The standard deviation is the positive square root of the variance; the greater the dispersion around the mean, the greater the standard deviation; is the most useful measure of variability in descriptive statistics; considers all scores in a distribution.

Inferential Statistics

Inferential statistics are used to make generalizations from the statistical sample to the general population. Good sampling techniques make the inferences more accurate.

I. The student's t-test is a procedure that is used to make comparisons between the means of two different studies; it determines the probability that the differences in the two means are real and are not caused by chance.

II. ANOVA is used in place of the t-test whenever more than two means must be compared.

III. The chi-square test compares the observed measurement of a given characteristic with the expected measurement for a sample. The chi-square statistic is a measure of the difference between the observed and expected measurements; is useful when studying categorical information.

IV. Correlation analysis involves the study of two variables and their effects on each other; is most useful when the number of pairs of variables is large (>30). The correlation coefficient is the number that summarizes the strength of the relationship between two variables; is denoted as $r = +1$ or -1; the closer the correlation coefficient is to 1, the stronger the relationship between two variables.

Epidemiology

Epidemiology is defined as the study of disease prevalence. It is conducted through systematic observation and is used in medicine, social and computer science, biology, and statistics. Epidemiologic methods can be applied in dentistry to evaluate the specific disease patterns and needs of a community. Comparisons can be made between groups of defined populations. To possess a firm grasp of epidemiologic concepts, one must be familiar with the various types of epidemiology and the common terms used in the field.

Types of Epidemiology

Epidemiology may be descriptive, analytic, or experimental.

I. Descriptive Epidemiology
   A. Is used to quantify and conceptualize the disease state of a particular community.

B. Evaluates disease status by examining the incidence and prevalence of disease in a given population.

C. An example is the record of the DMFT of children who are 10, 11, and 12 years of age in the Kansas City school district.

II. Analytic Epidemiology
   A. Is used to determine the etiology of diseases.
   B. Determines causal relationships between factors associated with a disease.
   C. An example is the study of the relationship between sugar consumption and decay.

III. Experimental Epidemiology
   A. Is used to determine the effectiveness of an oral health program or the therapeutic intervention of a disease.
   B. An example is the effectiveness of water fluoridation on the rate of caries in a population.

Terms

Incidence, prevalence, rate, morbidity, mortality, endemic, epidemic, and pandemic are common epidemiologic terms.

I. Incidence
   A. Is the rate at which a disease occurs.
   B. Is expressed as the number of *new* cases during a specific time.
      1. Incidence rate = The number of cases divided by individuals and time.

$$I_r = \frac{Cases}{Individual \text{ and } time}$$

   2. Example: 50 individuals in a community of 250,000 died of oral cancer during 1997.

$$I_r = \frac{50 \text{ deaths}}{250,000 \text{ individuals per year}}$$

II. Prevalence
   A. Is the total number of cases of disease in existence in a given population at a given time.
   B. Prevalence = The number of cases divided by population multiplied by 100.

$$P = \frac{Cases}{Population} \times 100$$

   C. Example: In 1996 there were 300 reported cases of ANUG among 1000 20-year-old college students examined.

$$\frac{300 \text{ ANUG cases}}{1000 \text{ students}} \times 100\% = 30\% \text{ prevalence of ANUG}$$

III. Rate
    A. Is expressed as a ratio (fraction).
    B. The numerator is the number of actual occurrences of a disease.
    C. The denominator is the number of possible occurrences of a disease.
    D. Rate = Actual occurrences divided by possible occurrences.

$$\text{Rate} = \frac{\text{Actual occurrences}}{\text{Possible occurrences}}$$

    E. Example: In 1997 there were 25 cases of gingivitis among 250 teenagers examined.

$$\frac{25 \text{ actual}}{250 \text{ possible}} = 10\% \text{ rate of gingivitis}$$

IV. Morbidity
    A. Refers to disease; can be expressed as a rate.
    B. The morbidity rate is the number of actual diseases divided by the number of possible diseases.
V. Mortality
    A. Refers to death; can be expressed as a rate.
    B. The mortality rate is the number of actual deaths divided by the number of possible deaths.
VI. Epidemic
    A. Is a significantly greater-than-normal incidence of a disease.
    B. Describes a disease that spreads rapidly through a particular segment of the population.
    C. Describes a disease that involves more cases than expected.
VII. Endemic
    A. Refers to a disease with an expected (typical) number of cases that continues over time.
    B. May be specific to a particular geographic area or population.
VIII. Pandemic
    A. Refers to a disease that occurs throughout the population of a country or people or the world.

Indices

An index is a systematic way of collecting and arranging data gathered from observations so that they can be quantified, analyzed, and understood. It is accomplished under specifically defined criteria and conditions. An example would be a record of data collected from periodontal probing.
I. Characteristics of a Good Index
    A. Reliable
    B. Reproducible
    C. Valid
    D. Easily understood and explained

Epidemiology of Caries

In 1996, the third National Health and Nutrition Examination Survey (NHANES III) reported dental caries in the permanent dentitions of adults in the United States. Surveys of adults 18 years of age and older were conducted between 1988 and 1991.[12, 13]
I. Statistics
    A. Coronal caries are present in 94% of dentate adults in the United States.
    B. Root caries are present in 22.5% of dentate adults in the United States; this percentage increases with age.
    C. Approximately 40.5% of the adult US population has at least one tooth surface that would benefit from dental treatment.
II. Trends
    A. Caries levels have been declining for more than 20 years in all age groups among insured Americans.[15]
    B. Untreated dental decay is increasing among young children.[16]
III. Specific Caries Indices
    A. DMF indices
        1. Provide a broad picture of caries activity in a specific population.
        2. Various components may be used to evaluate specific information that is needed.
        3. For example:
            a. DMFT = decayed, missing, filled *teeth*
            b. DMFS = decayed, missing, filled *surfaces*
        4. Deciduous teeth
            a. DEFT = decayed, extracted, filled *teeth*
            b. DEFS = decayed, extracted, filled *surfaces*
        5. Data collected from these indices can be used to determine community needs.
    B. Unmet treatment needs (UTN) index of a particular population
        1. UTN = mean number of decayed teeth divided by mean number of decayed and filled teeth multiplied by 100.

$$\text{UTN} = \frac{\text{mean number of decayed teeth}}{\text{mean number of decayed and filled teeth}} \times 100$$

        2. The UTN index also can be used to compare the treatment needs of one population with those of another (e.g., the UTN of a community with fluoridated water may be compared with the UTN of a community that does not have water fluoridation).
    C. RCI (root caries) index
        1. Evaluates the extent of root caries and a patient's risk for root caries disease.
        2. Includes only those root surfaces exposed to the oral environment by gingival recession.

$$RCI = \frac{(R{-}D) + (R{-}F)}{(R{-}D) + (R{-}F) + (R{-}N)}$$

Where

R = root surface

D = decayed root surface

F = filled root surface

N = intact, sound root surface

Epidemiology of Gingivitis and Periodontitis

Interpreting the results of epidemiologic studies of gingivitis, and particularly those of periodontitis, is extremely difficult. The prevalence of the disease must be measured in terms of the specific definition of each disease and the age group affected. For example, although periodontitis may be defined in one study as an attachment loss of 2 mm, it subsequently may be defined in another study as an attachment loss of 4 mm. Therefore describing the prevalence of periodontal disease in statistical terms can be difficult and misleading. The definition of disease must be determined before statistics are interpreted.

I. Statistics
   A. Gingivitis
      1. Often begins during early childhood, increases in severity during adolescence, and tapers off thereafter.
      2. National surveys report a prevalence of between 40% and 60% among US school children.[17]
      3. A recent study determined that more than 50% of adults have gingivitis that affects an average of 3 or 4 teeth.[18]
   B. Periodontitis
      1. Has decreased in severity during the past 25 years, with little change in prevalence.
      2. Pocketing of 4 mm or more in 3 or 4 teeth is exhibited by 30% of the US population; severe pocketing (6 mm or more) occurs in less than 5% of the population.[18]
      3. 40% of US adults have loss of attachment of 3 mm or more.[18]
      4. Early-onset periodontitis affects 1% of individuals between the ages of 14 and 17, and 3.6% of individuals between the ages of 18 and 34.[18]
      5. Severe and extensive periodontitis is more likely to be associated with lower SES, minority status, lower educational levels, infrequent dental care, subgingival calculus, smoking, and uncontrolled diabetes.[18, 19]
      6. Risk factors can be defined as unmodifiable or modifiable.[20, 21]
         a. Unmodifiable risk factors
            1) Age
            2) Race
            3) Gender
            4) Genetic disorders
            5) Genetics
         b. Modifiable risk factors
            1) Tobacco
            2) Systemic disease
            3) Cardiovascular disease
            4) Medications
            5) Socioeconomic status
            6) Nutrition

II. Specific Plaque Indices
   A. O'Leary plaque index
      1. Monitors oral hygiene performance.
      2. Indicates the location of plaque.
      3. Assists in the visualization of a patient's home care progress.
      4. Assists clinicians in emphasizing specific areas of need and tailoring home care with alternative plaque control aides.
      5. Does not quantify plaque.
      6. Directions for use
         a. Cross out all missing teeth.
         b. Divide the teeth into four parts (facial, lingual, distal, mesial) and the mouth into four quadrants.
         c. Apply disclosing solution and have patient rinse.
         d. Evaluate the presence of plaque using air, a mouth mirror, and an explorer.

$$\frac{\text{Number of plaque surfaces present}}{\text{Total number of tooth surfaces examined}} \times 100 = \% \text{ plaque}$$

   B. Oral hygiene index—simplified (OHI-S)
      1. Was developed in 1960 by Greene and Vermillion; was modified 4 years later.
         a. The two components, debris index (plaque, materia alba, and food) and the calculus index, are added together to obtain a single score.
         b. Is useful for large populations.
         c. Only facial and lingual surfaces are scored; includes facial surfaces of teeth #3, 8, 14, and 24, and lingual surfaces of teeth #19 and 30.
         d. Scoring criteria
            1) 0 = No debris or stain present.
            2) 1 = Soft debris covering not more than one third of tooth surface.
            3) 2 = Soft debris covering more than one third but not more than two thirds of tooth surface.
            4) 3 = Soft debris covering more than two thirds of tooth surface.
         e. The debris and calculus scores are combined and the total is divided by the number of surfaces examined to obtain the average OHI-S.
   C. Personal hygiene performance index-modified (PHP-M)
      1. Was developed by Podshadley and Haley and subsequently modified by Martens and Meskin.

2. Is used primarily to provide patients with information about their plaque that will assist in the improvement of their oral health.
3. The teeth that are selected during the initial visit are used for comparison during subsequent visits.
4. Criteria for use
   a. Select six teeth, divide each of them into five areas, and label areas a, b, c, d, and e on both facial and lingual surfaces.
   b. Record the presence of plaque in each of the lettered areas and give one point for each area of plaque.
   c. Scores range from 0 to 60 (best to worst).

D. Plaque index (PI)
1. Was developed in 1967 by Silness and Loe.
2. Assesses the thickness of plaque on teeth at the gingival margin.
3. Often is used in conjunction with the gingival index (GI) by the same authors.
4. Specific teeth or the entire dentition can be assessed using the distal, mesial, facial, and lingual surfaces of the teeth.
5. Scoring criteria:
   a. Visually examine plaque or use a probe to swipe along the cervical third of the teeth; a disclosing agent can be used.
   b. Score:
      1) 0 = no plaque adheres or is visible at gingival third.
      2) 1 = plaque adheres at gingival third; is visible with an explorer.
      3) 2 = moderate amounts of plaque are visible in the sulcus or at the gingival margin.
      4) 3 = heavy amounts of plaque are visible in the sulcus or at the gingival margin.
6. Criteria for use:
   a. For individual teeth, total the score for each of the four surfaces (mesial, distal, facial, lingual) of the tooth and divide by four.
   b. For groups of teeth, total the individual scores for all teeth in the group and divide by the number of teeth in the group; is used for comparing areas of the mouth.
   c. For individual dentition, total the individual scores for all teeth in the dentition and divide by the number of teeth in the dentition.
   d. For groups of individuals, total the individual dentition scores and divide by the number of members in the group.

E. Gingival index (GI; Loe and Silness)
1. Is the index most frequently used to evaluate gingivitis; bleeding is the most critical factor.
2. Assesses bleeding, color, contour, and ulceration of tissue.

3. Criteria for use
   a. Use on all or six selected teeth.
   b. Divide the teeth into four areas (facial, lingual, distal, and mesial).
   c. Total the scores from these four areas and divide by the number of surfaces examined.
   d. Scoring
      1) 0 = Normal gingiva
      2) 1 = Mild inflammation, slight change in color, slight edema, and no bleeding on probing
      3) 2 = Moderate inflammation, redness, edema, glazing, and bleeding on probing
      4) 3 = Severe inflammation, marked redness, edema, ulceration, and a tendency toward spontaneous bleeding

F. Gingival bleeding index (Ainamo and Bay)
1. Assesses bleeding of the gingival margin in response to gentle probing.
2. Is used as an indicator of gingival health or disease.
3. Criteria for use
   a. Divide the total number of areas that bleed by the number of gingival margins examined; subsequently multiply the result by 100 to arrive at a score (percentage).
4. Scoring
   a. Of gently probed areas
      1) + = bleeding within 10 seconds after gentle probing
      2) − = the absence of bleeding after 10 seconds after probing
   b. A positive score indicates the percentage of all gingival areas explored that bleed in response to probing.

G. Russell's periodontal index (PI)
1. Assesses the progressive stages of periodontal disease and the amount of attachment loss present on each tooth.
2. Is relatively easy to use and understand; results are comparative.
3. Is primarily used for major population groups.
4. Criteria for use
   a. Attachment loss is defined as the sum of the clinical probe depth and gingival recession; recession is measured from the cemento-enamel junction (CEJ) to the gingival margin.
   b. Tissues are examined for gingival inflammation, pocket formation (with a noncalibrated probe), and masticatory function and given a score.
5. Scoring
   a. Criteria
      1) 0 = *Negative:* No overt inflammation in investing tissues or loss of function from destruction of supporting tissues.

2) 1 = *Mild gingivitis:* An overt area of inflammation is present in free gingiva but the area does not circumscribe the tooth.

3) 2 = *Gingivitis:* Inflammation completely circumscribes tooth; no apparent break in epithelial attachment.

4) 6 = *Gingivitis with pocket formation:* Epithelial attachment has been breached and pocketing exists; no interference with normal masticatory function; tooth is firm in its socket, no drifting is discernible.

5) 8 = *Advanced destruction with loss of masticatory function:* Tooth may be loose, drifting, or dull on percussion, or may be depressed in its socket.

b. Findings

1) For individuals:

$$PI = \frac{\text{Sum of individual scores}}{\text{Number of teeth scored}}$$

2) For groups:

$$\text{Group PI} = \frac{\text{Total of individual scores}}{\text{Number of individuals examined}}$$

c. Clinical conditions and group PI score ranges

1) Indicates clinically normal tissues (0.0 to 0.2).

2) Indicates simple gingivitis (0.3 to 0.9).

3) Indicates incipient destructive periodontal disease (0.7 to 1.9).

4) Indicates established destructive periodontal disease (1.6 to 5.0).

5) Indicates terminal stages of periodontal disease (3.8 to 8.0).

H. Ramfjord's periodontal disease index (PDI)

1. Evaluates gingival health, probing depths, and plaque and calculus deposits.

2. Is used for the Ramfjord teeth (#3, 9, 12, 19, 25, and 28); these teeth often are used in clinical studies as a representative sample of the entire dentition.

3. The gingiva is given a score between 0 and 3, depending on the severity of inflammation.

4. Pockets are probed on the mesial and facial surfaces and are given a score between 4 and 6.

5. The critical measurement is the distance from the CEJ to the base of the sulcus.

6. Scoring

a. 0 = Absence of inflammatory signs

b. 1 = Mild-to-moderate inflammatory gingival change that does not extend around the tooth

c. 2 = Mild-to-moderately severe gingivitis that extends around the tooth

d. 3 = Severe gingivitis characterized by marked redness, swelling, and the tendency to bleed and ulcerate

e. 4 = Gingival crevice extends apically past the CEJ but not more than 3 mm

f. 5 = Gingival crevice extends apically 3 to 6 mm past the CEJ

g. 6 = Gingival crevice extends apically more than 6 mm from the CEJ

7. Combined gingival and pocket scores reflect an individual's periodontal status.

I. Community periodontal index of treatment needs (CPITN)

1. Was developed by the Fédération Dentaire Internationale and the World Health Organization to assess the treatment needs of specific groups.

2. Evaluates pockets, bleeding, and plaque retention factors.

3. Evaluates six sextants; one score from each sextant is used.

4. Excludes third molars unless they function as second molars.

5. Probing is performed with the CPITN-E probe.

6. First and second molars in posterior sextants are examined and only the worst of the two scores is recorded; one maxillary tooth and one mandibular anterior tooth also are scored for a total of six scores.

7. Scoring uses a five-point Likert scale (0 = no signs of periodontal disease and 4 = periodontal pockets of 6 mm or more).

8. Scores are converted to a four-point treatment needs (TN) classification.

a. TN 0 = No treatment is needed

b. TN 1 = Requires improved oral hygiene

c. TN 2 = Requires improved oral hygiene and scaling

d. TN 3 = Requires improved oral hygiene, scaling, and complex treatment

Prevention and Control of Dental Disease

Previously, dentistry was a purely reparative craft. However, with the advent of advanced technology, a greater understanding of oral disease, and well controlled scientific research, dentistry has made the leap to become a scientifically oriented profession. Fluorides, sealants, diet counseling, specific periodontal care, and an array of oral health care aides have made it possible for the dental professional, the community, and individuals to work together to identify and meet the oral health needs of the entire community. Caries and periodontal disease continue to be the two most significant oral health problems. Many risk factors recently have been identified and associated with these diseases. Factors such as tobacco use, oral cancer, and xerostomia are gaining greater attention. Providers currently are incorporating these factors into treatment planning efforts.

Prevention and Control of Caries

Caries can be controlled though the use of fluorides, pit and fissure sealants, and diet counseling.

I. Fluoride
   A. A primary preventive oral care service to reduce or prevent dental caries; can be given either systemically or topically.
   B. Community water fluoridation
      1. Is defined as the addition of fluoride compounds to the community water supply; the amount is maintained at an optimum level to decrease caries without causing dental fluorosis.
      2. The amount added to the water supply is dependent on the average temperature or climate of the particular community. Individuals in hotter climates are likely to drink more water and thus receive more fluoride.
         a. Optimally ranges from 0.7 parts per million (ppm) in hotter climates (115°F) to 1.2 ppm in cooler climates (53°F).
      3. 1 ppm = 1 mg fluoride/liter; is the standard concentration.
      4. Fluoride has been shown to be beneficial for older adults as well as for teens and young children.
      5. Meets all the characteristics of an ideal public health measure.
      6. In 1993, 232.4 million individuals in the United States were served by public water systems; 62.2% of those were served by fluoridated drinking systems.[3]
      7. In 1995, fluoridated water systems provided fluoridation to 42% of American Indian and Native Alaskan populations.[22]
      8. Has resulted in caries reduction in children,[1] including:
         a. A 15% to 35% reduction in permanent teeth.
         b. A 30% to 60% reduction in deciduous teeth.
         c. A 20% to 40% reduction in mixed dentitions.
      9. Has resulted in caries reduction in adults, including:
         a. A 20% to 30% reduction in coronal and root caries.
      10. Is very cost-effective; costs range from $0.12 to $1.16 per individual per year.
   C. School water fluoridation
      1. Is used primarily in rural areas, where elementary, junior high school, and high school students attend school together or in adjacent buildings with the same water supply; is an excellent vehicle for reaching a large group at one time.
      2. Is provided at a greater than optimum concentration because students have access to the water supply only on school days; 4.5 times the optimum level of fluoride is added to a school's water supply when the community water is not fluoridated.
      3. Caries reduction ranges from 22% to 48%.
   D. Fluoride supplements
      1. Are used when water fluoridation is not possible or is not implemented.
      2. Are available in various forms, including tablets, drops, lozenges, rinses, and vitamins.
      3. Are administered at home or through a school-sponsored program.
      4. Have topical and systemic effects.
      5. Cannot be added to milk; milk binds with fluoride and decreases its effectiveness.
      6. Dosages recommended by the American Academy of Pediatrics (revised in 1994) are dependent on the amount of fluoride in the community water supply (Table 16–2).
         a. For a child who is 3 years old, an oral care provider would recommend the dosage schedule for children between the ages of 3 and 6; a child who is 6 years old should receive the dosage recommended by the schedule for children between the ages of 6 and 16.
      7. Reduce caries by 25% to 65%.
      8. Provide the greatest caries reduction when started in infancy and taken consistently through age 16.
      9. School supplements can be prescribed by a local dentist; are easily administered by non-dental personnel, typically the school nurse. Schools are an excellent place for fluoride and oral health programs because a large population can be reached at one time.

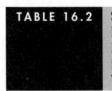

TABLE 16.2	Supplemental Fluoride Dosage Schedule by Parts Per Million (ppm) in the Community Water Supply		
Age	**Less than 0.3 ppm (mg)**	**Between 0.3 and 0.6 ppm (mg)**	**More than 0.6 ppm (mg)**
6 months-3 years	0.25	0	0
3–6 years	0.50	0.25	0
6–16 years	1.0	0.50	0

10. Home supplements are slightly more effective when started at 6 months of age and continued through the teen years; however, compliance typically is poor.

E. Fluoride mouth rinses

   1. Rinsing (swishing) with dilute formulations of sodium (NaF), stannous (SnF_2), or acidulated phosphate (APF) fluoride daily or weekly.

   2. Rinsing with a 10-mL solution for 1 minute provides a topical effect.

   3. Can be used at home or in a school-sponsored program.

   4. Percentages and caries reduction (Table 16–3)[1]

   5. School programs

     a. Can be administered by nondental personnel and/or volunteers.

     b. Range in cost from $0.52 to $1.78 per child per year; the average cost is $1.00 per child per year.[1]

     c. Cost is dependent on the type of supervision employed and whether or not school volunteers are used.

F. Topical fluorides are used in the form of rinses, gels, and prophylaxis pastes. Some are available only from an oral health care professional and are applied in the office; others are designed for application by the individual at home.

   1. Professionally applied forms

     a. Solutions

       1) Include 1.2% NaF, 8% SnF_2, and 1.23% APF.

       2) All provide a similar reduction in caries (approximately 30%).

     b. Gels and foams

       1) Have become more popular in recent years and have replaced solutions used in offices.

       2) Provide a reduction in caries that is comparable to that of solutions.

       3) Require 4-minute application for full benefit; some companies recommend 1-minute application because the majority of uptake occurs during the first minute.

     c. Prophylaxis pastes

       1) Most contain fluoride.

       2) Are beneficial in replenishing fluoride removed during polishing; if used alone during preventive appointments, are not sufficient to protect teeth.

   2. Individually applied forms

     a. Mouth rinses

       1) Are recommended for patients with an increased rate of caries and for orthodontic patients with banded, bonded, or removable appliances.

       2) Are used in both optimally fluoridated and fluoride-deficient communities.

       3) Products

         a) ACT and Fluorigard (0.05% NaF)

         b) Stancare (0.1% SnF_2)

       4) Involve swishing with a 5- or 10-mL solution for 1 minute once daily.

       5) Provide a reduction in caries of approximately 25% to 30% when used in combination with a fluoride dentifrice.

       6) Are not recommended for children under 6 years of age because they are unable to swish for 1 minute and may swallow the solution.

     b. Fluoride gels

       1) Include 0.1% SnF_2, applied with a toothbrush.

       2) Include 0.5% NaF, applied either with a toothbrush or in a custom polyvinyl mouth tray.

       3) Are recommended for use once daily; are applied for 1 minute with a toothbrush or for 5 minutes with a tray.

       4) Have the same indications as mouth rinses.

       5) Are not recommended for children under 6 years of age.

     c. Fluoride varnishes[1]

       1) Are used heavily in European countries, where their effects are examined in many clinical studies.

       2) Originally were designed to increase the fluoride uptake by enamel.

       3) Have a wide range of effectiveness (7% to 74%).

     d. Fluoride toothpastes (see Chapters 11 and 12).

II. Sealants

A. Are plastic dental resins that are professionally applied to pits and fissures on surfaces of teeth to isolate them from the caries-producing oral environment; pit and fissure enamel surfaces are protected least by fluorides.

TABLE 16.3 Percentages and Caries Reduction of Topical Fluorides[1]		
Fluoride Type	Concentration (%) and Time	Caries Reduction (%)
NaF	2/weekly	25–28
NaF	0.05/daily	20–35
APF	1.23/daily	20–30
SnF_2	0.1/daily	20–30

B. Sealants are placed in liquid form, enter the micropores, and subsequently are hardened (cured) by either ultraviolet (UV) light or chemical activation.

C. Sealant types
   1. UV-light-cured forms are first generation sealants.
      a. Are cured by exposure to UV light for a specific amount of time.
   2. Chemically cured forms are second generation sealants.
      a. Are cured by the mixture of the polymer and catalyst; require a specific amount of time before the sealant hardens; undergo a process called autopolymerization.
   3. Visible-light-cured forms are third generation sealants.
      a. Are cured by exposure to visible light for a specific amount of time.
      b. A visible light source is considerably smaller and easier to manipulate than UV light; also is less expensive.

D. Indications for sealants
   1. Unrestored pits and fissures
   2. Highest to lowest surfaces at risk for caries
      a. First and second permanent molars
      b. First and second primary molars
      c. First and second premolars
      d. Third molars
   3. Other pit and fissure sites that can benefit from sealants include:
      a. Lingual pits of permanent maxillary incisors.
      b. Buccal pits of mandibular molars.
      c. Lingual pits of maxillary molars.
   4. The selection of teeth for sealant placement should be based on:
      a. The tooth morphology of occlusal surfaces (e.g., deep incline pits and fissures are at greater caries risk than shallow cusps).
      b. The caries activity of the patient (those with previous caries history are in greatest need, except for those with rampant caries).
      c. Questionable surfaces
         1) The explorer "sticks" in the surface but other defining evidence is not present.
         2) Incipient caries
         3) Questionable surfaces are ideal for sealant placement because sealants can halt the progression of caries.
   5. Placement process
      a. Cleanse the tooth surface with an oil-free, nonfluoride agent.
      b. Isolate teeth with cotton rolls and salivary gland barriers.
      c. Dry the tooth surface for 30 seconds.
      d. Apply tooth conditioner (phosphoric acid etch) for 60 seconds.
      e. Rinse the tooth surface for 30 seconds.
      f. Dry the tooth surface for 30 seconds.
      g. Inspect the surface for a "chalky" white, frosted, etched appearance; re-etch for 10 seconds if necessary.
      h. Apply the sealant material without overflow.
      i. Cure the sealant with a light source or wait the appropriate amount of time (suggested by the manufacturer) for self-curing sealants.
      j. Maintain a dry field until the sealant is completely cured and examined.
      k. Examine the sealant for retention, adequate coverage, a lack of voids and bubbles, and a clear contact area.
   6. Cost effectiveness
      a. Research regarding the cost-effectiveness of sealants
         1) A 1995 survey by the ADA found that the average cost of a sealant was less than half the cost ($24.00) of a one-surface restoration ($54.00).[23]
         2) In a study of 600 children, Ismail and Gagnon determined that 74% of teeth remained fully sealed 2 years after sealant application; moreover, the fully sealed teeth were 75% more likely to remain restoration-free than were sound, unsealed molars.[24]
         3) Weintraub and colleagues conducted a comprehensive study on the retention and effectiveness of sealants and found the following[24]:
            a) Children and young adults have a high rate of pit and fissure caries (80% to 90%) and a low rate of interproximal caries (10% to 20%).
            b) Benefits of sealant programs decrease with the increasing age of the participants.
            c) The effectiveness and retention of sealants decrease after the first application.
            d) No difference in the benefits of sealants exists between fluoridated and nonfluoridated communities.
            e) Reapplication is required to ensure the preventive effect of the sealant over time.
            f) Retained sealants prevent decay; lost sealants should be replaced.
      b. Sealants used in combination with fluoride can markedly decrease caries; they enhance each other because fluoride decreases smooth surface caries and sealants decrease pit and fissure caries.
         1) The Healthy Individuals 2000 mid-

decade assessment found that the numbers of children's teeth being sealed are increasing.[16]

    2) The NHNES study found that among children, 83% of caries were in pits and fissures, yet few children had sealants placed in permanent teeth.[23] Among children between the ages of 8 and 14:

        a) 27% to 36% of Caucasians had at least one sealant.

        b) 5% to 9% of Blacks had at least one sealant.

        c) 10% to 11% of Hispanics had at least one sealant.

    3) Caries affects half of young children (early elementary age) and two thirds of 15 year olds.[23]

    4) Poor children have no more caries than other children but are less likely to have caries filled.[23]

III. Diet Counseling

  A. Is an avenue for helping to control dental caries in patients with high sugar consumption, high rates of caries, or salivary flow problems.

  B. Is recommended for:

    1. All school children.

    2. Children, adolescents, and adults with high rates of caries.

    3. Medically compromised patients.

    4. Patients with decreased salivary flow or salivary gland dysfunction.

  C. Characteristics of diet counseling

    1. Assesses a patient's cariogenic food intake by means of a diet diary.

    2. Identifies cariogenic foods and makes recommendations for alternative food choices without significantly changing the patient's diet.

    3. Allows the patient and/or guardian to play a role in alternative food selections; also allows consideration of a patient's likes and dislikes.

    4. Success is dependent on four elements:

      a. The motivation and cooperation of the patient

      b. The establishment of a professional rapport

      c. The consideration and fulfillment of the patient's individual needs

      d. The completion of a follow-up assessment and evaluation

Prevention and Control of Gingivitis and Periodontal Disease

The prevention and control of gingivitis and periodontal disease has traditionally focused on the mechanical removal of plaque and calculus deposits. This process is accomplished by supragingival plaque removal, daily toothbrushing and flossing, the use of mouth rinses, regular supragingival and subgingival removal of deposits by a dental hygienist and/or dentist, and the use of chemotherapeutic agents. Future treatment may increase the patient's host/immune response, identify susceptibility and risk for periodontal disease, and focus on the elimination of specific bacteria.

I. Individual Oral Hygiene Practices (self-care)

  A. Toothbrushing

    1. Frequency

      a. Traditionally has been recommended after each meal, which does not correspond well with most individual routines.

      b. Brushing thoroughly every 24 hours is in line with current research and theory on plaque maturity, which indicates that plaque develops slowly and increases in growth after 3 days; moreover, brushing thoroughly once a day corresponds more closely with most individual lifestyles.

    2. Toothbrush types

      a. Manual

        1) Designs vary according to size of head, bristle type, and length of handle; designs are constantly changing and there is little evidence that one manual toothbrush is superior to another.

        2) Recommendations regarding size and softness should be based on:

          a) The patient's manual dexterity.

          b) The size of the patient's mouth.

          c) The patient's motivation.

          d) The patient's oral health status.

      b. Power toothbrushes

        1) Are equally effective compared with manual toothbrushes.

        2) Are indicated for individuals with manual dexterity problems and/or a physical disability.

        3) Are indicated for individuals who do not brush long enough or well enough with manual toothbrushes.

  B. Interdental cleaning

    1. Is the mechanical removal of plaque interproximally and subgingivally, where a toothbrush cannot reach.

    2. Types of interdental cleaners

      a. Floss (waxed and unwaxed) is used for removing plaque interproximally and subgingivally; waxed floss may be more suitable for beginners because it typically shreds less.

      b. Dental tape is used for removing plaque interproximally and subgingivally; is an alternative to regular floss; covers a larger surface area.

      c. Interdental brushes are used for large embrasure spaces.

      d. A toothpick tip helps the patient access and remove plaque from deeper pockets and along the gingival margin.

e. Textured floss is excellent for use under bridgework and for flossing larger areas.

f. Floss threaders are used to thread floss under tight-fitting contacts or orthodontic wires.

g. Wood stick or rubber stimulators are used to remove plaque from between teeth; wood sticks do not remove plaque below the gumline.

3. Is recommended daily.

C. Mouth rinses

1. Cosmetic rinses contain oxygenating compounds and flavorings that deodorize the breath and remove gross debris; have limited use and effectiveness.

2. Therapeutic rinses are aimed at decreasing the number of microorganisms in the oral cavity.

a. Antiplaque agents

1) Should be used several times per day to produce a significant change. Examples include:

a) Oxygenating compounds.

b) Quaternary ammonium compounds.

c) Phenolic compounds.

d) Sanguinarine.

b. Antigingivitis rinses

1) Chlorhexidine gluconate is a prescription mouth rinse designed to control gingivitis; its effects last longer than those of other compounds.

a) Patient rinses for 30 seconds with 2 ounces, twice a day.

II. Professional Oral Hygiene Care

A. Regular professional removal of soft and hard deposits controls the disease process; however, its success primarily depends on the patient's commitment to a daily oral hygiene regimen.

B. Routine prophylaxis

1. Professional prophylaxis with oral hygiene instruction every 4 to 6 months reduces plaque and gingivitis and prevents periodontitis.

2. Daily, thorough self-care is the most critical factor in the successful outcome of professional treatment.

3. Recall is dependent on the following:

a. The patient's ability to remove and control plaque.

b. The patient's oral health/disease state.

c. The patient's risk for periodontal disease.

d. The patient's response to prophylaxis and debridement.

C. Chemotherapeutic methods

1. Chlorhexidine

a. In mouth rinse form (0.2%) is used twice daily.

b. In gel form (1% to 2%) is used daily.

c. In dentifrice form (0.4% to 1.0%) is used daily.

2. Anticalculus dentifrices

a. Are marketed by several companies.

b. Contain a 3.3% pyrophosphate concentration.

c. Work by inhibiting the deposition of new supragingival calculus.

d. Are most effective if used directly after professional oral prophylaxis.

Prevention and Control of Oral Cancer

The dental professional must conduct thorough head and neck examinations of patients and become familiar with the characteristics, risk factors, and prevalence of oral cancer. Dental professionals should identify, document, and refer patients with leukoplakia and mucosal erythroplasia lesions.

Oral Cancer

Oral cancer is limited to cancers of the lip, tongue, buccal mucosa, floor of the mouth, and pharynx. Oral cancer does not include cancer of the throat.

I. Oral Cancer Statistics

A. Mortality

1. Current oral cancer survival rates are no better than rates of the previous 20 years; 8,000 Americans die each year of oral cancer.[25]

2. Of the 30,000 new cases of oral cancer diagnosed annually, only half of the affected individuals will survive longer than 5 years.[26]

3. 3% of new cancers diagnosed in men and 2% of new cancers diagnosed in women are oral or pharyngeal cancers (Table 16–4).[26]

B. Occurrence of oral cancer (Table 16–5)

1. Varies widely throughout the world, depending on affected sites in the mouth and various environmental factors associated with oral cancer (e.g., between 1990 and 1993, death rates among males in the Netherlands were 2.8 per 100,000, compared with 12.9 per 100,000 in France).[26]

2. Men have more lip and pharyngeal cancers and women have more cancers of the tongue and mouth.

C. Prevalence

1. Occurs two times more often in males than in females.

2. Increases with age.

II. Prevention and Control

A. Early diagnosis increases the survival rate; thorough examinations of the head, neck, and oral cavity can help identify early lesions.

TABLE 16.4	Oral Cancer Death Rates per 100,000 Individuals	
Gender	Death Rate 1953–1955	Death Rate 1983–1985
Male	6.0	3.6
Female	1.5	1.3

TABLE 16.5	Incidence Rates of Oral Cancer per 100,000 Individuals	
Oral Cancer Site	Male	Female
Lip	2.7	0.3
Tongue	3.3	1.4
Mouth	1.9	0.7
Pharynx	5.7	1.9

B. Individuals with confined, localized lesions have a much higher survival rate than those with lesions that have spread to another region; individuals with lip cancer have a 91% survival rate.[28]

C. Risk factors

1. Tobacco use[3]

a. 4.4% of men and 0.1% of women smoke cigars.

b. 2.7% of men and 0.0% of women smoke pipes.

c. 27.7% of men and 22.5% of women smoke tobacco.

1) During the past 30 years, a significant drop in the number of individuals who smoke has occurred; in 1965, 42.4% of the US population smoked but in 1993, only 25.5% did.

2) 15.8% of women smoke during pregnancy.

3) 26.1% of Blacks, 24.9% of Caucasians, and 20.4% of Hispanics smoke.

4) 25.8% of individuals between the ages of 18 and 24 smoke; 29.2% of those between the ages of 25 and 44 smoke, 26.0% of those between the ages of 45 and 65 smoke, and 11.8% of those older than 65 years of age smoke.

5) Individuals who have quit smoking (former smokers) include: 7.2% of individuals between the ages of 18 and 24, 18.6% of those between the ages of 25 and 44, 33.9% of those between the ages of 45 and 65, and 38.4% of those older than 65 years of age.

6) Among smokers, 22.7% have less than 12 years of education, 21.4% have 12 years of education, 19.4% have 13 to 15 years of education, and 17.2% have 16 or more years of education.

d. 9% of males and 0.6% of females chew tobacco or use snuff; 20% of boys in grades 9 through 12 used smokeless tobacco in the past month.

2. Smoking; is more closely associated with lip and pharyngeal cancer.

3. Alcohol consumption, especially in combination with tobacco use.

4. Painful and ill-fitting dentures.

5. Excessive exposure to sunlight; is more closely associated with lip cancer.

6. Chronic inflammation.

7. Smokeless tobacco; is most strongly associated with cancer of the buccal mucosa.

 Clinical Case **STUDY**

A *junior high school counselor contacted local dental and medical professionals regarding a perceived increase in the number of girls with eating disorders in her school. Several local dental hygienists decided to develop a program for raising the awareness of the dangers of eating disorders for this population of students. To determine the current level of awareness, the dental hygienists developed a pretest that elicited information regarding facts and fallacies related to eating disorders; it also asked students whether they had an eating disorder and whether they knew of a classmate with an eating disorder. The pretest was voluntarily taken by 410 girls in grades 7 through 9. One week later, the participants gathered in an auditorium, where they listened to information about different eating disorders, their treatment, and the dental and medical effects of the disorders. The participants subsequently watched a 20-minute video of personal accounts of battles against anorexia and bulimia. One week after the presentation, the 410 participants were given a posttest that covered the information on the pretest. Participants scored significantly higher on the facts and fallacies section of the posttest than they did on the pretest.*

Clinical Case **QUESTIONS**

1. What type of sampling was used in this study?

2. What type of research does this project involve?

3. What are the oral manifestations of eating disorders?

4. The results of the study showed that students scored much higher on the posttest than on the pretest. What does this indicate?

Clinical Case **RATIONALES**

1. This study used a convenience sample (all female students in a school were chosen). A random study is one in which every element in a population has an equal chance of selection. A stratified sample involves selecting members from the subpopulations of a group. Single-subject sampling involves one or a few subjects who exhibit a special condition.

2. This study is an example of educational or behavioral research because it (1) assesses and evaluates the

application of an educational or behavioral technique in dentistry or dental hygiene to an individual or group; (2) focuses on knowledge, attitudes, and behaviors regarding oral health and disease; and (3) is conducted during a short period of time. Unlike this study, educational or behavioral studies typically involve smaller populations than experimental studies.

3. The oral manifestations of eating disorders include enamel erosion (perimolysis), cheilitis, parotid gland enlargement, palatal bruising, thermal sensitivity, and enlarged interdental papilla (see Chapter 6).

4. The fact that students scored much higher on the posttest than on the pretest indicates that learning occurred as a result of the information presented. However, an increase in knowledge may not lead to a change in behavior.

Research in Community Dentistry

Research can be defined as a continual search for truth by means of the scientific method. Research in community dentistry is categorized as biomedical research, which encompasses basic laboratory and clinical research, behavioral science, research regarding educational techniques, and administrative and evaluative research of community dental programs.

Types of Research

Research in community dentistry involves clinical/experimental, educational/behavioral, and administrative/evaluative research.

I. Clinical/Experimental Research
  A. Typically involves clinical trials.
    1. Are used to evaluate specific dental/dental hygiene techniques and therapeutic agents.
    2. Involve the use and application of epidemiology and basic laboratory research.
    3. Investigational new drug (IND) number
      a. Must be obtained before assessing and evaluating a drug that has not been tested on a human population.
      b. Is obtained from the Food and Drug Administration (FDA).
  B. Requires review by an Institutional Review Board (IRB).
    1. Is a committee that reviews proposed research protocols involving human subjects for the protection, safety, and privacy of participants.
    2. All institutions that conduct research must have an IRB.
    3. The committee must include the following:
      a. A minimum of 5 members.
      b. Male and female members.
      c. Professional representation by:
        1) At least one nonscientific professional.
        2) At least one consumer or lay individual not directly involved with the institution.
  C. Comprises three categories.
    1. True experimental research
      a. Involves random selection; all subjects in the sample have an independent and equal chance of being selected; all elements are selected at random. (e.g., numbers are drawn from a hat and replaced before each consecutive drawing).
      b. Involves random assignment; population subjects are assigned to each group at random.
    2. Quasi-experimental research
      a. Does not involve random selection; the subjects are selected as groups.
      b. Involves random assignment.
    3. Single-subject research
      a. Are studies that outline only one or a few subjects who may have a special problem or disorder rarely described in the literature.
  D. Important components
    1. Reliability; is a measure of accuracy (e.g., does the test, instrument, inventory, or questionnaire give the same results each time?).
    2. Inter-rater reliability; is a measure of reliability among two or more evaluators over time; calibration is conducted periodically during the study to check concurrence among examiners.
    3. Intra-rater reliability; is a measure of the reliability of one evaluator over time; calibration of individual examiners is conducted throughout a study to ensure that diagnostic technique does not change.
    4. Calibration; is a method of unifying examiners in the diagnostic technique; is accomplished by having examiners engage in trial runs on several sample cases and comparing findings of and between examiners; the process is repeated until all examiners concur; should be checked and recalibrated during the study.
    5. Validity; is a measure of accuracy (e.g., does the test, instrument, inventory, or questionnaire measure what it is intended to measure).

II. Educational/Behavioral Research
  A. Assesses and evaluates the application of an educational or behavioral technique in dentistry or dental hygiene to an individual or group.
  B. Focuses on knowledge, attitudes, and behaviors regarding oral health and disease.
  C. Typically involves studies of short duration.
  D. Typically involves smaller populations than experimental studies.

III. Administrative/Evaluative Research
  A. Is used for program evaluation in community dentistry.

1. Assesses a program's operation, effectiveness, and need for improvements.
2. Determines how the newest innovation has been accepted and used in the professional dental community (e.g., placement of sealants over incipient decay).

B. Often involves questionnaire surveys
   1. The survey instrument is a set of specifically designed questions that are carefully planned and tested in terms of context, structure, and appearance.
   2. Are used to gain knowledge from a particular population regarding information that is useful to the researcher.
   3. The number of subjects depends on the complexity of the study.
   4. The goals of the study should be well defined; its ability to evaluate the differences among groups should be tested.
   5. Survey questions types
      a. Dichotomous response involves yes/no or true/false questions
      b. Multiple choice involves a list of possible answers
      c. Quantifiable number response—answers involve a specific number (e.g., number of days per week, month, or year)
      d. Written response involves subjective answers to questions (is difficult to interpret)
      e. The Likert scale often is used to elicit feelings not mere facts.
   6. Pretesting
      a. Involves testing the survey instrument on a small group of individuals who are not part of, but have characteristics similar to, the study sample.
      b. Assists in gathering information and comments regarding the questionnaire itself.
      c. Allows errors, inconsistencies, misunderstandings, and the length of the questionnaire to be commented on and corrected before the study takes place.

 ## Clinical Case STUDY

Omar University has just been awarded funds to conduct research in an elementary school setting that targets fifth and sixth grade children. The dental hygiene professors at the university developed the research design and submitted a plan regarding the research and education they would provide. The target elementary school was located in a nonfluoridated, rural community. After examining the data collection, researchers found that the incidence of caries, plaque, and gingivitis was high. The researchers

planned intervention that includes oral health education, school water fluoridation, and sealant placement.

Clinical Case QUESTIONS

1. What type of extramural research and approval, funding, and announcement process did Omar University use to obtain funding?
2. What primary limitation is involved in the implementation of a school water fluoridation program?
3. After the oral health education program has been implemented, how can the presenters best evaluate whether the desired outcomes of the program were accomplished?
4. Explain why many dental public health education programs are conducted in the elementary school setting.

Clinical Case RATIONALES

1. The extramural research and approval, funding, and announcement process that Omar University used to obtain funding involved a grant and request for application (RFA). Grants are awarded to individuals or institutions who develop their own protocol for a specific research area. The money is applied for through a RFA.
2. The primary limitation of a school water fluoridation program is that the children are already 5 to 6 years of age when fluoridation begins, which decreases the beneficial effects on their teeth. However, the fluoride level of water is adjusted to 4.5 ppm for school fluoridation, which is not harmful because children are at school only part-time. School water fluoridation decreases caries by as much as 22% to 48%. Children must drink enough water to reap the benefits.
3. The best way for the presenters to evaluate whether the desired outcomes have been accomplished is by evaluating the extent to which the objectives were met. One must compare the objectives to the actual content delivered.
4. Many oral health education programs are conducted in school settings because the information can be delivered to large groups of students at once. The use of a school typically is the most time- and cost-effective approach and a school often is selected because of location and availability.

The Government's Role in Community Dental Research

Much of the money spent on community dental research is provided by the National Institute of Dental Research (NIDR). In 1990, the NIDR had an operating budget of $130 million. Research is funded according to the current priorities of the NIDR. Both intramural and extramural research is funded.

I. Intramural Research
   A. Is conducted within a facility by in-house researchers employed by that facility (e.g., NIDR).

II. Extramural Research
  A. Involves an agreement between the federal government and an outside institution to conduct the identified research.
  B. Two types of extramural research
    1. Grants
      a. Research money is awarded to an individual or institution to conduct a research protocol.
      b. The protocol has been developed and defined by the individual or institution requesting money.
    2. Contracts
      a. Research money is awarded to an individual or institution to conduct a research protocol.
      b. Differs from a grant in that the protocol has been defined by the federal government, not by the researcher.
      c. Researchers do *not* develop their own protocols; they consent to conduct research that already has been defined by the federal government.

Announcement and Application of Grants and Contracts

I. Two Types of Announcements
  A. Requests for Application (RFAs)
    1. The federal government announces a general area of research priority.
    2. Researchers who desire to apply submit a grant with a protocol that addresses the priority area.
    3. Researchers may define and develop their own goals and protocols for conducting the research.
  B. Requests for Proposal (RFPs)
    1. The federal government develops a detailed definition of the research goals and protocol.
    2. Researchers and institutions interested in the defined protocol are invited to apply through a contract.
    3. Interested researchers must describe methods for meeting the specific protocol terms.

Ethics and Privacy In Research

I. Nuremberg Code of Ethics
  A. Nuremberg War Crimes Tribunal
    1. A code of ethics that was developed in response to medical research conducted by the Nazis during World War II.
    2. Established guidelines and principles for conducting human research while protecting the rights and privacy of subjects.
  B. Institutional Review Board (IRB)
    1. Was established to monitor research on human subjects.
    2. Reviews all proposed research for evidence of the protection of each subject's rights and privacy.

II. Informed Consent
  A. Is consent given by an individual to a researcher or provider to conduct defined research or administer a treatment.
    1. Is mandatory whenever an individual participates in an experimental study.
  B. Characteristics and criteria
    1. Must include an explanation and definition of the following:
      a. Purpose of the research to be conducted
      b. Procedures and treatment
      c. Expected discomforts associated with the treatment
      d. Benefits of the treatment
      e. Risks associated with treatment
      f. Alternative procedures available
      g. Confidentiality
      h. Compensation for participation
      i. The names and phone numbers of individuals to contact regarding questions or concerns during the study period
      j. The ability to withdraw from the study at any time, without prejudice to the subject.

Clinical Case STUDY

A dental hygienist prepared an oral health education program regarding smokeless tobacco for a sixth-grade class. One of the objectives of the program was as follows: "After the lecture and videotape, Big Dipper, the student will list and describe three ingredients in a can of chew." The major points of the lecture were presented. The dental hygienist related specific information in the content to personal experiences with patients.

Clinical Case QUESTIONS

1. Describe the "condition element" of the instructional objective.
2. Identify how the dental hygienist can best evaluate the learning of the sixth-grade class.
3. During the lecture, the dental hygienist presented the major points and related specific information to personal experiences. Which part of the lecture was being delivered?
4. Oral cancer is prevalent among users of cigarettes and smokeless tobacco. Which is the most common site of oral cancer in both males and females? Which oral cancer is most closely associated with the use of smokeless tobacco?

Clinical Case RATIONALES

1. "After the lecture and videotape" best describes the condition element of the instructional objective. It gives the stipulation of the objective. "The student" refers to the audience; "will describe and list" is a behavior required of the student; and "three ingredi-

ents" describes the degree element, or how many the student must be able to list in order to pass.

2. The dental hygienist can best evaluate the learning of the sixth-grade class through testing.

3. Presenting the major points of the lecture and relating specific information to personal experiences occurs in the body of the lecture. The other components of the lecture format include the set, during which materials are introduced, and the closure, during which information is summarized and no new material is presented.

4. Cancer of the mouth is most prevalent among male and female users of tobacco products. Men have more lip and pharyngeal cancers and women exhibit more cancers of the tongue and pharynx. Cancer of the buccal mucosa is most closely associated with the use of smokeless tobacco.

Developing Community Oral Health Programs

Developing community oral health programs involves assessment, planning, implementation, and evaluation. In addition, developers must possess the skills and knowledge of communication and educational principles necessary to develop and practice the teaching and presentation of oral health education programs.

Assessing the Population

Population assessment is an organized, systematic approach to identifying a group with an oral health need.

I. Characteristics of an Assessment
   A. Defines the oral health problem
   B. Identifies the extent and severity of the problem
   C. Assists in the development of a community profile
   D. Collects data in several ways (survey questionnaire, clinical examination, or personal communications)

Developing a Community (Population) Profile

A community profile is developed by gathering comprehensive facts about a particular community regarding income, education, size, location, disease, health, and other characteristics.

I. Community profiles are developed from population characteristics that are determined by studying the following information:
   A. Number of individuals in a population
   B. Geographic distribution of the population
   C. Growth rate of the population
   D. Density of the population
   E. Urbanization vs rural areas
   F. Ethnicity of the population
   G. Socioeconomic status of the population
   H. Nutritional status of the population
   I. Types of housing available and standard of living (number of upper, middle, and lower class)

J. Public services and utility types
K. General health status

II. The dental disease profiles indicate patterns and distributions of disease, which are evaluated by the following:
   A. Clinical examination
   B. A review of patient dental records
   C. National health surveys

III. Dental program profiles include assessment of the:
   A. Histories and types of currently existing programs.
      1. Preventive
      2. Treatment oriented
      3. Educational
      4. Research
   B. Individual or organization responsible for each program.
   C. Success of the programs.
   D. Community's acceptance of the programs.

IV. Policy- and decision-making profiles include information on the:
   A. Occupations of financial leaders.
   B. Community's policy makers.
   C. Community's organizational structure.
   D. Oral health attitudes of community leaders.

V. The community resources profile includes an assessment of:
   A. Funding
      1. Availability of state and local funding for oral care
      2. Third party coverage
      3. Availability of federal funding
      4. Number of private funds through endowments or foundations
   B. Facilities
      1. Location of the closest major medical center
      2. Specialty services available at local medical center
      3. The number, type, and locations of dental facilities
      4. The use, accessibility, and provision of available dental services
      5. Whether OSHA guidelines are in place at each facility
      6. The adequacy and efficiency of dental equipment
      7. Number of available operatories in each facility
      8. Number of dental laboratories available
   C. Labor
      1. Number of active, licensed dentists and dental hygienists, and number of dental assistants and laboratory technicians in the area
      2. Availability and location of dental and dental hygiene schools in the immediate and surrounding areas
      3. Number of active nurse aides in the community

4. Number of public health nurses, public health dental hygienists, voluntary health agencies, and nutritionists available

VI. The fluoridated water profile includes the:
   A. Type of drinking water available (well-water versus central community water supplies).
   B. Fluoride content of the water supply and whether or not it is optimal.
   C. History of water fluoridation in the community.
   D. Attitudes concerning water fluoridation held by the community, dental professionals, and decision makers.
   E. Existence of fluoridation laws and referendum availability.
   F. Fluoride status of the school water supply.

VII. The profile of professionally applied fluorides assesses the:
   A. Fluoride supplement prescription recommendations of community dentists and physicians.
   B. Fluoride supplement or rinse programs available in community schools.
   C. Status of fluoride administration at health centers and/or hospitals.
   D. Toothbrushing program implementation in schools.
   E. Use of fluoride toothpaste and frequency of brushing in these programs.
   F. Success of all programs.

Interpretation of Community Profile Data

I. After all of the information regarding the community profile is gathered, current oral health needs and priorities are established.

II. Program goals and objectives subsequently are developed and are aimed at meeting the specific needs identified.

Planning the Program[29]

Program planning involves developing a lesson plan and defining goals and objectives.

I. Goals
   A. Are general statements that describe the major purpose of a program, lecture, course, or unit of instruction.
   B. Characteristics
      1. Are broad statements of direction or intent.
      2. Provide direction for devising instructional objectives.
      3. Are long-range targets.
      4. Clarify areas that need emphasis.
   C. Limitations
      1. Do not include specific achievements that can be assessed.
      2. Are timeless.
      3. Are open to various interpretations.

II. Objectives
   A. Are very specific, precise, and immediate steps to achieving a goal.

B. Characteristics
   1. Are specific, precise, and immediate.
   2. Are short-term.
   3. Lead to results that can be assessed and evaluated.
   4. Build to a goal.
   5. Include specific content and behavior.
      a. The content dimension includes the specific areas of content to be addressed and developed.
      b. The behavioral dimension includes the specific behavior the student or participant is expected to do with the content.

C. Characteristics of a good instructional objective
   1. Contains specific content that will be covered.
   2. Contains specific behavior desired as a result of learning the content.
   3. Is clear and concise.
   4. Includes precise terms.
   5. Is meaningful to learning and instruction.

D. Four elements of instructional objectives[30]
   1. Audience
      a. Refers to "who" will act as a result of the learning.
      b. Includes subjects (e.g., students, fifth-grade boys, adult learners).
      c. Example: After the demonstration on sulcular toothbrushing, the "fifth-grade boys" will be able to demonstrate the proper angulation of the toothbrush for removing plaque thoroughly.
   2. Behavior
      a. Refers to what the learner will be able to do as a result of the learning process.
      b. Is an action that the student must be able to perform or a behavioral verb that tells what the learner is to perform or exhibit.
      c. Includes verbs such as identify, write, describe, solve, label, list, and classify.
      d. Example: After the presentation on sulcular toothbrushing, the fifth-grade boys will be able "to demonstrate" the proper angulation of the toothbrush for removing plaque thoroughly.
      e. Also may include actions that are not observable, such as thinking or feeling; these behavioral elements must be specified by a performance or product that indicates an attitude or thought process.
         1) Example: After the presentation on developing a dental health education program, the student "will exhibit interest" in children's dental health month by designing a poster, producing a skit, or speaking at an elementary school.
   3. Condition
      a. Refers to the stipulations, restrictions, or requirements that the student must ob-

serve as he or she attempts to meet the objective.

  b. Examples:
    1) After viewing the videotape "Big Dipper," the student will describe three ingredients in a can of chew.
    2) Using a classmate as a patient, the student will demonstrate the proper angulation and insertion for the probe with a 90% accuracy.
  4. Degree
    a. Refers to how well the student must achieve an objective in order for his or her performance to be judged satisfactory.
    b. Involves limitations, range of accuracy, and/or the number of correct responses.
    c. Example: After viewing the videotape "Big Dipper," the student will describe "three ingredients" in a can of chew.
E. Example of an instructional objective that contains all four elements
  1. *After viewing the videotape* on sealant application, *the student* will be able to *list* the *five steps* necessary for placing a sealant that is well-bonded.
  2. The elements of this objective include:
    a. The audience (the student).
    b. The behavior (list).
    c. The condition (after viewing the videotape).
    d. The degree (5 steps).
III. The Lesson Plan[30]
  A. Three basic components
    1. The instructional "set"
      a. Introduces content procedures.
      b. Indicates the value and usefulness of information about to be presented.
      c. Motivates and arouses student interest by making it real.
      d. Ascertains the knowledge base of the audience by presenting information that brings the entire audience to the same level; involves administering a quiz or discussing material from the last presentation.
      e. States objectives for the presentation.
      f. Establishes the mood or climate.
    2. Lecture "body"
      a. Delivers the bulk of the information.
      b. Presents the major points.
      c. Relates information to personal experiences.
      d. Solicits audience participation and uses appropriate humor.
    3. The "closure"
      a. Summarizes material presented in the "body."
      b. Provides a sense of cohesiveness, purpose, and accomplishment of stated objectives.
      c. Reviews and summarizes major principles and key points.

  d. Does not introduce new material.
  e. Involves taking questions from the audience and giving announcements.
  f. Provides the audience with a sense of achievement; involves thanking the group for their attention and participation.

Program Implementation

Program implementation is the process by which a program is conducted and involves the participants, their roles, and the program specifics.
I. Implementation[29]
  A. Integrates all external variables.
  B. Involves team work.
  C. Includes the operation of the plan.
  D. Involves following a list of steps in the exact order in which they should occur.
  E. Involves assigning each individual to a specific task.
  F. Defines who does what, when, where, and how.
  G. Specifies the time allotment for each task or activity.

Program Evaluation[30]

The evaluation of a program involves defining the program purpose and evaluating the plan, the delivery, and the test results.
I. Purpose of Evaluation
  A. Three uses for evaluation
    1. To assess and determine the health needs of an individual, group, or population; directly determines the content of the health instruction and ensures that the information will be meaningful to the specific group identified.
    2. To determine the strengths and weaknesses of the teaching personnel, the teaching strategies, and the organization of the instruction.
    3. To assess the desired outcomes of oral health programs and the extent to which program objectives are met, and to determine a range of cognitive and behavioral outcomes.
  B. Defining the purpose of evaluation requires determining the following:
    1. *What* should be evaluated?
    2. *Who* should be evaluated?
    3. *Who* should administer the evaluation?
    4. *When* should the evaluation be conducted?
    5. *How* should the evaluation be conducted?
  C. Evaluating the plan
    1. Information to review
      a. The presenter should be thoroughly familiar with the subject matter.
      b. The material should be current and accurate.
      c. The information should be appropriate to the level and needs of the audience.
      d. The introduction ("set") should be interesting and appropriate.
      e. The bulk ("body") of the lecture should be organized and logical.

f. A plan for explaining important points fully and thoroughly should be established.

g. Supplementary materials must be as current as possible.

h. Technical terms must be defined.

i. Transitions from one piece of information to another should be smooth.

j. Audiovisual materials should help illustrate and enhance the main points.

k. Points in the program for assessing the audience's understanding of the information presented should be identified.

l. The ending ("closure") should be effective and include no new material.

m. Lecture notes should be easy to read.

n. The information presented should allow students to reach the stated instructional objectives.

D. Evaluating the delivery

1. Can be accomplished by reviewing a videotape of the presentation and gathering feedback from the audience and peers.

2. All parts of the presentation must be assessed, including content, organization, and style.

3. The following items should be evaluated:

    a. Clarity of speech

    b. Enthusiasm and body/facial expression

    c. Positive response to audience questions

    d. Maintenance of eye contact

    e. Smooth implementation of audiovisual materials

    f. Appropriate physical movement when communicating

    g. Organization of presentation

    h. Comfortable, appropriate atmosphere

    i. Allotment of appropriate time for entire presentation

    j. Minimal use of notes

    k. Provision of transitions and summaries

E. Evaluating test results

1. Instructional objectives serve as a guide for the lecture.

2. Exams and quizzes are developed to correlate with stated objectives.

3. Exams and quizzes subsequently can be used for evaluation; should accurately reflect the effectiveness of instruction.

4. Student feedback can provide information for the revision of future lessons.

Clinical Case STUDY

The activities coordinator of a senior citizens' center in a rural community asked the dental hygiene program director to present a 1-hour dental program. Eighty-eight senior citizens attend the local senior center. The program director decided to survey the attendees to determine their dental concerns and possible needs before developing the program. Twelve dental hygiene students volunteered to gather the information. An eight-item survey was developed that requested information regarding age, the number of remaining natural teeth, whether dentures are worn, whether the senior citizen has difficulty eating, swallowing, or speaking, the perceived cause of any difficulties, and perceived needs. Eighty-one seniors were surveyed. Table 16–6 summarizes the results.

Clinical Case QUESTIONS

1. What is the mean number of teeth for seniors 65 to 69 years of age? 70 to 74 years of age? 75 to 79 years of age?

2. Based on the results of the survey, which one of these statements could be made: a) These senior citizens have fewer teeth than the general population; b) Most of these senior citizens wear dentures; c) These senior

---

TABLE 16.6 Senior Citizen Survey Results

Item	Age		
	65–69 (46 persons)	70–74 (33 respondents)	75–79 (2 respondents)
Average number of remaining teeth	16	13	5
Wear dentures	78%	87%	100%
Difficulty swallowing	52%	67%	50%
Difficulty speaking	23%	28%	50%
Difficulty eating	44%	33%	100%
Cause of difficulty	Dry mouth, loose dentures	Dry mouth, loose dentures, stroke	Dry mouth
Perceived needs	Loose dentures, bad breath, yellow teeth	Cleaning dentures, loose dentures, toothpaste selection, yellow teeth	Preventing denture sores, bad breath

citizens have more bad breath than other groups; or d) The senior citizens between the ages of 70 and 74 are more likely to suffer a stroke.

3. Based on the results of the survey, what should be the emphasis of the 1-hour dental presentation for senior citizens?

4. What recommendations would help the senior citizens who are having difficulty swallowing?

Clinical Case RATIONALES

1. The mean number of teeth remaining in seniors between the ages of 65 and 69 is 16, between the ages of 70 and 74 is 13, and between the ages of 75 and 79 is 5.

2. According to the results of the survey, most of these senior citizens wear dentures. General population data is not available for comparison to determine whether these senior citizens have fewer teeth or more bad breath than others. No information is provided that allows assumptions regarding the likelihood of strokes in this group.

3. Based on the results of the survey, the emphasis of the 1-hour dental presentation should be on loose dentures. Two of the three groups had perceived needs involving loose dentures. The third group indicated that denture sores were problematic and these may be related to loose dentures.

4. Because many seniors feel dry mouth contributes to their difficulty, the following recommendations may help senior citizens who have difficulty with swallowing and with other problems (denture fit, speaking, and so on): oral lubricants, a liquid diet, sipping water, air humidification, chewing gum, and sugar-free candy. A referral to a physician is recommended if moistening therapies do not help the problem.

∼ CONTENT REVIEW QUESTIONS ∼

1. Facilitating a voluntary adaptation of health behaviors through learning opportunities, such as a behavior change through advice and counseling, is best described by which of the following terms?
   A. health promotion •
   B. health education
   C. health
   D. community oral health

2. Placing an amalgam restoration after removing caries from the tooth surface is an example of:
   A. health promotion
   B. primary prevention
   C. secondary prevention •
   D. tertiary prevention

3. The number of individuals in a given population who received dental care services during a specific time period refers to:
   A. demand
   B. need
   C. use
   D. normative need

4. Which of the following statements is NOT correct?
   A. more women than men use dental services
   B. as an individual's socioeconomic status (SES) rises, his or her use of dental services increases
   C. Caucasians use dental services more often than African Americans or Hispanic Americans
   D. individuals with poor general health are more likely to use dental services

5. Which factor below is interrelated with all of the factors that influence the use of dental care services?
   A. age
   B. ethnicity
   C. gender
   D. socioeconomic status

6. Which of the following has NOT influenced the rising cost of health care?
   A. decreased income of health care workers
   B. an increase in the elderly segment of the population
   C. technologic advancements in health care
   D. increased cost of third party payment

7. Which of the following is a contract between the patient, the dental office, and the insurance company?
   A. fee for service on 1 traditional
   B. indemnity plan – traditional
   C. third party plan
   D. capitation plan

8. Which statement below BEST describes the term *reasonable fee*?
   A. the actual fee charged by the provider for a rendered service
   B. the most frequently charged fee for a particular service usual fee
   C. a minimum fee set by the dental insurance company or plan
   D. a charged fee that exceeds the fee set by an insurance company

9. The Dental Service Corporation that was established in 1954 by the International Longshoreman and Warehouseman Union-Pacific Maritime Association currently is known as the:
   A. capitation plan
   B. direct reimbursement
   C. indemnity plan
   D. Delta Dental Plan

10. An insurance plan that gives a fixed, monthly payment to a dentist provider, whether or not an individual assigned to that dentist receives care, is BEST described by which of the following terms?
   A. third party plan
   B. indemnity plan
   C. capitation plan
   D. Delta Dental Plan

11. Which of the following is NOT true? Direct reimbursement occurs when:
    A. an insurance company directly reimburses an individual for a fee paid to a provider
    (B) an employer directly reimburses an employee for dental services paid for out of his or her pocket
    C. a fixed, monthly fee is paid to a providing dentist
    D. an actual fee exceeds the fee set by an insurance company

12. A group of researchers evaluated the incidence and prevalence of oral cancer among individuals between the ages of 50 and 65 in the Navajo Indian population. This type of epidemiologic study may be described as: *cause of disease*
    A. analytical
    B. descriptive *- incidence o prevalence*
    C. experimental
    D. proportional

13. In 1992, 250 cases of squamous cell carcinoma were reported among a group of 10,000 18 year olds examined in Fort Rock, Arizona. This is an example of:
    A. rate *ratio of actual to possible cases*
    B. incidence *new*
    C. prevalence *total # of cases in a time*
    D. morbidity
    E. mortality

14. Which of the following epidemiologic indices would be best for evaluating caries in a group of adults between the ages of 70 and 85 who experience gingival recession, inflammation, and bleeding?
    A. DMFT *⎫ same thing*
    B. DMFS *⎬*
    C. UTN *-unmet treatmt. needs*
    D. RCI *-root caries / recession*

15. Joe Black presents with generalized, moderate marginal plaque, inflammation, and bleeding. He indicates that he brushes once a day and flosses when food is caught between his teeth. Which of the following indices would be best for monitoring Joe's oral hygiene performance, indicating specific areas of need, and helping Joe with his oral care at home?
    A. OHI-S *- large population / debris + calc*
    B. PHP *- 6 selected teeth*
    C. GI
    D. O'Leary plaque index *location of plaque*

16. Which of the following indices uses the selection of six teeth to compare plaque removal performance at each subsequent visit and helps move a patient toward better oral health?
    A. OHI-S
    B. PHP
    C. GI
    D. Russell's periodontal index (PI)

17. Which of the following indices contains both a debris index and a calculus index, which are summed for a single score?
    A. OHI-S *debris + calc.*

B. PHP
C. GI
D. PI

18. The ideal epidemiologic index for evaluating specific oral disease is one in which:
    A. elaborate mechanisms are used to evaluate all aspects of the disease *difficult*
    B. simple indices, which are easily understood and explained, are used
    C. the index is not reproducible
    D. all possible factors are recorded

19. After the gingival health of Tom Cook, a 43-year-old business man, is evaluated, his teeth are divided into facial, lingual, distal, and mesial areas and the tissue is assessed for color, contour, bleeding, and ulceration. Which of the following indices is being used?
    A. O'Leary plaque index
    B. PHP
    C. PI
    D. Ramfjord's periodontal disease index (PDI)
    E. GI

20. Which of the following indices evaluates attachment loss and the progressive stages of periodontal disease?
    A. PI
    B. PDI
    C. CPITN
    D. GI

21. A public health dental hygienist has been asked to assess the periodontal status and treatment needs of the older adult patients in an assisted living community. To collect this information, the dental hygienist would use which index?
    A. PI
    B. PDI
    C. CPITN
    D. GI

22. Which of the following is NOT a true statement about water fluoridation?
    A. has been shown to be effective against decay
    B. requires no individual effort
    C. is relatively expensive to administer
    D. is a safe measure against caries

23. Mr. and Mrs. Jones and their children, ages 4 and 6, are moving to Watertown, New York during the winter holiday break. Their new community has fluoridated water. How many parts per million (ppm) of fluoride should be present in the Jones' drinking water?
    A. 0.3 to 0.7
    B. 0.7 to 1.0
    C. 1.0 to 1.2
    D. 1.3 to 1.8

24. What is the primary limitation of a school water fluoridation program?
    A. it decreases caries by only 25%
    B. the dosage must be increased to 4.5 times the optimum level

C. children are already between the ages of 5 and 6 when water fluoridation begins

D. children do not drink much water during school hours

25. The prescription of fluoride supplements such as tablets, drops, and vitamins is based on all of the following, EXCEPT:
A. the oral health of the patient
B. the age of the patient
C. the amount of fluoride in the patient's drinking water
D. thorough history of dietary supplementation

26. Mr. and Mrs. Calvin recently moved to Oak Woods, Missouri, a community with 0.3 ppm of naturally occurring fluoride in the drinking water. Their son, Jon, is 7 years old. Mrs. Calvin asks for prescription supplemental fluoride tablets. The correct dosage should be:
A. 0.25 mg/day
B. 0.50 mg/day
C. 1 mg/day
D. Jon should not take supplemental fluoride at this time.

27. Which of the following is NOT a true statement concerning school-sponsored fluoride mouth-rinse programs?
A. can achieve maximum effectiveness with monthly application *weekly*
B. can be easily implemented by nondental personnel
C. reduce caries by 20% to 30%
D. are very inexpensive to administer

28. Which home-care fluoride would give Karen, a 35-year-old with 2 to 3 mm of generalized gingival recession, the best results in terms of decreasing her sensitivity and her risk of caries?
A. 0.05% neutral sodium in an over-the-counter rinse
B. a 0.5% neutral sodium gel
C. either A or B
D. none of the above

29. Sealant placement is:
A. recommended for children and young adults living in fluoridated or nonfluoridated communities
B. recommended for all age groups in fluoridated and nonfluoridated communities
C. recommended for all age groups in nonfluoridated communities only
D. limited in its use and is applied only by a dentist
E. limited in its use because of low rates of retention and efficacy

30. Roselyn, a 16 year old, presents with several carious lesions on occlusal surfaces. She lives in a community with 0.7 ppm of fluoride in the drinking water. Which of the following would be the best oral health measure for preventing further decay?
A. sealants

B. fluoride mouth rinse
C. diet counseling
D. fluoride supplements

31. Which of the following is NOT necessary for successful diet counseling?
A. evaluation and counseling regarding food consumption are conducted in the same manner with all patients
B. patients exhibit cooperation and motivation
C. rapport has been established between the oral health professional and the patient
D. reevaluation and assessment have been completed

32. Mary, a 76-year-old woman with arthritis, presents for routine oral care. Her home care is good but she is having some difficulty with the lingual of the mandibular molars. Based on this information, how many times a day should Mary brush and with what type of toothbrush?
A. two times a day with a manual toothbrush
B. two times a day with a power driven toothbrush
C. once a day with a manual toothbrush
D. once a day with a power driven toothbrush

33. Harold, a 54-year-old businessman, presents for oral hygiene instruction. He has a three-unit bridge on teeth #13 through 15, tooth #14 is missing, and teeth #13 and 15 are pontics. In addition, large embrasure spaces on all posterior teeth are noted. Deep pockets are noted on DF #30, MF #31, and DF #18. Based on these findings, which of the following interdental plaque removal aides would be the best choice for Harold?
A. textured floss, rubber tip stimulator, dental tape, and floss threaders
B. waxed floss, floss threaders, toothpick tip, and interproximal brush
C. unwaxed floss, threaders, interproximal brush, and woodstick (wedge stimulator)
D. dental tape, threaders, woodstick, and toothpick tip

34. Approximately 2 weeks ago, four quadrants of periodontal debridement were completed on Catherine, a 34-year-old woman with diabetes and a mother of two young children. She presents for her reevaluation, during which an appropriate maintenance (recall) interval will be determined. Catherine is removing plaque fairly well and her gingival tissue has improved, as evidenced by decreased bleeding, inflammation, and pocketing. Slight marginal redness remains on the lingual surface of the mandibular molars. A 3-month maintenance interval is recommended. What factor was the primary reason for this recommendation?
A. response to the individualized debridement
B. plaque removal ability
C. current oral health/disease state
D. periodontal disease risk factors

35. When research is conducted in a university setting, a project must receive which of the following before research is begun?
    A. IND
    B. IRB approval
    C. informed consent
    D. FDA approval
36. The IRB is primarily responsible for:
    A. approving research on human subjects
    B. practically applying research
    C. regulating administrative procedures
    D. approving and improving the operation of a program
37. The University of Troy has proposed a study to evaluate the effects of a new antigingivitis drug, which has not been tested in a human population. To conduct this study, researchers must first obtain:
    A. approval from the IRB
    B. an IND number
    C. FDA approval
    D. informed consent
38. Which type of clinical trial research exhibits properties of both random assignment and random selection?
    A. true experimental
    B. quasi-experimental
    C. single-subject
    D. questionnaire survey
39. After the implementation of a baby bottle tooth decay (BBTD) program for low income mothers, data was collected to determine the program's effectiveness. This study is an example of:
    A. clinical trial research
    B. administrative/evaluative research
    C. educational/behavioral research
    D. experimental research
40. A dental hygienist wishes to assess the current skill level of a group of school nurses regarding the administration of a fluoride mouth-rinse program in the local elementary schools. Which of the following is the suggested method for collecting data regarding the skill level of these nurses?
    A. interview
    B. written questionnaire
    C. interviews with the school principals
    D. direct observation
41. When conducting a questionnaire survey, it is important to:
    A. have respondents include their names on returned questionnaires
    B. use questions that require a written response of feelings
    C. identify specific populations who possess information that is useful to the survey
    D. send the questionnaire to as many individuals as possible
42. Foster University recently was awarded money to conduct research concerning the geriatric population. The professors at Foster developed the research design and submitted a plan to address the oral health needs of the geriatric population in their state. Which type of extramural research and approval, funding, and announcement process did Foster University undergo to receive this money?
    A. grant, RFA
    B. grant, RFP
    C. contract, RFA
    D. contract, RFP
43. Which of the following is NOT a characteristic of informed consent?
    A. each subject is guaranteed confidentiality
    B. subjects are penalized for withdrawal
    C. an explanation of the purpose of the research is given
    D. an explanation of procedures and treatments is given
44. Information regarding the growth rate, geographic distribution, ethnicity, and socioeconomic status of a population refers to which component of the community profile?
    A. community resources
    B. population characteristics
    C. dental disease
    D. policies and decision making
45. In the community resources component of the community profile, which of the following terms best describes the use, accessibility, and provision of available dental services?
    A. labor
    B. funds
    C. facilities
    D. fluorides
46. A student is providing a lecture on smokeless tobacco. She presents the major principles and key points of her lecture. Which part of the lecture (program) is the student delivering?
    A. the set
    B. the body
    C. the closure
    D. the introduction
47. A public health dental hygienist has designed an educational program on baby bottle tooth decay for expectant parents. Information regarding the audience's current knowledge of the disease is gathered by means of a quiz administered at the beginning of the presentation. The administration of the quiz occurs during which part of the program?
    A. the set
    B. the body
    C. the closure
    D. the introduction
48. Which element of an instructional objective provides the stipulation, restriction, or requirement for a student?
    A. audience
    B. behavior

C. condition

D. degree

49. After reading the textbook chapter entitled "Developing Community Oral Health Programs," the student will be able to list and describe the four steps for developing and implementing an oral health education program.Which of the following describes the degree element of this instructional objective?

A. after reading the textbook chapter

B. four steps necessary

C. the student

D. list and describe

50. Two students are reviewing a videotape of their presentation. These students are evaluating:

A. the plan

B. the delivery

C. the learning

D. the plan and the delivery

E. the plan, the delivery, and the learning

51. It is most advantageous to conduct evaluation during which part of oral health education?

A. the plan

B. the delivery

C. the learning

D. the plan and the delivery

E. the plan, the delivery, and the learning

52. How can a program presenter best evaluate the desired outcome of his or her oral health education program?

A. by evaluating the extent to which the objectives were met

B. by evaluating the teaching strategies used

C. by evaluating the organization of the instruction

D. by evaluating the format and style of the presenter

53. Which of the following is a criteria for determining whether a particular disease constitutes a public health problem?

A. the knowledge of how to alleviate the problem is not being applied

B. the disease is widespread

C. the disease can be prevented, alleviated, or cured

D. all of the above

E. none of the above

54. Which teeth are known as the Ramfjord teeth?

A. 2, 6, 12, 19, 25, and 31

B. 2, 8, 13, 18, 26, and 29

C. 3, 9, 12, 19, 25, and 28

D. 3, 10, 13, 17, 24, and 30

55. Which of the following was developed in 1965 by the Office of Economic Opportunity and provides services to low income preschool children?

A. Medicaid

B. Medicare

C. HeadStart

D. Maternal and Child Health Services

56. Which of the following best describes dental services rendered through the Indian Health Service?

A. are provided by dentists and auxiliaries who are employed by the federal government

B. are provided by dentists and auxiliaries and are financed by the patient or through other means

C. are provided by dentists and auxiliaries who are not government employees

D. are provided by dentists and auxiliaries who are in a group practice with a Health Maintenance Organization

57. Dental education and services research, regulations and compliance functions, and biological research is governed by which of the following Health and Human Services groups?

A. the group concerned with the provision of dental services

B. the group concerned with improving the nation's capability to provide better oral health protection

C. the group concerned with maternal and child health

D. the group concerned with the elderly population

58. Troy, Colorado, is a rural mountain town of approximately 400 people. The town has inadequate dental services and the closest town with comprehensive dental services is 180 miles away. The federal government sends commissioned and civil service dental professionals to the area to meet the dental needs of this community. This service is provided by:

A. Maternal and Child Health services

B. National Health Services Corps

C. State Health Agency services

D. Medicaid services

59. Which program includes an early periodic screening, diagnosis, and treatment component?

A. Medicaid

B. HeadStart

C. Medicare

D. Maternal and Child Health Services

60. A neoplasm of which area of the head and neck is NOT an oral cancer?

A. buccal mucosa

B. floor of the mouth

C. throat

D. lip

E. tongue

61. Men have more of which type of oral cancer?

A. buccal mucosa

B. lip

C. tongue

D. floor of the mouth

62. Smoking is more closely associated with which of the following types of oral cancer?

A. floor of the mouth

B. pharyngeal

C. buccal mucosa

D. tongue

63. Which of the following was the PRIMARY goal of the health maintenance organizations (HMOs)?

A. to provide a range of health care services to its participants
B. to help lower the costs of health care
C. to increase competition for patients
D. to enable patients to have a wider choice of providers

64. A contract between several practitioners and an insurer to provide health care services for lower-than-average fees is referred to as a(n):
A. HMO
B. capitation plan
C. group practice
D. preferred provider organization (PPO)

REVIEW QUESTION RATIONALES

1. **A** Health promotion best describes a voluntary adaptation of health behaviors though learning opportunities because it includes a behavior change that is facilitated by a combination of learning activities, advice, and counseling. Health education only provides information, health is an ever-changing state, and community oral health addresses the oral health needs of a community.

2. **C** Placing an amalgam is a secondary prevention technique, which is designed to terminate a disease (e.g., caries) and restore tissues to near normal function (e.g., amalgam restoration). Primary prevention prevents, reverses, or arrests disease before treatment is needed. Tertiary prevention replaces lost tissues and rehabilitates to near-normal function. Health promotion refers to an individual's health–related behavior change.

3. **C** The use of dental services is defined as the proportion of a population who receive dental care services within a given period of time. Demand is a combination of perceiving need and seeking services. Need is the identification of an oral disease and normative need is the amount of oral care needed to keep a community healthy.

4. **D** The statement that "individuals with poor general health are more likely to use dental services" is false. Those who do not seek routine, preventive care for their general health are not likely to seek care for their oral health. All other statements are true.

5. **D** Socioeconomic status, which is a measure of both income and education, is interrelated with all of the other factors that affect an individual's use of dental services. The other factors (age, ethnicity, and gender) are not interrelated with regard to their effect on an individual's use of dental services.

6. **A** Health care workers' incomes have increased (not decreased), adding to the rise in costs of health care. The increase in health care worker income, coupled with other factors (rising elderly population, technological advances, and increased third-party payments), has impacted the rising cost of health care.

7. **C** Third-party payment plans are an insurance contract between the dental office, the patient, and the insurance company. Fee-for-service is a two-party plan whereby the patient pays an out-of-pocket fee to the provider. Indemnity plans operate in the same way as traditional insurance. Capitation plans refer to contracts between dentists and insurance companies to provide services to patients.

8. **A** Reasonable fees are the actual fees charged by the dental provider. These fees are modified according to each patient's individual need. These fees may or may not exceed the dentist's usual fee and/or the customary fee allowed by an insurance company. The most frequently charged fee is called the usual fee. The customary fee is the maximum benefit payable under a particular plan.

9. **D** The Delta Dental Plan was derived from the International Longshoremen and Warehousemen Union-Pacific Maritime Association, who joined forces with the Seattle District Dental Society to develop and implement a comprehensive dental program for children under 14 years of age. A capitation plan pays a fixed fee to a provider to deliver care to participants. Direct reimbursement occurs when an employer reimburses an employee for services paid out-of-pocket, and indemnity plans are traditional insurance plans that operate according to a submission and reimbursement method.

10. **C** A capitation plan is defined as a fixed monthly payment based on the number of patients assigned to a dentist. The insurance company takes into account that some patients will seek a significant amount of care and that others will not seek any care. A third-party plan is a contract between a dental office, a patient, and an insurance company. Indemnity plans are traditional insurance plans with submittal and reimbursement, and Delta Dental provides dental care contracts through a customary fee structure.

11. **B** Direct reimbursement occurs when an employer agrees to pay a portion of an employee's dental services. The employee seeks care and pays the dentist directly and the employer reimburses the employee for those services. When an insurance company directly reimburses an individual it is through an indemnity plan. Capitation refers to a fixed monthly fee that is paid to a providing dentist. An actual fee charged by the dentist/provider can exceed the fee set by the insurance company and is referred to as customary, however, the patient typically pays the difference.

12. **B** This research study is described as descriptive epidemiology and is used to evaluate the incidence and prevalence of a particular disease in a specific population. Analytical epidemiology refers to causal relationships among factors associated with a disease. Experimental research is used to evaluate a therapeutic intervention. Proportional is not a term that is used to describe a type of research.

13. **D** Prevalence is the term that describes 250 cases of squamous cell carcinoma in a group of 10,000 18 year olds in 1992. It is defined as the total number of cases of disease in a given population at a specific time. Rate refers to a ratio of actual to possible cases. Incidence is the number of new cases of a disease. Morbidity refers to disease and mortality refers to death; both typically are described as rates.

14. **D** The root caries index evaluates both the risk and extent of root caries in areas exposed by gingival recession and would be the best index for a group of adults between the ages of 70 and 85 who exhibit recession, inflammation, and bleeding. DMFT and DMFS indices evaluate decayed, missing, and filled teeth or surfaces, respectfully. The UTN index divides the mean number of decayed teeth by the mean number of decayed and filled teeth to determine the percentage of teeth that need treatment. The DMFT, DMFS, and UTN indices do not address root caries.

15. **D** The O'Leary plaque index would be the best selection for monitoring Joe's oral hygiene performance by indicating the location of plaque. It would enable him to visualize areas that need concentration and areas of thorough plaque removal. The OHI-S evaluates both debris and calculus and is used on large populations. The GI evaluates gingivitis and the PHP evaluates plaque on six selected teeth.

16. **B** The PHP index evaluates plaque on six selected teeth; it gives specific information about a patient's plaque removal ability and can be used during subsequent visits to demonstrate improvement over time. The OHI-S evaluates both debris and calculus for large populations. The GI evaluates gingivitis, and Russell's PI assesses the progressive stages of periodontal disease and attachment loss.

17. **A** The OHI-S contains both debris and calculus components and examines the facial surfaces of teeth #3, #8, #14, and #24 and the lingual surfaces of teeth #19 and #30 (see rationale for question 16).

18. **B** An ideal index is reliable, reproducible, valid, easily understood, and easily explained. Elaborate mechanisms that evaluate several factors are more difficult to understand and reproduce. Indices should be able to be replicated easily and only necessary factors should be recorded for the study.

19. **E** The GI is primarily used to evaluate gingivitis by assessing tissue for bleeding, color, contour, and ulceration. The O'Leary PI only records the location of plaque. The PHP assesses soft and hard debris and deposits. Russell's PI assesses periodontal disease and attachment loss, and Ramfjord's index evaluates gingival plaque, probing depths, and calculus.

20. **A** Russell's PI is primarily used to evaluate the progressive stages of periodontal disease and attachment loss in major populations. Scores range from 0 to 8 in severity. Ramfjord's PDI evaluates gingival plaque, probing depths, and calculus. The CPITN evaluates pockets, bleeding, and plaque in six sextants and is primarily used to identify the treatment needs of specific groups. The GI evaluates gingivitis.

21. **C** The CPITN would be most appropriate for the older adult patients in the assisted living community. It was developed by the World Health Organization to assess pocketing, bleeding, and plaque retention. This information is used to determine the specific periodontal treatment needs of a given population. The other indices are not designed to determine the specific needs of a population.

22. **C** Water fluoridation is not expensive to administer; it is very inexpensive and ranges in cost from $0.12 to $1.16 per individual per year. The other statements are true.

23. **C** 1.0 to 1.2 ppm should be used in cooler climates, such as in New York during the winter. The amount of fluoride added to the water is dependent on the climate; it ranges from 0.7 ppm in hotter climates (115° F) to 1.2 ppm in cooler climates (53° F). Fluoride levels of 0.3 to 0.7 ppm have no measurable effect; the ppm must be at least 0.7 to have a beneficial effect. Fluoride levels greater than 1.2 ppm do not offer more beneficial effects than those between 0.7 and 1.2 ppm and may be harmful.

24. **C** The primary limitation of school water fluoridation is that children do not begin drinking it until they are at least 5 or 6 years of age. The dosage is increased 4.5 times because children are at school only part of the day. School water fluoridation effectively reduces caries by 22% to 48%.

25. **A** Recommended fluoride dosages should be determined and adjusted according to the current level of fluoride in the water supply and the age of the patient. A thorough health history that reflects all dietary fluoride supplements is critical to prescribing the proper supplemental dosage. It is difficult to remove bacteria from the pit and fissures of teeth, even in individuals with excellent oral health. Fluoride, given systemically, helps reduce caries in pit and fissure surfaces.

26. **B** Jon should take 0.50 mg per day of supplemental fluoride. This dosage is recommended by the American Academy of Pediatrics for children between the ages of 6 and 16 years who live in an area that contains 0.3 to 0.6 ppm fluoride in the drinking water. No supplemental fluoride would be given if the child were 6 months to 3 years of age. If the child were 3 to 6 years old, 0.25 mg would be given.

27. **A** Fluoride mouth-rinse programs typically occur weekly, rather than monthly; some are provided on a daily basis. Fluoride mouth-rinse programs are easily implemented by nondental personnel, reduce caries by 20% to 30%, and are inexpensive.

28. **B** 0.5% NaF gel applied daily with a toothbrush can decrease sensitivity and decalcification in

areas of gingival recession. An over-the-counter 0.05% neutral sodium rinse is better for caries reduction.

29. **A** Sealants are recommended for children and young adults in fluoridated and nonfluoridated communities. They can be applied by dentists and dental hygienists and have excellent retention and efficacy against decay.

30. **C** Diet counseling is indicated when a patient has a high rate of caries and is taking the appropriate amount of fluoride. The age of the patient (16) indicates the possible consumption of highly cariogenic foods. Sealants are not indicated for carious lesions. She is receiving the appropriate amount of fluoride from the water, therefore supplemental tablets are not indicated.

31. **A** Success requires that patients are evaluated and counseled according to their specific needs and not in the same manner as other patients. Recommendations should be different for each patient. When successful counseling takes place, patients exhibit cooperation and motivation, especially when rapport has been established. Reevaluation and assessment also must take place after the patient implements new recommendations.

32. **D** Although toothbrushing traditionally has been recommended after each meal, current research suggests the need for thorough plaque removal once a day. Because Mary has arthritis, a power driven toothbrush may be easier for her to manipulate.

33. **B** Waxed (or unwaxed) floss and floss threaders can be used to clean the bridge. Textured floss also is useful for cleaning under bridges. A toothpick tip can be used for teeth with deeper pockets and an interproximal brush can be used for large embrasure spaces. Rubber tip stimulators and wood sticks do not remove plaque under the gumline or between large spaces. Dental tape is excellent for contacts that are not tight.

34. **D** A patient with insulin-dependent diabetes has a compromised immune system, especially if his or her glucose levels are unstable. A 3-month recall is recommended because diabetes is a risk factor for periodontal disease. Further periodontal destruction may result if therapy is not provided at frequent intervals. Catherine's response to treatment will be short-term, depending on her plaque removal ability, the length of recall, and her control of her diabetes. Her risk factors play the most important role in determining a maintenance phase.

35. **B** IRB approval is necessary before any research is conducted on human subjects. An IND number is obtained before evaluating new drugs never tested on human populations. Informed consent occurs after IRB approval and refers to obtaining the consent of the patient enrolled in a research study. FDA approval is required to market a new drug after research has been conducted.

36. **A** The primary responsibility of the IRB is to review and approve research on human subjects in order to protect their privacy and safety.

37. **B** The University of Troy must obtain an IND number through the FDA if the drug being evaluated has not been tested in a human population. The IRB reviews proposed research on human subjects to protect their safety and privacy. Patients must give their informed consent to participate in a study.

38. **A** True experimental research includes both random selection and random assignment; quasi-experimental research does not involve random selection. Single-subject studies are conducted on one or a few subjects who exhibit a rare or specific condition. Questionnaire surveys refer to research through written or verbal response.

39. **B** Data collected to determine a program's effectiveness best describes administrative and evaluative research, which evaluates the operation and effectiveness of and the need for improvement in an oral health education program. Clinical trials evaluate techniques or therapeutic interventions. Education/behavioral research assesses behavioral education techniques and focuses on knowledge, attitudes, and behaviors. Experimental research involves clinical trials or experiments.

40. **D** Direct observation would be the best method for learning about the school nurses' skill level in fluoride administration. It would enable the researcher to identify any inconsistencies and/or needs for improvement. Interviewing would provide only self-reported information, a written questionnaire would limit actual implementation techniques, and interviewing the principals would not gather information from the individuals directly involved.

41. **C** Questionnaire surveys should be sent to subjects who possess specific information that the researcher wants to capture. Having the individuals write their names would violate confidentiality, a response of feelings is difficult to interpret, and sending the questionnaires to as many individuals as possible would elicit unwanted information.

42. **A** A grant is awarded to researchers to conduct a research protocol that has been defined by the party receiving the award. Grants are applied for through a request for application (RFA), in which a plan for meeting the priority area is submitted. A contract is awarded to an individual or institution, and the protocol already is defined by the government agency awarding the money. A contract is applied for through an RFP (request for proposal).

43. **B** Subjects are not penalized for withdrawing from a study; rather, all subjects are guaranteed the ability to withdraw at any time without prejudice or repercussion. Confidentiality is kept throughout the study. The purpose of the research and its procedures and treatments are fully explained to each participant.

44. **B** The population characteristics of a community profile include: the number of individuals in the population and their geographic distribution, growth rate, population density, urban vs. rural areas, ethnicity, SES, nutrition and diet, types of housing availability, standard of living, public services, utilities, and general health status. Community resources include funds, facilities, and labor available for use in the community. Dental disease tracks the patterns and distribution of disease. Policy and decision making outline the community's organizational structure and the oral health attitudes of its leaders.

45. **C** Facilities describe the use, accessibility, and provision of dental services, including the location of the closest major medical center in a community, the specialty services available, the number, type, and location of dental facilities, the number of operatories and laboratories available, and the adequacy of equipment. Labor describes the number of active dental and other health care workers. Funds encompass all available monetary resources, and fluorides refer to both water fluoridation and professionally applied fluorides in the community.

46. **B** The "body" portion of a presentation provides the major points and key principles. The "set" introduces content and establishes mood. The "closure" summarizes the body and does not provide new material. "Introductions" are similar to the set.

47. **A** The instructional set of a presentation introduces the content or procedure to be discussed, describes the usefulness of the information, motivates the student and arouses the student's interest, can be used to assess the audience's knowledge base by administering a quiz or reviewing previous material, states the objectives, and establishes a mood for the presentation (see the rationale for question 26).

48. **C** The condition element of an instructional objective describes the stipulations, restrictions, and/or requirements needed to meet the objective (e.g., after viewing the video, after reading the text, after the presentation). The audience is "who" will act as a result of learning the objective satisfactorily. "Behavior" is what the learner will do as a result of learning, and "degree" refers to how well the student needs to perform to achieve the objective satisfactorily.

49. **B** The "four steps necessary" (degree element) describe how well the student needs to achieve an objective. It includes the limitations, range of accuracy, and number of correct responses. "After reading the textbook" is the condition. "The student" refers to the audience, and "list and describe" is the behavior element of the instructional objective.

50. **B** Evaluating the delivery of one's presentation can be accomplished by reviewing a videotape and/or by gathering feedback from the audience or peers. The student's learning can be evaluated through testing and the plan is evaluated by comparing it with the stated objectives.

51. **D** Evaluation should take place during all steps of developing an oral health education program.

52. **A** Evaluating the outcome of a program can be conducted by comparing the objectives with the outcome and assessing the degree to which each objective was met. Evaluating teaching strategies gives information on the delivery and plan, the organization, and the presentation format and style.

53. **D** A public health problem must meet the following three criteria: (1) the disease is widespread, (2) the disease can be prevented, alleviated, or cured, and (3) knowledge of how to alleviate the problem is not being applied.

54. **C** The Ramfjord teeth are teeth #3, 9, 12, 19, 25, and 28. These teeth often are used in clinical trial research as a representative sample of the entire dentition.

55. **C** Head Start was developed in 1965 by the Office of Economic Opportunity as a result of the Economic Opportunity Act of 1964. Its primary purpose was to provide social services and health education to low-income preschool children so that they would be able to enter school on equal ground with higher-income peers.

56. **A** Dental services rendered by the Indian Health Service are provided by dentists and auxiliaries who are employed by the PHS. These providers are commissioned officers of the Dental Service Corps. The other answers do not fit this description.

57. **B** Two categories of dental activities are handled by the federal government. The group that conducts dental education and services research, regulation and compliance functions, and biological research is headed under the group concerned with improving the nation's capability to provide better oral health protection. The groups concerned with the provision of dental services are programs delivered by the PHS. Federally-funded programs include Maternal and Child Health Services.

58. **B** The National Health Services Corps is a federal health labor deployment program. It provides commissioned officers and civil service individuals of the PHS to areas where there are inadequate health services because of shortages. The federal government provides Maternal and Child Health Services for women of childbearing age with low incomes and for children under 21 years of age. State health agencies provide services locally in each state and Medicaid provides health care to those under 21 years of age who are in a "needy" group.

59. **A** Medicaid administers the early periodic screening, diagnosis, and treatment program. Medicaid services are provided to specific needy people. Head Start is a federally-funded program distributed by the Office of Economic Opportunity to provide educational and social services to low-income preschool children. Medicare offers health insurance to individuals 65 years of age and older. Maternal and Child Health Services provide health services for women

of childbearing age and for children under 21 years of age.

60. **C** Cancer of the throat is not an oral cancer. Oral cancers include those of the lip, tongue, buccal mucosa, floor of the mouth, and pharynx.

61. **B** Men have more lip and pharyngeal cancers than women; women exhibit more tongue and pharynx cancers. Cancer of the buccal mucosa is more closely associated with the use of smokeless tobacco.

62. **B** Smoking is more closely associated with pharyngeal and lip cancers. Smokeless tobacco is more closely linked with cancer of the buccal mucosa.

63. **B** HMOs were developed primarily to help lower the costs of health care. A range of services, competition, and a choice of providers are available without an HMO.

64. **D** A PPO is a contract between several practitioners and an insurer to provide health care services for lower-than-average fees. Participants in HMOs pay a fixed fee for health care and choose physicians within their HMO. A capitation plan pays a fixed fee to a provider to deliver care to participants who are assigned for care. A group practice refers to a group of several health care professionals who provide services together.

References

1. Gluck GM, Morganstein WM: Jong's Community Dental Health, 4th ed. St. Louis, Mosby-Year Book, 1998.
2. Harris NO, Christen AG: Primary Preventive Dentistry, 4th ed. Norwalk, Appleton and Lange, 1995.
3. Darnay AJ, Fisher HS: Statistical Record of Health and Medicine, 2nd ed. Detroit, Gale Research, 1998.
4. Pamuk E, Makuc D, Heck K et al: Socioeconomic Status and Health Chartbook, United States, 1998. Hyattsville, Maryland, National Center for Health Statistics, 1998.
5. Davidson PL, Andersen RM: Determinants of dental care use for diverse ethnic and age groups. Adv Dent Res 11(2): 254–62, May 1997.
6. Burt BA, Eklund SA: Dentistry, Dental Practice, and the Community, 4th ed. Philadelphia, WB Saunders, 1992.
7. Larach-Robinson D: Factors associated with dental services use among Mexican Americans in the United States. AHSR FHSR Annual Meeting Abstract Book 12:111, 1995.
8. Nakazono TT, Davidson PL, Andersen RM: Oral health beliefs in diverse populations. Adv Dent Res 11(2):235–44, May 1997.
9. Gemignani J: Access causes a dental revolution. National Institute of Dental Research Report, Business and Health, 14(4): 65, 1996.
10. Source Book of Health Insurance Data, 1997–1998. Washington, DC, Health Insurance Association of America (HIAA), 1998.
11. Centers for Disease Control and Prevention: Dental Service Use and Dental Insurance Coverage, United States, Behavioral Risk Factor Surveillance System, 1995. MMWR 46(50), December 19, 1997.
12. 1988–1991: First three years of the third national health and nutrition examination survey. J Dent Res (special issue) 75, February, 1996.
13. Cherner LL: The Universal Healthcare Almanac. Phoenix, Silver and Cherner, 1998.
14. Brown LJ, Winn DM, White BA: Dental caries, restorations and tooth conditions in US adults, 1988–1991. J Am Dent Assoc 127:1315–1325, September 1996.
15. Eklund SA, Pittman JL, Smith RC: Trends in dental care among insured Americans: 1980 to 1995. J Am Dent Assoc 128(2):171–8, February 1997.
16. Gift HC, Drury TF, Nowjack-Raymer RE, Selwitz RH: The state of the nation's oral health: Mid-decade assessment of Healthy People 2000. J Public Health Dent 56(2):84–91, Spring 1996.
17. Burt BA: Epidemiology of periodontal diseases: A position paper. J Periodontol 67:935–945, 1996.
18. Oliver RC, Brown LJ, Loe H: Periodontal diseases in the United States population. J Periodontol 69(2):269–79, February 1998.
19. Taylor GW: Severe periodontitis and risk for poor glycemic control in patients with noninsulin-dependent diabetes mellitus. J Periodontol 67(Supp. 10): 1085–1093, October 1996.
20. Bray KK: Periodontal disease is risky business: Assessing factors to improve patient care. Part I: Unmodifiable risk factors. Access (special children's issue) 11(8):12–15, 1997.
21. Bray KK: Periodontal disease is risky business: Assessing factors to improve patient care. Part II: Modifiable risk factors. Access 11(9):12–16, 1997.
22. Trends in Indian Health 1996: Patient Care Statistics, US Department of Health and Human Services, 1996.
23. Siegal MD, Farquhar CL, Bouchard JM: Dental sealants: Who needs them. Public Health Rep Mar/Apr 112(2), 1997.
24. Gilpin JL: Pit and fissure sealants: A review of the literature. J Dent Hyg 71(4), Summer 1997.
25. Voelker R: Medical news and perspectives: October 9, 1996. New strategies to fight oral cancer. JAMA 276:1121, 1996.
26. Parker SD et al: Cancer statistics. CA Cancer J Clin 46:5–28, January/February 1996.
27. US Department of Health and Human Services: Cancers of the oral cavity and pharynx: A statistics review monograph 1973–1987. Atlanta, Centers for Disease Control and Prevention, 1991.
28. Hoffman HT, Karnell LH, Funk GF et al: The national cancer data base report on cancer of the head and neck. Arch Otolaryngol Head Neck Surg 124:951–962, 1998.
29. Fodor JT, Dalis GT, Giarrantano SC: Health Instruction, Theory, and Application, 5th ed. Baltimore, Williams and Wilkins, 1995.
30. Teacher Improvement Project System. Lexington, Kentucky, University of Kentucky, College of Allied Health Professions, Medical Center Annex #3.
31. Medical news and perspectives: New strategies to fight oral cancer. JAMA October 9, 1996.

Additional Readings

Burt BA, Eklund SA: Dentistry, Dental Practice, and the Community. 4th ed. Philadelphia, WB Saunders, 1992.

Gluck GM, Morganstein WM: Jong's Community Dental Health. 4th ed. St. Louis, Mosby-Year Book, 1998.

Harris NO, Christen AG: Primary Preventive Dentistry. 4th ed. Norwalk, Appleton and Lange, 1995.

Chapter SEVENTEEN

Ethics and Jurisprudence

Mary Danusis Cooper, R.D.H., M.S. Ed.

 Clinical Case **STUDY**

Dr. Smith receives a letter from an attorney stating that his client, a patient of Dr. Smith's, has contracted subacute bacterial endocarditis from a routine oral prophylaxis appointment 6 months ago. The dentist reviews the patient's medical history from the last visit and finds no indication on the record of any medical problems. The record of treatment indicates that the patient had moderate subgingival calculus and that home care instruction was given because of excess calculus, the condition of the patient's tissue, and excess bleeding. The chart also indicates that the patient was scheduled to have tooth #31 extracted by an oral surgeon the day after her oral prophylaxis appointment.

Clinical Case QUESTIONS

1. What suit will the attorney most likely file against the dentist?
2. Is this suit processed under civil or criminal law?
3. Is the dentist and/or dental hygienist liable for this suit?
4. What can the dentist do to help prove that the patient may not have contracted subacute bacterial endocarditis from her visit to Dr. Smith's office?

Clinical Case RATIONALES

1. Negligence/malpractice. Negligence implies carelessness without the intent of harming a patient.
2. Negligence is categorized under tort law, which is a branch of civil law (actions causing harm to an individual).
3. Possibly. However, there are four factors that must be present before the dentist and/or dental hygienist are liable for negligence: (1) the health care provider must have undertaken the care of the patient; (2) the health care provider must have breached a duty that was owed to the patient; (3) harm or damage to the patient must be proven; and (4) the harm must be related to the breach of duty. If any one of these four factors is missing, the ruling will be in favor of the dentist/dental hygienist.
4. Two considerations may be used to spare the dentist from judgment. First, the dentist may try to prove *contributory negligence*. The patient may have knowingly failed to inform the dentist or note on her medical history that she has mitral valve prolapse or some other heart condition that poses a risk for bacterial endocarditis. She also may have contributed to the negligence by not taking the premedication that her physician prescribed for her. Second, the dentist may try to prove *proximate cause*. The cause of the patient's subacute bacterial endocarditis may have been her visit to the oral surgeon because the tooth extraction may have necessitated antibiotic premedication. For these reasons, the dentist and other members of the dental team must make sure that a patient's medical history is updated regularly. Moreover all records must be complete.

Content Review

Ethics in Dentistry

The study of ethics in dental hygiene involves an understanding of the concepts of ethics, morals, mores, and values.

Terminology

Ethics—Issues of right and wrong with regard to conduct and character.

Morals—Specific judgments about right and wrong; are often but not always based on strong religious convictions.

Moral evaluation—Evaluation of the actions or character of an individual.

Ultimacy—A judgment that has no higher standard.

Universality—The principle by which it is determined that a good reason for one individual's behavior is a good reason for others to act the same way.

Altruism or neutralism—A moral evaluation that is not based exclusively on self-interest (i.e., "it may not be good for me . . . but it may be good for someone else").

Publicity—One publicly states evaluation and how this evaluation is based.

Ordering—Rules or principles that provide a basis for resolving conflict.

Mores—Established practices of a group or society.

Values—Beliefs and attitudes; often are established through societal, parental, and/or religious upbringing.

Relativism in Ethics

Relativism in ethics involves issues of behavior and belief. What is judged to be right varies among individuals, situations, and cultures.

I. Cultural relativism is moral rightness and wrongness based on cultural beliefs (often is referred to as common or social morality).

II. Descriptive relativism is the belief that people from different cultures have different views regarding morals.

III. Normative relativism is the belief that ultimately all ethical judgments are arbitrary and not justifiable.

IV. Personal relativism is the belief that an individual determines what is right or wrong according to his or her own personal standards of goodness and not according to cultural influences.

Ethical Theories

Ethical theories form the basis of principles and rules.

I. Utilitarian Theory
   A. Encompasses "the greatest good for the greatest number"; addresses consequences; also is known as Mills' "greatest happiness" theory.
      1. Act: the right act will result in the best consequences.
      2. Rule: actions are right or wrong based on their consequences.
      3. Value: value depends on whether something is determined to be good or harmful.

II. Deontologic Theory
   A. Focuses on the action, rule, or practice of an act rather than on the consequences; involves performing the right action regardless of the consequences; also is known as Kantian theory.

III. Virtue Theory
   A. Focuses on judging traits of character as good or bad; promotes good choices; is associated with the works of Aristotle and Plato.

Ethical Principles

Ethical principles are the laws or doctrines of ethics.

I. Autonomy means that everyone has the right to hold and act on personal values and beliefs such as the right to privacy, freedom of choice, and accepting responsibility for one's actions as long as harm is not inflicted on others.

II. Nonmaleficence means that an action is wrong if harm is inflicted on others.

III. Beneficence means that an action is moral if it is good and helps a person or enhances the welfare of person.
   A. Rules of beneficence (four elements)
      1. Avoid inflicting harm (principle of nonmaleficence).
      2. Prevent harm.
      3. Remove harm.
      4. Promote or do good.
   B. Problems in dentistry related to beneficence
      1. Balancing good against harm for the patient.
      2. Conflicts between patients and health care providers as to what is a good treatment record result.
      3. The influence of a third party (e.g., a caretaker, insurance carrier) on the nature of a dentist's beneficence.
      4. Conflicts that occur when patients refuse or disagree with treatment.
   C. Paternalism refers to acting as a parent would; includes overriding an autonomous decision for the good of a patient.

IV. Justice
   A. Refers to treating individuals fairly; involves giving patients their due or what is owed to them; is known as the "golden rule."
      1. Distributive justice applies to the proper and fair allocation of many aspects of society (e.g., political rights such as voting privileges, and the rights of women and minorities).
      2. The formal principle of justice or equality means that "equals must be treated equally, unequals treated unequally."
      3. Theories of distribution
         a. The utilitarian theory combines the principles of beneficence and nonmaleficence; aims to maximize the good and minimize the bad.
         b. The libertarian theory offers health care on the basis of respecting autonomy; need is not a factor; giving charitably.
         c. The egalitarian theory emphasizes equality; is based on the idea that everything is for everyone.

V. Veracity
   A. The health care provider has an obligation to:
      1. Speak the truth.
      2. Disclose information that is necessary for the patient to make sound treatment decisions.

VI. Fidelity
   A. The moral obligation to keep promises and other commitments.
   B. Duty on confidentiality—health care provider must keep confidential the information provided by the patient.

Ethical Dilemma

An ethical dilemma occurs when two or more ethical principles are morally justifiable but only one is acted on. The outcome of such a situation varies according to the principle that is chosen.

Ethical Decision Making

Ethical decision making involves several steps of analysis.
I. Relevant facts must be gathered; making a decision before receiving information should be avoided.
II. Values must be identified. For the dentist and dental hygienist these involve:
   A. Granting patient autonomy; allowing the patient to actively participate in decision making regarding treatment; allowing the patient the right to consent to or refuse treatment.
   B. Avoiding harm to others according to the principle of nonmaleficence.
   C. Having respect for the dental profession.
   D. Being true to oneself; following one's conscience.
   E. Following the law.
   F. Generating options and reviewing available options.
   G. Choosing an option and justifying it.
III. American Dental Hygienists Association's Code of Ethics (Box 17-1)

 ***Clinical Case* STUDY**

Naomi Farr, the dental hygienist, is completing an oral prophylaxis on a new patient. While she is retrieving a posterior scaler from her tray, the instrument slips from her hand and lands on her patient's head. The instrument tip embeds in the scalp tissues. Naomi carefully removes the instrument, cleanses the wound with antibacterial soap, applies pressure to stop the bleeding, and apologizes for the injury. The patient remains calm and says "Don't worry about it." Naomi documents the incident in the patient's record.

Clinical Case QUESTIONS

1. Is this an incidence of negligence? Why or why not?
2. Did Naomi handle the situation appropriately?
3. What types of information regarding the incident should Naomi include in the patient's record?

Clinical Case RATIONALES

1. This is not an incidence of negligence because there is no indication that the accident was caused by a particular action, such as not using a fulcrum. If Naomi had indicated to the patient that there was a particular cause for the incident (admission against interest), a case could be made for negligence, which is grounds for malpractice.
2. No one wishes to injure a patient; however, accidents do occur. Naomi showed concern for her patient by taking immediate care of the wound. She handled the situation well. There is evidence that concern and care on the part of the clinician can greatly reduce the incidence of litigation by a patient.
3. The patient's record should include the date and time of the incident, a detailed description of what occurred, the hygienist's actions, and the patient's actions and reactions.

Liabilities in Dentistry

Understanding the types of law and methods of avoiding lawsuits is vitally important in the practice of dental hygiene.

Jurisprudence

Jurisprudence is the philosophy of law.

Types of Law

Civil law, which includes contract law and tort law, and criminal law are the two major types of law.
I. Civil law
   A. Involves crime against a person; is concerned with actions that cause harm to an individual.
   B. An individual files suit with a private attorney; response to damages is typically measured in terms of money.
II. Contract law (form of civil law)
   A. Involves a breach of contract; involves the breaking of a contract by either party (health care provider or patient) or failing to keep one's part of the contract (e.g., the provider does not provide the care discussed, the patient does not pay, or services take too long to complete).
III. Tort law (form of civil law)
   A. Involves a civil wrong or injury to another person.
      1. Technical assault/battery is a wrongful act that is not consented to; includes performing a procedure that has not been agreed upon (e.g., unlawful touching, such as placing an instrument on a patient's chest).
      2. Maligning a patient involves saying or writing something that may damage a patient's reputation; includes slander and libel.

BOX 17.1 Code of Ethics for Dental Hygienists

1. Preamble
As dental hygienists, we are a community of professionals devoted to the prevention of disease and the promotion and improvement of the public's health. We are preventive oral health professionals who provide educational, clinical, and therapeutic services to the public. We strive to live meaningful, productive, satisfying lives that simultaneously serve us, our profession, our society, and the world. Our actions, behaviors, and attitudes are consistent with our commitment to public service. We endorse and incorporate the Code into our daily lives.

2. Purpose
The purpose of a professional code of ethics is to achieve high levels of ethical consciousness, decision making, and practice by the members of the profession. Specific objectives of the Dental Hygiene Code of Ethics are:
- to increase our professional and ethical consciousness and sense of ethical responsibility.
- to lead us to recognize ethical issues and choices and to guide us in making more informed ethical decisions.
- to establish a standard for professional judgment and conduct.
- to provide a statement of the ethical behavior the public can expect from us.

The Dental Hygiene Code of Ethics is meant to influence us throughout our careers. It stimulates our continuing study of ethical issues and challenges us to explore our ethical responsibilities. The Code establishes concise standards of behavior to guide the public's expectations of our profession and supports existing dental hygiene practice, laws, and regulations. By holding ourselves accountable to meeting the standards stated in the Code, we enhance the public's trust on which our professional privilege and status are founded.

3. Key Concepts
Our beliefs, principles, values, and ethics are concepts reflected in the Code. They are the essential elements of our comprehensive and definitive code of ethics, and are interrelated and mutually dependent.

4. Basic Beliefs
We recognize the importance of the following beliefs that guide our practice and provide context for our ethics:
- The services we provide contribute to the health and well-being of society.
- Our education and licensure qualify us to serve the public by preventing and treating oral disease and helping individuals achieve and maintain optimal health.
- Individuals have intrinsic worth, are responsible for their own health, and are entitled to make choices regarding their health.
- Dental hygiene care is an essential component of overall healthcare and we function interdependently with other healthcare providers.
- All people should have access to healthcare, including oral healthcare.
- We are individually responsible for our actions and the quality of care we provide.

5. Fundamental Principles
These fundamental principles, universal concepts, and general laws of conduct provide the foundation for our ethics.

Universality
The principle of universality assumes that if one individual judges an action to be right or wrong in a given situation, other people considering the same action in the same situation would make the same judgment.

Complementarity
The principle of complementarity assumes the existence of an obligation to justice and basic human rights. It requires us to act toward others in the same way they would act toward us if roles were reversed. In all relationships, it means considering the values and perspective of others before making decisions or taking actions affecting them.

Ethics
Ethics are the general standards of right and wrong that guide behavior within society. As generally accepted actions, they can be judged by determining the extent to which they promote good and minimize harm. Ethics compel us to engage in health promotion/disease prevention activities.

Community
This principle expresses our concern for the bond between individuals, the community, and society in general. It leads us to preserve natural resources and inspires us to show concern for the global environment.

Responsibility
Responsibility is central to our ethics. We recognize that there are guidelines for making ethical choices and accept responsibility for knowing and applying them. We accept the consequences of our actions or the failure to act and are willing to make ethical choices and publicly affirm them.

6. Core Values
We acknowledge these values as general guides for our choices and actions.

Individual autonomy and respect for human beings
People have the right to be treated with respect. People have the right to informed consent prior to treatment, and they have the right to full disclosure of all relevant information so that they can make informed choices about their care.

Confidentiality
We respect the confidentiality of client information and relationships as a demonstration of the value we place on individual autonomy. We acknowledge our obligation to justify any violation of a confidence.

Societal Trust
We value client trust and understand that public trust in our profession is based on our actions and behavior.

Nonmaleficence
We accept our fundamental obligation to provide services in a manner that protects all clients and minimizes harm to them and others involved in their treatment.

Beneficence
We have a primary role in promoting the well-being of individuals and the public by engaging in heath promotion/disease prevention activities.

BOX 17.1 Code of Ethics for Dental Hygienists *Continued*

Justice and Fairness
We value justice and support the fair and equitable distribution of healthcare resources. We believe all people should have access to high-quality, affordable oral healthcare.

Veracity
We accept our obligation to tell the truth and assume that others will do the same. We value self-knowledge and seek truth and honesty in all relationships.

7. Standards of Professional Responsibility
We are obligated to practice our profession in a manner that supports our purpose, beliefs, and values in accordance with the fundamental principles that support our ethics. We acknowledge the following responsibilities:

To Ourselves as Individuals . . .
- Avoid self-deception, and continually strive for knowledge and personal growth.
- Establish and maintain a lifestyle that supports optimal health.
- Create a safe work environment.
- Assert our own interests in ways that are fair and equitable.
- Seek the advice and counsel of others when challenged with ethical dilemmas.
- Have realistic expectations of ourselves and recognize our limitations.

To Ourselves as Professionals . . .
- Enhance professional competencies through continuous learning in order to practice according to high standards of care.
- Support dental hygiene peer-review systems and quality-assurance measures.
- Develop collaborative professional relationships and exchange knowledge to enhance our own lifelong professional development.

To Family and Friends . . .
- Support the efforts of others to establish and maintain healthy lifestyles and respect the rights of friends and family.

To Clients . . .
- Provide oral healthcare utilizing high levels of professional knowledge, judgment, and skill.
- Maintain a work environment that minimizes the risk of harm.
- Serve all clients without discrimination and avoid action toward any individual or group that may be interpreted as discriminatory.
- Hold professional client relationships confidential.
- Communicate with clients in a respectful manner.
- Promote ethical behavior and standards of care by all dental hygienists.
- Serve as an advocate for the welfare of clients.
- Provide clients with the information necessary to make informed decisions about their oral health and encourage their full participation in treatment decisions and goals.
- Refer clients to other healthcare providers when their needs are beyond our ability or scope of practice.
- Educate clients about high-quality oral healthcare.

To Colleagues . . .
- Conduct professional activities and programs, and develop relationships in ways that are honest, responsible, and appropriately open and candid.

- Encourage a work environment that promotes individual professional growth and development.
- Collaborate with others to create a work environment that minimizes risk to the personal health and safety of our colleagues.
- Manage conflicts constructively.
- Support the efforts of other dental hygienists to communicate the dental hygiene philosophy of preventive oral care.
- Inform other healthcare professionals about the relationship between general and oral health.
- Promote human relationships that are mutually beneficial, including those with other healthcare professionals.

To Employees and Employers . . .
- Conduct professional activities and programs, and develop relationships in ways that are honest, responsible, open, and candid.
- Manage conflicts constructively.
- Support the right of our employees and employers to work in an environment that promotes wellness.
- Respect the employment rights of our employers and employees.

To the Dental Hygiene Profession . . .
- Participate in the development and advancement of our profession.
- Avoid conflicts of interest and declare them when they occur.
- Seek opportunities to increase public awareness and understanding of oral health practices.
- Act in ways that bring credit to our profession while demonstrating appropriate respect for colleagues in other professions.
- Contribute time, talent, and financial resources to support and promote our profession.
- Promote a positive image for our profession.
- Promote a framework for professional education that develops dental hygiene competencies to meet the oral and overall health needs of the public.

To the Community and Society . . .
- Recognize and uphold the laws and regulations governing our profession.
- Document and report inappropriate, inadequate, or substandard care and/or illegal activities by any healthcare provider to the responsible authorities.
- Use peer review as a mechanism for identifying inappropriate, inadequate, or substandard care and for modifying and improving the care provided by dental hygienists.
- Comply with local, state, and federal statutes that promote public health and safety.
- Develop support systems and quality-assurance programs in the workplace to assist dental hygienists in providing the appropriate standard of care.
- Promote access to dental hygiene services for all, supporting justice and fairness in the distribution of healthcare resources.
- Act consistently with the ethics of the global scientific community of which our profession is a part.
- Create a healthful workplace ecosystem to support a healthy environment.
- Recognize and uphold our obligation to provide pro bona service.

Box continued on following page

BOX 17.1 Code of Ethics for Dental Hygienists *Continued*

To Scientific Investigation . . .
We accept responsibility for conducting research according to the fundamental principles underlying our ethical beliefs in compliance with universal codes, governmental standards, and professional guidelines for the care and management of experimental subjects. We acknowledge our ethical obligations to the scientific community:

- Conduct research that contributes knowledge that is valid and useful to our clients and society.
- Use research methods that meet accepted scientific standards.
- Use research resources appropriately.
- Systematically review and justify research in progress to ensure the most favorable benefit-to-risk ratio to research subjects.
- Submit all proposals involving human subjects to an appropriate human subject review committee.
- Secure appropriate institutional committee approval for the conduct of research involving animals.

- Obtain informed consent from human subjects participating in research that is based on specifications published in Title 21 Code of Federal Regulations Part 46.
- Respect the confidentiality and privacy of data.
- Seek opportunities to advance dental hygiene knowledge through research by providing financial, human, and technical resources whenever possible.
- Report research results in a timely manner.
- Report research findings completely and honestly, drawing only those conclusions that are supported by the data presented.
- Report the names of investigators fairly and accurately.
- Interpret the research and the research of others accurately and objectively, drawing conclusions that are supported by the data presented and seeking clarity when uncertain.
- Critically evaluate research methods and results before applying new theory and technology in practice.
- Be knowledgeable concerning currently accepted preventive and therapeutic methods, products, and technology and their application to our practice.

From Journal of Dental Hygiene 69(4): 159–162, 1995.
The 1995 ADHA House of Delegates has approved and ratified the *Code of Ethics for Dental Hygienists.* Six years in the making, acknowledgment and appreciation go to the Special Committee on Ethics—including Gail Bemis, RDH, chair; Karla Girts, BSDH, RDH; Merry Jo Thoele, RDH, BA; and Beverly Whitford, RDH, BS—plus consultant, Mary Alice Gaston, RDH, MS, for their efforts and dedication.

    a. Slander is saying something that may destroy someone's reputation.
    b. Libel is writing something that may destroy someone's reputation.

3. Negligence (often considered synonymous with malpractice) is carelessness, without the intent to harm a patient; occurs when the appropriate standard of care is not met and some damage results (e.g., dentist knowingly permits a hazard to exist in the office and consequently a patient is injured).
    a. Liability for negligence requires the existence of four factors.
      1) The health care provider undertakes care of the patient; a duty to the patient results.
      2) The health care provider breaches a duty owed to the patient.
      3) Damage or harm to the patient must be evident.
      4) The harm or damage to the patient must be related to the breach of duty.
    b. Grounds for malpractice
      1) *A failure to sterilize*; sterilization practices should be in accordance with OSHA and ADA recommendations.
      2) *A failure to radiograph or produce adequate radiographs*; this may involve:
        a) A failure to radiograph when a radiograph is indicated.
        b) The unskillful use or improper processing of a radiograph, which jeopardizes diagnosis.
        c) Refusal by the patient; if a patient refuses to have a radiograph, a written release form should be signed by the patient; a refusal *must* be noted in the patient's chart; radiographs are used for diagnosis and therefore must remain a part of a patient's record.
      3) *A failure to refer*; a patient should be referred to a specialist when the "average" dentist knows that procedure is complex.
      4) *Trauma*; the slipping of an instrument alone does not constitute negligence; however, making a statement that may indicate that an error was made by the health care provider (e.g., "I should have had a fulcrum") is known as *admission against interest*—a statement, spoken or written, that may prove the opposite of what one contends in court.
      5) *A failure to inform*; a patient must be informed before he or she can give consent.

IV. Criminal law
    A. Pertains to actions that constitute a wrong against society (e.g., practicing the profession of dental hygiene without a license).
    B. The state responds to such actions, which are punishable upon conviction by death, imprisonment, fine, or removal from office.

Clinical Case **STUDY**

Phyllis Day is a 47-year-old patient in the practice. A thorough periodontal evaluation reveals AAP Class-IV periodontitis. The dental hygienist explains treatment options to Ms. Day and asks her whether she has further questions. A series of four scaling and root planing appointments is scheduled. Ms. Day completes the series of appointments and agrees to return in 6 weeks for a reevaluation of her treatment.

Clinical Case QUESTIONS

1. Did Ms. Day give consent for her treatment? If so, what type of consent did she give?
2. The dental hygienist asks Ms. Day to allow her case to be used as a teaching tool in the practice, which would involve both extraoral and intraoral photographs of her face and mouth and a full-mouth series of x-rays. What type of consent is required before the photographs are taken?
3. If, after thorough treatment of her periodontal condition, further loss of alveolar bone is detected, what should be done?

Clinical Case RATIONALES

1. Ms. Day gave consent for treatment when she agreed to schedule the scaling and root planing appointments and agreed to return for reevaluation. This type of consent is called implied consent.
2. Written, mandatory consent is required in situations in which new drugs are used, recognizable photographs of a patient are used, general anesthetics are administered, or when treatment takes longer than 1 year to complete.
3. If the treatment performed is unsuccessful (as evidenced by further progression of the disease), the patient should be referred to an appropriate specialist, which in this case would be a periodontist.

Preventing a Lawsuit

Measures that are used to help avoid legal action include the reasonably prudent practitioner, admissions against interest, res ipsa loquitur, and proper documentation.

I. Be aware that the *reasonably prudent practitioner* measure is used by the law to determine whether the provider has exercised reasonable care.

II. Avoid *admissions against interest*, or making a statement that serves to defeat one's own interest; such admissions are legally admissible in court.
   A. The admission of negligence by an employee occurs when the health care provider admits to improper conduct.

   B. *Res gestae* means "part of the action" and refers to a statement made during the time of the negligent act.

III. Avoid *res ipsa loquitur*, or "a matter that speaks for itself," refers to an injury that is directly related to an instance of negligence (e.g., health care provider fails to take a medical history or renders services while intoxicated).

IV. Prove contributory negligence—that the patient has contributed to the harmful result.

V. Identify another proximate cause; reveal that the harm to the patient may have resulted from another incident.

VI. Keep accurate and complete patient records, the single most important factor in the defense of most malpractice cases; record information in indelible ink; if an error is made in a patient's chart, mark one line through the statement and place one's initials next to the area (do not erase, black-out, or use correction fluid).
   A. The medical history should be current, include the patient's signature, and be reviewed at each visit.
   B. The diagnosis should be recorded.
   C. Treatment plan(s) should include *all* options given to the patient.
   D. The record of treatment should include the date(s) of treatment, the procedure(s) performed, and the medications used and/or administered; also should indicate canceled and broken appointments.
   E. Copies of all correspondence regarding patients should be kept, together with receipts of registered mail.
   F. Radiographs
      1. Processed properly to avoid deterioration with age.
      2. Carefully labeled with the patient's name, the date taken, and the dentist's name.
      3. Taken properly so that they are diagnostically acceptable.
      4. Retained for the minimum length of time required by the statute of limitations in a state.
   G. Letters to patients (correspondence) should be carefully worded to ensure understanding and minimize the chance for libel.

VII. Transfer of Records
   A. For an inactive patient, records typically are kept for the length of time required by the statute of limitations.
   B. For active patients, records are kept by the dentist unless they are requested by another dentist.
      1. Steps for requesting a transfer of records:
         a. Always keep on record the letter(s) requesting records.
         b. Send copies of records via registered mail; request a receipt.

c. Request that records be returned to the office after their use.

VIII. Insurance claims include records only of performed procedures; falsifying information is fraudulent and may result in a legal action.

IX. The statute of limitations is the legal time in which a lawsuit (civil) for a wrong must be filed.

A. A malpractice suit, in most states, must be initiated within 2 years of the time that the wrongful act was committed.

B. The limitation for filing a breach of contract suit typically is 6 years; it is recommended that records be retained for a minimum of 10 years.

X. Liability insurance should be carried by each licensed professional.

A. Professional reliability: every professional has the responsibility to provide good dental care.

B. Respondeat superior: the employer often is named in a suit in which an employee caused harm to a patient.

XI. Informed Consent (in a contractual relationship) means that a patient has given a health care provider permission to perform certain procedure(s).

A. To give consent and avoid breach of contract, a patient must understand the following:
  1. The nature of his/her condition.
  2. The treatment proposed.
  3. Any risks involved or chances of failure.
  4. Possible results of not treating the condition.
  5. Any alternative procedures that may be necessary.

B. To validate consent, the following requirements must be met:
  1. Consent must be informed.
  2. Consent must be given for specific treatment(s).
  3. The individual giving consent must be legally competent.
  4. The treatments consented to must be legal.
  5. Consent must not have been obtained through deceit or fraud.

C. Types of consent or refusal
  1. Implied consent is implied by the actions of the patient (e.g., a patient comes to the office for an examination and consultation, therefore consent is established by the actions of the provider).
    a. Quasi-consent is a type of implied consent; the patient is in danger of injury or death and the patient is unable to give consent; emergency treatment is given.
  2. Expressed consent is informed consent that is given verbally or in writing (provides the most protection).
  3. Parental/guardian consent is required when a minor or an individual who is not mentally competent to give consent needs treatment;

typically is provided by a parent or other legal caretaker, preferably in writing.

  4. Written mandatory consent must be given for the following situations:
    a. Administration of new drugs.
    b. Use of a patient's photograph (must be recognizable).
    c. Administration of general anesthesia.
    d. Treatment will take longer than 1 year to complete.
    e. Treatment of children in a public program.
  5. Informed refusal occurs when a patient declines treatment after the treatment plan is presented.

Legal Responsibilities

Legal responsibilities in the dental practice include the duties of the health care provider and the patient.

Duties

Duties are the obligations that one person owes another.

I. Duties of the health care provider

A. Hold licensure; the health care provider must have a valid license to practice.

B. Protect and respect the personal and property rights of the patient; includes respecting a patient's right to the ownership of dentures, even if the patient has not paid for them. The health care provider should avoid asking patients personal questions; the patient has a right to confidentiality; photographs of patients cannot be displayed and/or published without written permission from the patient; any discussion in the office between the health care provider and the patient is considered *privileged communication*.
  1. Two exceptions to privileged communication
    a. Child abuse
    b. Communicable diseases

C. Provide only care that is necessary and to which the patient has agreed.

D. Exercise reasonable skill, care, and judgment.
  1. Reasonable skill involves not only having knowledge but the ability to use such knowledge.
  2. Reasonable care relates to how skill is used; the health care provider should use the degree of care that a reasonably prudent practitioner would use under similar circumstances.
  3. Reasonable judgment involves making the best decision(s) possible regarding the procedures performed.

E. Do not abandon the patient after the individual becomes a patient of record.
  1. Abandonment is desertion; involves a failure to provide services and needs to be agreed upon by the health care provider and the patient; applies to a practitioner who is not available.
  2. Withdrawal from a contract:

    a. Is a written letter of intent to withdraw that is sent to the patient by certified or registered mail (with return receipt).

    b. Contains a statement of the care that must be completed.

    c. Suggests to the patient how care can be obtained.

  F. Use standard materials, techniques, and drugs; any experimental procedures, techniques, or drugs used for treatment require the patient's *informed consent*.

  G. Charge reasonable fees; a charge is reasonable when it is customary and ordinary for a service in the same or a similar community.

  H. Keep the patient informed of the progress of treatment; give adequate and understandable instructions to the patient so they can be followed.

  I. Achieve reasonable results; the health care provider has a legal duty to provide standard care but does not have to obtain perfect results.

  J. Arrange for care during any temporary absence; if a health care provider is unavailable to treat the patient, competent care must be available (e.g., a dentist who goes on vacation arranges to have someone available for emergency care); failure to do so may result in abandonment.

  K. Refer the patient to a specialist when a patient's needs cannot be met; referral should be made when a case is particularly difficult or beyond one's capabilities.

  L. Complete care within a reasonable amount of time; if the completion of treatment exceeds 1 year, the patient must give *written consent*.

II. Duties of the patient

  A. Pay reasonable fees; fees should be paid within a reasonable length of time.

  B. Cooperate during treatment; involves following instructions given by the health care provider and keeping appointments.

Clinical Case STUDY

Dave Madsen recently graduated from a dental hygiene program and has completed all requirements for licensure. The State Board of Dental Examiners will meet in 6 weeks to issue new licenses. A local dentist has just hired Dave and would like him to begin practicing immediately.

Clinical Case QUESTIONS

1. What government regulation defines the requirements that an individual must meet in order to practice dental hygiene in a given state?
2. What is the State Board of Dental Examiners and what are their duties?
3. Can Dave begin practicing before obtaining his professional license if he has met the requirements for licensure?

Clinical Case RATIONALES

1. The Dental Practice Act is the government regulation that defines the practice of dental hygiene and how an individual can be granted a license to practice in the state.
2. The State Board of Dental Examiners is a group of appointed or elected members (dentists, dental hygienists, and/or consumers) who administer the practice act, issue and revoke licenses, investigate complaints, take disciplinary action, and measure the competence of graduates through state boards.
3. Dave would violate the Dental Practice Act, a crime against society, if he began practicing his profession without a license. If he were convicted of such a violation, he would be subject to punishment.

Government Regulations

The dental profession is regulated by the government regulations of the state dental practice acts.

Dental Practice Act

The dental practice act defines the practice of the dental profession and indicates how an individual may be granted a license to practice within a given state. Practice acts vary from state to state.

I. Purpose

  A. Protects the public from incompetent practitioners.

  B. Prohibits individuals from practicing in the profession before meeting certain qualifications.

  C. Gives authority to state boards of dentistry/dental examiners to issue or deny licensure.

  D. Empowers state boards of dentistry/dental examiners to suspend or revoke licenses.

II. Violations of the Dental Practice Act

  A. Are crimes against society; involve any acts in violation of the practice act.

  B. Subject an individual to punishment if convicted.

  C. Include illegal acts that do not necessarily result in physical harm (e.g., a dental hygienist performs an oral prophylaxis before receiving licensure). Examples of infractions include:

    1. Sex offenses against patients or employees.

    2. The illegal prescription of narcotics.

    3. Insurance fraud.

    4. Tax evasion.

III. State Board of Dental Examiners

  A. Members are appointed or elected and may include dentists, dental hygienists (in most states), and consumers (in many states).

  B. Duties

1. Administering the written word of the state's practice act.
2. Issuing and revoking licenses.
3. Investigating complaints and taking disciplinary action when necessary.
4. Measuring the competence of graduates via state board examinations.

∾ CONTENT REVIEW QUESTIONS ∾

1. The study of conduct, which is based on right and wrong issues, is:
   A. morals
   B. mores
   C. ethics
   D. values

2. The moral evaluation that because it is acceptable for one individual to act a particular way it is therefore acceptable for others to act in the same way is referred to as:
   A. publicity
   B. ultimacy
   C. neutrality
   D. universality

3. An individual who focuses on which actions are right is known as a(n):
   A. action utilitarian
   B. value utilitarian
   C. consequential utilitarian
   D. deontologist
   E. actiontologist

4. Treating others fairly and living by the "golden rule" is known as:
   A. justice
   B. nonmaleficence
   C. beneficence
   D. paternalism

5. A health care provider is responsible for speaking the truth and giving a patient adequate information to allow for sound decisions regarding treatment. This is referred to as:
   A. fidelity
   B. reparation
   C. gratitude
   D. veracity

6. When an ethical decision must be made, all of the following steps are recommended, EXCEPT:
   A. granting patient autonomy
   B. following an employer's directive
   C. avoiding harm
   D. respecting the profession

7. When a dental hygienist does not perform a procedure included in the contract with a patient, it is referred to as:
   A. technical battery
   B. breach of contract
   C. malpractice
   D. negligence

8. Saying or writing something that may damage a patient's reputation is:
   A. breach of contract
   B. technical assault
   C. maligning
   D. negligence

9. Malpractice is one type of:
   A. tort law
   B. breach of contract
   C. criminal law
   D. technical battery

10. When an individual commits a wrongful act against society, it is considered an offense of:
    A. tort law
    B. civil law
    C. contract law
    D. criminal law

11. Failure on the part of the patient to follow instructions given by the dentist during and after treatment is an example of:
    A. contributory negligence
    B. respondeat superior
    C. res gestae
    D. admission against interest

12. All of the following are true regarding patient records, EXCEPT:
    A. are kept for 1 year
    B. include diagnoses
    C. are recorded in ink
    D. include treatment plans

13. The principle that makes the dentist responsible for injuries caused by employees is:
    A. admission against interest
    B. respondeat superior
    C. res gestae
    D. professional reliability

14. A contract initiated by the actions of the parties concerned, in absence of a legally binding contract, is a(n):
    A. parental contract
    B. expressed contract
    C. written contract
    D. implied contract

15. Information acquired about a patient during the course of treatment is considered *privileged communication*, even in a court of law. Exceptions to this rule are made when patients exhibit signs or symptoms of (1) alcoholism; (2) child abuse; (3) illegal drug use; or (4) communicable disease.
    A. 1 and 2
    B. 2 and 3
    C. 1 and 3
    D. 2 and 4
    E. 3 and 4

16. When a dentist is unavailable to a patient at any time during treatment, it may be considered an act of:
    A. withdrawal
    B. abandonment

C. neglect

D. technical assault

17. A patient should give written consent to continue dental treatment if the treatment extends beyond:

A. 3 months

B. 6 months

C. 1 year

D. 2 years

18. Violations of legal principles are handled by the:

A. State Board of Dental Examiners

B. American Dental Association

C. State Practice Act

D. American Dental Hygienists' Association

REVIEW QUESTION RATIONALES

1. **C**   Ethics deals with right and wrong issues regarding conduct and character. Mores are the customs of a group. Morals are standards of thought or specific judgments that are typically, but not always, based on strong religious beliefs. Values are beliefs and attitudes that often are established by an individual's upbringing or religious affiliation.

2. **D**   Universality stresses that if it is good for an individual to act a certain way, it must be acceptable for others to act in the same way. With the moral evaluation of publicity, one publicly states his or her evaluation and how it is based. Neutralism is based on how an evaluation is best for someone else and ultimacy is a judgment based on a moral evaluation that has no higher standard.

3. **A**   The action utilitarian deals with the actions of what is right and is responsible for the consequences of those actions. The value utilitarian focuses on what counts as a good or a harm. A consequential utilitarian decides that an action is right or wrong based on the consequences of the action. The deontologist focuses on the action of an act without worrying about its consequences. There is no such thing as an action-tologist.

4. **A**   Treating others fairly and giving them their just due is known as justice. Nonmaleficence is identifying an action as wrong if harm is inflicted on an individual. Beneficence defines an action as moral if it is good and helps a person. Paternalism involves acting as a parent would, including overriding a decision for the good of an individual.

5. **D**   Veracity claims that a health care provider has an obligation to speak the truth and keep the patient abreast of all information that is needed to make sound decisions during treatment. Fidelity stresses the duty to maintain confidentiality. Reparation is the act of making amends to an individual who was harmed and gratitude is the act of showing respect to someone who has helped you.

6. **B**   When making an ethical decision, it is important to evaluate one's values. Granting a patient's autonomy is a necessary part of the process. The patient can be active in determining his or her treatment and can participate in the decision making regarding the treatment plan. It also is vital to avoid harm to others. The health care provider should have a conscience and a respect for the profession. An employer's direction may not offer the appropriate guidelines for making a decision.

7. **B**   Breach of contract involves the breaking of a contract (an agreement) by either party involved. Technical battery is an act performed that was not agreed on by the patient. Malpractice, often considered synonymous with negligence, is a form of carelessness that brings harm to a patient. The act that results in harm to the patient does not have to be intentional.

8. **C**   Maligning an individual involves saying or writing something that can damage that individual's reputation. Slander involves saying something that can destroy an individual's reputation and libel involves writing something that yields the same result.

9. **A**   Malpractice is a civil wrong that is handled under tort law. It involves an injury to a patient that occurs without an intent to harm. Such injuries typically are a result of carelessness. Criminal law involves wrongs against society. In such cases, the state takes action against the health care provider.

10. **D**   A criminal law pertains to a criminal action that is a wrong against society (e.g., an individual practicing dental hygiene without a license). Tort and contract laws are examples of civil law; lawsuits are filed with a private attorney and damages typically are measured monetarily.

11. **A**   Contributory negligence describes a patient's contribution to the harm. An example follows: a patient has periodontal problems and is advised to follow a 3-month oral prophylaxis maintenance program. However, the patient has failed to keep his appointments for the past 2 years. When he finally does keep an oral prophylaxis appointment, his condition is worse. Because the broken appointments were recorded in the patient's chart, one can claim that the patient contributed to the negligence. Respondeat superior indicates that the dentist is responsible for the wrongful actions of his or her employees. Res gestae is a statement that an individual makes during a negligent act and that can be used against him or her in a lawsuit. Admission against interest is a statement made at any time that goes against the legal interest of that patient.

12. **A**   Patient records should be kept on file for the length of the statute of limitations within a state. They always should be neatly recorded in ink and should include a complete record of the diagnosis, treatment plans, updated medical history, correspondence, radiographs, and record of treatment.

13. **B**   Respondeat superior is the principle that makes the dentist responsible for a wrongful action that caused harm to a patient. Admission against interest is a statement that is made, verbally or in writing, that

may prove to be the opposite of what one is contending in court and can be used in a lawsuit. Professional reliability states that every professional has the responsibility to provide good dental care to patients.

14. **D** An implied contract is established by certain actions on the part of the health care provider or patient. An expressed contract is informed consent given in writing or verbally. Parental/guardian consent is given when the patient is a minor or is mentally incompetent to give consent. Written consent provides the most protection for the patient and is a form of expressed consent.

15. **D** Privileged communication grants the patient autonomy. What the patient confides in the office must remain confidential. However, there are two exceptions. When suspected child abuse or communicable disease has not been reported, the proper authorities must be contacted.

16. **B** Abandonment is the result of desertion. The health care provider fails to provide services that the two parties had agreed upon. If the dentist is on vacation, provisions must be made for the period of absence. Withdrawal is the act of terminating treatment before it is completed. Neglect is failure to meet the appropriate standard of care and technical assault is a wrongful act that has not been agreed on.

17. **C** Treatment should be completed within 1 year of its initiation. If it extends beyond that time, the patient should give written consent.

18. **A** The State Board of Dental Examiners are appointed or elected members who are responsible for administering the written law of a state, or its practice act. They also are responsible for issuing and revoking licenses and investigating any complaints submitted to them. The American Dental Association and the American Dental Hygienists' Association do not administer any legal actions. The state practice act defines the practice of the dental profession and provides guidelines regarding licensure within the state.

Reference

1. American Dental Hygienists Association: Code of ethics for dental hygienists. J Dent Hyg 69(4):159–162, 1995.

Additional Readings

Becker LC, Becker CB: Encyclopedia of Ethics, 1st ed. New York, Garland, 1992.

Beauchamp TL, Walters L: Contemporary Issues in Bioethics, 4th ed. Belmont, Calif, Wadsworth, 1994.

Rule JT, Veatch RM: Ethical Questions in Dentistry, 1st ed. Carol Stream, Ill, Quintessence, 1993.

Weinstein BD: Dental Ethics, 1st ed. Philadelphia, Lea and Febiger, 1993.

Woodall IR: Legal, Ethical, and Management Aspects of the Dental Care System, 3rd ed. St. Louis, Mosby, 1987.

Simulated National Board Dental Hygiene Examination

This simulated examination consists of two parts. Part A contains 200 randomly-ordered multiple choice questions, answers, and rationales, and Part B contains 150 case-based questions, answers, and rationales. Read each question carefully and select the BEST answer choice. There is only one correct answer per question. Once the examination is completed, answer selections may be compared with the correct choices listed in the rationale section at the end of the examination section.

Part A: QUESTIONS

1. Sensory impulses from a toothache are likely to be transmitted on:
   A. cranial nerve I
   B. cranial nerve III
   C. cranial nerve V
   D. cranial nerve VII

2. Viruses can be distinguished from all other microorganisms by virtue of their:
   A. ability to be isolated from the blood
   B. necessity to replicate intracellularly
   C. resistance to antibodies
   D. possession of only one type of nucleic acid

3. Too little vertical angulation will result in:
   A. cone-cut
   B. elongation
   C. overlapping
   D. foreshortening

4. Which of the following describes a Class I furcation involvement?
   A. a slight concavity is detectable, but no radiolucency is visible on the radiograph
   B. a concavity is detectable, but does not extend between the facial and lingual; a slight radiolucency is visible on the radiograph
   C. a concavity is detectable, but does not extend between the mesial and distal; a large radiolucency is visible on the radiograph
   D. a concavity is detectable and extends between the facial and lingual; a large radioluecency is visible on the radiograph

5. Systemic diseases associated with early onset periodontitis include:
   A. Down syndrome, hypophosphatasia, diabetes

   B. Chediak-Higashi syndrome, Papillon-Lefèvre syndrome, hypophosphatasia
   C. Papillon-Lefèvre syndrome, AIDS, Chediak-Higashi syndrome
   D. diabetes, leukemia, Papillon-Lefèvre, hypophosphatasia

6. Kaposi's sarcoma is most commonly located on the:
   A. palate
   B. tongue
   C. fauces
   D. floor of the mouth

7. Which of the following could be used for removal of tenacious subgingival calculus in deep, narrow pockets with firm, fibrotic tissue?
   A. sickle scaler
   B. periodontal file
   C. hoe
   D. chisel
   E. universal curet

8. Oral manifestations of bulimia include all of the following, EXCEPT one. Which one is the EXCEPTION?
   A. dental erosion
   B. enlarged parotid glands
   C. inflamed interdental papillae
   D. thermal sensitivity
   E. leukoedema

9. Subgingival calculus gets it mineral content from
   A. crevicular fluid
   B. food nutrients
   C. blood products
   D. saliva

10. A dense, fibrous, raised, skin-colored lesion located on the buccal mucosa at the height of the occlusal plane is most likely a

A. hematoma
B. sponge nevus
C. granuloma
D. fibroma

11. The appearance of spongy rolled gingival margins and bulbous gingival papilla are the result of
    A. fibroblastic proliferation
    B. vascular hyperemia
    C. accumulation of tissue fluid
    D. micro ulceration of the epithelial attachment

12. When duplicating radiographs, the duplicating film is placed closest to the light source. The greatest density of the duplicated image will occur with the longest exposure to the light source.
    A. both statements are TRUE
    B. both statements are FALSE
    C. the first statement is TRUE, the second statement is FALSE
    D. the first statement is FALSE, the second statement is TRUE

13. Periodontal debridement of the maxillary left quadrant will require administration of a local anesthetic. Which nerve block injection will NOT provide anesthesia to the area?
    A. inferior alveolar
    B. greater palatine
    C. incisive
    D. posterior superior alveolar

14. Proper ultrasonic scaling technique is best described by which of the following?
    A. light stroke pressure and horizontal strokes
    B. light stroke pressure and multidirectional strokes
    C. adaptation on the point of the tip and multidirectional strokes
    D. adaptation on the point of the tip and horizontal strokes

15. Infection of a deciduous tooth may cause
    A. commissural lip pits
    B. static bone cyst
    C. hypodontia
    D. Turner's spot

16. Alginate impressions are displaced from the mouth in a quick, continuous movement to prevent
    A. distortion of the impression
    B. trauma to the oral tissues
    C. gagging by the patient
    D. loss of impression detail

17. When placing pit and fissure sealants, a topical fluoride
    A. should be applied immediately before the sealant is placed
    B. should be applied immediately after the sealant is placed
    C. should be applied one month post sealant placement
    D. is contraindicated whenever sealants are placed

18. Facial asymmetry is commonly associated with
    A. lupus erythematosus
    B. Lyme disease
    C. hypothyroidism
    D. Tourette's syndrome
    E. Bell's palsy

19. The predominant bacteria in adult periodontitis is
    A. *P. gingivalis*
    B. Eubacterium
    C. *A. actinomycetemcomitans*
    D. *Streptococcus* spp.

20. Silver halide crystals are placed in the film emulsion BECAUSE the crystals protect the film from heat, moisture, and chemicals.
    A. both the statement and reason are correct and related.
    B. both the statement and reason are correct but NOT related
    C. the statement is correct, but the reason is NOT
    D. the statement is NOT correct, but the reason is correct
    E. NEITHER the statement NOR the reason is correct

21. A person with an oral herpes lesion of the lip should do all of the following, EXCEPT one. Which one is the EXCEPTION?
    A. reschedule appointment for two weeks
    B. avoid intimate contact with others
    C. get plenty of bed rest
    D. spent more time in the sun
    E. increase intake of Vitamin C

22. A patient with congestive heart failure will most likely require
    A. an upright seating position
    B. nitroglycerin tablets
    C. longer appointments
    D. antibiotic premedication

23. All of the following are characteristics of a root planing technique EXCEPT one. Which one is the EXCEPTION?
    A. stroke length becomes progressively longer
    B. strokes are multidirectional and cross-hatched
    C. lateral pressure becomes progressively heavier
    D. grasp on the instrument is moderate to light

24. The continuing care schedule for a periodontal patient should be determined by
    A. the amount of calculus build-up
    B. the patient's income or desire
    C. the amount of inflammation seen
    D. the standard office recall schedule

25. All of the following drugs are antifungal and are used to treat candidiasis, EXCEPT one. Which one is the EXCEPTION?
    A. nystatin (Mycostatin)
    B. clotrimazole (Gyne-Lotrimin)
    C. ketoconazole (Nizoral)
    D. fluconazole (Diflucan)
    E. didanosine (ddl)

26. Parent supervision of fluoride use by small children is important to prevent which of the following
    A. chronic toxicity

B. fluorosis on primary teeth

C. green stain on permanent teeth

D. extra cusp formation on permanent teeth

27. Which defect is the result of failure of the maxillary processes to fuse with the median nasal processes?

A. unilateral cleft lip

B. bilateral cleft lip

C. partial cleft palate

D. complete cleft palate

28. Complications of AIDS-associated Necrotizing Ulcerative Periodontitis (NUP) which differentiate it from the conventional non-AIDS associated form of NUP may include

A. deep crater-like osseous lesions

B. sequestration of bone fragments

C. lack of conventional periodontal pockets

D. gangrenous stomatitis

29. The TMJ disk is attached to the

A. temporal bone

B. mandibular condyle

C. ethmoid bone

D. zygomatic process

30. A patient taking amphetamines is likely to exhibit all of the following EXCEPT one. Which one is the EXCEPTION?

A. hyperactivity

B. increased blood pressure

C. appetite suppression

D. mental depression

31. During periodontal therapy, the dental hygienist discussed the importance of daily plaque removal with the patient and modified the patient's flossing technique. At the continuing care appointment, the dental hygienist notes generalized bleeding and heavy plaque and calculus accumulation interproximally. Failure on the part of the patient to follow instructions given by the dentist hygienist is an example of

A. contributory negligence

B. *res gestae*

C. *respondeat superior*

D. admission against interest.

32. Zinc polycarboxylate cements are used to bond enamel. Their advantage over zinc phosphate cements is their adhesive property with calcium and carboxylate groups.

A. both statements are TRUE

B. both statements are FALSE

C. the first statement is TRUE, the second is FALSE

D. the first statement is FALSE, the second is TRUE

33. A well-defined red band of marginal gingiva adjacent to a base metal crown is likely to be caused by all of the following, EXCEPT one. Which one is the EXCEPTION?

A. inadequate oral hygiene

B. reactivity of metals in the crown

C. crown infringement on biological width

D. food impaction

E. overcontoured crown

34. When evaluating the relationship between sugar in the patient's diet and level of decay, the most important factor to determine in the patient's diet diary is

A. the type of sugar consumed.

B. the quantity of sugar consumed.

C. the consistency of sugar consumed.

D. the frequency of sugar consumed.

35. All of the following are true regarding power toothbrushes EXCEPT one. Which one is the EXCEPTION?

A. brushing technique is product dependent

B. removes more plaque than manual brush

C. brush motion can be rotational

D. recommended for patients with grasping difficulties

36. When an infrabony periodontal pocket forms, the junctional epithelium

A. is positioned apical to the CEJ.

B. migrates coronally

C. is coronal to the CEJ and the crest of the alveolar bone

D. is apical to the crest of the alveolar bone.

37. Utilizing G.V. Black's carious lesion classification system, a Class III lesion would involve the:

A. gingival 1/3 of the facial or lingual surfaces of an anterior or posterior tooth

B. proximal surface and incisal edge of an anterior tooth

C. proximal surface of an anterior or posterior tooth

D. proximal surface of a central, lateral, or cuspid

E. lingual surface of an anterior tooth

38. Patients taking antihistamines for allergy symptoms may exhibit

A. irritability

B. anxiety

C. sedation

D. trembling

39. Alcoholism is treated pharmacologically with

A. disulfiram (Antabuse)

B. diflunisal (Dolobid)

C. albuterol (Proventil)

D. methadone HCl (Dolophine)

40. The initial vascular response during acute inflammation is initiated by the release of

A. prostaglandins

B. histamine

C. kinins

D. lysosomes

41. The following are major cause(s) of temporomandibular joint disorder, EXCEPT one, Which one is the EXCEPTION?

A. stress

B. arthritis

C. trauma

D. trismus

42. Which one of the following collimator types can most effectively reduce scatter radiation to the patient?

A. long round

B. pointed plastic
C. rectangular
D. short round

43. Sufficient frictional heat can be generated by rubber-up polishing to cause discomfort to a patient. Frictional heat can be controlled (reduced) by using the rubber cup with a light touch, rapid patting or sweeping motion, high speed, and wet abrasive agent.
   A. both statements are TRUE
   B. both statements are FALSE
   C. the first statement is TRUE, the second is FALSE
   D. the first statement is FALSE, the second is TRUE

44. When taking radiographs during the first dental visit of a five-year-old with clinical signs of decay and anterior crowding, the bitewing radiographs should be exposed before the occlusal films. Positioning for the mandibular occlusal radiograph requires the patient's head be tipped back approximately 90 degrees.
   A. both statements are TRUE
   B. both statements are FALSE
   C. the first statement is TRUE, the second is FALSE
   D. the first statement is FALSE, the second is TRUE

45. When suspicious of abuse of a child or dependent adult, what should one do first?
   A. report suspicions to the local authorities, such as Social Services
   B. ask the parent for permission to photograph the dependent
   C. discuss abuse with the caregiver and try to get a confession
   D. report the incident if it is a second suspicious occurrence

46. On the day an HIV+ patient is scheduled for an oral prophylaxis, the dental hygienist feigns illness and goes home. This is an example of
   A. malpractice
   B. breach of contract
   C. negligence
   D. unethical conduct
   E. nonmaleficence

47. A radiographic sign of periodontal breakdown is the presence of
   A. fuzziness of the alveolar crests
   B. intact lamina dura
   C. radiolucency of the periodontal ligament space
   D. breakdown of the facial and lingual cortical plates

48. Which of the following microorganisms has been shown to predominate in Localized Juvenile Periodontitis?
   A. *A. actinomycetemcomitans*
   B. *P. gingivalis*
   C. *P. intermedia*
   D. *E. corrodens*

49. Immune protection of mucous membranes from infection is most closely associated with
   A. IgA antibodies

B. IgE antibodies
C. cytotoxic T cells
D. complement

50. A new patient presents with a suspicious lesion covering one half of the floor of the mouth and part of the ventral surface of the tongue. The lesion presents as a mixture of velvety-red areas and white hyperkeratotic-appearing areas. The most likely course of action would be to recommend
   A. reevaluation in 3 weeks
   B. excisional biopsy
   C. incisional biopsy
   D. exfoliative cytology

51. Which would be the most appropriate treatment for a health care worker who is the victim of a needle-stick injury involving a hepatitis B-positive patient?
   A. active immunization with hepatitis B vaccine
   B. passive immunization with pooled human gamma globulin
   C. active immunization with pertussis vaccine
   D. conservative therapy of the wound with hexachlorophene

52. The principal origin of the middle and lower face is the
   A. globular process
   B. median nasal process
   C. maxillary process
   D. mandibular arch

53. The active ingredient in many prescription in-home bleaching kits is
   A. sodium citrate
   B. carbamide peroxide
   C. sodium hypochlorite
   D. zinc-oxide eugenol

54. Primary herpetic gingivostomatitis
   A. occurs primarily in older adults
   B. presents with fever, ulcerating vesicles and pain
   C. typically involves the buccal mucosa and chin
   D. is a severe outbreak of apthous ulcers

55. A patient has a nondraining periapical abscess and reminds the dentist that she is allergic to penicillin. The following drug can be prescribed as an adjunct to safely manage the patient's abscess
   A. cloxacillin (Cloxapen)
   B. amoxicillin (Amoxil)
   C. terfenadine (Seldane)
   D. doxycycline (Doxycin)
   E. diflunisal (Dolobid)

56. Radiographically, a jaw fracture will appear as a radiolucent line. Internal resorption appears as a radiolucency within the pulp or dentin of a tooth.
   A. both statements are TRUE
   B. both statements are FALSE
   C. the first statement is TRUE, the second is FALSE
   D. the first statement is FALSE, the second is TRUE

57. For a patient taking medication daily for hypertension and no other conditions, the concern dentally is
   A. the medication may mask inflammation

B. the greater chance of syncope

C. the diuretic medication may alter clotting time

D. the increased risk of congestive heart failure

58. While walking a patient from the reception area to the operatory, the patient becomes noticeably out of breath. Which of the following actions should occur next?

A. begin cardiopulmonary resuscitation efforts immediately after calling for emergency medical assistance

B. rush the patient to the operatory, seat him in a supine position, and take his pulse, blood pressure, and respirations

C. reschedule the patient for an appointment later in the week before walking him slowly to his car

D. allow the patient to rest for a few minutes before proceeding to the chair, review his medical history and make treatment decisions based on additional information obtained from patient and/or physician consultation.

59. The dental hygienist has been asked to discontinue instrument sharpening because of cost concerns. All of the following are concerns associated with use of dull instruments, EXCEPT one. Which one is the EXCEPTION?

A. safety

B. effectiveness

C. patient comfort

D. debris detection

E. infection control

60. All of the following are true of pit and fissure sealants, EXCEPT one. Which one is the EXCEPTION?

A. seals out bacteria and nutrients

B. prevents further decay

C. indicated when proximal decay exists

D. made of Bis-GMA organic monomer

E. added fillers may be glass particles

61. After completion of a periodontal debridement session, the instrument cutting edges are covered with dried blood. What should be done first to prepare them for sterilization?

A. scrub the cutting edges with a stiff-bristle brush

B. soak the instruments in water with detergent

C. place the instruments in an ultrasonic cleaner

D. dip the cutting edges in 70% isopropyl alcohol

62. Oral irrigators are effective for all of the following EXCEPT one. Which one is the EXCEPTION?

A. removing attached plaque

B. reducing gingivitis

C. reducing plaque toxicity

D. delivering antimicrobial agents

63. Of the following permanent teeth, which one is MOST frequently congenitally missing?

A. maxillary second molar

B. mandibular canine

C. maxillary central incisor

D. mandibular second premolar

64. During an extra-oral inspection, swollen lymph nodes are detected beneath the chin. Which lymph nodes are these?

A. submandibular

B. preauricular

C. cervical

D. submental

65. The maximum absorbed dose of radiation that a 38 year-old dental hygienist should receive is

A. 35 R

B. 72 R

C. 100 R

D. 175 R

66. The ideal angle for insertion of a curet into a periodontal pocket in preparation for a scaling stroke is

A. 0 degrees

B. 15 degrees

C. 40 degrees

D. 90 degrees

67. The need to increase the dose of a drug to produce the same drug effect is called

A. drug dependence

B. physical dependence

C. drug tolerance

D. addiction

E. drug abuse

68. An isolated port-hole defect in bone which exposes the underlying root of the tooth is referred to as a

A. fenestration

B. dehiscence

C. buttress

D. festoon

69. Blood-soaked gauze is considered biomedical waste and must be sterilized or incinerated. Blood and saliva contaminated gloves must be washed before disposing of in the trash.

A. both statements are TRUE

B. both statements are FALSE

C. first statement is TRUE, the second is FALSE

D. first statement is FALSE, the second is TRUE

70. The triceps brachii muscle functions to straighten (extend) the elbow joints. This muscle:

A. inserts on a bone of the forearm, the ulna

B. originates on a bone of the forearm, the radius

C. inserts on the humerus

D. is an agonist of the biceps brachii

71. Treatment for xerostomia may include:

A. anticholinergics

B. antihistamines

C. diuretics

D. antipsychotics

72. For which emergency situation would it be better NOT to use oxygen?

A. syncope

B. diabetic coma

C. asthma attack

D. hyperventilation

73. *Candida albicans* is known or suspected to cause all of

the following denture-related problems EXCEPT one. Which one is the EXCEPTION?

A. denture stomatitis
B. epulis fissuratum
C. papillary hyperplasia
D. angular cheilitis

74. A patient completing a two-week regimen of amoxicillin for a periapical abscess complains of a sore mouth. The examination reveals a thick whitish coating on the palate and buccal mucosa. This coating is most likely

A. linea albicans
B. lichen planus
C. hairy leukoplakia
D. candidiasis

75. Stenosis of the bicuspid valve is likely to initially cause a backup of blood in the:

A. inferior and superior vena cava
B. left ventricle and systemic arteries
C. right atrium and systemic veins
D. left atrium, pulmonary veins, and lungs

76. All of the following affect image sharpness, EXCEPT one. Which one is the EXCEPTION?

A. focal spot size
B. object to film distance
C. film speed
D. source to object distance
E. exposure time

77. Embryonic cells trapped in fusion lines during facial development may become

A. cysts
B. clefts
C. granulomas
D. cementomas
E. supernumerary teeth

78. A patient indicates a current history of shingles. What is this condition?

A. hemorrhoids
B. herpes zoster
C. psoriasis
D. eczema

79. Hypothyroidism can result in:

A. an elevated metabolic rate
B. an increased heart rate
C. slow tooth eruption
D. increased numbers of catecholaminergic receptors

80. Which one of the following is the BEST aid for plaque and debris removal in an area where the papilla is missing?

A. oral irrigator
B. waxed floss
C. dental tape
D. interdental brush

81. Glycolysis is:

A. the pathway for breaking-down glucose to pyruvate
B. the pathway for conversion of pyruvate into acetyl CoA

C. the pathway for production of both NADH and $FADH_2$
D. the pathway for donating electrons for production of ATP

82. During the intra and extra-oral examination, which of the following findings would be of greatest concern?

A. pea-sized, soft, movable nodule on the superficial cervical lymph nodes
B. several brown pigmentations on the lip of a person of Hispanic descent
C. fixed, non-movable mass of the deep cervical lymph nodes
D. mucous retention cyst on the floor of the mouth
E. limited tongue movement resulting in a speech disorder

83. The largest group of Principal Fibers of the periodontal ligament which prevents tilting and dislocation of the tooth is the

A. alveolar crest group
B. horizontal group
C. oblique group
D. apical group

84. All of the following are effects of periodontal pocket lavage by an ultrasonic scaler, EXCEPT one. Which one is the EXCEPTION?

A. acoustic microstreaming
B. lysing and killing of bacterial cells
C. flushing away blood and debris
D. creating a smooth root surface

85. When taking blood pressure the "auscultatory gap" indicates an irregular heart beat. Having the patient raise his/her arm for several seconds before inflating the cuff can eliminate the "auscultatory gap."

A. both statements are TRUE
B. both statements are FALSE
C. first statement is TRUE, the second if FALSE
D. first statement is FALSE, the second is TRUE

86. During a review of the patient's dental experience, you learn that tooth #8 was traumatized during a bicycle accident about 6 months ago. The tooth was sensitive for a week but is not sensitive now. Teeth #'s 7, 8, and 9 all respond similarly when you test them with palpation, percussion, and cold. It would be reasonable to conclude that at this time, the tooth pulp

A. is normal
B. has reversible pulpitis
C. has irreversible pulpitis
D. is necrotic

87. A patient is a Hepatitis B carrier. Which one of the following is an appropriate way to prevent cross-contamination?

A. wear double gloves
B. avoid ultrasonic scaler
C. HBV immunization
D. reschedule patient

88. Professional treatment of root sensitivity may include all of the following, EXCEPT one. Which one is the EXCEPTION?
    A. fluoride varnishes
    B. mineral solutions
    C. dentin sealers
    D. iontophoresis
    E. zinc-oxide eugenol

89. When a radiograph is only partially immersed in developer, but fully immersed in fixer, the resultant processed film will exhibit a black area. Radiographs that are inadequately rinsed following fixing will develop yellow-brown stains later.
    A. both statements are TRUE
    B. both statements are FALSE
    C. first statement is TRUE, the second is FALSE
    D. first statement is FALSE, the second is TRUE

90. Which of the following palpation techniques best describes bidigital palpation?
    A. all fingers of one hand are used to grasp tissues
    B. one finger is used to examine tissues
    C. fingers move in a circular motion while applying pressure to the issues
    D. tissues are grasped between finger(s) and thumb to examine tissues

91. An infrabony pocket in which facial and lingual alveolar bone is missing is classified as a (an)
    A. one-walled pocket
    B. two-walled pocket
    C. three-walled pocket
    D. four-walled pocket

92. For removal of a heavy ledge of calculus on the lingual surface of the mandibular anterior teeth, which of the following is the best tip and power combination?
    A. slim/thin style tip at medium to high power
    B. slim/thin style tip at low to medium power
    C. standard tip at medium to high power
    D. standard tip at low to medium power

93. Polishing of amalgams helps prevent corrosion and improves longevity of amalgam restorations. Overheating of the amalgam during polishing can result in damage to odontoblasts.
    A. both statements are TRUE
    B. both statements are FALSE
    C. first statement is TRUE, the second is FALSE
    D. first statement is FALSE, the second is TRUE

94. Endogenous intrinsic stain is associated with all of the following, EXCEPT one. Which one is the EXCEPTION?
    A. fluorosis
    B. traumatized pulp
    C. tetracycline ingestion
    D. genetic anomalies
    E. caries

95. Nicotine stomatitis presents itself as
    A. ulcerated fluid-filled lesions with red halos
    B. pimple-like lesions with diffuse purplish coating

C. tiny nodules with red center and diffuse grayish-white coating
    D. varicosities across the palate and buccal mucosa

96. Following injection of the posterior superior alveolar nerve, a patient complains of inadequate "numbing" and receives additional cartridges of 2% lidocaine with 1:100,000 epinephrine. The patient begins to talk incessantly, exhibits restlessness and becomes drowsy, and then suffers a convulsion. These symptoms are MOST likely a(an)
    A. fear reaction to the injection procedures
    B. toxicity reaction to the local anesthetic agent
    C. synergistic effect between the local anesthetic and the vasoconstrictor
    D. anaphylactic reaction to the vasoconstricting agent

97. Sulcular epithelium is generally
    A. keratinized
    B. ortho-keratinized
    C. para-keratinized
    D. non-keratinized

98. A newly processed radiograph appears light. This is most likely due to
    A. contaminated fixing solution
    B. insufficient fixing time
    C. overexposure to developing solution
    D. cold developing solution

99. Cushing's syndrome is associated with obesity, hirsutism, and moon face. This condition is caused by
    A. overproduction of ACTH
    B. excessive production of GH
    C. undersecretion of TSH
    D. inadequate production of FSH

100. A patient requires a prophylactic antibiotic regimen due to a history of infective endocarditis. He is allergic to penicillin and takes astemizole (Hismanal). The American Heart Association (AHA) anti-infective agent regimen-of-choice for this patient is
    A. amoxicillin (Amoxil)
    B. azithromycin (Zithromax)
    C. clindamycin (Cleocin)
    D. tetracycline (Tetracyn)

101. Opsonins are
    A. cytokines produced by B cells
    B. antigens that directly neutralize viruses
    C. antibodies deficient in the Fc region
    D. molecules that stimulate phagocytosis

102. If a deposit of calculus is difficult to remove with an ultrasonic scaler, which of the following should be adjusted?
    A. water flow
    B. power level
    C. lateral pressure
    D. air intake

103. Which of the following conditions is NOT associated with tongue thrusting?
    A. overjet
    B. gingival recession

C. open bite

D. protrusive lower lip

104. Essential amino acids are defined as such because they
   A. are vital to the production of lipids
   B. cannot be synthesized by the body
   C. are needed to regulate blood pressure
   D. are necessary for immune defenses

105. Patients with fixed orthodontic appliances often need extensive instruction in plaque control methods in order to remove the more virulent bacterial plaque they develop. A daily self-applied fluoride treatment should be a standard recommendation for these patients to prevent decalcification and caries.
   A. both statements are TRUE
   B. both statements are FALSE
   C. first statement is TRUE, the second is FALSE
   D. first statement is FALSE, the second is TRUE

106. A film has good density when produced at 10 mA and 6/10 seconds. At 15 mA, what exposure time is need to maintain the density?
   A. 0.4 seconds
   B. 0.8 seconds
   C. 1.2 seconds
   D. 1.6 seconds

107. Which one of the following will produce a film with low contrast?
   A. high kVp
   B. low kVp
   C. high mA
   D. low mA

108. Hormones produced by the pancreas include:
   A. insulin and glucagon
   B. insulin and thyroxine
   C. glucagon and cortisol
   D. epinephrine and norepinephrine

109. To correct closed contacts on a radiograph, one would adjust
   A. horizontal angulation
   B. patient positioning
   C. vertical angulation
   D. film placement

110. Which external landmark helps determine central ray placement when exposing a radiograph of a maxillary canine?
   A. outer corner of the eye
   B. ala of the nose
   C. nasal septum
   D. tragus-ala line

111. Junctional epithelium
   A. separates the periodontal ligament from the oral environment
   B. is called gingival connective tissue
   C. is made up of five distinct fiber bundle groups
   D. defines the coronal margin of the gingival sulcus

112. Area-specific curet V has a shank with complex angles and is designed for use in periodontal pocket of 5 mm or less in depth. What design characteristic would need to be changed in order for instrument V to work well in pockets over 5 mm in depth?
   A. shank thickness
   B. terminal shank length
   C. blade width
   D. lateral surface curvature
   E. blade back

113. A fracture of the zygomatic bone is a fracture of
   A. the cranium
   B. the face
   C. the wrist
   D. the appendicular skeleton

114. Which one of the following nerves is a branch of the mandibular nerve?
   A. posterior superior alveolar
   B. inferior alveolar
   C. infraorbital
   D. anterior superior alveolar

115. A component of gram-negative bacteria that functions as a potent endotoxin is
   A. lipoteicoic acid
   B. lipoprotein
   C. lipopolysaccharide
   D. mycolic acid

116. When placing a periodontal dressing over a surgical site, the pack material should be pressed into the interproximal spaces. No pack material should be placed above the height of contour of the teeth.
   A. both statements are TRUE
   B. both statements are FALSE
   C. first statement is TRUE, the second is FALSE
   D. first statement if FALSE, the second is TRUE

117. Which vitamin deficiency during pregnancy may contribute to a spinal birth defect in the infant?
   A. cobalamin
   B. folate
   C. biotin
   D. pantothenic acid

118. Stressed college-students may develop this bacillus-type bacterial infection. Symptoms include oral ulceration, pain, and fever.
   A. primary herpetic gingivostomatitis
   B. gingival hyperplasia
   C. steroid-hormone-induced gingivitis
   D. acute necrotizing ulcerative gingivitis

119. A structure comprised of polysaccharides molecules that is responsible for adherence of bacteria to surfaces such as teeth is called a
   A. flagellum
   B. glycocalyx
   C. capsule
   D. plasmid

120. What viral disease exhibits fever, lymphadenopathy, malaise, and palatal petechiae?
   A. histoplasmosis
   B. tuberculosis
   C. moniliasis
   D. mononucleosis

121. A malignant tumor with etiology directly related to exposure to sunlight is a
    A. basal cell carcinoma
    B. juvenile melanoma
    C. squamous carcinoma
    D. intradermal nevus

122. All of the following are true about anaphylaxis, EXCEPT one. Which ONE is the exception?
    A. occurs only in adults
    B. describes an allergic reaction
    C. may be induced by contact with latex
    D. is treated by injection with epinephrine

123. Signs, symptoms, and side effects of diabetes mellitus include all of the following, EXCEPT one. Which one is the EXCEPTION?
    A. parotid gland enlargement and xerostomia
    B. confusion, slurred speech, and clammy skin
    C. increased incidence or oral and other infections
    D. heart, kidney, eye, and neurological problems
    E. rapid weight gain and increased salivation

124. The swelling associated with an infection involving the lingual of a maxillary second molar is often located in the submental space. Ludwig's angina is a cellulitis that can be caused by the spread of a dental infection from the submental space.
    A. both statements are TRUE
    B. both statements are FALSE
    C. first statement is TRUE, the second is FALSE
    D. first statement is FALSE, the second is TRUE

125. Proper control of infection when producing a study model requires
    A. patient rinsing with chlorhexidine gluconate
    B. disinfection of the impression
    C. steam heating the dental plaster
    D. dry heat sterilization of the model

126. Hutchinson's triad is a result of congenital infection with
    A. *Treponema pallidum*
    B. Epstein-Barr virus
    C. *Neisseria gonorrhea*
    D. Histoplasmosis encapsulatum

127. A patient with a midline shift on opening that continues to increase as the mandible opens has
    A. deflection
    B. crepitus
    C. deviation
    D. trismus

128. The initial vascular response during acute inflammation is initiated by the release of
    A. prostaglandins
    B. histamine
    C. kinins
    D. lysosomes

129. Which one of the following bacteria influences root caries?
    A. *Actinomyces viscosus*
    B. *Prevotella intermedia*

C. *Fusobacterium species*
D. gram-positive cocci

130. When etching a tooth for sealant placement, deciduous teeth are etched for a longer period of time than are permanent teeth. Rinsing a saliva-contaminated etched surface immediately prior to sealant placement will remove the contamination.
    A. both statements are TRUE
    B. both statements are FALSE
    C. first statement is TRUE, the second is FALSE
    D. first statement is FALSE, the second is TRUE

131. Bis-GMA is the
    A. resin in pit and fissure sealants
    B. glass filler in composites
    C. mercury component in amalgams
    D. powder component in cements

132. During exploratory strokes made with either a curet or explorer, the modified pen grasp should be kept very light in order to feel the vibration created as the instrument moves over the tooth. There is a correlation between the tightness of the grasp on the instrument and the amount of lateral pressure applied against the tooth.
    A. both statements are TRUE
    B. both statements are FALSE
    C. first statement is TRUE, the second is FALSE
    D. first statement is FALSE, the second is TRUE

133. Which one of the following is a coating material on dental implants that improves bonding with bone?
    A. strontium chloride
    B. hydroxyapatite
    C. chlorhexidine gluconate
    D. calcium carbonate

134. When the directional migration of PMNLs toward attracting molecules such as bacteria is impaired, the condition is referred to as a(n)
    A. adherence defect
    B. chemotactic defect
    C. leukopenic defect
    D. migration defect

135. All of the following muscles are responsible for opening and closing the jaws, EXCEPT one. Which one is the EXCEPTION?
    A. thyrohyoid
    B. suprahyoid
    C. pterygoid
    D. temporalis
    E. masseter

136. Bifurcated roots are common to maxillary first premolars. Mandibular second premolars often have three cusps.
    A. both statements are TRUE
    B. both statements are FALSE
    C. first statement is TRUE, the second is FALSE
    D. first statement is FALSE, the second is TRUE

137. What characteristic do adult periodontitis and localized juvenile periodontitis share?
    A. age of onset

B. rate of tissue destruction
C. immune system defects
D. specific bacteria as causative agents
E. loss of attachment

138. Secretions of the parotid gland are
A. primarily serous
B. primarily mucous
C. both serous and mucous
D. neither serous nor mucous

139. Mrs. Smith has a history of hypertension and takes medication to treat it. She complains that her gums look swollen and an intraoral exam reveals gingival overgrowth. The medication causing this adverse reaction is most likely
A. furosemide (Lasix)
B. hydrochlorothiazide (Hydro-Chlor)
C. captopril (Capoten)
D. nifedipine (Procardia)

140. In 10% of periodontal cases, standard professional therapy and home care do not improve or stop the progression of the disease. What is this condition?
A. recurrent periodontitis
B. rapidly progressive periodontitis
C. refractory periodontitis
D. acute necrotizing periodontitis

141. Which of the following oral manifestations, when it persists longer than one month in the oral cavity, is recognized by the Centers for Disease Control and Prevention to be AIDS-defining?
A. oral candidiasis
B. herpes simplex virus lesions
C. oral hairy leukoplakia
D. Kaposi's sarcoma

142. With which condition is Sjögren's syndrome most commonly associated?
A. xerostomia
B. median rhomboid glossitis
C. leukoedema
D. geographic tongue

143. Mucosa of the oral cavity floor is considered
A. lining mucosa
B. specialized mucosa
C. masticatory mucosa
D. secretory mucosa

144. For a mandibular removable partial denture with calculus on the anterior replacement teeth, the preferred method of professional cleaning would be
A. scale as for natural teeth with sickles and curets
B. use an ultrasonic bath with a tarter remover solution
C. polish with a rag wheel on a dental lathe
D. use a denture brush with an abrasive cleaner

145. John tested negative for HIV 6 months after an exposure to the virus. When tested again 6 months later, the results were positive. If in error, the first test is
A. negative
B. false negative
C. positive
D. false positive

146. A collimator
A. increases the number of divergent rays
B. removes longer x-ray wavelengths
C. is made of aluminum or copper disks
D. restricts the size of the x-ray beam

147. Purpura describes a
A. reddish-purple discoloration
B. nipple-like growth
C. rippled surface
D. tissue overgrowth

148. On a permanent mandibular first molar, a furcation is located
A. in the apical third of the root, distally
B. in the middle third of the root, mesially
C. in the middle third of the root, lingually
D. in the cervical third of the root, buccally

149. Magnification on dental radiographs can be decreased by
A. using a shorter collimator
B. increasing focal spot size
C. placing the film farther from the tooth
D. increasing the source-object distance

150. The process of copying genetic information from DNA to RNA is called
A. mutagenesis
B. genetic engineering
C. translation
D. transcription

151. Accurate shadow casting requires meeting all of the following rules, EXCEPT one. Which one is the EXCEPTION?
A. greatest target-object distance
B. parallelism of the film to tooth
C. central ray 90 degrees to the film
D. greatest tooth-film distance

152. Use of an air powder abrasive polishing system is contraindicated because of the possible systemic absorption of sodium bicarbonate for patients with all of the following conditions EXCEPT one. Which one is the EXCEPTION?
A. immunosuppression
B. hypertension
C. metabolic alkalosis
D. renal insufficiency

153. Providing the patient active involvement in treatment decisions is an example of
A. *respondeat superior*
B. justice
C. autonomy
D. *res gestae*

154. At the posttreatment evaluation after initial debridement therapy of 12 periodontal pockets of 5–6 mm depth, two areas of bleeding are found. The next step should be
A. immediate referral of the patient to the periodontist

B. retreatment of bleeding areas and reevaluation in a month

C. reevaluation at the 3 month continuing care appointment

D. systemic antibiotic coverage for two weeks

155. After quadrant scaling and root planing, the patient is unable to close his jaw and complains of severe pain. This condition is called
A. lateral deviation
B. deflection
C. mandibular protrusion
D. subluxation

156. One can be assured instruments are being properly sterilized if
A. indicator tapes turn dark
B. autoclave timer is set for 45 minutes
C. biological indicators test negative
D. instruments are wrapped loosely

157. The order of hardness of gypsum products, from softest to hardest, is
A. model plaster, dental stone, die stone, impression plaster
B. impression plaster, model plaster, dental stone, die stone
C. dental stone, die stone, impression plaster, model plaster
D. die stone, impression plaster, model plaster, dental stone

158. Immediate (Type I) hypersensitivity is associated with all of the following, EXCEPT one. Which one is the EXCEPTION?
A. release of T cell chemical mediators
B. histamine
C. smooth muscle contraction
D. immunoglobulin E

159. The number of furcations in a maxillary first molar is
A. one
B. two
C. three
D. four

160. When a patient experiences a seizure, all of the following should be done, EXCEPT one. Which one is the EXCEPTION?
A. restrain the patient to minimize movement
B. clear the area surrounding the patient
C. maintain the airway if unconscious
D. remove dental instruments from the patient's mouth as possible

161. Gingival hyperplasia is NOT caused by
A. channel blockers
B. diuretics
C. antidysrythmatics
D. anticonvulsants

162. Epstein-Barr virus is the causative agent in verruca vulgaris and condyloma acuminatum. Surgical excision is the primary treatment modality.
A. both statements are TRUE
B. both statements are FALSE

C. first statement is TRUE, the second is FALSE
D. first statement is FALSE, the second is TRUE

163. The calculus-controlling ingredient in some tarter control toothpastes is
A. potassium nitrate
B. monofluorophosphate
C. strontium chloride
D. pyrophosphate

164. A patient who receives radiation therapy to the oral cavity and salivary glands will experience lifelong
A. mucositis and loss of taste
B. salivary gland dysfunction and risk of osteoradionecrosis
C. salivary gland dysfunction, mucositis, and risk of osteoradionecrosis
D. salivary gland dysfunction, mucositis, risk of osteoradionecrosis, and loss of taste

165. All of the following are true of localized juvenile periodontitis, EXCEPT one. Which one is the EXCEPTION?
A. bone loss is severe and involves permanent incisors and first molars
B. defective PMNLs cause increased susceptibility to infection
C. *A. actinomycetemcomitans* is the predominant causative agent
D. heavy plaque build-up and inflammation are evident
E. prognosis is poor without treatment

166. Although epithelial healing after surgery takes place in approximately 7 days, complete osseous healing may take up to
A. 2–4 weeks
B. 1–2 months
C. 2–4 months
D. 4–6 months

167. A composite restoration of the mesial contact area of tooth #11 is a
A. Class I restoration
B. Class II restoration
C. Class III restoration
D. Class IV restoration
E. Class V restoration

168. Panoramic radiographs are LEAST useful for detecting
A. fractures of the mandible
B. impacted maxillary canines
C. interproximal bone loss
D. unerupted third molars

169. An alcoholic with chronic liver disease needs anesthesia for periodontal debridement. Which is the safest local anesthetic for this patient?
A. lidocaine
B. mepivacaine
C. prilocaine
D. etidocaine

170. An advantage of glass ionomer cement over composite restorations is

A. higher thermal insulation
B. greater aesthetic value
C. better cervical retention
D. higher compressive strength

171. Lactose intolerance is a condition caused by a deficiency in the enzyme lactase. Lactase has the ability to break down lactose into
A. glucose and sucrose
B. glucose and galactose
C. glucose and fructose
D. two molecules of glucose

172. Which film speed requires the LEAST exposure time?
A. A
B. B
C. C
D. D
E. E

173. Which allergic reaction may be characterized by laryngeal edema, nausea, hypotension, and diarrhea?
A. anaphylaxis
B. asthma attack
C. urticaria
D. pruritus

174. Which salts deposit in bacterial plaque to form calculus?
A. potassium and zinc
B. calcium and selenium
C. phosphate and calcium
D. hydroxyapatite and phosphorus

175. When transferring a patient from a dental chair to the wheelchair, the dental chair should be _____ the wheelchair.
A. 6 or more inches higher than
B. 6 or more inches lower than
C. the same height or slightly lower than
D. perpendicular to

176. Which one of the following statements regarding the subgingival environment is TRUE?
A. bacteria living in this environment need oxygen to survive
B. saliva bathes the environment and carries in bacteria for colonization
C. normal oral cleansing mechanisms cause the bacterial makeup to change often
D. nutrients for subgingival plaque are derived from crevicular fluid and blood products

177. All of the following instrument types should be avoided on dental implants, EXCEPT one. Which one is the EXCEPTION?
A. plastic instruments
B. metal instruments
C. ultrasonic instruments
D. air polishing instruments

178. T lymphocytes are
A. required for immune responses to all antigens
B. necessary only for humoral responses to injected antigens
C. found only in the thymus

D. bound to antigens with their membrane-associated T cell receptor

179. A retrognathic jaw position with anterior overjet is referred to as:
A. Class I
B. Class II, division I
C. Class II, division II
D. Class III

180. Which of the following best describes effective adaptation of the curet against a tooth surface?
A. face-to-tooth angle is close to 70 degrees
B. instrument is placed at 0 degrees
C. lighter grasp is needed during the exploratory phase
D. toe third of the blade contacts the tooth at all times

■ Testlet 1 ■

Residents in this middle-class, East Coast community have an average annual income of $27,000. Public facilities include a regional medical center, skilled nursing facilities, nursing homes, home health services, dental clinics, and a psychiatric facility. There are 12 elementary, 2 middle, and 3 high schools, as well as a vocational/technical school, a community college, and a university.

Ten years ago, antifluoridation legislation was passed and the city water fluoridation was discontinued. Currently, the water contains less than 0.3 ppm natural fluoride. The local elementary schools participate in a weekly fluoride mouth-rinsing program. Local dentists and pediatricians commonly prescribe fluoride supplements, but compliance is low.

181. A study to determine the caries and periodontal status of community residents by age is being planned. The age groups to be studied are listed in Table T–1. Which sampling method can best accomplish this task?
A. random
B. stratified
C. stratified random
D. convenience
E. systematic

TABLE T.1	Community Residents by Age	
AGE		**NUMBER**
Under 18 years		12,522
18–24 years		12,892
25–44 years		16,172
45–64 years		5,783
65 years and over		1,983
Total population		**49,352**

182. Which epidemiological index would be the BEST choice for evaluating caries prevalence of the senior population?
    A. decayed, missing, and filled teeth (DMFT) index
    B. root caries index (RCI)
    C. community periodontal index of treatment needs (CPITN)
    D. decayed, missing, and filled surfaces (DMFS)

183. What is the recommended dosage of supplemental fluoride for a 5-year-old child in this community?
    A. no supplemental fluoride is needed
    B. 0.25 mg/day
    C. 0.50 mg/day
    D. 1.0 mg/day

184. Prior to assessing the dental needs of the residents, two examiners practice performing the index on four volunteers. The examiners compare their techniques and results with each other until both examiners feel their techniques are equivalent. This is an example of:
    A. reliability
    B. inter-rater reliability
    C. intra-rater reliability
    D. calibration

185. A comparison of the dental caries rate in two groups of students (those who received a prescription supplemental fluoride and those who did not) found a three times higher rate of caries in those who did not receive supplemental fluoride than in those who did. This is an example of:
    A. standard deviation
    B. nominal data
    C. correlation analysis
    D. analysis of variance

186. Which one of the following has the MOST influence on dental utilization rates?
    A. race
    B. gender
    C. ethnicity
    D. geographic location
    E. socioeconomic status

187. When Influenza X reached the East Coast this week, thousands of school-aged children and institutionalized elders were hospitalized with high fevers, dehydration, and pneumonia. The BEST epidemiologic term to describe this occurrence is
    A. pandemic
    B. incidence
    C. epidemic
    D. endemic
    E. prevalence

▪ Testlet **2** ▪

The city homeless shelter houses 559 adult males, 124 adult females, and 97 children under the age of 18 years. Fewer than 2% of sheltered adults hold full-time employment. City officials have recently implemented an employment-training project for the homeless. Based on results of a survey of prospective employers, the project will provide participants with assistance in reading and writing skills, resume and interview preparation, personal hygiene, appropriate attire, and working skills. Several dental hygienists and dentists have volunteered to assess the oral health needs of project participants using the OHI-S.

188. The OHI-S is used to measure all of the following, EXCEPT one. Which one is the EXCEPTION?
    A. plaque
    B. materia alba
    C. calculus
    D. demineralization
    E. stain

189. Every ninth adult listed on the alphabetized roster of shelter residents will be selected for assessment of oral hygiene needs. This sampling method is known as:
    A. convenience
    B. stratified
    C. random
    D. systematic

190. All project participants received a toothbrush and toothpaste. What is the MOST efficient way to provide oral hygiene instruction to participants?
    A. pamphlets
    B. videotaped presentation
    C. lecture and demonstration
    D. individualized instruction

191. After watching a toothbrushing demonstration, the residents will be able to perform the Modified Stillman's toothbrushing technique. The "condition element" of this objective is
    A. after watching a toothbrushing demonstration
    B. the residents
    C. will be able to perform
    D. the Modified Stillman's toothbrushing technique

192. A resident's behavior is modified when the resident
    A. becomes involved in patient education discussions
    B. is interested in improving his/her oral health
    C. habitually brushes and flosses daily
    D. understands flossing removes disease-causing bacteria

193. Nearly 46% of project participants gained full-time employment within 3 months of project completion. Eighty-two percent of those remained employed for at least two years. This is an example of project
    A. assessment
    B. evaluation
    C. implementation
    D. supervision

194. The BEST measure of the effect of an oral health program is
    A. total cost
    B. change in attitude

C. health improvement
D. social chance

■ Testlet 3 ■

A middle-school administrator is concerned about the increased frequency of cigarette smoking among the sixth through eighth grade students in her school. She asks her dental hygienist to develop a program for raising the awareness of the dangers of smoking. To determine the current level of smoking behavior and awareness of the danger of smoking, the dental hygienist asked each student in the seventh grade to answer a six-item questionnaire. Two weeks later, the dental hygienist gave a presentation on the general and oral health dangers of cigarette smoking to all seventh grade students. Two weeks following the presentation, the seventh grade students were given a questionnaire containing the same items as on the pre-test.

195. The questionnaire given to students prior to the presentation on smoking dangers serves as the
    A. subject
    B. control
    C. population
    D. standard deviation

196. Which one of the following inferences can be made from this study?
    A. there is a significant reduction in the number of students who smoked 15 or more cigarettes in the past month
    B. significant learning occurred regarding the relationship of smoking to infant birth-weight
    C. there is a significant reduction in the rate at which middle-school students begin smoking
    D. significant learning occurred regarding the relationship of smoking to lung cancer

197. Discussion of which one of the following smoking-

	Pre-Test	Post-Test
1. Have you ever smoked?	Yes 16% No 84%	Yes 17% No 83%
2. How many cigarettes have you smoked in the past month?		
0	89%	94%
5	5%	2%
10	2%	1%
15	3%	2%
20	0	0
More than 20	1%	1%
True or False		
3. Cigarettes cause lung cancer	T 86% F 14%	T 93% F 7%
4. Women who smoke have smaller babies	T 28% F 72%	T 92% F 8%
5. Breathing-in second-hand smoke can be just as dangerous as smoking cigarettes	T 15% F 85%	T 90% F 10%
6. People who smoke have a greater risk of loosing their teeth due to gum disease	T 33% F 67%	T 89% F 11%

related issues would MOST appeal to this population?
    A. tooth loss
    B. heart disease
    C. emphysema
    D. halitosis

198. Educating children about tobacco use and its effects is an excellent way of teaching children the dangers of smoking. This will ensure that the children will avoid cigarette smoking in the future.
    A. both statements are TRUE
    B. both statements are FALSE
    C. first statement is true, the second is FALSE
    D. first statement is FALSE, the second is TRUE

199. The number of middle-school students who began smoking in 1998 is considered its
    A. morbidity
    B. prevalence
    C. index
    D. incidence

200. Students who attend the "dangers of cigarette smoking" presentation will decrease their use of cigarettes. This statement is an example of a (an)
    A. objective
    B. hypothesis
    C. observation
    D. instruction

Part A: ANSWER KEY AND RATIONALES

1. **C** The trigeminal nerve, cranial nerve V, has three branches (ophthalmic, maxillary, and mandibular). The maxillary branch transmits impulses from the teeth of the upper jaw, while the mandibular branch transmits impulses from the mandibular teeth. Cranial nerve I transmits smell from the nasal mucosa to the brain. The facial nerve (cranial nerve VII) innervates many muscles of the face and neck, while cranial nerve III innervates the eye muscles which move the eyeball.

2. **D** A distinguishing feature of viruses is that they contain either type of nucleic acid (DNA or RNA) but not both as do cellular life forms. They are able to replicate themselves from information contained in the DNA or information in their RNA.

3. **B** Elongation is caused by too little vertical angulation. Too much vertical angulation causes foreshortening. Cone cuts and overlapping of contacts are due to improper cone placement and horizontal angulation, respectively.

4. **A** Class I furcation is a slightly detectable concavity that cannot be seen on the radiograph. A Class II furcation involves a detectable concavity that does not extend between the facial and lingual of the roots and is just visible on the radiograph. A Class III furcation is a detectable concavity that extends between the facial and lingual and is very visible on the radiograph.

5. **B** Chediak-Higashi syndrome, Papillon-Lefèvre syndrome, leukemia, and hypophosphatasia have been directly implicated in early onset periodontitis. Diabetes, Down syndrome, and AIDS may increase the risk and severity of periodontal destruction, but are not considered forms of early-onset periodontitis.

6. **A** Kaposi's sarcoma, a vascular bluish-red lesion, is most commonly located on the palate and gingiva.

7. **B** Periodontal files have a strong, thick shank and working end that allows the removal of tenacious deposits. It will also fit in deep, narrow areas because of the thinness of the working end in all dimensions. Sickle scalers, hoes, and chisels are all good choices for supragingival gross deposit removal. Area-specific curets are good choices for all types of calculus removal but have limited access to narrow, tight pockets that are deeper than the length of their working end (about 3–4 mm).

8. **E** Leukoedema is an opalescent appearance of buccal and labial mucosa not associated with eating disorders. Since most individuals with bulimia are not easily detected due to a normal body weight, oral manifestations may be the only way to detect this disorder. The individual will usually show signs of dental erosion on the lingual surfaces of the maxillary teeth due to the exposure to acid from vomiting. The amalgams may appear 'raised' from the tooth, again from the erosion to the enamel. The patient may complain of thermal sensitivity and show evidence of enlarged parotid glands. There may also be evidence of cheilosis and inflamed interdental papillae as a result of the vomiting.

9. **A** Crevicular fluid is the major source of minerals for subgingival calculus development.

10. **D** Fibromas are dense, raised lesions of normal color that are located along the occlusal plane on the gingiva. They are likely associated with trauma from mastication and are often located near the lip commissures. Hematomas are blood-filled traumatic lesions that appear purplish in color. Sponge nevus is an inherited disorder demonstrated by white, folded mucosa in the oral cavity. A granuloma is a traumatic ulcer that can mimic the appearance of squamous cell carcinoma.

11. **C** Changes in the gingival contour resulting in rolled margins and bulbous gingival papilla are usually the result of either an accumulation of tissue fluid or tissue proliferation. Sponginess is more indicative of an accumulation of tissue fluid while cellular proliferation causes firm, fibrotic tissue. Vascular hyperemia and attachment microulceration do not typically result in gingival contour changes.

12. **B** When duplicating radiographs, the original film is placed closest to the light source and the duplicate film placed on top of the original so the light passes through the original to make an image on the duplicate. Density of the duplicate film is controlled by the length of exposure to the light source. A longer exposure results in less density in a duplicated film. The opposite occurs during exposure of an original radiograph; a longer exposure results in greater density.

13. **A** The inferior alveolar nerve block will not anesthetize the maxillary arch. Instead, it is responsible for anesthesia of the mandible. Full anesthesia to the maxillary left quadrant is provided by the greater palatine, incisive, and posterior, middle, and anterior superior alveolar nerve blocks.

14. **B** The best ultrasonic scaling results are achieved with multidirectional working strokes and light pressure of the tip against the tooth. While strokes in any direction are effective, multidirectional strokes best assure complete coverage of the surface being treated. The effective width of ultrasonic strokes is similar to manual instrumentation, so overlapping of strokes is important. The point of the tip should never be adapted to the tooth as it can damage the tooth surface.

15. **D** Turner's spot is enamel hypoplasia of a permanent tooth as a result of local trauma or infection of a deciduous tooth. The trauma or infection halts the work of ameloblasts and results in poorly formed enamel in the area. Commissural lip pits are a developmental anomaly caused by incomplete fusion of the mandibular and maxillary processes. or inadequate development of the horizontal facial cleft. A static bone cyst is a not a true cyst and appears radiographically as a radiolucency in the mandible. Hypodontia is a developmental anomaly whereby one or more teeth are missing. Common teeth affected are the maxillary lateral incisors, third molars, and mandibular second premolars.

16. **A** The quick removal of alginate impressions helps prevent distortion. Trauma to oral tissues can result from improper tray size and rough manipulation of the tray. Gagging usually occurs during the placement and setting of the impression. Loss of impression detail is most likely with removal of the impression before the alginate completely sets.

17. **B** Topical fluoride should be applied immediately following rather than polymerization of the pit and fissure sealant because fluoride will interfere with the action of the etchant on the tooth surface. Fluoride treatments are not contraindicated when placing sealants. There is no reason to wait one month after sealant placement to give a fluoride.

18. **E** Bell's palsy is the usually temporary paralysis of the facial nerve that results in facial asymmetry associated with unilateral drooping of the eyelid and mouth. This condition is often due to viral or bacterial infection or trauma from surgical procedures. Lupus erythematosus, lyme disease, hypothyroidism, and Tourette's syndrome are not associated with facial asymmetry.

19. **A** Porphorymonas Gingivalis is the predominant bacteria in adult periodontitis. Eubacterium are found in small numbers in adult periodontitis. While

A. actinomycetemcomitans predominates in localized juvenile periodontitis, it is also found in adult periodontitis. *Streptococcus* organisms are common oral flora in both healthy and inflamed gingival sulci.

20. **C** Silver halide crystals are placed in the gelatinous film emulsion because they are sensitive to light or radiation. Therefore these crystals are vital to x-ray production. The black paper and outer wrapping protect the film from heat, moisture, and chemicals.

21. **D** Oral herpes lesions often occur in response to sun or wind exposure, so spending more time in the sun would not be a good choice. The HSV remain latent on the nerve branch and re-activates in response to trauma or immune suppression. Because the virus is contagious, the patient should avoid intimate contact with others and cancel the appointment. The appointment can be rescheduled in two weeks when the lesion(s) are healed. Plenty of bed rest and proper nutrient intake (especially Vitamin C) will encourage healing and strenghten the immune system.

22. **A** The congestive heart failure patient usually has difficulty breathing when placed in a supine position, so sitting in an upright position will be necessary. Shorter appointments, rather than longer, are more comfortable for this patient. Nitroglycerin tablets are recommended for the patient with angina, not congestive heart failure. Antibiotic premedication is not indicated unless the patient has some other condition putting him at risk of infection from dental procedures.

23. **C** During root planing, lateral pressure becomes progressively lighter rather than heavier. The final root planing strokes are intended to polish the root surface and remove scratches. In addition, during root-planing, the grasp is moderate to light and strokes are long and multidirectional.

24. **C** The amount of inflammation present should determine an individual's continuing care schedule. For most periodontal patients, this recall period is 3–4 months. The calculus build-up, patient income or desire, and standard office schedule are secondary to the presence of infection.

25. **E** Didanosine (ddI) is not an antifungal agent. Rather, it is an antiviral agent used to treat patients with advanced HIV infection who have been on previous prolonged zidovudine (AZT) therapy for HIV infection. Nystatin (Mycostatin), Clotrimazole (Gyne-Lotrimin), Ketoconazole (Nizoral), and Fluconazole (Diflucan) are all antifungal agents used to treat candidiasis.

26. **A** When a young child swallows too much fluoridated toothpaste or fluoridate rinse, a chronic toxicity may occur. Fluorosis would not occur on primary teeth because the enamel has already formed by the time the teeth have erupted and toothbrushing begins. Excessive fluoride does not cause green stain or extra cusp formation.

27. **B** Failure of the fusion of the both right and left maxillary processes with the globular process results in a bilateral cleft lip. When the left or the right maxillary process fails to fuse with the globular process, a unilateral cleft results. A partial or complete cleft palate occurs when the lateral palatine processes fail to fuse to each other or to the premaxilla.

28. **B** Both forms of necrotic ulcerative periodontitis (NUP) may include deep crater-like osseous lesions, gangrenous stomatitis and lack of periodontal pockets, however, sequestration of bone fragments occurs only in AIDS-associated NUP.

29. **B** The disk of the TMJ is attached to the mandibular condyle and forms an articulation with the temporal bone and mandible. The ethmoid bone makes up the medial wall of the eye orbit. The zygomatic process is a part of the temporal bone.

30. **D** Mental depression is NOT a characteristic of amphetamine use. Amphetamines are potent CNS stimulants and as such, will cause increases in blood pressure and activity but suppress the appetite. They are used in the treatment of narcolepsy and depression. They have limited success as appetite suppressants.

31. **A** When a patient contributes to his own harm (as in not following home care instructions), this is termed contributory negligence. *Respondeat superior* indicates that the dentist is responsible for the wrongful actions of employees. *Res gestae* is a statement that an individual makes during a negligent act and can be used against him/her in a lawsuit. Admission against interest is a statement made at any time which goes against the legal interest of that patient.

32. **A** Zinc polycarboxylate cements are used to chemically bond to enamel and dentin by adhering to the calcium and carboxylate groups in the tooth structure. They are also considered very biocompatible materials due to the quick loss of acidity after placement.

33. **D** Food impaction causes a localized area of inflammation, often interproximally, that is not well-defined nor specifically adjacent to base metal crown margins. Infringement on the biological width can cause a band of localized inflammation in the area of the crown, as can inadequate oral hygiene, reactivity of some metals in crowns, and overcontouring of crowns.

34. **D** Although the consistency of the cariogenic food is a factor in the decay process, the between-meal snacking of sugar is most prevalent in the caries process. Eating sweets with a meal is less cariogenic.

35. **B** Power toothbrushes are only effective in removing plaque if used properly. Placing a power toothbrush into one's mouth does not guarantee better plaque removal. Many people do a better job of plaque removal with a powered toothbrush because of built-in timers, not the type of brush itself. Power

toothbrushes are recommended for a variety of patients but are especially good for arthritic patients and those with grasping difficulties. The brush heads or tufts can move in a rotational or counter rotational, oscillating or sonic motion. The brushing technique is product dependent.

36. **D** When an infrabony periodontal pockets forms the junctional epithelial tissue is apical to the crest of the alveolar bone. In a suprabony pocket, the junctional epithelium is apical to the CEJ and coronal to the crest of the alveolar bone. In a gingival pocket, the gingiva proliferates in a coronal direction with no apical migration of the attachment.

37. **D** A Class III lesion involves the proximal surfaces of a central, lateral or cuspid. Class IV lesions involve proximal surfaces and incisal edges of anterior teeth. Lesions of proximal surfaces of posterior teeth are considered. Class II, while Class I lesions involve the lingual surfaces of anterior teeth as well as other pit and fissure areas of posterior teeth. Class V lesions are located at the gingival third of facial and lingual surfaces.

38. **C** The most common side effect of antihistamine use is excessive sedation. Other side effects include dizziness, blurred vision, and fatigue. Irritability, anxiety, and trembling are not side effects of antihistamine use.

39. **A** Antabuse is used in the treatment of chronic alcoholism; Dolobid is an NSAID used for pain of rheumatoid arthritis and osteoarthritis; Proventil is a bronchodilator used by asthmatics; Dolophine is a controlled substance used in opiod withdrawal programs.

40. **B** The initial vascular response is produced by the release of histamine and serotonin by mast cells located in the lamina propria. The release of prostaglandins and kinins follows later to assist in sustaining the vascular permeability initiated by the histamine. Lysosomes are cellular organelles that contain proteolytic enzymes and are found primarily in phagocytic cells.

41. **D** Trismus may be a symptom of TMJ disorder but is not a cause. The causes of TMJ disorders are multifactorial and may include stress, arthritis, and macro or micro trauma to the joint, but may also include other factors.

42. **C** Scatter radiation is produced when x-rays strike matter. Use of the rectangular collimator decreases patient dose approximately 55% when compared with round collimators, resulting in less scatter radiation. Pointed cones are large sources of scatter radiation.

43. **C** Patients can feel frictional heat if poor technique is used. Frictional heat is reduced by slow, not high, speed of the cup and also by light pressure, brief duration of contact, and a wet, abrasive agent.

44. **B** When radiographs are indicated during a child's first dental visit, occlusal films should be taken before the bitewing radiographs as a means of introducing radiology to the patient. Occlusal films are easier for the patient to adapt to because of area and ease of placement. When positioning the child patient for a mandibular occlusal radiograph, the patient sits upright and the central ray is at approximately –55 degrees.

45. **A** When suspicious of abuse of a child or dependent adult, one should report suspicions to the local authorities, such as Social Services, while the patient is in the operatory. In suspected cases of abuse, photographing signs of abuse on the dependent does not require parental or caregiver permission. Never discuss abuse with the caregiver or try to get a confession. Leave that to the authorities. The incident should be documented in the patient's file immediately, along with reporting the incident. Do not wait for a second incident to occur before reporting this incident.

46. **D** Refusal to treat a patient with a life-threatening disease, such as AIDS, is considered unethical conduct. Unethical conduct may include disrespect, unfair treatment, untruthfulness, or lack of health promotion to a patient. Malpractice involves the failure of the health care provider to exercise due care in provision of services which then results in injury to the patient. Breach of contract is the failure to perform the terms of an expressed contract. Negligence is a breaching of duty and is also called malpractice. Nonmaleficence is the obligation to prevent harm to a patient.

47. **A** Radiographically, fuzziness of the alveolar crests and breaks in the integrity of the lamina dura are initial signs of periodontal breakdown. The periodontal ligament space is normally radiolucent while facial and lingual cortical plates are not visible in routine radiographic exposures.

48. **A** In localized juvenile periodontitis, the predominant microorganism in up to 90% of the total cultivable microflora is *A. actinomycetemcomitans*.

49. **A** IgA antibodies predominate at mucosal sites, such as the respiratory, gastrointestinal, and genitourinary sites. Although other antibody classes, cytotoxic T cells, and complement proteins are found at these sites, IgA has been most-strongly linked to mucous membrane protection.

50. **C** The lesion, as it is described for this patient, is serious and potentially life-threatening. The exact nature of the lesion needs to be known as soon as possible. Incisional biopsy is preferred over excisional biopsy in this case because of the size of the lesion. Neither a reexamination in a few weeks or exfoliative cytology would give the timely or definitive answer needed.

51. **B** Needlestick exposure requires rapid prophylactic treatment, but development of immunity after active

immunization is too slow to prevent clinical infection. Therefore, passive immunization with preformed anti-viral antibodies is the mainstay of preventive therapy. Pooled human IgG, containing high titers of antibodies against various pathogens, can provide temporary protection against hepatitis B, hepatitis A, and some other diseases, if it is injected soon after exposure. Cleansing the wound with hexachlorophene is too conservative for the risk. Active immunization with pertussis vaccine would not protect the injured against Hepatitis B.

52. **D** The mandibular arch is the principal origin of the middle and lower face, forming the lower cheek, the lower lip, the lower jaw, and part of the tongue. The globular process forms the philtrum (center) of the upper lip. The maxillary process forms the palate, upper cheeks, and sides of the upper lip. The medial nasal process is responsible for development of the center and tip of the nose.

53. **B** Home bleaching kits usually contain a 10% or greater solution of carbamide peroxide or a 1.5–6% solution of hydrogen peroxide. Sodium citrate is the active ingredient in some tooth desensitizing products. Sodium hypochlorite is common household bleach and is not used for intra-oral bleaching. Zinc-oxide eugenol is a compound found in dental cements and impression materials.

54. **B** Primary herpetic gingivostomatitis is a viral infection that usually results in fever and pain from vesicles on the oral tissues, such as the palate, gingiva, tongue, and lips. Recurrent herpes outbreaks tend to be located on intraoral soft tissues covering bone (palate, gingiva) or the lips. It occurs most often in young adults and is unrelated to apthous ulcers.

55. **D** Doxycycline (Doxycin), a tetracycline, is used as an alternative drug choice when pen VK or amoxicillin (Amoxil) cannot be used due to penicillin allergy. Cloxacillin (Cloxapen), a penicillinase-resistant penicillin, terfenadine (Seldane), an antihistamine, and diflunisal (Dolobid), a NSAIA analgesic, are also not appropriate for this patient's condition.

56. **A** Both statements are true. Both a jaw fracture and internal resorption appear radiolucent on a radiograph.

57. **B** For the patient taking hypertensive medication, there is a greater chance of syncope occurring due to the orthostatic hypotension which may occur during dental treatment. After elevating from the supine position, it is important to allow the patient several minutes in an upright position before leaving and avoid the chance for syncope to occur. The other foils do not relate to hypertensive medication.

58. **D** Have the patient rest and then proceed to the chair to collect appropriate medical information. This will give you the information needed to make a decision whether to provide treatment, consult with

the physician and/or to reschedule the patient appointment.

59. **E** Dull instruments are not an infection control issue. However, use of dull instruments are a safey and patient comfort concern, since heavier pressure is needed to remove calculus and slipping commonly occurs. The ability to both detect and remove calculus and other debris is decreased when dull cutting edges decrease tactile sense.

60. **C** Placement of pit and fissure sealants is not indicated on smooth surfaces, such as decayed proximal surfaces. They are most effective in sealing out bacteria and nutrients and preventing further decay when placed in pits and fissures. Sealants are Bis-GMA organic monomers that may also be filled with glass particles to make them stronger and better able to withstand the rigors of mastication.

61. **B** Dried blood on instruments is best removed by presoaking in a mixture of water and detergent before sonicating and sterilizing the instruments. Scrubbing instruments should be avoided whenever possible to reduce the risk of accidental injury. Dipping the cutting edges in alcohol is not a recommended procedure and will not remove the dried blood. Some commercial presoaks are available that have the ability to destroy the proteins in blood and may be used in place of the detergent/water presoak.

62. **A** Oral irrigators are not effective at removing attached plaque, but will removed unattached or loosely-attached bacteria and large debris. Removal of unattached plaque, which contains motile bacteria, is associated with reducing gingivitis and reducing plaque toxicity. Oral irrigators also effectively deliver antimicrobial agents.

63. **D** Of the choices listed, the permanent mandibular second premolar is the most frequently congenitally missing. The most frequently missing teeth are the maxillary and mandibular third molars. Permanent maxillary lateral incisors are also frequently congenitally missing.

64. **D** Submental lymph nodes are located below the chin. Submandibular nodes are located more posteriorly, while cervical nodes can be palpated along the sternocleidomastoid muscle. Preauricular nodes are located near the TMJ.

65. **C** The maximum absorbed dose of radiation that a 38-year-old dental hygienist should receive is 100 Rad. This is figured by: 38 yrs. of age – 18 yrs. of age = 20 years; 20 yrs. × 5 (maximum annual permissible dose) = 100 Rad.

66. **A** For insertion of a cutting blade into a pocket, the angle should be as close to 0 degrees as possible to make the placement as easy and comfortable as possible.

67. **C** Tolerance to a drug occurs when an abuser needs a higher dose of a drug to achieve the same effect. Drug dependence is the use of a drug for its effects

or to avoid discomfort associated with it absence; physical dependence is a physical craving or need for a drug. Addiction is the same as drug dependence, while drug abuse is self-administration and excessive use of any drug without regard for its proper medical use.

68. **A** Isolated porthole defects located on the facial surfaces of the alveolar bone are window-like exposures of small portions of the tooth root and are named after the French name for window "fenetre", thus fenestration. Dehiscenses are vertical areas of denuded bone also occurring on facial surfaces. Buttressing bone is an abnormal thickening of bone in areas where trabeculae have been weakened by resorption while festoons are wavy contours of bone found between the teeth. A festoon is a lifesaver-like enlargement of the marginal gingiva, not a bony defect.

69. **C** Blood contaminated gauze and gloves are considered biomedical waste and must either to sterilized or placed in properly labeled biohazard bags for storage until incinerated. Contaminated gloves should not be washed after use, but instead should be carefully removed by pulling the cuff toward the finger tips and allowing the glove to turn inside-out. The gloves are then placed in a biohazard bag.

70. **A** The origin of a muscle is the stable attachment and the insertion is the movable attachment. The forearm moves with flexion and extension of the elbow joint. The origin cannot be on the radius because the forearm moves. The humerus does not move in this action so it cannot be the insertion. Since the triceps brachii extends the elbow joint, thus moving the forearm, it must have its insertion on a bone of the forearm, specifically the ulna. An agonist is a prime mover, in this case, the triceps brachii. The biceps brachii has an opposite action, therefore it is an antagonist.

71. **A** Anticholinergics are sometimes used to stimulate salivary glands to produce more saliva. Antihistimines, diuretics, and antipsychotics will worsen xerostomia.

72. **D** Oxygen will not benefit the patient who is hyperventilating. In this situation, the increased number of respirations results in a shortage of carbon dioxide causing the patient to work hard at breathing. Treatment involves calming the patient and restoring the carbon dioxide level by having the patient breath into a paper bag.

73. **B** Epulis fissuratum or denture irritation hyperplasia is caused by long-term irritation from an ill-fitting denture. Denture stomatitis, papillary hyperplasia and angular cheilitis are all believed to have candida albicans as one of the etiologic agents.

74. **D** Candidiasis, a fungal infection, is associated with antibiotic use and resembles a cottage-cheesy coating on the oral mucosa. The coating can be removed

and exhibits reddened tissue beneath. Discomfort may be associated with candida. Linea albican is hyperkeratinized buccal mucosa adjacent to the occlusal plane. Lichen planus has a lacy, white, and raised appearance on the buccal and occasionally gingival tissues. Hairy leukoplakia is a raised white lesion commonly found on the lateral borders of the tone and associated with AIDS and other immune-suppressing diseases.

75. **D** The bicuspid, or mitral, valve is located between the left atrium and left ventricle. Stenosis of this valve inhibits the flow of blood from the left atrium into the left ventricle, causing the blood to accumulate in the left atrium, pulmonary veins, and lungs.

76. **E** Exposure time affects density of a film, but has no effect on image sharpness. The focal spot size, object to film distance, source to object distance, and film speed all influence image sharpness.

77. **A** Cysts form where embryonic cells are trapped in fusion lines during facial development. Clefts occur during facial development when globular and maxillary processes do not fuse. Granulomas are masses of inflammatory cells and are not associated with facial development. Cementomas, also known as periapical cemental dysplasia, appear as well-circumscribed, radiolucent lesions on radiographs. Over time, they calcify and become more radiopaque. When extra tooth buds form or when tooth buds divide, they form supernumerary teeth.

78. **B** Shingles is also called herpes zoster. It is a painful, unilateral eruption of herpetic lesions along a sensory nerve that occurs in persons who are immuno-deficient or have other serious conditions, such as leukemia. Hemorrhoids are outpouchings of blood vessels in the rectal area, while psoriasis and eczema are skin conditions.

79. **C** Slow tooth eruption in children is associated with hypothyroidism. All of the others occur in hyperthyroidism.

80. **D** The interdental brush is very good in removing plaque and debris from large embrasures. Oral irrigators are good for removing loosely attached bacteria and debris. Waxed floss and dental tape work best in smaller embrasure spaces when teeth are in proximal contact.

81. **A** Glycolysis is the pathway for breaking-down the simple sugar glucose to pyruvate. The conversion of pyruvate into acetyl CoA is by the enzyme pyruvate dehydrogenase. Tricarboxylic Acid Cycle (TCA) is the pathway that results in production of NADH and $FADH_2$, which later donate their electrons to the electron transport chain.

82. **C** A fixed, nonmoveable mass of the deep cervical nodes may prove to be carcinoma which could be life threatening. The other choices should be noted for further investigation, but are not potentially life-threatening.

83. **C** The oblique group of periodontal fibers of the PDL is the largest group and is responsible for preventing tilting and dislocation of the tooth. The alveolar crest group runs from the alveolar crest to the cementum and opposes lateral forces while holding the tooth in the socket. The horizontal group controls lateral movement, while the apical fibers surround the apex of the root and provide resistance to tipping and dislocation along with protection of the pulp.

84. **D** The lavage created by an ultrasonic does not affect the root surface either by making it smoother or rougher. Fluid lavage has a number of therapeutic benefits due to acoustic microstreaming, primarily its effect in damaging bacteria and flushing the area of bacteria, fractured calculus, and blood.

85. **D** Auscultatory gap is a loss of heart sounds when taking blood pressure. It can be eliminated by having the patient raise their arm prior to inflating the cuff or having the patient open and close their fist 4–5 times after the cuff has been inflated.

86. **A** Three different pulpal tests all gave a similar and normal response for the injured tooth and the adjacent and like-kind teeth. This is consistent with an interpretation that the pulp is normal.

87. **B** When treating a patient who carries HBV, one should avoid the use of ultrasonic scalers since they create aerosols and have the potential to contaminate surfaces and humans. Double-gloving is not proper unless the clinician wears them for each and every patient. All HCW's should be immunized against HBV, however, care is still needed when treating HBV carriers to prevent contaminating surfaces that the non-immunized may contact. Rescheduling the patient is unnecessary if universal precautions and reasonable care are taken to prevent cross-contamination.

88. **E** Zinc-oxide eugenol is a cement and is not used to treat root hypersensitivity. Common treatments are fluoride varnishes, dentin sealers, mineral solutions (potassium nitrate, sodium citrate, strontium chloride), and iontophoresis (electrical deposition of fl⁻ ions).

89. **D** Films partially immersed in developer and completely immersed in fixer will exhibit a clear area where the developer was not allowed to react with the silver halide crystals to produce an image. Inadequate rinsing following fixing will result in yellow-brown staining of the films months later.

90. **D** To palpate tissue bidigitally the tissues are held between the thumb and one or more fingers. Manual palpation is using all the fingers of one hand to grasp and palpate tissues. Digital palpation is using one finger to examine tissues. Circular compression requires moving fingers in a circular motion while applying pressure to the tissues.

91. **A** Infrabony pockets are classified according to the number of existing walls of bone that surround them. If the facial and lingual bone is missing, only one

wall, the interproximal wall, will be present. This would be labeled a one-walled pocket.

92. **C** To remove heavy calculus, the best choice is the thicker standard tip at a medium to high power. The tip is bulky and strong. At medium to high power, the larger tip movements are most likely to be effective. The lowest power that will effectively remove the deposit should be used. At medium to high power, the thinner tips would have very large movements, which could cause discomfort to the tooth and damage to the instrument tip.

93. **A** Amalgam polishing helps prevent corrosion and improves the longevity of amalgam restorations. Polishing amalgams without water cooling of the amalgam can lead to odontoblast damage. Continuous rotation of the burr on the amalgam surface without cooling causes heat build-up and release of mercury from the amalgam.

94. **E** Caries can cause exogenous intrinsic stain. Fluorosis, traumatized pulp, tetracycline and genetic anomalies are all classified as endogenous intrinsic stain.

95. **C** Nicotine stomatitis is associated with tiny nodules with red centers on the palate. The tissue appears diffuse grayish white. It indicates an inflamed minor salivary gland. Ulcerated fluid-filled lesions with red halos are associated with apthous ulcers or burns. Varicosities on the underside of the tongue are associated with the elderly. Pimple-like lesions are associated with abscesses. Recession on the linguals of maxillary anterior teeth may be related to periodontal disease.

96. **B** Signs of mild to moderate overdose (toxic) reaction to local anesthetic include talkativeness, excitedness, slurred speech, apprehension, stuttering, increased blood pressure, increased heart rate, increased respiration, light headedness, dizziness, and drowsiness. When the blood level of local anesthetic is high, the CNS is both depressed and then stimulated to produce convulsions. A fearful person may exhibit some of the same reactions, but will not convulse. Anaphylactic shock is the most severe form of an allergic, not overdose, reaction. Synergistic effect between vasoconstrictor and local anesthetic does not occur.

97. **D** Sulcular epithelium is typically non-keratinized, which is one reason why it is particularly susceptible to periodontal infection. Keratinized tissues, like the gingiva and dorsal surface of the tongue, are the toughest soft tissues. A tobacco-chewer's lesion is an example of an ortho-keratinized tissue. Buccal mucosa is generally non-keratinized, although it may become para-keratinized due to masticatory activities. Parakeratinization is located between non- and ortho-keratinization.

98. **D** A film placed in developing solution at too low of a temperature will appear lighter than normal (cooler temperatures require longer processing time). Film

insufficiently fixed (inadequate time) or placed in contaminated fixing solutions will result in films with a brown cast (incomplete fixing). Films left in a developer too long will be darker than normal.

99. **A** Overproduction of adrenocorticotrophic hormone (ACTH) leads to Cushing's syndrome. Underproduction of ACTH causes Addison's disease. Excessive growth hormone (GH) production results in acromegaly or gigantism. Undersecretion of thyroid stimulating hormone (TSH) results in hypothyroidism, while low follicle-stimulating hormone (FSH) affects reproductive ability.

100. **C** Clindamycin is a drug-of-choice in the AHA prophylactic antibiotic regimen and the only choice for this patient. Since the patient is allergic to penicillin, the AHA's first antibiotic choice, amoxicillin (Amoxil), a penicillin, cannot be prescribed. Azithromycin (Zithromax), a macrolide antibiotic, is a drug choice of the AHA's regimen, however, when combined with Hismanal, an increase in cardiac dysrhythmias occurs. Tetracycline is not a drug choice in the AHA regimen.

101. **D** Antibodies and/or complement molecules that stimulate phagocytosis are called opsonins. Antibodies deficient in the Fc region could not be effective opsonins, since they would not react with Fc receptors on the surface of phagocytic cells. Direct neutralization of viruses does not depend on phagocytosis.

102. **B** Increasing the power level increases the size (amplitude) of instrument tip movement and makes the tip more effective in fracturing and removing heavy calculus. Due to increased chances of tip breakage at high power levels, only standard tips should be used. Increasing the water flow would not affect calculus removal. Increasing the lateral pressure would dampen the action of the tip and reduce calculus removal. There is no air intake on ultrasonic units.

103. **B** Gingival recession is not associated with tongue thrusting. Because of the extreme force of the tongue against the anterior teeth (rather than palate) during tongue thrusting, the central and lateral incisors are forced anteriorly (overjet) and into an open bite. The protrusive lower lip is caused by overdeveloped facial muscles as a result of the deviant swallowing.

104. **B** Essential amino acids must be provided by the diet since the body cannot make them in sufficient amounts to provide for physiological needs. There are 9 amino acids that are considered essential and 11 that are considered nonessential—ones the body can synthesize and do not need to be provided through the diet.

105. **D** The tooth surface adjacent to the bracket is prone to decalcification because it is a more difficult area to clean, not because the quality of plaque is different. Daily home fluoride should be the standard recommendation for individuals with fixed orthodontic appliances.

106. **A** 10 mA × 0.6 seconds = 6.0 mA; therefore 15 mA × 0.4 seconds = 6 mA.

107. **A** A high kVp will produce a film with low contrast, while a low kVp will produce one with high contrast. MA affects the density of the film, not the contrast.

108. **A** Insulin and glucagon are produced by cells of the islets of Langerhans in the pancreas. Thyroxine is produced by the thyroid gland, cortisol by the adrenal cortex, and epinephrine and norepinephrine by the medulla of the adrenal gland.

109. **A** Overlapped contacts on radiographs are due to improper horizontal angulation. Vertical angulation affects the appearance of tooth length (elongation and foreshortening) as do patient positioning and film placement.

110. **B** The ala of the nose is used to determine placement of the cental ray when exposing a maxillary canine. The outer corner of the eye is used when exposing molars, the tragus-ala line assists in determining patient positioning, and the nasal septum is a landmark for placement for maxillary central periapicals.

111. **A** The junctional epithelium separates the periodontal ligament from the oral environment. Gingival connective tissue is another name for the lamina propria. The periodontal ligament is made up of five principal fiber groups or bundles. The JE is at the apical margin, rather than coronal margin, or the gingival sulcus.

112. **B** The length of the lower or terminal shank of an instrument most directly influences the reach of the instrument. A longer shanked instrument can gain access to a deeper pocket. Another factor that can influence an instrument's access to a deep pocket is the size of the working end. Deep pockets tend to be narrower, making it hard to adapt and maneuver a wide instrument. Although they were not given as an option in the question, this is why short curets (minis) and files work well in deep pockets.

113. **B** The fourteen bones of the face include the two zygomatic bones. While both the cranium and face are part of the skull, the cranium is the portion that surrounds the brain. The wrist is part of the appendicular skeleton.

114. **B** The mandibular nerve is comprised of the inferior alveolar, lingual, buccal, mental, and incisive branches.

115. **C** Lipopolysaccharides are components of Gram negative bacterial cell walls. These molecules are potent endotoxins and are responsible for severe food poisoning reactions due to organisms, such as *Salmonella* spp. and *Escherichia coli*. Lipoprotein is also a component of the Gram negative wall, while lipoteicoic acids are found in Gram positive walls, and mycoloic acids are specifically associated with Mycobacteria.

116. **A** To prevent dislodging the pack during mastication, periodontal dressings are pressed into the interproximal spaces to encourage mechanical adherence and should not be placed above the height of contour of the teeth.

117. **B** A deficiency in folate increases the risk of certain birth defects. During pregnancy, the body is being challenged by greater cell division and, in turn, greater DNA synthesis. Therefore, the pregnant woman is in need of an increase in folate intake. Often times, a physician will prescribe folate supplements even prior to the pregnancy to help prevent birth defects.

118. **D** Acute necrotizing ulcerative gingivitis, a bacillus-type infection, occurs most commonly in college-age students who are at risk. Strong malodor is associated with ANUG. Risk factors include: emotional stress, smoking, poor diet, lack of sleep, and poor oral hygiene. College students are also prone to primary herpetic gingivostomatitis, a viral infection, which has similar symptoms. Gingival hyperplasia is not age nor stress associated. Steroid hormone induced gingivitis does not exhibit fever nor obvious ulceration.

119. **B** The glycocalyx functions in attachment (adherence) to surfaces. Flagella function in motility, capsules surround the surface of some bacteria, and plasmids are involved in gene transfer between bacteria.

120. **D** Infectious mononucleosis is a viral (Epstein-Barr) disease that presents with prodromal (initial) palatal petechiae, malaise, fever, and lymphadenopathy. Histoplasmosis is a fungal disease caused by exposure to bird droppings and tuberculosis is a bacterial infection of the respiratory tract. Moniliasis is a yeast infection that is also called candidiasis.

121. **A** A malignant lesion that is associated with the skin being exposed to the sun is a basal cell carcinoma. Squamous cell carcinoma is associated with smoking, alcohol, and syphilis. Juvenile melanoma and intradermal nevus are not malignant lesions.

122. **A** Anaphylaxis can occur at any age. Epinephrine injection is the mainstay of treatment for this medical emergency, an allergic reaction, which can occur at any age. There seems to be a recent upswing in the number of anaphylactic reactions to latex antigens present in some rubber gloves and other rubber products.

123. **E** Rapid weight gain and increased salivation are NOT associated with diabetes mellitus. The opposite it true. Uncontrolled diabetics often loose weight when the body is unable to utilize blood sugar to feed itself. Decreased salivation (xerostomia) is common as are parotid gland enlargement, confusion, slurred speech, clammy skin, infections, and organ damage.

124. **D** An infection associated with the buccal of a maxillary second molar will be located in the vestibular space of the maxilla, rather than the submental space. Ludwig's angina, called cellulitis, is associated with infection of a mandibular tooth that spreads to the submandibular space (often via the sublingual and submental spaces) and creates a dental emergency requiring hospitalization.

125. **B** Before producing study casts or models from a saliva-contaminated impression, the impression must be disinfected. Materials that have contacted mucous membranes must be sterilized or disinfected with a high-level disinfectant. Because impression materials cannot withstand sterilization, disinfectants are the best choice. Having the patient rinse with an antimicrobial such as chlorhexidine gluconate will help reduce contamination but will not adequately disinfect the impression. Dental plaster and models cannot withstand the heat of sterilization.

126. **A** Maternal infection with *Treponema pallidum*, a spirochete, may result in Hutchinson's triad in the offspring. The triad consists of mulberry molars, notched incisors, and eighth nerve deafness.

127. **A** Deflection is a lateral mandibular shifting on opening that increases as the mandible opens and decreases as it closes. A deviation is a lateral shift from and to centric during both opening and closing. Creptus is joint sounds. Trismus is a muscular spasm causing restricted opening.

128. **B** The initial vasoactive response is produced by the release of histamine and serotonin by mast cells located in the lamina propria. The release of prostaglandins and kinins follows later to assist in sustaining the vascular permeability initiated by the histamine. Lysosomes are cellular organelles which contain proteolytic enzymes and are found primarily in phagocytic cells.

129. **A** *Actinomyces viscosus* are associated with the development of root surface caries. *Prevotella intermedia*, *Fusobacterium* spp., and gram positive cocci are associated with periodontal disease.

130. **C** Deciduous teeth must be etched for a longer period of time than permanent teeth because of the prismic shape of the enamel rods. A saliva or moisture-contaminated etched surface must be re-etched, rinsed and dried before placing a sealant. Rinsing alone will not reverse the mineralization that takes place when the surface is contaminated with saliva.

131. **A** Bis-GMA is the resin component in pit and fissure sealants. It holds the glass filler used in some sealants and in composites. In some cements, it is the liquid component. It is not found in amalgams.

132. **A** Both statements are true. A light grasp is used during assessment and a moderate to firm grasp is used during a working stroke. A tighter grasp results in more lateral pressure.

133. **B** Hydroxyapatite is the ceramic coating material used on implants to improve biocompatability. It

produces a chemical bonding between the bone and implant. Strontium chloride is a compound found in desensitizing toothpastes. Chlorhexidine gluconate, an antimicrobial solution, is often used to control bacterial growth around implants. Calcium carbonate is a chalk used as a mild abrasive in prophylactic pastes.

134. **B** The term *chemotaxis* refers to the directional migration of PMNLs toward attracting molecules such as bacteria. Thus the appropriate term for impairment in this ability would be a chemotactic defect. Adherence defects and leukopenic defects do not involve directional migration but instead are defects of adhesion and leukocytes respectively.

135. **A** The thyrohyoid muscle does not open and close the jaws, rather, it depresses the hyoid bone and raises the thyroid cartilage and larynx. The temporalis, masseter, and medial pterygoid muscles are all involved in jaw closure, while the suprahyoid and inferior heads of the lateral pterygoid open the jaws.

136. **A** Maxillary first premolars often have bifurcated roots, while mandibular second premolars often have three cusps (1 buccal and 2 lingual).

137. **E** Adult periodontitis and localized juvenile periodontitis both exhibit loss of attachment. The adult form appears in middle-aged and older adults, progresses slowly, and is a multi-bacterial infection with *P. gingivalis* predominating. LJP appears in children and adolescents, is rapidly progressing, is associated with immune defect, and is predominantly associated with *A. actinomycetemcomitans*.

138. **A** Parotid gland secretions are serous, as are secretions of the middle tongue. Secretions of the submandibular and sublingual glands are a combination of serous and mucous. The sublingual glands, palate, and posterior tongue produce mucous secretions.

139. **D** Nifedipine (Procardia), a calcium channel blocker, is used to treat hypertension and angina pectoris. One of its adverse reactions is gingival hyperplasia. Furosemide (Lasix) , a loop diuretic, hydrochlorothiazide (Hydro-Chlor), a thiazide diuretic, and captopril (Capoten), an angiotensin-converting enzyme (ACE) inhibitior, have not been associated with gingival hyperplasia as an adverse reaction.

140. **C** Ten percent of periodontal cares are considered refractory since they do not respond to traditional therapy. Many of these cases occur in cigarette smokers. Recurrent periodontitis is a reoccurence of the disease after successful treatment. Rapidly progressive periodontitis is associated with immune defect or systemic disease and is characterized by fast and severe periodontal destruction, such as occurs with acute necrotizing periodontitis (as seen in AIDS patients).

141. **B** The Centers for Disease Control and Prevention have declared herpetic lesions that persist intraorally for one month or longer as AIDS-defining.

Although candidiasis, oral hairy leukoplakia and Kaposi's sarcoma are often found in the AIDS-infected individual, none of them have been determined to be AIDS-defining.

142. **A** Xerostomia is a common oral manifestation of Sjögren's syndrome due to disease of the salivary and lacrimal glands. The syndrome may accompany rheumatoid arthritis or systemic lupus erythematosus. Median rhomboid glossitis is associated with candidiasis and appears as a denuded area near the midline on the posterior tongue. Leukoedema is a benign, opaque white lesion of the buccal mucosa, while geographic tongue appears as denuded patches on the tongue.

143. **A** Lining mucosa is present in non-masticatory regions such as the floor of the mouth, ventral surface of the tongue, soft palate, cheeks, lips, and alveolar mucosa. This typically non-keratinized tissue in not firmly attached to bone. Specialized mucosa applies to the covering of the dorsal surface of the tongue, which forms papilla and taste organs. Masticatory mucosa covers the hard palate and gingiva and are usually keratinized and firmly attached to underlying bone. Secretory mucosa secretes substances, such as occurs with intestinal mucosa which secretes mucous.

144. **B** The vibrations of the ultrasonic bath plus the chemical tartar remover are generally effective and non-damaging to the plastic or metal surfaces of a partial denture. The acrylic can be easily scratched with sickles and even curets or an abrasive cleaner applied with a denture brush. A rag wheel on a dental lathe has a high potential of damaging the clasps that secure the partial denture and is not recommended for cleaning.

145. **B** The first test is an example of a false negative test result. Many things can cause false (negative or positive) test results. These include poor testing technique, contamination of testing materials, improper handling or storage of test materials, low sensitivity of tests, and inadequate levels of disease (virus, protein, antibodies, etc.) for testing. In John's case, there may not have been enough antivirus in his system during the first 6 months for the test to detect it. A negative test result occurs when someone is tested for a disease they don't have and the result is negative. A positive test result occurs when someone is tested for a disease they have and the result is positive. A false positive test result occurs when someone is tested for a disease they don't have and the test result is positive.

146. **D** A collimator restricts the size of the x-ray beam and will decrease the number of divergent rays. Filters are made of aluminum or copper disks and are responsible for removing longer x-ray wavelengths.

147. **A** Purpura is a red-purple discoloration greater than 0.5 cm. Papillomatous lesions are nipple-like

growths. Corrugated surfaces are rippled in appearance. Tissue overgrowth is also known as hyperplastic tissue.

148. **D** Furcations on permanent mandibular first molars are located in the cervical third of the root (buccally and lingually).

149. **D** The use of a longer cone (increased source-object distance) will decrease magnification. A large focal spot size, short collimator, and film placement far from the tooth all act to increase magnification.

150. **D** The process of copying genetic information from DNA to RNA is called transcription. Translation is the process of transferring genetic information from mRNA to synthesis of protein. Mutagenesis is a DNA alteration that changes encoded genetic information. Genetic engineering is the process of using specific techniques to manipulate genetic information.

151. **D** The rules of accurate shadow casting do NOT include a greatest tooth to film distance. The CR directed 90 degrees to the film and the teeth, having the greatest target/object distance possible, and keeping the film parallel to the teeth being exposed are all rules of accurate shadow casting.

152. **A** Patients who are immunosuppressed or compromised should not be exposed to air-powder polish because they will inhale the microbial aerosol and not because of the absorption of the sodium bicarbonate. Hypertension, metabolic alkalosis and renal insufficiency are all contra indications for use of an air polishing abrasive system.

153. **C** Autonomy is a moral principle which includes respect for patient opinions and beliefs regarding treatment. *Respondeat superior* is a doctrine which holds the employer liable for negligent acts of employees. Justice is the fair and equal treatment of others. *Res gestae* is a statement made during the occurence of a negligent act that can be used against the speaker in a lawsuit.

154. **B** The initial periodontal therapy was successful for 10 of the 12 treated pockets. The two bleeding sites should be carefully checked for residual plaque and calculus, retreated, and reevaluated in 4–6 weeks. Bleeding pockets should not be ignored for 3 months. Referral to the periodontist is recommended when retreatment is not successful or when loss of attachment continues regardless of non-surgical treament provided. Systemic antibiotic coverage is generally reserved for individuals with immune suppression or chronic disease that prevents healing.

155. **D** Prolonged opening of the jaws allows the head of each condyle to move too far anteriorly on the articular eminence. Muscle spasticity causes the condylar heads to lock in position. This prevents the jaws from closing, a condition called subluxation. Lateral deviation occurs when the mandible shifts to the side and back to centric during both opening and closing movements. Deflection is the movement of the mandible to the side during opening and back to centric during closing movements. Mandibular protrusion is a normal incisor-guided movement.

156. **C** Biologic indicators are the best method of determining if instruments are being sterilized because they contain bacterial spores that will die when exposed to proper sterilizing conditions. Indicator tapes are useful for indicating which instruments have or haven't been exposed to the high heat of a sterilizer, but do not ensure adequate sterilization. The length of time sterilizers run, alone, will not ensure that the proper pressure and heat is present to sterilize, any more than the looseness of instrument wraps does.

157. **B** From softest to hardest, the order of hardness of gypsum products is: impression plaster, model plaster, dental stone, and die stone. Dental stone is approximately three times harder than plaster. The hardness of the product is related to the water/powder ratio which is determined by the manufacturing process differences between stones and plasters.

158. **A** Type I hypersensitivity is not associated with release of T-cell chemical mediators. Histamine and other chemical mediators found in mast cells and basophils, but not T cells, cause smooth muscle contraction and other symptoms of Type I hypersensitivity, which is triggered when IgE molecules are cross-linked by antigen on the surface of mast cells or basophils.

159. **C** The three furcations of a maxillary first molar (and all maxillary molars) are located mid-mesially, mid-distally, and mid-buccally. Mandibular molars have two furcations located buccally and lingually.

160. **A** During an epileptic seizure, no attempt should be made to restrain the patient. The main objectives are to keep the patient from hurting himself and to provide support following seizure activity. It will be necessary to clear the area surrounding the patient and to remove any dental instruments from the oral cavity if possible. If the patient becomes unconscious, the airway must be maintained.

161. **B** Diuretics do NOT cause gingival overgrowth as do calcium channel blockers, anticonvulsants, antidysrhythmics, and antihistamines.

162. **D** The papillomavirus, not the Epstein-Barr virus, is the cause of verruca vulgaris (common wart) and condyloma acuminatum. Surgical excision warts is required to prevent reinoculation or spread of the virus.

163. **D** Pyrophosphates are the ingredients in tarter-control toothpastes that reduce supragingival calculus deposition by inhibiting development of the crystalline structure of calculus. Potassium nitrate and strontium chloride are desensitizing agents used in desensitizing toothpastes. Monofluorophosphate, when combined with sodium, is an anti-caries ingredient found in many fluoridated toothpastes.

164. **B** Salivary gland dysfunction and risk of osteoradionecrosis are lifelong side effects of radiation therapy to the oral cavity. Mucositis and taste loss resolve within weeks to months after completion of radiation therapy to the oral cavity. Sometimes patients complain of a change in tasting ability compared to pre-radiation experience, but nearly all patients regain some taste. Mucositis resolves after mucosal tissues regenerate following radiation therapy.

165. **D** Heavy plaque build-up and inflammation are NOT associated with LJP. To the contrary, this disease is often present in very clean mouths with little inflammation. The patient has an inherited PMN defect which prevents inhibition of *A. actinomycetemcomitans* and leads to severe destruction of periodontium surrounding newly erupted permanent teeth. The destruction may stop if the patient is able to produce antibodies to *A. actinomycetemcomitans*, which will prevent periodontal destruction of tissues surrounding future erupting teeth. Without treatment, the prognosis is poor for affected sites.

166. **D** Although epithelial healing after surgery takes approximately 7 days, bone does not begin to heal for at least 4 weeks and may take up to 6 months for complete osseous healing and remodeling to take place.

167. **C** The restoration of a mesial contact area on an anterior tooth (#11) is considered a Class III restoration (M or D). A Class I restoration covers the occlusal pit and fissure surfaces (O). Class II restorations involve the occlusal and proximal surfaces of posterior teeth (MOD, DO), while Class IV restorations involve proximal and incisal surfaces of anterior teeth (MI, DIL). Cervical restorations are considered Class V restorations.

168. **C** Panoramic radiographs, like other extraoral radiographs, do not have the detail to adequately detect interproximal bone loss (especially slight to moderate levels) or other fine changes. They are useful for viewing large areas of the maxilla or mandible on a single film.

169. **C** Prilocaine is the only amide anesthetic listed that is metabolized in the lung, rather than the liver. Patients with liver disease should not receive anesthetics or other drugs that are metabolized in the liver.

170. **C** Glass ionomer restorative materials have better cervical retention due to their adhesive qualities than do composite restoratives. In addition, the ionomer restorations have an anticaries effect due to leaching of fluoride from the restorations. Composite restoratives provide better thermal insulation, have greater esthetic value, and higher compressive strength than glass ionomers.

171. **B** Lactose intolerance is an intestinal condition that causes such symptoms as cramping, abdominal distention, and gas symptoms. Associated with lactose intolerance is the body's absence of the enzyme lactase—which breaks down lactose into glucose and galactose. Without this process, the lactose descends directly to the large intestine where intestinal bacteria break it down into acids and gas, causing abdominal discomfort.

172. **E** Film speed E is the fastest film, meaning it reacts quickly to radiation and thus requires less time exposure. Film speed A is the slowest reacting, followed by B, C, and D.

173. **A** Anaphylaxis or anaphylactic shock affects different body systems individually or simultaneously. Urticaria and pruritus may be exhibited as part of the skin's response to this severe allergic reaction. An asthmatic attack most commonly affects the respiratory system.

174. **C** Primary calculus forming salts in bacterial plaque are phosphates and calcium.

175. **C** When transferring a patient from wheelchair to dental chair or dental chair to wheelchair, the dental chair should be at the same height as or slightly lower than that of the wheelchair.

176. **D** Nutrients for subgingival plaque are derived from crevicular fluid and blood products. Anaerobic bacteria thrive in this oxygen-deficient area. Sulcular fluid, not saliva, bathes the environment. Oral cleansing mechanisms have little effect on bacterial makeup in subgingival regions.

177. **A** The only instruments currently recommended for implant use are plastic instruments. Ultrasonic, air polishing and metallic instruments have all been shown to produce significant damage to the implant surface.

178. **D** T lymphocytes are bound to antigens with their membrane-associated T cell receptor. Some antigens (e.g., bacterial lipopolysaccharides) are T-independent, and do not require T cells in order to stimulate antibodies. Although T cells are necessary for full-blown antibody (humoral) immunity to most antigens, T cells also are critical in the generation of cell-mediated immunity. T cells are found at many body sites, e.g. they circulate in the blood and are present in lymph nodes.

179. **B** A retrognathic jaw position with anterior overjet is referred to as Class II, Division I occlusion. Class I occlusion is mesiognathic and Class III is prognathic.

180. **D** Adaptation relates to the relationship of the entire working end of the instrument to the tooth. Adaptation does not address the angle between the face and tooth during the placement or working phase of the stroke nor does it address issues of grasp.

181. **C** The stratified random sampling method can best accomplish the task of determining the dental needs of community residents because it randomly selects a specific number of residents from each of the age groups listed, thus allowing a representative sample of the actual population to be included. A random sample would allow each resident an equal opportunity to be selected but would not guarantee

proportional representation from each age group. A stratified sample would allow proportional representation from each age group but would not allow each member within each group an equal change of selection. A convenience sample is the least representative method of sampling as it would entail selecting a sample, such as elderly residents at a senior citizen center, and would not necessarily be representative of the total population being studied. A systematic sample would select each nth resident and would not allow each resident an equal opportunity to be selected.

182. **B** The Root Caries Index (RCI) is the epidemiological index that is the BEST choice for evaluating caries prevalence in the senior population of this community because older adults are at greatest risk of developing root caries. The DMFT and DMFS do not assess root surface caries. The CPITN assesses periodontal treatment needs, not restorative needs of populations.

183. **D** The recommended dosage of supplemental fluoride for a 5-year-old child in this community (natural fluoride concentration is less than 0.3 mg) is 1.0 mg.

184. **B** Calibration is the method of practicing and making comparisons (trial runs) of assessments on a sample (volunteers) until all evaluators are comparable in technique. Reliability is a measure of whether a test measures what it is meant to measure. Inter-rater reliability is reliability between 2 or more evaluators over time and occurs throughout the course of the study. Intra-rater reliability is reliability within an evaluator over time and is conducted through the course of the study to make sure an evaluator consistently measures the same thing the same way.

185. **C** Correlation analysis is the study of two variables (caries rate and use of prescription fluoride supplementation) and their effect on each other. The stronger the relationship, the stronger the correlation. In this case, there is a strong negative correlation between caries rate and use of prescription fluoride supplements. Standard deviation is a means of describing the dispersion of scores around a mean. Nominal data are categorized data that indicate frequencies of occurrence of the categories. Analysis of variance is used to make comparisons between more than two means.

186. **E** While all of the answer choices are factors in dental utilization, socioeconomic status (SES) is the MOST important influence on dental utilization rates. Persons with higher SES (education and income), regardless of age, race, gender, location, or ethnicity, seek dental services at a higher rate than those of lower SES. Those with higher SES also are more likely to have dental insurance.

187. **C** An epidemic is a rapid increase in the number of cases of a disease within a particular population, as in the Influenza X example. Incidence is the rate at which a disease occurs, while prevalence is the total number of cases of disease in a given population. A pandemic is a disease that occurs throughout a population of a country, people, or world. An endemic is a slightly higher-than-normal incidence of a disease.

188. **D** The OHI-S is used to measure debris (plaque, stain, material alba, and food) and calculus on specific tooth surfaces, not tooth demineralization. The debris and calculus levels are scores (scale of 1–3) on six surfaces of six teeth and are averaged to provide the average OHI-S.

189. **D** Systematic sampling is exemplified by selecting every 9th adult listed on the alphabetized roster of shelter residents for assessment of oral hygiene needs. A convenience sample is the least representative method of sampling as it would entail selecting a sample, such as elderly residents at a senior citizen center, that is not necessarily representative of the total population being studied. A stratified sample would allow proportional representation from each age group but would not allow each member within each group an equal chance of selection. A random sample would allow each resident an equal opportunity to be selected but would not guarantee proportional representation from each age group.

190. **C** The MOST efficient way to provide oral hygiene instruction to large numbers of project participants is through lecture and demonstration. This means allows the speaker to adjust the pace and content of the presentation for the audience and allows participants to ask questions. A videotaped presentation also allows large groups to hear instruction and see demonstration but does not allow interaction. Pamphlets containing oral hygiene instruction are best used as a take-home tool after formal instruction. Individualized instruction is ideal but impractical when dealing with educating large groups of people.

191. **A** The "condition element" of an instructional objective restricts or guides the participants as they attempt to meet the objective. In this example, "after watching a toothbrushing demonstration" is the condition the participant must meet. The "audience element" of the objective is the residents who are the subjects, while the "behavior element" is they will be able to perform. The Modified Stillman toothbrushing technique is an example of the "degree element" of the objective since it describes the level of achievement expected of the participant.

192. **C** A resident's behavior is modified when the resident habitually brushes and flosses daily. A habit is formed when behavior is modified. Awareness, understanding, self-interest, and involvement are all steps to forming a habit.

193. **B** Project evaluation or appraisal is a judgment of the worth of a project. One way to make this judgment is to compare baseline data (<2% homeless fully employed) with results obtained during and after the project is completed (nearly 46% of homeless fully-

employed within 3 months of project completion and eighty-two percent of those remain employed for at least two years). Assessment is the tool used to determine the needs of the population and the outcomes of the project. Implementation is putting the program into action. Supervision is the administration or overseeing of a project.

194. **C** Improvement in oral health is the BEST measure of the effect of an oral health program. Costs are a measure of the program efficiency. Changes in attitude measure affect but may not result in a health change. Social change may be an effect of an oral health care program, but not enough information is know about the type of change to indicate it is the best measure.

195. **B** The questionnaire given to students prior to the presentation on smoking dangers serves as the control, since the questionnaire itself does not change when administered again (only the results change). A sample is a selected number of persons from the population that represents the population itself. The population is the larger pool of persons that is being studied and from which a sample is taken. Standard deviation is a measure of variability of scores around the mean.

196. **B** The only inference that can be made from this study is that significant learning occurred regarding the relationship of smoking to infant birth-weight. Little change occurred between pre-test and post-test regarding the number of students who smoked 15 or more cigarettes in the past month, the rate at which middle-school students began smoking, and learning regarding the relationship of smoking to lung cancer.

197. **D** Discussion of halitosis as a smoking-related issue would MOST appeal to this middle-school-aged population, since adolescents are often concerned with appearances and acceptance by their peers. Issues such as heart disease, emphysema, and tooth loss are less likely to appeal to adolescents since they tend to occur much later in life.

198. **C** Educating children about tobacco use and its effects will raise awareness of its dangerous affects and its addictive properties, however, a raised awareness does not always result in the desired behavior (avoiding tobacco use in the future).

199. **D** The number of middle-school students who began smoking in 1998 is considered it incidence. Prevalence is the total number of cases in a given population in a given period of time (number of middle-school students who smoked in the time period of January 1997 to January 1999). An index is a systematic way of collecting data so it can be analyzed. Morbidity is a number representing the number of actual diseases in relation to the number of possible diseases.

200. **B** A hypothesis is a statement of expected outcomes of a study, such as "Students who attend the Dangers of Cigarette Smoking presentation will decrease their use of cigarettes". An objective has a similar form but contains a measurable end result, such as "at the completion of the presentation, 96% of students will decrease their daily use of cigarettes by 10%". An observation describes an action that takes place. An instruction includes guidelines, rules, and limits for performing a function.

618 • Saunders Review of Dental Hygiene

Part B: QUESTIONS

Case Study A: Illustrations on pages I-2 and I-3 refer to this case.

1. Taking into consideration the severity and age of onset of condition, oral hygiene, and risk factors, what is the most likely diagnosis of this condition?
   A. moderate adult periodontitis
   B. rapidly progressive periodontitis
   C. acute necrotizing ulcerative periodontitis
   D. juvenile periodontitis

2. What is the estimated attachment loss on the mesiobuccal of teeth #3?
   A. <2 mm
   B. 2–4 mm
   C. 5–7 mm
   D. >7 mm

3. Which environmental factor MOST contributed to this patient's periodontal breakdown?
   A. cigarette smoking
   B. malocclusion
   C. defective restorations
   D. emotional stress

4. The radiolucency in the center of the root of tooth #31 is indicative of:
   A. periodontal abscess
   B. furcation involvement
   C. periapical abscess
   D. enamel pearl

5. Based on radiographic evidence in the region of the anterior teeth, which of the following would one expect clinical evidence of?
   A. globulomaxillary cyst
   B. drifting of the teeth
   C. tooth sensitivity
   D. periodontal abscess

6. What does the significant widening of the periodontal ligament space on the mesial of tooth #5 indicate?
   A. root fracture
   B. occlusal trauma
   C. disuse atrophy
   D. hypofunction

7. Which of the following treatment plans is MOST appropriate for his periodontal condition?
   A. a 1-hour appointment of scaling to remove calculus and stain followed by a maintenance appointment in 6 months
   B. two 1-hour appointments for scaling and root planing followed by a maintenance appointment in 6 months
   C. four 1-hour appointments for scaling and root planing followed by a reevaluation in 3 months
   D. four 1-hour appointments for scaling and root planing with anesthesia followed by a reevaluation in 4–6 weeks

8. One week after treatment, the patient complains of sensitivity to cold temperatures. An appropriate desensitization protocol would include all of the following, EXCEPT one. Which one is the EXCEPTION?
   A. potassium nitrate-based toothpaste
   B. professionally applied dentin sealer
   C. evaluation of plaque removal
   D. increased intake of citrus foods

9. All of the following adjunctive therapies should be considered for this patient, EXCEPT one. Which one is the EXCEPTION?
   A. desensitization of exposed root surfaces
   B. prescription of chlorhexidine mouthrinse
   C. professional bleaching of the teeth
   D. selective polishing to remove tobacco stain

10. After completion of initial therapy, presuming a positive tissue response, what sequence of supportive care would be the most appropriate for this patient?
   A. 1 month
   B. 3 months
   C. 6 months
   D. 12 months

11. Which factor will inhibit healing of the periodontal pocket on the distal of tooth #14?
   A. overhanging restoration
   B. occlusal trauma
   C. furcation involvement
   D. inflamed tissues

12. Which oral hygiene device can BEST remove plaque on the distal of tooth #14?
   A. oral irrigator
   B. dental floss
   C. end-tuft brush
   D. interproximal brush

13. What is the MOST likely reason for the whitish coloration of the palatal tissues?
   A. leukoplakia
   B. normal coloration
   C. hyperkeratinization
   D. candidiasis
   E. leukoedema

Case Study B: Illustrations on pages I-4 and I-5 refer to this case.

14. What is the appropriate classification for the restoration on tooth #30?
   A. Class I
   B. Class II
   C. Class III
   D. Class IV

15. Which of the following BEST describes the patient's occlusion?
   A. Class I
   B. Class II, division I
   C. Class II, division II
   D. Class III

16. What is the MOST likely cause for the radiolucent area at the apex of tooth #28?
    A. periapical abscess
    B. mental foramen
    C. mandibular canal
    D. bone cyst

17. What is the MOST likely cause of the appearance of radiolucent areas on the crown surfaces of tooth #5 and 12?
    A. coronal caries
    B. tooth fracture
    C. fixer spots
    D. enamel erosion

18. Which one of the following is the MAJOR cause of the patient's chief complaint?
    A. occlusal trauma
    B. incipient caries
    C. enamel erosion
    D. toothbrush abrasion

19. The patient's hypersensitivity will be treated by daily fluoride application. Which type of fluoride product should be recommended?
    A. acidulated phosphate fluoride
    B. fluoride varnish
    C. neutral sodium fluoride
    D. stannous fluoride

20. Which clinical sign is this patient MOST likely to exhibit?
    A. lanugo
    B. ideal body weight
    C. reduced body weight
    D. loss of menstrual periods

21. This patient may show evidence of all the following conditions, EXCEPT one. Which one is the EXCEPTION?
    A. swollen glands
    B. decreased heart rate
    C. bleeding esophagus
    D. thermal sensitivity of teeth

22. Which of the following is MOST likely to cause health problems for this patient?
    A. purging
    B. weight loss
    C. inadequate diet
    D. binge eating

Case Study C: Illustrations on pages I-6 and I-7 refer to this case.

23. This patient's periodontal condition has continued to decline after extensive periodontal treatment and frequent continuing care. What is the appropriate term for this form of periodontitis?
    A. localized juvenile periodontitis
    B. chronic adult periodontitis
    C. refractory periodontitis
    D. hormone-induced periodontitis

24. The patient complains of having a dry mouth, which began in the past year or two. What is the MOST probable cause of this condition?
    A. medication
    B. cigarette smoking
    C. menopause
    D. periodontitis

25. Cigarette smoking increases the incidence of all of the following oral conditions, EXCEPT one. Which one is the EXCEPTION?
    A. bone loss
    B. calculus
    C. caries
    D. stomatitis

26. What is the MOST likely cause of the root exposures apparent on the photograph of the right side?
    A. toothbrush trauma
    B. periodontal surgery
    C. age-related recession
    D. anterior crowding

27. Which one of the following is the MOST descriptive of the appearance of inflamed gingival tissues adjacent to tooth #9?
    A. acute papillary
    B. acute marginal
    C. chronic diffuse
    D. chronic papillary

28. After a thorough assessment, which teeth indicate a WORST prognosis?
    A. maxillary right posterior
    B. mandibular anterior
    C. maxillary anterior
    D. maxillary left posterior

29. What is the cause of the radiopaque area identified by an arrow on the maxillary right canine radiograph?
    A. cone cut
    B. maxillary sinus
    C. bent film
    D. nasal fossa wall

30. Which of the following is descriptive of the legal relationship that is established between the patient and her current dentist?
    A. written contract
    B. expressed contract
    C. guardian contract
    D. implied contract

31. When the periodontal chart and full-mouth radiographs were requested of the patient's current dentist, none were available. What might failure to record a periodontal chart and take full-mouth radiographs be indicative of?
    A. breach of contract
    B. negligence
    C. contract assault
    D. technical battery

32. What auxiliary aid will BEST remove plaque between teeth #10 and 11?

A. oral irrigating device
B. interdental brush
C. interdental tip stimulator
D. toothpick

Case Study D: Illustrations on pages I-8 and I-9 refer to this case.

33. Which of the following is TRUE regarding the patient's blood pressure measurement?
    A. Both the systolic and diastolic measurements are within normal limits
    B. Neither the systolic nor diastolic measurements are within normal limits
    C. The systolic measurement is within normal limits, but the diastolic is NOT
    D. The diastolic measurement is within normal limits, but the systolic is NOT

34. Which of the following organisms causes genital warts?
    A. Epstein-Barr virus
    B. *Staphylococcus epidermitis*
    C. *Helicobacter pylori*
    D. Human papilloma virus

35. What is the BEST description for this patient's interdental tissues?
    A. localized knifelike papilla
    B. generalized knifelike papilla
    C. localized blunted papilla
    D. generalized blunted papilla

36. Which of the following BEST describes the contour of the facial gingival margin of tooth #24?
    A. rolled
    B. festooned
    C. clefted
    D. ulcerated

37. What does an examination of the hard palate reveal?
    A. irritation fibroma
    B. papilloma
    C. torus palatinus
    D. pyogenic granuloma

38. What is the MOST likely cause of the radiolucent lesions found on teeth # 3, 4, and 30?
    A. high sugar intake
    B. periodontal involvement
    C. medication use
    D. normal anatomy

39. Which one of the following is indicated by radiographic interpretation of the posterior alveolar bone?
    A. localized vertical bone loss
    B. generalized vertical bone loss
    C. localized horizontal bone loss
    D. generalized horizontal bone loss

40. What is the MOST likely cause of the brown lesion on the buccal of tooth #19?
    A. fluorosis
    B. decay

C. demineralization
D. recession

41. What is the black band-like line that follows the contour of the gingiva on the lingual surfaces of teeth #11, 13, and 14?
    A. cervical decay
    B. stained composite resin
    C. metal substructure of bridge
    D. Class V amalgam

42. Because of rheumatoid arthritis, the patient finds it impossible to manipulate dental floss or an interdental brush at times. What other home care aid is an appropriate recommendation?
    A. powered toothbrush
    B. antimicrobial mouthrinse
    C. neutral sodium fluoride gel
    D. toothpick in holder

43. Dental hygiene treatment of the Class I and II furcations is best accomplished with which of the following?
    A. ultrasonic scaler
    B. periodontal probe
    C. air abrasive polishing
    D. sickle scaler

44. Which professionally-applied fluoride is indicated for this patient?
    A. neutral sodium gel (NaF)
    B. acidulated phosphate gel (APF)
    C. stannous gel (SnF)
    D. acidulated phosphate/stannous rinse

45. The patient contracted hepatitis A while on vacation in Mexico. She was ill for 2 to 3 weeks and became jaundiced. What is the MOST common means of contracting this disease?
    A. contaminated food
    B. unprotected sex
    C. sharing needles
    D. blood contact

Case Study E: Illustrations on pages I-10 and I-11 refer to this case.

46. The patient complains about food impaction in the maxillary posterior areas of her mouth. Which one of the following is LEAST likely to cause food impaction?
    A. periodontal pocketing
    B. three unit bridge
    C. open contacts
    D. gingivitis

47. The patient is concerned about sensitivity to scaling procedures in the mandibular anterior incisor area. What is MOST likely to cause this sensitivity?
    A. gingival recession
    B. pulpitis
    C. periapical abscess
    D. attrition

48. The pulse rate of this patient is 120 and her blood pressure is 140/85. What is the MOST likely reason for these readings?

Clinical Case Studies A-O

On the following pages are the case histories, charting forms, radiographs, and clinical photographs referred to in Part B: Case Studies A-O of the Simulated National Board Dental Hygiene Examination. The questions, answers, and rationales are located on pages 618 to 637.

CASE STUDY A

SYNOPSIS OF PATIENT HISTORY		
Age	40	
Gender	M	
Height	5'8"	
Weight	140 lbs.	

VITAL SIGNS

Blood pressure	136/82
Pulse rate	84
Respiration rate	18

1. Under care of physician
   Yes ___ No **X** Condition: _____

2. Hospitalized within the last 5 years
   Yes ___ No **X** Reason: _____

3. Has or had the following conditions
   Arthritis in knees and elbows _____
   Blindness in left eye _____

4. Current medications
   Aspirin occasionally for arthritis pain _____

5. Smokes or uses tobacco products
   Yes **X** No ___

6. Is pregnant
   Yes ___ No ___ NA **X**

MEDICAL HISTORY: Has a smoker's cough. Is legally blind in his left eye due to cortisone use 10 years earlier. Family history of cervical and lung cancer.

DENTAL HISTORY: He has known of his periodontal disease condition for 15 years but could not afford treatment. His last "cleaning" was 3 months ago. He brushes 3–4 × daily with a soft-bristled brush and uses an end-tuft brush, interdental brush, and floss daily. Tooth #2 was extracted due to periodontal disease. He has generalized sensitivity to cold, heat, and sweets.

SOCIAL HISTORY: Divorced father of two; has smoked 1 to 2 packs of cigarettes daily for 24 years; feels stressed (father is dying of lung cancer).

CHIEF COMPLAINT: "I need to get my deep pockets treated."

NOTE:

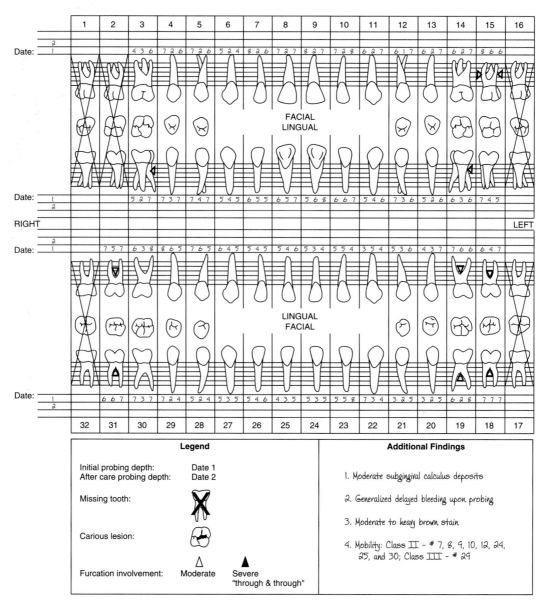

Legend

Initial probing depth: Date 1
After care probing depth: Date 2

Missing tooth:

Carious lesion:

Furcation involvement: △ Moderate ▲ Severe "through & through"

Additional Findings

1. Moderate subgingival calculus deposits

2. Generalized delayed bleeding upon probing

3. Moderate to heavy brown stain

4. Mobility: Class II – # 7, 8, 9, 10, 12, 24, 25, and 30; Class III – # 29

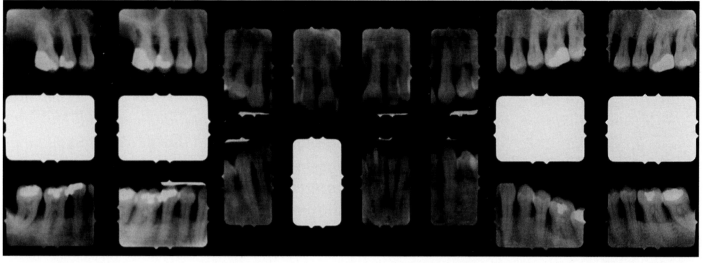

R   L

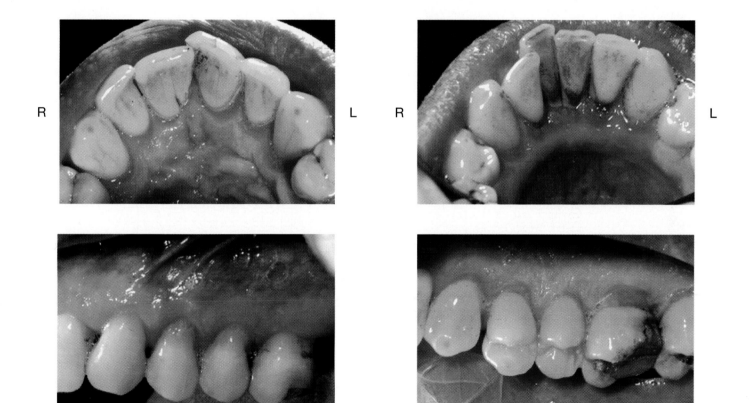

R   L   R   L

Maxillary Right Buccal   Maxillary Left Lingual

CASE STUDY B

SYNOPSIS OF PATIENT HISTORY

Age	32
Gender	F
Height	5'8"
Weight	145 lbs.

VITAL SIGNS

Blood pressure	108/70
Pulse rate	70
Respiration rate	16

1. Under care of physician
   Yes   No   Condition: _____
               X

2. Hospitalized within the last 5 years
   Yes   No   Reason: _____
               X

3. Has or had the following conditions

4. Current medications

5. Smokes or uses tobacco products
   Yes   No
          X

6. Is pregnant
   Yes   No   NA
          X

MEDICAL HISTORY: Unremarkable.

DENTAL HISTORY: The patient has a dental examination and oral prophylaxis annually. She brushes 2–3 × daily.

SOCIAL HISTORY: Is currently a full-time student in her junior year of college.

CHIEF COMPLAINT: "My upper teeth are sensitive to cold."

NOTE: Has excellent oral hygiene. Calluses are noted on the knuckles of her right hand. Patient appears anxious. Is currently receiving counseling for eating disorder.

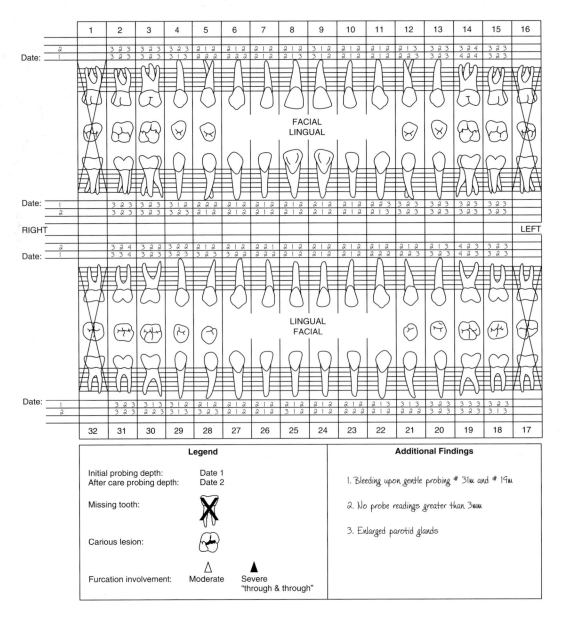

Legend

Initial probing depth: Date 1
After care probing depth: Date 2

Missing tooth:

Carious lesion:

Furcation involvement: Moderate △   Severe ▲ "through & through"

Additional Findings

1. Bleeding upon gentle probing # 31m and # 19m

2. No probe readings greater than 3mm

3. Enlarged parotid glands

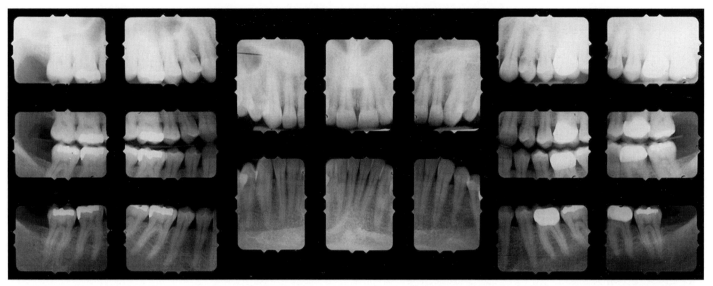

R   L

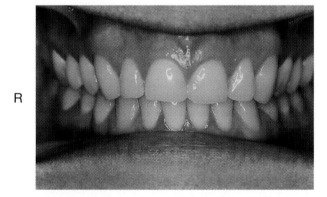

R   L

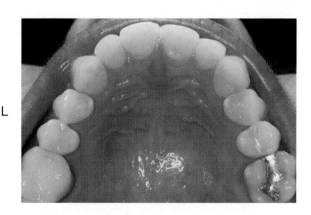

L   R

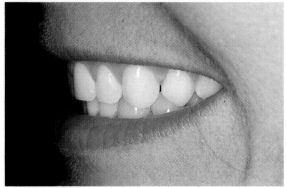

Left Side

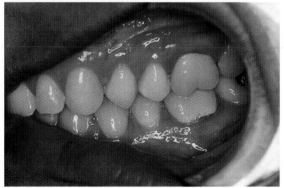

Left Side

CASE STUDY C

SYNOPSIS OF PATIENT HISTORY

Age	51	
Gender	F	
Height	5'5"	
Weight	135 lbs.	

VITAL SIGNS

Blood pressure	110/76
Pulse rate	70
Respiration rate	16

1. Under care of physician
   Yes   No   Condition: Depression
   X

2. Hospitalized within the last 5 years
   Yes   No   Reason:
        X

3. Has or had the following conditions
   Depression

4. Current medications
   Estradiol (Estraderm); Nortriptyline HCL (Pamelor)

5. Smokes or uses tobacco products
   Yes   No
   X

6. Is pregnant
   Yes   No   NA
        X

MEDICAL HISTORY: Under care for treatment of depression for 18 months.

DENTAL HISTORY: Ten years earlier, she had a gingivectomy and was told to get her teeth cleaned every 3-months. Soon after, she relocated and has been visiting her current dentist for oral prophylaxis every 3 months. She brushes 2 × daily and flosses 3–4 × a week.

SOCIAL HISTORY: Patient is a homemaker and mother of three teenagers. She has smoked 1 pack of cigarettes daily for 32 years.

CHIEF COMPLAINT: "Two of my front teeth are really loose. I'm concerned about losing my teeth, but my current dentist insists my mouth is fine."

NOTE: Patient is seeking a second opinion regarding the condition of her oral health. Her upper front teeth are loose, but her current dentist is not concerned.

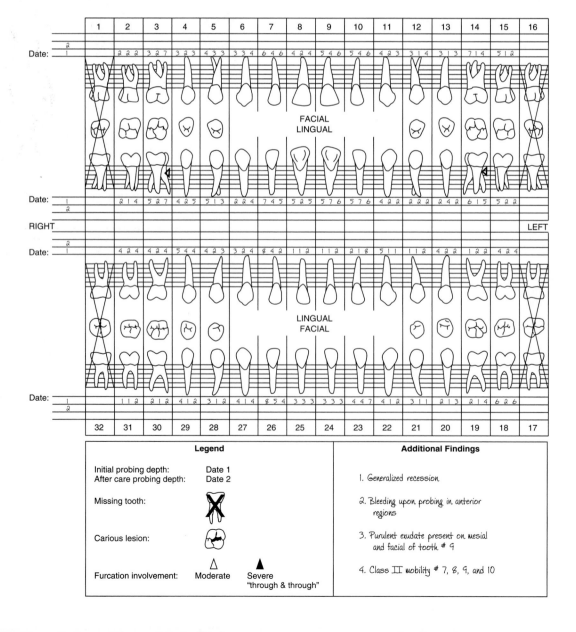

Legend

Initial probing depth:	Date 1
After care probing depth:	Date 2
Missing tooth:	
Carious lesion:	
Furcation involvement:	Moderate Severe "through & through"

Additional Findings

1. Generalized recession

2. Bleeding upon probing in anterior regions

3. Purulent exudate present on mesial and facial of tooth # 9

4. Class II mobility # 7, 8, 9, and 10

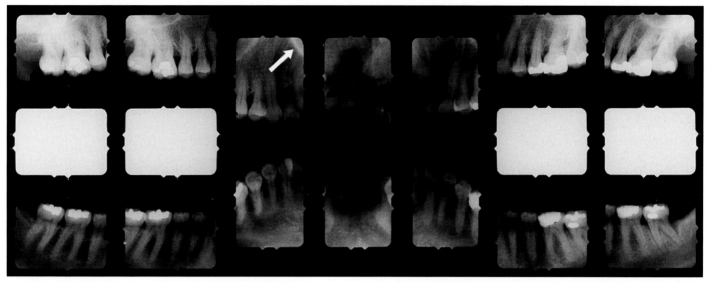

R   L

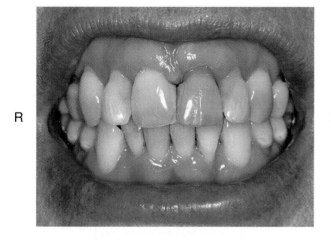

R   L   L

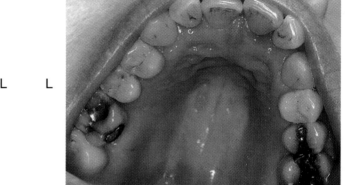

R

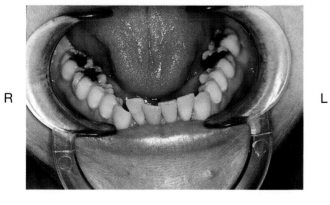

R   L

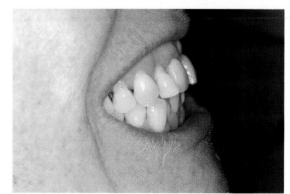

Right Side

CASE STUDY D

SYNOPSIS OF PATIENT HISTORY

Age	37
Gender	F
Height	5'6"
Weight	250 lbs.

Vital Signs

Blood pressure	137/92
Pulse rate	68
Respiration rate	20

1. Under care of physician
   Yes — X   No   Condition: Rheumatoid arthritis

2. Hospitalized within the last 5 years
   Yes — X   No   Reason: hysterectomy at age 35

3. Has or had the following conditions
   Hepatitis A; asthma; arthritis in hands, knees and neck; hysterectomy; genital warts; depression

4. Current medications
   Albuterol (Proventil); Naproxen sodium (Aleve); Prednisone (Deltasone); Sertraline (Zoloft); Trazadone HCL (Trialodine); Conjugated estrogen (Premarin)

5. Smokes or uses tobacco products
   Yes — X   No

6. Is pregnant
   Yes   No — X   NA

MEDICAL HISTORY: Patient takes Proventil for asthma, Aleve daily and prednisone every other day for arthritis, Zoloft and Trazadone for depression, Premarin for estrogen replacement.

DENTAL HISTORY: Has had sporadic dental care. Until last dental visit 3 months ago, it had been 10 years. Plaque index is 30%, she brushes 2 × daily and uses floss and interdental brush sporadically. Is highly fearful of dental/dental hygiene procedures. Reports dry mouth.

SOCIAL HISTORY: Attended college 1 year, then took position as a telephone operator.

CHIEF COMPLAINT: "I don't like the way my teeth look."

NOTE: Smokes 1 pack of cigarettes daily. Drinks 3 cups of regular coffee and two 20 oz. diet colas daily. Plaque index at previous appointment was 85%.

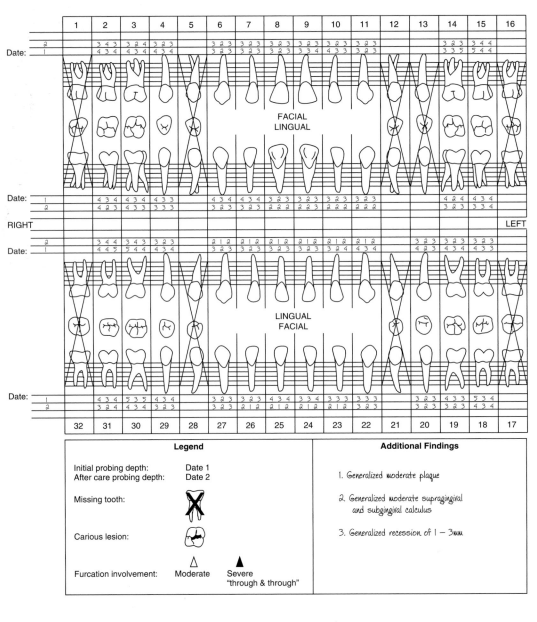

Legend

Initial probing depth: Date 1
After care probing depth: Date 2

Missing tooth:

Carious lesion:

Furcation involvement: Moderate △ Severe ▲ "through & through"

Additional Findings

1. Generalized moderate plaque

2. Generalized moderate supragingival and subgingival calculus

3. Generalized recession of 1 – 3mm

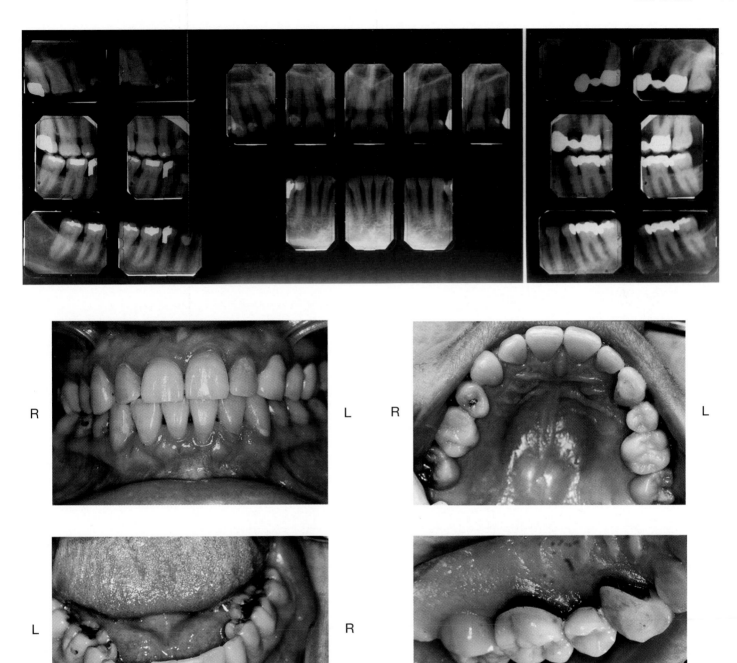

Maxillary Left Lingual

CASE STUDY E

SYNOPSIS OF PATIENT HISTORY

Age	48
Gender	F
Height	5'1"
Weight	135 lbs.

VITAL SIGNS

Blood pressure	140/85
Pulse rate	120
Respiration rate	25

1. Under care of physician
   Yes X No Condition: menopause

2. Hospitalized within the last 5 years
   Yes No X Reason:

3. Has or had the following conditions
   Eye surgery 3 times to correct muscle imbalance;
   tubal ligation

4. Current medications
   Estradiol transdermal (Climera)
   Medroxyprogesterone acetate (Provera)

5. Smokes or uses tobacco products
   Yes No X

6. Is pregnant
   Yes No X NA

MEDICAL HISTORY: Is allergic to codeine, menopausal; has annual physical; generally healthy.

DENTAL HISTORY: Last visit was 6 months ago for placement of a crown; has a great fear of dentists; 7 years since last oral prophylaxis; participates in research studies on calculus formation.

SOCIAL HISTORY: Is employed as a dental clinic manager.

CHIEF COMPLAINT: "There is a feeling of thickness on my palate behind my upper front teeth. My lower front teeth are sensitive and getting loose."

NOTE: Is afraid of "needles."

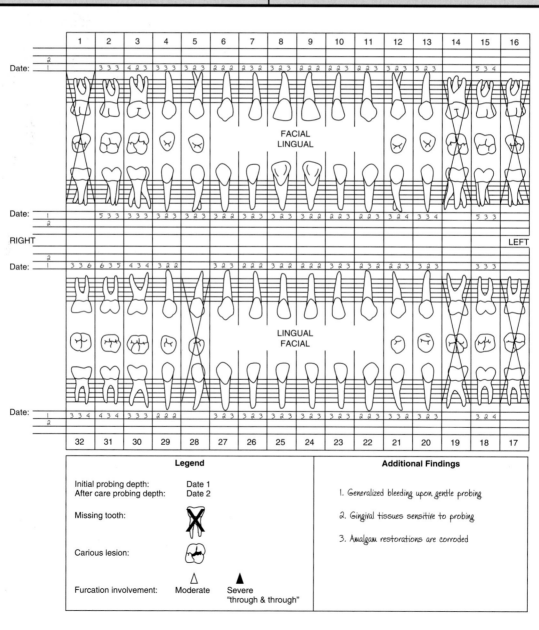

Legend

Initial probing depth:	Date 1
After care probing depth:	Date 2
Missing tooth:	✗
Carious lesion:	
Furcation involvement:	△ Moderate ▲ Severe "through & through"

Additional Findings

1. Generalized bleeding upon gentle probing
2. Gingival tissues sensitive to probing
3. Amalgam restorations are corroded

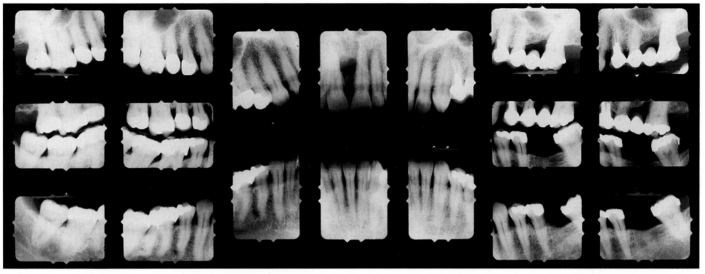

R   L

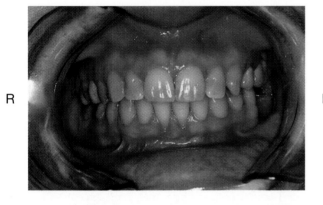

R   L

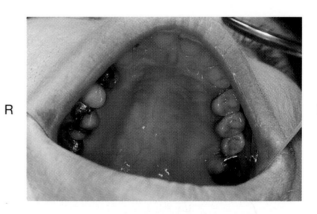

R   L

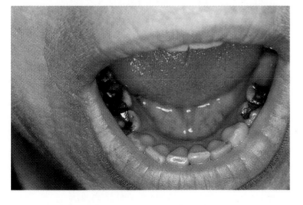

R   L

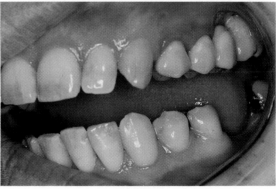

Left Side

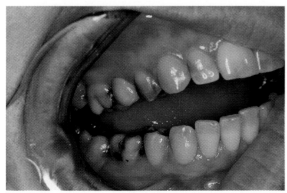

Right Side

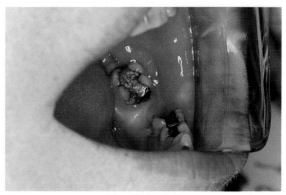

Mandibular Left

CASE STUDY F

SYNOPSIS OF PATIENT HISTORY

Age	7
Gender	M
Height	3'7"
Weight	55 lbs.

VITAL SIGNS

Blood pressure	90/56
Pulse rate	90
Respiration rate	22

1. Under care of physician
   Yes ___ No X ___ Condition: _____

2. Hospitalized within the last 5 years
   Yes X ___ No ___ Reason: Repair of cleft palate and lip

3. Has or had the following conditions
   Cleft palate and lip

4. Current medications

5. Smokes or uses tobacco products
   Yes ___ No X

6. Is pregnant
   Yes ___ No ___ NA X

MEDICAL HISTORY: Treated for bilateral cleft palate and lip shortly after birth; has had frequent ear and respiratory infections.

DENTAL HISTORY: Has had annual dental care since birth. Patient brushes his own teeth once a day.

SOCIAL HISTORY: Is having a difficult time making friends.

CHIEF COMPLAINT: "Kids at school tease me because my teeth are yellow."

NOTE: Mother was hospitalized in her fourth month of pregnancy and received a variety of medications. Photos were taken prior to eruption of permanent mandibular first molars.

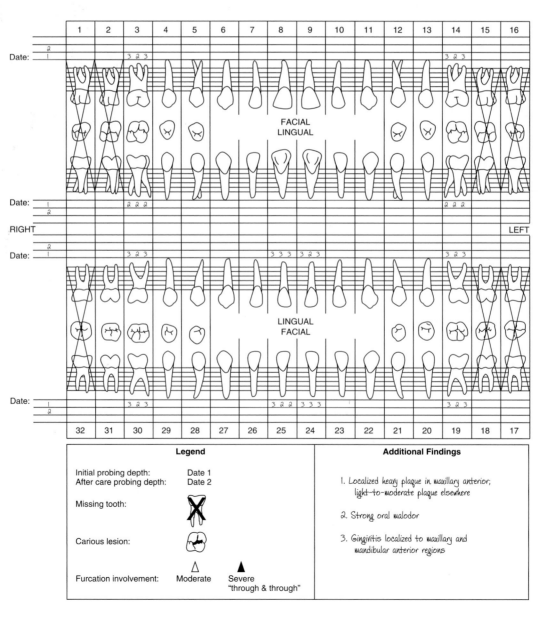

Legend

Initial probing depth:	Date 1
After care probing depth:	Date 2
Missing tooth:	✗
Carious lesion:	
Furcation involvement:	△ Moderate ▲ Severe "through & through"

Additional Findings

1. Localized heavy plaque in maxillary anterior; light-to-moderate plaque elsewhere

2. Strong oral malodor

3. Gingivitis localized to maxillary and mandibular anterior regions

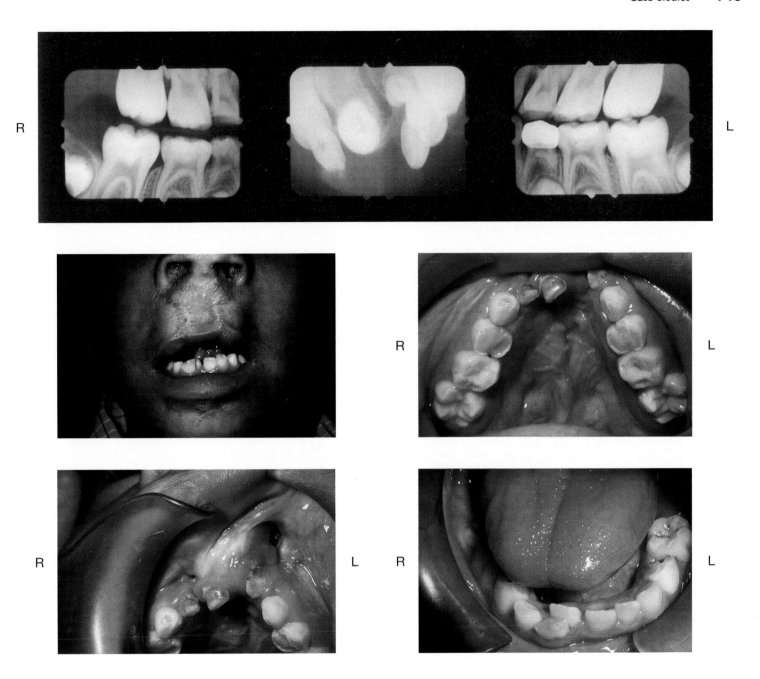

Illustrations for Case Study F courtesy Dr. Gayle Nelson, Sioux Falls, SD.

CASE STUDY G

SYNOPSIS OF PATIENT HISTORY

Age	4
Gender	M
Height	3'4"
Weight	32 lbs.

VITAL SIGNS

Blood pressure	86/60
Pulse rate	96
Respiration rate	24

1. Under care of physician
   Yes   No X   Condition: _____

2. Hospitalized within the last 5 years
   Yes X   No   Reason: _Adenoidectomy and myringotomy_

3. Has or had the following conditions
   Numerous ear infections; allergy to mold, cats, eggs

4. Current medications

5. Smokes or uses tobacco products
   Yes   No X

6. Is pregnant
   Yes   No   NA X

MEDICAL HISTORY: Tube placed in right ear and adenoids removed at age 3.

DENTAL HISTORY: This is his first dental visit.

SOCIAL HISTORY: Shy child; enjoys attending preschool 2 mornings/week.

CHIEF COMPLAINT: Mother wants to know "Is there anything that will get rid of the brown stains on his front teeth?"

NOTE:

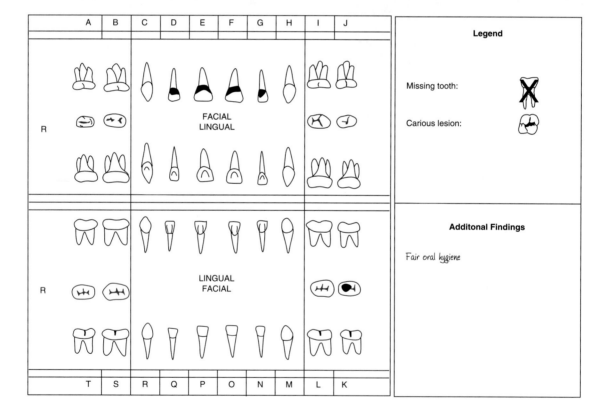

Legend

Missing tooth:

Carious lesion:

Additional Findings

Fair oral hygiene

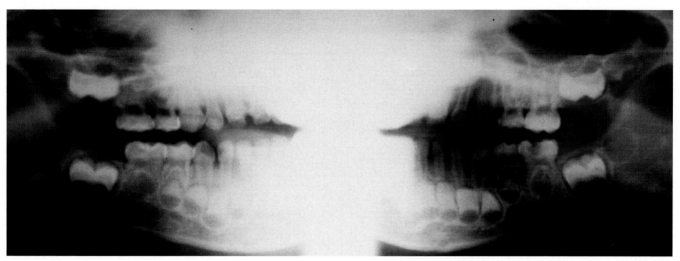

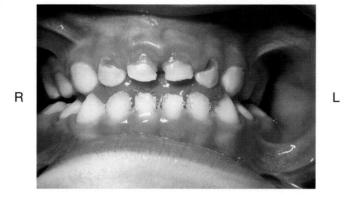

Illustrations for Case Study G courtesy Dr. Gayle Nelson, Sioux Falls, SD.

CASE STUDY H

SYNOPSIS OF PATIENT HISTORY

Age	56
Gender	F
Height	5'11"
Weight	182 lbs.

VITAL SIGNS

Blood pressure	110/70
Pulse rate	68
Respiration rate	16

1. Under care of physician
   Yes No Condition: _____
          X

2. Hospitalized within the last 5 years
   Yes No Reason: _____
          X

3. Has or had the following conditions:
   Frequent headaches in morning

4. Current medications
   Fluoxetine (Prozac); Amoxicillin trihydrate (Amoxil)

5. Smokes or uses tobacco products
   Yes No
          X

6. Is pregnant
   Yes No NA
              X

MEDICAL HISTORY: Currently taking Prozac for depression and Amoxil for sinus infection of 2 months duration.

DENTAL HISTORY: Has received routine dental examination and oral prophylaxis annually for 5 years. Prior to that time, dental care was infrequent.

SOCIAL HISTORY: Lives with elderly mother in rural community and has little social outlet.

CHIEF COMPLAINT: "My mouth is very sore and my upper back teeth hurt".

NOTE: Biopsy of oral lesions reveals lichen planus.

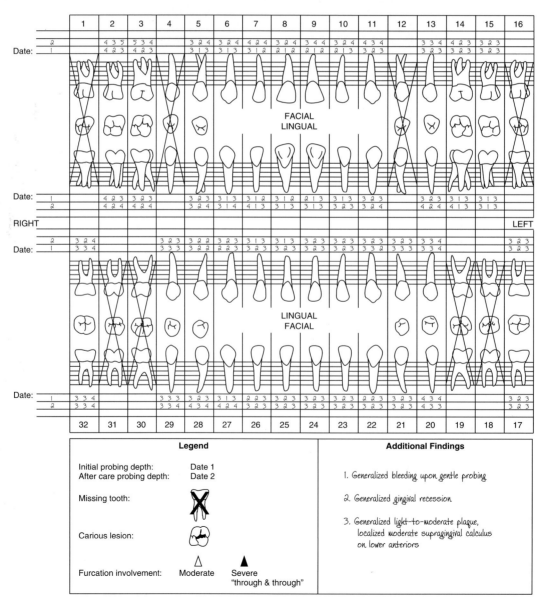

Legend

Initial probing depth: Date 1
After care probing depth: Date 2

Missing tooth:

Carious lesion:

Furcation involvement: Moderate △   Severe ▲ "through & through"

Additional Findings

1. Generalized bleeding upon gentle probing

2. Generalized gingival recession

3. Generalized light-to-moderate plaque, localized moderate supragingival calculus on lower anteriors

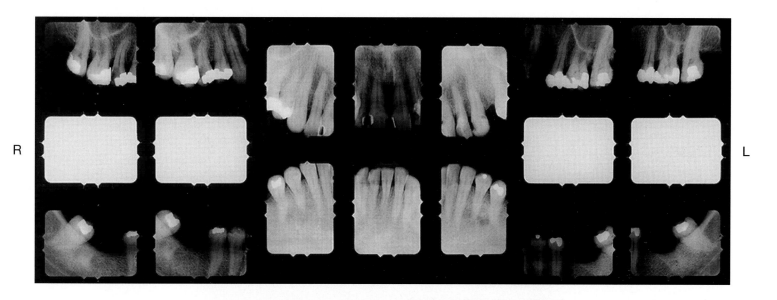

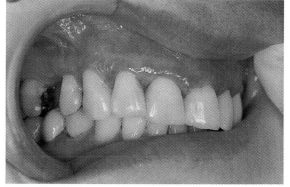

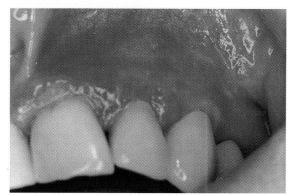

Right Side

Maxillary Left Buccal

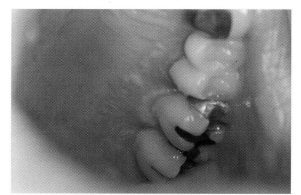

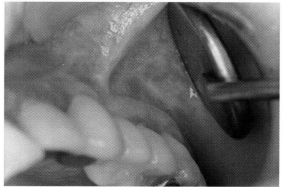

Maxillary Left Lingual

Maxillary Left Buccal

Illustrations for Case Study H courtesy Dr. Gordon Schulte, Canton, SD.

CASE STUDY I

SYNOPSIS OF PATIENT HISTORY		

Age	12
Gender	F
Height	4'11"
Weight	90 lbs.

VITAL SIGNS

Blood pressure	110/68
Pulse rate	80
Respiration rate	16

1. Under care of physician
   Yes   No X   Condition: _____

2. Hospitalized within the last 5 years
   Yes   No X   Reason: Compound fracture of tibia

3. Has or had the following conditions

4. Current medications

5. Smokes or uses tobacco products
   Yes   No X

6. Is pregnant
   Yes   No X   NA

MEDICAL HISTORY: Compound fracture healed properly. Recently completed prescription for doxycycline for nonspecific throat infection.

DENTAL HISTORY: Receives dental examination biannually.

SOCIAL HISTORY: Is a sixth grade student in an urban area. Is self-conscious of her teeth.

CHIEF COMPLAINT: "How long will it be before I can have the rest of my front teeth capped?"

NOTE: Has two sisters with same teeth condition, brother does not.

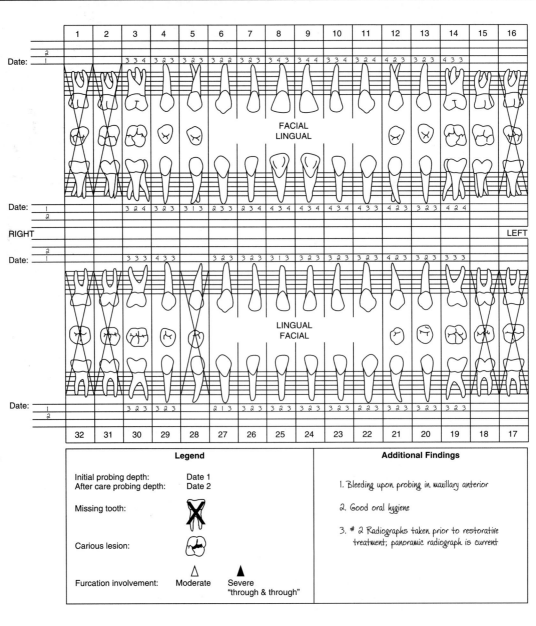

Legend

Initial probing depth: Date 1
After care probing depth: Date 2

Missing tooth:

Carious lesion:

Furcation involvement: Moderate   Severe "through & through"

Additional Findings

1. Bleeding upon probing in maxillary anterior
2. Good oral hygiene
3. # 2 Radiographs taken prior to restorative treatment; panoramic radiograph is current

Illustrations for Case Study I courtesy Dr. Gayle Nelson, Sioux Falls, SD.

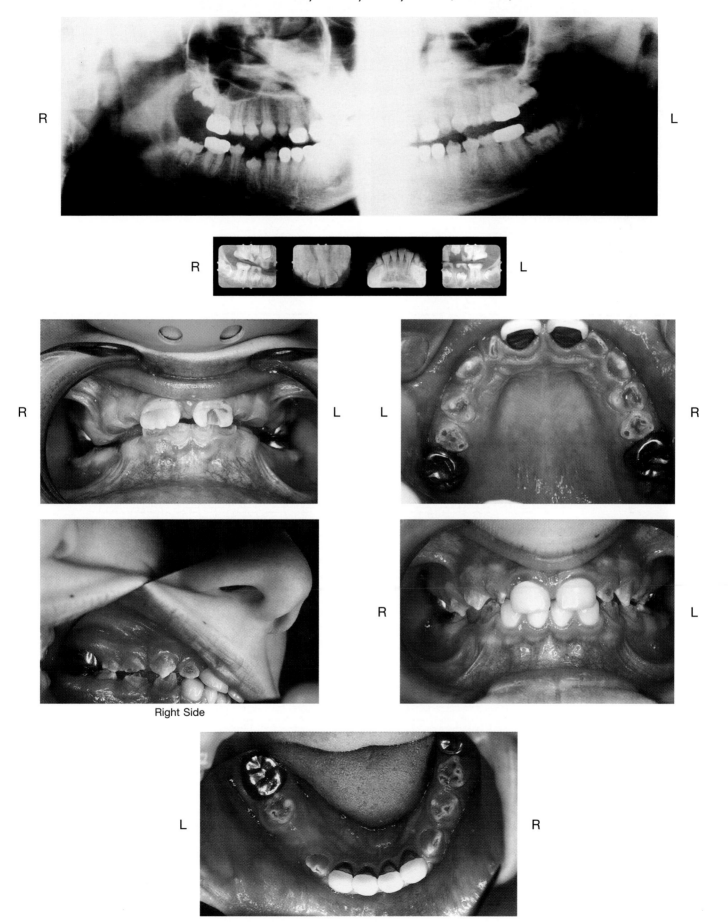

Right Side

CASE STUDY J

SYNOPSIS OF PATIENT HISTORY	Age	74	VITAL SIGNS	
	Gender	M	Blood pressure	148/94
	Height	5'10"	Pulse rate	78
	Weight	280 lbs.	Respiration rate	16

1. Under care of physician
   Yes ___ No ___ Condition: High blood pressure, diabetes
   X

2. Hospitalized within the last 5 years
   Yes ___ No ___ Reason: Minor stroke 3 years ago
   X

3. Has or had the following conditions
   Heart attack, age 30 and age 60; stroke, age 71;
   diagnosed with Type II diabetes age 65

4. Current medications
   Glipizide (Glucotrol); Amlodipine besylate (Norvasc); aspirin

5. Smokes or uses tobacco products
   Yes ___ No ___
   X

6. Is pregnant
   Yes ___ No ___ NA ___
   X

MEDICAL HISTORY: Has hard-to-control blood pressure; Norvasc has been most successful; takes Glucotrol and a single aspirin daily; does not carefully monitor blood sugar nor practice diet and exercise modification.

DENTAL HISTORY: Usually receives dental examination and oral prophylaxis every year or two. Last full-mouth series of radiographs was 2 years ago. Brushes 1–2 × daily, doesn't floss.

SOCIAL HISTORY: Is semi-retired farmer; does not have active social life.

CHIEF COMPLAINT: "My gums are really swollen but they don't hurt"

NOTE: Patient walks in a slow, shuffling manner and has difficulty climbing stairs.

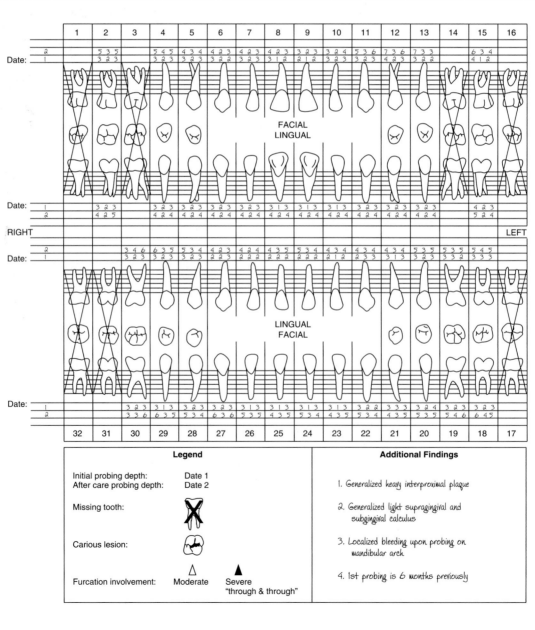

	Legend		
Initial probing depth:	Date 1		
After care probing depth:	Date 2		
Missing tooth:			
Carious lesion:			
Furcation involvement:	Moderate △	Severe ▲ "through & through"	

Additional Findings

1. Generalized heavy interproximal plaque

2. Generalized light supragingival and subgingival calculus

3. Localized bleeding upon probing on mandibular arch

4. 1st probing is 6 months previously

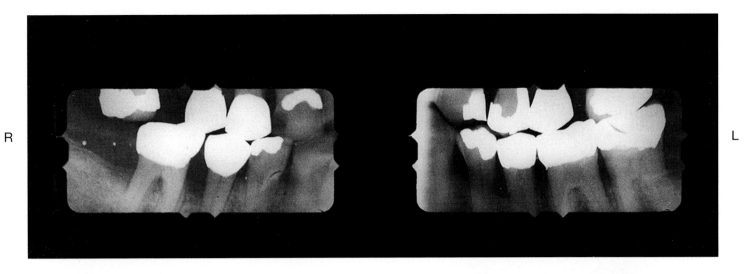

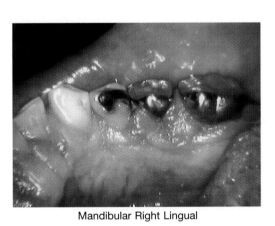

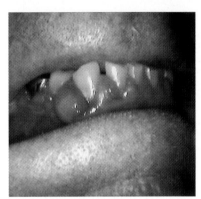

Mandibular Right Buccal

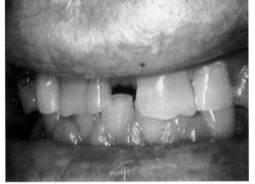

Mandibular Right Lingual

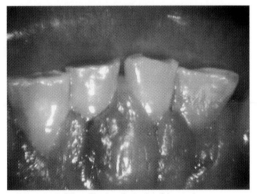

Mandibular Anterior Lingual

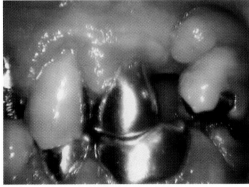

Left Side Buccal

CASE STUDY K

SYNOPSIS OF PATIENT HISTORY

Age	36
Gender	M
Height	5'9"
Weight	165 lbs.

VITAL SIGNS

Blood pressure	118/78
Pulse rate	80
Respiration rate	14

1. Under care of physician
   Yes   No   Condition: _Hypertension_
   X

2. Hospitalized within the last 5 years
   Yes   No   Reason: _____
   X

3. Has or had the following conditions
   Hypertension for 6 years

4. Current medications
   Furosemide (Lasix)

5. Smokes or uses tobacco products
   Yes   No
   X

6. Is pregnant
   Yes   No   NA
                 X

MEDICAL HISTORY: Hypertension is well controlled with Lasix; no drug allergies; alcohol and cocaine dependency.

DENTAL HISTORY: Seeks dental care approximately every 2–3 years, when something bothers him.

SOCIAL HISTORY: Former abuser of cocaine and alcohol, has been "clean" for 2 years; on probation and performing community service for vandalism while under the influence.

CHIEF COMPLAINT: "My new girlfriend doesn't like the stains on my teeth."

NOTE: Patient smokes 2 packs of unfiltered cigarettes per day.

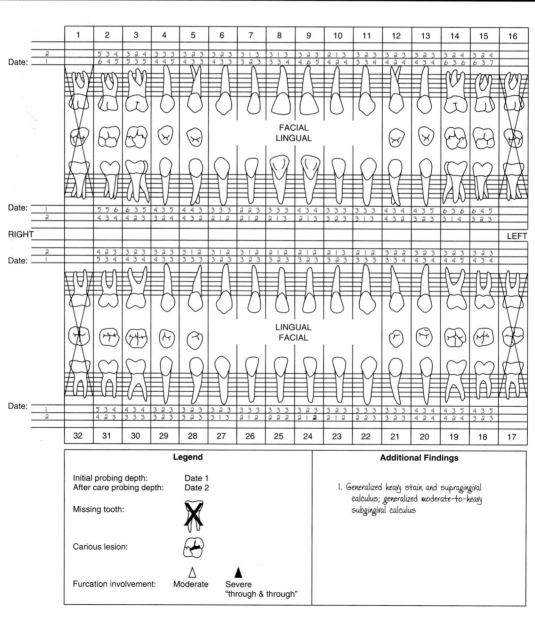

Legend

Initial probing depth: Date 1
After care probing depth: Date 2

Missing tooth:

Carious lesion:

Furcation involvement: △ Moderate   ▲ Severe "through & through"

Additional Findings

1. Generalized heavy stain and supragingival calculus; generalized moderate-to-heavy subgingival calculus

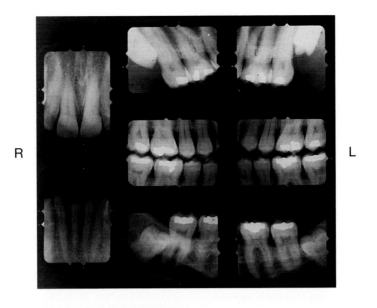

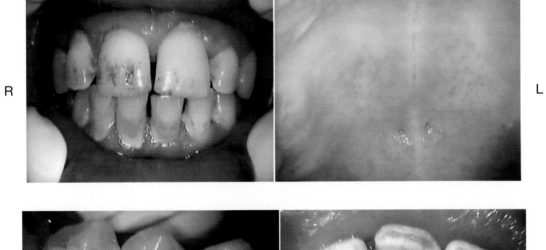

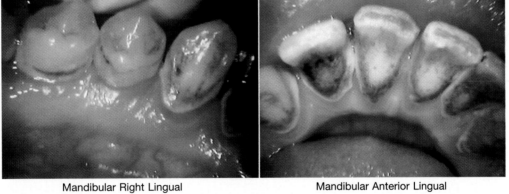

Mandibular Right Lingual   Mandibular Anterior Lingual

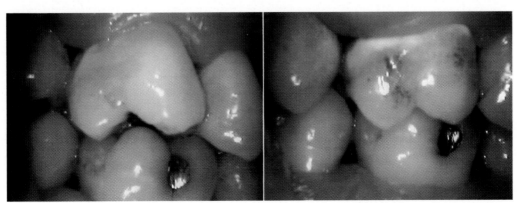

Left Side   Right Side

CASE STUDY L

SYNOPSIS OF PATIENT HISTORY

Age	14
Gender	F
Height	5'2"
Weight	110 lbs.

VITAL SIGNS

Blood pressure	90/72
Pulse rate	60
Respiration rate	14

1. Under care of physician
   Yes ___ No X ___ Condition: _____

2. Hospitalized within the last 5 years
   Yes ___ No X ___ Reason: _____

3. Has or had the following conditions
   _____
   _____

4. Current medications
   _____
   _____

5. Smokes or uses tobacco products
   Yes ___ No X ___

6. Is pregnant
   Yes ___ No X ___ NA ___

MEDICAL HISTORY: Unremarkable.

DENTAL HISTORY: Has dental examination and oral prophylaxis biannually.

SOCIAL HISTORY: 8th grade student; active in athletics; outgoing personality.

CHIEF COMPLAINT: "My teeth are so crowded, I hate them."

NOTE: Patient's mother indicates the patient frequently bruxes at night. Has strong gag reflex, especially to bitewing radiographs.

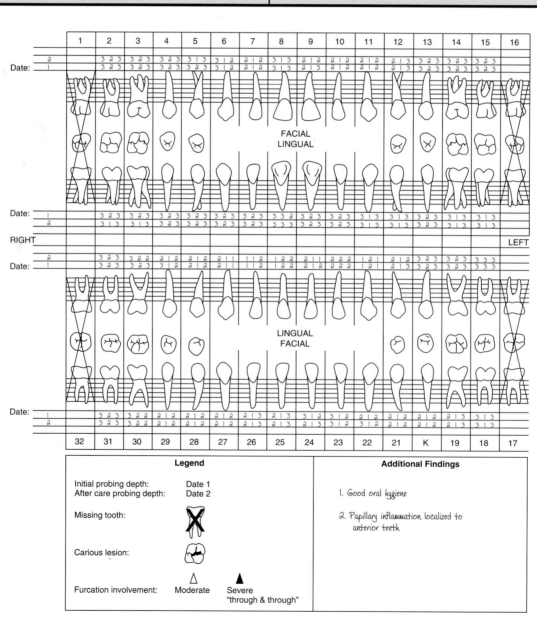

Legend

Initial probing depth: Date 1
After care probing depth: Date 2

Missing tooth:

Carious lesion:

Furcation involvement: △ Moderate ▲ Severe "through & through"

Additional Findings

1. Good oral hygiene

2. Papillary inflammation localized to anterior teeth

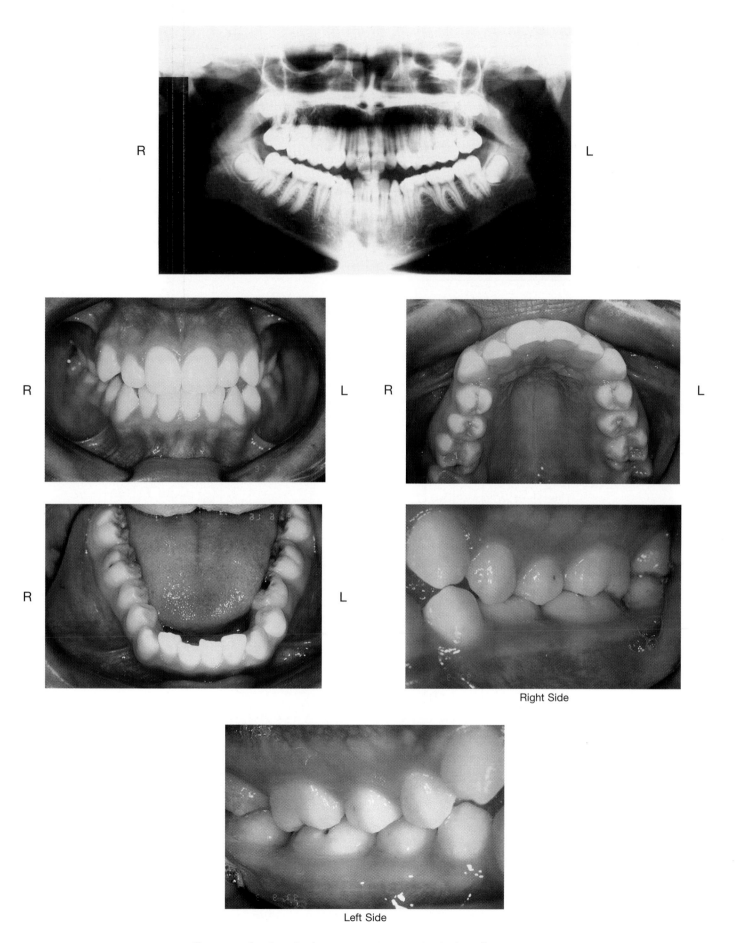

R   L

R   L

R   L

R   L

Right Side

Left Side

Illustrations for Case Study L courtesy Dr. Dona M. Seely, Bellevue, WA.

CASE STUDY M

SYNOPSIS OF PATIENT HISTORY

Age	59
Gender	F
Height	5'2"
Weight	176 lbs.

VITAL SIGNS

Blood pressure	138/76
Pulse rate	82
Respiration rate	18

1. Under care of physician
   Yes X   No   Condition: Sleep apnea, heart disease, diabetes

2. Hospitalized within the last 5 years
   Yes X   No   Reason: Heart attack, bypass surgery (triple)

3. Has or had the following conditions
   Insulin-dependent diabetes mellitus; breast cancer
   10 years ago; high cholesterol; depression

4. Current medications
   Aspirin; insulin; levothyroxine sodium (Synthroid); lovastatin (Mevacor); lisinopril (Prinivil); nitroglycerin spray (Nitrolingual); sertraline (Zoloft); trazodone (Trazon)

5. Smokes or uses tobacco products
   Yes   No X

6. Is pregnant
   Yes   No X   NA

MEDICAL HISTORY: Injects insulin daily for control of diabetes; hypertension is controlled by lisinopril; has sleep apnea; had triple bypass surgery after a heart attack 3 years ago; thyroidectomy 20 years ago.

DENTAL HISTORY: Dental care is infrequent, usually every 2–4 years; multiple stress fractures in premolar and anterior teeth.

SOCIAL HISTORY: Retired after heart surgery, formerly a postal worker for 20 years.

CHIEF COMPLAINT: "My gums bleed when I brush my teeth."

NOTE: Coffee and tea drinker; uses medium-bristled toothbrush.

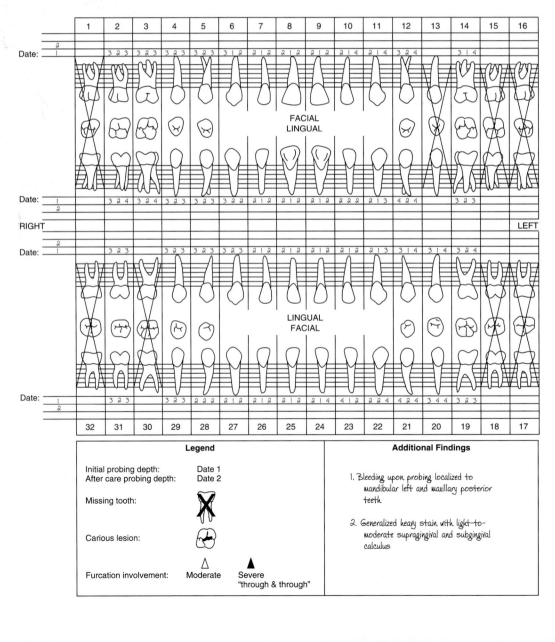

Legend

Initial probing depth: Date 1
After care probing depth: Date 2

Missing tooth: ✗

Carious lesion:

Furcation involvement: △ Moderate ▲ Severe "through & through"

Additional Findings

1. Bleeding upon probing localized to mandibular left and maxillary posterior teeth.

2. Generalized heavy stain with light-to-moderate supragingival and subgingival calculus

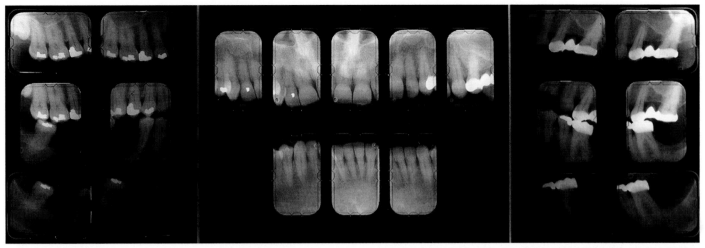

R   L

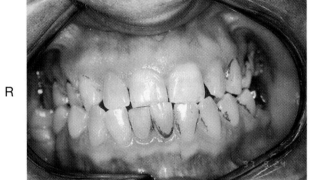

R   L

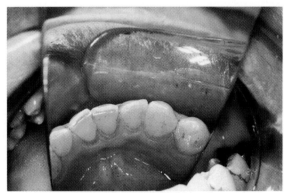

Mandibular Anterior Lingual

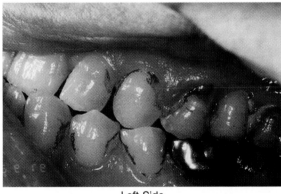

Left Side

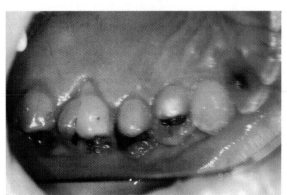

Maxillary Right Lingual

CASE STUDY N

SYNOPSIS OF PATIENT HISTORY

Age	33
Gender	F
Height	5'6"
Weight	130 lbs.

VITAL SIGNS

Blood pressure	116/72
Pulse rate	72
Respiration rate	16

1. Under care of physician
   Yes   No   Condition: _____
          X

2. Hospitalized within the last 5 years
   Yes   No   Reason: _____
          X

3. Has or had the following conditions
   _____
   _____

4. Current medications
   _____
   _____

5. Smokes or uses tobacco products
   Yes   No
          X

6. Is pregnant
   Yes   No   NA
          X

MEDICAL HISTORY: Unremarkable; family history of cancer.

DENTAL HISTORY: Had orthodontic treatment while her periodontal condition was unstable. Was informed by her orthodontist of the need for frequent, meticulous home and professional oral care, but until now had not had dental hygiene therapy for 6 years. Patient recently had first full-mouth series of radiographs and periodontal debridement was begun; patient brushes 2 × daily and flosses occasionally.

SOCIAL HISTORY: Employed by US Navy; attending college in evenings.

CHIEF COMPLAINT: "My teeth are ugly."

NOTE: Teeth #15 and 18 are scheduled for extraction; questionable prognosis on teeth #2, 3, and 30; lingual splint placed on maxillary anterior teeth recently; heavy calculus at initial visit.

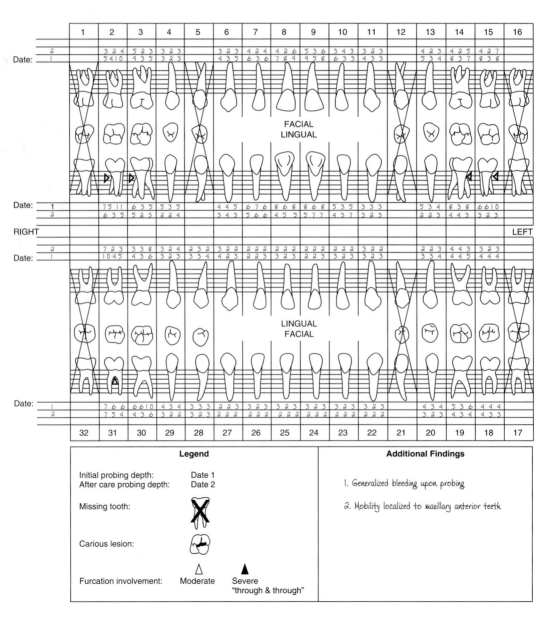

Legend

Initial probing depth: Date 1
After care probing depth: Date 2

Missing tooth: ✗

Carious lesion:

Furcation involvement: △ Moderate   ▲ Severe "through & through"

Additional Findings

1. Generalized bleeding upon probing

2. Mobility localized to maxillary anterior teeth

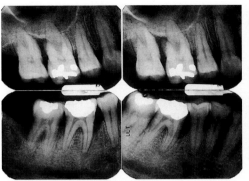
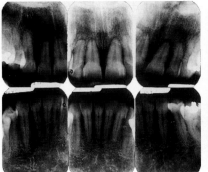
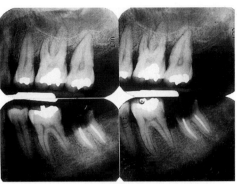

Right Post

Anterior

Left Post

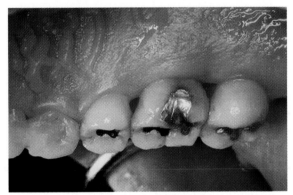

Maxillary Anterior Lingual

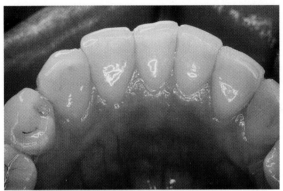

Mandibular Anterior Lingual

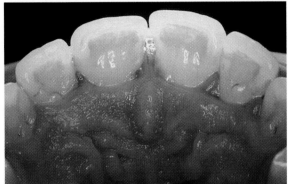

Maxillary Left Lingual

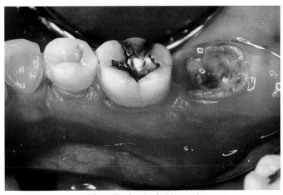

Mandibular Left Lingual

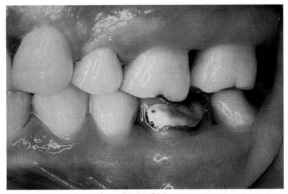

Right Side

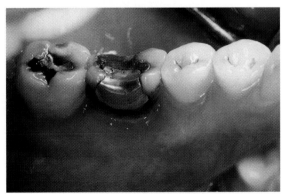

Mandibular Right Lingual

CASE STUDY O

SYNOPSIS OF PATIENT HISTORY		
Age	40	
Gender	M	
Height	5'9"	
Weight	148 lbs.	

VITAL SIGNS

Blood pressure	118/74
Pulse rate	84
Respiration rate	16

1. Under care of physician
   Yes   No   Condition: _____
           X

2. Hospitalized within the last 5 years
   Yes   No   Reason: _____
           X

3. Has or had the following conditions
   Latex sensitivity

4. Current medications
   Aspirin occasionally for headaches

5. Smokes or uses tobacco products
   Yes   No
    X

6. Is pregnant
   Yes   No   NA
                 X

MEDICAL HISTORY: Had blood transfusion after car accident 8 years ago; has frequent cold sores associated with stress; allergy to latex.

DENTAL HISTORY: Last oral prophylaxis was 8 years ago when third molars were removed; brushes 2 × daily with fluoridated toothpaste; is concerned that space between front teeth may be widening; gums bleed occasionally when brushing.

SOCIAL HISTORY: Divorced father of one son; works full-time as short-order cook; lots of stress in life over last 2–3 years; smokes 3 pack of cigarettes a day.

CHIEF COMPLAINT: "I get lots of tartar on my teeth and my gums are receding."

NOTE: Is nervous about dental treatment.

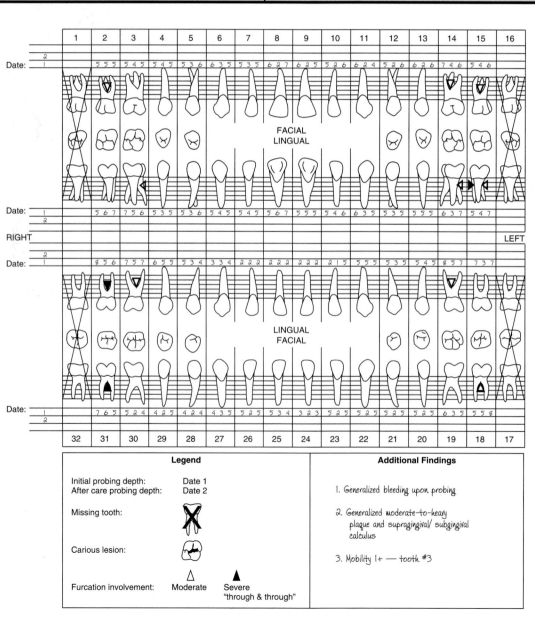

Legend

Initial probing depth: Date 1
After care probing depth: Date 2

Missing tooth:

Carious lesion:

Furcation involvement: Moderate △   Severe ▲ "through & through"

Additional Findings

1. Generalized bleeding upon probing

2. Generalized moderate-to-heavy plaque and supragingival/ subgingival calculus

3. Mobility 1+ — tooth #3

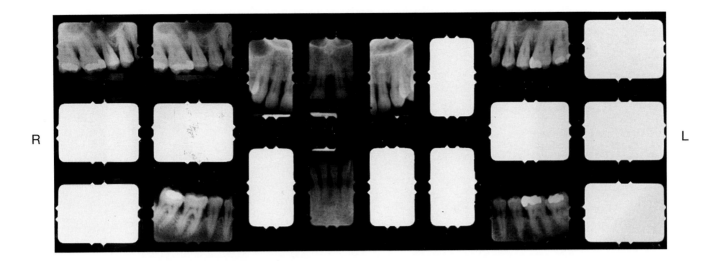

R   L

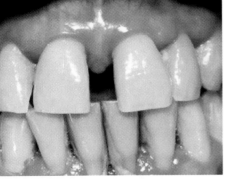

R   L

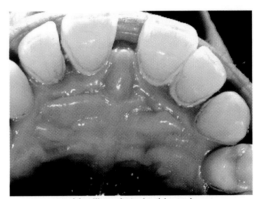

Maxillary Anterior Lingual

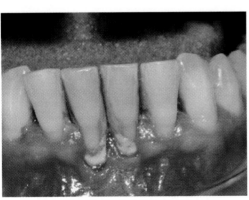

Mandibular Anterior Facial

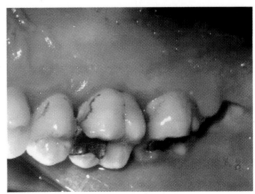

Maxillary Left Lingual

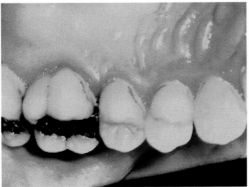

Maxillary Right Lingual

A. age

B. weight

C. employment status

D. dental phobia

49. The patient complains of a swollen palate. On clinical examination, a slight swelling along the midline of the palate behind the maxillary incisors is noted. What is the MOST likely cause of the radiolucent area between the roots of teeth #8 and #9?

A. incisive foramen

B. nasopalatine duct cyst

C. mental foramen

D. median palatal suture

50. Which one of the following is indicated by the radiolucent area at the apex of tooth #13?

A. maxillary foramen

B. periapical cyst

C. periapical abscess

D. maxillary sinus

51. Which type of radiograph will BEST display the alveolar crest of bone in posterior areas?

A. occlusal radiographs

B. vertical bitewing radiographs

C. panoramic radiographs

D. cross-sectional radiographs

52. Clinical examination reveals attrition on teeth #24 and #25, with excessive attrition present on the lingual surfaces of teeth #8 and #9. What is the likely cause of the attrition?

A. Class III occlusion

B. occlusal trauma

C. gingival recession

D. periodontal involvement

53. What is the instrument of choice for root planing on the mesio-lingual of teeth #32 and #15?

A. Gracey 3–4

B. Gracey 7–8

C. Gracey 13–14

D. Gracey 15–16

54. During the periodontal examination procedures, the patient expresses discomfort and becomes anxious. How BEST might one handle the situation?

A. reschedule her appointment

B. explain the pain is due to infection

C. offer nitrous oxide analgesia

D. administer local anesthetics

55. What is the MOST appropriate recommendation for treatment of tooth #18?

A. amalgam polishing

B. overhang removal

C. restoration replacement

D. tooth extraction

56. What is the grayish-blue coloration on the buccal gingiva adjacent to tooth #13?

A. amalgam tattoo

B. melanin pigmentation

C. freckling

D. bruising

Case Study F: Illustrations on pages I-12 and I-13 refer to this case.

57. Which permanent teeth are MOST likely to be missing from his dentition?

A. central incisors

B. lateral incisors

C. canines

D. premolars

58. Which embryonic processes did not fuse during development of the face and resulted in bilateral clefting of the lips?

A. right and left maxillary processes

B. maxillary processes and the globular process

C. median nasal process and the lateral nasal process

D. lateral processes and the globular process

59. Which of the following is NOT a likely cause of this patient's clefts?

A. medications at fourth month in utero

B. hereditary factors

C. inadequate prenatal nutrition

D. exposure to cigarette smoke

60. Which one of the following is FALSE regarding cleft lips and palates?

A. occur more commonly on the right side

B. make infant-feeding a difficult task

C. occur more frequently in males

D. often requires orthodontic treatment

61. What histologic changes are likely to occur with this patient's gingivitis?

A. vasoconstriction and leukocyte infiltration

B. vascular proliferation with increase in leukocytes and gingival crevicular flow

C. vascular proliferation, leukocyte infiltration and decrease in gingival crevicular flow

D. vascular proliferation and increase in leukocyte and osteoclast activity

62. A foul malodor is noted when examining the patient. What is a common cause of oral malodor in those with cleft palates?

A. poor oral hygiene

B. dental decay

C. nasal drainage

D. food debris

63. The brown coloration on the occlusal surface of tooth I is:

A. fluoride mottling

B. exposed dentin

C. occlusal decay

D. extrinsic stain

64. Tooth #25 is situated in:

A. lingual-version

B. buccal-version

C. torso-version

D. mesial-version

65. When scaling the maxillary arch, one should avoid fulcruming on the maxillary:

A. first molars

B. canines

C. second premolars

D. central incisors

66. A major risk for this patient associated with prophylaxis procedures is:
    A. bacterial endocarditis
    B. debris lodged in the cleft
    C. difficulty breathing in supine position
    D. profuse bleeding in maxillary anterior

67. At what age is the final reconstructive surgery and replacement of missing teeth commonly done?
    A. 1–5 years
    B. 6–10 years
    C. 11–15 years
    D. 16–20 years

Case Study G: Illustrations on pages I-14 and I-15 refer to this case.

68. What is the MOST likely cause of the anterior tooth decay?
    A. high sugar intake
    B. amelogenesis imperfecta
    C. poor oral hygiene
    D. prolonged night feeding

69. What are the radiolucencies on the crowns of teeth Q and R?
    A. interproximal caries
    B. cervical burn-out
    C. processing artifact
    D. composite restoration

70. Why is the inferior border of the mandible not continuous on the panoramic radiograph?
    A. patient was seated too low
    B. patient was slumped
    C. patient wasn't centered
    D. patient moved

71. The mother wishes to have tooth "K" extracted rather than restored. What is the BEST reason the tooth should be restored rather than extracted?
    A. restoration will be more cost-effective
    B. discomfort will be lessened for the child
    C. its permanent replacement is years from erupting
    D. jaw development will not be delayed

72. What professional plaque removal method is BEST for this patient?
    A. tooth brush
    B. rubber cup polish
    C. antimicrobial rinse
    D. ultrasonic scaler

73. When teaching the mother and son about proper care of the child's teeth, which of the following should NOT be recommended?
    A. limit toothpaste to a pea-sized amount
    B. use the Fones toothbrushing method
    C. brush the teeth at least twice daily
    D. swish twice daily with fluoridated mouthrinse
    E. limit frequency of simple carbohydrates

74. What is the MOST likely reason this child has numerous ear infections and had surgery to remove adenoids and place an ear tube?
    A. deficient immune system
    B. poor body hygiene
    C. numerous allergies
    D. congenital defect

75. Earlier this year, the child had a high fever for several days. Which teeth are MOST likely to show enamel disruption upon eruption?
    A. primary mandibular canines
    B. primary mandibular second molars
    C. permanent maxillary central incisors
    D. permanent maxillary second molars

Case Study H: Illustrations on pages I-16 and I-17 refer to this case.

76. What are the white raised areas on the buccal, gingival, and palatal soft tissues?
    A. Wickham's straie
    B. fungal infection
    C. hyperkeratosis
    D. linea albicans
    E. oral leukoplakia

77. The patient complains of a sore mouth. What is the MOST likely reason for the soreness?
    A. gingival recession
    B. dental restorations
    C. erosive lesions
    D. psychosomatic symptomology

78. The patient has been taking Amoxil for two months. What oral manifestation is associated with long-term use of this drug?
    A. candidiasis
    B. apthous ulcers
    C. petechiae
    D. angular cheilitis

79. Prozac causes depression of the central nervous system. Which of the following is NOT a side effect of Prozac use?
    A. orthostatic hypotension
    B. sinus headache
    C. salivary flow reduction
    D. light sensitivity
    E. mental illness

80. Lichen planus affects approximately 1 percent of the population. Which one of the following BEST describes this inflammatory disease?
    A. acute and infectious
    B. acute and noninfectious
    C. chronic and infectious
    D. chronic and noninfectious

81. During exacerbations of lichen planus, the patient should:
    A. avoid hot and spicy foods
    B. reduce social activities
    C. take systemic antibiotics
    D. avoid intimate contact

82. What is the radiopaque structure in the alveolar bone located anterior to tooth #32 on the older radiographs?
    A. root fragment
    B. sclerotic bone
    C. hypercementosis
    D. dens in dente
83. On the older radiographs, which teeth have calculus spurs?
    A. 2 and 3
    B. 7 and 8
    C. 13 and 14
    D. 24 and 25
84. The patient complains her upper back teeth hurt. What is the MOST likely reason for this complaint?
    A. dental caries
    B. galvanic reaction
    C. sinus infection
    D. chronic clenching
85. What is the MOST obvious reason for the increased probing depths at this continuing care appointment?
    A. gingival recession
    B. gingival inflammation
    C. attachment loss
    D. probing technique

Case Study I: Illustrations on pages I-18 and I-19 refer to this case.

86. As evidenced in the photos and radiographs, what condition is associated with the bluish-to-brownish opalescent hue of this patient's teeth?
    A. amelogenesis imperfecta
    B. dentinogenesis imperfecta
    C. severe fluorosis
    D. tetracycline staining
87. At what age can tetracyclines and their derivatives be safely prescribed to avoid staining of the enamel?
    A. No age
    B. 4 years of age
    C. 6 years of age
    D. 8 years of age
    E. Any age
88. What is the result of faulty enamel or dentin development?
    A. atrophy
    B. dysplasia
    C. dystrophy
    D. hypertrophy
89. How BEST might the lingual gingival tissues adjacent to teeth #8 and 9 be described?
    A. rolled and cyanotic
    B. firm and fibrotic
    C. red and edematous
    D. blunted and pigmented
90. All of the following are likely sequela to this patient's teeth condition, EXCEPT one. Which one is the EXCEPTION?

A. sensitivity
B. attrition
C. anodontia
D. abrasion

91. A compound fracture of the tibia is a break of which bone?
    A. forearm
    B. upper arm
    C. thigh
    D. shin
92. Which of the following should be included in home care recommendations for this patient?
    A. vigorous tooth brushing
    B. acidulated phosphate fluoride gel
    C. desensitizing, fluoridated toothpaste
    D. teeth-whitening toothpaste
93. In the photograph taken before crown treatment of teeth #8 and 9, the deciduous teeth are visible only at the gingival margin. What is the MOST likely reason for their appearance?
    A. baby bottle decay
    B. severe attrition
    C. surgical removal of crown
    D. delayed eruption

Case Study J: Illustrations on pages I-20 and I-21 refer to this case.

94. What is the MOST likely cause of the gingival overgrowth seen on the photographs?
    A. toothbrush trauma
    B. medication use
    C. chronic inflammation
    D. poor oral hygiene
95. What is the BEST description for the mandibular anterior lingual soft tissues?
    A. festooned
    B. cratered
    C. bulbous
    D. clefted
    E. blunted
96. Which one of the following is a MAJOR difficulty associated with gingival overgrowth?
    A. effective plaque removal
    B. severe bleeding
    C. blunting of papilla
    D. root caries
97. The patient arrives promptly for his 11 am appointment. During the oral prophylaxis, the patient suddenly appears pale, sweaty, and confused. What should the dental hygienist do next?
    A. offer the patient a drink of water
    B. place nitroglycerin under his tongue
    C. administer some orange juice
    D. give the patient his oral insulin
98. The patient's gingival condition can influence his diabetes, because inflammation anywhere in the body will make blood glucose control more difficult.

A. statement and reason are both correct

B. statement and reason are both incorrect

C. statement is correct, but reason is incorrect

D. statement is incorrect, but reason is correct

99. Treatment planning for this patient should include all of the following EXCEPT one. Which one is the EXCEPTION?

A. gingivectomy

B. flossing instruction

C. overhang removal

D. periodontal debridement

E. root planing

100. The MOST likely cause of the vertical enamel fissure on tooth # 8 is:

A. enamel caries

B. age

C. occlusal trauma

D. composite restorative

101. Considering the patient's noncompliance with flossing recommendations, which adjunctive therapy will be most beneficial for controlling gingival overgrowth?

A. chlorhexidine gluconate rinse

B. stannous fluoride gel

C. hydrogen peroxide rinse

D. neutral sodium fluoride gel

E. sanguinaria rinse

102. Which type of radiographs should be taken at this appointment?

A. full-mouth series of radiographs

B. vertical #2 bitewing radiographs

C. horizontal #2 bitewing radiographs

D. horizontal #3 bitewing radiographs

E. panoramic radiograph

Case Study K: Illustrations on pages I-22 and I-23 refer to this case.

103. Given Jake's medical history, which of the following recommendations is advisable?

A. premedication with 2.0 g of amoxicillin 1 hour prior to his dental appointment

B. premedication with 2000 mg of amoxicillin 1 hour prior to appointment and an additional 1000 mg 6 hours after initial dose

C. premedication with 2.0 g of erythromycin

D. no premedication to prevent bacterial endocarditis is necessary

104. Which one of the following pathologic findings should be documented upon completion of the clinical examination?

A. maxillary tori

B. nicotinic stomatitis

C. high lingual frena

D. fissured tongue

E. palatal rugae

105. Which one of the following anomalies should be recorded for this patient?

A. enamel pearl on #19

B. dens in dente in maxillary anterior region

C. calcified pulp chamber on the maxillary central

D. congenitally missing maxillary laterals

E. supernumerary tooth between teeth #8 and #9

106. Which of the following is MOST descriptive of his gingival tissue?

A. scalloped margins with edematous papilla

B. edematous, red tissue with rolled margins, and blunted papilla

C. red marginal tissues with hyperkeratotic papilla

D. cyanotic tissue with blunted papilla

107. Most of this patient's bone loss can be described as horizontal. Vertical bone loss is apparent on the distal of tooth #30 and the mesial of tooth #31.

A. both statements are TRUE

B. both statements are FALSE

C. first statement is TRUE, the second is FALSE

D. first statement is FALSE, the second is TRUE

108. Which of the patient' teeth can be described as a full bony impaction?

A. teeth #1 and #17

B. teeth #1, #16, and #17

C. teeth #17 and #32

D. tooth #17 only

E. tooth #32 only

109. Based on the clinical findings, which oral hygiene aid would be the most effective for cleaning between teeth #14 and #15?

A. manual toothbrush

B. interproximal brush

C. orange-wood toothpick

D. waxed floss

110. What is the preferred method of stain removal for this patient?

A. toothbrush polish

B. air abrasive polish

C. rubber cup polish

D. ultrasonic debridement

111. What of the following MOST accurately describes this patient's hypertension?

A. essential hypertension

B. age-related hypertension

C. primary hypertension

D. secondary hypertension

112. Which teeth have radiographically visible calculus spurs?

A. teeth #2, 3 and 15

B. teeth #13 and 14

C. teeth #19, 20 and 21

D. teeth #28, 29 and 30

E. no calculus is visible on radiographs

113. The maxillary right posterior radiograph is elongated. To correct this error, the vertical angulation should be decreased.

A. both statements are TRUE

B. both statements are FALSE

C. first statement is TRUE, the second is FALSE

D. first statement is FALSE, the second is TRUE

114. What is the molar occlusion classification?
    A. Class I with 2 mm overbite
    B. Class I with teeth #10 and 23 in crossbite
    C. Class II division I
    D. Class II division II
    E. Class III
115. What is this patient's highest priority for dental care?
    A. stain removal
    B. improved oral hygiene self-care
    C. comprehensive periodontal debridement
    D. restoration of all caries
    E. arresting periodontal disease

Case Study L: Illustrations on pages I-24 and I-25 refer to this case.

116. Which of the following developmental disturbances is present in this patient?
    A. dens in dente
    B. focal microdontia
    C. partial anodontia
    D. supernumerary tooth
117. If the patient's gag reflex is triggered by placing pressure on the soft palate, what demarcates the soft palate from the hard palate?
    A. whiter hue of pink
    B. tighter tissue
    C. bluer hue of pink
    D. presence of uvula
118. Which nerve was anesthetized to ensure there would be no pulpal pain when the restoration was placed on this patient?
    A. long buccal nerve
    B. posterior superior alveolar nerve
    C. lingual nerve
    D. inferior alveolar nerve
119. While anesthetized, the patient chewed her lip. It later became infected. Which of the following lymph nodes would be affected initially by the infection?
    A. facial lymph nodes
    B. submandibular lymph nodes
    C. submental lymph nodes
    D. cervical lymph nodes
120. Which one of the patient's teeth has mesial, distal, central and buccal pits that may need an enamel sealant?
    A. tooth #3
    B. tooth #13
    C. tooth #21
    D. tooth #30
121. Which salivary gland produces most of the oral saliva and may complicate enamel sealant procedures on this patient?
    A. sublingual salivary gland
    B. submandibular salivary gland
    C. parotid salivary gland
    D. all glands produce the same amount
122. Which muscle is likely to become enlarged due to frequent night bruxing by the patient?

A. buccinator muscle
B. sternocleidomastoid muscle
C. orbicularis oris muscle
D. masseter muscle
123. Which sinus is present in a panoramic radiograph of the patient?
    A. sphenoid sinus
    B. maxillary sinus
    C. ethmoid sinus
    D. frontal sinus

Case Study M: Illustrations on pages I-26 and I-27 refer to this case.

124. The facial interdental papilla between teeth #11 and #12 can be described by
    A. edematous
    B. fibrotic
    C. flat
    D. cratered
125. Which condition is present on the lingual on tooth #3?
    A. abscess
    B. hyperplasia
    C. root caries
    D. gingival recession
126. Which of the patient's medications may pose an interaction problem if 2% lidocaine with 1:100,000 epinephrine is administered?
    A. trazodone (Trazon)
    B. insulin
    C. lisinopril(Prinivil)
    D. aspirin
127. Which oral health care aid would improve plaque removal under the pontic in the maxillary left posterior sextant?
    A. toothpick in holder
    B. floss and threader
    C. orange-wood toothpick
    D. interdental stimulator
128. During treatment, the patient complains of pain in her chest and left shoulder. What is the MOST likely explanation for the pain?
    A. anxiety attack
    B. myocardial infarction
    C. anginal attack
    D. stroke
129. What is the MOST likely cause of the gingival recession on the maxillary right lingual quadrant?
    A. occlusal trauma
    B. mesial drift
    C. periodontitis
    D. toothbrush abrasion
    E. prior periodontal treatment
130. Of the patient's medications, which one is LEAST likely to cause xerostomia?
    A. lisinopril (Prinivil)
    B. sertraline (Zoloft)

C. trazadone (Trazon)

D. nitroglycerin (Nitrolingual)

131. For what condition is the patient taking lisinopril?

A. hypertension

B. diabetes

C. thyroid disorder

D. angina

Case Study N: Illustrations on pages I-28 and I-29 refer to this case.

132. Which one of the following is the MOST likely cause of the condition of the root apices of teeth #8 and 9?

A. congenital abnormality

B. orthodontic treatment

C. periodontal therapy

D. root pathology

133. To adequately anesthetize the soft and hard tissues of the maxillary right posterior sextant in preparation for periodontal debridement, which injections must be given?

A. PSA, MSA, greater palatine, nasopalatine nerve injections

B. three (3) buccal infiltrations over the posterior teeth

C. PSA and infraorbital nerve injections

D. PSA, MSA, greater palatine nerve injections

134. Bone loss on the mesial of tooth #30 is of which type?

A. vertical

B. horizontal

C. both vertical and horizontal

D. three walled

135. If recession is noted around the disto-facial of tooth #3 during the periodontal reevaluation appointment, what is the most probable cause?

A. tissue shrinkage

B. occlusal trauma

C. clinician error

D. previous periodontal therapy

136. Following periodontal debridement, probing depths of most pockets were reduced. All of the following are likely to have caused a reduction in probing depths, EXCEPT one. Which one is the EXCEPTION?

A. long junctional epithelial attachment

B. gingival recession

C. healthier attachment apparatus

D. lighter probing pressure

137. To measure the loss of clinical attachment, the clinician first measures the distance from the CEJ to the epithelial attachment. Clinical attachment level is the distance from the CEJ to the gingival margin.

A. both statements are TRUE

B. both statements are FALSE

C. first statement is TRUE, the second is FALSE

D. first statement is FALSE, the second is TRUE

138. According to the patient's past dental history, the mobility associated with the maxillary anterior teeth most likely was caused by all of the following, EXCEPT one. Which one is the EXCEPTION?

A. orthodontic therapy

B. periodontal disease

C. loss of attachment levels

D. poor diet

139. The treatment plan for this patient should NOT include:

A. restorative treatment

B. antibiotic therapy

C. intentional curettage

D. periodontal debridement

140. Which of the following is a MAJOR factor in the decline in the periodontal health of this patient?

A. inappropriate dental treatment

B. lack of patient motivation

C. increased restorative needs

D. hereditary background

141. Incomplete debridement of tooth #7 might result in which of the following conditions?

A. periodontal abscess

B. periapical abscess

C. papilloma

D. mucositis

Case Study O: Illustrations on pages I-30 and I-31 refer to this case.

142. Which of the following BEST describes this patent's gingival condition?

A. acute gingivitis

B. chronic gingivitis

C. necrotic gingivitis

D. herpetic gingivostomatitis

143. What is the dark discoloration on the more posterior portion of the palate?

A. Kaposi's sarcoma

B. nicotine stomatitis

C. leukoplakia

D. herpetiform lesion

144. During the oral inspection, the patient breaks out in hives and has difficulty breathing. What is the MOST likely cause of this reaction?

A. angina

B. anxiety

C. embarrassment

D. allergy

145. Based on the clinical data, what is the appropriate AAP classification for this patient?

A. Case type I

B. Case type II

C. Case type III

D. Case type IV

146. Which one of the following did NOT contribute to this patient's periodontal disease?

A. poor plaque control

B. alcohol use

C. cigarette smoking

D. stress

E. calculus

147. The clinical attachment loss on the facial of tooth #25 is 8 mm. What is the total amount of recession in this area?

   A. 2 mm

   B. 3 mm

   C. 4 mm

   D. 5 mm

148. Considering both the clinical and radiographic evidence about tooth #25, all of the following complications are suspected, EXCEPT one. Which one is the EXCEPTION?

   A. tooth mobility

   B. mucogingival involvement

   C. occlusal trauma

   D. root sensitivity

149. Following initial therapy and reevaluation of tissue response, the next logical course of treatment is:

   A. referral for correction of mucogingival defect

   B. placement of tetracycline fibers in all four molar areas

   C. splinting of teeth #8 and 9 to prevent further drifting

   D. referral to a periodontist for possible surgical intervention

150. Which procedure should be performed to eliminate local contributing factors with the intent to prevent further disease progression?

   A. amalgam overhang reduction on tooth #14

   B. removal of all hard and soft deposits

   C. occlusal equilibration

   D. correction of malocclusion

Part B: ANSWER KEY AND RATIONALES

Case Study A

1. **B** Based on the generalized, severe bone loss, the early onset (age 20–30) of the disease, the presence of good oral hygiene, and a smoking habit, the most likely diagnosis is rapidly progressive periodontitis. Most persons with this disease have a neutrophil chemotaxis disorder that puts them at great risk of rapid periodontal destruction. The bone loss is too severe for moderate adult periodontitis. Acute necrotizing ulcerative periodontitis is found in persons with severely weakened immune systems (such as those with AIDS) and is a generalized, rapid, severe destruction of the periodontal tissues. Juvenile periodontitis is generally limited to anterior teeth and first molars.

2. **D** The clinical attachment loss present on the mesiobuccal of tooth #3 is >7 mm based on a probing depth of 6 mm and the visual presence of several millimeter of recession.

3. **A** The environmental factor that MOST contributed to this patient's periodontal breakdown is cigarette smoking. Emotional stress and defective restora-

tions play a lesser role. Malocclusion does not appear to influence his bone loss.

4. **B** The radiolucency in the center of the root of tooth #31 indicates a furcation involvement. The area appears radiolucent because bone has been lost from the area. A periodontal abscess may be present in conjunction with bone loss that appears as a discontinuation of the lamina propria along the root surface, while a periapical abscess would appear as a radiolucent area located at a root apex. An enamel pearl appears as a radiopaque area at the cervical third of the tooth.

5. **B** Based on the amount of radiographic bone loss visible in the anterior teeth, one would expect to observe drifting of the teeth.

6. **B** The significant widening of the periodontal ligament space on the mesial of tooth #5 indicates possible occlusal trauma. Both disuse atrophy and hypofunction would be demonstrated by a narrowed periodontal ligament space. A root fracture would appear as a radiolucent line through the opaque root.

7. **D** Based on the clinical and radiographic findings, this patient will require four 1-hour appointments for scaling and root planing with anesthesia. The deepness of the pocketing and the length of the procedure necessitate use of local anesthetics for patient comfort. Reevaluation of the pocket depths and bleeding should occur 4–6 weeks later.

8. **D** Root sensitivity is common after periodontal debridement due to the removal of debris from the root surface and subsequent exposure of the dentin tubules. Treatment should include professional application of a desensitizing agent or dentin sealer, daily use of desensitizing toothpaste (potassium nitrate, sodium citrate, strontium chloride), and thorough daily plaque removal. Citrus foods, because of their acidic nature, may worsen the condition.

9. **C** Other adjunctive therapies to be considered for this patient include desensitization of exposed root surfaces, prescription of chlorhexidine mouthrinses, and selective polishing to remove tobacco stain. Bleaching procedures are not indicated as they may increase root sensitivity and there is no indication the patient requests such a service.

10. **B** After completion of initial therapy, presuming a positive tissue response, supportive care for this patient should occur every 3 months. Research indicates that most periodontal patients need supportive care at 3-month intervals to maintain their periodontal health.

11. **C** The furcation involvement on the distal of #14 will inhibit healing of the periodontal pocket because it collects plaque and is difficult to clean. The restoration on the distal surface is not defective nor in close proximity to the gingival tissues, so it should not inhibit healing. There is no evidence of occlusal trauma. Inflamed tissues are an indication of inade-

quate plaque removal and will heal once plaque is removed.

12. **D** An interproximal brush is the best oral hygiene device to recommend for plaque removal on the distal of tooth #14. Dental floss will clean the smooth surfaces but not the furcation area, an end-tuft brush will not fit between teeth #14 and 15 and is more suited for terminal molars or furcations located on buccal and lingual surfaces. An oral irrigator will remove unattached plaque interproximally but will not disrupt established bacterial colonies in the furcation area.

13. **C** Based on given information, the whitish-colored palatal tissues are hyperkeratinized (increase in the fibrous layer of tissues) due to the chronic irritation of cigarette smoke. Leukoplakia (a thickening of the stratified squamous epithelium) and candidiasis (a fungal infection) are whitish plaques that can be found on the palate and other areas of the oral cavity. Normal palatal tissues are pink not white.

Case Study B

14. **B** The restoration on tooth #30 is classified as a Class II restoration. Class II restorations involve the proximal surfaces of premolars and molars. Class I includes a single surface area such as the occlusal surfaces of premolars and molars, the facial and lingual surfaces of molars, and the lingual surfaces of maxillary anteriors. Class III involves the proximal surfaces of anterior teeth, while Class IV involves the proximal and incisal angles of anterior teeth.

15. **A** The BEST description of this patient's occlusion is Class I. In this type of occlusion, the permanent maxillary canine is in occlusion with the distal half of the mandibular canine and the mesial half of the mandibular first premolar. Class II occlusion, division 1, displays the mandible in retrusion and all maxillary incisors protruded. In Class II, division 2, the mandible is once again protruded, however, at least one of the maxillary incisors is retruded. With a Class III occlusion, the distal portion of the mandibular canine is anterior to the mesial surface of the maxillary canine.

16. **B** The radiolucent area at the apex of #28 is most likely the mental foramen because of its location and lack of symptoms in the area. The mental foramen is an opening on the outer surface of the body of the mandible located below the second premolar area and is commonly mistaken for pathology. The mandibular canal is a passageway through the body of the mandible and appears as a horizontal radiolucent line in the posterior mandible. Most periapical abscesses and bone cysts appear as round radiolucent areas. Periapical pathology is generally located at the root apex and is associated with non-vital teeth. A bone cyst also appears as a round radiolucent area and may appear in any bony structure with or without symptoms.

17. **D** The radiolucent appearance of areas on the crown surfaces of teeth #5 and 12 is due to enamel erosion caused by purging. Coronal caries will appear with greater radiolucency and more pronounced margins. Tooth fracture is not evident clinically. Fixer spots will appear as whitish droplets on the film.

18. **C** The patient's chief complaint of sensitive teeth is due to the enamel erosion caused by vomit acid, as evidenced by the erosion on the linguals of the maxillary teeth. Erosion, a chemical process, appears on the linguals of palatal surfaces and may extend over the occlusal and incisal surfaces. Occlusal trauma will appear as wear facets on occlusal surfaces and will cause a localized sensitivity. Caries is common in bulimics, due to low pH of the mouth, and incipient caries may cause sensitivity, however in this case, no radiographic evidence exists of caries. Toothbrush abrasion is a loss of tooth structure as a result of a mechanical cause, such as brushing with a hard-bristled toothbrush. There is no evidence of ditching of the cervical areas on the buccal surfaces of teeth as is common with toothbrush abrasion.

19. **C** A neutral sodium fluoride is the recommended product for this patient's hypersensitivity because it is not acidic and can be used on a daily basis. The tray-applied fluoride will provide the best coverage; however, mouthrinses and gels are also acceptable. Both acidulated phosphate and stannous fluorides are acidic. Fluoride varnishes will help seal exposed dentin but must be professionally applied.

20. **B** Bulimics exhibit an ideal body weight (usually within 10–20 pounds of normal) and maintain that weight by vomiting (purging), excessive exercising, and/or use of diuretics and laxatives after eating large volumes of food. The clinical signs of lanugo (fine hair growth), reduced body weight, and lack of ovulation are associated with anorexia nervosa.

21. **B** A decreased heart rate is not associated with bulimia. Swollen parotid glands, a bleeding esophagus, and thermal sensitivity of teeth are common manifestations of bulimia.

22. **A** Purging causes the majority of health problems associated with bulimia because of the frequent vomit acid attacks to the esophagus, teeth and oral tissues. The diet of a patient with bulimia, though excessive in calories, often provides adequate nutrients and as such does not cause health problems. Weight loss is not excessive because of the large number of calories consumed prior to purging. Binge eating can result in the intake of thousands of calories at one time, but by itself does not cause the majority of health problems identified in bulimics.

Case Study C

23. **C** Refractory periodontitis is the periodontal condition that continues to decline following extensive periodontal treatment and frequent continuing care.

Localized juvenile periodontitis will result in severe bone loss also, but has a good prognosis with proper treatment. Chronic adult periodontitis responds well to periodontal therapy. Hormone-induced periodontitis is treated with scaling and root planing and may require modification of hormone therapy or medication.

24. **A** The most likely cause of the recent xerostomia (dry mouth) is the patient's prescription antidepressant medication, Pamalor (nortriptyline HCL). Cigarette smoking also causes dry mouth, but this xerostomia developed recently, so is not likely to be related to the smoking. Menopause and periodontitis are not associated with causing xerostomia.

25. **C** Cigarette smoking does NOT increase the incidence of caries, however, it is associated with increased bone loss, increased calculus formation, and nicotine stomatitis.

26. **B** The root exposures apparent on the photograph of the right side are the result of periodontal surgery (gingivectomy) done ten years earlier. Toothbrush trauma can cause recession but is also associated with abrasion of the root surface. Recession is not age-related. Anterior crowding may be a factor in development of recession due to inadequate plaque removal, however, this patient's recession is not limited to anterior areas of crowding.

27. **C** The gingival tissues adjacent to tooth #9 can best be described with chronic diffuse inflammation, since the tissue is bluish-purple and the inflammation involves the papilla, margin and attached gingiva.

28. **C** The maxillary anterior teeth have the worst prognosis because of mobility associated with 5–7 mm pocketing in areas previously treated by gingivectomy. Prognosis of other areas is better due to less loss of bone and lack of mobility.

29. **D** The radiopaque area identified by an arrow on the maxillary right canine radiograph is the bony wall of the nasal fossa. The nasal fossa itself appears radiolucent. A cone cut appears as a circular or rectangular radiopacity. Bending a film causes a break in the film's emulsion and results in a radiolucent image the shape of the bend. The maxillary sinus appears as a radiolucency in maxillary posterior films.

30. **D** Once certain actions are performed by the dentist, an implied contract is established. An expressed contract is informed consent given in writing or verbally, while a written contract is a form of expressed consent and provides the most protection for the patient. Parental/guardian consent is provided when the patient is a minor or mentally incompetent to give consent.

31. **B** Failure of the dentist to record a periodontal chart and take full-mouth radiographs may indicate negligence. Negligence, often synonymous with malpractice, is defined as an act omitted or care not provided which can bring harm/damage to a patient.

Breach of contract is breaking an agreement by either party involved. Technical battery involves an act that was not agreed on.

32. **B** The interdental brush will most effectively remove plaque between teeth # 10 and 11 because the diastema provides sufficient space. An oral irrigating device will not remove attached plaque and an interdental tip stimulator is useful for gingival stimulation, not plaque removal. Use of a toothpick may cause further recession.

Case Study D

33. **C** A diastolic reading of 92 is abnormally high and is indicative of hypertension. An additional reading should be taken to verify. Because of the patient's risk factors for hypertension (smoking, overweight), the patient should be advised to monitor her blood pressure and seek consultation with her physician.

34. **D** The human papilloma virus (HPV) is responsible for causing venereal or genital warts (condyloma acuminatum). The Epstein-Barr virus is believed to be associated with a number of chronic health conditions, such as chronic fatigue syndrome. Staphylococcus epidermitis is the bacteria that causes styes, while *Helicobacter pylori* causes peptic ulcer disease.

35. **D** Because the interdental papilla are blunted in greater than 50% of the mouth, this indicates a generalized condition. Blunting is apparent on the majority of the teeth in the intra-oral photographs.

36. **A** Contour describes shape. The shape of gingiva on the facial surface of tooth #24 is rolled. Festooned describes larger, inner-tube shaped tissues, while clefted tissues exhibit a linear defect. The term ulcerated does not describe the contour or shape of the gingiva, but rather a condition.

37. **C** Bony exostoses in the midline of the hard palate are referred to as torus palatinus, or more commonly, maxillary torus. Most often tori and other exostoses require no treatment by the dental professional, however, if they interfere with a prosthetic appliance such as a partial or denture, removal may be indicated.

38. **C** The patient history indicates the use of two antidepressant medications, both of which cause xerostomia. Patients who take xerostomic medications and have areas of recession are very prone to cervical caries. Examination of the history does not show a high sugar intake, therefore the most likely cause of the caries is medication.

39. **D** Horizontal bone loss occurs in a plane parallel to the CEJ of adjacent teeth. Vertical bone loss occurs in a plane that is not parallel to the CEJ of adjacent teeth. Because the bone loss involves more that 50% of the teeth, it is classified as generalized horizontal bone loss.

40. **C** The intraoral photographs reveal many areas of demineralization. Demineralization results from a breakdown of the tooth structure with a subsequent

loss of mineral content. Demineralization can be detected clinically as chalky spots, or in the case of this patient, as brown spots as a result of discoloration from tobacco.

41. **C** The patient has a porcelain-fused-to-metal bridge on teeth #11, 13 and 14. The black bandlike line is the metal substructure to the bridge. In the lab, porcelain is fired to the metal in order to produce an esthetically pleasing restoration.

42. **B** The rheumatoid arthritis makes is difficult or impossible for the patient to manipulate small objects because of stiffness of joints and discomfort. An antimicrobial mouthrinse is the best choice for reducing the bacterial levels interproximally, although it will dry the mouth. The patient should still be encouraged to floss and use the interdental brush when possible. A powered toothbrush may be helpful in removing marginal plaque but is not very effective with interproximal plaque. Neutral sodium fluoride gels are used for prevention of caries and root sensitivity not plaque. A toothpick in holder is as difficult to handle as floss or interdental brush.

43. **A** The ultrasonic scaler provides increased access over traditional hand scaling due to its smaller working end. In addition, acoustic streaming and water lavage cause rupture of bacterial cell walls and flushing of debris from the pockets, respectively, which are health-promoting.

44. **A** Neutral sodium fluorides are the best choice because the patient's restorative work includes both porcelain and composite materials. Daily use of the fluoride gel will provide protection against caries due to medication-induced xerostomia. Both acidulated phosphate gels and rinses are contraindicated due to their ability to cause pitting and roughening of the porcelain and composite surfaces. Stannous gel is not desirable because of its potential for staining.

45. **A** The patient contracted Hepatitis A while on vacation. Fecal-oral, water-borne and food-borne are the most common routes of transmission for Hepatitis A and E. Transmission is thorough close contact in unsanitary conditions, i.e., unwashed hands of an infected person can contaminate anything touched. Contaminated water may carry hepatitis A virus directly to those using the water, or it may contaminate aquatic shellfish living in the water. The typical symptoms are flu-like in nature with abrupt onset and jaundice in adults. Unprotected sex, shared needles, and blood contact are associated with contraction of Hepatitis B, C, and D.

Case Study E

46. **D** Gingivitis is the least likely cause of food impaction in the maxillary posterior areas of her mouth. More likely causes are periodontal pocketing, the three-unit bridge, and open contacts in the area.

47. **A** The sensitivity in the mandibular anterior incisors is due to exposure of the dentinal tubules as a result of gingival recession. Pulpitis will result in an acute pain in a localized area, such as s single tooth, rather than involving several teeth. A periapical abscess will result in a deep pain but does not cause sensitivity. Attrition of the incisal edges may cause sensitivity, but usually not to instrumentation.

48. **D** Dental fear caused by dental phobia is the most likely reason for the unusually high pulse rate of this patient. Stress can cause an increase in blood pressure also. Age and employment status are not directly related to abnormal vital sign measurement. Excess weight can cause an increase in blood pressure and may be associated with faster heart rate when lack of exercise contributes to weight gain.

49. **B** The feeling of a swollen palate, swelling along the midline of the palate behind the maxillary incisors, the radiolucency seen between the roots of teeth #8 and 9, and the flaring of teeth #8 and 9 is indicative of a nasopalatine duct cyst (incisive canal cyst). This cyst forms from epithelial remnants of the nasopalatine duct, which disintegrates around the time of birth. The incisive foramen is a radiolucent object found between the apices of the maxillary central incisors. The mental foramen is a radiolucent round object generally located near the apices of mandibular premolars. The median palatal suture is a radiolucent line separating the palate between the right and left central incisors.

50. **D** The Maxillary sinus is the radiolucent area at the apex of tooth #13. The sinuses are normal structures that appear above the maxillary premolars and molars. There is no such thing as a maxillary foramen. A periapical abscess and cyst are radiolucent round images that are located in bone adjacent to the apex of a diseased tooth.

51. **B** Vertical bitewings provide the best view of the alveolar crest of bone because the technique allows a more anatomically and dimensionally correct image of a larger bone area. They are especially suited for periodontal patients. Occlusal radiographs are best for viewing large areas of the jaw but don't provide the most accurate image. The panoramic radiograph is designed to provide a full view of both arches but does not provide the clarity needed for viewing minor alveolar bone changes. Cross-sectional radiographs use a right-angle technique to determine if objects, such as impacted 3rd molars, are located facially or lingually.

52. **B** Occlusal trauma is the reason for the attrition on teeth #24, 25, 8, and 9.

53. **D** The instrument of choice for root planing on the mesio-lingual of teeth #32 and 15 is the Gracey 15–16. The Gracey 3–4 was designed to instrument the anterior teeth, while the Gracey 7–8 is best for the buccal and lingual surfaces of posterior teeth.

The Gracey 13–14 was designed to instrument the distal surfaces of posterior teeth.

54. **C** Anxious (dental phobic) patients have a heightened sense of pain caused by their fear. Nitrous oxide sedation is the best choice for the anxious patient. Rescheduling the appointment will only prolong the agony. Explanations of why there is pain do not alleviate the pain of fears. An anxious patient who if fearful of needles will continue to "feel" the pain since it is psychogenic—even if she allows the dental hygienist or dentist to administer the anesthetic.

55. **C** The MOST appropriate recommendation for treatment of tooth #18 is replacement of the restoration. The restoration is pitted, corroded, has a distal overhang, and appears to have a defective margin on its mesio-lingual surface. Polishing the amalgam will correct some of the corrosion but will not address the other issues. Removing the overhang alone will not address the issues of corrosion and leakage. There is no reason for the tooth to be extracted since it has adequate bone height and is asymptomatic.

56. **A** The grayish-blue coloration on the buccal gingiva adjacent to tooth #13 is indicative of an amalgam tattoo because of its location near restorative work. While preparing the porcelain-fused-to-metal bridge, a small piece of amalgam from an existing restoration found its way into the soft tissues adjacent to the bridge site. Other than coloration, the tattoo has no ill effects. Melanin pigmentation generally occurs bilaterally and may be localized or generalized brown to black coloration more common to individuals with heavily pigmented skin (Native Americans, Hispanics, Blacks). Freckling is usually brown to black and can occur anywhere in the mouth. Because this coloration is located near restorations, the amalgam tattoo is most likely. Bruising tends to have a more purplish-red-blue hue and would disappear within 2 weeks.

Case Study F

57. **B** The maxillary lateral incisor is the tooth most likely to be affected by a cleft. The site of fusion in the anterior palate is between the lateral and canine teeth and clefting can lead to tooth loss. The canine, premolar, or central incisor are much less likely to be affected, however, it is possible that they may also be missing or at least displaced from their normal position.

58. **B** The left and right maxillary processes did not properly fuse with the globular process and resulted in the bilateral cleft lip. The lack of fusion of the right and left maxillary processes results in a cleft palate. The median and lateral nasal processes are responsible for formation of the sides of the nose. The globular process is produced by an extension of the median nasal process and would not be responsible for a cleft formation.

59. **A** The fusion of the lip normally occurs by the eighth week and palatal closure is normally completed by the end of the twelfth week gestation, therefore the medications taken during the fourth month of pregnancy are not the likely cause of the clefting. Diet, hereditary factors, smoking, and other environmental factors have been associated with cleft formation.

60. **A** Cleft lips tend to occur more frequently on the left side, rather than the right. Cleft lip, with or without a cleft palate, is more common in males than females. They lead to tooth loss or tooth displacement, eating difficulties, and result in malocclusions which require orthodontic treatment.

61. **B** The histological changes typical of gingivitis are an increase in vascular proliferation leading to a red appearance, leukocyte infiltration, and an increase in crevicular fluid in the gingival sulcus. Osteoclast activity is associated with bone loss and is not found in gingivitis.

62. **C** Nasal drainage into the mouth is common when palatal closure is incomplete since the palatal bones serves as the floor of the nose. A foul malodor is a common occurrence and is controlled by frequent cleansing of the mouth and oral appliances. Poor oral hygiene, dental decay, and food debris can cause malodor but are not specific to those with clefting.

63. **B** The brown coloration on the occlusal surface of tooth I is exposed dentin from attrition. Fluoride mottling can be similar in color but would not be associated with worn surfaces. Occlusal decay would appear darker brown and pitted or ditched. Extrinsic stain is often brown in color and would generally be located on other surfaces of the teeth also.

64. **A** Tooth #25 is situated in lingual-version. Tooth #26 is in buccal-version. A tooth in torso-version is rotated in the socket but still lies within the occlusal plane. Mesial-version is the mesial placement of the tooth.

65. **D** When scaling the maxillary arch, one should avoid fulcruming on the maxillary central incisors since the patient has a free premaxilla due to the lack of bone fusion and the tissue will move. Fulcruming on any of the other tooth choices should not pose a problem.

66. **B** Plaque, calculus, or prophy paste introduced into the cleft during prophylaxis procedures is major risk of infection for this patient. Bacterial endocarditis, difficulty breathing in supine position, and profuse bleeding in the maxillary anterior are no more prevalent in those with clefts than those without.

67. **D** The final reconstructive surgery and replacement of missing teeth is commonly done after the age of 15, when physical growth is complete.

Case Study G

68. **D** The MOST likely cause of the anterior tooth decay is prolonged night feeding. This condition is commonly called nursing (or baby) bottle syndrome because it occurs in children who are either put to bed

with a bottle of milk or juice or are nursed frequently and for prolonged periods of time during the night. The infant (who is old enough to have teeth) falls asleep with liquid in the mouth, doesn't swallow, and the milk or juice ferments on the tooth.

69. **A** The radiolucencies on crowns of teeth "Q" and "R" are interproximal caries. Cervical burnout is typically located at the neck of the tooth. Composite restorations generally have more defined boundaries due to the removal of tooth structure. Processing artifacts tend to appear as brown or dark spots on the films and are not the likely choice because of the great number of carious lesions in the mouth.

70. **D** The inferior border of the mandible is not continuous on the panoramic radiograph because the patient moved during irradiation procedures. Seating the patient too low will result in loss of the inferior border on the film. A slumping patient will cause a ghost image of the spine in the film, while not centering the patient can cause teeth to appear larger on one side of the radiograph than the other.

71. **C** The BEST reason the tooth should be restored rather than extracted is because its permanent replacement, the mandibular second premolar, is years from erupting. While cost and discomfort are considerations in treating a child, it is not the MOST important consideration; restoration of a severely decayed tooth may or may not be more cost-effective than extraction and discomfort is not necessarily lessened for the child—although both are likely. Jaw development is generally not affected by either of the procedures.

72. **A** Professional plaque removal for this patient is BEST accomplished by tooth brush. Since there is so much caries and decalcification, the toothbrush polish will be the least abrasive to the already damaged tooth structure. A rubber cup polish with prophy paste can abrade damaged enamel. Antimicrobial rinses are for control of gingivitis, not for plaque removal. An ultrasonic scaler may cause damage to the tooth structure, frighten the child, and cause discomfort when water touches the decayed areas.

73. **D** When teaching the mother and son about proper care of the child's teeth, use of a fluoridated mouthrinse is contraindicated because of his age. Preschool–aged children are likely to swallow, rather than swish and expectorate the rinse. Because of the risk of toxicity, fluoride should only be applied by a parent in controlled amounts (by gel or paste to a toothbrush). Tooth pastes should be limited to a pea-sized amount on the brush because even if a child swallows this amount, it should not result in toxicity or severe fluorosis. The Fones toothbrushing method is a circular brushing method appropriate for small children. The teeth should be brushed at least twice daily and a reduction in amount and frequency of simple carbohydrates (sugars, sucrose) is needed.

74. **C** Allergies to mold, dust mites, animals, and foods are common causes of inner ear infections. Allergies cause swelling of the mucous membranes of the mouth and nose, which traps microorganisms in the Eustachian tubes and leads to infection. Placing ear tubes (called myringotomy) allows fluid to drain from the ear when the Eustachian tubes are blocked. A deficient immune system may predispose a child to any type of infection, but there is no evidence of this in his health history. There is no evidence that this child has poor body hygiene or a congenital defect that could predispose him to ear infections.

75. **D** A high fever of several days duration my cause "fever lines" or other disruption of enamel in teeth undergoing enamel deposition. At 4 years of age, this patient's permanent mandibular and maxillary second molars are undergoing enamel deposition and are at risk of dysplasia due to trauma. Since all primary teeth are fully formed and erupted by age four, they are not at risk from high fever. Enamel of the permanent maxillary central incisors is normally fully developed by ages 4–5, so those teeth are at low risk.

Case Study H

76. **A** The white raised areas on the buccal, gingival, and palatal soft tissues are Wickham's straie and are associated with lichen planus. Fungal infection, hyperkeratosis, linea albicans, and oral leukoplakia are all white but have different associations and are not lacy in appearance.

77. **C** The patient's sore mouth is most likely due to the erosive lesions of some forms of lichen planus. In the erosive form, the epithelium sloughs from the underlying tissue and leaves painful ulcerations.

78. **A** The most common oral manifestation associated with long-term use of any antibiotic is a fungal infection, candidiasis.

79. **E** Mental illness is not a side effect of Prozac use but instead may be a reason for its use. Orthostatic hypotension, sinus headache, salivary flow reduction, and light sensitivity are some of the many side effects of Prozac use.

80. **D** Lichen Planus is a benign, chronic, noninfectious disease of unknown origin.

81. **A** During exacerbations of lichen planus, the patient should avoid hot and spicy foods or other things that trigger pain.

82. **A** On the older radiographs, a root fragment appears as a radiopaque structure in the alveolar bone located anterior to tooth #32. In the current radiographs the fragment is missing, indicating it was removed prior to placement of the bridge. Sclerotic bone would appear similar but is usually not associated with bone where a tooth has been removed. Hypercementosis would appear as a radiopacity attached to the root surface of a tooth. Dens in Dente

is a tooth within a tooth and appears as a tear-drop shaped radiolucent image.

83. **A** On the older radiographs, calculus spurs are seen on teeth # 2 and 3.

84. **C** A sinus infection is the most likely cause of this patient's complaint of hurting teeth, particularly since the teeth involved are the maxillary molars, the radiographs show the root tips are within the sinus space, and she is undergoing long-term treatment for sinus infections. While previous radiographs show caries, current ones do not. A galvanic reaction caused when different metals in the mouth react and create an electrical current does not typically cause patient discomfort. There is no indication the patient chronically clenches her teeth.

85. **B** Gingival inflammation is the MOST obvious reason for the increased probing depths at this continuing care appointment. The patient's gingiva is very sore due to the acute erosive lesions, making it difficult to thoroughly clean her teeth. Gingival recession would not result in deeper probe readings. Attachment loss and probing technique can both result in deeper than usual probing depths, but are not as likely when once considers all clinical evidence.

Case Study I

86. **B** As evidenced in the photos and radiographs, the blue-gray to brown opalescent hue of this patient's teeth is associated with dentinogenesis imperfecta, an inherited disorder of dentin production that results in chipping of enamel, obliteration of pulp canals, blunting of roots, and increased incidence of attrition, abrasion sensitivity, and caries. Amelogenesis imperfecta may have a similar appearance but does not have a blue-gray to brown opalescent appearance and does not affect the root structure or function of the teeth. Severe fluorosis will result in gray to brown discoloration of the teeth and loss of tooth enamel, but does not affect the roots of the teeth. Tetracycline staining causes a grayish-brown staining of the enamel of teeth undergoing enamel deposition. Since this patient only recently received tetracycline, this is not a concern. Tetracycline (doxycycline) does not cause enamel dysplasia.

87. **D** Tetracyline and its derivatives can be safely prescribed for those age 8 and over to avoid staining of the enamel. At that time, enamel formation of all but the third molars is complete, so stain is not an aesthetic problem.

88. **B** When enamel or dentin development is faulty or disordered, the result is dysplasia (abnormal development of a tissue). Atrophy is a wasting, progressive loss of structure and function, while dystrophy is a progressive loss of function (usually associated with muscles or syndromes). Hypertrophy is an increase in size due to an increase in cell size.

89. **A** Lingual gingival tissues adjacent to teeth #8 and 9 are BEST described as rolled and cyanotic due to the thickening of the gingival margin and the bluish coloration associated with chronic inflammation.

90. **C** Anodontia, or lack of teeth, is not associated with dentinogenesis imperfecta. Sensitivity, attrition, and abrasion are commonly associated with the enamel loss and dentin exposure of this condition.

91. **D** A compound fracture of the tibia is a break of the shin bone, one of two bones of the lower leg.

92. **C** Home care recommendations for this patient should include use of a desensitizing, fluoridated toothpaste because of the extreme sensitivity these people experience due to loss of enamel. Vigorous tooth brushing can damage the already fragile tooth and acidulated phosphate fluorides are avoided because their acidity is unnecessary and will cause further erosion of the teeth and discomfort to the patient. Teeth-whitening toothpastes may be too abrasive or acidic and cause further damage to the tooth structure.

93. **B** The deciduous teeth are visible only at the gingival margin because of severe attrition. The weakness of the dentin puts the patient at extreme risk of enamel and dentin abrasion from chewing during eating. There is no history of baby bottle decay, nor is there any reason to surgically remove the deciduous crowns. Radiographic evidence does not indicate delayed eruption.

Case Study J

94. **B** The gingival overgrowth seen on the photographs is MOST likely due to medication use, such as Norvasc, a calcium channel blocker. Toothbrush trauma may cause localized thickened gingiva with a more linear appearance. Chronic inflammation can appear firm, rolled and fibrotic but not with the thickness seen in this case. Poor oral hygiene can lead to chronic inflammation and thickened gingiva, but by itself does not appear this overgrown. Poor oral hygiene, in conjunction with Norvasc, is a large factor in causing severe gingival overgrowth.

95. **D** The mandibular anterior lingual soft tissues are BEST described as clefted because of the linear grooves separating the enlarged gingiva. Festooned gingiva appears inner-tube shaped, while cratered gingiva appears as ulcerated or lost papilla. Bulbous tissues are enlarged and appear to bulge out of the interproximal spaces. Blunted tissues occur when bone is lost interproximally and the gingival papilla no longer fills the interdental space.

96. **A** The major difficulty with gingival overgrowth is effective plaque removal. Once the overgrowth is moderate or severe, plaque removal becomes very difficult since gingival sulci become much deeper and tooth structure is covered with gingival tissues. The overgrown gingiva does not usually bleed severely upon touching, nor is there blunting of papilla. Root caries is not usually a problem since the overgrowth is over the crown of the tooth and the

root structure is not exposed to the oral environment.

97. **C** When a diabetic patient suddenly appears pale, sweaty and confused, the dental hygienist should administer orange juice because low blood sugar (hypoglycemia) is likely due to the late hour of the appointment. Offering water will not help this medical emergency. Placing nitroglycerin under the tongue of a patient for whom it is not prescribed is not appropriate. Administering oral insulin would make matters worse as it would further reduce the blood glucose level.

98. **A** The patient's gingival condition can influence his diabetes, because inflammation anywhere in the body will make blood glucose control more difficult. Both statement and reason are true.

99. **E** Treatment planning for this patient should include all of the following except root planing, since the gingival overgrowth occurs primarily on the crown of the tooth rather than the root. Gingivectomy, flossing instruction, overhang removal, and periodontal debridement (plaque and calculus removal) will help the patient control the inflammation and gingival response to his medication.

100. **C** The MOST likely cause of the vertical enamel fissure on tooth # 8 is occlusal trauma. The patient has an edge-to-edge bite which places undo stress on the anterior teeth. Enamel caries will appear as a brown or black depression on the enamel surface. Age itself is not a cause of fissuring. A composite restorative will appear tooth-colored and will not have a linear appearance.

101. **A** Chlorhexidine gluconate rinse, an antimicrobial rinse with substantivity, is the adjunctive therapy most beneficial for controlling gingival overgrowth in patients with systemic and local conditions that predispose them to inflammation. Stannous fluoride and neutral sodium fluoride gel would not effectively control interproximal plaque because of their nature and viscosity. Hydrogen peroxide rinses are not recommended for long-term use and are most beneficial for ANUG because of its oxygenating effect. Sanguinaria rinses control plaque but not as effectively as chlorhexidine gluconate.

102. **B** Because the patient had a full-mouth series of radiographs only two years earlier, vertical bitewing radiographs should be taken at this appointment (Four posterior and 2–3 anterior). The vertical bitewing radiographs will allow a better view of bone surrounding the teeth. As seen in the current radiographs, #3 bitewing films do not allow viewing of the crestal bone in patients with bone loss. Horizontal #2 bitewing radiographs will also prevent viewing of the crestal bone in patients with bone loss. A panoramic radiograph does not have the clarity needed to monitor this patient's periodontal condition.

Case Study K

103. **D** This patient does not have a history of heart valve dysfunction. High blood pressure does not increase the risk for bacterial endocarditis. There is nothing in his medical history to indicate high risk for bacterial endocarditis.

104. **B** Nicotinic stomatitis is present on the soft palate and lightly on the posterior hard palate. Clinically it begins as inflammation of the minor salivary ducts. Look for diffuse grayish-white thickened epithelium adjacent to inflamed red orifices. The etiology is heavy smoking.

105. **C** The pulp chamber of tooth #9 is completely calcified and appears radiopaque. A normal healthy pulp chamber would be radiolucent.

106. **B** His gingival tissues are generally marginally red throughout his mouth. The gingival margin is rolled and the interdental papilla are blunted.

107. **C** The predominant bone loss pattern is horizontal. The bone loss pattern on teeth #30 & #31 is also horizontal. When the crestal bone is parallel to the adjacent CEJ of involved teeth, the loss is considered to be horizontal. Vertical bone loss is exhibited by loss of parallelism with the alveolar crestal bone.

108. **E** Tooth #32 is entirely submerged beneath the bone. Tooth #17 is a partial bony impaction and only partially submerged beneath bone. Teeth #1 and 16 are partially erupted and visible in the oral cavity.

109. **B** The interdental papilla are blunted and the embrasure space is a large triangular shape making it ideal for an interproximal brush. An orange-wood toothpick is difficult to maneuver so far posteriorly. Floss works best in smaller embrasure spaces with more knife-edged papilla.

110. **D** Debridement with ultrasonic instruments is ideal (faster and more effective) for removing heavy stain, especially when calculus is also present. Toothbrush polishing would be inadequate for removing tobacco stain. Due to the patient's history of high blood pressure, air abrasive polishing is contraindicated because of the sodium bicarbonate content of the powder. A rubber cup polish works well for minor stain removal and when aerosols can't be produced or little calculus is present.

111. **D** Secondary hypertension is hypertension of unknown etiology. Since the patient's medical history is negative for kidney or renal disease, primary (essential) hypertension can be ruled out. Age is a risk, not a hypertension category.

112. **A** Radiographic calculus is only visible on the mesial of tooth #2, the distal of tooth #3, the mesial of tooth #15, and the distal of tooth #14.

113. **C** The radiograph is elongated, making the tooth image appear abnormally long. To correct this error, the vertical angulation of the x-ray beam should be increased.

114. **A** The maxillary first molar's mesio-buccal cusp tip occludes with the mandibular 1st molar's buccal groove, indicating a Class I occlusion. The anterior overbite is normal (~2 mm). In a Class II division I occlusion, the mesio-buccal cusp tip occludes anterior to the buccal grove and the maxillary anterior teeth are protruded. In Class II division II, the maxillary anterior teeth are retruded. In a Class II occlusion, the maxillary first molar's mesio-buccal cusp tip occludes distal to the mandibular first molar's buccal groove.

115. **A** The patient's chief complaint is stain on his teeth. Satisfying the patient's needs is always a high priority. A comprehensive exam and diagnosis with subsequent treatment plan are also needed after the patient's first priority is addressed.

Case Study L

116. **C** The developmental disturbance present in this patient is partial anodontia, as evidenced by missing tooth #20. Dens in dente is a tooth within a tooth and appears as a radiolucent area within another tooth. Focal microdontia is an unusually small tooth, while a supernumerary tooth is an extra tooth typically found in the third molar and maxillary regions of the mouth.

117. **D** The uvula demarcates the soft palate from the hard palate, so the patient's gag reflex can be avoided by eliminating pressure to the soft tissues near the uvula. The hard palate is a whiter or bluer hue of pink and is tightly bound to the hard tissue.

118. **D** The inferior alveolar nerve was anesthetized when the restoration was placed on this patient to insure there would not be any pulpal pain. The long buccal nerve innervates the buccal soft tissues of the mandibular posterior teeth, while the posterior superior alveolar nerve innervates the maxillary molars and their periodontium. The lingual nerve will anesthetize the lingual soft tissues of the mandibular teeth.

119. **C** If after the initial extraction appointment, the patient chews her lip and it becomes infected, the submental lymph nodes will initially be affected. The facial lymph nodes are a superficial group of nodes located along the facial vein and are responsible for draining the skin and mucous membranes in their area. The submandibular lymph nodes are located beneath the posterior mandible and would eventually handle drainage of the submental and facial lymph nodes. The cervical lymph nodes drain regions of the neck.

120. **D** Tooth #30 has mesial, distal, central and buccal pits that may need an enamel sealant.

121. **B** The submandibular salivary gland produces the highest percentage (~65%) of total oral saliva, possibly complicating enamel sealant procedures on this patient. The sublingual salivary gland produces approximately 10% of the total salivary volume, while the parotid salivary gland produces about 25%.

122. **D** Bruxism works the masseter muscles and can cause their enlargement. The buccinator muscle assists the muscles of mastication by moving the lip and cheek muscles during mastication. The sternocleidomastoid muscles are located on both sides of the neck and are responsible for turning the head laterally. The orbicularis oris muscle is responsible for closing the lips.

123. **B** The maxillary sinus is present in a panoramic radiograph of the patient and is observed as radiolucent structures above the zygoma and the root apices of the maxillary molars. The sphenoid sinus is located in the body of the sphenoid bone near the occipital bone. The ethmoid sinuses are very small and are located on the side of the ethmoid bones. The frontal sinuses are located within the frontal bone of the forehead.

Case Study M

124. **A** The tissue exhibits swelling due to edema. It does not appear fibrotic (firm, leathery) and the papilla is not flat or cratered.

125. **D** Gingival recession is seen when the junctional epithelium migrates apically on the tooth and a portion of the root becomes exposed. An abscess, if seen clinically, will be draining via a fistula on the gingiva. Hyperplasia is exhibited by an overgrowth of tissue. Root caries is seen as a soft lesion of cementum and dentin that may be yellow to brown to black in color.

126. **B** Epinephrine may decrease the hypoglycemic effect of insulin. Epinephrine with trazodone, lisinopril, and aspirin presents no known interaction problems. Lidocaine with any of these drugs presents no known interaction problems.

127. **B** The easiest way to remove plaque from the undersurface of a pontic is by using floss that is threaded under the pontic. This can be done with a floss and floss threader or by specialty texture floss that incorporates a stiff self-threading end (such as Superfloss). A toothpick in holder (such as the Perio-aid) and orange-wood toothpick (such as Stimudent) are utilized more in areas of gingival recession and not under pontics. The interdental stimulator is utilized more for interdental areas in embrasures and under contacts.

128. **C** This patient has a history of angina pectoris and takes nitrogylcerin, which is an antianginal medication. She is most likely to experience an anginal attack, which has similar symptoms to a myocardial infarction, which will be relieved by spraying nitroglycerin beneath the tongue. If symptoms do not abate quickly, a myocardial infarction must be suspected and further emergency care provided. An

anxiety attack often results in hyperventilation. A stroke results in paralysis on one side.

129. **D** Toothbrush abrasion is the most likely cause of the gingival recession seen in this patient's mouth because she uses a medium-bristled toothbrush rather than a soft brush. This patient has no known occlusal trauma and the mesial drift is localized. The patient reports no history of periodontal treatment or gingival surgery that would cause recession.

130. **D** Nitroglycerin is the least likely drug to cause this patient xerostomia. Although the drug has a drying effect, it is used infrequently. Lisinopril, Sertraline, and Trazadone are used daily and all have xerostomia as a side effect.

131. **A** Lisinopril is an angiotensin-converting enzyme (ACE) inhibitor that is used to treat hypertension. The other medications this patient is taking are insulin (antidiabetic agent for the treatment of diabetes), levothyroxine (for thyroid disorder),and nitroglycerine (for angina).

Case Study N

132. **B** Orthodontic treatment is the most likely cause of the blunted root apices evident in the radiographs. There is no evidence that congenital abnormality, root pathology, or periodontal therapy caused root blunting in this case.

133. **D** PSA (posterior superior alveolar), MSA (middle superior alveolar) and the greater palatine nerve injections are the best choice, as only those injections that will provide anesthesia to the posterior sextant should be given. Lingual pocket depths are deep enough to warrant the greater palatine nerve injection. The nasopalatine and infraorbital injections do not anesthetize tissues in the maxillary posterior regions so should not be chosen. Three buccal infiltrations over the posterior teeth will not anesthetize the lingual tissues so are not appropriate in this case.

134. **B** The bone loss mesial to tooth #30 is horizontal. Although the defect at first appears to be vertical, a line connecting the CEJ of teeth #29 and 30 closely parallels the bone defect, thus making it a horizontal bone loss.

135. **A** Edematous tissue, especially in deeper pocket areas, usually shrinks after periodontal therapy and results in recession. For the most part, probe readings showed a decrease when recorded at the one-month tissue evaluation appointment as is indicative of tissue shrinkage. Occlusal trauma, clinician error, and previous periodontal therapy can all result in recession but are not likely contributing factors in this case.

136. **D** While using a heavier probing pressure in diseased tissues may result in deeper probing depths, when used on healthy tissues, any reasonable probe pressure should make no difference. Development

of a long junctional epithelial attachment, gingival recession, and a healthier attachment apparatus (eliminates probing through the fragile, diseased attachment) are all likely reasons for the reduction in probing depths.

137. **C** Clinical attachment level is the distance from the CEJ to the epithelial attachment.

138. **D** Since the dietary habits of the patient are not presented, her diet is not a likely cause. The history of orthodontic therapy and the radiographic evidence of periodontal disease and significant bone loss are the obvious cause of the mobility.

139. **C** Intentional curettage is contraindicated in areas of infrabony pockets. Infrabony defects occur when the pocket extends apically beyond the crest of the alveolar bone.

140. **B** The major factor influencing the decline in this patient's periodontal health is the patient's lack of motivation. The 6-year interval between dental hygiene therapy appointments and lack of flossing are indicative of lack of motivation. Orthodontic treatment is not contraindicated as long as the patient stabilized his/her periodontal condition by frequent oral prophylaxis and thorough daily plaque removal. The restorative needs and hereditary background of the patient are not major factors, if at all.

141. **A** A periodontal abscess can be initiated by incomplete removal of deposits that harbor pathologic bacteria in a periodontal pocket. The most coronal tissue in the periodontal pocket tightens around the tooth and does not allow the exudate (bacterial byproducts) to exit the pocket, thus causing the abscess. A periapical abscess result from inflammation and death of the pulpal tissues. A papilloma is a small, raised, benign tissue mass that is not specifically-associated with periodontal therapy. Mucositis is inflammation of the oral mucosa and occurs as a result of systemic disease, medication, and cancer therapy.

Case Study O

142. **B** Based on the appearance of the gingival tissues, particularly the redness and edema in the linguals of the mandibular anteriors, this patient most likely has chronic gingivitis. Acute gingivitis, necrotic gingivitis and herpetic gingivitis can all be ruled out as the patient has not complained of pain which would be present in all three conditions. Furthermore, no ulcerations have been noted which would be present in the latter two conditions.

143. **B** The palatal discoloration is nicotine stomatitis due to the patient's heavy smoking habit. Kaposi's sarcoma is associated with later stages of AIDS and is usually confined to the gingiva although it can occur anywhere in the oral cavity. Leukoplakia is a white or speckled plaque-like lesion commonly found on the

floor of the mouth, lateral border of the tongue, or the retromolar pad. Herpetiform lesions are small individual reddish ulcerations often found on the palate or the gingiva.

144. **D** Allergy to the latex gloves the operator is wearing can cause a serious allergic reaction in sensitive patients that can range from local (hives or contact dermatitis) to systemic (anaphylaxis) reactions. Angina presents as chest, neck, and shoulder pain that disappears in minutes. Anxiety can result in hyperventilation, rashes, and fainting. Embarrassment is typically noted by a reddened face.

145. **D** Based on pocket depths ranging from 2–8 mm with furcation involvements in several teeth and numerous mobilities present, Case type IV would be the appropriate AAP classification. Case type I does not involve bone loss while type II is associated with minor bone loss or early periodontitis. Type III involves moderate bone loss of moderate periodontitis.

146. **B** Poor plaque control, cigarette smoking, stress, and calculus have all been identified in this patient's history and are recognized as risk factors for periodontal disease. Although alcohol is a major risk factor for the development of oral cancer, it has not been identified as a risk factor for periodontal disease nor does this patient have a history of excessive alcohol consumption.

147. **D** The pocket depth on the facial of tooth #25 is recorded as 3 mm. Since the total attachment loss is 8 mm, the recession is 5 mm.

148. **C** Due to the 5-mm recession and lack of attached gingiva, a mucogingival defect has been identified. Mobility of 1+ has also been recorded. The 5-mm recession is likely to cause root sensitivity, however no evidence of occlusal trauma, i.e., widening of the periodontal ligament space, can be seen radiographically.

149. **D** In advanced cases such as this one, referral to a periodontist after completion of initial therapy and re-evaluation, should always be considered. Surgical intervention may include repair of the mucogingival defect but may also include other procedures to reduce pocket depths and improve accessibility for home care procedures. Tetracycline fibers have been shown to have best results in specific problem sites rather then for resolution of advanced cases.

150. **B** The prime etiologic and local contributing factors present in this patient are bacterial plaque and calculus. No overhanging margin can be detected on tooth # 14 and malocclusion and major occlusal disharmonies have not been noted.

Index